COMPREHENSIVE GYNECOLOGY

COMPREHENSIVE GYNECOLOGY

WILLIAM DROEGEMUELLER, M.D.
Robert A. Ross Distinguished Professor and
Chairman of Obstetrics and Gynecology,
University of North Carolina School of Medicine,
Chapel Hill, North Carolina

ARTHUR L. HERBST, M.D.
Joseph Bolivar DeLee
Distinguished Service Professor and Chairman,
Department of Obstetrics and Gynecology,
University of Chicago,
Chicago, Illinois

DANIEL R. MISHELL, Jr., M.D.
Professor and Chairman,
Department of Obstetrics and Gynecology,
University of Southern California School of Medicine,
Los Angeles, California

MORTON A. STENCHEVER, M.D.
Professor and Chairman,
Department of Obstetrics and Gynecology,
University of Washington School of Medicine,
Seattle, Washington

with 838 illustrations

The C. V. Mosby Company

ST. LOUIS • WASHINGTON, D.C. • TORONTO

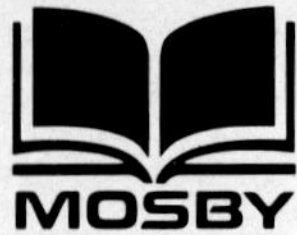

MOSBY

A TRADITION OF PUBLISHING EXCELLENCE

Editor: Thomas A. Manning
Developmental Editor: Elaine Steinborn
Assistant Editor: Beth Campbell
Project Editor: Mark Spann
Editing and Production: CRACOM Corporation

Great care has been used in compiling and checking the information
in this book to ensure its accuracy. However, because of changing technology,
new discoveries, and individualization of patient care, the uses, effects,
and dosages of drugs may vary from those given here. The medications
discussed do not necessarily have specific approval by the Food and Drug
Administration for use in the diseases and dosages for which they are recommended.

Printed in the United States of America

The C.V. Mosby Company
11830 Westline Industrial Drive, St. Louis, Missouri 63146

Library of Congress Cataloging-in-Publication Data

Comprehensive gynecology.

   Includes bibliographies and index.
   1. Gynecology.   I. Title.   II. Droegemueller,
William, 1934-   . [DNLM: 1. Genital Diseases,
Female.   2. Genital Neoplasms, Female.   WP 140 C737]
RG101.C726   1987   618.1   87-5508
ISBN 0-8016-1929-7

C/MV/MV   9   8   7   6   5   02/B/216

PREFACE

Comprehensive Gynecology is the culmination of efforts of the four authors to develop a textbook that provides all the information needed to understand the physiologic and pathologic principles of gynecology. The format for presenting this contemporary information allows the clinician to easily apply it when caring for the female patient. A special effort has been made to incorporate current insights into the psychosocial aspects of gynecologic practice, information that has great importance for the clinician. The book is written especially for use by the resident training in gynecology; in addition, it presents material of interest to the medical student. It also provides sufficient detail for the practitioner to make appropriate diagnoses and institute treatment.

This book explores the areas of gynecologic oncology and reproductive endocrinology in depth. It also details current information on infections, family planning, breast disease, and pregnancy termination, all within a framework that emphasizes sensitivity to the individual patient. It is truly comprehensive.

Among the unique features in this book are the lists of key terms and definitions at the beginning of each chapter. These lists allow the reader to quickly become acquainted with terms used in the chapter discussion and provide a valuable review tool. Pertinent information is also presented in the many boxes and tables highlighting the text. In addition, the key points listed at the end of each chapter give the reader a synopsis of the important facts about the topic discussed. Each of these teaching aids will help the student master the complexities of gynecology.

Over the past few years the four authors have worked closely together to produce this text. In contrast to other textbooks with many authors, each chapter in this book was written by one author and then reviewed and revised by the other authors. This method was chosen to provide a comprehensive approach and allow the reader to benefit from our diverse backgrounds, interests, and experiences as well as our widely separate geographic locations. Our goal has been to synthesize the current approaches to gynecologic problems. Since the four authors contributed equally to the text, there is no senior author. Thus the names are listed alphabetically on the title page. It is planned to rotate the sequence of names in future editions of the book.

We especially thank our families and particularly our wives for their patience and support during the long hours we have spent developing this book. We are also delighted that, despite frequently candid and occasionally heated discussions, we have remained a cohesive unit and close friends.

William Droegemueller
Arthur L. Herbst
Daniel R. Mishell, Jr.
Morton A. Stenchever

CONTENTS

COMPREHENSIVE GYNECOLOGY

BASIC SCIENCES

Embryology

———————— KEY TERMS AND DEFINITIONS ————————

Acrosome Reaction. The process by which the cap over the head of the sperm, the acrosome, is removed to expose the portion of the sperm head containing the hydrolytic enzymes, which will make it possible for the sperm to penetrate the cells and structures investing the egg. This process is involved in capacitation but is not necessarily the same response as capacitation.

Anlage. The cell mass that gives rise to a specific organ or structure.

Bivalent. Homologous chromosomes that become paired during meiosis.

Blastula. The stage of embryonic development that follows the morula stage. At this stage a cyst (blastocyst) forms within the cell mass and early differentiation begins.

Capacitation. The morphologic, physiologic, and biochemical changes that a sperm goes through to be capable of penetrating the cumulus oophorus, corona radiata, and zona pellucida of the egg. It involves the sequentially timed release of a series of hydrolytic enzymes, which allows the sperm to digest a passage through the aforementioned structures.

Chiasmata. Points of attachment of homologous chromosomes during meiosis, where the exchange of genetic material occurs.

Cleavage. The first cell division of the fertilized ovum (zygote).

Cumulus Oophorus. The cell mass that invests the egg. It is a remnant of the primitive sex cords of the embryonic ovary.

Gartner's Duct. Remnants of the mesonephric (wolffian) duct system often found in the broad ligament and beside the uterus, cervix, and vagina of the adult woman.

H-Y antigen. A cell surface antigen that will lead to male differentiation of the gonad.

Implantation. The process by which the early embryo burrows within the endometrial lining of the uterus.

Mesonephros. The mesodermal anlage of the male sexual duct system.

Metanephros. The anlage of the adult kidney.

Morula. A ball of cells composing the early embryo that will produce both the embryo and the placenta and membranes. Each cell is totipotential.

Oogenesis. The development of the ovum from an oogonium by meiosis.

Paramesonephric (Müllerian) Duct. The anlage of the female sex duct system that will give rise to the fallopian tube, uterus, and cervix in the adult woman.

Polar Body. The daughter cell produced during oogenesis at first and second meiotic division (first and second polar body); it contains a nucleus and minimal cytoplasm. For each polar body the nuclear material is similar to the nucleus of the ovum at the same stage.

Primordium. An early embryonic structure that will further differentiate into an adult structure.

Sister Chromatid Exchange. The exchange of chromosomal material between the homologous arms of a chromosome that has already divided all of its structure except its centromere.

Spermatogenesis. The development of mature sperm from spermatogonia by meiosis.

Synapsis. The pairing process that brings together homologous chromosomes of maternal and paternal origin during meiosis.

Teratogen. An endogenous or exogenous substance that causes the formation of an anomaly.

Teratogenesis. The process of developing an anomaly of an organ or organs.

Zona Pellucida. The translucent belt consisting of a noncellular layer of mucopolysaccharide that is deposited at the periphery of the ovum while it is in the ovary and continues to surround the egg, the conceptus, and the morula until the stage of implantation.

Two areas of investigation within the field of gynecology have refocused attention on the process of fertilization and embryonic development: teratology and in vitro fertilization. The process under which eggs and sperm are produced and fertilization occurs is gaining close scrutiny. Likewise, the preimplantation, implantation, and embryonic stages of development in the human can be studied because of the development of newer techniques and pursuits. This chapter considers the processes of oocyte meiosis, fertilization and early cleavage, implantation, development of the genitourinary system, and sex differentiation.

OOCYTE MEIOSIS

The oocyte is a unique and extremely specialized cell. During the process of oocyte meiosis, genetic variability of the species is ensured. Later the oocyte develops the ability to facilitate fertilization and to provide the energy system to support the early embryonic development of the new individual.

Primordial germ cells in both males and females are large eosinophilic cells derived from endoderm in the wall of the yolk sac. These cells migrate to the germinal ridge by way of the dorsal mesentery of the hind gut by ameboid action. Here they undergo a period of intense mitotic activity in which their numbers increase to 6 to 7 million. By 20 weeks' gestation, this rapid multiplication has ended, and indeed the numbers rapidly fall off, being about 2 to 4 million at birth and about 400,000 at menarche. By 5 months' gestation, surviving oocytes enter the process of meiosis and progress to the prophase of the first meiotic division before entering an arrest period that lasts many years. After puberty, a few oocytes mature during each ovarian cycle. The numbers vary from species to species, being one or two in the human. Maturation then continues to the second meiotic metaphase, when once again arrest of meiosis occurs unless the oocyte is activated by fertilization.

Fig. 1-1 illustrates the steps of meiosis through both the first and second meiotic divisions. Prophase of the first meiotic division is divided into several phases. The earliest, the leptotene stage, is associated with condensation of the chromatin, which becomes visible as single elongated, threadlike structures. The next stage, zygotene, features the migration of these single threadlike chromosomes toward the equatorial plate of the nucleus. Homologous chromosomes arrange themselves close to one another to form bivalents. At the end of this stage, tight pairing of the chromosomes along their entire length, synapsis, takes place. The pachytene stage follows, during which the chromosome pairs contact one another and become shorter and thicker. During this stage, each chromosome splits longitudinally, and two chromatids are produced that are united at the centromere. Thus the bivalent is now a structure composed of four closely opposed chromatids, or tetrads. The human ovum at pachytene demonstrates 23 tetrads. In the next stage, diplotene, the member chromosomes of the bivalents are held together only at certain points. At these terminal bridges, called chiasmata, the crossing over of genetic material takes place. The sister chromatids are still joined at the centromere, and crossing takes place only between the chromatids of homolo-

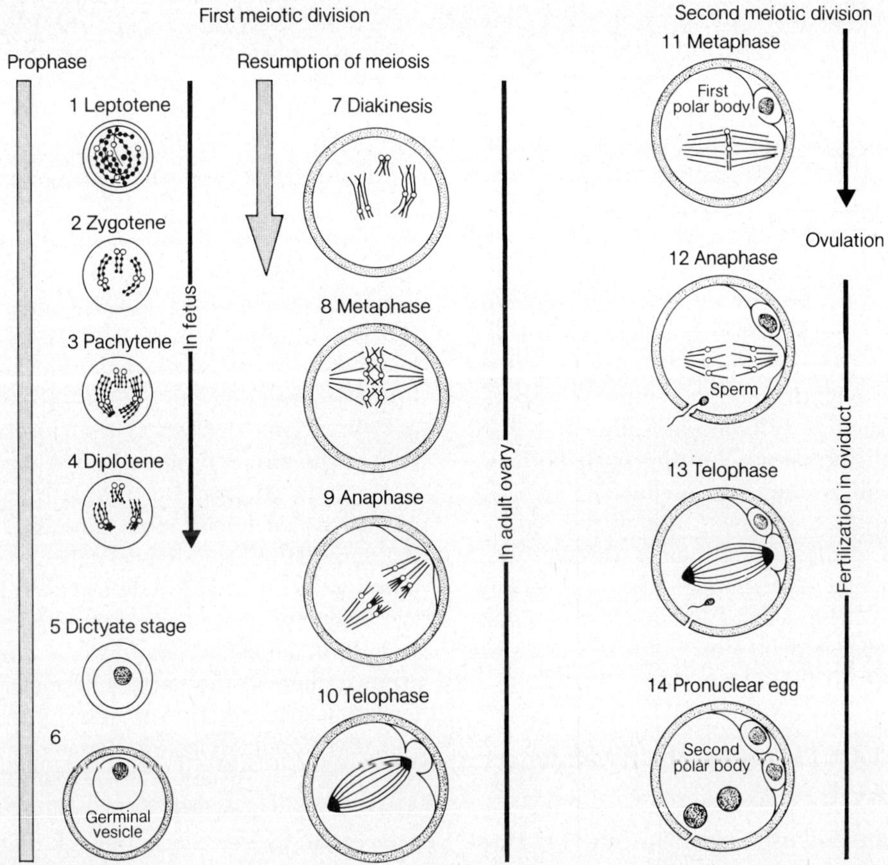

FIGURE 1-1

Diagram of oocyte meiosis. For simplicity, only three pairs of chromosomes are depicted. *1-4*, Prophase stages of the first meiotic division which occur in most mammals during fetal life. The meiotic process is arrested at the diplotene stage ("first meiotic arrest") and the oocyte enters the dictyate stages (*5-6*). When meiosis is resumed, the first maturation division is completed (*7-11*). Ovulation occurs usually at the metaphase II stage (*11*) and the second meiotic division (*12-14*) takes place in the oviduct only following sperm penetration. (From Tsafriri A: Oocyte maturation in mammals. In Jones RE, ed: The vertebrate ovary. New York, Plenum Publishing Corp., 1978.)

gous chromosomes and not between identical sister chromatids. The ovum then enters the dictyate stage and meiosis is arrested. Ova at this stage usually form germinal vesicles. It has been shown that initiation of the meiotic process occurs because of stimulation by a substance known as meiotic-inducing substance, which originates in the rete cords derived from the developing mesonephric tubules. A second substance, probably produced by the granulosa cells of the differentiated ovarian follicle, acts as a countersubstance to inhibit meiosis (meiosis-preventing substance). Apparently the interaction of these two substance regulates meiosis in the developing gonad. Once the ovum at the dictyate stage is encapsulated in granulosa cells, oogenesis is arrested because of the interruption of contact with the rete ovarii and the meiosis-preventing substance becomes dominant.

After puberty, with follicle ripening, meiosis resumes in a few follicles during each cycle with the formation of the diakinesis stage. Here the bivalents contract and the chiasmata move toward the end of the chromosomes. The homologs pull apart and the nuclear membrane disappears, ending prophase I. Metaphase I then occurs. The bivalents, which are highly contracted, align themselves along the equatorial plate of the cell. Chromosomes derived from paternal and maternal sources line up completely at random to each other, and in the following stage, anaphase I, the homologous chromosomes of the bivalent pairs separate. Telophase I is similar to telophase in the mitotic process except that one daughter cell receives the majority of the cytoplasm and the second daughter cell becomes the first polar body. Both the oocyte and the polar body are present within the zona pellucida covering. The oocyte then advances immediately to mataphase II of the second meiotic division, during which time ovulation occurs. The remaining steps of the second meiotic division take place in the oviduct after sperm penetration takes place.

FERTILIZATION AND EARLY CLEAVAGE

In humans and most mammals, the egg is released from the ovary in the metaphase II stage. At the time it enters the fallopian tube, it is surrounded by a cumulus of granulosa cells (cumulus oophorus) and intimately surrounded by a clear zona pellucida. Within the zona pellucida are both the egg and the first polar body. Meanwhile, spermatozoa are transported through the cervical mucus and the uterus and into the fallopian tubes. During this transport period they undergo two changes, capacitation and acrosome reaction, which essentially activate enzyme systems within the sperm head and make it possible for the sperm to transgress the cumulus oophorus and the zona pellucida. Once the sperm has passed the barrier of the zona pellucida, it attaches to the cell membrane of the egg and then enters the cytoplasm. When the sperm enters the cytoplasm, intracytoplasmic structures, the coronal granules, arrange themselves in an orderly fashion around the outmost portion of the cytoplasm just beneath the cytoplasmic membrane, and the sperm head swells and gives rise to the male pronucleus. The egg completes its second meiotic division, casting off the second polar body to a position also beneath the zona pellucida. The female pronucleus swells as well. In most mammals the male pronucleus can be recognized as the larger of the two. The pronuclei, which contain the haploid sets of chromosomes of maternal and paternal origin, do not fuse in mammals. However, the nuclear membranes surrounding them disappear, and the chromosomes contained within each arrange themselves on the developing spindle of the first mitotic division. In this way the diploid complement of chromosomes is reestablished, completing the process of fertilization.

Cell division (cleavage) then occurs, giving rise to the two-cell embryo. The first division takes about 20 hours to complete, and the actual phase of fertilization generally occurs in the ampulla of the fallopian tube. A significant number of fertilized ova do not complete cleavage. This may be due to a number of reasons, including failure of appropriate chromosome arrangement on the spindle, specific gene defects that prevent the formation of the spindle, and environmental factors. Teratogens acting at this point are usually either completely destructive or cause little or no effect. Twinning may occur by the separation of the two cells produced by cleavage, each of which has the potential to develop into a separate embryo. Twinning may occur at any stage until the formation of the blastula, since each cell is totipotential. Both genetic and environmental factors are probably involved in the causation of twinning.

Morula and Blastula Stage— Early Differentiation

After the first mitotic division the cells continue to divide as the embryo passes along the fallopian tube and enters the uterus. This process takes 3 to 4 days after fertilization in the human, and the embryo may arrive at the uterus in any form, from 32 cells to the early blastula stage. In the human, implantation generally takes place 3 days after the embryo enters the uterus.

Implantation depends on the development of early trophoblastic cells during the blastula stage. These cells digest away the zona pellucida and allow the embryo to fix to the wall of the uterus and subsequently to burrow within

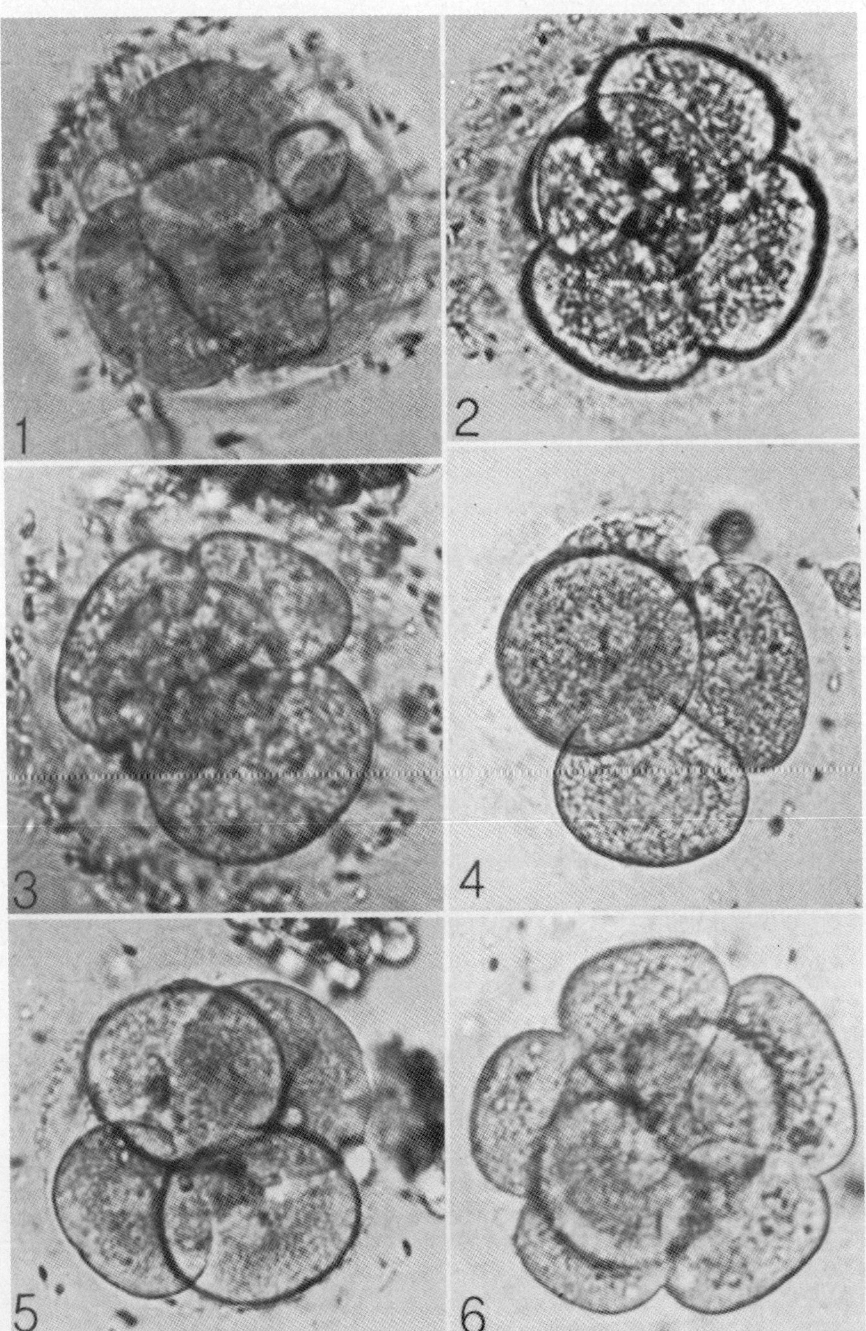

FIGURE 1-2
Six photomicrographs of fresh unmounted human embryos. The first five show four-cell human embryos at various grades of development. **1,** Poor; note the misshapen blastomeres and fragments. **2,** Fair to poor; note single fragments. **3,** Fair; note slightly uneven blastomere size and some small fragments. **4,** Fair to good. **5,** Good; note the large, spherical blastomeres of even density and size. **6,** A good eight-cell embryo. (From Mohr LR, Trounson AO, Leeton JF, Wood C: Evaluation of normal and abnormal human embryo development during procedures in-vitro. In Beier HM, Lindner HR, eds: Fertilization of human egg in-vitro. Berlin, Springer-Verlag, 1983.)

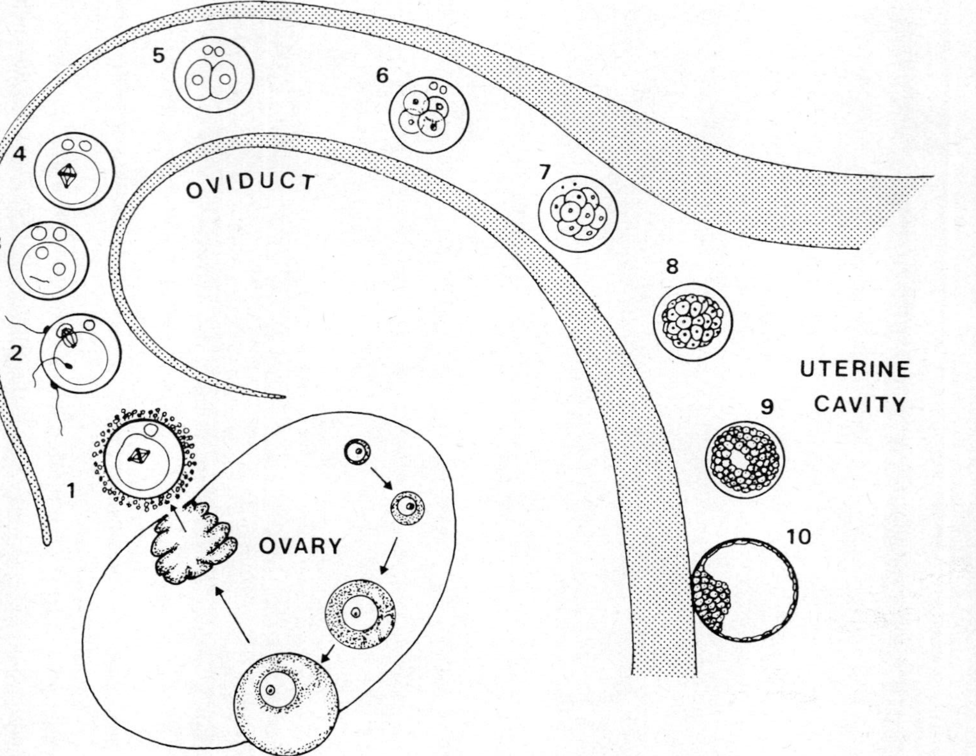

FIGURE 1-3
Diagrammatic representation of follicle growth, ovulation, fertilization, and preimplantation. (From Whittingham DG: Br Med Bull 35:105, 1979.)

the endometrium. The development of the blastula and the separation of the embryonic disk cells from the developing trophoblastic cells together make up the first stage of differentiation in the embryo. Again, at this stage of development, teratogens will generally either be completely destructive or have little or no effect, since each of the cells of the early embryonic disk are multipotential. Differentiation within the embryonic disk, however, proceeds fairly rapidly, and if separation of cells and twinning occur at this point, the twins will frequently be conjoined in some fashion. Fig. 1-2 presents photomicrographs of several fresh human embryos obtained during in vitro fertilization. These embryos have been graded poor to good and probably relate to the possibility of future successful implantation and development. Fig. 1-3 schematically demonstrates the process of follicle growth, ovulation, fertilization, and preimplantation.

IMPLANTATION

Implantation has been noted to occur in the human embryo as early as day 6 after ovulation. For implantation to take place, the zona pellucida must be removed from the developing blastocyst, which occurs because of enzyme action produced either by cells of the blastocyst or by some endometrial enzymes. Endometrial capillaries in contact with the invading syncytiotrophoblast are engulfed to form venous sinuses at or about 7½ days after conception and are seen abundantly by day 9. Endometrial spiral arteries are not invaded at this point. The endoplasmic reticulum of the syncytiotrophoblast is probably responsible for the synthesis of chorionic gonadotrophin, which is well developed by 11 days after ovulation. Transfer is probably through the venous sinuses before intact circulation to the developing embryo has been established. It is important that chorionic gonadotrophin be transmitted to maternal circulation by one means or another, since it is responsible for maintaining the corpus luteum. Chorionic gonadotrophin has been detected in the peripheral blood of the mother as early as 6 days postovulation but is always seen by the twelfth day. The concentration doubles every 1.2 to 2 days, reaching its highest point at 7 to 9 weeks of pregnancy.

Discussion of implantation is not complete without at least considering why the fetus is not immunologically rejected by the mother. Although it is not completely understood why rejection does not occur, some theories have been advanced. One considers the fact that some substance or substances suppress lymphocyte transformation in the mother. Such substances could be any that are produced by the embryo, including chorionic gonadotrophin. Other theories include the production of suppressor T lymphocytes by the fetus, which could inhibit maternal lymphocyte transformation by secreting an inhibitory substance that crosses the placenta. Finally, the phenomenon of enhancement, which states that weakly antigenic sites on the trophoblast are blocked by maternal antibodies, thereby rendering them unavailable to circulating T cells, is also a possibility.

Table 1-1 describes the events of implantation.

TABLE 1-1
Events of Implantation

Event	Days After Ovulation
Zona pellucida disappears	4-5
Blastocyst attaches to epithelial surface of endometrium	6
Trophoblast erodes into endometrial stroma	7
Trophoblast differentiates into cytotrophoblastic and syncytial trophoblastic layers	7-8
Lacunae appear around trophoblast	8-9
Blastocyst burrows beneath endometrial surface	9-10
Lacunar network forms	10-11
Trophoblast invades endometrial sinusoids, establishing a uteroplacental circulation	11-12
Endometrial epithelium completely covers blastocyst	12-13
Strong decidual reaction occurs in stroma	13-14

Early Organogenesis in the Embryonic Period

During the third week after fertilization, the primitive streak forms in the caudal portion of the embryonic disk and the embryonic disk begins to grow and change from a circular configuration to one that is pear shaped. At that point the epithelium facing superiorly is considered ectoderm and will eventually give rise to the developing central nervous system, and the epithelium facing downward toward the yolk sac is endoderm. During this week the neuroplate develops with its associated notochordal process. By the sixteenth day after conception the third primitive germ layer, the intraembryonic mesoderm, begins to form between the ectoderm and endoderm. Early mesoderm migrates cranially, passing on either side of the notochordal process to meet in front in the formation of the cardiogenic area. The heart will soon develop from this area. Later in the third week, extraembryonic mesoderm joins with the yolk sac and the developing amnion to contribute to the developing membranes. An intraembryonic mesoderm develops on each side of the notochord and neural tube to form longitudinal columns, the paraxial mesoderm. Each paraxial column thins laterally into the lateral plate mesoderm, which is continuous with the extraembryonic mesoderm of the yolk sac and the amnion. The lateral plate mesoderm is separated from the paraxial mesoderm by a continuous tract of mesoderm called the intermediate mesoderm. By the twentieth day, paraxial mesoderm begins to divide into paired linear bodies known as somites. About 38 pairs of somites form during the next 10 days. Eventually a total of 42 to 44 pairs will develop, and these will eventually give rise to body musculature.

Angiogenesis, or blood vessel formation, can be seen in the extraembryonic mesoderm of the yolk sac by day 15 or 16. Embryonic vessels can be seen about 2 days later. They develop when mesenchymal cells known as angioblasts aggregate to form masses and cords called blood islands. Spaces will then appear within these islands, and the angioblasts will arrange themselves around these spaces to form primitive endothelium. Isolated vessels form channels, and then grow into adjacent areas by endothelial budding. Primitive blood cells develop from endothelial cells as the vessels develop on the yolk sac and allantois. However, blood formation does not begin within the embryo until the second month of gestation, occurring first in the developing liver and later in the spleen, bone marrow, and lymph nodes. Separate mesenchymal cells surrounding the primitive endothelial vessels differentiate into muscular and connective tissue elements. The primitive heart forms in a similar manner from mesenchymal cells in the cardiogenic area. Paired endothelial channels called heart tubes develop by the end of the third week and fuse to form the primitive heart. By the twenty-first day, this primitive heart has linked up with blood vessels of the embryo, forming a primitive cardiovascular system. Blood circulation starts about this time, and the cardiovascular system becomes the first functioning organ system within the embryo.

From the fourth to the seventh week of gestation, all the organ systems are formed. Only the genitourinary system will be considered in detail later in this chapter.

A teratogenic event that takes place during the embryonic period will give rise to a constellation of malformations related to the organ systems that are actively developing at that particular time. Thus cardiovascular malformations tend to occur because of teratogenic events early in the embryonic period, whereas genitourinary abnormalities tend to occur because of events that occur later. Fig. 1-4 demonstrates the malformations that were seen when thalidomide was applied to a human population during gestational days 35 to 50. Teratogenic effects prior to implantation will often cause death but not malformations.

In general, the effects of a given teratogen depend on the genetic makeup of the individual, other environmental factors in play at the time, the stage during embryonic development that the teratogen is applied, and in some cases the dose of the teratogen and the duration that it is allowed to act. Some teratogens in and of themselves are harmless, but their metabolites cause the damage. Teratogens may be chemical substances and their by-products, or they may be physical entities, such as temperature elevation and irradiation. Teratogenic agents applied after the forty-ninth day of gestation may injure or kill the embryo or cause developmen-

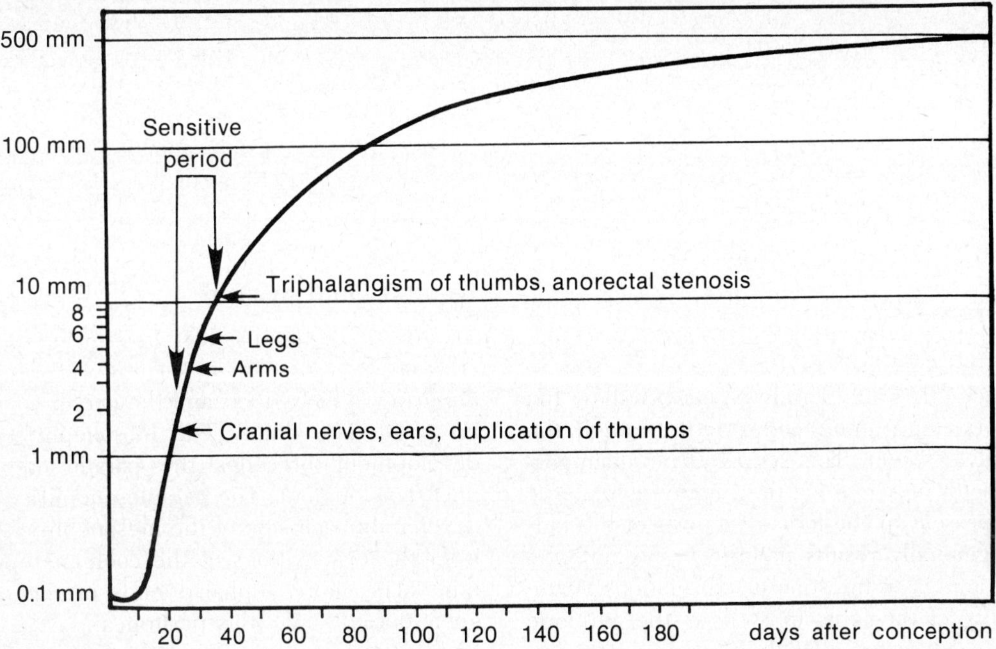

FIGURE 1-4

Schematic drawing of sensitive period for teratogenic effect of thalidomide with corresponding length of embryo. (From Lenz W: Chemicals and malformations in man. In Fishbein M, ed: Second International Conference on Congenital Malformations. New York, International Medical Congress, 1964.)

tal and growth retardation but usually will not be responsible for specific malformations. The period of embryonic development is said to be complete when the embryo attains a crown-rump length of 30 mm. It corresponds in most cases to day 49 after conception.

DEVELOPMENT OF THE GENITOURINARY SYSTEM

Excretory System

Nephrogenic cords develop from the intermediate mesoderm as early as the 2 mm embryo stage, beginning in the more cephalad portions of the embryo. Three sets of excretory ducts and tubules develop, each bilaterally. The first, the pronephros, with its pronephric ducts forms in the most cranial portion of the embryo at about the beginning of the fourth week after conception. The tubules associated with the duct probably have no excretory function in the human. Late in the fourth week a second set of tubules, the mesonephric tu-

bules, and their accompanying mesonephric ducts begin to develop. These are associated with tufts of capillaries, or glomeruli, and tubules for excretory purposes. Thus the mesonephros functions as a fetal kidney, producing urine for about 2 or 3 weeks. As new tubules develop, those derived from the more cephalad tubules degenerate. There are usually about 40 mesonephric tubules functioning on either side of the embryo at any given time.

The metanephros, or permanent kidney, begins its development early in the fifth week of gestation and starts to function late in the seventh or early in the eighth week. The metanephros develops both from the metanephrogenic mass of mesoderm, which is the most caudal portion of the nephrogenic cord, and its duct system, which is derived from the metanephric diverticulum (ureteric bud) and is a cranially growing outpouching of the mesonephric duct close to where it enters the cloaca. The latter will give rise to the ureter, the renal pelvis, the calyces, and the collecting tubules of the adult kidney. A critical process

gland, known as the prostatic utricle. Occasionally the prostatic utricle is developed to the point where it will excrete a small amount of blood and cause hematuria in adult life.

Female Genital Ducts

In the presence of ovaries or of no gonads at all, the mesonephric ducts regress and the paramesonephric ducts will develop into the female genital tract. This process begins at about 6 weeks and proceeds in a cephalad and caudal fashion. The more cephalad portions of the paramesonephric ducts, which open directly into peritoneal cavity, will form the fallopian tubes. The fused portion, or uterovaginal primordium, will give rise to the epithelium and glands of the uterus and cervix. Endometrial stroma and myometrium will be derived from adjacent mesenchyme.

Failure of development of the paramesonephric ducts will lead to agenesis of the cervix and the uterus. Failure of fusion of the caudal portion of these ducts may lead to a variety of anomalies of the uterus, including complete duplication of the uterus and cervix or partial duplication of a variety of types, which will be outlined in Chapter 9.

Peritoneal reflections in the area adjacent to the fusion of the two paramesonephric ducts give rise to the formation of the broad ligaments. Mesenchymal tissue here develops into the parametrium.

The vagina develops from paired solid outgrowths of endoderm of the urogenital sinus, the sinovaginal bulbs. These grow caudally as a solid core toward the end of the uterovaginal primordium. This core constitutes the fibromuscular portion of the vagina. The sinovaginal bulbs then canalize to form the vagina. However, abnormalities in this process may lead to either transverse or horizontal vaginal septi. The junction of the sinovaginal bulbs with the urogenital sinus remains as the vaginal plate, which forms the hymen. This remains imperforate until late in embryonic life. Occasionally, perforation does not take place normally (imperforate hymen).

Failure of the sinovaginal bulbs to form will lead to agenesis of the vagina. The precise boundary between the paramesonephric and urogenital sinus portions of the vagina has not been established.

Auxiliary genital glands in the female form from buds that grow out of the urethra. They derive contributions from the surrounding mesenchyme and form the urethral glands and the paraurethral glands (Skene's glands). These correspond to the prostate gland in males. Similar outgrowths of the urogenital sinus form the vestibular glands (Bartholin's glands), which are homologous to the bulbourethral glands in the male.

The remnants of the mesonephric duct in the female include a small structure called the appendix vesiculosa, a few blind tubules in the broad ligaments, the epoophoron, and a few blind tubules adjacent to the uterus collectively called the paroophoron. Remnants of the mesonephric duct system are often present in the broad ligaments or are adjacent to the uterus or the vagina as Gartner's duct cysts. The epoophoron or paroophoron may develop into cysts. Cysts of the epoophoron are known as paraovarian cysts.

Remnants of the paramesonephric duct in the female may be seen as a small, blind cystic structure attached by a pedicle to the distal end of the fallopian tube, the hydatid of Morgagni. Table 1-2 categorizes the adult derivatives and residual remnants of the urogenital structures in both the male and the female. Fig. 1-6 outlines schematically the development of the internal sexual organs in both sexes.

External Genitalia

In the fourth week after fertilization, the genital tubercle develops at the ventral tip of the cloacal membrane. Two sets of lateral bodies, the labioscrotal swellings and urogenital folds, develop soon after on either side of the cloacal membrane. The genital tubercle then elongates to form a phallus in both males and females. By the end of the sixth week, the cloacal membrane is joined by the urorectal septum. The septum separates the cloaca into the urogenital sinus ventrally and the anal canal and rectum dorsally. The point on the cloacal membrane where the urorectal septum fuses becomes the location of the perineal body in later development. The cloacal membrane is then divided into the ventral urogenital membrane and the dorsal anal membrane. These membranes then rupture, opening the vulva

TABLE 1-2
Male and Female Derivatives of Embryonic Urogenital Structures

Embryonic Structure	Derivatives	
	Male	**Female**
Labioscrotal swellings	Scrotum	Labia majora
Urogenital folds	Ventral portion of penis	Labia minora

Phallus	Penis
	  Glans, corpora cavernosa penis,
	  and corpus spongiosum
		Clitoris
		  Glans, corpora cavernosa,
		  bulb of the vestibule

Urogenital sinus	Urinary bladder Prostate gland Prostatic utricle Bulbourethral glands Seminal colliculus	Urinary bladder Urethral and paraurethral glands Vagina Greater vestibular glands Hymen
Paramesonephric duct	Appendix of testes	Hydatid of Morgagni Uterus and cervix Fallopian tubes
Mesonephric duct	Appendix of epididymis Ductus epididymis Ductus deferens Ejaculatory duct and seminal vesicle	Appendix vesiculosis Duct of epoophoron Gartner's duct —

Metanephric duct	Ureter, renal pelvis, calyces, and
	  collecting system
		Ureter, renal pelvis, calyces,
		  and collecting system

Mesonephric tubules	Ductuli efferentes Paradidymis	Epoophoron Paroophoron
Undifferentiated gonad	Testis	Ovary
Cortex	Seminiferous tubules	Ovarian follicles
Medulla	— Rete testis	Medulla Rete ovarii
Gubernaculum	Gubernaculum testis	Round ligament of uterus

and the anal canal. Failure of the anal membrane to rupture will give rise to an imperforate anus. With the opening of the urogenital membrane, a urethral groove forms on the undersurface of the phallus, completing the undifferentiated portion of external genital development. Differences between male and female embryos can be noted as early as the ninth week, but the distinct final forms are not noted until 12 weeks.

Androgens produced by the testes are responsible for the masculinization of the undifferentiated external genitalia. The phallus will grow in length to form a penis, and the urogenital folds are pulled forward to form the lateral walls of the urethral groove on the undersurface of the penis. These folds then fuse to form the penile urethra. Defects in fusion of various amounts give rise to various degrees of hypospadias. The skin at the distal margin of the penis grows over the glans to form the prepuce (foreskin). The vascular portion of the penis (corpora cavernosa penis and corpus cavernosum urethrae) arise from the mesenchymal tissue of the phallus. Finally, the labioscrotal swellings grow toward each other and fuse in the midline to form the scrotum. Later in embryonic life the testes descend through the inguinal canal guided by the gubernaculum. This event occurs at about the twenty-eighth week.

In the absence of androgen stimulation, feminization of the undifferentiated external geni-

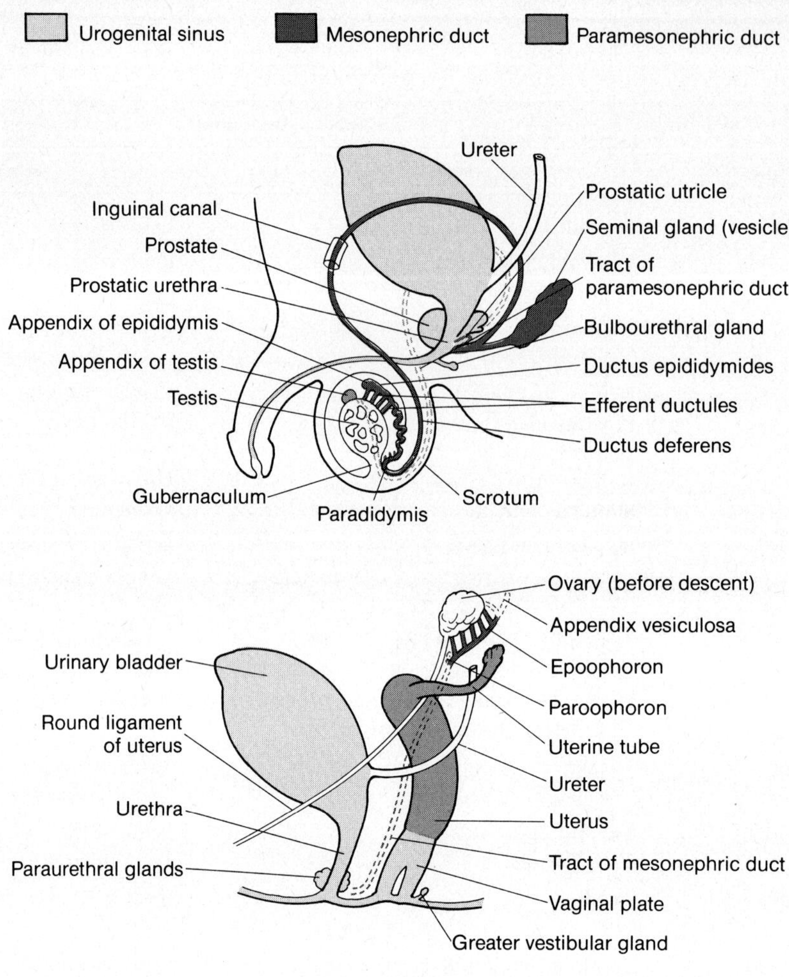

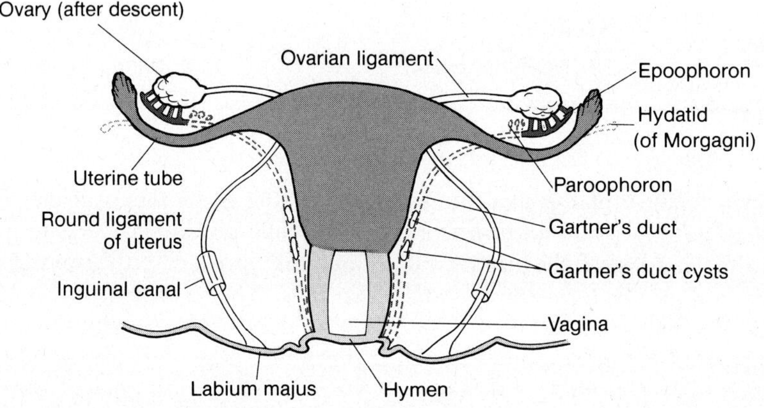

FIGURE 1-6

Schematic drawings illustrating development of male and female reproductive systems from the primitive genital ducts. Vestigial structures are also shown. **A,** Reproductive system in a newborn male. **B,** Reproductive system in a female fetus at 12 weeks. **C,** Reproductive system in a newborn female. (From Moore KL: The developing human, clinically oriented embryology. Philadelphia, W.B. Saunders Co., 1973.)

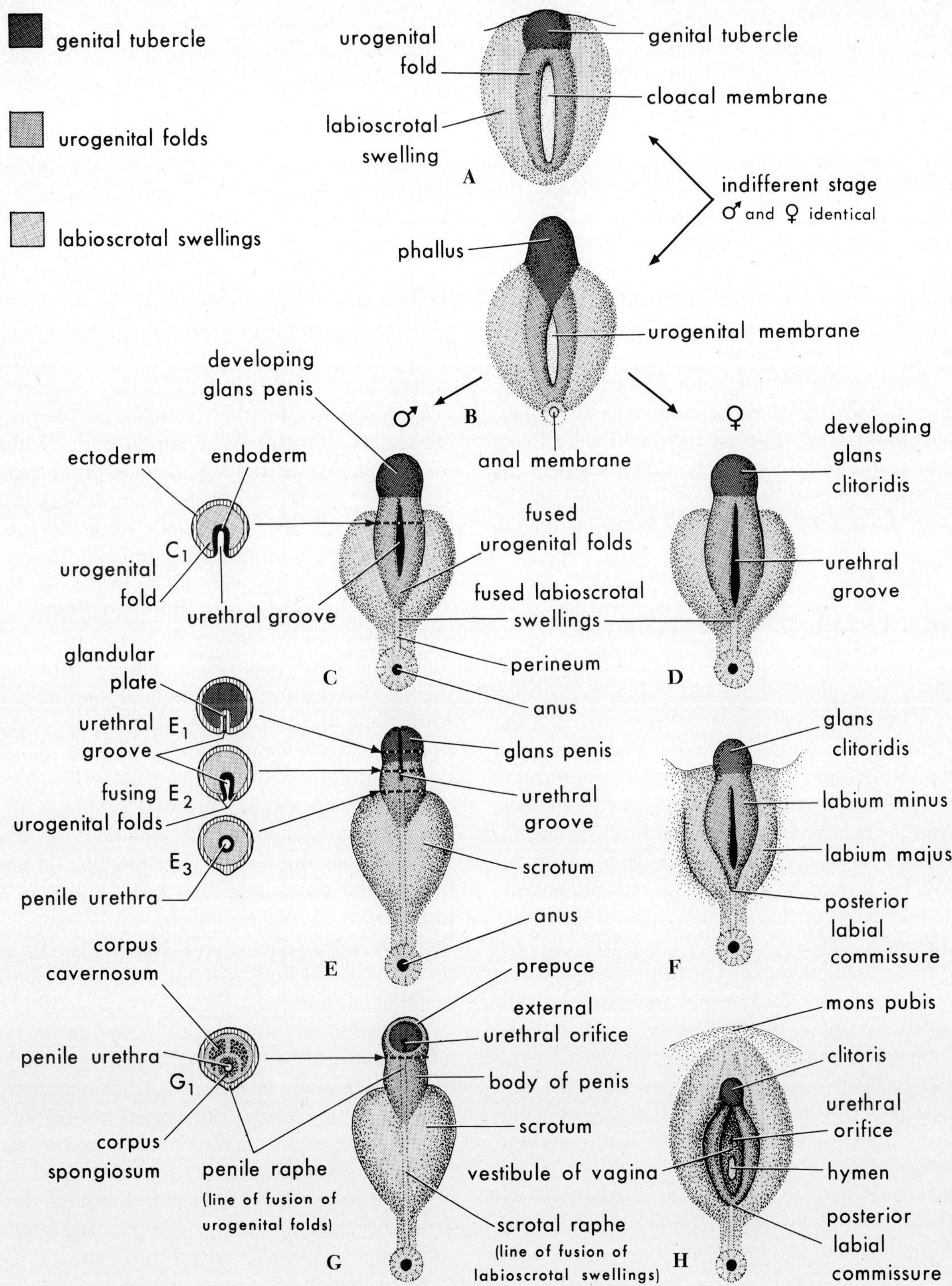

FIGURE 1-7

A and **B**, Development of the external genitalia in different stages (4 to 7 weeks). **C**, **E**, and **G**, Stages in the development of the external male genitalia at about 9, 11, and 12 weeks, respectively. To the left are schematic transverse sections (C_1, E_1 to E_3, and G_1) through the developing penis, illustrating formation of the penile urethra. **D**, **F**, and **H**, Stages in the development of the female external genitalia at 9, 11, and 12 weeks, respectively. (From Moore KL: The developing human: Clinically oriented embryology, 3rd ed., 1982. Courtesy W.B. Saunders Co.)

talia occurs. The embryonic phallus does not demonstrate rapid growth and becomes the clitoris. Urogenital folds do not fuse except in front of the anus. The unfused urogenital folds form the labia minora. The labioscrotal folds fuse posteriorly in the area of the perineal body but laterally remain as the labia majora. The labioscrotal folds do fuse anteriorly to form the mons pubis. A portion of the urogenital sinus between the level of the hymen and the labia develops into the vestibule of the vagina, into which the urethra, the vagina, and the ducts of Bartholin's glands enter.

The ovaries do not descend into the labioscrotal folds. A structure similar to the gubernaculum develops in the inguinal canal, giving rise to the round ligaments, which suspend the uterus in the adult. Fig. 1-7 summarizes the development of the external genitalia in each sex.

SEX DIFFERENTIATION

Genetic sex is determined at the time of conception. In general, a Y chromosome is necessary for the development of the testes, and the testes are responsible for the organization of the sexual duct system to a male configuration and for the suppression of the paramesonephric system. In the absence of a Y chromosome, indeed, in the absence of a gonad, development will be female in nature. General phenotypic development of the female seems to be a neutral event.

Genes coded on the Y chromosome are either responsible for the development of a cell-specific protein, the H-Y antigen, or for activator genes that will stimulate the gene for the H-Y antigen on another chromosome. In rare cases a Y chromosome may be absent, but the H-Y antigen may express itself. In theory, one could speculate that in such cases the H-Y antigen was indeed present on another chromosome, most likely the X chromosome, and that either an activator gene or some other gene that acts as an activator is capable of stimulating its response.

During the fifth week after conception, coelomic epithelium, later known as germinal epithelium, thickens in the area of the medial aspect of the mesonephros. As germinal epithelial cells proliferate, they invade the underlying mesenchyme, producing a prominence known as the gonadal ridge. In the sixth week the primordial germ cells, which have formed at about week 4 in the wall of the yolk sac, migrate up the dorsal mesentery of the hind gut and enter the undifferentiated gonad. For the formation of a testis, H-Y antigen must be activated. A gene or genes in the area of the centromere of the Y chromosome cause the somatic cells of the primitive gonadal ridge to differentiate into interstitial cells (Leydig cells) and Sertoli cells. As they do so, the primordial germ cells and Sertoli cells become enclosed within seminiferous tubules. The interstitial cells remain outside these tubules. H-Y antigen can be demonstrated in Sertoli cells at this stage but not in the developing germ cells. However, the H-Y antigen activity is passed to the germ cells by Sertoli cells when they are encased in the seminiferous tubules. This occurs in the seventh and eighth weeks. In the eighth week, Leydig cells differentiate and begin to produce testosterone. At this point the mesonephric (wolffian) duct differentiates into the vas deferens, epididymis, and seminal vesicles while the paramesonephric duct is suppressed. Suppression occurs because of the action of müllerian inhibiting factor (MIF).

Primary sex cords, meanwhile, have condensed and extended to the medullary portion of the developing testes. They branch and join to form the rete testes. The testis therefore is primarily a medullary organ, and eventually the rete testes connect with the tubules of the mesonephric system and join the developing epididymal duct.

In specific androgen target areas, testosterone is converted to 5-α-dihydrotestosterone by the microsomal enzyme Δ-4-5-α-reductase. Data suggest that two androgens, testosterone and its metabolite, dihydrotestosterone, are involved in sexual differentiation in the male fetus, with selective roles for each hormone during embryogenesis; that is, dihydrotestosterone stimulates the testes and scrotum, and testosterone stimulates the prostate gland.

Androgen action must be initiated at the target areas. Testosterone enters the cell and either is bound to a cytoplasmic receptor or, in certain target tissue, is converted to dihydrotestosterone. Dihydrotestosterone in such cells would then bind to a cytoplasmic receptor. Af-

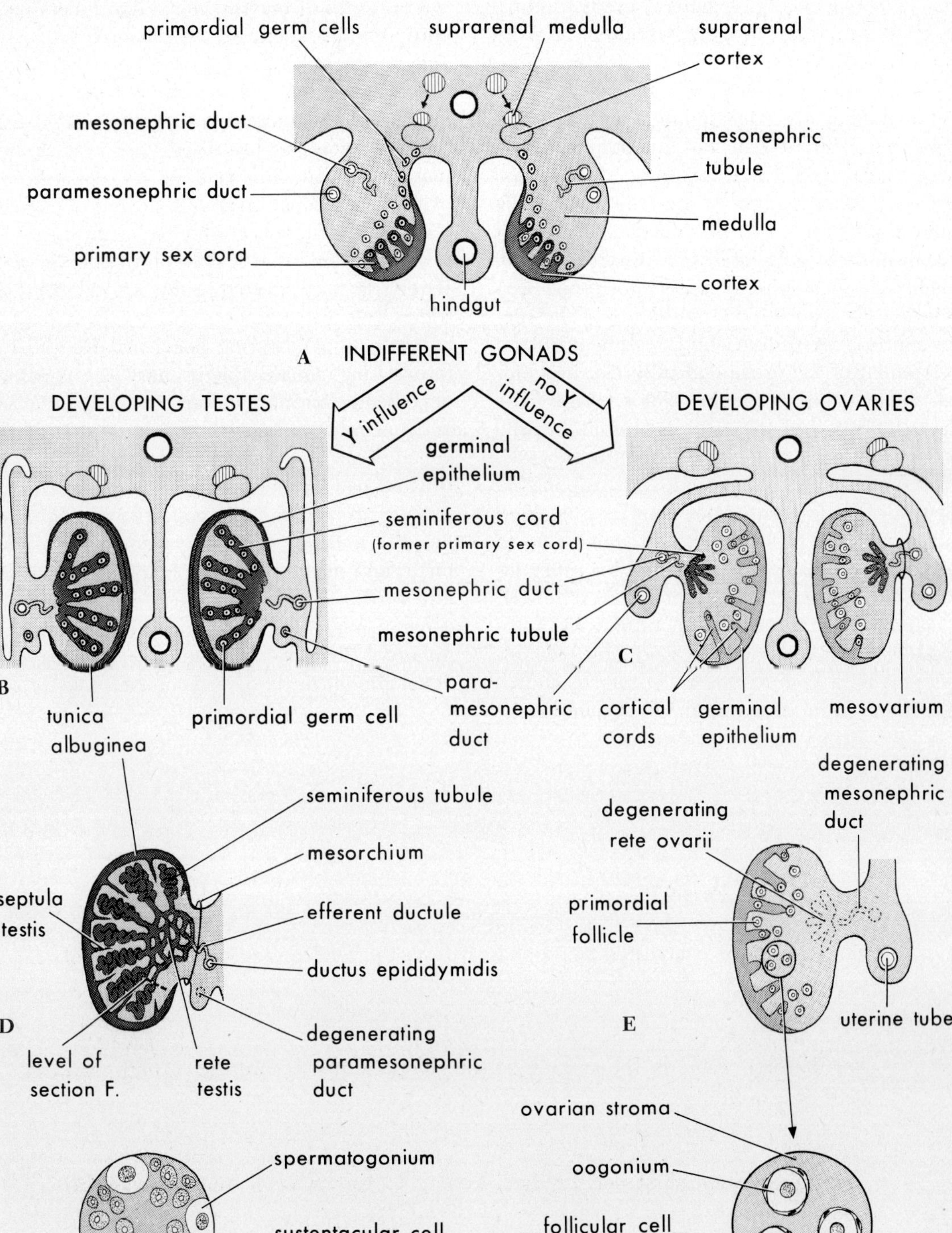

FIGURE 1-8

Differences in development in gonads of each sex. (From Moore KL: The developing human: Clinically oriented embryology, 3rd ed., 1982. Courtesy W.B. Saunders Co.)

terward, the androgen-receptor complex gains access to the nucleus, where it binds to chromatin and initiates the transcription of messenger ribonucleic acid. This leads to the metabolic process of androgen action.

For normal male development in utero, the testes must differentiate and function normally. At a critical point, MIF is produced by Sertoli cells and testosterone is secreted by Leydig cells. Both must be produced in sufficient amounts. MIF acts locally in suppressing the müllerian duct system, and testosterone acts systemically, causing differentiation of the mesonephric duct system and affecting male development of the urogenital tubercle, urogenital sinus, and urogenital folds. Thus the masculinization of the fetus is a multifactorial process under a variety of genetic controls. Genes on the Y chromosome are responsible for testicular differentiation. Enzymes involved in testosterone biosynthesis and conversion to dihydrotestosterone are regulated by genes located on autosomes. The ability to secrete MIF is a recessive trait coded on either the autosome or the X chromosome, and genes for development of cytoplasmic receptors of androgens seem to be coded on the X chromosome.

Development of the ovary occurs at about the eleventh or twelfth week. Two functional X chromosomes seem necessary for optimal development of the ovary. The effect of an X chromosome deficiency is most severe in species in which there is a long period between the formation and use of oocytes (i.e., the human). Thus in 45,X and 46,XY females, the ovaries are almost invariably devoid of oocytes. On the other hand, germ cells in the testes do best when only one X chromosome is present. Rarely do they survive in the XX or XXY condition.

When non-Y-bearing oocytes enter the differentiating gonad, the primary sex cords do not become prominent but, instead, break up and encircle the oocytes in the cortex of the gonad. This occurs at about 16 weeks, and the isolated cell clusters derived from the cortical cords that surround the oocytes are called primordial follicles. No new oogonia form after birth, and many of the oogonia degenerate before birth. Those which remain grow and become primary follicles to be stimulated after puberty. Fig. 1-8 illustrates the differences in development in the gonads of each sex.

_______________ KEY POINTS _______________

- Oocyte meiosis is arrested at prophase I from the fetal period until the time of ovulation.

- Fertilization occurs in the ampulla of the fallopian tube before the second polar body is cast off.

- After fertilization, first cell division leading to the two-cell embryo takes 20 hours.

- The human embryo enters the uterus somewhere between 3 and 4 days after conception. At this point it will be between the 32-cell and blastocyst stages of development.

- Implantation occurs when trophoblastic cells contact endometrium and burrow beneath the surface by enzymatic action. This generally takes place 3 days after the embryo enters the uterus.

- Twinning may occur at any time until the formation of the blastula, after which time each cell is no longer multipotential.

- The earliest fetal epithelium to develop is the ectoderm, the second is the entoderm, and the third is the mesoderm.

- Chorionic gonadotrophin is secreted by the syncytiotrophoblast at about the time of implantation. It doubles in quantity every 1.2 to 2 days and until 7 to 9 weeks of gestation.

- Angiogenesis is seen by day 15 or 16. Embryonic heart function begins in the third week of gestation.

- Organogenesis is complete by day 49.

- The mesonephric duct system gives rise in the male to the epididymis, vas deferens, and seminal vesicles. Remnants of the mesonephric duct system in the female remain as parovarian cysts and Gartner's duct.

- The paramesonephric duct system develops in the female to give rise to the fallopian tube, uterus, and cervix. Remnants give rise to the hydatid of Morgagni at the end of the fallopian tubes. Remnants in the male remain as the appendix of the testes and prostatic utricle.

- The vagina develops from the sinovaginal bulbs, which are outgrowths of the urogenital sinus. Failure of these bulbs to form leads to agenesis of the vagina.

- The adult kidney develops from the metanephros, and its collecting system (ureter and caliceal system) develops from the metanephric (ureteric) bud from the mesonephric duct.

- The urinary bladder develops from the urogenital sinus.

affected. A recessive characteristic requires the same mutant gene on both paired chromosomes for expression.

Nondisjunction. The failure of a pair of chromosomes to separate during meiosis or mitosis. In meiosis, if one daughter cell receives both members of the chromosome pair, then after fertilization a triple number of each chromosome, or a trisomic state, exists in each cell.

Penetrance. The percentage of individuals in a population with a mutation that actually demonstrates a phenotypic change.

RNA (Ribonucleic Acid). A single-helix nuclear protein that serves several purposes in the cell. It is composed of a sugar (ribose), a phosphate, and a purine or pyrimidine base.

Translocation. The rearrangement of two chromosomes involving the exchange of chromosome material. Balanced translocation is one in which no active genetic material is lost.

A large number of illnesses and conditions have a genetic basis. In some cases the problem arises from a single-point mutation within a gene, whereas others may involve changes in multiple genes or in an interreaction of genes and environmental factors. Finally, some conditions are the result of chromosome abnormalities of a variety of types. Although this chapter cannot provide a complete course in genetics, it will attempt to offer an understanding of the genetic basis of conditions of particular interest to the gynecologist.

GENES AND GENE ACTION

Genes consist of deoxyribonucleic acid (DNA) molecules, which are made up of a linear sequence of nucleotides, each of which is composed of a pentose sugar, a phosphate, and a nitrogenous base. Four such bases are found in a DNA molecule. They are two purines, adenine (A) and guanine (G), and two pyrimidines, thymine (T) and cytosine (C). It has been shown that the total amount of purine in DNA molecules equals the total amount of pyrimidine, and the pairings of A to T and G to C always occur in the two strands of the double helix. These associations allow for accuracy both in the replication of the DNA molecule and in the translation of a genetic message from the DNA molecule to the development of a single-strand ribonucleic acid (RNA) molecule

known as messenger RNA. The message is transmitted in such a fashion that a configuration with three bases in sequence represents a code for an amino acid. This has been called the genetic code. With the message of the gene encoded on the messenger RNA, the latter leaves the nucleus of the cell, attaches to a cytoplasmic structure (the ribosome), and then attracts amino acids by means of smaller RNA molecules known as transfer RNA. Transfer RNA molecules each carry a specific amino acid and have three bases, which match the code of the messenger RNA, following the A to T and G to C pairings. In the RNA molecule, uracil (U) is substituted for thymine. When all segments of the message are covered, the amino acids are spliced together and the protein determined by the message is complete and free for use in the cell and for transport from the cell. Fig. 2-1 schematically demonstrates this process.

GENE MUTATION

Conditions that change the sequence of bases in the genetic code may cause a mutation. The mutation may involve a single point, that is, the changing of a single base, or a larger segment, in which the bases are removed or replaced. Mutation may occur spontaneously by the accidental replacement of one base with another during replication of DNA,

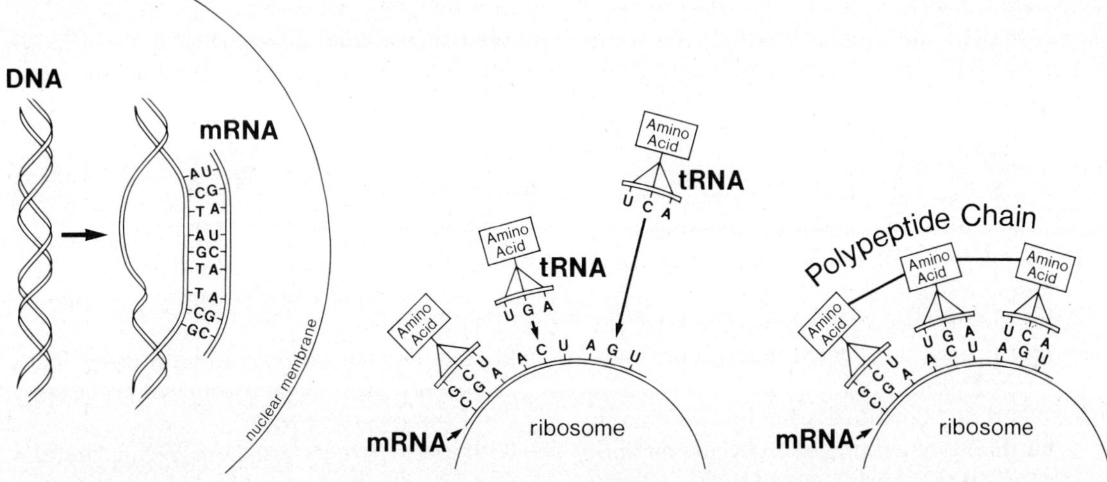

FIGURE 2-1

Schematic representation of protein production from genetic message on the DNA molecule to the final product.

by the incorporation of an inappropriate base during repair of a DNA molecule, or by an intermediate replacement with a substance similar to a usual base but capable of entering the DNA molecule and later attracting an inappropriate base in the next replication. Agents such as x-rays or other forms of irradiation may break a DNA strand, leading to the loss of one or more bases and a complete change in the sequence or to a replacement with an inappropriate base during healing. Even a single-point mutation will lead to the production of a modified protein that may be responsible for an abnormal expression of a trait. Fig. 2-2 demonstrates such an occurrence for a group of hemoglobinopathies caused by the substitution of a single base at a single point.

	Possible Mutation 1	Possible Mutation 2
Hgb A (glutamic acid)	CTT	CTC
Hgb S (valine)	CAT	CAC
Hgb C (lysine)	TTT	TTC

FIGURE 2-2

Point mutation in a DNA molecule causing a single amino acid substitution and conversion of hemoglobin A to hemoglobin S or hemoglobin C.

TYPES OF INHERITANCE

Autosomal Dominant Trait

If only one gene of a pair is mutated, and if the altered protein produced by the mutated gene brings about a phenotypic change, the condition is said to be autosomal dominant. If both genes of a pair must carry the mutation for the phenotypic characteristic to occur, the condition is said to be autosomal recessive. Usually, if 50% of the protein produced by the gene pair is enough to give the usual phenotype, the condition is dominant. However, phenotypic expression of a mutation may occasionally occur under unusual circumstances. For example, a patient with sickle cell trait will usually not experience red blood cell sickling at sea level with normal oxygen saturation but may do so at high altitudes or in cases of decreased oxygen saturation such as may occur with pneumonia. Thus the presence of hemoglobin S in the red blood cell in equal proportions to hemoglobin A will usually not lead to the expression of sickling unless oxygen saturation is decreased.

With respect to autosomal dominant conditions, the concept of *penetrance* and *expressivity* must be introduced to explain some variations noted. Penetrance is the percentage of individuals in a population with the mutation that actually demonstrate the phenotypic change. Expressivity is the degree to which the phenotypic change occurs in the affected individual, that is, the degree to which the gene expresses itself. Penetrance and expressivity are dependent on the action of other genes and on environmental factors that may modify the action of the mutated gene.

The following general statements can be made about autosomal dominant mutations:

1. Phenotypic expression appears with equal frequency in both sexes.
2. For inheritance to take place, at least one parent must be affected unless a new mutation has occurred.
3. When an individual who is homozygous for the mutation (mutation occurs on both genes of the pair) is mated with a normal individual, all offspring will carry the trait. When a heterozygous individual is mated with a normal individual, 50% of the offspring will demonstrate the trait.
4. If the trait is rare in the population, most individuals demonstrating it will be heterozygous.

The following is a list of a number of autosomal dominant conditions:

Achondroplasia
Angioedema, hereditary
Craniofacial dysostosis
Dupuytren's contracture
Ehlers-Danlos syndrome
Facial palsy, congenital
Huntington's chorea
Intestinal polyposis
Keloid formation
Marfan's syndrome
Mitral valve prolapse
Muscular dystrophy
Neurofibromatosis (von Recklinghausen's disease)
Night blindness
Otosclerosis
Pectus excavatum
Renal disease, polycystic, adult type
Tuberous sclerosis
von Willebrand's disease
Wolff-Parkinson-White syndrome (some cases)

When one parent demonstrates one of these conditions, appropriate counseling would be that 50% of future offspring could be expected to demonstrate the condition as well. When neither parent demonstrates the condition but when a child is born with such a condition, it can be assumed that the problem is caused by a new mutation. In such cases, future progeny of the couple would be expected to be no more likely to have the condition than would occur by chance mutation.

Autosomal Recessive Trait

The following general statements can be made about an autosomal recessive trait:

1. The characteristic will occur equally in both sexes.
2. For the characteristic to be present, both parents must demonstrate or be carriers of the recessive trait.
3. If both parents are homozygous for the trait, all offspring will demonstrate it.
4. If both parents are heterozygous (carrier) for the trait, 25% of the offspring will have the trait and 50% will be carriers. The remaining 25% will be free of the trait.
5. Consanguinity is often present in families demonstrating frequent occurrences of rare recessive traits.

The following lists a number of common autosomal recessive conditions:

Acid maltase deficiency
Alkaptonuria
Ataxia-telangectasia
Bloom's syndrome
Color blindness (total)
Cystic fibrosis
Cystinosis
Cystinuria
Deafness (many variants)
Dysautonomia
Galactosemia
Gaucher's disease
Glaucoma (congenital)
Homocystinuria
Maple syrup urine disease
Mucolipidosis I, II, III
Mucopolysaccharidosis I-H, I-S, III, IV, VI, VII
Muscular dystrophy (autosomal recessive)
Niemann-Pick disease
Phenylketonuria
Sickle cell anemia
11β-hydroxylase deficiency
21-hydroxylase deficiency
Tay-Sachs disease
Wilson's disease

In counseling a couple who have produced a child with such a characteristic, it is appropriate to tell them that 25% of future offspring will have the condition and 50% will be carriers. If a prenatal diagnostic test is available, it should be offered. One autosomal recessive condition, Tay-Sachs disease, is the subject of a large national screening program to determine carriers. Since the condition usually occurs in Jews of Eastern European origin, such individuals should certainly be offered screening.

X-linked Trait

Most X-linked conditions are recessive in type, since female carriers do not demonstrate the trait. A few conditions belie this rule, however, and are really X-linked dominant conditions. For the X-linked recessive trait the following statements are true:

1. The condition occurs more commonly in males.
2. If both parents are free of the trait and a male is produced with the trait, it must be assumed that the mother is a carrier.
3. If the father is affected and an affected male is produced, it must be assumed that the mother is at least a carrier of the trait.
4. If a female is produced who exhibits the X-linked trait, she may do so for one of two reasons. First, she may have received the mutant gene from both the mother and father and thereby is homozygous for the trait. Generally this would imply the presence of an affected father and a carrier mother. Second, she may exhibit the trait as a function of the *Lyon hypothesis*, which states that in a female heterozygous for the trait, each cell of the developing embryo from about the time of implantation selects and uses one X chromosome only. Thereafter all developing cells from these particular cells use the same X chromosome. Thus a female is mosaic for her two X chromosomes, with some cells using the paternal X and some the maternal X chromosome. Since this selection occurs on a random basis, some females will be produced who use an X chromosome predominantly from one parent. If the X chromosome has the mutation, the female will exhibit the trait because of the

quantitative influence of that chromosome. Thus the female may be genotypically heterozygous but still exhibit the trait.

In the case of X-linked dominant traits the following may be said:

1. They occur in both males and females with equal frequency.
2. An affected male mated to a normal female will produce offspring with the trait 50% of the time, but all female offspring will be affected.
3. An affected homozygous female mated to a normal male will produce offspring with the trait 100% of the time.
4. Occasional heterozygous females will not exhibit the trait on the basis of the Lyon hypothesis.

The following lists several X-linked recessive conditions:

Agammaglobulinemia, X-linked, infantile
Androgen insensitivity syndrome, complete
Androgen insensitivity syndrome, incomplete
Color blindness, several varieties
Diabetes insipidus, some varieties
Fabry's disease
Glucose-6-phosphate dehydrogenase deficiency
Gonadal dysgenesis, XY type (probable)
Gout, some types
Factor VIII disease
Factor IX disease
Lesch-Nyhan syndrome
Mucopolysaccharidosis II
Muscular dystrophy, Duchenne type

Some X-linked dominant conditions are as follows:

Aero-osteolysis, dominant type
Cervico-oculo-acoustic syndrome
Hyperammonemia
Orofaciodigital syndrome I
Tubular stenosis (possible)

Multifactorial Inheritance

Multifactorial inheritance is defined as traits or characteristics produced by the action of several genes, with or without the interplay of environmental factors. A number of structural abnormalities such as cleft palate and harelip, open neural tube disease (including anencephaly and spina bifida), and several orthopedic defects are examples of such conditions. When both parents are normal and an affected child is produced, the chance of recurrence is generally between 2% and 5% for any given pregnancy. These risk rates, however, are modified when one or both parents are affected with the condition or when close relatives are also affected. Many multifactorial diseases and conditions are more common in offspring when transmitted via the mother, and in general, when more than one offspring is affected in a family, the chances that subsequent offspring will be affected are greater.

Open neural tube disease (NTD) is a good example of a multifactorial defect. When a couple produces such a child, appropriate counseling is important. In the case of this condition the observation that alpha-fetoprotein is increased both in the amniotic fluid and in the maternal serum in affected offspring is helpful in making a prenatal diagnosis of the condition. Ultrasound examination is also helpful in making a specific diagnosis. It is of interest that although the diagnosis can be made prenatally if looked for, 9 of 10 cases will occur spontaneously in the offspring of couples who have no previous family or personal history. This observation has led to the suggestion that all pregnancies be screened with maternal serum alpha-fetoprotein determinations to uncover such cases antenatally. At present, screening programs are common, and patients should probably be offered the option of being studied even if there is no history of open neural tube disease in the family. The screening of 1000 pregnant women will uncover about 50 who have maternal serum alpha-fetoprotein determinations in excess of 2.5 times the mean for values considered normal for their specific week of gestation. Although a number of instances of multiple gestation, Turner's syndrome, other anomalies, and fetal demise may be uncovered, only about 1 of these 50 women will actually prove to be carrying a fetus with NTD.

Chromosome Abnormalities

A variety of chromosome abnormalities may occur during meiosis or mitosis (see Chapter 1). They fall into several general categories, and many clinical conditions are associated with each type. Although it is impossible to discuss every clinical condition associated with a known chromosome abnormality within the scope of this chapter, an attempt will be made to categorize the specific types of anomalies and the more common problems seen by obstetricians and gynecologists that relate to these anomalies. Several will be dealt with in more detail in other chapters of this book.

Nondisjunctional Events and Deletion

A nondisjunctional event is the faulty separation of chromosome pairs at anaphase in either meiosis or mitosis. The final result in meiosis is that the daughter cell receives either both chromosomes of the pair or neither. At

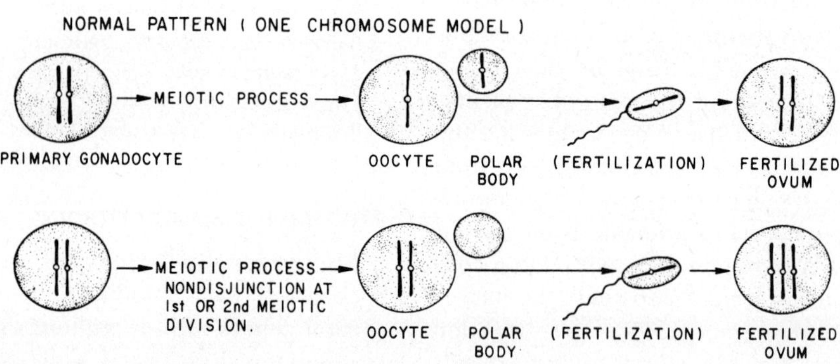

FIGURE 2-3
Meiotic nondisjunction, graphic representation. (Reproduced with permission from Stenchever MA: Human cytogenetics: A workbook in reproductive biology. Copyright © 1973 by Year Book Medical Publishers, Inc., Chicago.)

the time of fertilization, with the addition of another haploid set of chromosomes, the resulting individual will have either three chromosomes at that particular position or only one (Fig. 2-3). In normal mitosis, after division of the chromosomes at anaphase, a complete pair goes to each daughter cell. If nondisjunction occurs, three chromosomes go to one daughter cell and one to the other.

Deletion is the simple loss of a chromosome

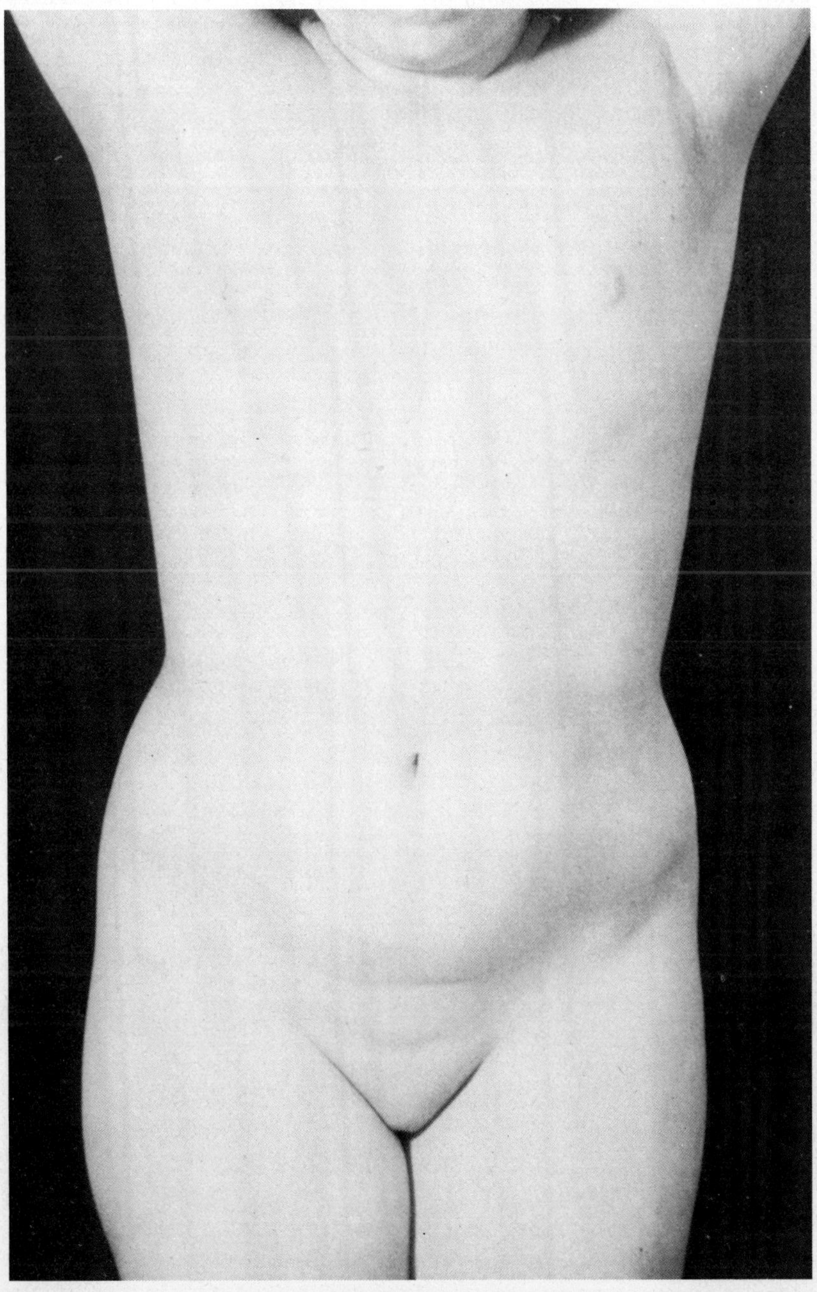

FIGURE 2-4
Torso of an individual with Turner's syndrome. (From Stenchever MA: Chromosome evaluation: Clinical applications. In Taymor MC, Green TH, eds: Progress in gynecology, vol. VI. New York, Grune & Stratton, 1975.)

at anaphase because of either anaphase lag or nondisjunction. In this instance the new cell receives only one chromosome of the pair and is essentially monosomic for that chromosome. Monosomic states involving autosomes are extremely rare and generally lethal. With respect to the sex chromosomes, monosomy of the Y chromosome without the presence of an X chromosome is likewise lethal and has never been seen in a clinical situation or even in an abortus. Monosomy of the X chromosome, however, is the typical finding in the condition known as Turner's syndrome. This condition is likewise lethal, with as many as 24 of each 25 of such conceptuses being aborted. When an infant is born alive with a 45,X karyotype, the common denominators of shortness of stature and sexual infantilism are seen, and many abnormalities involving most of the organ systems may likewise occur. One frequent occurrence (about 50% of cases) is webbing of the neck, which is the end product of hygromas seen during embryologic development (Fig. 2-4).

Nondisjunctional events involving the autosomes have been seen in abortus material in all but chromosomes 1 and 17. However, in infants born alive, only trisomy states of chromosomes 13, 18, 21, and 22 and an occasional C group chromosome have been seen. Trisomy of chromosome 13 (Patau's syndrome) results in

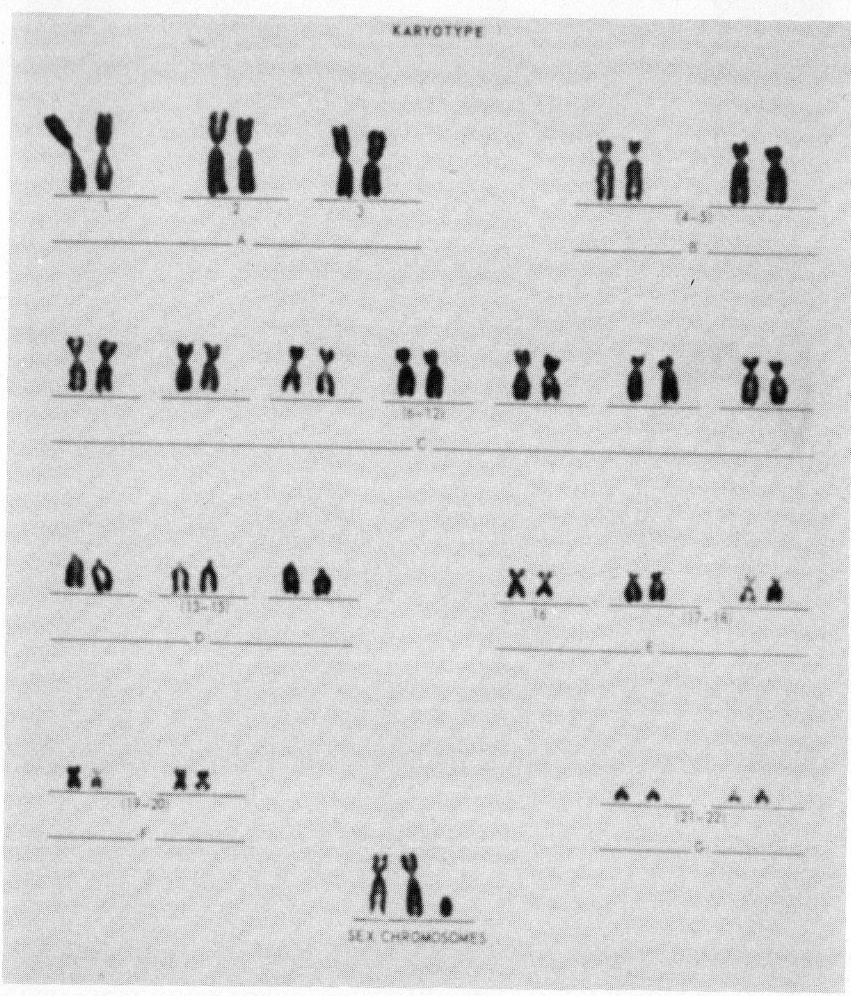

FIGURE 2-5
Karyotype 47,XXY—Klinefelter's syndrome. (From Stenchever MA: Chromosome evaluation: Clinical applications. In Taymor MC, Green TH, eds: Progress in gynecology, vol. VI. New York, Grune & Stratton, 1975.)

gross multiple structural defects that are usually incompatible with extended life. Trisomy of chromosome 18 likewise leads to a syndrome (Edwards' syndrome) that has a characteristic group of structural abnormalities, again generally not compatible with long life. Trisomy 21 is classic Down syndrome, and trisomy 22 has been seen in a few live-born individuals but is associated with severe retardation.

Trisomy involving the sex chromosomes has been seen in circumstances relating to both X and the Y chromosome. Nondisjunctional events involving both oogenesis and spermatogenesis can be responsible, as in autosomal trisomy.

If trisomy X is the result, a female with a reasonably normal phenotype is produced. Mild mental retardation is occasionally present, but fertility is present in at least 50% of such individuals. Although most of the offspring produced are normal chromosomally, there is a slight increase of offspring with nondisjunctional events involving both the sex chromosomes and the autosomes.

Individuals with a 47,XXY karyotype are likewise produced as the result of a nondisjunctional event involving the sex chromosomes that may occur by an error in either oogenesis or spermatogenesis (Fig. 2-5). This leads to the clinical state of Klinefelter's syndrome. The classic finding in these individuals is that they are usually tall of stature and suffer from azoospermia caused by sclerosis of the seminiferous tubules. Other mild phenotypic anomalies may be present. One of these, gynecomastia, is present in about one third of the cases (Fig. 2-6). Men with Klinefelter's syndrome have primary infertility.

Nondisjunction during spermatogenesis involving the Y chromosome can lead to the karyotype 47,XYY (Fig. 2-7). Such individuals may be entirely normal phenotypically but generally are tall of stature, and many have aggressive personalities. For this reason a number have been found in prisons and mental hospitals, but just as many have been found among the normal population. Although such men are fertile, their female partners often suffer from reproductive wastage problems, and this may be the means of identifying such cases. In addition, they often produce offspring with normal karyotypes but may produce conceptuses

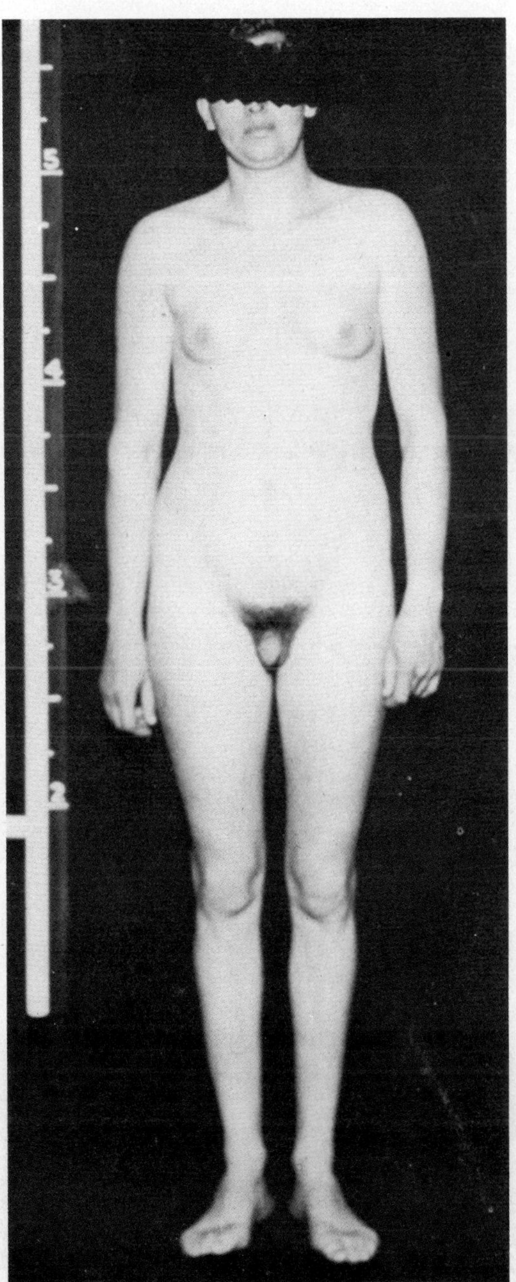

FIGURE 2-6
An individual with Klinefelter's syndrome demonstrating gynecomastia. (From Stenchever MA: Chromosome evaluation: Clinical applications. In Taymor MC, Green TH, eds: Progress in gynecology, vol. VI. New York, Grune & Stratton, 1975.)

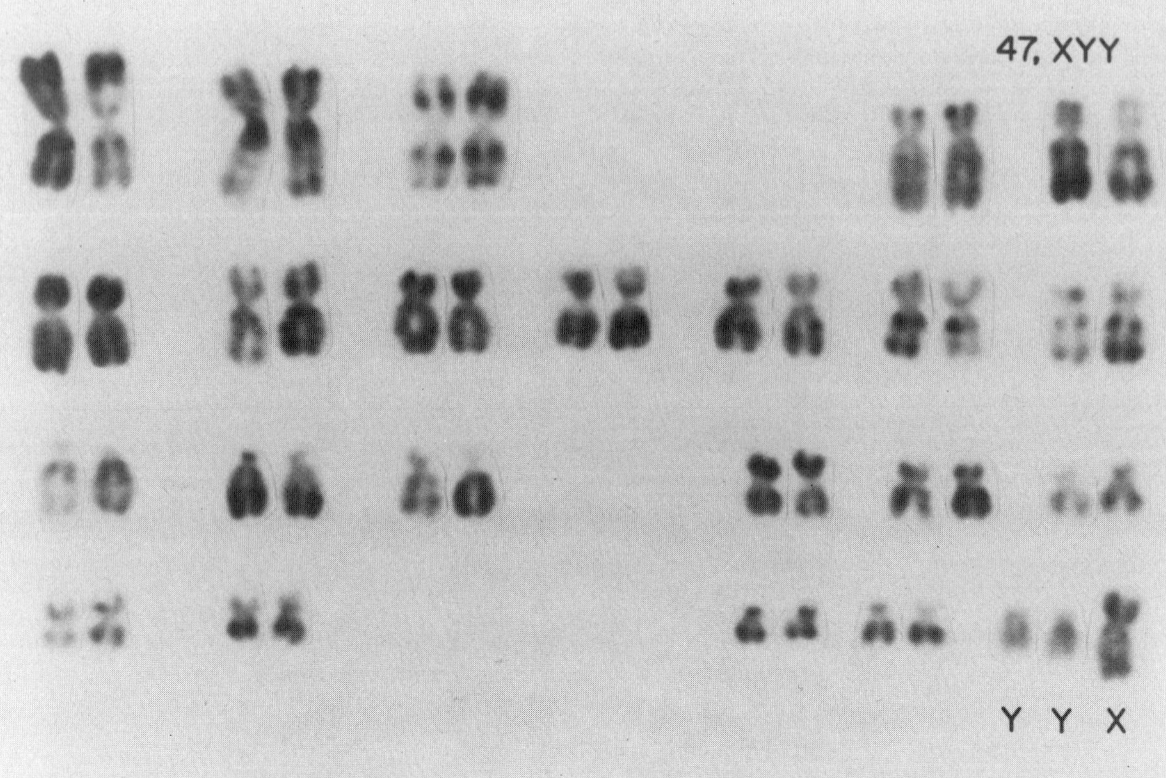

FIGURE 2-7

Karyotype 47,XYY. (From Stenchever MA: Chromosome evaluation: Clinical applications. In Taymor MC, Green TH, eds: Progress in gynecology, vol. VI. New York, Grune & Stratton, 1975.)

with trisomic problems involving both autosomes and the sex chromosomes.

Nondisjunctional events during mitosis in the early embryo will frequently produce individuals with cell populations containing different chromosome numbers. This condition is known as *mosaicism* and may be seen involving any of the members of the autosome complement or the sex chromosomes. The actual phenotype produced depends on the number of cells present with an abnormal complement and on the tissue in which these cells have the opportunity to express themselves.

Chromosome Breaks and Rearrangements

Chromosome breaks and rearrangements may be brought about by damage to the chromosome caused by irradiation of many different types, by viruses, or by other changes within the cell or within its environment that can damage the chromosome structure or the DNA molecule within the chromosome. When these breaks occur, a number of things can happen. The break may simply heal, with or without a point mutation at the point of breakage. If a segment of the chromosome is lost during this healing process, partial deletion of chromatin material may take place. If two chromosomes break, they may exchange chromosome arms and give rise to a translocation. In karyotypes, translocations have been seen involving various combinations of all the chromosomes. They are probably a chance occurrence, although there may be some active areas on various chromosomes that make such events more common. Rearranged chromosomes at first are generally balanced with respect to gene complement, and the individual so affected is referred to as a carrier of the translocation and can expect in most cases to be phenotypically normal. About 10% of new translocations, even though balanced, are associated with mental retardation and other mild anomalies. These carrier individuals, however, have difficulty when meiosis occurs in gametogenesis. With the production of the gametes the stage might be set for reassortment of chromosomes in such a way that normal chromosomes pair with abnormal chromosomes, leading to partial trisomy or partial monosomy of various chromatin materials. Such individuals are said to be unbalanced and will generally have relatively severe phenotypic abnormalities. Roughly 3% to 4% of all abortuses have unbalanced chromosome rearrangements. In addition, some live-born infants have unbalanced translocations.

Fig. 2-8 demonstrates two possible ways that such translocations can come about. The first involves the fusion of two acrocentric chromosomes in which the short arms of both and the centromere of one are lost, with the production of a chromosome that essentially has the long arm of each of these two chromosomes and an overall reduction of the chromosome number by one. Thus the balanced carrier has 45 chromosomes with the loss of one normal chromosome from each pair involved and the formation of one translocated chromosome. This is known as *Robertsonian fusion.* Gametes produced by such an individual will be either normal in chromosome configuration, balanced as in the parent, unbalanced because the translocated chromosome and one or the other of the normal chromosomes of the pairs involved are included, or monosomic because only one of the chromosomes is present and not the translocated chromosome. After fertilization, one would expect that 25% of the offspring would

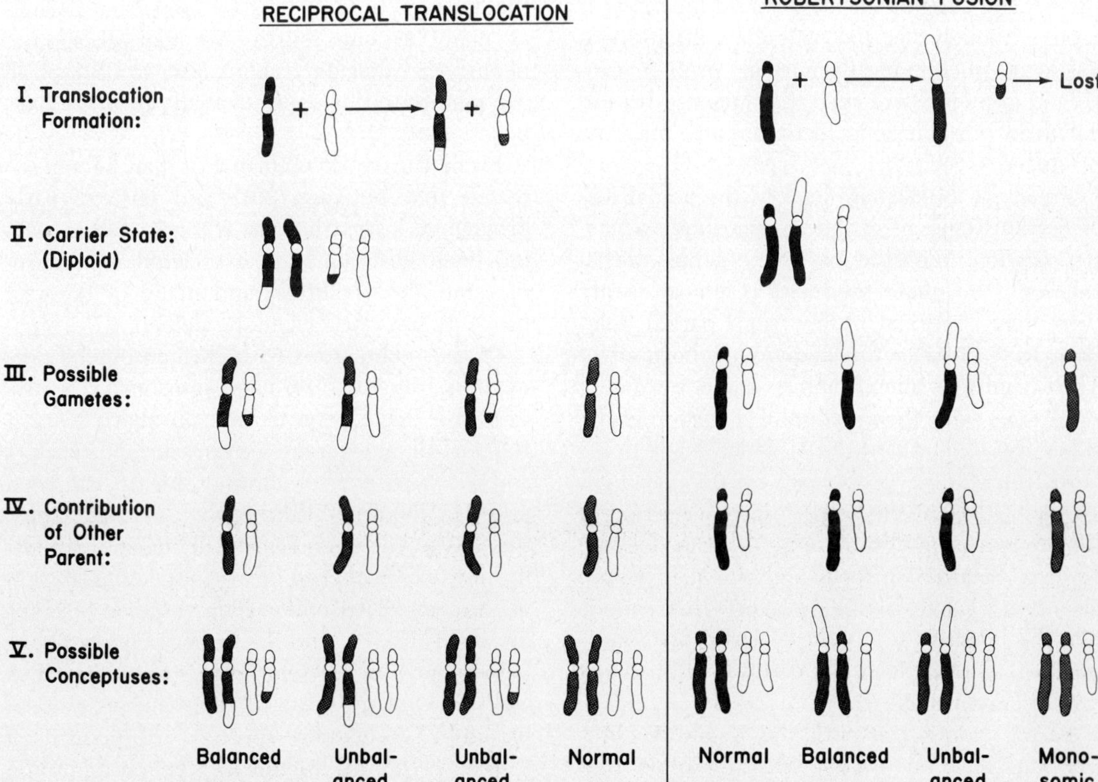

FIGURE 2-8

Schematic representation of translocation formation, including reciprocal translocation and Robertsonian fusion. (From Stenchever MA: Contemp OB/GYN 16:24, Sept. 1980.)

be normal, 25% carriers, 25% unbalanced and affected, and 25% monosomic and probably would be aborted.

The other means of translocation is the reciprocal translocation, in which chromatin material is exchanged between chromosomes but the chromosome number does not change. In this case, two new chromosomes are essentially produced, and with gamete formation one can expect either a normal gamete, a gamete with the two balanced translocated chromosomes, or two possibilities in which a normal chromosome of one pair is matched with one of the translocated chromosomes. About 25% of the offspring could be expected to be normal, 25% balanced carriers, and 50% unbalanced and abnormal. Indeed, women with the carrier state of reciprocal translocation are frequently found among those with recurrent abortions.

If one chromosome breaks at two points, the broken segment may turn on its axis, leading to an *inversion*. If the centromere is present in the broken segment, a *pericentric inversion* is seen. Although this, too, will allow the individual to be phenotypically normal, problems involved in meiosis are such that infants with unbalanced chromosome components may be produced.

Finally, a break may lead to the actual loss of a small segment of the chromosome, a *partial deletion*. With the loss of the genes on that segment, the infant produced is almost always extremely abnormal. A few such partial deletions have been seen in individuals born alive. The resulting abnormalities include Wolf's syndrome, with the deletion of a portion of the short arm of chromosome 4, which leads to severe retardation problems; cri-du-chat syndrome, which involves the loss of a portion of the short arm of chromosome 5, again leading to gross retardation in an individual in whom laryngeal changes result in a cry that sounds like the plaintive cry of a cat; and gross abnormalities resulting from the deletion of the short arm of chromosome 18.

Partial deletion of both the X and Y chromosomes have been seen. With the loss of part or all of the short arm (Xp−) of the X chromosome, many of the findings of Turner's syndrome, including shortness of stature, have been noted. With the loss of all or part of the long arm of the X chromosome (Xq−), some of the findings of Turner's syndrome have been seen, but not shortness of stature.

Chromosome Abnormalities and Abortion

Hertig and Rock observed, as early as 1949, that many early gestations were obviously defective and that a genetic defect might be responsible. When it became possible to karyotype these abortuses, a number of investigators verified this theory by finding specific chromosome anomalies of a variety of types. Now with banding techniques, specific chromosomes can be identified and the abnormalities more accurately categorized.

With the use of the data from a number of different studies, it has been estimated that about 15% of ova penetrated by sperm fail to divide. Another 15% fail to implant, and 25% to 30% are aborted spontaneously at previllous stages. Of the roughly 40% of fertilized ova that survive the first missed menstrual period, as many as one fourth are aborted spontaneously, so that only about 30% to 35% of all ova penetrated by sperm actually result in liveborn infants.

From the work of many, it has been estimated that between 30% and 60% of early pregnancy losses that are recognizable as having been gestations are associated with chromosome abnormalities, and many of the rest probably have other genetic defects.

Of those abortuses with chromosome abnormalities, roughly 50% have autosomal trisomy. Trisomies have been defined in abortus material for all autosomes except chromosomes 1 and 17. A trisomy of chromosome 16 has been noted in about one third of the cases, and since this has never been seen in living individuals, it must be considered universally lethal (Fig. 2-9). Autosomal trisomies such as those of chromosomes 13, 18, and 21 do occur in live-born babies but may be seen in abortus material as well. It is of interest that as many as 80% of trisomy 21 fetuses are aborted. The error itself is that of nondisjunction of the chromosome pair at anaphase in either the first or second meiotic division. Because the risk of repeating a nondisjunctional event is greater than in the general population, a woman who is known to have produced a trisomic abortus should be of-

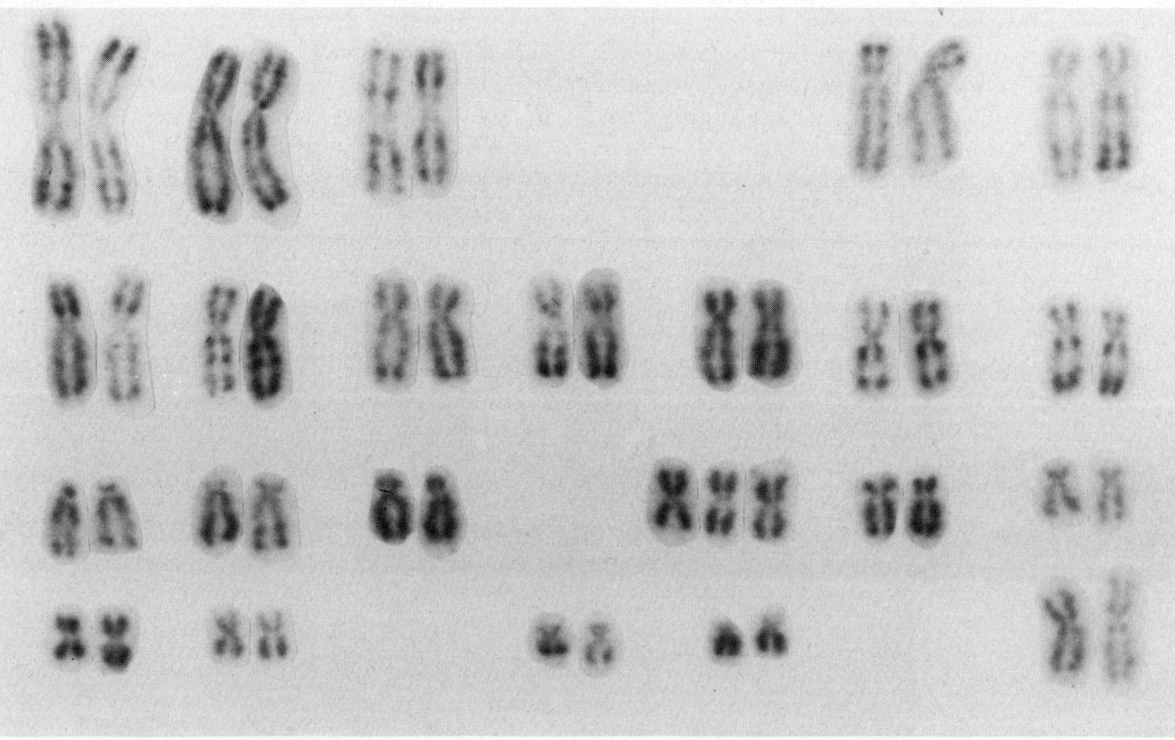

FIGURE 2-9
Karyotype of an abortus with 47,XX,16+. (From Stenchever MA: Contemp OB/
GYN 17:38, April 1981.)

fered prenatal diagnosis by amniocentesis in much the same fashion as she would be if she had previously produced a live-born infant with a trisomy. In women who have produced a conceptus that is trisomic, the risk of subsequent trisomy is 2% to 5%.

Roughly 20% of the chromosomally aborted abnormal fetuses have the karyotype 45,X. Only about 5% of such conceptuses are born alive, and these have the characteristic findings of Turner's syndrome. The mechanism responsible for this condition seems to be the loss of a sex chromosome at zygote formation, but the loss of a chromosome via the mechanism of nondisjunction is also possible. The error leading to the problem may occur in either male or female meiosis, and a variety of mosaic patterns have been seen, indicating that errors in mitosis after fertilization may also occur. Data obtained from studies using as a marker the Xg blood group, which is coded on the X-chromosome, suggest that about three fourths of living 45,X individuals use the X chromosome derived from the mother.

Sex chromosome trisomies such as 47,XXX, 47,XXY, and 47,XYY are rarely found in abortus material. The relative lethality of such karyotypes is probably minor, and most individuals are born alive. Each birth occurs at a rate of about once per thousand live births of infants of the appropriate sex.

Triploidy occurs in between 14% and 19% of abortuses with chromosome abnormalities and apparently results from errors in meiosis or from double fertilization of a single ovum. It has been seen in live-born infants only as a mosaic when a normal cell line is also present. Using special chromosome banding techniques, Kajii and Nikawa demonstrated that triploidy occurs by a variety of mechanisms. This phenomenon has been seen in artificially bred cattle and in other animals as well. It is thought to be the result of late insemination in some cases. In such situations, double fertilization in an egg that has lost its selectivity for penetration by normal sperm may be the mechanism. Triploid abortuses frequently are associated with multiple anomalies as well as hydropic degeneration of the placenta (Fig. 2-10). Some hydatidiform moles, therefore, have a triploid karyotype.

Tetraploidy, or a mean chromosome count of 92, occurs in 3% to 6% of all chromosomally abnormal abortuses. This condition is undoubtedly lethal, since it has never been seen in living individuals. It probably occurs when chromosome division is not followed by cytoplasmic division in the initial cell division of the zygote.

Rearrangements, primarily translocations and inversions, are noted in about 3% of all chromosomally abnormal abortuses. According to Creasy and associates, most but definitely not all of these are unbalanced translocations. Although most unbalanced translocations in conceptuses result in abortion, some individuals are born alive.

A discussion of chromosome abnormalities among early abortuses is not complete without mentioning the findings in a series of stillbirths. Shepard and Fantel noted that of 283 stillborn infants, 17 had chromosome abnormalities, a rate of 6%. Trisomies occurred in 58.8% of these chromosomally abnormal fetuses. Sex chromosome abnormalities occurred

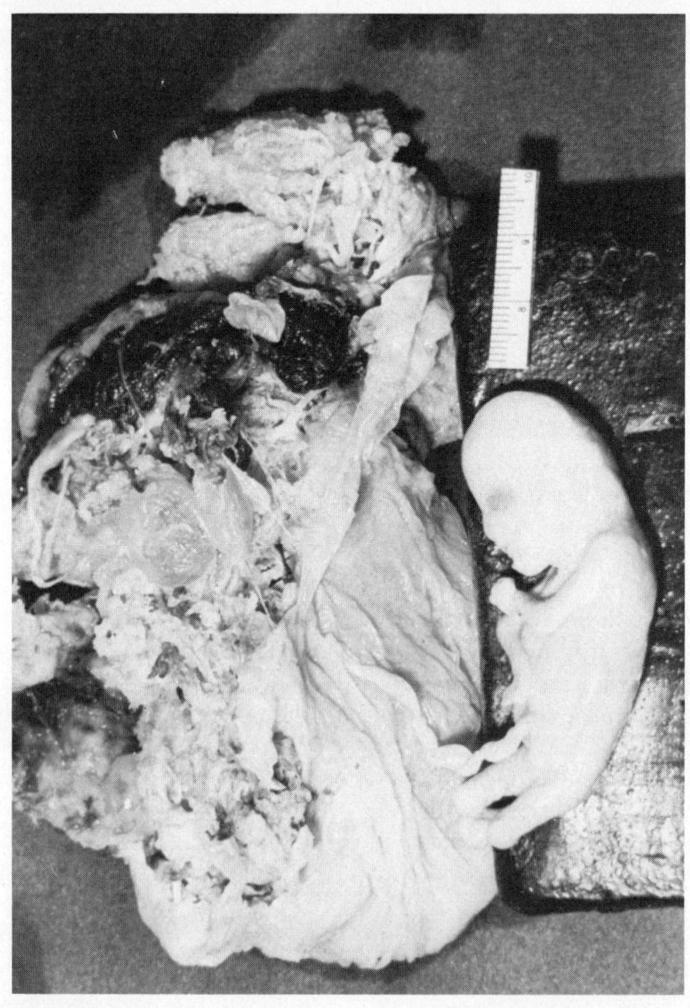

FIGURE 2-10
Abortus with triploid karyotype. Note hydropic degeneration of the placenta. (From Stenchever MA: Contemp OB/GYN 17:38, April 1981.)

in 29.4%, but none had a karyotype of 45,X. There was one instance of translocation and one of triploidy among the stillborn infants.

It is interesting to compare the findings of chromosome abnormalities among spontaneous abortuses with those seen among consecutive live-born infants. In a series of 43,558 live-born infants reported by Ratcliff, 247 (0.56%) had chromosome abnormalities. Of these, two (0.8%) had a karyotype of 45,X, 36.8% had other sex chromosome abnormalities, and 21.1% had autosomal trisomies of chromosomes 13, 18, and 21. The latter abnormality was by far the most common. Balanced chromosomal translocations were found in 32.4% of chromosomally abnormal individuals, and unbalanced translocations were present in 3.2%. The remaining abnormalities were classified as miscellaneous. In a comparison of chromosome abnormalities in live-born infants with those in abortuses and stillborn infants, a concept of lethality can be noted.

Recurrent Abortion

Roughly one in every 200 couples suffers from multiple abortion or multiple pregnancy wastage. Depending on how the problem is defined, one individual of the couple will be found to have a chromosome abnormality in somewhere between 6% and 25% of couples. Recently a review of the world literature by Simpson revealed that the prevalence of chromosome abnormalities in women with chronic spontaneous abortion problems was about twice that in men (4.8% versus 2.4%). Although occasional sex chromosome abnormalities such as 47,XXX and 47,XYY, as well as a

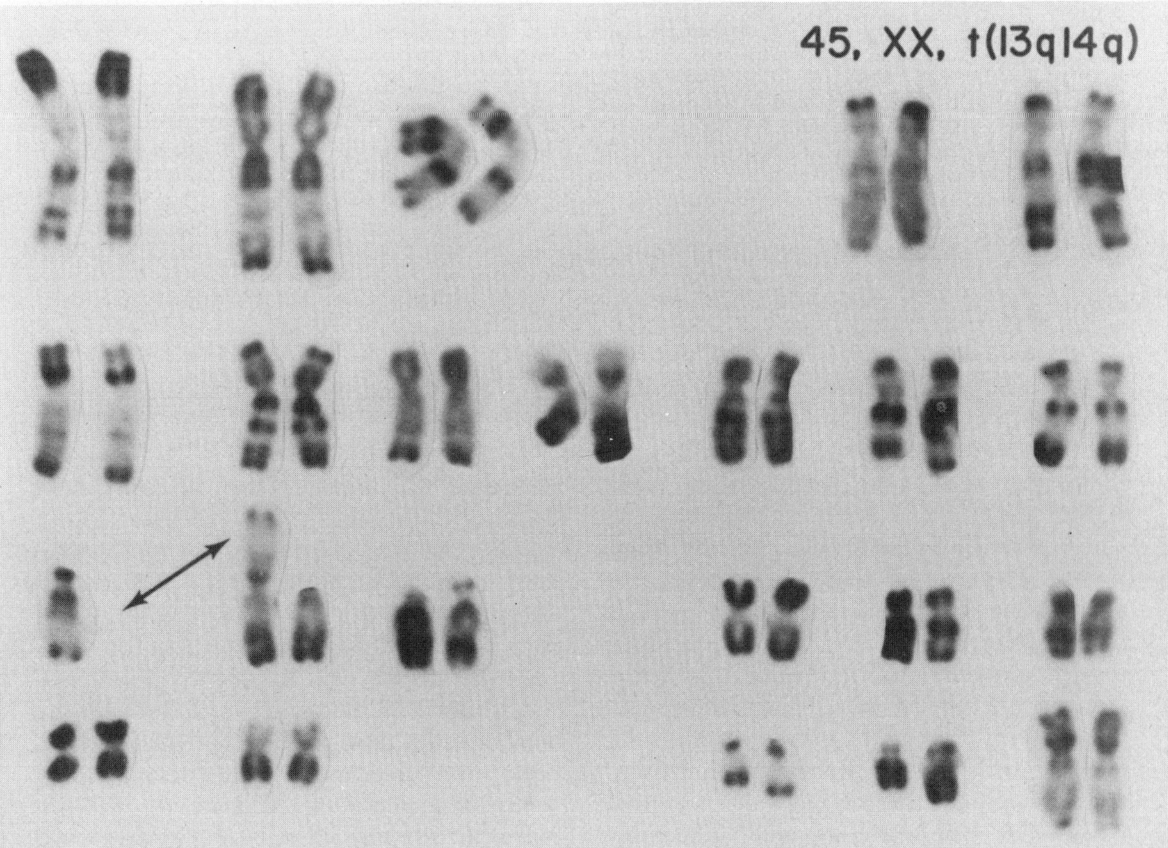

FIGURE 2-11
Karyotype of patient with 13-14 translocation who had a history of three spontaneous first-trimester abortions. (From Stenchever MA: Contemp OB/GYN 17:38, April 1981.)

variety of mosaic representations, are seen among such couples, the majority demonstrate either balanced reciprocal translocations or Robertsonian fusion problems (Fig. 2-11).

The diagnosis of a chromosome abnormality in couples with chronic pregnancy wastage is important for two reasons. The first is to rule out an abnormality incompatible with normal gestation. Examples would be homologous translocations between identical members of the same group of chromosomes, such as 13-13, 14-14, 15-15, 21-21, and 22-22. Individuals with other types of reciprocal translocations or Robertsonian fusion may have a normal pregnancy in which the chromosome makeup reflects either a normal karyotype or a balanced carrier state. However, such individuals may produce a conceptus with an unbalanced translocation, which would not be normal. In addition, chromosomally abnormal individuals are more likely to produce offspring with chromosome abnormalities. In some cases in which the father is the carrier of a chromosome abnormality, particularly when the abnormality is incompatible with normal gestation, artificial insemination with donor sperm may be offered. The technique of embryo transplant may offer potential help to the woman with such a chromosomal problem.

Hydatidiform Mole

The two common karyotypes noted in hydatidiform moles, and indeed in other trophoblastic disease, are 46,XX and triploidy. With the use of Q and R banding techniques, it has been shown that most moles have a karyotype of 46,XX, and all homologous chromosomes are homozygous for banding polymorphism. Thus, although the moles are diploid in number, the chromosomes arise from a haploid set from one parent. In each case that parent proved to be the father. Thus it appears likely that in the formation of a hydatidiform mole, the female pronucleus is lost and the male pronucleus duplicates, so that all the genetic material is foreign to the mother (Fig. 2-12).

The other type of chromosome abnormality seen in hydatidiform moles is triploidy. Frequently a fetus is present, and the problem is represented by a hydropic degeneration of the placenta. Although most choriocarcinomas are

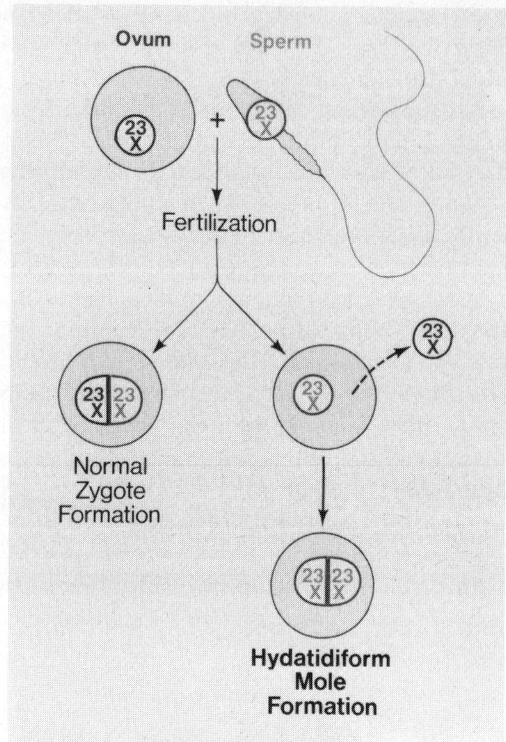

FIGURE 2-12
Diagram of possible development of 46,XX hydatidiform mole. (From Stenchever MA: Contemp OB/GYN 17:38, April 1981.)

derived from 46,XX moles, triploidy has occasionally been seen.

Chromosome Abnormalities in Cancer

A number of tumors have demonstrated aneuploidy, and many have been seen with marker chromosomes specific for that particular tumor. The best example is the Philadelphia chromosome, seen in chronic myelogenous leukemia. This minute chromosome disappears from peripheral circulation and from the bone marrow when therapy is effective and the patient's cancer is in remission. Space does not allow a categorization of each tumor that can occur in the human and its chromosome experience. It should be noted, however, that premalignant (dysplastic) cells of the cervix are generally aneuploid, as are the cells that compose invasive squamous cell carcinomas. This aneuploid distribution has been observed in cancers that arise in other organs as well but frequently is not observed in tumors arising in endocrine organs (endometrium, breast, thyroid, etc.).

A variety of cancers occur in individuals who have fragile chromosomes and may be associated with chromosome breaks and rearrangements or with mutations that occur when breaks take place and healing is faulty. Such conditions are seen in families with Bloom's syndrome, Fanconi's anemia, and ataxia-telangiectasia. In each case there is an increased percentage of individuals with a variety of cancers, and chromosome breaks are commonly seen in the cells of these individuals.

Hermaphroditism

TRUE HERMAPHRODITISM. This condition, which involves the presence of both male and female gonads within the same individual, is frequently associated with the karyotype 46,XX. However, a variety of other chromosome findings have been noted. One of these, 46,XX/46,XY, is a condition that most likely occurs when the fertilization of two eggs is followed by their fusion, resulting in chimerism within the individual. Chimerism is defined as the presence of two different cell populations from two separate conceptuses within the same individual. Other chromosome anomalies associated with true hermaphroditism include various mosaicisms involving 45,X/46,XY and 45,X/47,XYY karyotypes, as well as karyotypes with various translocations and deletions of the X and Y chromosomes. The influence of these chromosomes in the development of hermaphroditism will be discussed in detail elsewhere.

PSEUDOHERMAPHRODITISM.   Female pseudohermaphroditism is seen when a female is androgenized during embryonic life. The commonest such case is associated with congenital adrenal hyperplasia. This syndrome may come about because of a number of enzyme defects transmitted as autosomal recessive characteristics. The commonest is 21-hydroxylase deficiency, but 11-β-hydroxylase deficiency may also cause the syndrome. A third and rarer defect is the 18-hydroxysteroid dehydrogenase deficiency, which leads to aldosterone deficiency but no genital tract anomalies. In every case, such individuals have a 46,XX karyotype unless other conditions are associated by chance. These will be discussed in detail elsewhere.

Male pseudohermaphroditism occurs when the individual has a 46,XY karyotype and is genetically and gonadally male but phenotypically and psychologically female. The commonest condition in which this is found is the androgen insensitivity syndrome (testicular feminization syndrome).

In this condition the genetic error is transmitted as an X-linked recessive characteristic leading to a faulty androgen receptor on the cell membranes, preventing the cell from transporting testosterone or dihydrotestosterone into the cell. Both complete and incomplete forms exist. A related condition, 5α-reductase deficiency, prevents the conversion of testosterone to dihydrotestosterone. Since the latter is the form of testosterone that enters most cells, a defect of the enzyme mimics the findings of androgen insensitivity.

KEY POINTS

- Base pairing in DNA and RNA molecules is always A-T and G-C.

- When a heterozygous individual who has an autosomal dominant trait mates with a normal individual, 50% of their offspring will have the trait.

- When two individuals who carry an autosomal recessive trait mate, 25% of their offspring will demonstrate the trait and 50% will be carriers.

______________ **KEY POINTS, cont'd** ______________

- X-linked recessive characteristics are transmitted from maternal carriers to male offspring and will affect 50% of such male offspring.

- In general, if a couple produces an offspring with a multifactorial defect, and the problem has never occurred before in the family, it can be expected to be repeated in 2% to 5% of subsequent pregnancies.

- The findings always present in 45,X Turner's syndrome are shortness of stature and sexual infantilism.

- Nondisjunctional events have been described in every autosome except chromosomes 1 and 17. The risk of producing a second conceptus with a nondisjunctional event is 2% to 5%.

- Conditions always seen in individuals with Klinefelter's syndrome (47,XXY) are tallness of stature and azoospermia. One third will have gynecomastia.

- Of ova penetrated by sperm, 15% will fail to implant and 25% to 30% will be aborted spontaneously at a previllous stage. Of the 40% that survive the first missed menstrual period, as many as one fourth will abort spontaneously. From 30% to 35% of all ova penetrated by sperm actually end in live-born individuals.

- Between 30% and 60% of known aborted conceptuses have chromosome abnormalities. Half of these have autosomal trisomies; 20% 45,X; 14% to 19%, triploidy; 3% to 6%, tetraploidy; and 3% to 4%, chromosome rearrangements.

- Of live-born infants with chromosome abnormalities, about 0.8% to 1% have 45,X; 36.8% have other sex chromosome abnormalities; 21% have autosomal trisomies; and balanced chromosome translocations occur in 32.4%. About 3.2% have unbalanced translocation abnormalities.

- One in 200 couples suffers recurrent (three or more) abortions, with chromosome abnormalities occurring in about 4.8% of the mothers and 2.4% of the fathers.

- Hydatidiform mole will have a karyotype of 46,XX or of triploidy. Moles with 46,XX are derived from a single haploid set of chromosomes originating from the father.

BIBLIOGRAPHY

Boue J, Boue A, Lazar P: Retrospective and prospective epidemiological studies of 1500 karyotyped spontaneous human abortions. Teratology 12:11, 1975.

Creasy MR, Crolla JA, Alberman ED: A cytogenetic study of human spontaneous abortion using banding techniques. Hum Genet 31:177, 1976.

Dewhurst J: Fertility in 47,XXX and 45, X patients. J Med Genet 15:132, 1978.

Ford EHR: Human chromosomes. New York, Academic Press, 1973.

Hamerton JL, Canning N, Ray M, Smith S: A cytogenetic survey of 14,069 newborn infants. I. Incidence of chromosome abnormalities. Clin Genet 8:223, 1975.

Jones HW Jr, Scott WM: Hemaphroditism: Genital anomalies and related endocrine disorders. Baltimore, Williams & Wilkins, 1971.

Kajii T, Nikawa N: Origin of triploidy and tetraploidy in man: Cases with chromosome markers. Cytogenet Cell Genet 18:109, 1977.

Kajii T, Ohama K: Androgenetic origin of hydatidiform mole. Nature 268:633, 1977.

Lubinsky MS: Female pseudohermaphroditism and associated anomalies. Am J Med Genet 6:123, 1980.

McKusick VA: Mendelian inheritance in man. Baltimore, The Johns Hopkins Press, 1978.

Ratcliffe S: Postnatal chromosome abnormalities. In Boyce HJ, ed: Chromosome variations in human evolution. London, Taylor & Francis, 1975.

Schimke RN: Genetics and cancer in man. Edinburgh, Churchill Livingstone, 1980.

Shepard TH, Fantel AG: Embryonic and early fetal loss. Clin Perinatol 6:219, 1979.

Simpson JL: Disorders of sexual differentiation: Etiology and clinical delineation. New York, Academic Press, 1976.

Simpson JL: True hermaphroditism: Etiology and phenotypic considerations. Birth Defects 14:9, 1978.

Simpson JL: Repeated suboptimal pregnancy outcome. Birth Defects 17:113, 1981.

Simpson JL, Globus MS, Martin AO, Sarto GE: Genetics in obstetrics and gynecology. New York, Grune & Stratton, 1982.

Anatomy

<hr>

KEY TERMS AND DEFINITIONS

Bladder Neck. That part of the bladder which is continuous with the urethra.

Canal of Nuck. A tubular process of peritoneum that accompanies the round ligament into the inguinal canal. It is generally obliterated in the adult but sometimes remains patent.

Carunculae Myrtiformes. Small nodules of fibrous tissue at the vaginal orifice that are remnants of the hymen.

Cornua. The superolateral aspects of the uterine cavity, the anatomic areas where the oviducts enter the uterine cavity.

Cul-de-sac of Douglas. A deep pouch formed by the most caudal extent of the parietal peritoneum. It is anterior to the rectum, separating the uterus from the large intestine.

Fimbria Ovarica. One of the largest fingerlike projections of the distal end of the oviducts. The fimbria ovarica usually attaches the oviducts to the ovary.

Frankenhauser's Plexus. An extensive concentration of both myelinated and nonmyelinated nerve fibers located in the uterosacral ligaments and supplying primarily the uterus and the cervix.

Fundus. The dome-shaped top of the uterus.

Genitocrural Fold. The skin line dividing the external female genitalia and the medial aspects of the thigh.

Isthmus. The short area of constriction in the lower uterine segment.

Parametria. The extraperitoneal fatty and fibrous connective tissue immediately adjacent to the uterus. The parametria lie between the leaves of the broad ligament and in the contiguous area anteriorly between the cervix and the bladder.

Pelvic Diaphragm. A thin, muscular layer of tissue that forms the inferior border of the abdominal pelvic cavity. The primary muscles of the pelvic diaphragm are the levator ani and coccygeus muscles.

Perineum. The region between the thighs bounded anteriorly by the vulva and posteriorly by the anus.

Plexus. A mixture of preganglionic and postganglionic fibers, small, inconsistently placed nerve ganglia, and afferent sensory fibers. In the female pelvis a plexus also may be termed a nerve.

Plicae Palmatae. Longitudinal folds in the mucous membrane of the endocervical canal. The secondary branching folds are called arbor vitae.

Posterior Fourchette. The fold of skin that joins the labia minora at their inferior margins.

Presacral Nerve. Also termed the superior hypogastric plexus. It is found in the retroperitoneal connective tissue from the fourth lumbar vertebra to the hollow over the sacrum.

Rugae. Numerous transverse folds of the vagina in women of reproductive age.

Space of Retzius. The area lying between the bladder and symphysis pubis and bounded laterally by the obliterated hypogastric arteries.

Urachus. The adult remnant of the embryonic allantois.

Urogenital Diaphragm. A strong, muscular membrane that occupies the area between the symphysis pubis and the ischial tuberosities. Posteriorly, the urogenital diaphragm inserts into the central point of the perineum.

Vestibular Bulbs. Two elongated masses of erectile tissue situated on either side of the vaginal orifice. They are homologous to the bulb of the penis in the male.

The organs of the female reproductive tract are classically divided into the external and the internal genitalia. The external genital organs are present in the vulvar region and include the mons pubis, clitoris, urinary meatus, labia majora, labia minora, vestibule, Bartholin's glands, and periurethral glands. The internal genital organs are located in the true pelvis and include the vagina, uterus, cervix, oviducts, ovaries, and surrounding supporting structures. This chapter will attempt to integrate the basic anatomy of the female pelvis with clinical situations.

Embryologically the urinary, reproductive, and gastrointestinal tracts develop in close proximity. This relationship continues throughout a woman's life span. In the adult, the reproductive organs are in intimate contact with the lower urinary tract and large intestines. Because of the anatomic proximity of the genital and urinary systems, altered pathophysiology in one organ often produces symptoms in the other, adjacent organ. The gynecologic surgeon masters the intricacy of these anatomic relationships to avoid major surgical complications.

This chapter will not duplicate the completeness of anatomic texts or surgical atlases. It will concentrate on the norms of human anatomy. The reader must appreciate that wide individual differences in anatomic detail exist between patients. Understanding these variations is one of the greatest challenges of clinical medicine.

EXTERNAL GENITALIA

Vulva

The vulva, or pudendum, is a collective term for the external genital organs that are visible in the perineal area. The vulva consists of the following: the mons pubis, labia majora, labia minora, hymen, clitoris, vestibule, urethra, Skene's glands, Bartholin's glands, and the vestibular bulbs (Fig. 3-1).

The boundaries of the vulva extend from the mons pubis anteriorly to the rectum posteriorly and from one lateral genitocrural fold to the other. The entire vulvar area is covered by keratinized, stratified squamous epithelium. The further from the vagina, the thicker, more pigmented, and more keratinized is the skin. The skin closest to the vagina is the thinnest and has the least keratin.

Mons Pubis

The mons pubis is a rounded, cushionlike eminence that becomes hairy after puberty. It is directly anterior and superior to the symphysis pubis. The hair pattern, or escutcheon, of most women is triangular. Genetic and racial differences produce a variety of normal hair patterns, with approximately one in four women having a modified escutcheon that has a diamond (malelike) pattern.

Labia Majora

The labia majora are two large, longitudinal, cutaneous folds of adipose and fibrous tissue. Each labium majus is approximately 7 to 8 cm in length and 2 to 3 cm in width. The labia extend from the mons pubis anteriorly to become lost in the skin between the vagina and anus in the area of the posterior fourchette. The skin of the outer convex surface of the labia majora is pigmented and covered with hair follicles. The thin skin of the inner surface does not have hair follicles but has many sebaceous glands. Histologically the labia majora have both sweat and sebaceous glands (Fig. 3-2). The apocrine glands are similar to those of the breast and axillary areas. The size of the labia is related to fat content. Usually the labia atrophy following menopause. The labia majora are homologous to the scrotum in the male.

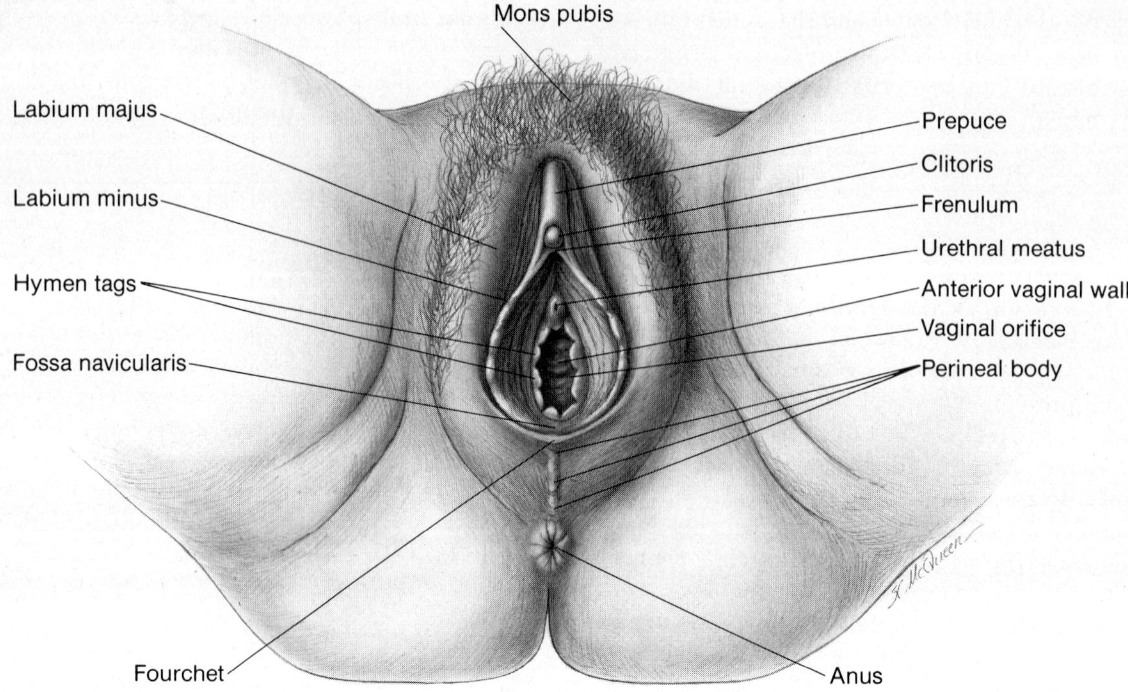

FIGURE 3-1
The structures of the external genitalia that are collectively called the vulva. (Redrawn from Pritchard JA, MacDonald PC, Gant NF: Williams' obstetrics, 17th ed. New York, Appleton-Century-Crofts, 1985, p. 8.)

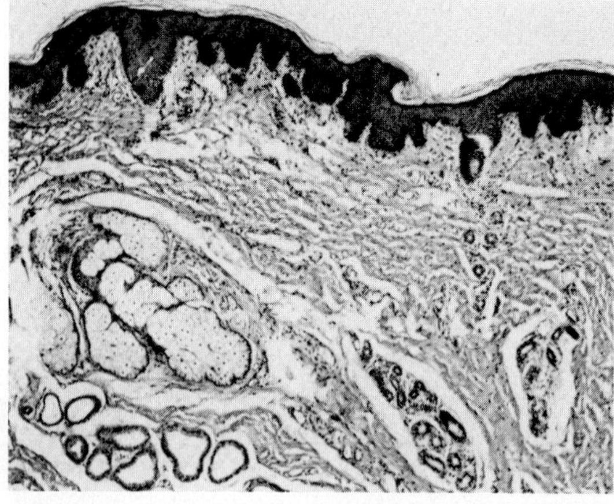

FIGURE 3-2
A histologic section from the labium majus. A cornified squamous epithelium covers the dermis, which contains eccrine, apocrine, and sebaceous glands. (H&E stain; ×77.) (Reproduced with permission from Kaufman RH: Anatomy of the vulva and vagina. In Gardner HL, Kaufman RH, eds: Benign disease of the vulva and vagina, 2nd ed. Copyright © 1981 by Year Book Medical Publishers, Inc., Chicago.)

Labia Minora

The labia minora, or nymphae, are two small, red cutaneous folds that are situated between the labia majora and the vaginal orifice. They are more delicate, shorter, and thinner than the labia majora. Anteriorly, they divide at the clitoris to form superiorly the prepuce and inferiorly the frenulum of the clitoris. Histologically, they are composed of dense connective tissue with erectile tissue and elastic fibers, rather than adipose tissue. The skin of the labia minora is less cornified and has many sebaceous glands but no hair follicles or sweat glands. The labia minora and the breasts are the only areas of the body rich in sebaceous glands without hair follicles. In women of reproductive age, there is considerable variation in the size of the labia minora. They are relatively more prominent in children and postmenopausal women. The labia minora are homologous to the penile urethra and part of the skin of the penis in males.

Hymen

The hymen is a thin, perforated membrane at the entrance of the vagina. There are many variations in the structure and shape of the hymen in the adult. The hymen histologically is covered by stratified squamous epithelium on both sides and consists of fibrous tissue with a few small blood vessels. Small tags, or nodules, of firm fibrous material, termed carunculae myrtiformes, are the remnants of the hymen identified in adult females.

Clitoris

The clitoris is a short, cylindrical, erectile organ at the superior portion of the vestibule. The average length of the clitoris is 1.5 to 2 cm. The normal adult clitoris has a diameter less than 1 cm. Usually, only the glans is visible, with the body of the clitoris positioned beneath the skin surface. The clitoris consists of a base of two crura, which attach to the periosteum of the symphysis pubis. The body has two cylindrical corpora cavernosa composed of thin-walled, vascular channels that function as erectile tissue. The distal one third of the clitoris is the glans, which has many nerve endings. The clitoris is the female homologue of the penis in the male.

Vestibule

The vestibule is the lowest portion of the embryonic urogenital sinus. It is the cleft between the labia minora that is visualized when the labia are held apart. The vestibule extends from the clitoris to the posterior fourchette. The orifices of the urethra and vagina and the ducts from Bartholin's glands open into the vestibule. Within the area of the vestibule are the remnants of the hymen and numerous mucinous glands.

Urethra

The urethra is a membranous conduit for urine from the urinary bladder to the vestibule. The female urethra measures 3.5 to 5 cm in length. The mucosa of the proximal two thirds of the urethra is composed of stratified transitional epithelium, whereas the distal one third is stratified squamous epithelium. The distal orifice is 4 to 6 mm in diameter, and the mucosal edges grossly appear everted.

Skene's Glands

Skene's glands, or paraurethral glands, are branched, tubular glands that are adjacent to the distal urethra. Usually Skene's ducts run parallel to the long axis of the urethra for approximately 1 cm before opening into the distal urethra. Sometimes the ducts open into the area just outside the urethral orifice. Skene's glands are the largest of the paraurethral glands; however, there are many smaller glands that empty into the urethra. Skene's glands are homologous to the prostate in the male.

Bartholin's Glands

Bartholin's glands are vulvovaginal glands that anatomically are located beneath the fascia at about 4 and 8 o'clock, respectively, on the posterolateral aspect of the vaginal orifice. Each lobulated, racemose gland is about the size of a pea. Histologically the gland is composed of cuboidal epithelium (Fig. 3-3, A). The duct from each gland is lined by transitional epithelium and is approximately 2 cm in length (Fig. 3-3, B). Bartholin's ducts open into a groove between the hymen and labia minora. Bartholin's glands are homologous to Cowper's glands in the male.

Vestibular Bulbs

The vestibular bulbs are two elongated masses of erectile tissue situated on either side of the vaginal orifice. Each bulb is immediately below the bulbocavernosus muscle. The distal end of the vestibular bulbs are adjacent to Bartholin's glands. They are homologous to the bulb of the penis in the male.

Clinical Correlations

The skin of the vulvar region is subject to both local and general dermatitis. The intertriginous areas of the vulva remain moist, and obese women are particularly susceptible to chronic infection. The vulvar vestibule is an area where small mucous glands frequently become cystic.

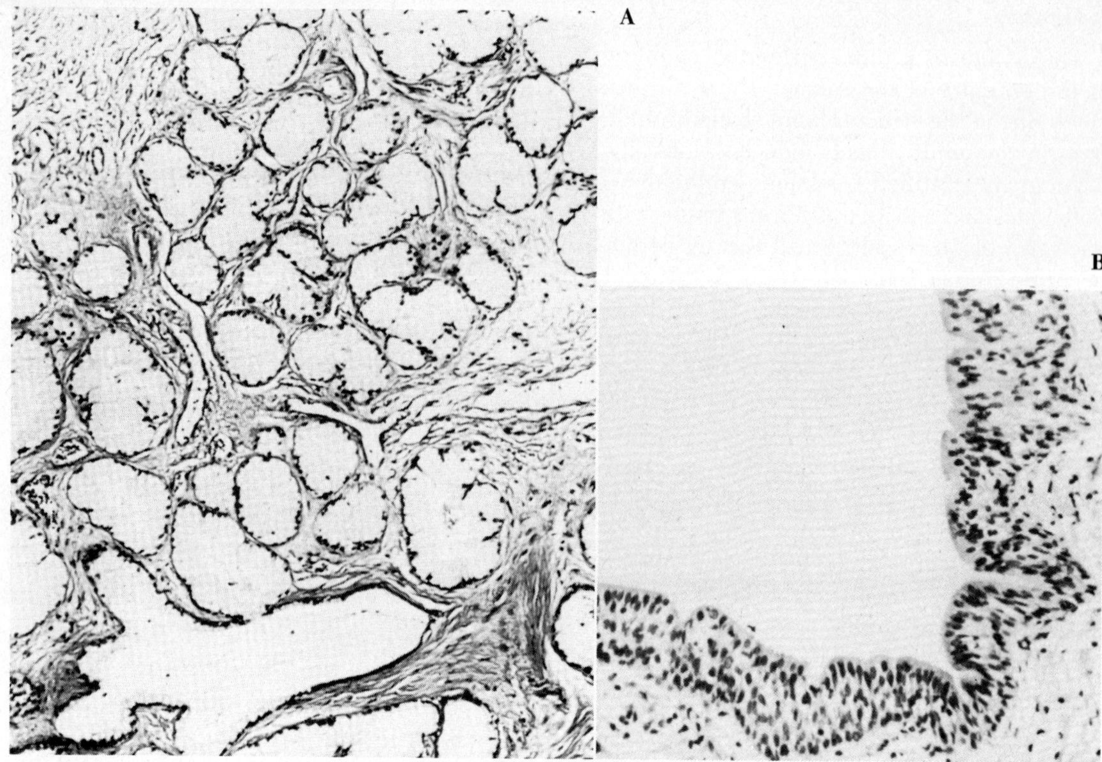

FIGURE 3-3
A, A histologic section of a Bartholin's gland, showing cuboidal epithelium lining acinar structures. (H&E stain; ×117.) **B,** A histologic section of the duct of the Bartholin's gland. The lining of the duct is transitional epithelium. (H&E stain; ×286.) (Reproduced with permission from Kaufman RH: Anatomy of the vulva and vagina. In Gardner HL, Kaufman FH, eds: Benign diseases of the vulva and vagina, 2nd ed. Copyright © 1981 by Year Book Medical Publishers, Inc., Chicago.)

A cyst of Nuck's canal may be confused with an indirect inguinal hernia. Vulvar trauma frequently results in a large hematoma or profuse external hemorrhage. The richness of the vascular supply and the absence of valves in vulvar veins both contribute to this complication.

VAGINA

The vagina is a thin-walled, distensible, fibromuscular tube that extends from the vestibule of the vulva to the uterus. The potential space of the vagina is larger in the middle and upper thirds. The walls of the vagina are normally in apposition and flattened in the anteroposterior diameter. Thus the vagina has the appearance of the letter **H** in cross-section (Fig. 3-4).

The axis of the upper portion of the vagina lies close to the horizontal plane when a woman is standing, the upper portion of the vagina curving toward the hollow of the sacrum. In most women an angle of at least 90 degrees is formed between the axis of the vagina and the axis of the uterus. The vagina is secured in its position by the surrounding endopelvic fascia and ligaments.

The lower third of the vagina is in close relationship with the urogenital and pelvic diaphragms. The middle third of the vagina is supported by the levator ani muscles and the lower portion of the cardinal ligaments. The upper third is supported by the upper portions of the cardinal ligaments and the parametria.

The vagina of reproductive-age women has numerous transverse folds, termed rugae. They

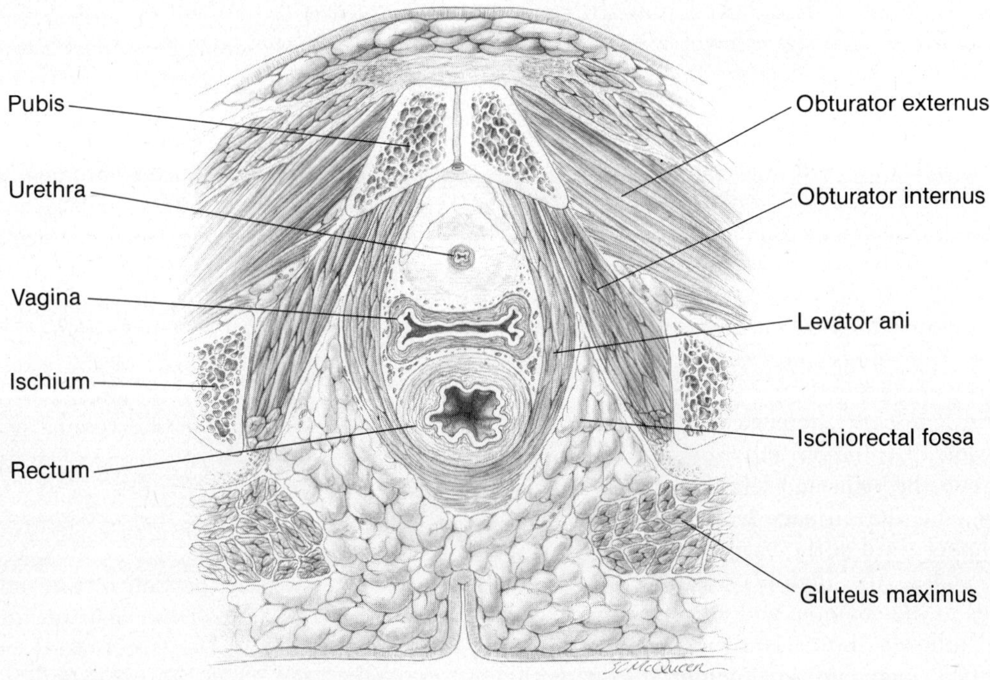

FIGURE 3-4
A schematic drawing of a cross section of the female pelvis, demonstrating the **H** shape of the vagina. Note the surrounding levator ani muscle. (Redrawn from Pritchard JA, MacDonald PC, Gant NF. Williams' obstetrics, 17th ed. New York, Appleton-Century-Crofts, 1985, p. 12.)

help provide accordian-like distensibility and are more prominent in the lower third of the vagina. The cervix extends into the upper part of the vagina. The spaces between the cervix and attachment of the vagina are called fornices. The posterior fornix is considerably larger than the anterior fornix; thus the anterior vaginal length is approximately 6 to 9 cm in comparison with a posterior vaginal length of 8 to 12 cm.

Histologically the vagina is composed of four distinct layers. The mucosa consists of a stratified, nonkeratinized squamous epithelium. If the environment of the vaginal mucosa is modified, as in uterine prolapse, then the epithelium may become keratinized. The squamous epithelium is similar microscopically to the exocervix, although the vagina has larger and more frequent papillae that extend into the connective tissue. The normal vagina does not have glands. The next layer is the lamina propria, or tunica. It is composed of fibrous connective tissue. Throughout this layer of collagen and elastic tissue is a rich supply of vascular and lymphatic channels. The density of the connective tissue in the endopelvic fascia varies throughout the longitudinal axis of the vagina. The muscular layer has many interlacing fibers. However, an inner circular layer and an outer longitudinal layer can be identified. The fourth layer consists of cellular areolar connective tissue and a large plexus of blood vessels.

The vascular system of the vagina is generously supplied with an extensive anastomotic network throughout its length. The vaginal artery originates either directly from the uterine artery or as a branch of the internal iliac artery arising posterior to the origin of the uterine and inferior vesical arteries. The vaginal artery may be multiple arteries on each side of the pelvis. There is an anastomosis with the cervical branch of the uterine artery to form the azygos arteries. Branches of the internal pudendal, inferior vesical, and middle hemorrhoidal arteries also contribute to the interconnecting network and the longitudinal azygos arteries.

The venous drainage is complex and accompanies the arterial system. Below the pelvic floor the principal venous drainage occurs via the pudendal veins. The vaginal, uterine, and vesical veins, as well as those around the rectosigmoid, all provide venous drainage of the venous plexuses surrounding the vagina.

The nerve supply of the vagina comes from the autonomic nervous system's vaginal plexus, and sensory fibers come from the pudendal nerve. Pain fibers enter the spinal cord in sacral segments 2 to 4.

The lymphatic drainage is characterized by its wide distribution and frequent crossovers between the right and left sides of the pelvis. In general the primary lymphatic drainage of the upper third of the vagina is to the external iliac nodes, the middle third of the vagina drains to the common and internal iliac nodes, and the lower third has a wide lymphatic distribution, including the common iliac, superficial inguinal, and perirectal nodes.

Clinical Correlations

In clinical practice, anatomic descriptions of pelvic organs are derived from Latin roots, such as "vagina," from the Latin word for sheath. In contrast, the names for surgical procedures of pelvic organs are derived from Greek roots. *Colpectomy, colporrhaphy,* and *colposcopy* are derived from *kolpos* (fold), the Greek word for the vagina.

The posterior fornix is an important surgical landmark, since it provides direct access to the cul-de-sac of Douglas. The distal course of the ureter and the changes in anatomic relationships produced by uterine prolapse are important considerations in vaginal surgery. Ureteral injury has occurred as a result of vaginally placed sutures to obtain hemostasis with vaginal lacerations. The anatomic proximity and interrelationships of the vascular and lymphatic networks of the bladder and vagina result in inflammation of one organ, often producing symptoms in the other. For example, vaginitis often produces urinary tract symptoms such as frequency and dysuria.

Gartner's duct cyst, a cystic dilation of the embryonic mesonephros, is usually present on the lateral wall of the vagina. However, in the lower third of the vagina, these cysts are present anteriorly and may be difficult to distinguish from a large urethral diverticulum.

An interesting phenomenon discovered by recent interest in sexual medicine is the source of vaginal lubrication during intercourse. For years there was speculation on how an organ without glands is able to "secrete" fluid. Vaginal lubrication occurs from a transudate produced by engorgement of the vascular plexuses that encircle the vagina. The anatomic relationship between the long axis of the vagina and other pelvic organs may be altered by pelvic relaxation resulting from the trauma of childbirth.

CERVIX

The lower, narrow portion of the uterus is the cervix. The word *cervix* originates from the Latin word for neck. The Greek word for neck is *trachēlos,* and when the cervix is removed, the surgical procedure is termed trachelectomy. The cervix varies in shape from cylindrical to conical. It is predominantly fibrous and is separated from the muscular corpus of the uterus by the internal os.

The vagina is attached obliquely around the middle of the cervix; this attachment divides the cervix into an upper, supravaginal portion and a lower segment in the vagina, called the portio vaginalis (Fig. 3-5). The supravaginal segment is covered by peritoneum posteriorly and is surrounded by loose, fatty connective tissue, the parametrium, anteriorly.

The canal of the cervix is fusiform, with the widest diameter in the middle. The length and width of the endocervical canal vary; it is usually 2.5 to 3 cm in length and 7 to 8 mm at its widest point. The width of the canal varies with changing hormonal levels. The cervical canal opens into the vaginal canal at the external os of the cervix, which is small and round in nulliparous women. The os is wider and gaping following vaginal delivery. Often lateral or stellate scars are residual marks of previous cervical lacerations. In the majority of women, the external os is in contact with the posterior vaginal wall.

The mucous membrane of the endocervical canal of nulliparous women is arranged in longitudinal folds, plicae palmatae, with secondary

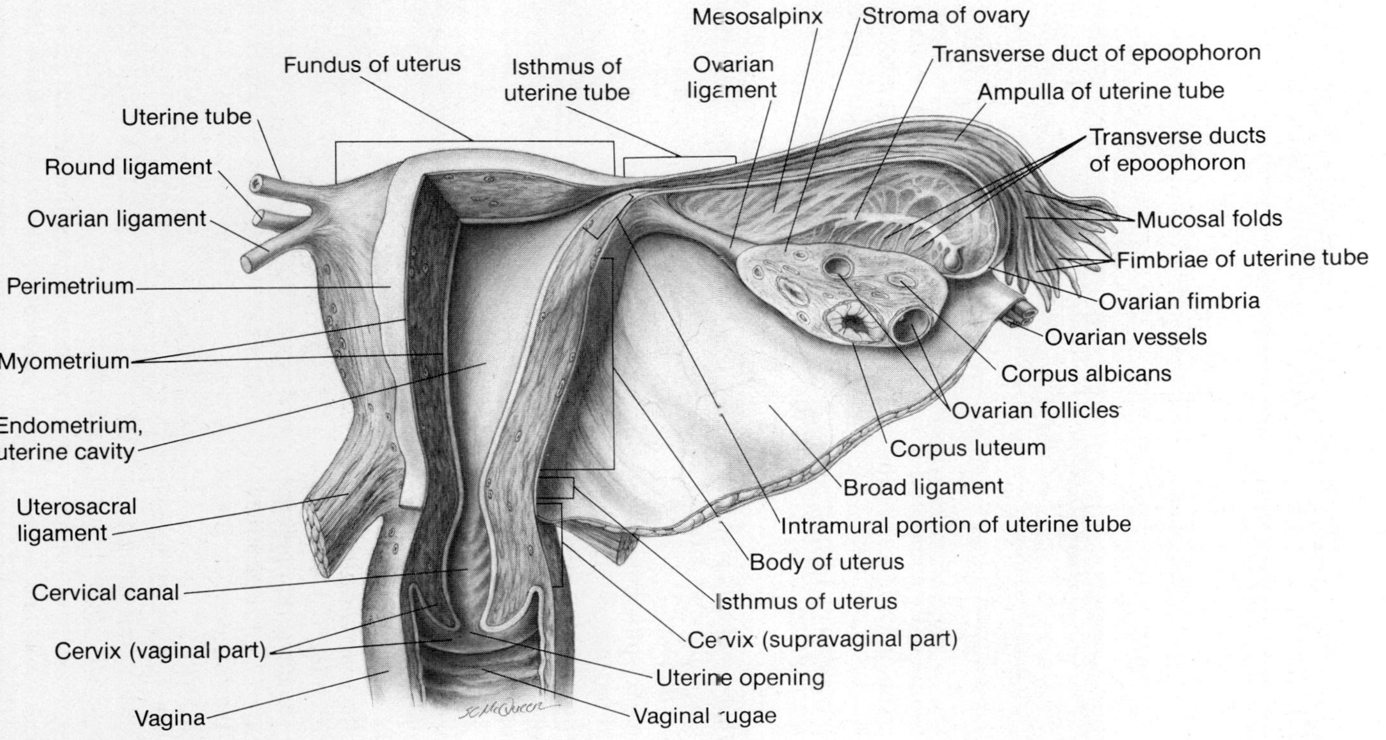

FIGURE 3-5

A schematic drawing of a posterior view of the cervix, uterus, fallopian tube, and ovary. Note that the cervix is divided by the vaginal attachment into an external portio segment and a supravaginal segment. Note that the uterus is composed of the dome-shaped fundus, the muscular body, and the narrow isthmus. Note the fimbria ovarica, or ovarian fimbria, attaching the oviduct to the ovary. (Redrawn from Clemente CD: Anatomy: A regional atlas of the human body © 1987, Urban & Schwarzenberg, Baltimore-Munich.)

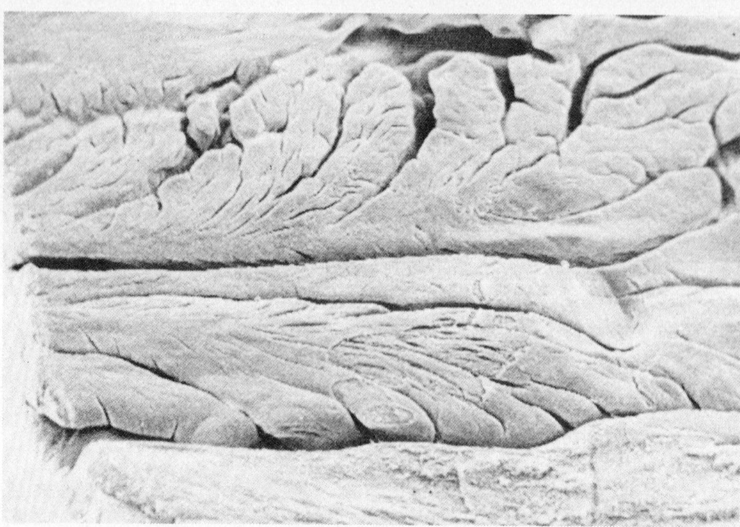

FIGURE 3-6
An electron micrograph of the endocervical canal, demonstrating the "arbor vitae."
These folds and crypts provide a reservoir for sperm. (From Singer A, Jordan JA:
The anatomy of the cervix. In Jordan JA, Singer A, eds: The cervix. Philadelphia,
W.B. Saunders Co., 1976, p. 18.)

branching folds, the arbor vitae (Fig. 3-6).
These folds, which form a herringbone pattern,
disappear following vaginal delivery.

A single layer of columnar epithelium lines
the endocervical canal and the underlying glandular structures. This specialized epithelium
secretes mucus, which facilitates sperm transport. Anatomically arranged crypts and villi
provide a reservoir for spermatozoa immediately following coitus. This epithelium contains
two types of columnar cells: nonciliated secretory cells and ciliated cells. An abrupt transformation usually is seen at the junction of the columnar epithelium of the endocervix and the
nonkeratinized stratified squamous epithelium
of the portio vaginalis (Fig. 3-7). The stratified
squamous epithelium of the exocervix is identical to the lining of the vagina.

The dense, fibromuscular cervical stroma is
composed primarily of collagenous connective
tissue and mucopolysaccharide ground substance. The connective tissue contains approximately 15% smooth muscle cells and a small
amount of elastic tissue. However, there are
few muscle fibers in the distal portions of the
cervix.

Because the cervix is the lower portion of the
uterus, it is not surprising that the cervical and

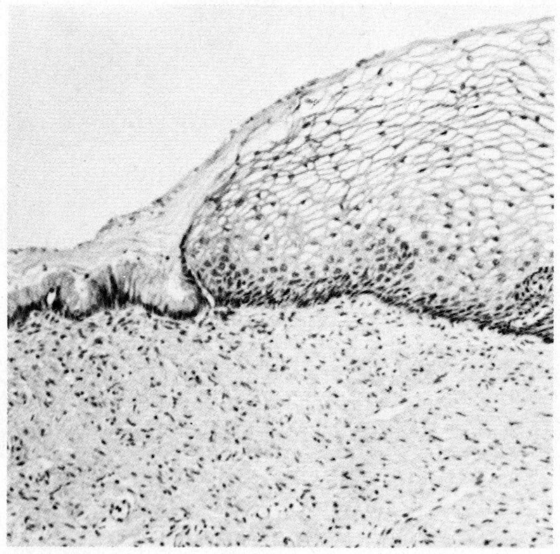

FIGURE 3-7
A histologic section through the squamocolumnar junction of the cervix. Note the abrupt
transformation from squamous to columnar epithelium. (From Ferenczy A: Anatomy and histology of the cervix. In Blaustein A, ed: Pathology of the female genital tract, 2nd ed. New
York, Springer-Verlag, 1982, p. 127.)

uterine vascular supplies are interrelated. The arterial supply of the cervix arises from the descending branch of the uterine artery. The cervical arteries run on the lateral side of the cervix and form the coronary artery, which encircles the cervix. The azygos arteries run longitudinally in the middle of the anterior and posterior aspects of the cervix and the vagina. There are numerous anastomoses between these vessels and the vaginal and middle hemorrhoidal arteries. The venous drainage accompanies these arteries. The lymphatic drainage of the cervix is complex, involving multiple chains of nodes. The principal regional lymph nodes are the obturator, common iliac, internal iliac, external iliac, and visceral nodes of the parametria. Other possible lymphatic drainage includes the following chains of nodes: superior and inferior gluteal, sacral, rectal, lumbar, aortic, and visceral nodes over the posterior surface of the urinary bladder. The stroma of the endocervix is rich in free nerve endings. Pain fibers accompany the parasympathetic fibers to the second, third, and fourth sacral segments.

Clinical Correlations

The major arterial supply to the cervix is located on the lateral cervical walls at the 3 and 9 o'clock positions, respectively. Therefore a deep figure-of-eight suture through the vaginal mucosa and cervical stroma helps to reduce blood loss during procedures such as cone biopsy. If the gynecologist is overzealous in placing such a hemostatic suture high in the vaginal fornix, it is possible to compromise the course of the distal ureter.

The endocervix is rich in free nerve endings. Occasionally, women experience a vagovagal response during transcervical instrumentation of the uterine cavity. Serial cardiac monitoring during insertion of intrauterine devices demonstrates a reflex bradycardia in some women. The sensory innervation of the exocervix is not as concentrated or sophisticated as that of the endocervix or external skin. Therefore the exocervix may be cauterized by either cold or heat with only minor discomfort to the patient.

UTERUS

The uterus is a thick-walled, hollow, muscular organ located centrally in the female pelvis. Adjacent to the uterus is the urinary bladder anteriorly, the rectum posteriorly, and the broad ligaments on either side (Fig. 3-8). The uterus is globular and slightly flattened anteriorly; it has the general configuration of an inverted pear. The short area of constriction in the lower uterine segment is termed the *isthmus* (see Fig. 3-5). The dome-shaped top of the uterus is termed the *fundus*. The lower edge of the fundus is described by an imaginary line drawn between the site of entrance of each oviduct. The size and weight of the uterus depend on previous pregnancies and the hormonal status of the individual. The uterus of a nulliparous woman is approximately 8 cm long, 5 cm wide, 2.5 cm thick, and weighs 40 to 50 g. In contrast, in a multiparous woman, each measurement is approximately 1.2 cm larger, and normal uterine weight is 20 to 30 g heavier. A recent study at the University of Southern California defines the upper limit for weight of a normal uterus as 110 g. The capacity of the uterus to enlarge during pregnancy results in a 10- to 20-fold increase in weight at term. Following menopause the uterus atrophies in both size and weight.

The cavity of the uterus is flattened and triangular. The oviducts enter the uterine cavity at the superolateral aspects of the cavity in the areas designated the cornua. In the majority of women, the long axis of the uterus is both anteverted in respect to the long axis of the vagina and anteflexed in relation to the long axis of the cervix. However, a retroflexed uterus is a normal variant found in approximately 25% of women.

The uterus has three layers, similar to other hollow abdominal and pelvic organs. The thin, external serosal layer comprises the visceral peritoneum. The peritoneum is firmly attached to the uterus in all areas except anteriorly at the level of the internal os of the cervix. The wide middle muscular layer is composed of three indistinct layers of smooth muscle. The outer longitudinal layer is contiguous with the muscle layers of the oviduct and vagina. The middle layer has interlacing oblique, spiral bundles of smooth muscle and large venous plexuses. The inner muscular layer is also longitudinal. The endometrium is a reddish mucous membrane that varies from 1 to 6 mm in thickness, depending on hormonal stimulation.

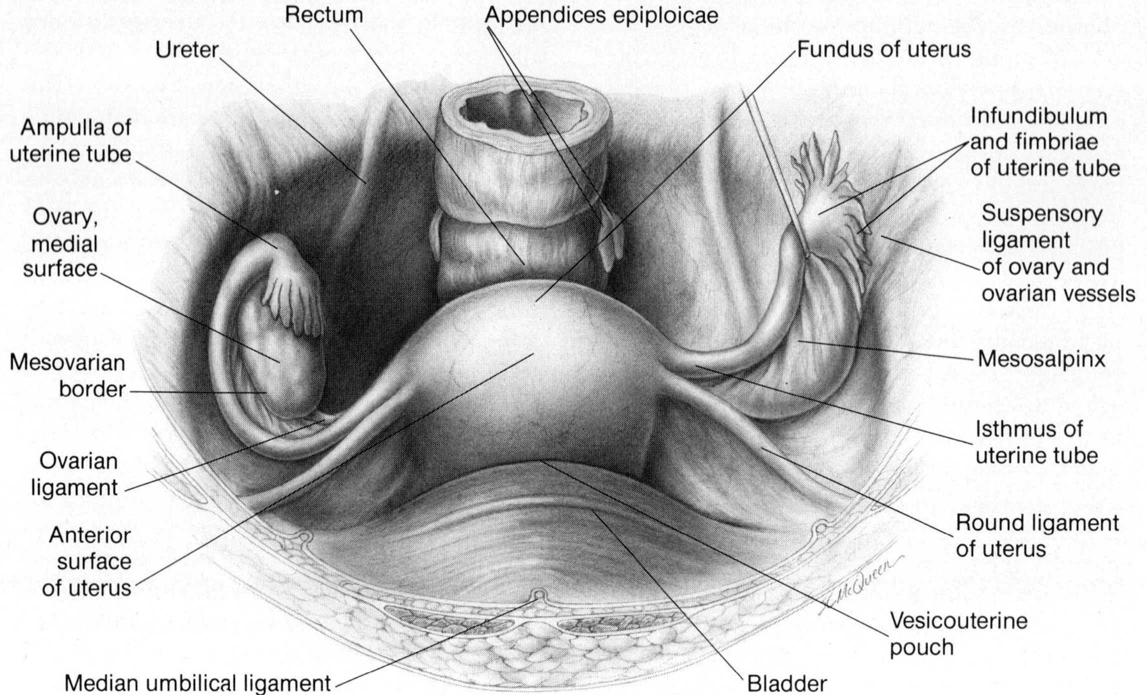

FIGURE 3-8
The organs of the female pelvis. The uterus is surrounded by the bladder anteriorly, the rectum posteriorly, and the folds of the broad ligaments laterally. (Redrawn from Clemente CD: Anatomy: A regional atlas of the human body © 1987, Urban & Schwarzenberg, Baltimore-Munich.)

The uterine glands are tubular and composed of tall columnar epithelium. The cells of the endometrial stroma resemble embryonic connective tissue with scant cytoplasm and large nuclei. The endometrium may be divided into an inner stratum basale and an outer stratum functionale. The stratum functionale may be further subdivided into an inner compact stratum and a more superficial spongy stratum. Only the stratum functionale responds to fluctuating hormonal levels (Fig. 3-9).

The arterial blood supply of the uterus is provided by the uterine and ovarian arteries. The uterine arteries are large branches of the hypogastric arteries, whereas the ovarian arteries originate directly from the aorta. The veins accompany the arteries. Therefore venous drainage from the fundus goes to the inferior vena cava, and blood from the corpus exits via the uterine veins into the iliac veins. The lymphatic drainage of the uterus is complex. The majority of lymphatics from the fundus and the body of the uterus go to the aortic, lumbar, and pelvic nodes surrounding the iliac vessels, especially the internal iliac nodes. However, it is possible for metastatic disease from the uterus to be found in the superior inguinal nodes transported via lymphatics in the round ligament.

In contrast to other pelvic organs, the afferent sensory nerve fibers from the uterus are in close proximity to the sympathetic nerves. Afferent nerve fibers from the uterus enter the spinal cord at the eleventh and twelfth thoracic segments. The sympathetic nerve supply to the uterus comes from the hypogastric and ovarian plexus. The parasympathetic fibers are largely derived from the pelvic nerve and from the second, third, and fourth sacral segments.

Clinical Correlations

Removal of the uterus is termed *hysterectomy,* which is derived from the Greek word

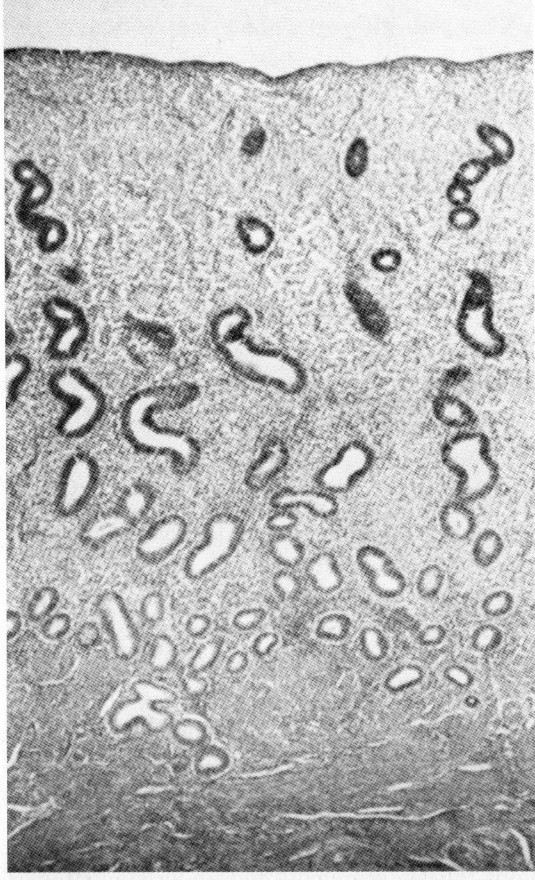

FIGURE 3-9
A histologic view of the endometrium during the proliferative phase, demonstrating the strata in the endometrium. (From Demopoulos RI: Normal endometrium. In Blaustein A, ed: Pathology of the female genital tract, 2nd ed. New York, Springer-Verlag, 1982, p. 216.)

hystera. The symptoms of primary dysmenorrhea are treated successfully in most women by prostaglandin synthetase inhibition. Rarely is a woman's pain not controlled by oral medication. However, it is possible to alleviate uterine pain by cutting the sensory nerves that accompany the sympathetic nerves. During this operation, a presacral neurectomy, the gynecologist must be careful not to injure the ureters.

The arterial blood supply enters the uterus on its lateral margins. This relationship allows morcellation of an enlarged uterus to facilitate removal of multiple myomas without appreciably increasing blood loss during vaginal hysterectomy.

Methods of transcervical female sterilization designed to occlude the tubal ostia at the uterine cornua have been attempted for many years. Procedures that blindly inject caustic solutions into the uterine cornua have a high percentage of failure. Individual differences in size and shape of the uterine cavity and muscular spasm of this region are the primary reasons that sufficient amounts of the caustic chemicals do not reach the fallopian tubes after approximately 20% of injections.

OVIDUCTS

The paired uterine tubes, more commonly referred to as the fallopian tubes or oviducts, extend outward from the superolateral portion of the uterus and end by curling around the ovary (see Fig. 3-5). The tubes are contained in a free edge of the superior portion of the broad ligament. The mesentery of the tubes, the mesosalpinx, contains the blood supply and nerves. The uterine tubes connect the cornua of the uterine cavity and the peritoneal cavity. The ostia into the endometrial cavity are 1.5 mm in diameter, whereas the ostia into the abdominal cavity are approximately 3 mm in diameter.

The oviducts are between 10 and 14 cm in length and slightly less than 1 cm in external diameter. Each tube is divided into four anatomic sections. The uterine intramural or interstitial segment is 1 to 2 cm in length and is surrounded by myometrium. The isthmic segment begins as the tube exits the uterus and is approximately 4 cm in length. This segment is narrow, 1 to 2 mm in inside diameter, and straight. The isthmic segment has the most highly developed musculature. The ampullary segment is 4 to 6 cm in length and approximately 6 mm in inside diameter. It is wider and more tortuous in its course than other segments. Fertilization normally occurs in the ampullary portion of the tube. The infundibulum is the distal trumpet-shaped portion of the oviduct. From 20 to 25 irregular fingerlike projections, termed *fimbriae,* surround the abdominal ostia of the tube. One of the largest fimbriae is attached to the ovary, the fimbria ovarica (see Fig. 3-5).

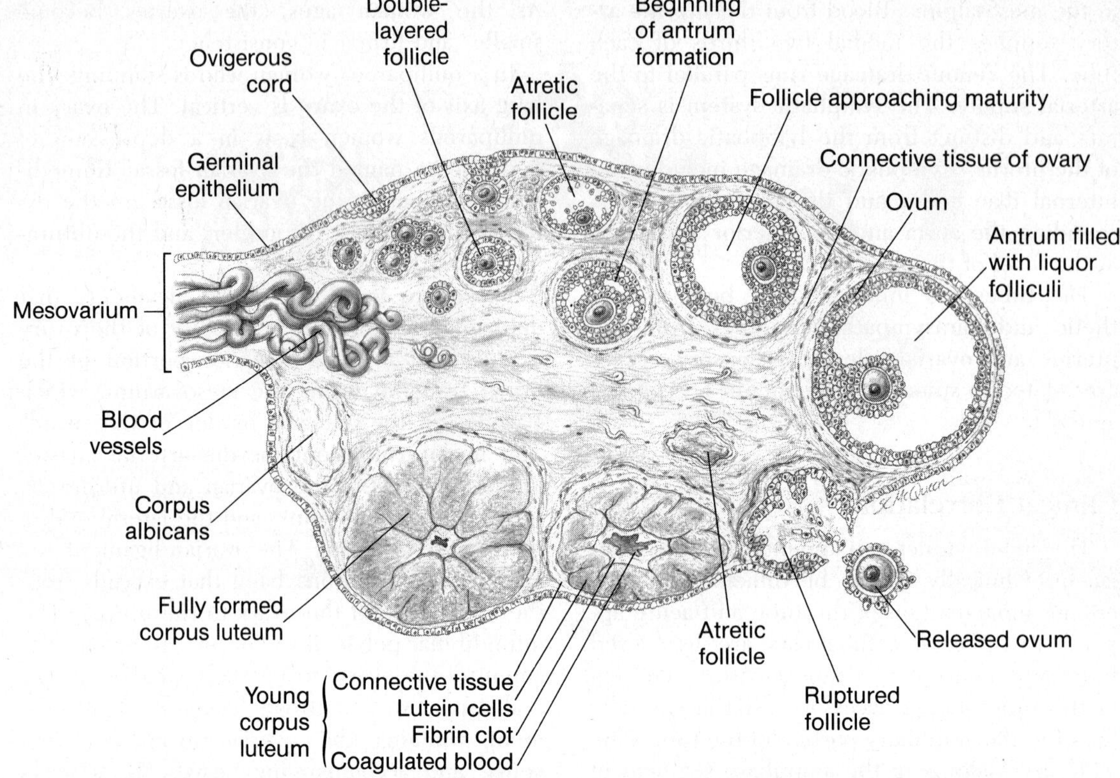

FIGURE 3-12

A schematic drawing of the ovary. Note the single layer of cuboidal epithelium called the germinal epithelium. Note the graafian follicles in different stages of development. Note the inner medullary region of stroma and blood vessels. (Adapted from Gray's Anatomy of the Human Body, 35th ed. Philadelphia, Lea & Febiger, 1973. Redrawn from Blaustein A: Anatomy and histology of the human ovary. In Blaustein A, ed: Pathology of the female genital tract, 2nd ed. New York, Springer-Verlag, 1982, p. 417.)

iliac vessels, and enter the infundibulopelvic ligaments, reaching the mesovarium in the broad ligament. The ovarian blood supply enters through the hilum of the ovary. The venous drainage of the ovary collects in the pampiniform plexus and consolidates into several large veins as it leaves the hilum of the ovary. The ovarian veins accompany the ovarian arteries, with the left ovarian vein draining into the left renal vein, whereas the right ovarian vein connects directly with the inferior vena cava.

The lymphatic drainage of the ovaries is primarily to the aortic nodes adjacent to the great vessels at the level of the renal veins. Metastatic disease from the ovary occasionally takes a shorter course to the iliac nodes. The autonomic and sensory nerve fibers accompany the ovarian vasculature in the infundibulopelvic ligament. They connect with the ovarian, hypogastric, and aortic plexuses.

Clinical Correlations

The size of the "normal" ovary during the reproductive years and the postmenopausal period is important in clinical practice. Before the menopause, a "normal" ovary may be up to 5 cm in length. Thus a small physiologic cyst may cause an ovary to be 6 to 7 cm in diameter. In contrast, the "normal" atrophic postmenopausal ovary usually cannot be palpated during pelvic examination. If an adnexal mass is palpated in a postmenopausal woman, an ovarian neoplasm should be suspected.

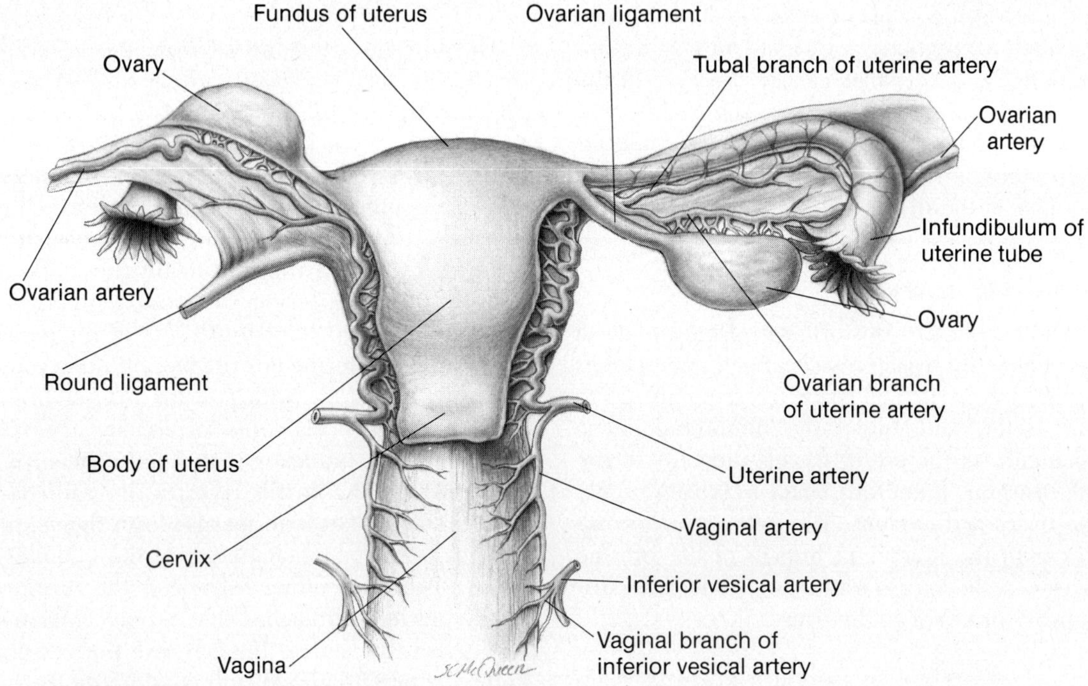

FIGURE 3-13
The arteries of the reproductive organs. Note the paired arteries entering laterally and freely anastomosing with each other. (Redrawn from Clemente CD: Anatomy: A regional atlas of the human body © 1987, Urban & Schwarzenberg, Baltimore-Munich.)

Attempts have been made to alleviate chronic pelvic pain by performing an ovarian denervation operation by cutting and ligating the infundibulopelvic ligaments. This operation has been abandoned because of the high incidence of cystic degeneration of the ovaries, which resulted from the interruption of their primary blood supply that accompanied the neurectomy procedure.

The close anatomic proximity of the ovary, ovarian fossa, and ureter is emphasized in surgery for severe endometriosis or pelvic inflammatory disease. It is important to identify the course of the ureter in order to facilitate removal of all of the ovarian capsule that is adherent to the peritoneum and to avoid both ureteral injury and residual ovarian remnants in the future.

VASCULAR SYSTEM OF THE PELVIS

In a description of the network of arteries that bring blood to the female reproductive organs, several generalizations should be made. The arteries are paired, are bilateral, and have multiple collaterals (Fig. 3-13). The arteries enter their respective organs laterally and then unite with anastomotic vessels from the other side of the pelvis near the midline. There has been a long-standing teaching generalization that the pelvic reproductive viscera lie within a loosely woven basket of large veins with numerous interconnecting venous plexuses. The arteries thread their way through this interwoven mesh of veins to reach the pelvic reproductive organs, giving off numerous branching arcades to provide a rich blood supply.

Arteries

Inferior Mesenteric Artery

The inferior mesenteric artery, a single artery, arises from the aorta approximately 3 cm above the aortic bifurcation. It supplies part of the transverse colon, the descending colon, the sigmoid colon, and the rectum and terminates as the superior hemorrhoidal artery. The inferior mesenteric artery is occasionally torn during node dissections performed in staging operations for gynecologic cancer. Because of the rich collateral circulation from the middle and inferior hemorrhoidal arteries, the inferior mesenteric artery can be ligated without compromise of the distal portion of the colon.

Ovarian Artery

The ovarian arteries originate from the aorta just below the renal vessels. Each one courses in the retroperitoneal space, crosses anterior to the ureter, and enters the infundibulopelvic ligament. As the artery travels medially in the mesovarium, numerous small branches supply the ovary and oviduct. The ovarian artery unites with the ascending branch of the uterine artery in the mesovarium just under the suspensory ligament of the ovary.

Common Iliac Artery

The bifurcation of the aorta occurs at the level of the fourth lumbar vertebra, forming the two common iliac arteries. Each common iliac artery is approximately 5 cm in length before the vessel divides into the external iliac and hypogastric arteries.

Hypogastric Artery (Internal Iliac Artery)

The hypogastric arteries are short vessels, each approximately 3 to 4 cm in length. Throughout their course they are in close proximity both to the ureters, which are anterior, and to the hypogastric veins, which are posterior. Each hypogastric artery branches into an anterior and a posterior division (or trunk). The posterior trunk gives off three parietal branches, the iliolumbar, lateral sacral, and superior gluteal arteries. The anterior trunk has nine branches. The three parietal branches are the obturator, internal pudendal, and inferior gluteal arteries. The six visceral branches include the umbilical, middle vesical, inferior vesical, middle hemorrhoidal, uterine, and vaginal arteries. The superior vesical artery usually arises from the umbilical artery. The individual branches of the hypogastric artery may vary from one woman to another.

Uterine Artery

The uterine artery arises from the anterior division of the hypogastric artery and courses medially toward the isthmus of the uterus. Approximately 2 cm lateral to the endocervix, it crosses over the ureter and reaches the sidewall of the uterus. The ascending branch of the uterine artery courses in the broad ligament, running a tortuous route to finally anastomose with the ovarian artery in the mesovarium (Fig. 3-14). Through its circuitous route in the parametrium, the uterine artery gives off numerous branches that unite with arcuate arteries from the other side. This series of arcuate arteries develop radial branches that supply the myometrium and the basalis layer of the endometrium. The arcuate arteries also form the spiral arteries of the functional layer of the endometrium. The descending branch of the uterine artery produces branches that supply both the cervix and the vagina. In each case the vessels enter the organ laterally and anastomose freely with vessels from the other side.

Vaginal Artery

The vaginal artery may arise either from the anterior trunk of the hypogastric artery or from the uterine artery. It supplies blood to the vagina, bladder, and rectum. There are extensive anastomoses with the vaginal branches of the uterine artery to form the azygos arteries of the cervix and vagina.

Internal Pudendal Artery

The internal pudendal artery is the terminal branch of the hypogastric artery and supplies branches to the rectum, labia, clitoris, and perineum.

Veins

The venous drainage of the pelvis begins in small sinusoids that drain to profuse venous plexuses contained within or immediately adjacent to the pelvic organs. Invariably there are numerous anastomoses between the parietal and visceral branches of the venous system. In general, the veins of the female pelvis and perineum are thin walled and have few valves.

The veins that drain the pelvic plexuses fol-

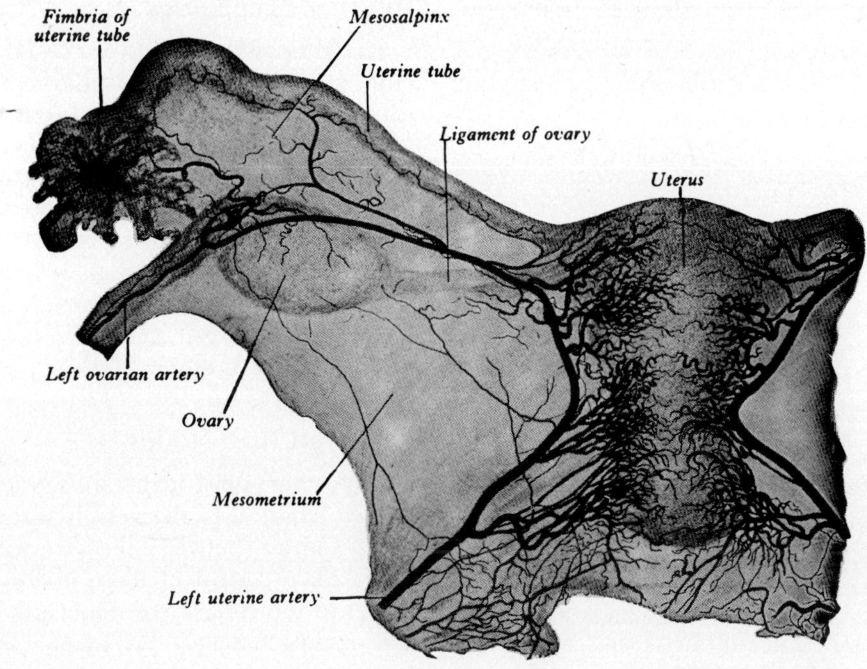

FIGURE 3-14
A photograph of an injected specimen demonstrating the rich anastomoses of the uterine and ovarian arteries. (From Warwick R, Williams PL: Gray's anatomy, 35th ed. Churchhill Livingstone, Edinburgh, 1973, p. 1361. Reprinted by permission.)

low the course of the arterial supply. Their names are similar to those of the accompanying arteries. Often multiple veins run alongside a single artery. The leading exception to these generalizations is the venous drainage of the ovaries. The left ovarian vein empties into the left renal vein, whereas the right ovarian vein connects directly with the inferior vena cava.

Clinical Correlations

In certain clinical situations associated with profuse hemorrhage from the female pelvis, hypogastric ligation is performed. Because of the extensive collateral circulation, this operation does not produce hypoxia of the pelvic viscera but reduces hemorrhage by decreasing the pulse pressure. The extent of collateral circulation following hypogastric artery ligation depends on the site of ligation and may be divided into three groups (Table 3-1).

In cases of intractable pelvic hemorrhage, it may be necessary to supplement the effects of bilateral hypogastric artery ligation with liga-

tion of the anastomotic sites between the ovarian and uterine vessels. Ligation of the terminal end of the ovarian artery preserves the direct blood supply to the ovaries, and there is no fear of the subsequent cystic degeneration of the ovaries that may occur following ligation of the vessels in the infundibulopelvic ligaments. An alternative approach is to embolize the bleeding vessel with Gelfoam. This is accomplished by direct canalization with fluoroscopy.

One of the treatments for repetitive embolization from the female pelvis is the placement of an umbrella, or ligation, of the inferior vena cava. Collateral circulation exists between the portal venous system of the gastrointestinal tract and the systemic venous circulation through anastomosis in the pelvis, especially in the hemorrhoidal plexus. The pelvic veins also anastomose with the presacral and lumbar veins. Therefore patients may develop trophoblastic emboli to the brain without the trophoblast's being filtered by the capillary system in the lungs.

TABLE 3-1
Collateral Arterial Circulation

Branches from the Aorta

Ovarian artery—anastomoses freely with uterine artery

Inferior mesenteric artery—continues as superior hemorrhoidal artery to anastomose with middle and inferior hemorrhoidal arteries from hypogastric and internal pudendal

Lumbar and vetebral arteries—anastomose with iliolumbar artery of hypogastric

Middle sacral artery—anastomoses with lateral sacral artery of hypogastric

Branches from External Iliac Artery

Deep iliac circumflex artery—anastomoses with iliolumbar and superior gluteal of hypogastric

Inferior epigastric artery—gives origin to obturator artery in 25% of cases, providing additional anastomoses of external iliac with medial femoral circumflex and communicating pelvic branches

Branches from Femoral Artery

Medial femoral circumflex artery—anastomoses with obturator and inferior gluteal arteries from hypogastric

Lateral femoral circumflex artery—anastomoses with superior gluteal and iliolumbar arteries from hypogastric

Reprinted with permission from Mattingly RF, Thompson JD: Te Linde's operative gynecology, 6th ed. Philadelphia, J.B. Lippincott Co., 1985, p. 53.

LYMPHATIC SYSTEM

External Iliac Nodes

The external iliac nodes are immediately adjacent to the external iliac artery and vein (Figs. 3-15 and 3-16). There are two distinct groups, one situated lateral to the vessels and the other posterior to the psoas muscle. The distal portion of the posterior group is enclosed in the femoral sheath. The majority of lymphatic channels to this group of nodes originate from the vulva, but there are also channels from the cervix and lower portion of the uterus. The external iliac nodes receive secondary drainage from the femoral and internal iliac nodes.

Internal Iliac Nodes

The internal iliac nodes are found in an anatomic triangle whose sides are composed of the external iliac artery, the hypogastric artery, and the pelvic sidewall. Included in this important area for biopsy are nodes with special designation, including the nodes of the femoral ring, the obturator nodes, and the nodes adjacent to the external iliac vessels. This rich collection of nodes receives channels from every internal pelvic organ and the vulva, including the clitoris and urethra.

Common Iliac Nodes

The common iliac nodes are a group of nodes located adjacent to the vessels that bear their name and are between the external iliac and aortic chains. Most of these nodes are found lateral to the vessels. To remove this chain, it is necessary to dissect the common iliac vessels away from their attachments to the psoas muscle. This group receives lymphatics from the cervix and the upper portion of the vagina. Secondary lymphatic drainage from the internal iliac, external iliac, superior gluteal, and inferior gluteal nodes is to the common iliac nodes.

Inferior Gluteal Nodes

A small group of lymph nodes, the inferior gluteal nodes, are located in the anatomic proximity of the ischial spines and are adjacent to the sacral plexus of nodes. It is difficult to remove these nodes surgically, and often they are considered inaccessible. The nodes receive lymphatics from the cervix, the lower portion of the vagina, and Bartholin's glands. This group of nodes secondarily drains to the internal iliac, common iliac, superior gluteal, and subaortic nodes.

Superior Gluteal Nodes

The superior gluteal nodes are a group of nodes found near the origin of the superior gluteal artery and adjacent to the medial and posterior aspects of the hypogastric vessels. The superior gluteal nodes receive primary lymphatic drainage from the cervix and the vagina. Efferent lymphatics from this chain drain to the common iliac, sacral, or subaortic nodes.

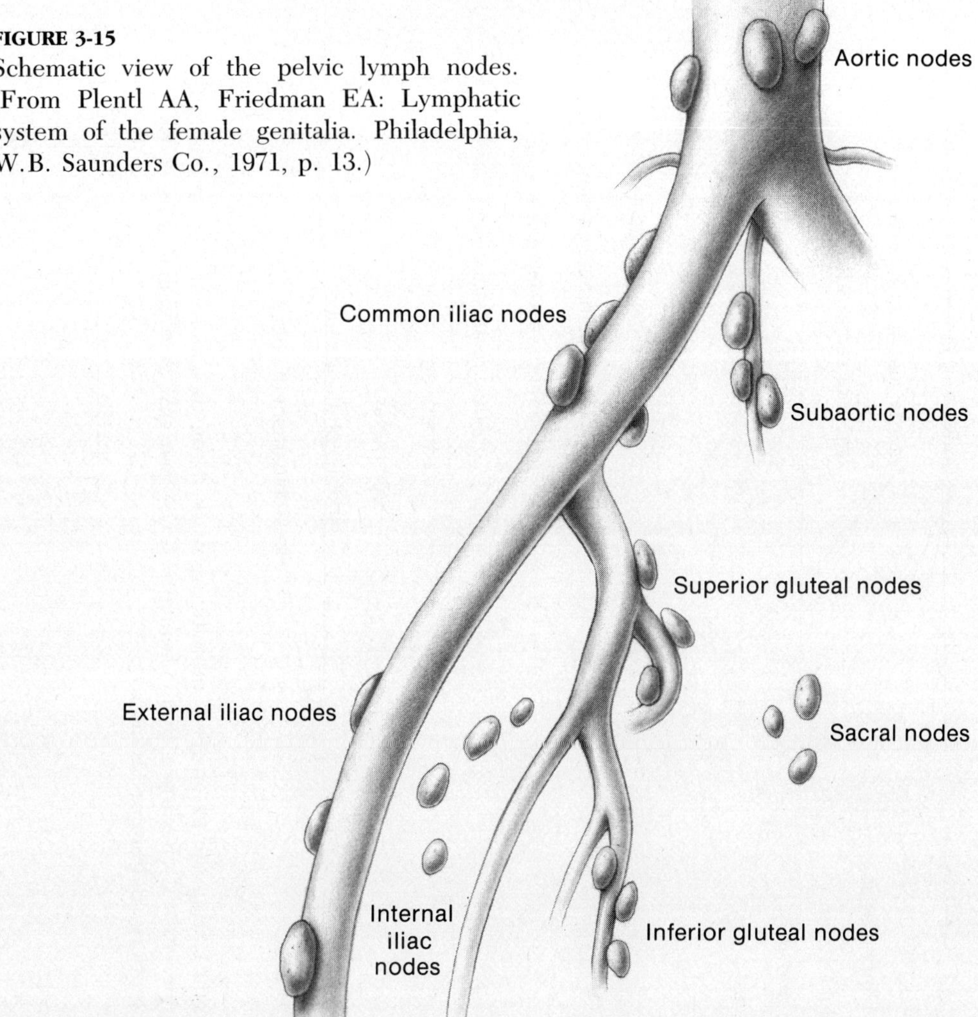

FIGURE 3-15
Schematic view of the pelvic lymph nodes.
(From Plentl AA, Friedman EA: Lymphatic
system of the female genitalia. Philadelphia,
W.B. Saunders Co., 1971, p. 13.)

Sacral Nodes

The sacral nodes are found over the middle
of the sacrum in a space bounded laterally by
the sacral foramina. These nodes receive lymphatic drainage from both the cervix and the
vagina. Secondary drainage from these nodes
run in a cephalad direction to the subaortic
nodes.

Subaortic Nodes

The subaortic nodes are arranged in a chain
and are located below the bifurcation of the
aorta, immediately anterior to the most caudal
portion of the inferior vena cava and over the
fifth lumbar vertebra. The primary drainage to
this chain of nodes is from the cervix, with a
few lymphatics from the vagina. This group is
the first secondary chain to receive the efferent
lymphatics as lymph flow progresses in a cephalad direction from the majority of other pelvic nodes.

Aortic Nodes

The many aortic nodes are immediately adjacent to the aorta on both its anterior and lateral aspects, predominantly in the furrow between the aorta and inferior vena cava. Primary
lymphatics drain from all the major pelvic organs, including the cervix, uterus, oviducts,
and especially the ovaries. The aortic chain receives secondary drainage from the pelvic

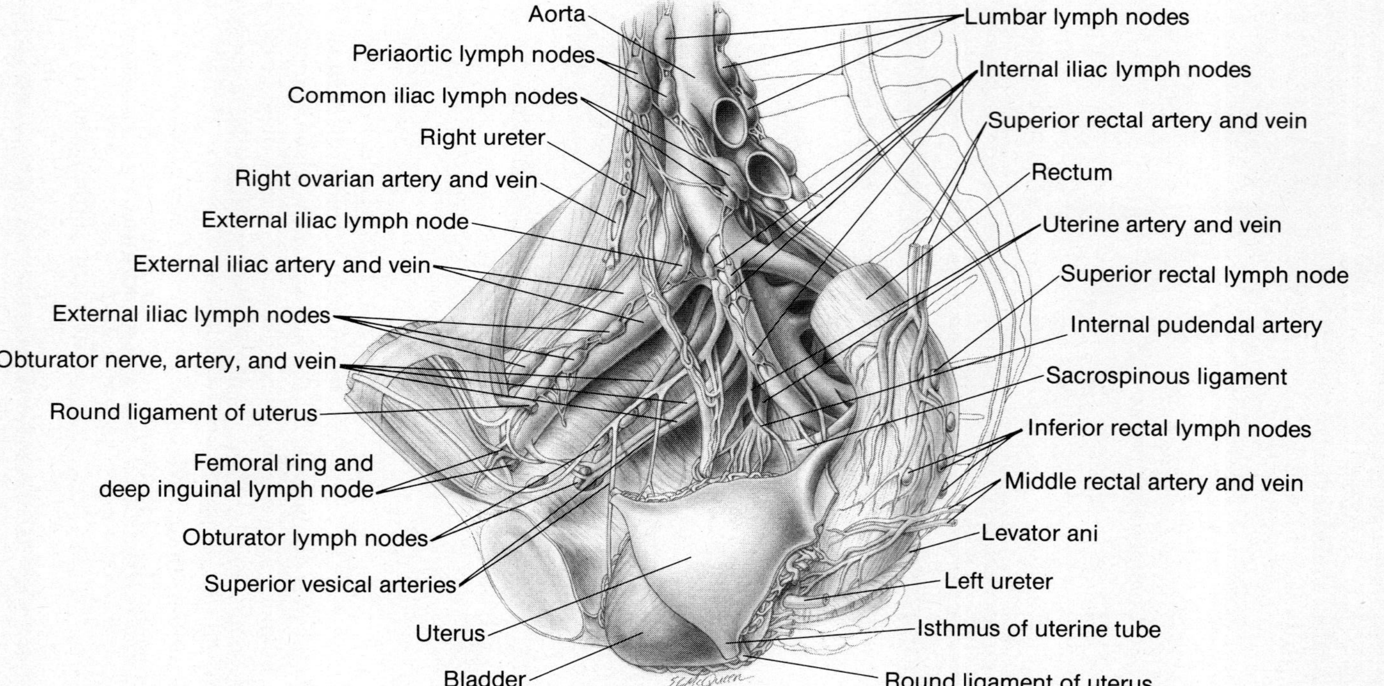

FIGURE 3-16
A lateral view of the female pelvis demonstrating the extensive lymphatic network. Note that most of the lymphatic channels follow the courses of the major vessels. (Redrawn from Clemente CD: Anatomy: A regional atlas of the human body © 1987, Urban & Schwarzenberg, Baltimore-Munich.)

nodes. In general, primary afferent lymphatics drain into the nodes over the anterior aspects of the aorta, whereas secondary efferent drainage from other pelvic nodes is found in those nodes situated lateral and posterior to the aorta.

Rectal Nodes

The chain of rectal nodes is found both subfascially and in the loose connective tissue surrounding the rectum. Primary drainage from the cervix flows to the superior rectal nodes, and drainage from the vagina appears in the rectal nodes in the anorectal region. Secondary drainage from the rectal nodes goes to the subaortic and aortic groups.

Parauterine Nodes

The number of lymph nodes in the group of parauterine nodes is small; most frequently there is a single node immediately lateral to each side of the cervix and close to the pelvic course of the ureter. Though anatomists frequently do not comment about the parauterine nodes, the group receives special attention in radical surgical operations for uterine or cervical malignancy. Primary drainage to this node originates in the vagina, cervix, and uterus. Secondary drainage from this node is to the internal iliac nodes on the same side of pelvis.

Superficial Femoral Nodes

The superficial femoral nodes are a group of nodes found in the loose, fatty connective tissue of the femoral triangle between the superficial and deep fascial layers. These lymph nodes receive lymphatic drainage from the external genitalia of the vulvar region, the gluteal region, and the entire leg, including the foot. Efferent lymphatics from this group of nodes penetrate the fascia lata to enter the deep fem-

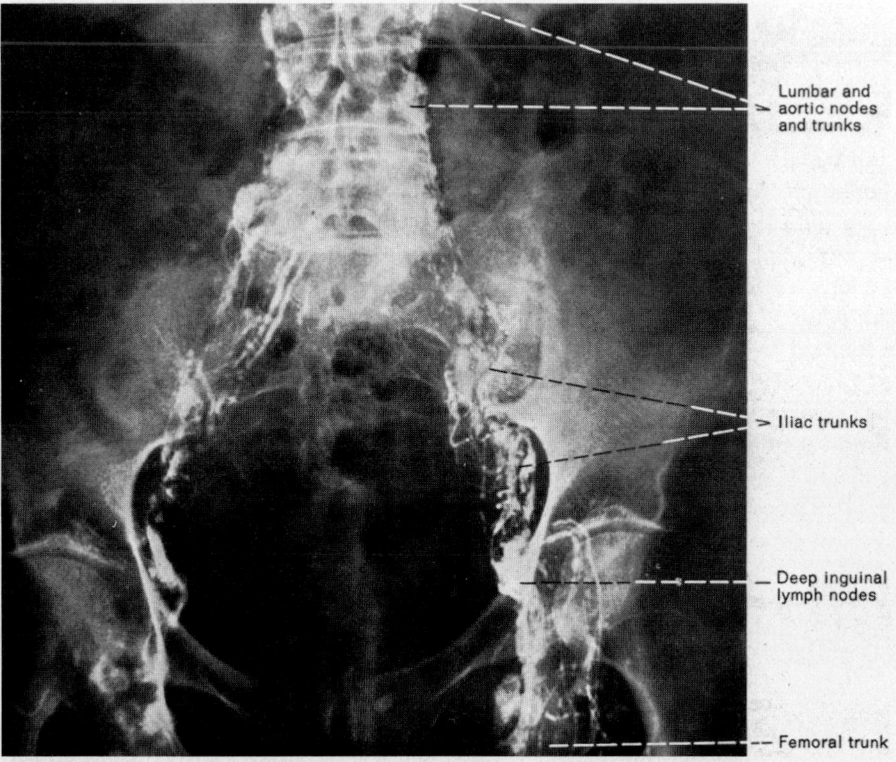

FIGURE 3-17
A lymphangiogram of the pelvis and lumbar areas. This x-ray film shows the course of the lymphatics from the deep femoral nodes into the iliac nodes. Note the extensive network of nodes in the inguinal region. (From Clemente CD: Anatomy: A regional atlas of the human body. Philadelphia, Lea & Febiger, 1975.)

oral nodes. Plentl and Freidman have stated that this area undoubtedly represents the greatest concentration of lymph nodes in the female (Fig. 3-17).

Deep Femoral Nodes

The deep femoral nodes are located within the femoral sheath, adjacent to both the femoral artery and the vein within the femoral triangle. This chain receives the primary lymphatics for the lower extremity and receives secondary efferent lymphatics from the superficial lymph nodes and thus the vulva. This group of lymph nodes is in direct continuity with the iliac and internal iliac chains.

Clinical Correlations

A precise knowledge of pelvic lymphatics is important for the gynecologic oncologist who is surgically determining the extent of spread of a pelvic malignancy. Plentl and Freidman give a detailed review of the lymphatic system of the female genitalia. The fact that most lymphatic metastatic spread from ovarian carcinoma occurs in a cephalad direction should be emphasized; it explains the primary importance of sampling aortic and subaortic nodes during second-look operations for ovarian cancer. In carcinoma of the vulva, lymphatic drainage may occur in either side of the pelvis. Thus bilateral node dissections are important.

For many years it was believed that all the superficial femoral nodes drained to a sentinel node called Cloquet's node. Cloquet's node, by the present classification system, would be the most distal and medial of the nodes in the external iliac chain. Cloquet's node is only of historical interest, since the assumption is neither anatomically nor clinically correct.

INNERVATION OF THE PELVIS

Internal Genitalia

The innervation of the internal genital organs is supplied primarily by the autonomic nervous system. The sympathetic portion of the autonomic nervous system originates in the thoracic and lumbar portions of the spinal cord, and sympathetic ganglia are located adjacent to the central nervous system. In contrast, the parasympathetic portion originates in cranial nerves and the middle three sacral segments of the cord, and the ganglia are located near the visceral organs. Although the fibers of both subdivisions of the autonomic nervous system frequently are intermingled in the same peripheral nerves, their physiologic actions are usually directly antagonistic. As a broad generalization, sympathetic fibers in the female pelvis produce muscular contractions and vasoconstriction, whereas parasympathetic fibers cause the opposite effect on muscles and vasodilation.

The semantics of pelvic innervation is confusing and imprecise. A plexus is a mixture of preganglionic and postganglionic fibers; small, inconsistently placed ganglia; and afferent (sensory) fibers. Throughout both the anatomic and surgical literature, a plexus may also be termed a nerve. For example, the superior hypogastric plexus is also called the presacral nerve.

Although autonomic nerve fibers enter the pelvis by several routes, the majority are contained in the superior hypogastric plexus, which is a caudal extension of the aortic and inferior mesenteric plexuses. The superior hypogastric plexus is found in the retroperitoneal connective tissue. It extends from the fourth lumbar vertebra to the hollow over the sacrum. In its lower portion the plexus divides into two parts to form the two hypogastric nerves, which run laterally and inferiorly. These nerves fan out to form the inferior hypogastric plexus in the area just below the bifurcation of the common iliac arteries. The nerve trunks then descend farther into the base of the broad ligament, where they join with parasympathetic fibers to form the pelvic plexus. Both motor fibers and accompanying sensory fibers reach the pelvic plexus from S2, S3, and S4 via the pelvic nerves, or nervi erigentes. From the pelvic plexus there are secondary plexuses adjacent to all pelvic viscera, namely, the rectum, anus, urinary bladder, vagina, and Frankenhäuser's plexus in the uterosacral ligaments. Frankenhäuser's plexus is extensive and contains both myelinated and nonmyelinated fibers passing primarily to the uterus and cervix, with a few fibers to the urinary bladder and vagina. The ovarian plexus, like the blood supply to the ovaries, is not part of the hypogastric system. The ovarian plexus is a downward extension of the aortic and renal plexuses.

It is impossible to separate afferent, sensory fibers from pelvic organs into morphologically independent tracts. The majority of fibers accompany the vascular system from the organ and then enter plexuses of the autonomic nervous system before eventually entering white rami communicates to the cell bodies in dorsal root ganglia of the spinal column. The major sensory fibers from the uterus accompany the sympathetic nerves, which enter the nerve roots of the spinal cord in segments T11 and T12. Thus referred uterine pain is often felt in the lower abdomen. In contrast, afferents from the cervix enter the spinal cord in nerve roots of S2, S3, and S4. Referred pain from cervical inflammation is characterized as low back pain in the lumbosacral region.

External Genitalia

The pudendal nerve and its branches supply the majority of both motor and sensory fibers to the muscles and skin of the vulvar region.

The pudendal nerve arises from the second, third, and fourth sacral roots. It has a complicated course in which it initially leaves the pelvis via the greater sciatic foramen. Next, it crosses beneath the ischial spine, running on the medial side of the internal pudendal artery. The pudendal nerve then reenters the pelvic cavity and travels in Alcock's canal, which runs along the lateral aspects of the ischial rectal fossa. As the nerve reaches the urogenital diaphragm, it divides into three branches: the inferior hemorrhoidal, the deep, and the superficial perineal (Fig. 3-18). The dorsal nerve of the clitoris is a terminal branch of the deep perineal nerve.

The skin of the anus, clitoris, and medial and inferior aspects of the vulva is supplied primarily by distal branches of the pudendal nerve. The vulvar region receives additional sensory fibers from three nerves. The anterior branch of the ilioinguinal nerve sends fibers to the mons pubis and the upper part of the labia majora. The genital femoral nerve supplies fibers

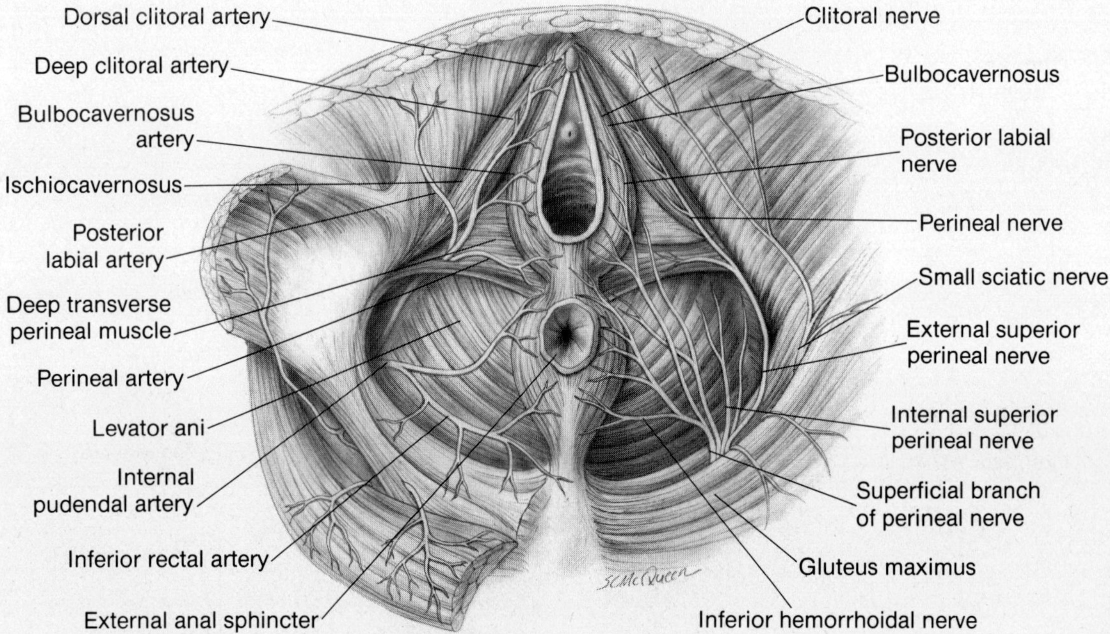

FIGURE 3-18
A posterior view of the female perineum, demonstrating the pudendal nerve emerging externally. The nerve divides into three segments as it passes out of the pelvis: the inferior hemorrhoidal nerve and the deep and superficial perineal nerves. The clitoral nerve is the terminal branch of the deep perineal nerve. (Redrawn from Mattingly RF, Thompson JD: Te Linde's operative gynecology, 6th ed. Philadelphia, J.B. Lippincott Co., 1985, p. 49.)

to the labia majora, and the posterior femoral cutaneous nerve supplies fibers to the infero-posterior aspects of the vulva.

Clinical Correlations

Because of the low density of nerve endings in the upper two thirds of the vagina, women are unable to determine the presence of a foreign body in this area. This explains how a "forgotten tampon" may remain unnoticed for several days in the upper part of the vagina until its presence results in a symptomatic discharge, abnormal bleeding, or odor. Infrequent but serious complications of pudendal nerve block are hematomas from trauma to the pudendal vessels and intravascular injection of anesthetic agents. The vessels and nerves are in close anatomic proximity to the ischial spine.

The fallopian tube is one of the most sensitive of the pelvic organs when crushed, cut, or distended, a fact that is appreciated in performing tubal ligations with the patient under local anesthesia. Damage to the obturator nerve during radical pelvic operations does not affect the pelvis directly. Although the nerve has an extensive pelvic course, its motor fibers supply the adductors of the thigh, and its sensory fibers innervate skin over the medial aspects of the thigh.

DIAPHRAGMS AND LIGAMENTS

Pelvic Diaphragm

The pelvic diaphragm is a wide but thin muscular layer of tissue that forms the inferior border of the abdominopelvic cavity. Composed of a broad, funnel-shaped sling of fascia and muscle, it extends from the symphysis pubis to the coccyx and from one lateral sidewall to the other. The primary muscles of the pelvic diaphragm are the levator ani and the coccygeus (Fig. 3-19). This structure is the evolutionary remnant of the tail-wagging muscles in lower animals.

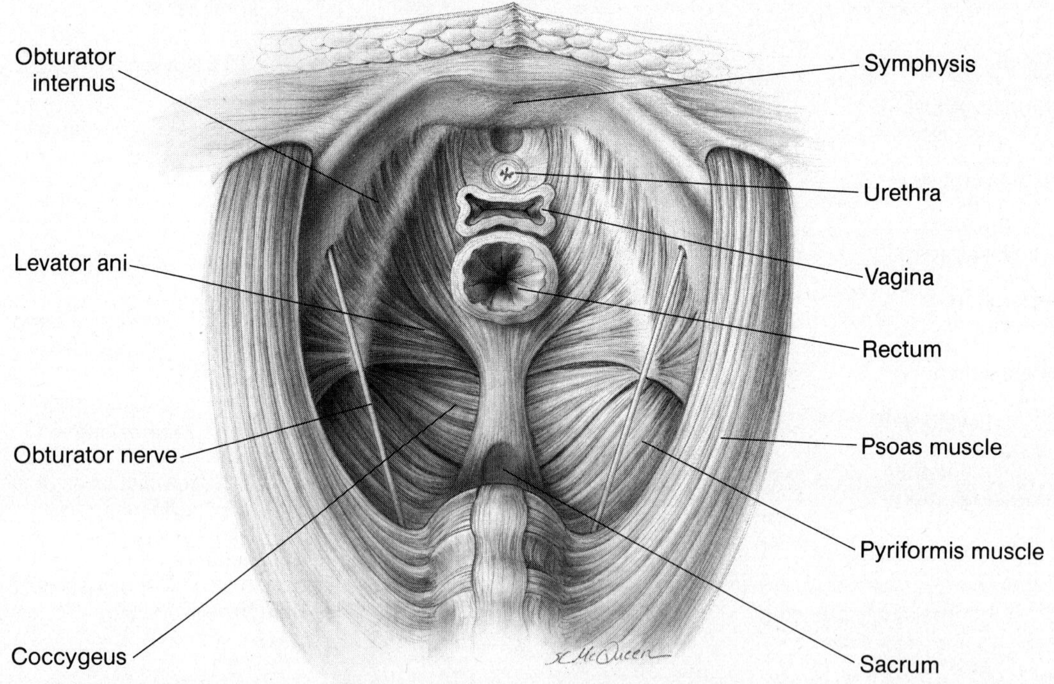

FIGURE 3-19
A superior view of the pelvic diaphragm of the pelvic floor. The primary muscles that compose this funnel-shaped sling are the coccygeus and the levator ani. (Redrawn from Mattingly RF, Thompson JD: Te Linde's operative gynecology, 6th ed. Philadelphia, J.B. Lippincott Co., p. 41.)

The muscles of the pelvic diaphragm are interwoven for strength, and a continuous muscle layer encircles the terminal portions of the urethra, vagina, and rectum. The levator ani muscles produce the greatest bulk of the pelvic diaphragm and are divided into three components, which are named after their origin and insertion: pubococcygeus, puborectalis, and iliococcygeus. The coccygeus is a triangular muscle that occupies the area between the ischial spine and the coccyx. The fascia of the pelvic diaphragm divides the extraperitoneal space around the rectum from the lower ischiorectal spine.

The paired levator ani muscles act as a single muscle and functionally are important in the control of urination, in parturition, and in maintaining fecal continence. The pelvic diaphragm is important in supporting both abdominal and pelvic viscera and facilitates equal distribution of intraabdominal pressure during activities such as coughing.

Urogenital Diaphragm

The urogenital diaphragm, also called the triangular ligament, is a strong, muscular membrane that occupies the area between the symphysis pubis and ischial tuberosities (Fig. 3-20). It stretches across the triangular anterior portion of the pelvic outlet. The urogenital diaphragm is external and inferior to the pelvic diaphragm. Anteriorly, the urethra is suspended from the pubic bone by continuations of the fascial layers of the urogenital diaphragm. The free edge of the diaphragm is strengthened by the superficial transverse perineal muscle. Posteriorly, the urogenital diaphragm inserts into the central point of the perineum. Situated farther posteriorly is the ischiorectal fossa. Located more superficially are the bulbocavernosus and ischiocavernosus muscles.

The urogenital diaphragm has two layers that enfold and cover the striated, deep transverse perineal muscle. The latter muscle surrounds both the vagina and the urethra, which pierce the diaphragm. The pudendal vessels and nerves, the external sphincter of the membranous urethra, and the dorsal nerve to the clitoris are also found within the urogenital diaphragm. The deep transverse perineal muscle

is innervated by branches of the pudendal nerve. The major function of the urogenital diaphragm is support of the urethra and maintenance of the urethrovesical junction.

Ligaments

The pelvic ligaments are not classic ligaments but are thickenings of retroperitoneal fascia and consist primarily of blood and lymphatic vessels, nerves, and fatty connective tissue. Anatomists call the retroperitoneal fascia *subserous fascia*, whereas surgeons refer to this fascial layer as *endopelvic fascia*. The connective tissue is denser immediately adjacent to the lateral walls of the cervix and the vagina.

Broad Ligaments

The broad ligaments are a thin, mesenteric-like double reflection of peritoneum from the lateral pelvic sidewalls to the uterus (Fig. 3-21). They become contiguous with the uterine serosa, and thus the uterus is contained within two folds of peritoneum. These peritoneal folds enclose the loose, fatty connective tissue termed the *parametrium*. The broad ligaments afford minor support to the uterus but are conduits for important anatomic structures. Within the broad ligaments are found the following structures: oviducts; ovarian and round ligaments; ureters; ovarian and uterine arteries and veins; parametrial tissue; embryonic remnants of the mesonephric duct, wolffian body, and secondary ligaments; mesovarium; and mesosalpinx. The round ligament is composed of fibrous tissue and muscle fibers. It attaches to the superoanterior aspect of the uterus, anterior and caudal to the oviduct, and runs via the broad ligament to the lateral pelvic wall. It, too, offers little support to the uterus. The round ligament crosses the external iliac vessels and enters the inguinal canal, ending by inserting into the labia majora in a fanlike fashion. In the fetus a small, fingerlike projection of the peritoneum accompanies the round ligament into the inguinal canal, Nuck's canal. Generally it is obliterated in the adult woman.

Cardinal Ligaments

The cardinal, or Mackenrodt's, ligaments extend from the lateral aspects of the upper part

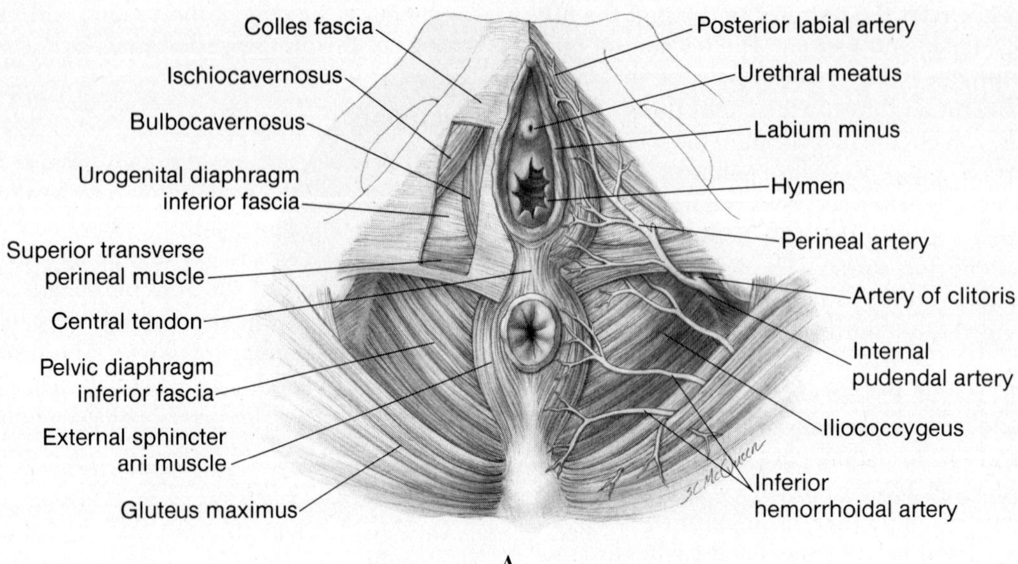

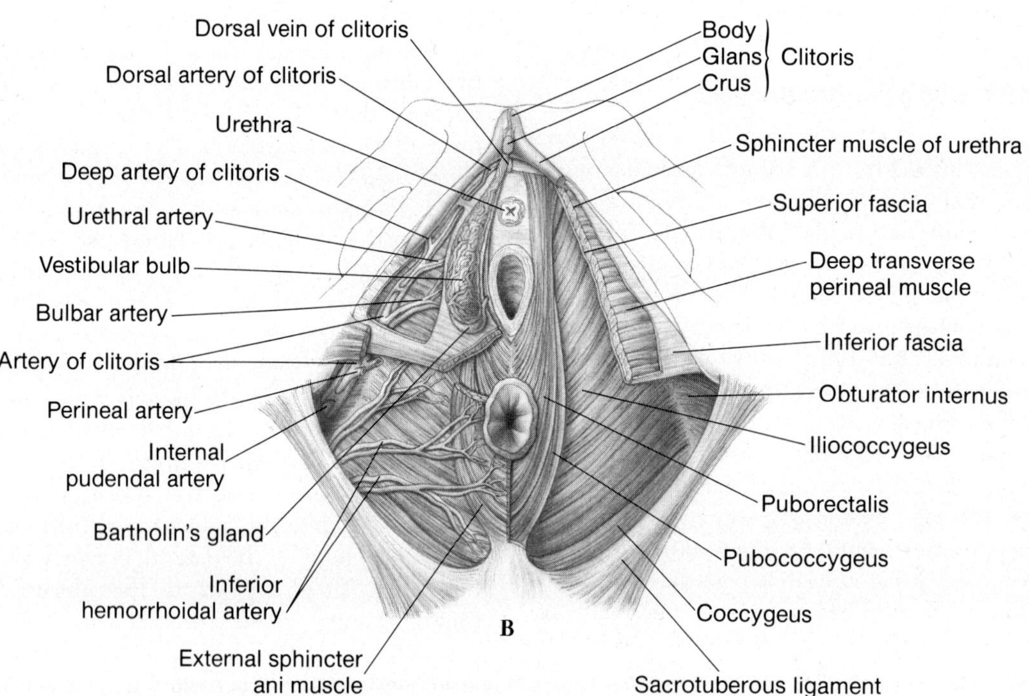

FIGURE 3-20

A, Schematic views of the perineum demonstrating superficial structures. Note the two layers of the urogenital diaphragm enfolding the deep transverse perineal muscle. **B,** Schematic views of the perineum demonstrating superficial structures and deeper structures. Note the pelvic diaphragm deep to the perineum, composed primarily of the levator ani and the coccygeus muscles. (Redrawn from Pritchard JA, MacDonald PC, Gant NF: Williams' obstetrics, 17th ed. New York, Appleton-Century-Crofts, 1985, p. 14.)

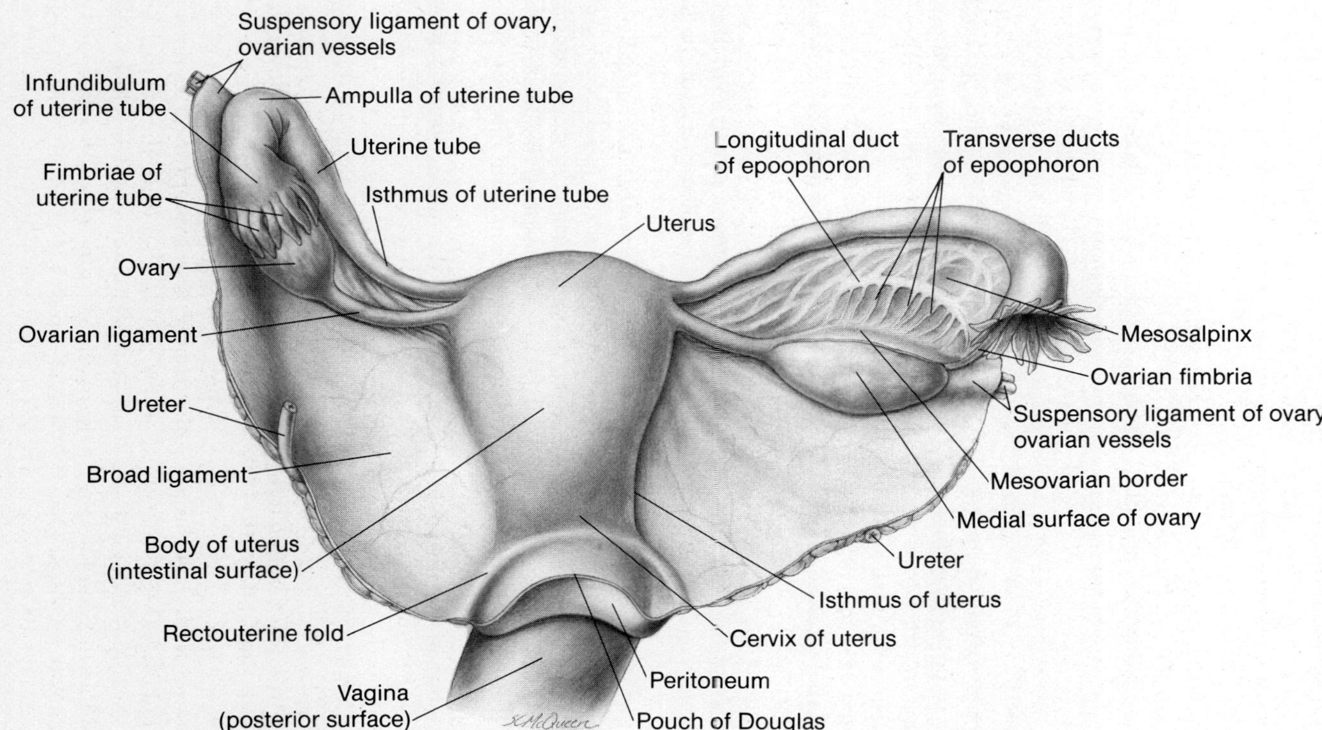

FIGURE 3-21
A schematic drawing of the broad ligament, posterior view. Note the many structures contained within the broad ligament. Note the posterior aspect of the rectouterine fold, called the cul-de-sac, or pouch, of Douglas. (Redrawn from Clemente CD: Anatomy: A regional atlas of the human body © 1987, Urban & Schwarzenberg, Baltimore-Munich.)

of the cervix and the vagina to the pelvic wall. They are a thickened condensation of the subserosal fascia and parametria between the interior portion of the two folds of peritoneum. The cardinal ligaments form the base of the broad ligaments, laterally being attached to the fascia over the pelvic diaphragm and medially merging with fibers of the endopelvic fascia. Within these ligaments are found blood vessels and smooth muscle. The cardinal ligaments help to maintain the anatomic position of the cervix and the upper part of the vagina and provide the major support of the uterus and cervix.

Uterosacral Ligaments

The uterosacral ligaments extend from the upper portion of the cervix posteriorly to the third sacral vertebra. They are thickened near the cervix and then run a curved course around each side of the rectum and subsequently thin out posteriorly. The external surface of the uterosacral ligaments is formed by an inferoposterior fold of peritoneum at the base of the broad ligaments. The middle of the uterosacral ligaments is composed primarily of nerve bundles. The uterosacral ligaments serve a minor role in the anatomic support of the cervix.

Clinical Correlations

The posterior fibers of the levator ani muscles encircle the rectum at its junction with the anal canal, thereby producing an abrupt angle that reinforces fecal continence. Surgical repair of a displacement or tear of the levator ani muscles resulting from childbirth is important during posterior colporrhaphy. Coccygodynia, a form of chronic low back pain, may be related to tearing of muscle fibers during childbirth.

An apron of omentum has been used to create a replacement for portions of the pelvic diaphragm removed during radical pelvic surgery.

The round ligament is an important surgical landmark in making the initial incision into the parietal peritoneum to gain extraperitoneal access to the hypogastric vessels.

During pelvic surgery, traction on the uterus will make the uterosacral and cardinal ligaments more prominent. There is a free space approximately 2 to 4 cm from the anterior edge of the broad ligament. In this "free space"

there are no blood vessels, and the two sides of the broad ligament are in close proximity. Gynecologic surgeons utilize blunt dissection of this area to facilitate clamping of the anastomosis between the uterine and ovarian arteries.

URETERS

The ureters are whitish, muscular tubes, 28 to 34 cm in length, extending from the renal pelves to the urinary bladder. The ureter is divided into abdominal and pelvic segments. The diameters vary. The abdominal segment is approximately 8 to 10 mm in diameter. The pelvic segment is approximately 4 to 6 mm. A congenital anomaly of a double, or bifid, ureter occurs in 1% to 4% of the population. Ectopic ureteral orifices may occur in either the urethra or the vagina.

The abdominal portion of the right ureter is lateral to the inferior vena cava. Four arteries and accompanying veins cross anterior to the right ureter: the right colic artery, the ovarian vessels, the ileocolic artery, and the superior mesenteric artery. The course of the left ureter is similar to its counterpart on the right side in that it runs downward and medially along the anterior surface of the psoas major muscle.

The iliopectineal line serves as the marker for the pelvic portion of the ureter. The ureters run along the common iliac artery and then cross over the iliac vessels as they enter the pelvis. There is a slight variation between the two sides of the female pelvis. The right ureter tends to cross at the bifurcation of the common iliac artery, whereas usually the left ureter crosses 1 to 2 cm above the bifurcation.

The ureters then follow the descending, convex curvature of the posterolateral pelvic wall toward the perineum. Throughout its course the ureter is retroperitoneal in location. The ureter can be found on the medial leaf of the parietal peritoneum and in close proximity to the ovarian, uterine, obturator, and superior vesical arteries (Fig. 3-22). The uterine artery lies on the anterolateral surface of the ureter for 2.5 to 3 cm. At approximately the level of the ischial spine, the ureter changes its course and runs forward and medially from the uterosacral ligaments to the base of the broad ligament. There the ureter enters into the cardinal ligaments. In this location the ureter is approximately 1 to 2 cm lateral to the uterine cervix and is surrounded by a plexus of veins. The ureter then runs upward and medially in the vesical uterine ligaments to obliquely pierce the bladder wall. Just before entering the base of the bladder, the ureter is in close contact with the anterior vaginal wall.

The ureter has a rich arterial supply with numerous anastomoses from many small vessels that form a longitudinal plexus in the adventitia of the ureter. Parent vessels that send branches to this arterial plexus surrounding the ureter include the renal, ovarian, common iliac, hypogastric, uterine, vaginal, vesical, middle hemorrhoidal, and superior gluteal arteries. The ureter is resistant to injury resulting from devascularization unless the surgeon strips the adventitia from the muscular conduit.

Urinary Bladder

The urinary bladder is a hollow muscular organ that lies between the symphysis pubis and the uterus. The size and shape of the bladder vary with the volume of urine it contains. Similarly, the anatomic proximity to other pelvic organs depends on whether the bladder is full or empty. The superior surface of the bladder is the only surface covered by peritoneum. The inferior portion is immediately adjacent to the uterus. The urachus is a fibrous cord extending from the apex of the bladder to the umbilicus. The urachus, which is the adult remnant of the embryonic allantois, is occasionally patent for part of its length. The base of the bladder lies directly adjacent to the endopelvic fascia over the anterior vaginal wall. The bladder neck and connecting urethra are attached to the symphysis pubis by fibrous ligaments. The prevesical or retropubic space of Retzius is the area lying between the bladder and symphysis pubis and is bounded laterally by the obliterated hypogastric arteries. This space extends from the fascia covering the pelvic diaphragm to the umbilicus between the peritoneum and transversalis fascia.

The mucosa of the anterior surface of the bladder is light red and has numerous folds. The inferoposterior surface delineated by the two ureteral orifices and the urethral orifice is the trigone. The trigone is a darker red than

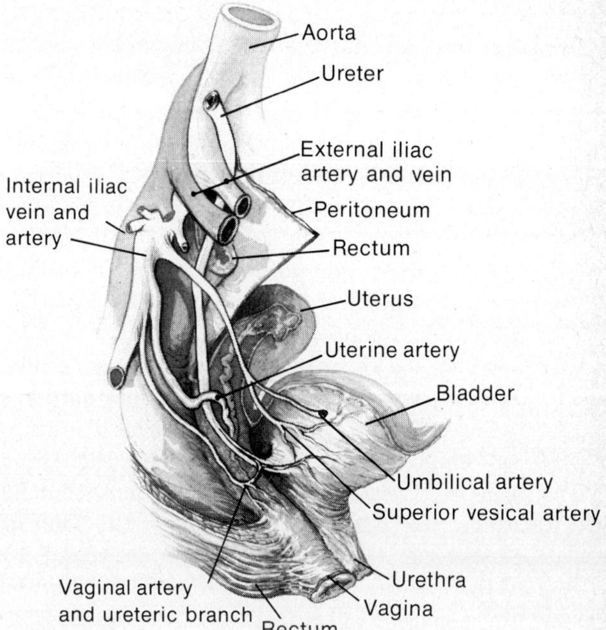

FIGURE 3-22
A schematic drawing of the female pelvis, lateral view, demonstrating the ureter's relation to the major arteries. Note the uterine artery crossing over the ureter. (From Buchsbaum HJ, Schmidt JD: Gynecologic and obstetric urology. Philadelphia, W.B. Saunders Co., 1978, p. 24.)

the rest of the bladder mucosa and is free of folds. When the bladder is empty, the ureteral orifices are approximately 2.5 cm apart. This distance increases to 5 cm when the bladder is distended. The muscular wall of the bladder, the detrusor muscles, is arranged in three layers. The arterial supply of the bladder originates from branches of the hypogastric artery: the superior vesical, inferior vesical, and middle hemorrhoidal arteries. The nerve supply to the bladder includes sympathetic and parasympathetic fibers, with the external sphincter being supplied by the pudendal nerve.

Rectum

The rectum is the terminal 12 to 14 cm of the large intestine. The rectum begins over the second or third sacral vertebra, where the sigmoid colon no longer has a mesentery. After the large intestine loses its mesentery, its anatomic posterior wall is in close proximity to the curvature of the sacrum. Anteriorly, peritoneum covers the upper and middle thirds of the rectum. The lowest one third is below the peritoneal reflection and is in close proximity to the posterior wall of the vagina.

The rectum empties into the anal canal, which is 2 to 4 cm in length. The anal canal is fixed by the surrounding levator ani musculature of the pelvic diaphragm (see Fig. 3-4). The external sphincter of the anal canal is a circular band of striated muscle. The rectum, unlike other areas of the large intestine, does not have teniae coli or appendices epiploicae. The arterial supply of the rectum is rich, originating from five arteries: the superior hemorrhoidal artery, which is a continuation of the inferior mesenteric; the two middle hemorrhoidal arteries; and the two inferior hemorrhoidal arteries.

Clinical Correlations

The anatomic proximity of the ureters, urinary bladder, and rectum to the female reproductive organs is a major consideration in most gynecologic operations. Surgical compromise of the ureter may occur during clamping or ligating of the infundibulopelvic vessels, clamping or ligating of the cardinal ligaments, reperitonealization of the lateral wall following hysterectomy, or wide suturing in the endopelvic fascia during an anterior repair.

For years teachers have referred to the area in the base of the broad ligament near the cervix where the uterine artery crosses the ureter as the area where "water flows under the bridge." A ureter may be differentiated from a large vessel in the retroperitoneal space by touching the wall of the ureter with a surgical instrument and observing for characteristic peristalsis.

The urinary bladder, if properly drained, will heal rapidly after a surgical insult if the blood supply to the bladder wall is not compromised. This capacity allows the gynecologist to insert a suprapubic cystostomy tube blindly without fear of fistula formation.

One of the surgical approaches for urinary stress incontinence is to suspend the periurethral tissue to either the symphysis pubis or to Cooper's ligaments. Occasionally, this surgical approach is complicated by significant postoperative venous bleeding. If the space of Retzius is not properly drained, a subfascial hematoma may extend as high as the umbilicus.

Rectal injury occurs most frequently during vaginal hysterectomy with associated posterior colporrhaphy. In the middle third of the vagina the distance between vaginal and rectal mucosa is only a few millimeters, and the connective tissue is densely adherent and must be separated by sharp dissection.

CUL-DE-SAC OF DOUGLAS

The cul-de-sac of Douglas is a deep pouch formed by the most caudal extent of the parietal peritoneum. The cul-de-sac is a potential space and also is called the rectouterine pouch or fold (see Fig. 3-21). It is anterior to the rectum, separating the uterus from the large intestine. The parietal peritoneum of the cul-de-sac covers the cervix and upper part of the posterior vaginal wall, then reflects to cover the anterior wall of the rectum. The pouch is bounded on the lateral sides by the peritoneal folds covering the uterosacral ligaments.

Parametria

The parametria are the extraperitoneal fatty and fibrous connective tissues adjacent to the uterus. The parametria lie between the leaves of the broad ligament and in the contiguous area anteriorly between the cervix and bladder. This connective tissue is thicker and denser adjacent to the cervix and vagina, where it becomes part of the connective tissue of the pelvic floor. The parametria may also thicken in response to radiation, pelvic cancer, infection, or endometriosis.

Clinical Correlations

The parametria and cul-de-sac of Douglas are important anatomic landmarks in advanced pelvic infection and neoplasia. Intrauterine infection and endometrial carcinoma may penetrate the myometrium and secondarily may invade the loose connective tissue of the parametria. Bleeding resulting from an anterior perforation of the lower uterine segment during dilation and curettage may produce a pelvic hematoma involving both broad ligaments because of the anatomic continuity of the two areas.

The pouch of Douglas is easily accessible in performing transvaginal surgical procedures. Vaginal tubal ligation may be the procedure of choice in massively obese women. Posterior colpotomy is frequently chosen for drainage of a pelvic abscess occurring in the posterior cul-de-sac.

Many women with uterine prolapse have an associated enterocoele, which is a hernial sac of parietal peritoneum that protrudes between the uterosacral ligaments. Surgical repair of an enterocoele includes removal of the sac of peritoneum and plication of the uterosacral ligaments. Occasionally the cul-de-sac of Douglas is obliterated by the inflammatory process associated with either endometriosis or advanced malignancy.

KEY POINTS

- The labia majora are homologous to the scrotum in the male. Skene's glands are homologous to the prostate gland in the male.

- The average length of the clitoris is 1.5 to 2 cm. Clinically, width is more important and should be less than 1 cm, for it is difficult to actually measure the length of the clitoris.

- The female urethra measures 3.5 to 5 cm in length. The mucosa of the proximal two thirds of the urethra is composed of stratified transitional epithelium, and the distal one third is stratified squamous epithelium.

- The middle third of the vagina is supported by the levator ani muscles and the lower portion of the cardinal ligaments.

- The primary lymphatic drainage of the upper third of the vagina is to the external iliac nodes, the middle third of the vagina drains to the common and internal iliac nodes, and the lower third has a wide lymphatic distribution, including the common iliac, superficial inguinal, and perirectal nodes.

- In a description of the clinical practice of gynecology, descriptive terms for pelvic organs are derived from the Latin root, whereas terms relating to surgical procedures are derived from the Greek root.

- The fibromuscular cervical stroma is composed primarily of collagenous connective tissue and ground substance. The connective tissue contains approximately 15% smooth muscle cells and a small amount of elastic tissue.

- The major arterial supply to the cervix is located on the lateral cervical walls at the 3 and 9 o'clock positions.

________ KEY POINTS, cont'd ________

- The pain fibers from the cervix accompany the parasympathetic fibers to S2, S3, and S4.

- The uterus of a nulliparous woman is approximately 8 cm long, 5 cm wide, and 2.5 cm thick and weighs 40 to 50 gm. In contrast, in a multiparous woman each measurement is approximately 1.2 cm larger and normal uterine weight is 20 to 30 gm heavier. The maximal weight of a normal uterus is 110 gm.

- In the majority of women, the long axis of the uterus is both anteverted in respect to the long axis of the vagina and anteflexed in relation to the long axis of the cervix. However, a retroflexed uterus is a normal variant found in approximately 25% of women.

- The cardinal ligaments provide the major support to the uterus.

- The endometrium varies from 1 to 6 mm in thickness, depending on hormonal stimulation. Both endometrial stroma and glands change in response to estrogen and progesterone.

- Afferent nerve fibers from the uterus enter the spinal cord at the eleventh and twelfth thoracic segments.

- The oviducts are 10 to 14 cm in length and are composed of four anatomic sections. Closest to the uterine cavity is the interstitial segment, followed by the narrow isthmic segment, then the wider ampullary segment, and distally the trumpet-shaped infundibular segment.

- During the reproductive years, the ovaries measure approximately 1.5 cm $\times$ 2.5 cm $\times$ 4 cm.

- The ovary in nulliparous women rests in a depression of peritoneum named the fossa ovarica. Immediately adjacent to the ovarian fossa are the external iliac vessels, the ureter, and the obturator vessels and nerves.

- The arterial supply of the pelvis is paired, bilateral, and has multiple collaterals and numerous anastomoses.

- The pudendal nerve and its branches supply the majority of both motor and sensory fibers to the muscles and skin of the vulvar region.

- The pelvic diaphragm is important in supporting both abdominal and pelvic viscera and facilitates equal distribution of intra-abdominal pressure during activities such as coughing.

- The major function of the urogenital diaphragm is support of the urethra and maintenance of the urethrovesical junction.

- A congenital anomaly of a double, or bifid, ureter occurs in 1% to 4% of the population.

- The distal ureter enters into the cardinal ligament. In this location the ureter is approximately 1 to 2 cm lateral to the uterine cervix and is surrounded by a plexus of veins.

- Surgical compromise of the ureters may occur during clamping or ligating of the infundibulopelvic vessels, clamping or ligating of the cardinal ligaments, reperitonealization of the lateral wall after hysterectomy, or wide suturing in the endopelvic fascia during an anterior repair.

BIBLIOGRAPHY

Boss JH, Scully RE, Wegner JH, et al: Structural variations in the adult ovary: Clinical significance. Obstet Gynecol 25:747, 1965.

Burchell RC: Physiology of internal iliac artery ligation. J Obstet Gynaecol Br Commnw 75:642, 1968.

Clemente CD: Gray's anatomy, 30th ed. Philadelphia, Lea & Febiger, 1985.

Cruikshank SH, Stoelk EM: Surgical control of pelvic hemorrhage: Method of bilateral ovarian artery ligation. Am J Obstet Gynecol 147:724, 1983.

Demopoulous RI: Normal endometrium. In Blaustein A. Pathology of the female genital tract. New York, Springer-Verlag, 1977.

Farrer-Brown G, Beilby JOW, Tarbit MH: The blood supply of the uterus. J Obstet Gynaecol Br Commnw 77:673, 1970.

Ferenczy A, Richart RM: Female reproductive system: Dynamics of scan and transmission microscopy. New York, John Wiley & Sons, 1974.

Finn CA, Porter DG: The uterus. Acton, Mass., Publishing Sciences Group, 1975.

Grant JCB: An atlas of anatomy, 7th ed. Baltimore, Williams & Wilkins, 1978.

Jordan JA, Singer A: The cervix. Philadelphia, W.B. Saunders Co., 1976.

Krantz KE: The anatomy of the urethra and anterior vaginal wall. Am J Obstet Gynecol 62:374, 1951.

Mahran M: The microscopic anatomy of the round ligament. J Obstet Gynaecol Br Commnw 72:614, 1965.

Milley PS, Nichols DH: The relationship between the pubo-urethral ligaments and the urogenital diaphragm in the human female. Anat Rec 170:281, 1971.

Neilson D, Jones GS, Woodruff JD, et al: The innervation of the ovary. Obstet Gynecol Surv 25:889, 1970.

Netter FH: Reproductive system, vol. 2. THE CIBA Collection of Medical Illustrations. Summit, N.J., CIBA Pharmaceutical Products, 1983.

Nichols DH, Milley PS: Surgical significance of the rectovaginal septum. Am J Obstet Gynecol 108:215, 1970.

Nichols DH, Randall CL: Vaginal surgery, 2nd ed. Baltimore, Williams & Wilkins, 1983.

Novak ER, Woodruff JD: Gynecologic and obstetric pathology, 7th ed. Philadelphia, W.B. Saunders Co., 1974.

Plentl AA, Freidman EA: Lymphatic system of the female genitalia. Philadelphia, W.B. Saunders Co., 1971.

Roberts WH, Habenicht J, Krishinger G: The pelvic and perineal fasciae and their neural and vascular relationships. Anat Rec 149:707, 1964.

Truex RC, Carpenter MB: Human neuroanatomy, 7th ed. Baltimore, Williams & Wilkins, 1976.

Zacharin RF: The suspensory mechanism of the female urethra. J Anat 97:423, 1963.

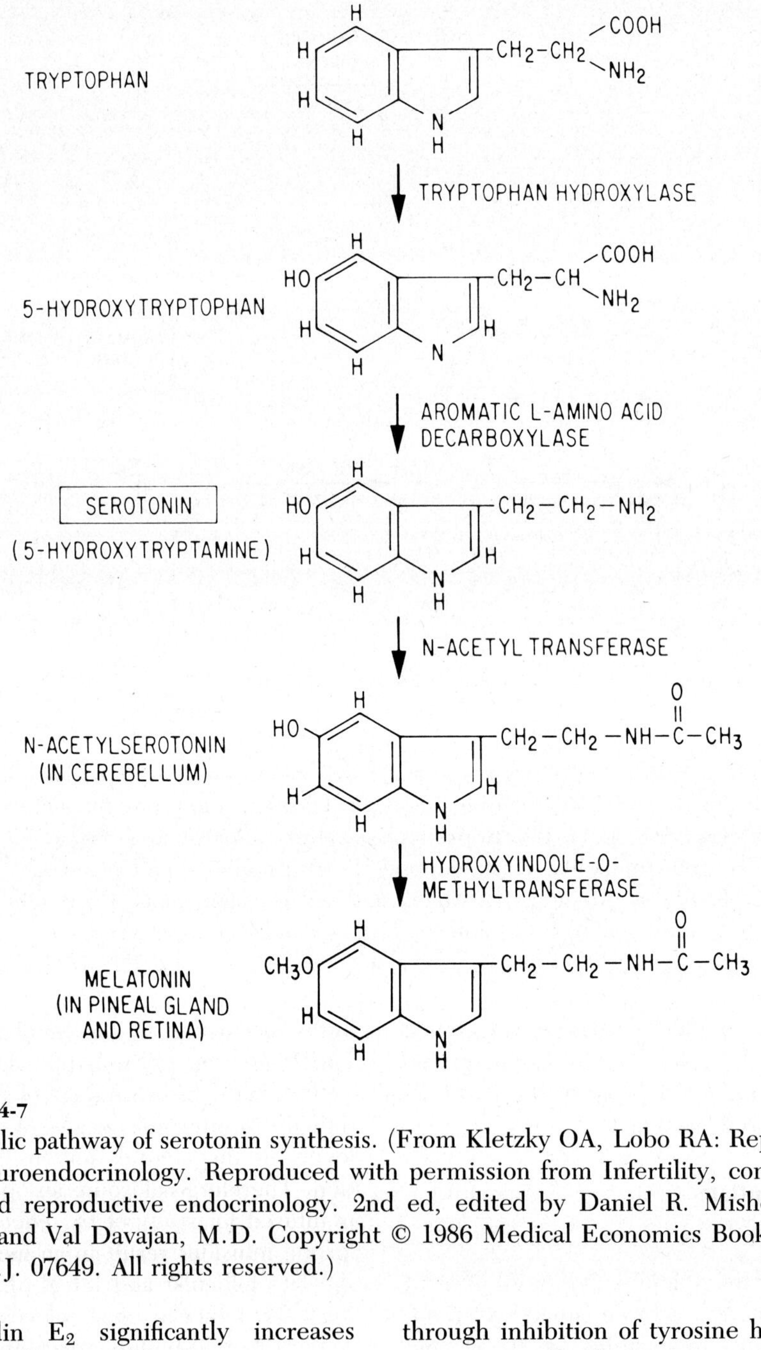

FIGURE 4-7

Metabolic pathway of serotonin synthesis. (From Kletzky OA, Lobo RA: Reproductive neuroendocrinology. Reproduced with permission from Infertility, contraception and reproductive endocrinology. 2nd ed, edited by Daniel R. Mishell, Jr., M.D., and Val Davajan, M.D. Copyright © 1986 Medical Economics Books, Oradell, N.J. 07649. All rights reserved.)

of prostaglandin E_2 significantly increases GnRH levels in the portal blood.

Catechol Estrogens

The compounds 2-hydroxyestradiol and 2-hydroxyestrone, as well as their 3-methyl derivatives, are present in higher concentrations in the hypothalamus than are prostaglandins E_1 and E_2. It has been hypothesized that these compounds may act as neuromodulators by modulating the function of catecholamines through inhibition of tyrosine hydroxylase and competition for the enzyme catechol-O-methyltransferase. However, the evidence that catechol estrogens have a major effect on neuromodulating reproductive function is insufficient.

GnRH ACTION

GnRH, when it reaches the anterior lobe of the pituitary, stimulates the synthesis and release of both LH and FSH from the same cell

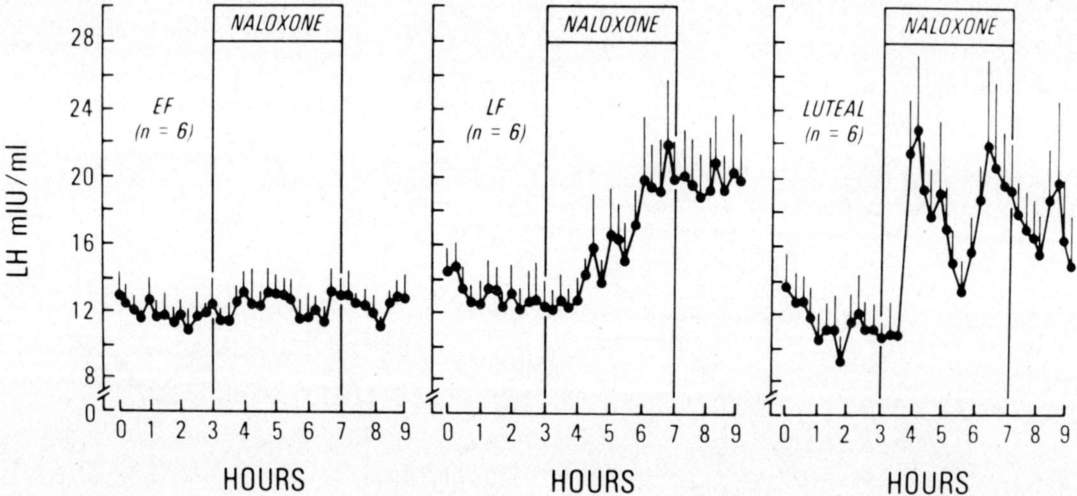

FIGURE 4-8

Infusion of naloxone, an opiate receptor antagonist, elicits incremental change of LH in subjects during late follicular and midluteal phases of cycle (but not in early follicular phase), indicating progressive increase in endogenous opioid inhibition of GnRH secretion, especially during luteal phase. (From Quigley ME, Yen SSC: J Clin Endocrinol Metab 51:179, 1980. © by The Endocrine Society, 1980.)

in the pituitary gland. Thus, whereas the hypothalamic control of prolactin is both inhibitory (dominant) and stimulatory, the hypothalamic control of gonadotrophins is only stimulatory. The peptide hormones, such as GnRH, bind to specific receptors on the surface membrane of the target cell, in contrast to steroid hormones, which pass through the cell membrane to bind to intracellular receptors.

Protein hormone receptors are of high molecular weight (200,000 to 300,000 daltons), and each receptor binds a single molecule of the protein. Peptide hormones, including LH, FSH, and prolactin, although highly soluble in aqueous media, have low solubility in lipids and thus do not readily pass the lipid barrier of the target cell's plasma membrane. Thus in order to act within the cell, after the protein binds to the membrane receptor, a second messenger needs to be activated to induce an intracellular biochemical effect. After the protein hormone binds to its receptor, the entire hormone receptor complex is brought into the cell membrane to protect it from other interactions. This process is called internalization.

When a protein hormone binds to its specific receptor, it activates or inhibits the enzyme adenyl cyclase, the second messenger, which in turn changes the concentration of adenosine 3'5'-cyclic monophosphate (cyclic AMP, cAMP) (Fig. 4-9). The cAMP then activates protein kinase in the cytoplasm by binding its regulatory subunit and thus dissociating this subunit from its catalytic subunit. When the regulatory subunit of the protein kinase is freed from the catalytic subunit, the latter subunit is able to transfer a phosphate from adenosine triphosphate (ATP) to the protein substrate. This action modifies the biologic function of the protein to produce a cellular response.

GnRH stimulates both the synthesis and the secretion of LH and FSH from the same cells in the pituitary. It appears that both calcium and prostaglandins facilitate the binding of GnRH to the cell membrane of these cells. After activation of the catalytic subunit of protein kinase by the mechanism just described, FSH and LH are synthesized in the ribosomes of the cell and then transferred first to the rough endoplasmic reticulum and then to the Golgi apparatus, where they are condensed into mature granules (Fig. 4-10). The granules then coalesce with the cell membrane and are transferred to an adjacent blood vessel by exocytosis.

When GnRH is administered to humans,

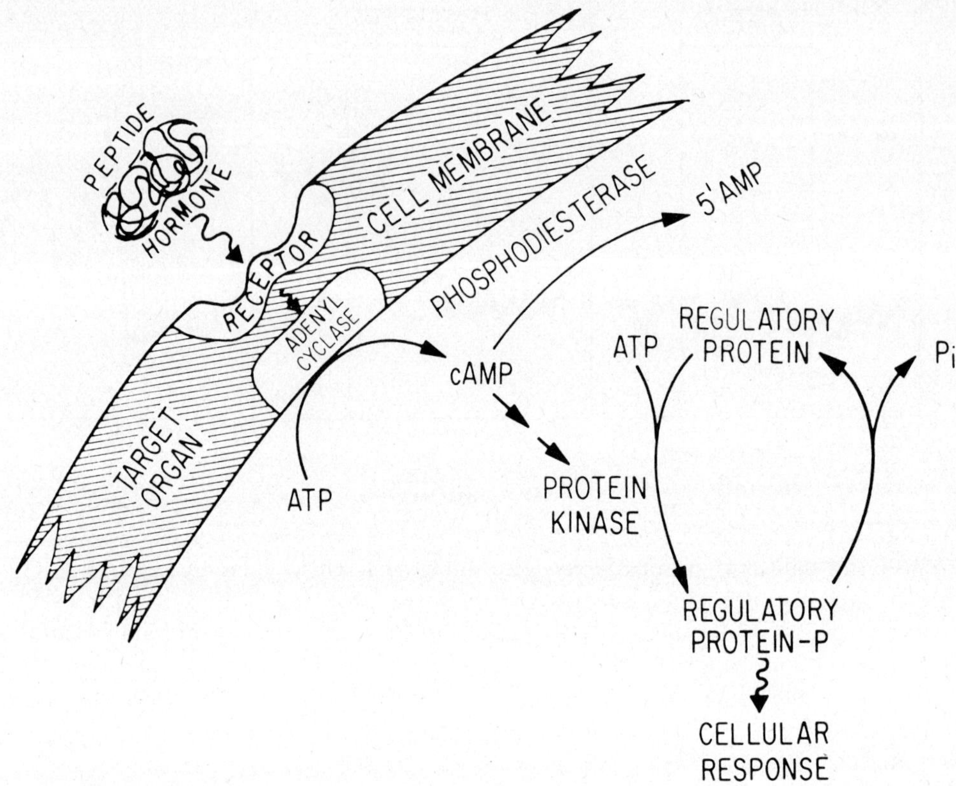

FIGURE 4-9
Second messenger model of peptide hormone action. Interaction of hormone with receptor leads to activation of membrane-bound adenylate cyclase, resulting in conversion of ATP to cyclic AMP (cAMP). Cyclic AMP then interacts with cyclic AMP–dependent protein kinase, causing activation of the enzyme and phosphorylation of intracellular regulatory protein substrates, with ATP as phosphate donor. *P*, Phosphate group; P_i, inorganic phosphate. Cyclic AMP is inactivated by conversion to 5′-AMP by phosphodiesterase. (From Gibbons WE, Battin DA, diZerega GS: Mechanisms of action of reproductive hormones. Reproduced with permission from Infertility, contraception and reproductive endocrinology, 2nd ed, edited by Daniel R. Mishell, Jr., M.D., and Val Davajan, M.D. Copyright © 1986 Medical Economics Books, Oradell, N.J. 07649. All rights reserved.)

there is a rapid increase in circulating levels of LH and FSH. Peak LH levels over 30 minutes and those of FSH 60 minutes after a single intravenous bolus of GnRH (Fig. 4-11). Levels of both LH and FSH return to baseline after 3 hours. With a constant infusion of GnRH, there is a biphasic release of LH but not FSH. The initial increase of LH occurs 30 minutes and the second 90 minutes after the start of the infusion (Fig. 4-12). Yen has theorized that the initial rise represents the release of previously synthesized LH (first pool), and the second rise represents the release of newly synthesized LH (second pool). The combined size of both pituitary sensitivity (first pool) and reserve (second pool) has been called the functional capacity of the gonadotrophes. However, if GnRH continues to be infused, gonadotrophin secretion is inhibited, probably because the receptors are saturated and are unable to continue to stimulate release of the second messenger (desensitization, or down regulation) (Fig. 4-13). Even though maximal hormonal stimulation occurs when only a small percentage of the target cell receptors are bound by hormone, when stimulation is maximal the unoccupied receptors become refractory to hormone binding for 12 to 72 hours. This phenomenon has allowed fre-

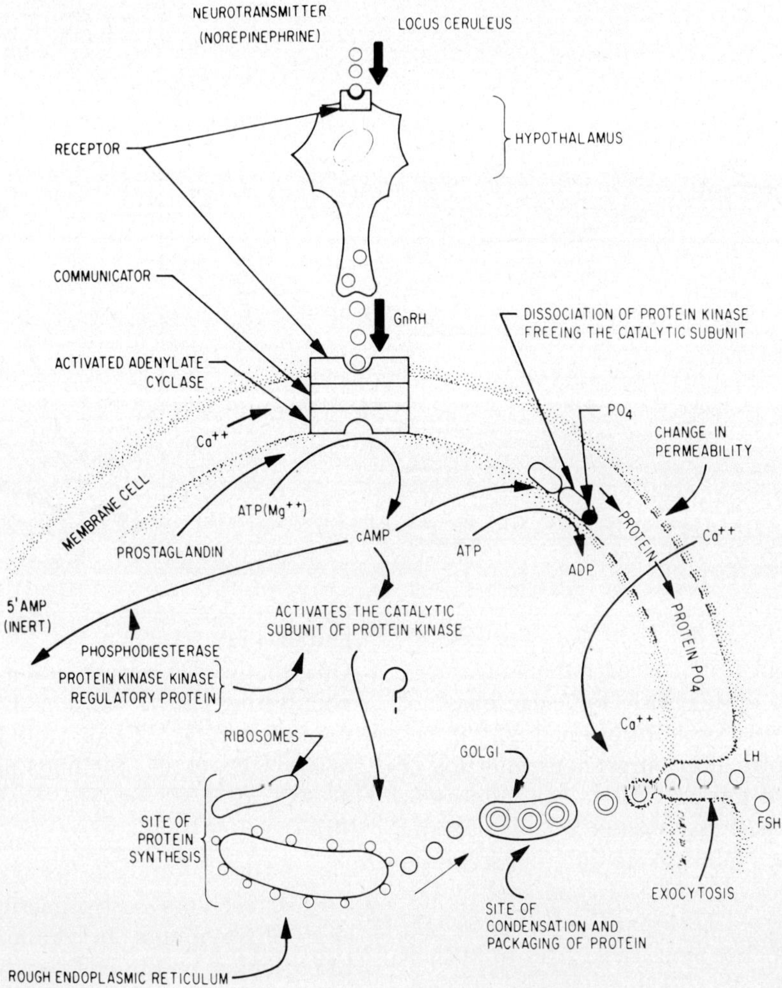

FIGURE 4-10
Effect of GnRH on synthesis and release of gonadotrophins. (From Kletzky OA, Lobo RA: Reproductive neuroendocrinology. Reproduced with permission from Infertility, contraception and reproductive endocrinology, 2nd ed, edited by Daniel R. Mishell, Jr., M.D., and Val Davajan, M.D. Copyright © 1986 Medical Economics Books, Oradell, N.J. 07649. All rights reserved.)

quent administration of GnRH analogs to be used clinically to inhibit FSH and LH levels and thus decrease steroidogenesis to treat hormone-dependent conditions such as endometriosis and leiomyoma.

GONADOTROPHIN STRUCTURE AND FUNCTION

LH and FSH are glycoproteins of high molecular weight, 28,000 and 37,000 daltons, respectively. They each have the same α subunit (14,000 daltons) of about 90 amino acids, which is similar in structure to the α subunit of thyroid-stimulating hormone and human chorionic gonadotrophin. The β subunits of all these hormones have different amino acids and carbohydrates and provide specific biologic activity. The α and β subunits are joined by disulfide bonds. The half-life of LH is shorter (30 minutes) than that of FSH (3.9 hours). In the female, although the two gonadotrophins act synergistically, LH acts primarily on the theca cells to induce steroidogenesis, whereas FSH acts primarily on the granulosa cells to stimulate follicular growth.

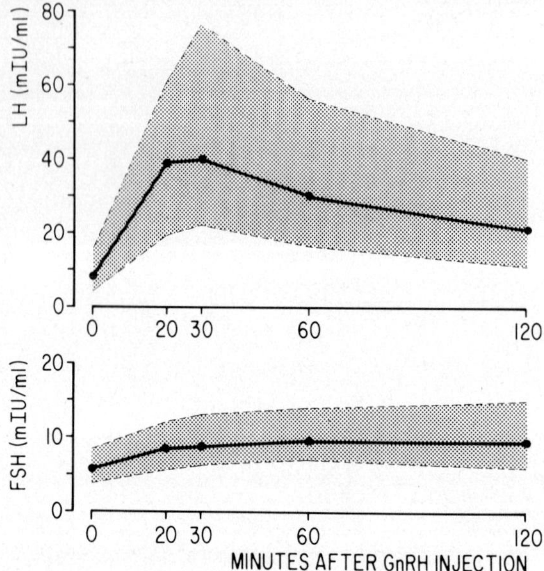
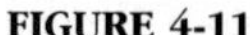

FIGURE 4-11

Serum LH and FSH concentrations measured in 10 women during early follicular phase of normal menstrual cycle before and 20, 30, 60, and 120 minutes after intravenous injection of single bolus of 150 μg GnRH. Dots represent geometric means, and shaded area depicts the 95% confidence limits. Note different scales on ordinates. (Drawn from data generated by Oscar A. Kletzky, M.D. From Goebelsmann UT, Mishell DR Jr: The menstrual cycle. In Mishell DR Jr, Davajan V, eds: Reproductive endocrinology, infertility and contraception. Philadelphia, F.A. Davis Co., 1979.)

Receptors for LH exist on the theca cells at all stages of the cycle; they are on granulosa cells after the follicle matures under the influence of FSH and estradiol, as well as on the corpus luteum. Each gonadal target tissue cell contains between 2000 and 30,000 membrane receptors. Maximal stimulation of hormonal activity occurs when less than 5% of these receptors are bound with hormone. The main action of LH is to stimulate androgen synthesis by the theca cells and progesterone synthesis by the corpus luteum through stimulation of intracellular cAMP production (Fig. 4-14). The precise action of LH on granulosa cells has not been determined, but it probably acts synergistically with FSH to help follicular maturation.

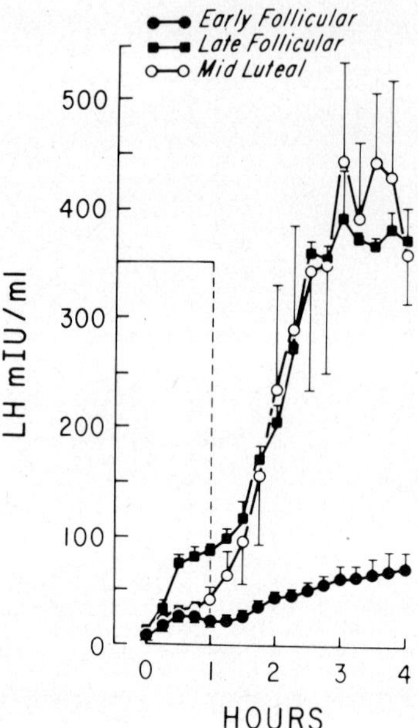

FIGURE 4-12

Quantitative LH release within first and second pool during GnRH infusion. Dotted line separates two pools. (From Hoff JD, Lasley BL, Wang CF, et al: J Clin Endocrinol Metab 44:302, 1977. © by The Endocrine Society, 1977.)

FSH receptors exist primarily on the granulosa cell membrane. In addition to stimulating LH receptors on this cell memberane, FSH activates the aromatase and the 3-hydroxysteroid dehydrogenase enzymes within the cell by increasing cAMP. FSH stimulation of isolated granulosa cells in vitro produces only small amounts of estrogen; however, when androgens or theca cells are added, large amounts of estrogen are produced. These data support the two-cell hypothesis of estrogen production. This hypothesis proposes that LH acts on the theca to produce androgens (androstenedione and testosterone), which are then transported to the granulosa cells, where they are aromatized to estrogens (estrone and estradiol) by the action of FSH (see Fig. 4-14). The aromatase enzyme catalyzes this conversion.

FSH also stimulates follicular growth by increasing both FSH and LH receptor content in granulosa cells. This action is enhanced by estrogen. After a sufficient number of LH receptors have been produced by the action of FSH and estradiol, LH acts directly on the granulosa

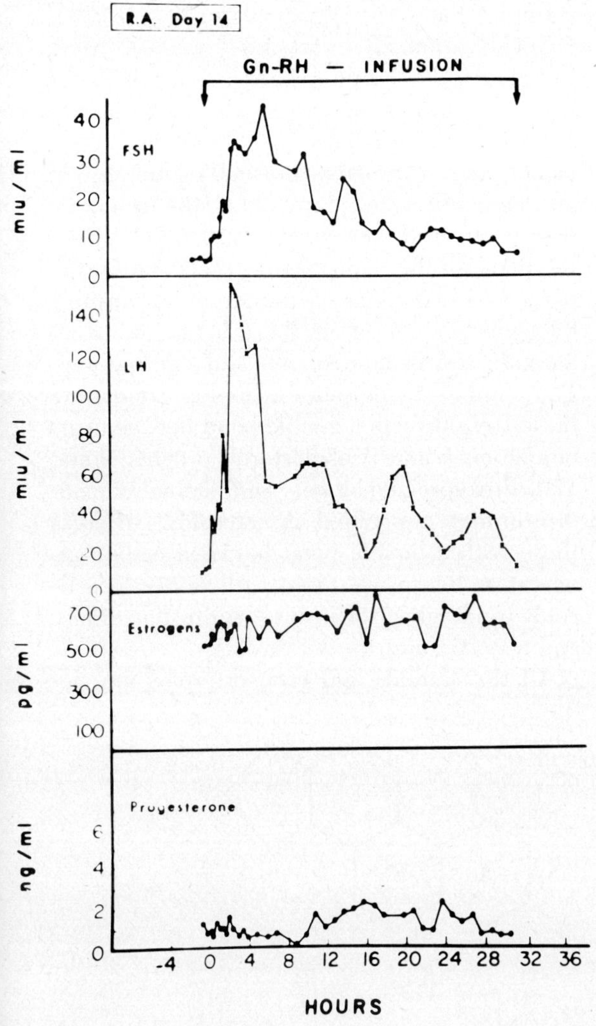

FIGURE 4-13
Mean serum FSH, LH, estrogen, and progesterone levels during 30-hour continuous infusions of GnRH at midcycle phase in three normal women. (From Jewelewicz R, Ferin M, Dyrenfurth I, et al: Long-term LH, RH infusions at various stages of the menstrual cycle in normal women. In Beling CG, Wenitz AC, eds: The LH-releasing hormone. New York, Masson Publishing, 1980.)

FIGURE 4-14
Action of gonadotrophins on ovary: LH stimulates theca cell to synthesize androgen by cyclic AMP (cAMP)–mediated action. FSH stimulates granulosa cell to activate aromatase via cyclic AMP–mediated action. Aromatase in granulosa cell converts androgen to estrogen, which is then utilized by target organs. Estrogen also stimulates granulosa cell proliferation. (From a concept in Schulster D, Burstein S, Cooke BA, eds: Control of gonadal steroidogenesis by FSH and LH. In Molecular endocrinology of the steroid hormones. London, John Wiley & Sons, Ltd., 1976.)

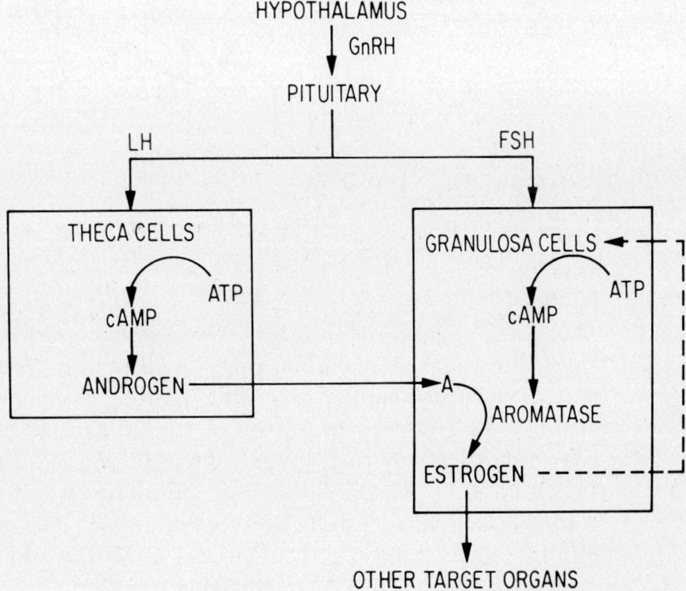

cells to cause luteinization and production of progesterone. LH also stimulates prostaglandin synthesis by intracellular production of cAMP. Prostaglandins are also involved in luteinization of the follicle and production of progesterone, as well as in performing an important function in the process of rupture of the follicle. The follicular content of prostaglandin increases markedly at the time of the midcycle LH surge, shortly before ovulation occurs.

OVARIAN STEROIDS

The ovary secretes three principal steroid hormones: estradiol from the follicle, progesterone from the corpus luteum, and androstenedione from the stroma. Steroid hormones, which have a low molecular weight (220 to 387 daltons), are lipidlike substances insoluble in water but soluble in organic solvents. Steroids have a basic cyclopentanoperhydrophenanthrene nucleus with three 6-carbon rings (*A,*

B, and *C*) and one 5-carbon ring *(D)* (Fig. 4-15). The carbon atoms are numbered according to a generally accepted system that is used to determine their systemic scientific names. Most steroid hormones have common (trivial) names, such as progesterone and estradiol, that are generally used instead of the scientific names. In addition, functional groups above the plane of the molecule are preceded by the β symbol and shown in the structural formula by a solid line, whereas those below the plane are indicated by an α symbol and a dotted line. The symbol Δ indicates a double bond, and those steroids with a double bond between carbon atoms 5 and 6 (cholesterol, pregnenolone, 17-hydroxypregnenolone, and dehydroepiandrosterone) are called Δ^5 steroids, whereas those with a double bond between carbon atoms 4 and 5 (progesterone, all mineralocorticoids and glucocorticoids, androstenedione, and testosterone) are Δ^4 steroids.

All sex steroids and corticosteroids are de-

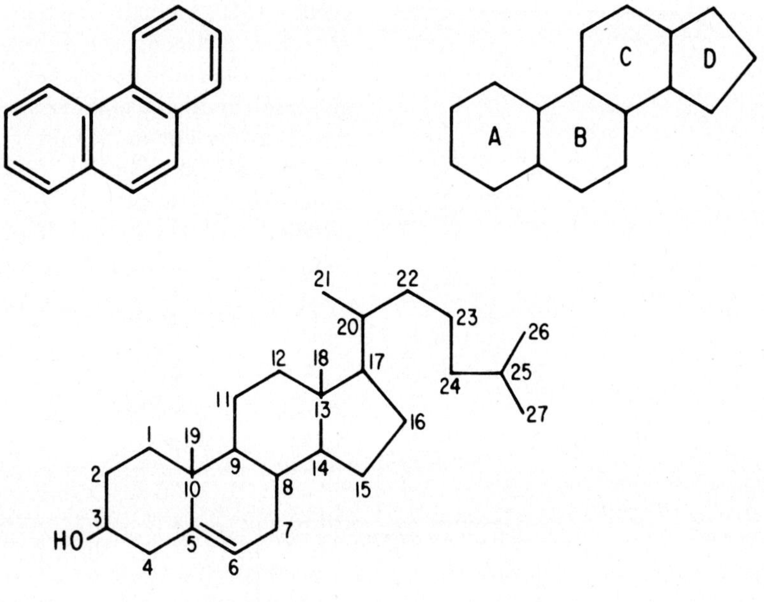

FIGURE 4-15

Phenanthrene nucleus *(top left).* Cyclopentanoperhydrophenanthrene nucleus *(top right),* in which the 6-carbon rings *(A, B,* and *C)* resemble the phenanthrene ring system and the 5-carbon ring *(D)* resembles cyclopentane. Cholesterol *(bottom)* is common biosynthetic precursor of steroid hormones. Numbers *1* to *27* indicate conventional numbering system of carbon atoms of steroid skeleton. (From Goebelsmann UT: Steroid hormones. Reproduced with permission from Infertility, contraception and reproductive endocrinology, 2nd ed, edited by Daniel R. Mishell, Jr., M.D., and Val Davajan, M.D. Copyright © 1986 Medical Economics Books, Oradell, N.J. 07649. All rights reserved.)

TABLE 4-1

Three-Way Cross-Classification of Steroid Hormones and Related Substances*

| | | Classification by Relation to Endocrine Effect | | | |
| | | Sexogens | | | |
Classification by Origin	Classification by Metabolic Stage	Androgens	Estrogens	Gestagens	Corticosteroids
Hormones	Agents	Testosterone	Estradiol-17β	Progesterone	Cortisol
	Metabolites	Androsterone	Estriol	"Pregnanediol"	"Tetrahydrocortisone"
Drugs	Agents	Methyltestosterone	Mestranol Diethylstilbestrol	Medroxyprogesterone	Prednisolone
	Metabolites	17α-Methyl-5β-androstane-3α, 17β-diol	D-Homo-estradiol	6α-Methyl-17α-acetoxy-6β, 21-dihydroxy-4-pregnene-3, 20-dione	17α, 20α, 21-trihydroxy-1, 4-pregnadiene-3, 11-dione

From Borth R: Generic names for steroid hormones and related substances [guest editorial]. Contraception 12:373, 1975.
*The compounds in the body of the table are examples.

rived by the stepwise degradation of cholesterol, which has 27 carbon atoms and has itself been synthesized from acetate. Corticosteroids, progesterone, pregnenolone, 17-hydroxypregnenolone, and 17-hydroxyprogesterone have 21 carbon atoms; androgens (testosterone and androstenedione) have 19 carbon atoms; and natural estrogens have 18 carbon atoms and a phenolic or aromatic ring A. Borth has shown that steroid hormones may be classified by origin, metabolic stage, and endocrine effect (Table 4-1).

The first step in ovarian steroid biosynthesis is the reduction of cholesterol to pregnenolone by hydroxylation of C-20 and C-22 and cleavage between these atoms. This process reduces the C-27 compound cholesterol to the C-21 compound pregnenolone. From pregnenolone, ovarian steroid biosynthesis proceeds along two major pathways under the influence of specific enzymes: (1) the Δ^5 pathway through 17-hydroxypregnenolone and dehydroepiandrostenedione to androstenedione and (2) the Δ^4 pathway through progesterone and 17-hydroxyprogesterone to androstenedione (Fig. 4-16). As mentioned earlier, LH stimulates this synthesis.

Androstenedione and testosterone are interconverted, and the former can be converted to estrone and the latter to estradiol, respectively, by 19-hydroxylation. This enzymatic process results in loss of the C-19 group and development of the phenolic, or aromatase A, ring (aromatization) in the C-18 steroid.

The ovary secretes three primary steroids: estradiol, progesterone, and androstenedione. It also secretes pregnenolone, 17-hydroxyprogesterone, testosterone, dehydroepiandrosterone (DHEA), and estrone. Because the ovaries lack the enzymes 21-hydroxylase, 11β-hydroxylase, and 18-hydroxylase reductase, they are unable to synthesize mineralocorticoids or glucocorticoids.

Each day the ovary secretes between 100 and 500 μg of estradiol, with the amount being lowest during menses and highest just before ovulation. Daily progesterone production varies from 4 mg in the follicular phase to 30 mg in the luteal phase. During the follicular phase, almost all progesterone is secreted from the adrenal gland and very little from the ovary. The ovary secretes between 1 and 2 mg of androstenedione, less than 1 mg of DHEA, and

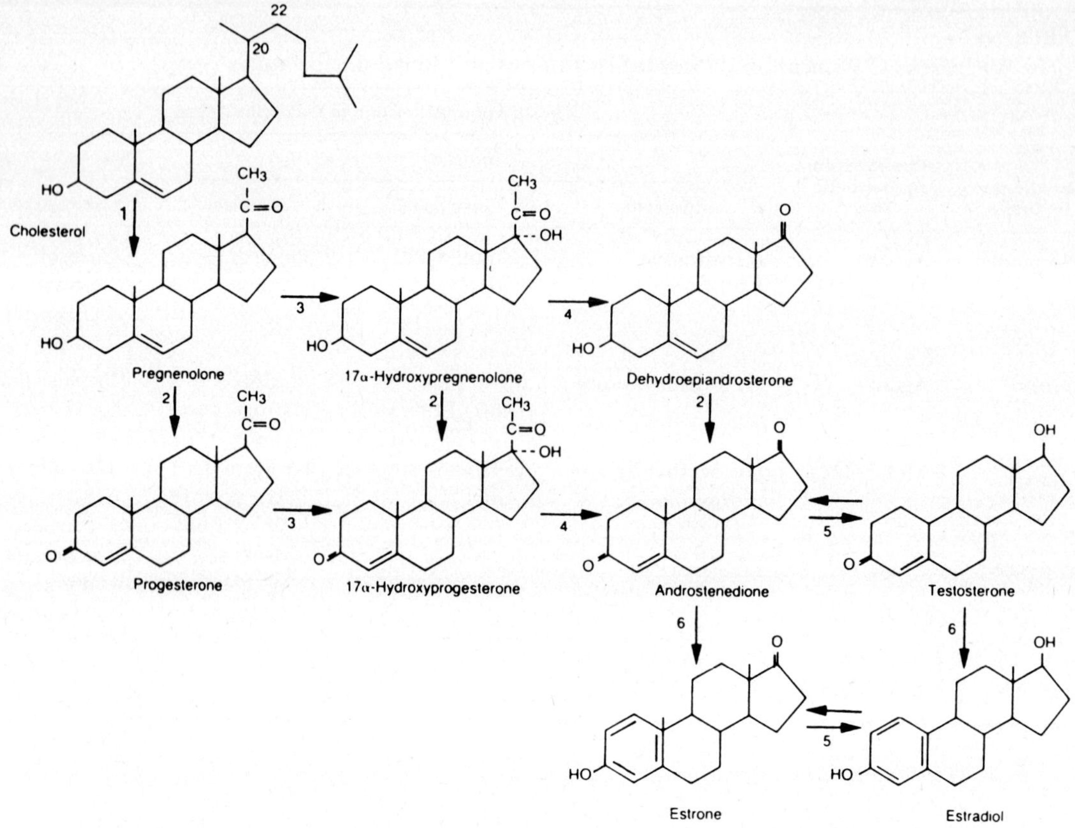

FIGURE 4-16

Ovarian steroid biosynthetic pathways. The following enzymes are required where indicated: *(1)* 20-hydroxylase, 22-hydroxylase, and 20,22-desmolase; *(2)* 3β-ol dehydrogenase and $\Delta^5 \rightarrow \Delta^4$-isomerase; *(3)* 17α-hydroxylase; *(4)* 17,20-desmolase; *(5)* 17β-ol dehydrogenase; and *(6)* aromatizing enzyme system. (From Goebelsmann UT: Steroid hormones. Reproduced with permission from Infertility, contraception and reproductive endocrinology, 2nd ed, edited by Daniel R. Mishell, Jr., M.D., and Val Davajan, M.D. Copyright © 1986 Medical Economics Books, Oradell, N.J. 07649. All rights reserved.)

about 0.1 mg of testosterone daily. Androgen metabolism and corticosteroid synthesis are discussed in Chapter 38.

In addition to gonadal steroid biosynthesis, extraglandular steroid metabolism occurs. Interconversion of androstenedione and testosterone, as well as estrone and estradiol, takes place outside the ovaries, mainly by oxidation of the latter steroids to the former, thus reducing their biologic potency. Estrone is then converted to estrone sulfate, which has a long half-life and is the largest component of the pool of circulating estrogens (Fig. 4-17). Estrone sulfate in turn may be converted to estrone and, to a lesser extent, to estradiol.

MacDonald et al showed that androstenedi-one is peripherally converted to estrone in adipose tissue. The greater the amount of fat tissue present, the greater the percentage of androstenedione that is converted to estrone. In a normal individual about 1.3% of the daily 3000 μg of androstenedione produced is converted to estrone (40 μg), whereas in an obese individual as much as 7% (200 μg) of the 3000 μg is converted.

Estradiol (E_2) and estrone (E_1) are converted in the liver to estriol (E_3). These three estrogens have been called the classic estrogens. Estradiol has the greatest biologic activity and is excreted in the least amount, estriol is the least potent and is excreted in the greatest amount, and estrone is intermediate in both categories.

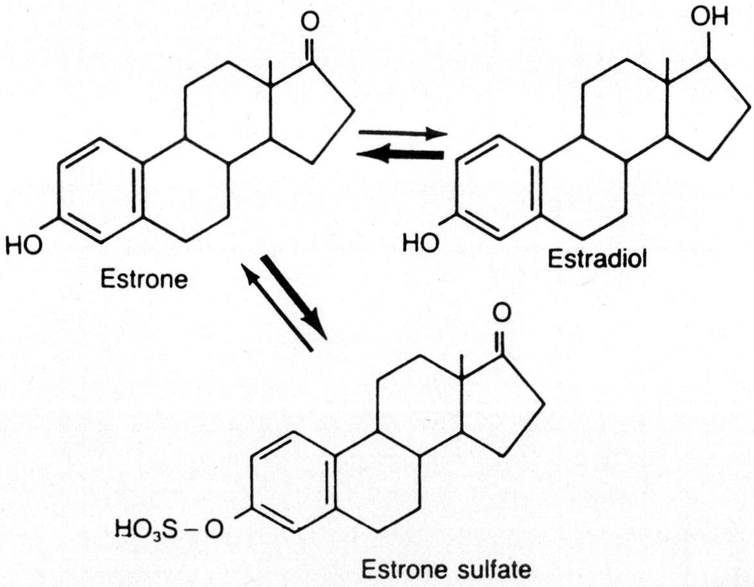

FIGURE 4-17
Interconversion of three principal circulating estrogens. (From Goebelsmann UT: Steroid hormones. Reproduced with permission from Infertility, contraception and reproductive endocrinology, 2nd ed, edited by Daniel R. Mishell, Jr., M.D., and Val Davajan, M.D. Copyright © 1986 Medical Economics Books, Oradell, N.J. 07649. All rights reserved.)

Before urinary excretion the sex steroids need to be conjugated so that they are soluble in water. Estrogens are conjugated by the liver and intestinal mucosa into sulfates, glucuronides, or other conjugates. About 10% to 15% of progesterone is conjugated to pregnanediol glucuronide.

The concentration of a steroid hormone in serum or plasma is dependent on its production rate (PR) and metabolic clearance rate (MCR). The MCR is determined by infusing a radioactively labeled steroid in tracer amounts at a constant rate over several hours. The MCR is calculated according to the following formula:

$$\text{MCR} = \frac{\text{Tracer administered/time}}{\text{Tracer concentration}}$$

$$= \frac{\text{Counts/min/day}}{\text{Counts/min/liter}} = \text{Liters/day}$$

The concentration (C) of steroid can be measured by radioimmunassay, and when both MCR and C are known, the PR is determined by multiplying the MCR × C. PR = MCR × C = liters/day × amount/liter = amount/day. Normal C, MCR, and PR of androgens, estrogens, and progesterone at different phases of the menstrual cycle have been calculated (Table 4-2).

Steroid hormones in the circulation either are bound to proteins or are unbound (free), with the majority of each hormone being bound. Sex steroids are loosely bound to albumin ($K_D = 10^{-6}$M), as well as tightly bound to a specific binding globulin ($K_D = 10^{-9}$ to 10^{-8}M). The specific binding globulin for both progesterone and cortisol is cortisol-binding globulin (CBG) (transcortin). Dihydrotestosterone, testosterone, and estradiol are bound specifically, in order of decreasing affinity, to sex hormone binding globulin (SHBG). Circulating levels of each of these globulins are increased by estrogen; SHBG levels are also increased by obesity and hyperthyroidism and lowered by androgens and hypothyroidism. Generally the majority of steroid in the circulation is bound to its specific globulin, a smaller percentage is bound to albumin, and less than 5% is free. It is controversial whether only the free steroid, the non–SHBG or CBG bound steroid, or all of the steroid in the circulation can enter the cell and attach to its specific receptor.

In contrast to the membrane receptors of

TABLE 4-2

Plasma Concentrations (C), Metabolic Clearance Rates (MCR), and Production Rates (PR) of Androgens, Estrogens, and Progesterone During Menstrual Cycle

Steroid Hormone	Phase of Cycle	Plasma Concentration*			Metabolic Clearance Rate Plasma* (L/day)	Production Rate (mg/day) (PR = C × MCR)	
		Mean	Range	Units		Mean	Range
Androstenedione	†	1.4	0.7-3.1	ng/ml	2000	2.8	1.4-6.2
Testosterone	†	0.35	0.15-0.55	ng/ml	700	0.25	0.1-0.4
Dehydroepiandrosterone	†	4.2	2.7-7.8	ng/ml	1600	6.7	4.8-12.5
Dehydroepiandrosterone sulfate	†	1.6	0.8-3.4	µg/ml	7	11.2	5.6-23.8
Estradiol	Follicular	44	20-120	pg/ml	1350	0.059	0.027-0.162
	Preovulatory	250	150-600	pg/ml	1350	0.338	0.203-0.810
	Luteal	110	40-300	pg/ml	1350	0.149	0.054-0.405
Estrone	Follicular	40		pg/ml	2200	0.088	
	Preovulatory	170		pg/ml	2200	0.374	
	Luteal	92		pg/ml	2200	0.202	
Estrone-sulfate	Follicular	470		pg/ml	146	0.069	
	Luteal	890		pg/ml	146	0.130	
Progesterone	Follicular	0.2	0.06-0.37	ng/ml	2300	0.46	0.14-0.85
	Luteal	8.9	4.3-19.4	ng/ml	2300	20.5	9.9-45.0

From Goebelsmann UT: Steroid hormones. Reproduced with permission from Infertility, contraception, and reproductive endocrinology, 2nd ed, edited by Daniel R. Mishell, Jr., M.D., and Val Davajan, M.D. Copyright © 1986 Medical Economics Books, Oradell, N.J. 07649. All rights reserved.
*These values may vary somewhat depending on investigator and method.
†Unspecified. No major changes during menstrual cycle.

protein hormones, steroid hormone receptors are intracellular. Steroid hormone receptors will bind a specific class of steroids. Thus estrogen receptors will bind natural and synthetic estrogens but not gestagens or androgens. The affinity of a receptor for a steroid correlates with its potency. Thus the estrogen receptor has a greater affinity for estradiol than estrone or estriol. After the steroid hormone (H) is bound to its receptor (R), a hormone-receptor (HR) complex forms. The steroid induces a change in receptor conformation that allows it to pass through the nuclear membrane (transformation). It was previously thought that the hormone receptor complex then passes from the cytoplasm through the nuclear membrane into the nucleus (translocation), but current information indicates that all steroid receptors are located in the nucleus. After transforma-

tion, messenger RNA is then generated from a segment of DNA (transcription). The messenger RNA migrates into the cytoplasm, where it attaches to ribosomes and translates information so that they synthesize new protein (Fig. 4-18).

The magnitude of the signal to the cell depends on the concentration of both hormones (H) and receptors (R), as well as on the affinity (K) of the hormone to the receptor. Thus the hormone effect may be altered by receptor concentration and affinity, as well as by concentration of the hormone in the circulation. Affinity is quantitatively characterized by a constant derived from the law of mass action.

$$H + R \underset{K_d}{\overset{K_a}{\rightleftharpoons}} HR$$

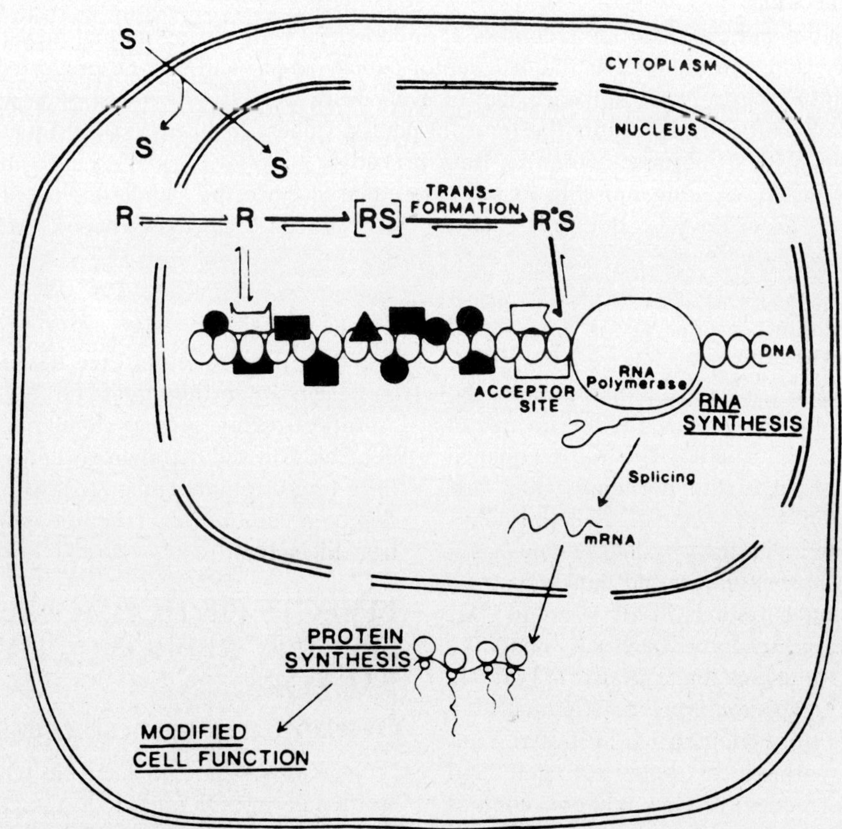

FIGURE 4-18
Revised model of steroid-receptor interaction and induction of cellular response. For simplicity, molecular aspects of receptor structure have been omitted. (From Walters MR: Endocrinol Rev 6:512, 1985.)

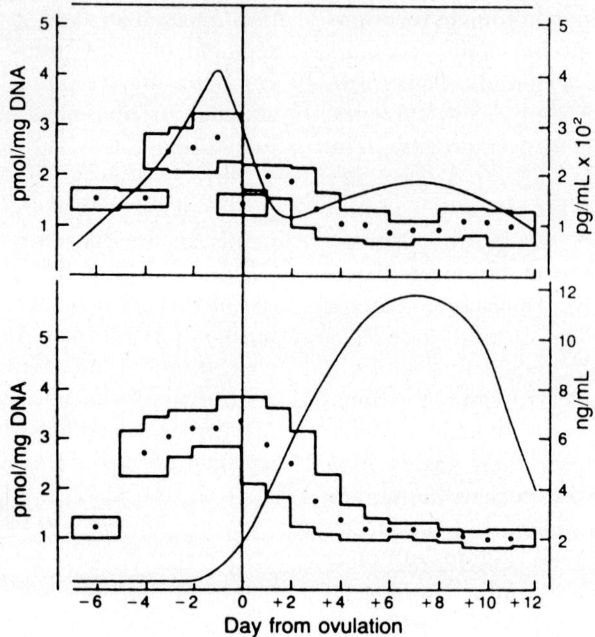

FIGURE 4-19

Estradiol and progesterone receptors in endometrial cells during normal menstrual cycle. Concentrations of estradiol receptor *(upper panel)* and of total progesterone receptor *(lower panel)* for each day of cycle were pooled with those of adjacent days. Each point represents the mean of pooled values. It is surrounded by a rectangle, with its abscissa extending from preceding to following day to account for imprecision of dating and with its ordinate equal to twice the standard error of the mean. (From Levy C, Robel P, Gautray JP, et al: Am J Obstet Gynecol 136:646, 1980.)

The association constant, K_a, is determined by dividing the rate constant for association, K_a, by the ratio constant for dissociation, K_d. The dissociation constant, K_d, is the inverse of K_a; therefore, $K_d = 1/K_a$. The K_d is equal to the concentration of the hormone when half the receptor sites are occupied. Receptor affinity is correlated with the physiologic concentration of the hormone. Steroid hormones are present in concentrations of 10^{-10} to $10^{-8}M$, and most steroid receptors have a K_d of 10^{-9}.

Estrogen stimulates the synthesis of both estrogen and progesterone receptors in target tissues such as the endometrium. Progestins inhibit the synthesis of both estrogen and progesterone receptors. Thus receptor content in the endometrium peaks about midcycle and then decreases (Fig. 4-19). Mitotic activity and endometrial growth rates therefore peak at midcycle. Progestins also increase the intracellular synthesis of estradiol dehydrogenase, which converts the more potent estradiol to the less potent estrone, further decreasing estrogenic activity in the target cell.

Antiestrogens, such as clomiphene or tamoxifen, bind to the estrogen receptor but initiate little transcription. Thus estrogen receptors are depleted without new receptor synthesis or estrogenic action.

EFFECTS OF HORMONES ON SPECIFIC REPRODUCTIVE FACTORS

Ovarian Gametogenesis (Oogenesis)

Oogenesis begins in fetal life when the primordial germ cells migrate to the genital ridge. These germ cells, oogonia, increase in number by mitotic division from about 600,000 in the second month to 7 million in the seventh month of fetal life. The oogonia then begin meiotic division and are called primary oo-

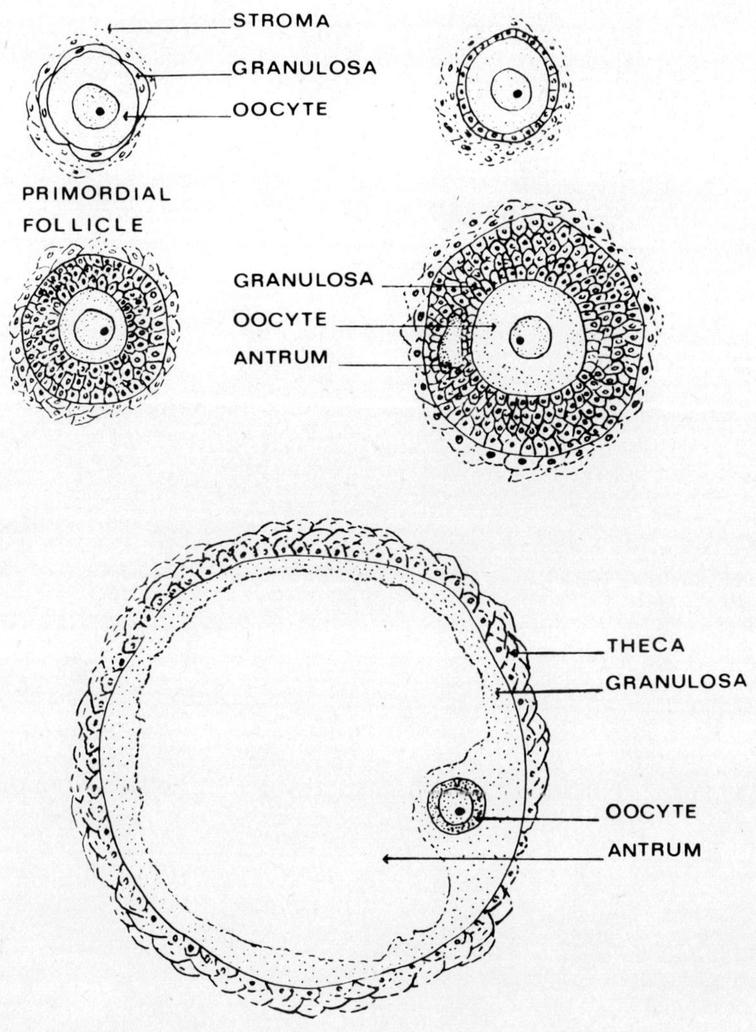

FIGURE 4-20
Changes occurring during follicular maturation. (From Shea BF, Baker RD, Latour
JPA: Oogenesis, folliculogenesis and maturation of follicular oocytes. In Hafez ES,
ed: Human ovulation: Mechanism, prediction, detection, and induction. New York,
Elsevier/North-Holland Biomedical Press, 1979.)

cytes. Just prior to birth the primary oocytes, which now number 10 million, reach the diplotene stage of development, also called the germinal vesicle stage. At this stage they stay quiescent or undergo atresia until puberty, at which time some of the oocytes mature and complete their meiotic division.

The primary oocyte that is still in the diplotene stage of its first meiotic division is covered by a single layer of granulosa cells and constitutes the primordial follicle. Even without gonadotrophin stimulation, some primordial follicles develop into (primary) preantral follicles, which are oocytes covered by multiple layers of granulosa cells (Fig. 4-20). This process occurs in all premenopausal women during childhood, pregnancy, and with the use of oral contraceptives, as well as during ovulatory cycles. Nearly all these follicles become atretic, but under the influence of FSH in ovulatory cycles, some of them develop to the antrum stage.

Under the influence of FSH the number of granulosa cells in the primordial follicle increases dramatically, and the follicle matures

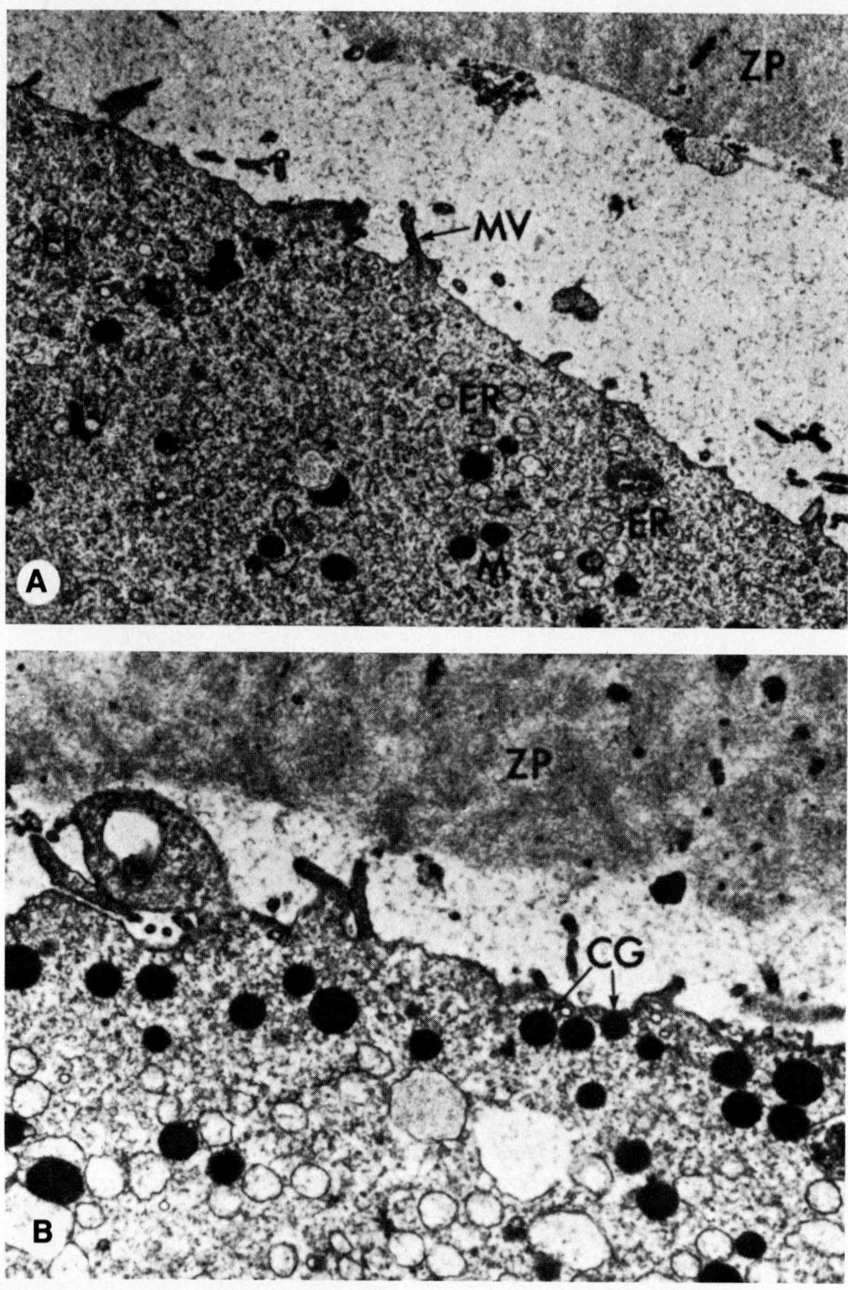

FIGURE 4-21

A, Surface of fertilized ovum, showing absence of cortical granules. A few microvilli *(MV)* are projecting into perivitelline space, which has been widened by retraction of ooplasm from zona pellucida *(ZP)*. Dense mitochondria *(M)* and large vesicular components of endoplasmic reticulum *(ER)* are visible in ooplasm. The egg was fixed 3 hours after insemination in vitro. (×15,400.) **B,** Surface of unfertilized ovum that had been inseminated for 3 hours. Numerous extremely electron-dense cortical granules *(CG)* are present beneath vitelline membrane. Zona pellucida *(ZP)* has a fine fibrilar appearance. (×19,600.) (From Lopata A, Sathananthan AM, McBain JC, et al: Fertil Steril 33:12, 1980. Reproduced with permission of the publisher, The American Fertility Society.)

into a primary (preantral) follicle. As the number of granulosa cells increases under the influence of LH and FSH, there is a concomitant parallel increase in estradiol production and secretion. Estradiol stimulates preantral follicle growth, reduces follicle atresia, and increases FSH action on the granulosa cells. Testosterone, on the other hand, increases follicle atresia and prevents preantral follicle growth. Ross et al suggested that local concentration of estrogens and androgens within the follicle determines whether a specific follicle grows or becomes atretic.

The follicle destined to become dominant secretes the greatest amount of estradiol, which in turn increases the density of FSH receptors. Thus mitotic activity and the number of granulosa cells also increase. In addition, the rising concentration of estradiol exerts a negative feedback effect of FSH release from the pituitary, which halts development of all the other follicles so that they become atretic. In addition, granulosa cells secrete a nonsteroidal substance, inhibin, which also suppresses FSH secretion. The dominant follicle continues to develop because it has a greater density of FSH receptors and is more vascularized than the other follicles, allowing more FSH to reach its receptors.

As the oocyte develops, it becomes surrounded by the zona pellucida, and fluid accumulates in the follicle. The zona pellucida is a mucopolysaccaride coat that allows only spermatozoa of the same species to penetrate and fertilize the ovum. Underneath the zona pellucida is the vitelline membrane, which surrounds the ooplasm. Cortical granules form in this membrane as the oocyte matures. Once the zona pellucida has been penetrated by a single sperm cell, these granules are released and block further sperm penetration (Fig. 4-21). The follicular fluid contains estrogens, androgens, and various proteins. Several of these proteins are now being characterized, and they, in addition to the steroids, appear to help regulate follicle maturation by acting within the follicle to alter gonadotrophin action. As the granulosa cells proliferate, LH receptors appear on their surface membrane; when LH binds to these receptors, granulosa cell proliferation ceases and the cells begin to secrete progesterone.

The pattern of follicular growth, as determined by ultrasonography, has been correlated with the endocrine pattern in several studies. Eissa et al., as well as Zegers-Hochschild et al., correlated these parameters in 43 cycles in which conception occurred. Both these groups found a steady increase in follicular diameter and volume that parallels the rise in estradiol (Fig. 4-22).

As determined by ultrasonography, the dominant follicle has a maximal mean diameter of about 19.5 mm, with a range of 18 to 25 mm just before ovulation. The mean maximal follicular volume is 3.8 ml, with a range of 3.1 to 8.2 ml. These investigators, as well as others, have shown that the maximal size of the dominant follicle can vary among different women. LeMay et al have shown that the mean maximal diameter of the preovulatory follicle can vary in the same woman in different cycles.

About 80% of the approximately 500 mg of estradiol produced daily just before ovulation comes from the dominant follicle. The rapidly rising estradiol levels, in combination with a small but significant increase in progesterone produced by the dominant follicle, serve as the signal to the hypothalamic-pituitary axis that the follicle is ready to ovulate. When estradiol levels rise substantially at midcycle, to about 200 pg/ml or higher for 2 or more days, LH secretion is stimulated (positive feedback) (Fig. 4-23). Apparently the small preovulatory increase in progesterone also stimulates the release of LH and may be responsible for the midcycle FSH surge. Thus by a positive feedback, these steroids elicit a surge in LH and FSH release from the pituitary. The midcycle gonadotrophin surge initiates the ovulatory process.

A task force of the World Health Organization correlated the temporal relation of changes in hormone levels with the time of ovulation as determined by histologic examination of the maturity of the corpus luteum, which had been removed at the time of subsequent laparotomy in 78 women. With the use of those parameters, it was determined that ovulation occurs about 24 hours after the estradiol peak. Ovulation occurs about 32 hours after the initial rise in LH levels and about 12 to 16 hours after the peak of LH levels in serum (Table 4-3). Using ultrasonography to detect the time of ovula-

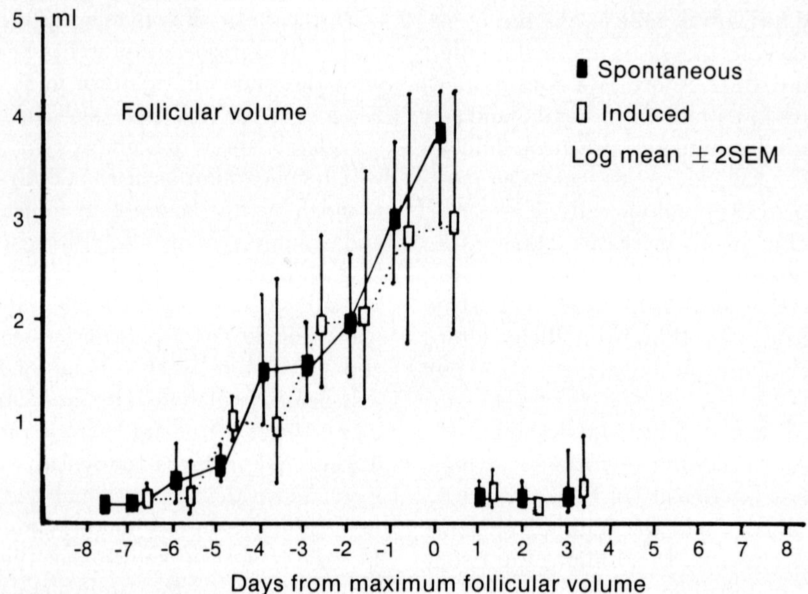

FIGURE 4-22
For legend see opposite page.

tion, LeMay et al. reported that ovulation occurs between 18 and 48 hours after the initial rise in LH levels. With serial ultrasound definition and LH measurements, Eissa et al. and Zegers-Hochschild et al. reported that in conception cycles, ovulation usually occurs within 24 hours and always within 48 hours after the LH peak.

TABLE 4-3
Range of Observed Times from Defined Hormonal Events and Time of Ovulation*

| | Time of Ovulation (h) from Rise to Peak | | | |
| | First Significant Rise | | Peak | |
Hormone	Median	Range	Median	Range
17β-Estradiol	82.5	48-168	24.0	0-48
LH	32.0	24-56	16.5	8-40
FSH	21.1	8-24	15.3	8-40
Progesterone	7.8	0-32	—	

*From World Health Organization. Temporal relationships between ovulation and defined changes in the concentration of plasma estradiol-17β, luteinizing hormone, follicle-stimulating hormone, and progesterone. Am J Obstet Gynecol 138:383, 1980.

The midcycle LH surge initiates germinal vesicle disruption, and metaphase I is completed. As the oocyte enters metaphase II, the first polar body appears. Completion of meiosis and extrusion of the second polar body occur only when a spermatozoon penetrates the ovum. In preparation for follicular rupture, LH stimulates synthesis of both prostaglandins and proteolytic enzymes. The rise in FSH levels stimulates production of a plasminogen activator, which converts plasminogen to the proteolytic enzyme plasmin. Plasmin helps to detach the cumulus from the parietal granulosa cells and thus aids in the process of extrusion of the egg and cumulus at the time of follicle rupture.

After the oocyte is extruded, the amount of follicular fluid is markedly reduced, the follicular wall becomes convoluted, and the follicular diameter and volume greatly decrease. These changes are detectable by ultrasonography (Fig. 4-24). As the granulosa and theca cells become luteinized, they take up lipids and lutein pigment, giving them a yellow coloration. The granulosa cells become vascularized only after ovulation. Under the influence of LH, the corpus luteum produces progesterone in amounts of about 20 mg/24 hr and also secretes estradiol.

Levels of progesterone steadily increase in

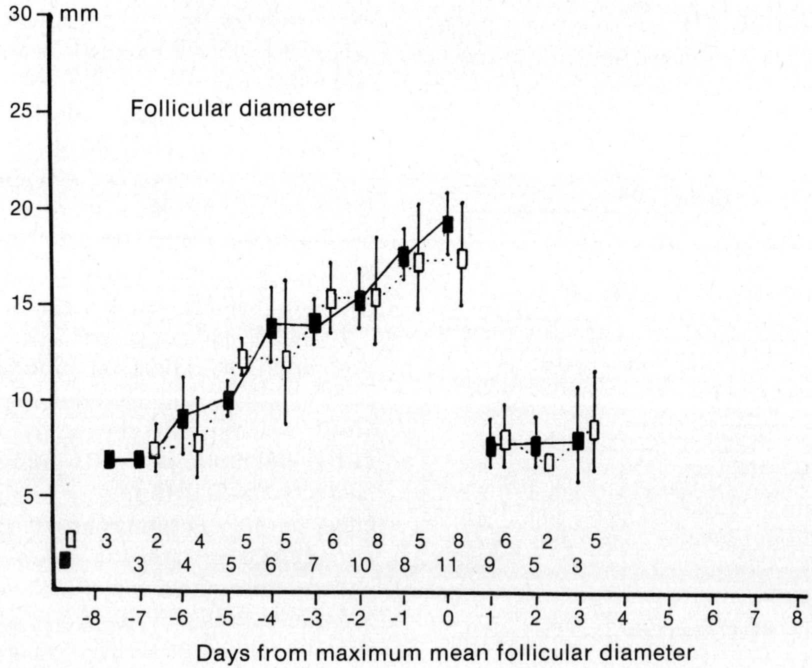

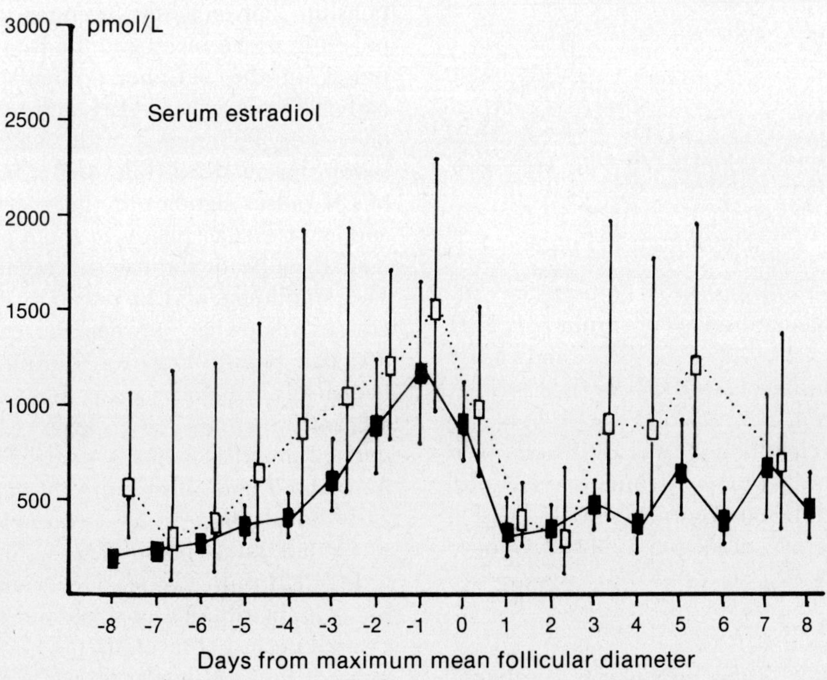

FIGURE 4-22

Correlation of follicular diameter with follicular growth and volume with estradiol in 11 spontaneous and 8 induced conception cycles. (Redrawn from Eissa MK, Obhrai MS, Docker MF, et al: Fertil Steril 45:191, 1986. Reproduced with permission of the publisher, The American Fertility Society.)

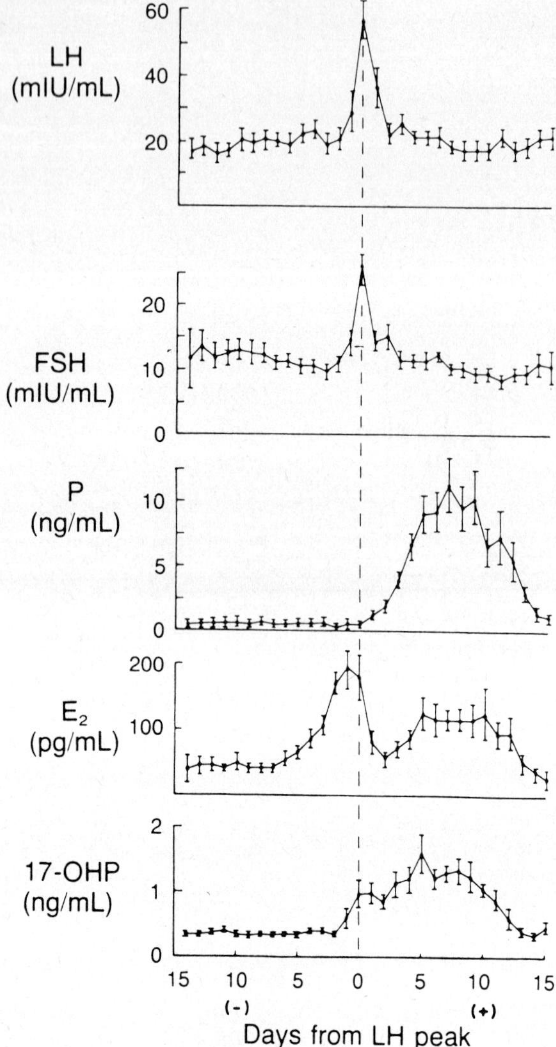

FIGURE 4-23
Means and standard errors of serum *LH*, *FSH*, progesterone *(P)*, estradiol *(E₂)*, and 17-hydroxyprogesterone *(17-OHP)* levels measured in nine women daily during entire ovulatory menstrual cycle. Individual daily results were grouped according to day of midcycle LH peak and averaged. (From Thorneycroft IH, Mishell DR Jr, Stone SC, et al: Am J Obstet Gynecol 111:947, 1971.)

the serum after ovulation and plateau about 1 week later, after which they decline unless pregnancy occurs. The increasing levels of progesterone and estradiol exert a negative feedback on FSH and LH secretion. Estradiol inhibits mainly FSH (negative feedback), whereas progesterone inhibits mainly LH. There is

also evidence that the luteal estradiol production exerts a local luteolytic action. It is postulated that increased intraovarian progesterone concentration prevents follicle maturation in that ovary in the subsequent cycle.

As luteolysis occurs and estradiol and progesterone levels decline, there is less negative feedback. Therefore FSH and LH levels begin to rise before the onset of menstruation to stimulate follicular growth for the next cycle.

Estradiol and progesterone exert both a direct inhibitory effect on pituitary gonadotrophin synthesis and secretion and an effect on GnRH release, altering the frequency as well as the amplitude of GnRH pulses. The steroid feedback on GnRH release occurs by a direct effect on the neurotransmitters (dopamine and norepinephrine) and the neuromodulators (β-endorphin) in the arcuate nucleus.

Recent studies by Reame et al., Crowley et al., and Filicori et al. have shown that the frequency of LH peaks, and presumably of GnRH pulses, when blood sampling was performed every 10 minutes, changes throughout the menstrual cycle. In sheep there is a close relationship between the frequency of GnRH pulses in portal blood and the frequency of LH pulses in the peripheral circulation. In the early follicular phase, LH pulses occur about once every 90 minutes, with an absence of pulsation during sleep (Fig. 4-25). The frequency of LH pulses significantly increases in the mid and late follicular phases to about one pulse per hour throughout the day and night (Fig. 4-26). The amplitude of LH pulses is low and decreases somewhat between the early and mid follicular phases; however, during the late follicular (preovulatory) phase, LH amplitude significantly increases (Fig. 4-27). LH pulse frequency progressively slows in the luteal phase from about one pulse every 90 minutes in the early luteal phase to about one every 3 hours in the late luteal phase (Fig. 4-28). The amplitude of LH pulses varies after ovulation, with a bimodal distribution of small and large pulses. Overall mean LH levels are higher in the luteal phase than the follicular phase (Fig. 4-29). Similar changes in FSH pulsation in peripheral blood do not occur, probably because of its longer half-life.

The increase in frequency of LH pulses during the late follicular phase is probably important in stimulating follicular secretion of estra-

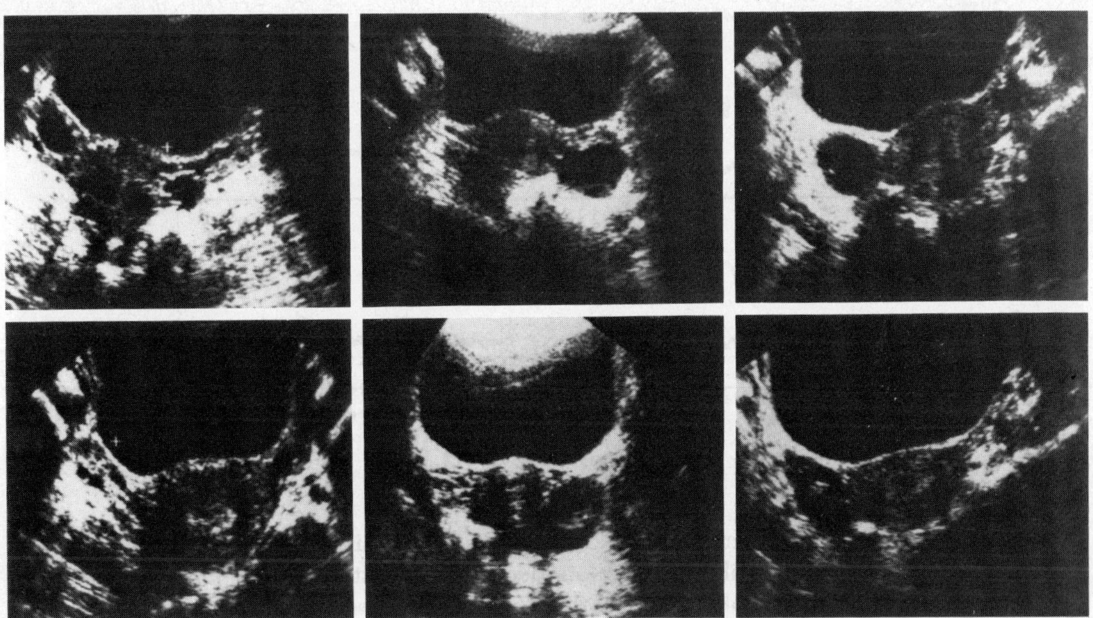

FIGURE 4-24
Ultrasonographic signs of ovulation: complete disappearance *(left)*, loss of volume and thickening of wall *(middle)*, and replacement by irregular spongy area *(right)*. (From Wetzels LCG, Hoogland HJ: Fertil Steril 37:336, 1982. Reproduced with permission of the publisher, The American Fertility Society.)

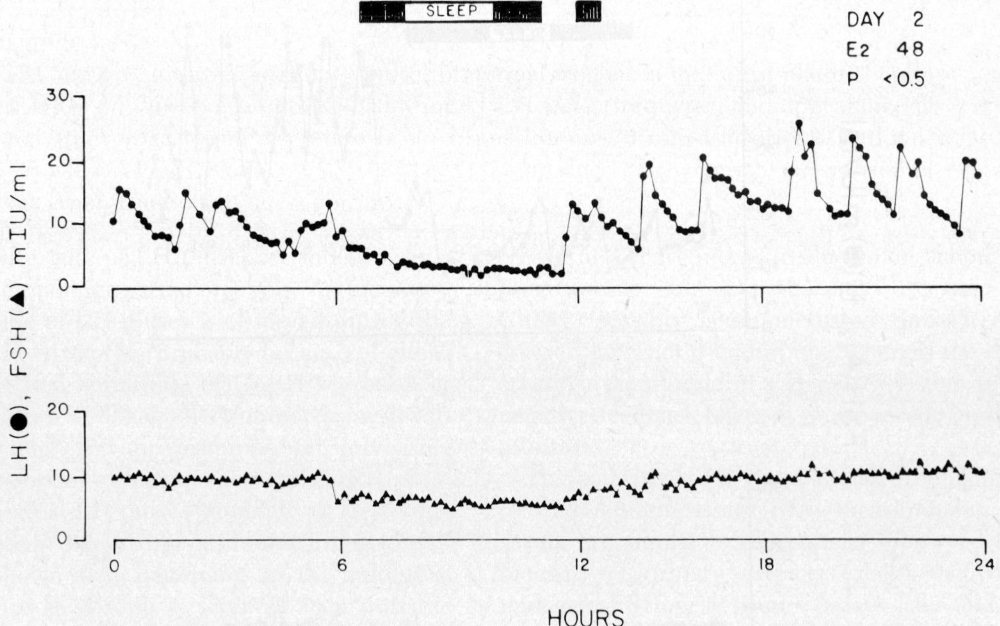

FIGURE 4-25
Twenty-four-hour gonadotrophin secretory pattern (sampling at 10-minute intervals) of woman in early follicular phase (day 2) of menstrual cycle. Notice nearly total suspension of LH secretory activity during sleep in early follicular phase. (From Crowley WF, Filicori M, Spratt DI, et al: Recent Prog Horm Res 41:473, 1985.)

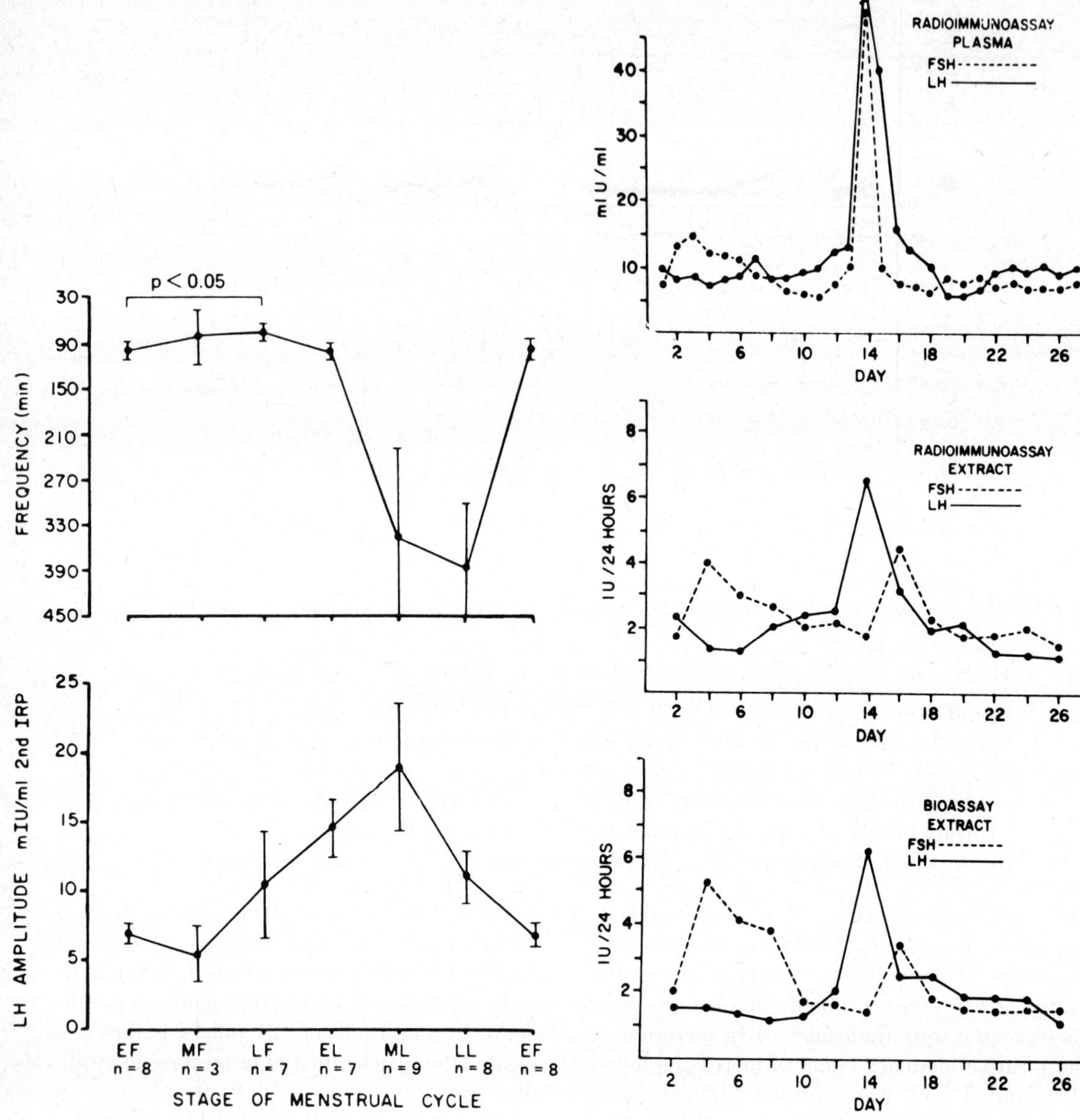

FIGURE 4-29

Summary of frequency and amplitude of episodic gonadotrophin release over normal menstrual cycle. (From Crowley WF, Filicori M, Spratt DI, et al: Recent Prog Horm Res 41:473, 1985.)

FIGURE 4-30

Serum FSH and LH measured by radioimmunoassay (RIA) and urinary FSH and LH measured by both RIA and bioassay through an entire ovulatory menstrual cycle. (From Stevens VC: J Clin Endocrinol Metab 29:904, 1969. © by The Endocrine Society, 1969.)

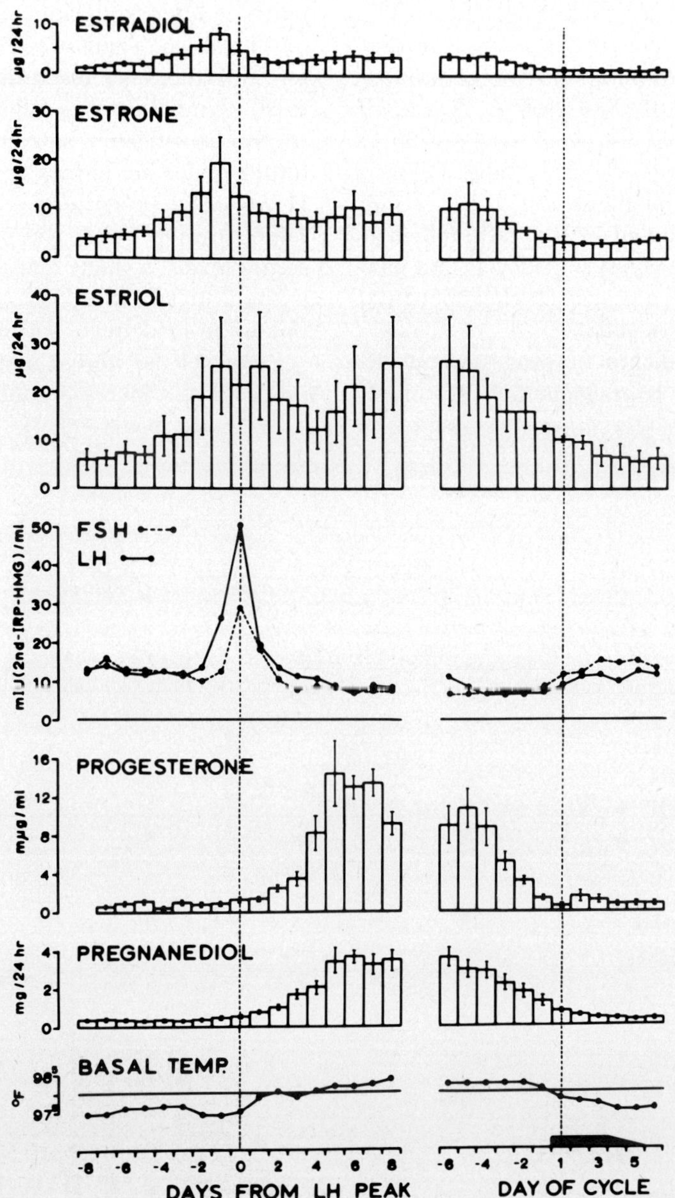

FIGURE 4-31

Mean serum FSH and LH levels, urinary estrogen levels, pregnanediol excretion, and basal body temperatures measured daily in five women during ovulatory menstrual cycle. Bars depict standard errors. Individual results were grouped according to day of midcycle LH surge *(left)* or first day of menstruation *(right)* and averaged. (From Goebelsmann UT, Midgey AR Jr, Jaffe RB: J Clin Endocrinol Metab 29:1222, 1969. © by The Endocrine Society, 1969.)

trone, estradiol, and estriol, is lowest during the early follicular phase, peaks just before LH peaks, decreases shortly thereafter, and rises in the luteal phase, after which it falls again. The luteal-phase rise of these estrogens is of smaller amplitude but longer duration than the preovulatory peak (Fig. 4-31). Midcycle peak urinary excretion of all three estrogens is about 50 to 75 μg/24 h. Serum levels of estradiol follow a similar pattern throughout the cycle, rising from less than 50 pg/ml in the early follicular phase to 200 to 500 pg/ml at midcycle and having a broad luteal-phase peak level of about 100 to 150 pg/ml (see Fig. 4-23).

The major metabolite of progesterone excreted in the urine is pregnanediol (PD). Levels of pregnanediol are less than 0.9 μg/24 h before ovulation (mean, 0.4 μg/24 h) and consistently greater than 1 μg/24 h (mean, 3 to 4 μg/24 h) after ovulation (Fig. 4-32). Progesterone levels in serum are less than 1 ng/ml before ovulation and reach midluteal levels of 10 to 20 ng/ml. In cycles followed by conception, several investigators have reported that progesterone levels are always greater than 9 mg/ml. However, as progesterone is secreted in a pulsatile manner with wide fluctuations in its serum levels, a single low serum value may not be indicative of a lack of corpus luteum formation or an inadequate corpus luteum.

Levels of the steroid metabolite 17-hydroxyprogesterone increase concomitantly with the

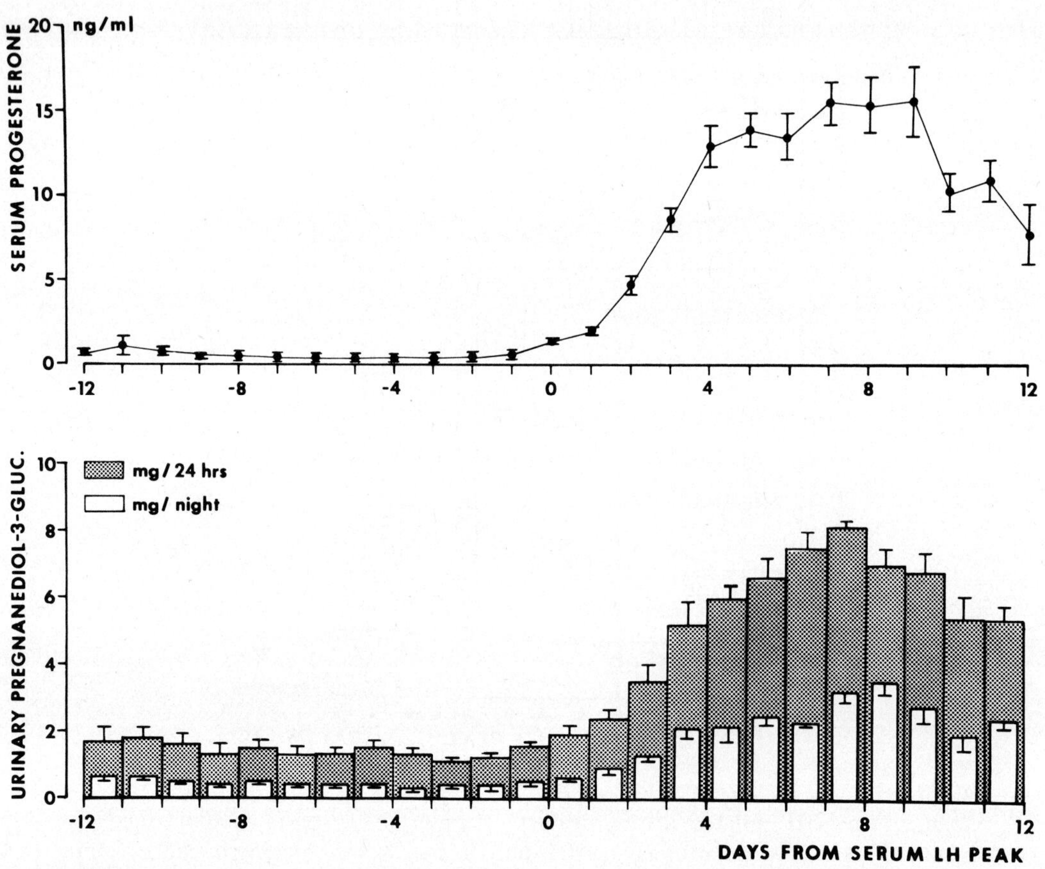

FIGURE 4-32

Means and standard errors of daily 8 AM serum progesterone concentrations and 24-hour (8 AM to 8 AM) and overnight urinary excretion of radioimmunoassayable pregnanediol-3-glucuronide in seven women during entire menstrual cycle. Data obtained in individual subjects were grouped according to day of midcycle LH peak and averaged. (From Stanczyk FZ, Miyakama I, Goebelsmann UT: Am J Obstet Gynecol 137:443, 1980.)

increase of the LH surge, indicating a shift of steroidogenesis from the Δ^5 to the Δ^4 pathway (see Fig. 4-23). Levels of 17-hydroxyprogesterone then fall and rise again in the midluteal phase as progesterone and estradiol levels increase. About 4 to 6 days before the onset of menses, levels of estradiol, progesterone, and 17-hydroxyprogesterone all begin to decline.

During midcycle the first event is a rise in estradiol. When estradiol reaches peak levels, there is an abrupt increase (surge) in LH and FSH (Fig. 4-33). The increase in LH reaches a peak in about 18 hours, and peak levels plateau for about 14 hours, after which there is a decline. The mean duration of the LH surge is about 24 hours. Beginning about 12 hours before the onset of the LH surge, there is an increase of both progesterone and 17-hydroxyprogesterone. With the occurrence of the LH peak there is a decline in estradiol and a further increase in progesterone. This shift in steroidogenesis in favor of progesterone instead of estradiol production is brought about by the luteinization of the granulosa cells produced by LH.

Levels of numerous other hormones have been measured in serum throughout the cycle and summarized in the excellent review by Diczfalusy and Landgren. Serum levels of androstenedione and testosterone change little during the cycle, but mean levels are slightly higher during the follicular than the luteal phase (Fig. 4-34). Serum thyroid-stimulating hormone (TSH) levels also remain relatively constant, while adrenocorticotropic hormone (ACTH) and growth hormone (GH) have a preovulatory peak. Prolactin levels appear to be slightly higher in the luteal phase. Steroid hormone metabolites of estradiol, progesterone, and 17-hydroxyprogesterone follow cyclic changes similar to those of the parent hormone. Pregnenolone, 17α-hydroxypregnenolone, and dehydroepidandrostenedione all have a circadian variation, but only pregnenolone

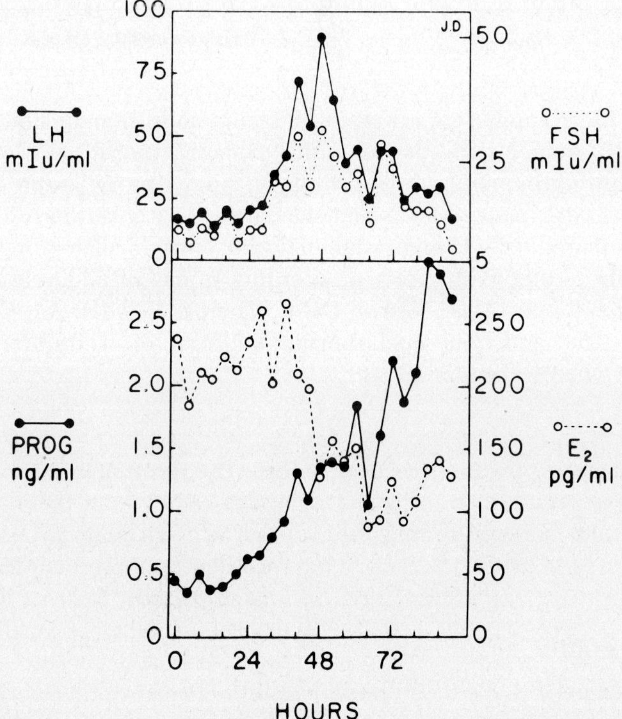

FIGURE 4-33
Serum FSH, LH, estradiol *(E₂)*, and progesterone *(PROG)* levels around midcycle. (From Thorneycroft IH, Sribyatta B, Tom WK, et al: J Clin Endocrinol Metab 39:754, 1974. © by The Endocrine Society, 1974.)

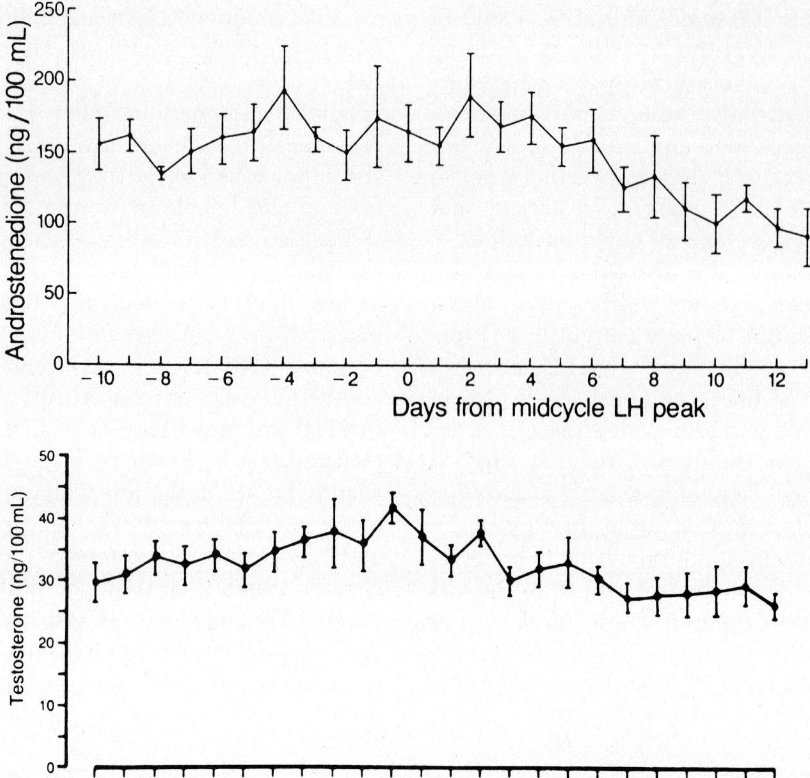

FIGURE 4-34

Upper panel: Means and standard errors of serum androstenedione concentrations measured in six women daily during entire ovulatory menstrual cycle. Individual daily results were grouped according to day of preovulatory serum estradiol peak and averaged. *Lower panel:* Means and standard errors of serum testosterone concentrations measured daily in eight women during entire ovulatory menstrual cycle. Individual daily results were grouped according to day of midcycle LH peak and averaged. (From Ribeiro WO, Mishell DR Jr, Thorneycroft IH: Am J Obstet Gynecol 119:1026, 1974, and from Goebelsmann UT, Arce JJ, Thorneycroft IH, et al: Am J Obstet Gynecol 119:445, 1974.)

rises during the luteal phase. Cortisol, corticosteroid, and aldosterone, in addition to having a circadian variation, also increase during the luteal phase.

Menstrual Cycle Length

The mean age of menarche is about 13 years, and the mean age of menopause is about 51 years. Therefore women have menses for a duration of about 38 years. Menstrual cycle length varies among different women and for an individual woman at different times of her life. The most information regarding menstrual cycles comes from the classic study of Treolar et al, who analyzed 275,947 menstrual intervals recorded by more than 2700 women over prolonged periods. Analysis of these data revealed that menstrual cycle length is most irregular in the 2 years after menarche and the 3 years before menopause, times of life during which anovulatory cycles are most frequent (Table 4-4). During these times of life, both shortened and prolonged cycle lengths are common, with the latter being more frequent (Fig. 4-35).

Menstrual cycle length is least variable be-

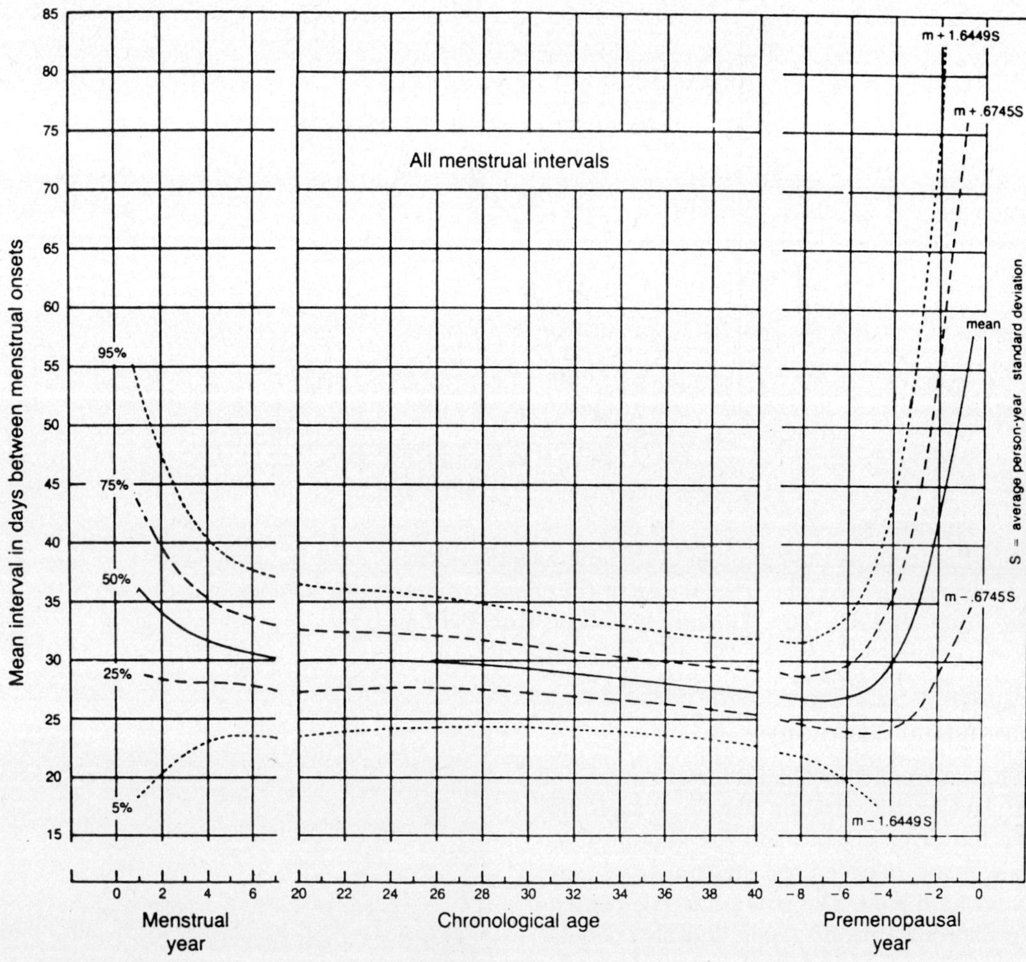

FIGURE 4-35

Normal curve contours for distribution of menstrual intervals in three zones of menstrual life. (From Treloar AE, Boynton RE, Borghild BG, et al: Int J Fertil 12:77, 1967.)

TABLE 4-4

Means and Standard Deviations in Days for Menstrual Intervals at Selected Ages*

Age	Mean (Days)	Standard Deviation (Days)
2 yr after menarche	32.20	8.38
20 yr	30.09	3.94
25 yr	29.84	3.45
30 yr	29.30	3.16
35 yr	28.22	2.67
40 yr	27.26	2.83
3 yr before menopause	33.20	14.24

*Data from Treloar AE, Boynton RE, Borghild BG, et al: Variation of the human menstrual cycle through reproductive life. Int J Fertil 12:77, 1967.

tween the ages of 20 and 40 years. During this time there is a gradual decrease of mean cycle length. However, between these ages, menstrual cycle length still varies in an individual woman, as shown by the variation in cycle length recorded by the women with the most regular duration of menstrual cycles among the several thousand studied by Vollman for many years (Fig. 4-36). It is generally accepted that the mean duration of menstrual cycle length is 28 ± 7 days, with the occurrence of shorter cycles (<21 days) being called polymenorrhea and that of longer cycles (>35 days) being called oligomenorrhea. The mean duration of menstrual flow is 4 ± 2 days.

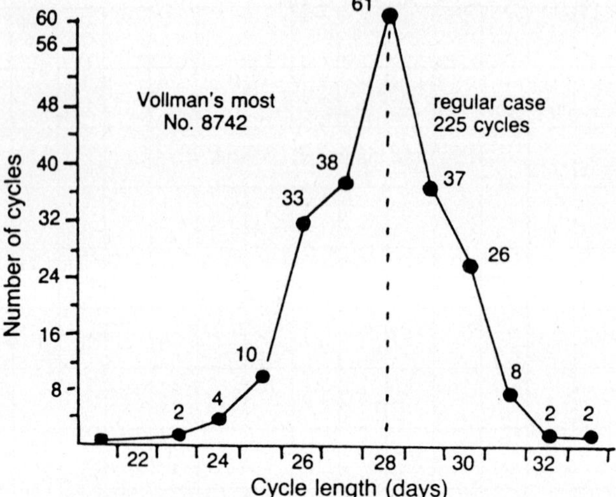

FIGURE 4-36

Frequency distribution of cycle lengths of Vollman's "most regular" subject. (From Hartman CG: The irregularity of the menstrual cycle. In Science and the safe period. © 1966, The Williams & Wilkins Co., Baltimore.)

Endometrial Histology

The human endometrium is made up of two basic layers: the stratum basale, which lies above the myometrium, and the stratum functionale, lying between the stratum basale and the uterine lumen. The stratum basale consists of primordial glands and densely cellular stroma, which changes little throughout the menstrual cycle and does not desquamate at the time of menstruation. The stratum functionale is divided into two layers. The superficial, narrow stratum compactum consists of the necks of the glands and densely populated stromal cells. The underlying, broader stratum spongiosum consists primarily of glands with less densely populated stroma and large amounts of interstitial tissue. The stratum functionale grows during the cycle, and a portion of it desquamates at the time of menses.

After menstruation the endometrium is only 1 to 2 mm thick and consists mainly of the stratum basale and a portion of the spongiosum. Under the influence of estrogen the stratum functionale proliferates greatly by multiplication of both glandular and stromal cells. Mitotic figures are abundant. In the late follicular phase, glycogen begins to be stored in the glands, which become more tortuous in appearance. Just before ovulation, as estrogen

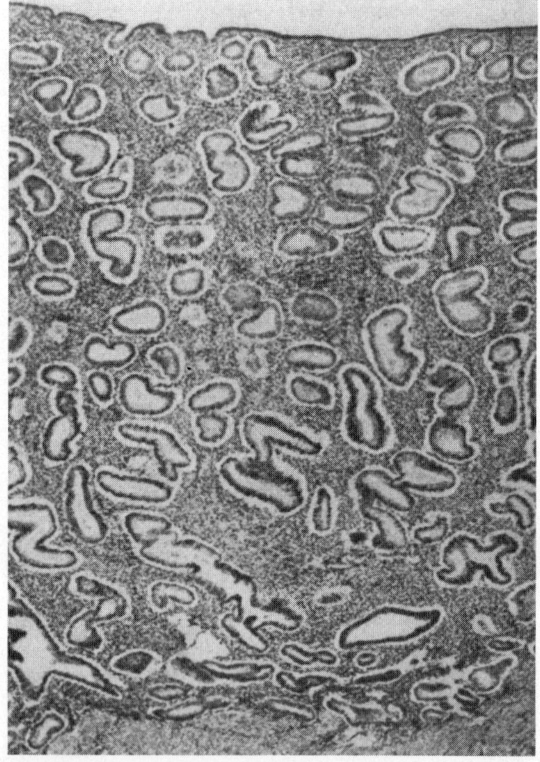

FIGURE 4-37

Early-interval endometrium. (From Novak E, Novak ER, eds: Textbook of gynecology, 4th ed. © 1952, The Williams & Wilkins Co., Baltimore.)

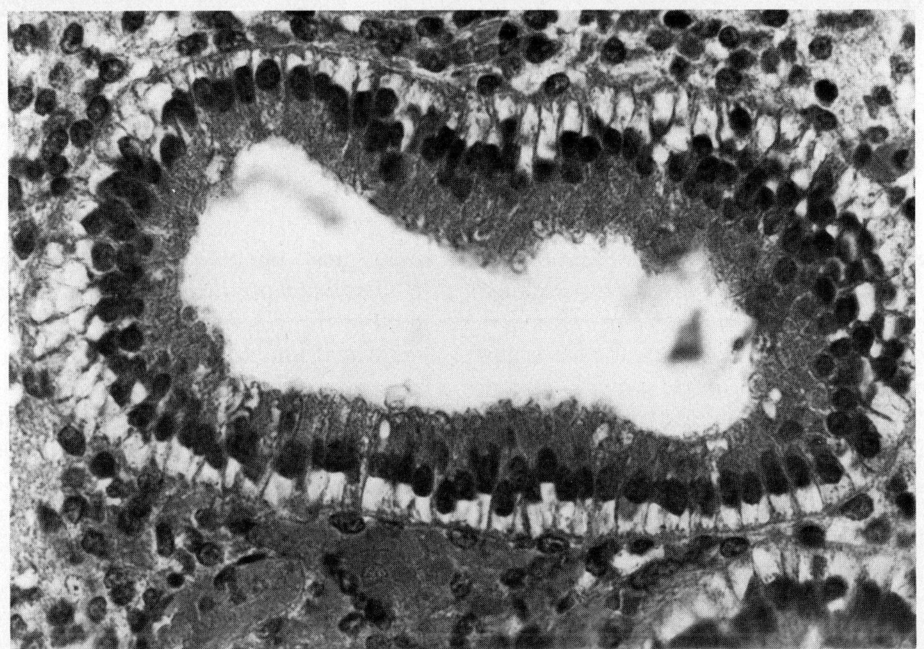

FIGURE 4-38
Subnuclear vacuoles lining base of endometrial gland 2 to 3 days after ovulation. (×500; reduced by 22%.) (From March CM: The endometrium in the menstrual cycle. Reproduced with permission from Infertility, contraception and reproductive endocrinology, 2nd ed, edited by Daniel R. Mishell, Jr., M.D., and Val Davajan, M.D. Copyright © 1986 Medical Economics Books, Oradell, N.J. 07649. All rights reserved.)

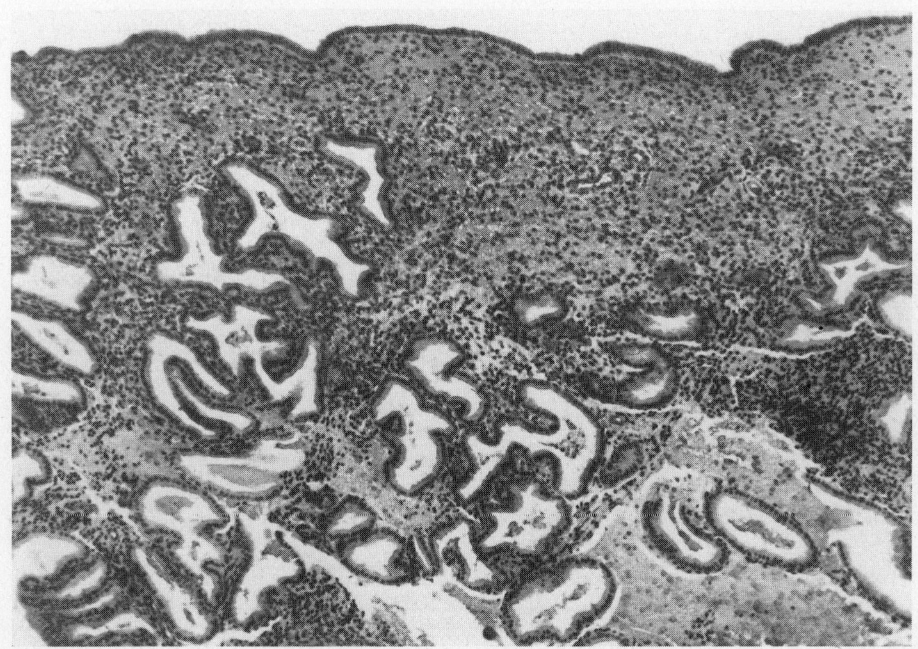

FIGURE 4-39
Maximal secretory activity characteristic of 7 to 8 days after ovulation. (×90; reduced by 22%). (From March CM: The endometrium in the menstrual cycle. Reproduced with permission from Infertility, contraception and reproductive endocrinology, 2nd ed, edited by Daniel R. Mishell, Jr., M.D., and Val Davajan, M.D. Copyright © 1986 Medical Economics Books, Oradell, N.J. 07649. All rights reserved.)

levels peak, the cells lining the gland lumina undergo pseudostratification (Fig. 4-37).

Just after ovulation, glycogen-rich subnuclear vacuoles appear in the base of the cells lining the glands (Fig. 4-38). This subnuclear vacuolization is the first histologic indication of the effect of progesterone but is not evidence that ovulation has occurred. As progesterone levels increase in the early luteal phase, the glycogen-containing vacuoles ascend toward the gland lumina. Soon thereafter the contents of the glands are released into the endometrial cavity to provide energy to the free-floating blastocyst, which reaches the endometrial cavity about 3½ days after fertilization but does not implant until 1 week after fertilization.

In the midluteal phase the glands become increasingly tortuous and the stroma becomes more edematous and vascular (Fig. 4-39). As steroid levels begin to wane in the late luteal phase, if implantation of the blastocyst does not occur and human chorionic gonadotrophin (HCG) is not produced to maintain the corpus luteum, the glands begin to collapse and fragment, and infiltration of the glands and stroma by polymorphonuclear leukocytes and monocytes occurs. Autolysis of the functional zone of the endometrium occurs and desquamation begins. The histologic pattern of the endometrium has been correlated with the phase of the menstrual cycle in the classic study of Noyes et al (Fig. 4-40).

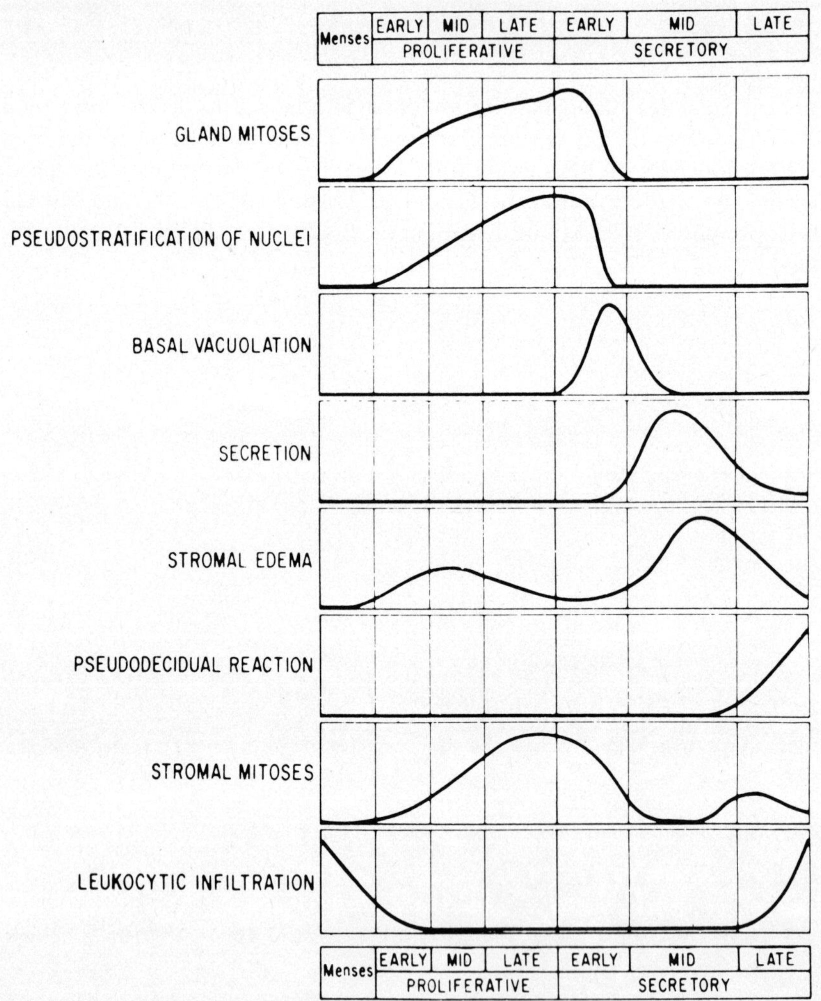

FIGURE 4-40
Patterns of histologic changes throughout menstrual cycle. (Modified from Noyes RW, Hertig AT, Rock J: Fertil Steril 1:3, 1950. Reproduced with permission of the publisher, The American Fertility Society.)

Menstruation

There has been relatively little research regarding the mechanism of menstruation since the classic studies of Markee and those of Bartermez in the 1930s and 1940s. In Markee's classic study, endometria from rhesus monkeys were transplanted into the anterior chamber of the eye of the same animal from which the tissue was obtained. He observed that during the cycle the transplants underwent four periods of change: (1) the period of rest (occurring just after menses), (2) the first period of growth (in the follicular phase, during which the size of the transplant doubled), (3) the second period of growth (after ovulation, during which the transplants doubled in size again), and (4) the period of regression (during which menstruation occurred) (Fig. 4-41). Markee noted that as steroid levels fell several days before menstruation, there was regression in size of the transplants, resulting in coiling of the spiral arteries and slowing of the blood flow within them. This vascular stasis was followed 4 to 24 hours before menstruation by vasoconstriction of the coiled arteries. About 4 to 24 hours after

vasoconstriction began, the coiled arteries relaxed, blood escaped from them, and menstruation began. Only the spiral arteries that supply the upper two thirds of the endometrium became coiled and constricted. The straight arteries supplying the stratum basale did not constrict.

Thus the regression in size of the endometrium brought about by decreasing steroid levels leads to increased coiling and constriction of the spiral arteries, possibly because of decreased cellular monoamine oxidase levels. The resultant decreased blood flow to the functional portion of the endometrium causes ischemia of this tissue. The epithelial and stromal cells show ultrastructural changes of degeneration and autodegradation. With this autolysis, hydrolases and other lysosomal enzymes are released into the interstitium. These enzymes degrade the substances that make up the supporting growth substance of the endometrium, the mucopolysaccharides, collagen, and reticulum. The resulting degraded endometrial tissue is desquamated into the uterine cavity.

Both Markee and Bartlemez, who performed

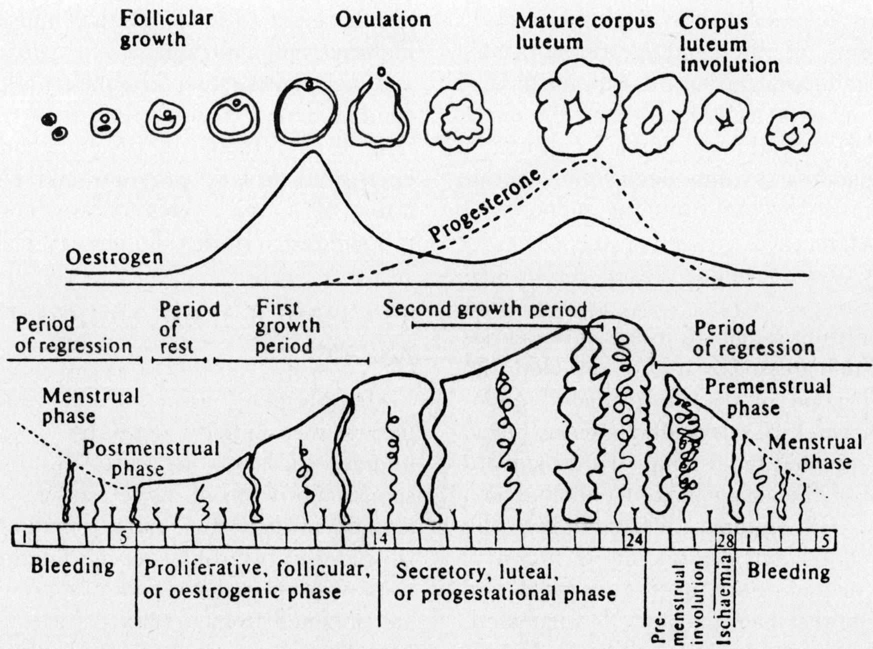

FIGURE 4-41
Diagram of changes in normal human ovarian and endometrial cycles. (From Shaw ST Jr, Roche PC. Menstruation. In: Finn CA, ed. Oxford reviews of reproduction and endocrinology, Vol. 2. London, Oxford University Press, 1980, p. 41.)

histologic studies on uteri removed by hysterectomy in the 1930s, concluded that menstruation begins in different areas of the uterus at different times and that all the extravasation of blood begins in the first 2 days of menses.

Although the classic belief that all tissue of the stratum functional is exfoliated, leaving only the stratum basale remaining at the end of menstruation, is written in many textbooks of gynecology, Bartelmez reported that only the entire stratum compactum is uniformly shed, with variable amounts of the stratum spongiosum being desquamated. McLennan and Rydell confirmed this finding in their 1965 study and showed that regeneration of the endometrium comes from cells in the spongiosum that were previously a portion of the secretory endometrium, and not from the stratum basale, as was previously believed. These investigators also found extreme variations in the amount of endometrial shedding in different areas of the same uterus, as well as variations among different uteri removed by hysterectomy.

Nogales-Ortiz et al also found extreme variability in the extent of endometrial exfoliation. In their study they found that usually only the entire compactum and some parts of the spongiosum were shed, but in some areas nearly the entire endometrium was desquamated. Desquamation of the endometrium occurs mainly in the fundus, not in the isthmus or cornual areas. As early as 36 hours after the onset of menses, regeneration of surface epithelium from the glandular stumps begins and continues to occur at the same time as endometrial shedding occurs.

Ferenczy, using scanning as well as transmission electron microscopy, also reported that the endometrium remained intact in the cervical and isthmic areas. His studies revealed that reepithelialization of the desquamated endometrium began 2 to 3 days after menses began and was completed in 48 hours. He concluded that repair of the desquamated endometrium occurred by both epithelial outgrowth from the mouths of the basal glands and by ingrowth from the endometrium in the cervical and isthmic areas that had not been desquamated. Ferenczy and co-workers also performed historadioautography studies that resulted in these findings: they believe that regeneration of the endometrial surface occurs as a local reaction to injury and is not mediated by ovarian steroid hormones. Circulatory estrogen levels are very low at this time of the cycle.

In 1978 Flowers and Wilborn performed a histologic, histochemical, and ultrastructural study of endometrial biopsy specimens obtained from a group of menstruating women. In these detailed studies they also found that the only cells that become desquamated are from the compactum and upper spongiosum layers and that very few endometrial cells undergo necrosis. Instead, the majority of cells in the endometrium survive, but they undergo regression in size by autophagocytosis, heterophagocytosis, and release of enzymes. Endometrial autophagocytosis is carried out by lysosomes, which digest the cytoplasm; heterophagocytosis is performed by macrophages, which phagocytose debris from stromal tissue; and the enzymes digest reticular fibers. After the regression of cell size, the cells are reorganized in structure and participate in the new proliferative process. Thus the same cells that previously formed the secretory endometrium also form the new proliferative endometrium. It has been postulated that a process called apoptosis is the mechanism whereby controlled cell deletion and tissue regression are followed by reorganization of cells so that large secretory glands revert to small glands found in the proliferative endometrium.

Thus menstruation in humans is probably a combination of (1) some superficial tissue shedding, brought about by ischemia and the presence of hydrolytic enzymes and possibly relaxin, (2) tissue regression (mainly), and (3) reorganization of the endometrial cells.

TECHNIQUE OF HORMONE ASSAY

Measurement (assay) of reproductive hormones was initially done by bioassay techniques. Bioassays measure the biologic response (growth) of target organs of certain animals (usually rats, rabbits, or mice), which is produced by administering different concentrations of the substances to be assayed, which are obtained from urinary extracts. First, various dilutions of a known (standard) preparation of hormone are administered. The varying increases in weight of the target organ in the animal are then used to develop a dose-response curve against which the response of the unknown urinary extract is determined. These bioassay techniques were mainly used to quantify gonadotrophins.

Chemical methods were developed to measure sex steroid levels in women. Before chemical assay, three basic preparatory steps are performed. First, the steroids need to undergo hydrolysis to remove the conjugate. Second, they need to be extracted by organic solvents from the urinary hydrolysate. The final basic step is purification of the steroid by column chromatography. The amount of steroid is then quantitated by measurement of the color reaction, either colorimetry or the more sensitive fluorimetry. The most sensitive chemical method of measurement of steroids is gas chromatography, an extremely tedious procedure.

In 1959 Yalow and Berson developed the technique of radioimmunoassay, which provided the method of measuring extremely small amounts of hormone in serum or plasma. Use of this technique has greatly increased the knowledge of reproductive endocrinology. Radioimmunoassay allows a much greater number of assays to be performed than does bioassay or chemical assay, in addition to having much greater sensitivity and needing less than 1 ml of serum or plasma for testing. However, this technique measures only the immunologic property of a hormone, not its biologic effects. The two effects frequently differ in magnitude.

The basic principle of radioimmunoassay involves the competition between a radioactively labeled and an unlabeled antigen for binding sites on an antibody. To produce a standard curve that permits measurement of a hormone in the serum or plasma, the investigator uses a standard preparation of the hormone to be measured (antigen). Varying known amounts of the unlabeled (cold) antigen and the labeled (hot) antigen are incubated with an antibody raised specifically against the antigen to be measured for a period, and an antigen-antibody complex is formed (Fig. 4-42). Since there is always an excess of labeled and unlabeled antigen in the reaction, some of each type of antigen is always bound to the antibody and some always remains free in solution after the incubation. After the bound complex is separated from the excess free antigen in solution, usually by the addition of an antibody (second antibody) raised against the first antibody, the amount of tracer present in either the bound or free component, usually the bound complex, is measured by a radioactive analyzer (counter). A standard curve is then constructed by plotting the counts per minute measured in the various dilutions of the standard preparation against the mass of antigen used. The type of curve varies with the scale of the abscissa (Fig. 4-43).

For measurement of the amount of hormone in the unknown specimen, excess labeled antigen is added to an aliquot of the unknown specimen, and after incubation and separation, the amount of tracer that is bound in the antigen-antibody complex is also counted. The number of counts per minute on the ordinate is intersected on the standard curve, and a perpendicular is dropped to the abscissa to deter-

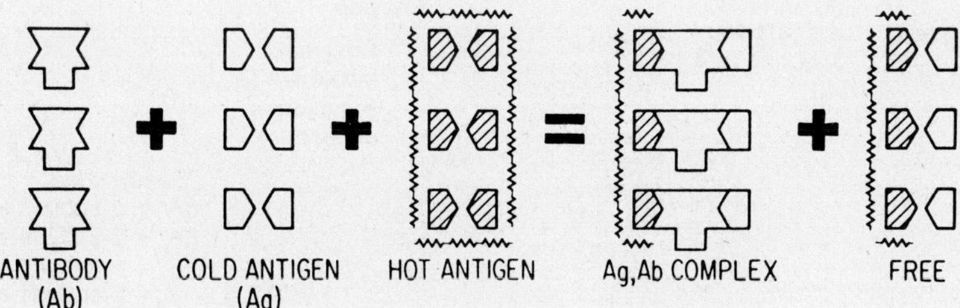

FIGURE 4-42

Schematic representation of antigen-antibody reaction in radioimmunoassay. For final analysis, free component must be separated from the antigen-antibody complex. (From Kletzky OA, Nakamura RM: Measurement of hormones. Reproduced with permission from Infertility, contraception and reproductive endocrinology, 2nd ed, edited by Daniel R. Mishell, Jr., M.D., and Val Davajan, M.D. Copyright © 1986 Medical Economics Books, Oradell, N.J. 07649. All rights reserved.)

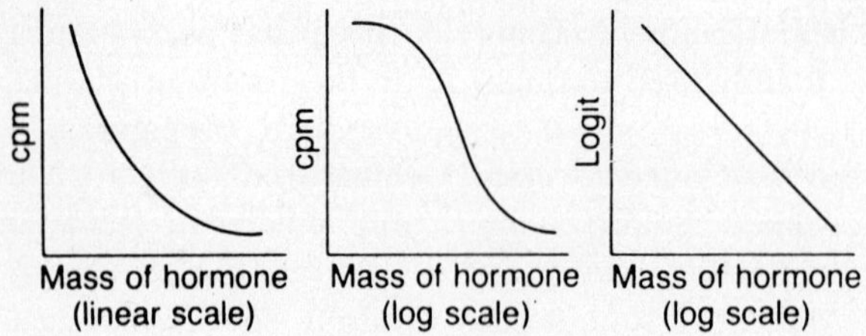

FIGURE 4-43

Standard curve using linear scale *(left)* or log scale *(center and right)* for the abscissa and linear *(left and center)* or logit *(right)* for the ordinate. (From Kletzky OA, Nakamura RM: Measurement of hormones. Reproduced with permission from Infertility, contraception and reproductive endocrinology, 2nd ed, edited by Daniel R. Mishell, Jr., M.D., and Val Davajan, M.D. Copyright © 1986 Medical Economics Books, Oradell, N.J. 07649. All rights reserved.)

mine the amount of hormone in the unknown specimen.

Another sensitive assay is the enzyme immunoassay (EIA), in which an enzyme is coupled to the antibody instead of to unbound antigen. The reaction is read by spectrophotometry and avoids all radioactivity. Recently, enzyme-linked immunosorbent assay (ELISA), or "sandwich," techniques have been developed to measure protein hormones by means of monoclonal antibodies against the α and β subunits (Fig. 4-44). The end point is a color reaction and can be read in a spectrophotometer. A standard curve is constructed in the usual manner, and the amount of hormone in the unknown is measured without needing radioactivity. The new generation of alternative immunoassays includes tests that are even more rapid and sensitive than radioimmunoassay. These techniques are time-resolved immunofluorometric assay (IMFA), which is based on the use of pulsed light and fluorescent

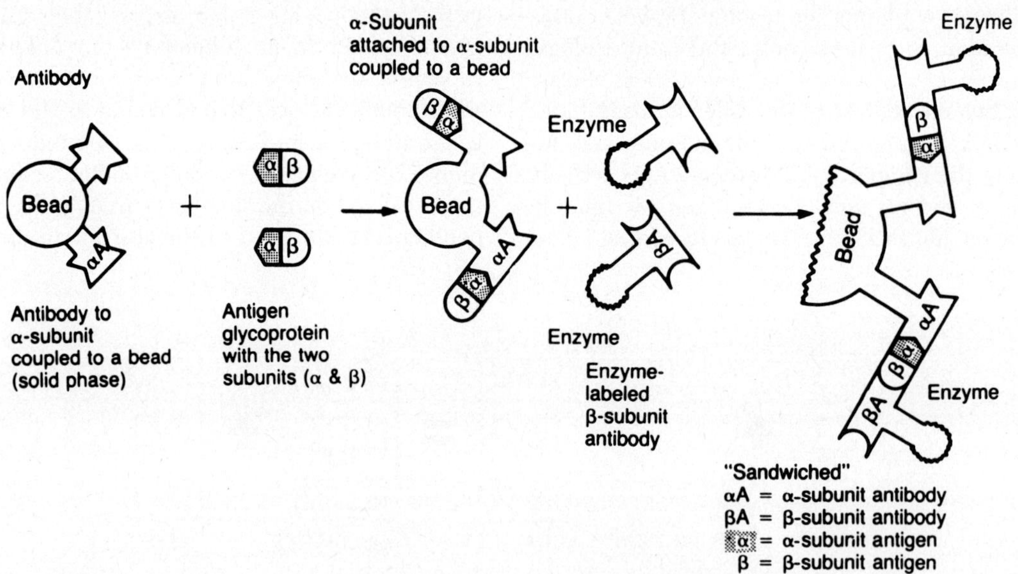

FIGURE 4-44

Schematic representation of enzyme-linked immunosorbent assay (ELISA), or "sandwich," technique. (From Kletzky OA, Nakamura RM: Measurement of hormones. Reproduced with permission from Infertility, contraception and reproductive endocrinology, 2nd ed, edited by Daniel R. Mishell, Jr., M.D., and Val Davajan, M.D. Copyright © 1986 Medical Economics Books, Oradell, N.J. 07649. All rights reserved.)

labels, and chemoluminescence immunoassay (CIA). The chemoluminescent label has the ability to convert energy produced by a chemical reaction into light energy, similar to that performed by the firefly.

These techniques, as well as ELISA, need a high concentration of specifically labeled antibody. Thus the use of these assays has been made possible by the development of monoclonal antibodies. All these assays require short incubation times, approximately 30 minutes or less, and avoid the use of radioisotopes and expensive radioactive counters. Therefore the clinical usefulness of hormone measurement by these techniques will certainly increase.

Since all these techniques measure the immunologic properties of the hormone, bioassay techniques that measure the effect of LH on testicular homogenates to produce testosterone and of FSH on granulosa cells to produce estradiol have been developed to aid investigative efforts. These techniques combine bioassays and radioimmunoassay, since the amount of steroid produced is measured by radioimmunoassay.

Four characteristics of assays apply to each of these techniques: sensitivity, specificity, accuracy, and precision. Sensitivity is the least amount of substance that can be measured in the assay. Specificity is the ability of the assay to measure only one substance and not allow the measurement to be altered by the presence of other substances (cross-reaction). Accuracy is the ability to measure the exact amount of substance in the sample; thus specimens containing known low and high values of the substance to be measured are always included in each assay. Precision is the ability of the assay to consistently reproduce the same results. Precision is determined by measuring the within-assay, or intraassay, coefficient of variation (CV) and the between-assay, or interassay, CV. The intraassay CV is calculated by determining the amounts of a known sample measured in about 10 replicates in the same assay.

$$CV = \frac{\text{Standard deviation}}{\text{Mean}} \times 100$$

The interassay CV is determined by measuring the same unknown sample on different days. The intrassay CV should be less than 10%, and the interassay CV should be less than 15% for satisfactory precision of the assay.

The protein hormones themselves are antigenic and can produce antibody formation. Either the entire hormone or, preferably, the specific β subunit can be used as the antigen. Since steroids are haptens and are not antigenic by themselves, they need to be attached to a carrier protein (usually bovine serum albumin) to induce antibody formation. Even with the injection of purified antigens, there is a degree of cross-reaction of most hormone antibodies with other hormones. Monoclonal antibodies are now being produced to eliminate

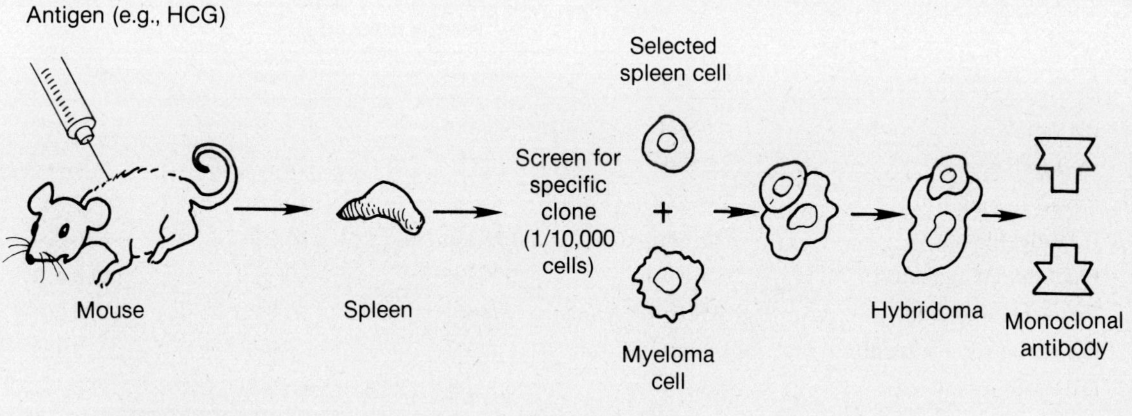

FIGURE 4-45

Schematic representation of monoclonal antibody production. (From Kletzky OA, Nakamura RM: Measurement of hormones. Reproduced with permission from Infertility, contraception and reproductive endocrinology, 2nd ed, edited by Daniel R. Mishell, Jr., M.D., and Val Davajan, M.D. Copyright © 1986 Medical Economics Books, Oradell, N.J. 07649. All rights reserved.)

the variability and heterogeneity of antibodies produced by several injections of antigen and thus to increase the specificity of the assay. Monoclonal antibodies are produced by first injecting the antigen into a mouse to induce an immunologic reaction in its spleen (Fig. 4-45). The spleen cells are screened to find those particular ones (clones) capable of secreting a single antibody type. These cells are then fused with a myeloma cell from the same species to form a hybrid or hybridoma cell. Because of the immortality of the myeloma cell in culture, the hybridoma continually secretes antibodies characteristic of the selected spleen cell. This clone line is maintained in culture to provide homogenous monoclonal antibody molecules, which are used for sensitive specific immunoassays of protein hormones.

To produce standard curves, varying amounts of known preparations of hormone need to be utilized. Since steroid hormones are available as chemically pure preparations, the amount added to form the standard curve and determine the amount in the unknown can be expressed in terms of absolute mass or weight, such as nanograms (10^{-9}) or picograms (10^{-12}). Thus the results obtained from different laboratories should be constant. However, most European laboratories express the results in terms of nanomoles instead of nanograms. For most steroids, about 3 nmol/L are equivalent to 1 ng/ml.

Protein hormones, however, being of high molecular weight, are not circulated in pure form, and therefore the results of measuring unknown samples need to be expressed in terms of the amount of a standard reference preparation obtained from standard extracts of the hormone from collections of urine, serum, or pituitary glands. Therefore the levels of hormone measured by laboratories using different standards do not always agree, and clinicians should be aware of the normal levels used by these laboratories. The standard is frequently an international reference preparation, and the results are usually expressed in international units.

The normal range of values of hormones in normal women is frequently expressed in terms of the mean level plus the mathematically calculated 95% confidence limits (± 2 SD). However, the distributions of hormone levels in the menstrual cycles of a group of women with normal ovulation follow a log-normal distribution instead of a gaussian (normal) distribution. Although results of normal values usually vary from laboratory to laboratory, the 95% confidence limits of measurement of reproductive hormones among women in our laboratory are listed in Table 4-5 as a guide of normality.

TABLE 4-5
95% Confidence Limits of Hormones Used in Reproduction

Hormone	Follicular	Midcycle	Luteal	Menopause
		Phase of Menstrual Cycle		
LH (mIU/ml)	4.0-20.0	43-145	3-18	>40
FSH (mIU/ml)	3.2-9.0	10-18	3-9	>30
Prolactin (ng/ml)	8.0-20.0	0-22	10-30	8-25
Estradiol (pg/ml)	30-140	150-480	50-250	10-30
Progesterone (ng/ml)	0.5-1.0	0.8-2.0	3.0-31	0.5-1.0
Testosterone (ng/dl)	20-85	20-85	20-85	8-30*
Free testosterone (ng/dl)	1.2-9.9	1.2-9.9	1.2-9.9	3-13†
DHEA-S (µg/ml)	0.5-2.8	0.5-2.8	0.5-2.8	0.2-1.5

From Kletzky OA, Nakamura RM: Measurement of hormones. Reproduced with permission from Infertility, contraception, and reproductive endocrinology, 2nd ed, edited by Daniel R. Mishell, Jr., M.D., and Val Davajan, M.D. Copyright © 1986 Medical Economics Books, Oradell, N.J. 07649. All rights reserved.
*In oophorectomized women the range is 4 to 18 ng/dl.
†In oophorectomized women the range is 1 to 10 ng/dl.

KEY POINTS

- The hypothalamic hormone that controls gonadotrophin release is a decapeptide, gonadotrophin-releasing hormone (GnRH).

- The cell bodies of the hypothalamic neurons that produce GnRH are concentrated mainly in two areas: the anterior hypothalamus and the medial basal (tuberal) hypothalamus.

- GnRH can be released both in large amounts periodically via the tuberoinfundibular tract (cyclic release) and in a low-grade continuous transependymal fashion (tonic release) via the tanycytes.

- GnRH is secreted in a pulsatile manner. The amplitude and frequency of the pulse vary throughout the menstrual cycle. The frequency is rapid in the follicular phase, about one pulse per hour, and slower in the luteal phase, about one pulse every 2 or 3 hours.

- The most important neurotransmitters involved in reproductive neuroendocrinology are two catecholamines, dopamine and norepinephrine, as well as an indolamine, serotonin.

- Infusion of β endorphin results in an increase in prolactin and a decrease in LH, the latter occurring by an inhibitory effect on GnRH neurons in the hypothalamus.

- The peptide hormones, such as GnRH, bind to specific receptors on the surface membrane of the target cell, in contrast to steroid hormones, which pass through the cell membrane to bind to intracellular receptors.

- When a protein hormone binds to its specific receptor, it activates or inhibits the enzyme adenyl cyclase, the second messenger, which in turn changes the concentration of adenosine 3′, 5′-cyclic monophosphate (cyclic AMP, cAMP).

- Following a single intravenous bolus of GnRH, the LH levels peak in 30 minutes and FSH in 60 minutes.

- With a constant infusion of GnRH there is a biphasic release of LH but not FSH. The initial increase of LH occurs 30 minutes and the second 90 minutes after the start of the infusion.

History and Examination of the Patient

<hr>

KEY TERMS AND DEFINITIONS

Anovulatory Cycle. Menstrual cycle when ovulation does not occur.

Dyspareunia. Painful intercourse.

Ectropion. The presence of endocervical (glandular) epithelium on the portio vaginalis of cervix. It may result from scarring of the external os or may be congenital.

LMP. Last menstrual period.

Menstrual Formula. Age of menarche × number of days of cycle × number of days of menstrual flow (e.g., 13 × 28 × 5).

Normal Transformation Zone. Area of columnar epithelium and squamous metaplasia in the vagina or on the cervix that has normal colposcopic patterns.

PMP. Previous menstrual period.

Sexual Dysfunction. A psychological or physiologic problem or condition that prevents the usual full participation and enjoyment of coitus.

<hr>

The first contact a physician has with a patient is critical. It allows an initial bond of trust to be developed on which the future relationship may be built. The patient will share sensitive information, feelings, and fears. The physician will gain her confidence by the understanding and nonjudgmental manner in which he or she collects these data. In such a way, rapport is established.

The first contact generally involves taking a complete history, performing a complete physical examination, and ordering appropriate initial laboratory tests. In such a way the physician gains impressions of the patient's problems and needs and develops a plan for solutions. A gynecologic history includes a complete general history and adds information of gynecologic importance. In like manner the physical examination should be complete. No corners should be cut. The physician practicing obstetrics and gynecology should not assume that the patient's general medical needs are cared for by others even if the patient has a personal family physician.

This chapter will focus on the appropriate manner that a gynecologic physician should use to conduct a history and physical examination.

DIRECT OBSERVATIONS BEFORE SPEAKING TO PATIENT (NONVERBAL CLUES)

When meeting a patient it is important to *look* at her even before speaking. Some experienced physicians will observe patients sitting in their waiting rooms before actually beginning personal contact. The general demeanor of the patient should be evaluated. Basically there are five general impressions that can be transmitted both by facial expression and by posture. These are happiness, apathy, fear, anger, and sadness.

A patient who is happy, self-assured, and in good personal control will generally have a relaxed face with a smile and a sparkle in her eyes. She is generally sitting relaxed and will offer the physician a warm and friendly greeting. Many new patients are apprehensive about meeting a new physician, and this apprehension may modify their usual expression of good spirits. Even under these circumstances, however, their warmth shows. Happy patients returning for visits after having established a relationship with a physician will usually be warm, relaxed, and responsive.

Apathetic patients generally have a blank facial expression. The eyes lack sparkle, there is little muscular movement of the face, and the mouth is generally thin and in a neutral position, neither turned up nor down. The posture may be somewhat slouched, the handshake weak, and answers to verbal questions short and unemotional. While apathetic patients may have severe emotional illness, they may also be demonstrating resignation to an imagined or real serious condition, or they may be responding to multiple problems, which make them feel overwhelmed.

The frightened patient will frequently have a tense expression on her face; her mouth will be tight and the eyes darting and narrow. She may be perspiring but have a dry mouth. Her posture demonstrates forward leaning, and there is often endless hand activity. When she reacts, it may be grossly out of proportion to offered stimuli.

The angry patient will frequently have narrowed eyes, furrowed brows, and narrow, tight lips. She may be sitting on the edge of her chair, leaning forward as if to pounce. Unlike the frightened patient, whose pose may be quite defensive, the angry patient radiates aggression. Her voice is usually harsh, and her overreaction to questions usually involves short, threatening phrases.

The sad patient generally sits with slouched shoulders, large, sad eyes, and a turned-down mouth. The eyes may glisten, and there may be tears. This patient is most likely depressed, and her speech reflects remorse and hopelessness.

By making observations of these nonverbal clues, the physician prepares for the way in which the interview will need to be conducted. Often an opening remark appropriate to the patient's demeanor may be useful, such as, "You seem sad today, Ms. Jones," or, "I detect a note of anger in your voice, Ms. Smith. Can you tell me why that is?" By so doing, the physician projects sensitivity to the patient's feelings and genuine care with respect to her circumstances. This is a good way to start.

HISTORY OUTLINE

   I. Observation—nonverbal clues
  II. Chief complaint
 III. History of gynecologic problem(s)
    A. Menstrual history—LMP, PMP
    B. Pregnancy history
    C. Vaginal and pelvic infections
    D. Gynecologic surgical procedures
    E. Urologic history
    F. Pelvic pain
    G. Vaginal bleeding
    H. Sexual status
    I. Contraceptive status
  IV. Significant health problems
    A. Systemic illnesses
    B. Surgical procedures
    C. Other hospitalizations
   V. Medications, habits, and allergies
    A. Medications taken
    B. Medication and other allergies
    C. Smoking history
    D. Alcohol usage
    E. Illicit drug usage
  VI. Bleeding problems
 VII. Family history
    A. Illnesses and causes of death of first-order relatives
    B. Congenital malformations, mental retardation, and reproductive wastage
VIII. Occupational and avocational history
  IX. Social history
   X. Review of systems
    A. Head
    B. Cardiovascular-respiratory
    C. Gastrointestinal
    D. Genitourinary
    E. Neuromuscular
    F. Psychiatric
      1. Physical abuse
      2. Sexual abuse
        a. Incest
        b. Rape

ESSENCE OF THE GYNECOLOGIC HISTORY

Chief Complaint

The patient should be encouraged to tell the physician why she has sought help. Questions such as, "What is the nature of the problem that brought you to me?" or, "How may I help you?" are good ways to begin. The patient should be able to present the problem as she sees it, in her own words, and should be interrupted only for specific clarification of points or to offer direction if she digresses too far. During the interview the physician should face the patient with direct eye contact and acknowledge important points of the history either by nodding or by a word or two. Such an approach allows the physician to be involved in the problem and demonstrates a degree of caring to the patient. When the patient has completed the history of her current problem, pertinent openended questions should be asked with respect to specific points made by the patient. This process will allow the physician to develop a more detailed data base. Directed questions may be asked where pertinent to clarify points. In general, however, the patient should be encouraged to tell her story as she sees it rather than to react with short answers to very specific questions. Under the latter circumstance the physician may get the answers he or she is looking for, but they may not be accurate answers.

A general outline for a gynecologic and general history is given in the box on p. 132. The outline is given in a specific order for general orientation. The information, however, may be collected through any comfortable discussion with the patient that seems appropriate in the circumstances. It is important that all aspects be covered.

Pertinent Gynecologic History

A pertinent gynecologic history can be divided into several parts. It begins with a menstrual history. The age of menarche should be noted, as should the duration of each monthly cycle and the number of days during which menses occur. The regularity of the menstrual cycles should be noted, and the dates of the last menstrual period and previous menstrual period should be obtained. In addition, the characteristics of the menstrual flow, including the color, the amount of flow, and accompanying symptoms such as cramping, sweating, headache, or diarrhea should be noted. In general, menstruation that occurs monthly (range 21 to 40 days), lasts 4 to 7 days, is bright red and is often accompanied by cramping on the day preceding and the first day of the period is characteristic of an ovulatory cycle. Menstruation that is irregular, often dark in color, painless, and frequently short or very long may indicate lack of ovulation. The first few cycles in teenagers or cycles in premenopausal women will frequently be anovulatory and as a result may come at irregular intervals.

The second pertinent point in the gynecologic history is that of previous pregnancies. The patient should be asked specifically to list pregnancies that she has experienced, including the year of the pregnancy, the duration, the type of delivery, the size, sex, and current condition of the baby, any complications that may have occurred, and whether the infant was breast fed and, if so, for how long. Elective terminations of pregnancy and spontaneous abortions should also be noted, including the time of gestation that they occurred and the circumstances under which they took place. Ectopic or molar pregnancies should also be noted, including the type of therapy that was given. When such events have occurred, obtaining old records for review is appropriate. Any pregnancy should be discussed with respect to excessive bleeding, chills, fever, known infection, or other complicating events. It is also appropriate to ask the patient about the individual who fathered each of these pregnancies so that the physician may determine the number of sexual partners the patient has had.

A history of vaginal and pelvic infections should be obtained. The patient should be asked what types of infection she has had in the past, what treatment was received, and what complications were suffered. All hospitalizations should be reviewed as to cause and outcome.

All instances of gynecologic surgical procedures should be noted. This would include minor operations such as endometrial biopsies; vulvar, vaginal, or cervical biopsies; dilation and curettage; laparoscopic examinations; and

---

IMPORTANT POINTS OF SEXUAL HISTORY

1. Sexual activity (presence of)
2. Types of relationships
3. Individual(s) involved
4. Satisfaction?
   a. Orgasmic?
5. Dyspareunia
6. Sexual dysfunction
   a. Patient
   b. Partner

---

any major procedure that the patient may have undergone. When such data are elicited, dates, types of procedures, diagnosis, and significant complications should be noted. In cases where pertinent, past records should be sought.

A careful urologic history should be taken. A history of bladder dysfunction, loss of urine, acute or chronic bladder or kidney infections, or other urologic problems such as hematuria or the passage of urinary stones should be noted.

Symptoms of pelvic pain or discomfort should be discussed fully. The pain should be described, noting the presence or absence of a relationship to the menstrual cycle and its association with other events such as coitus or bleeding.

If vaginal bleeding not related to menses has occurred, it should be noted as well as its relationship to the menstrual cycle and to other events such as coitus, the use of tampons, or the use of a contraceptive device.

A complete sexual history should be obtained (see box above). It should include whether the patient is sexually active, the types of relationships that she has, whether she is orgasmic, whether she experiences pain or discomfort with coitus (dyspareunia), and whether she or her partner is experiencing problems with sexual performance (sexual dysfunction). Specific problems should be evaluated. It is important that the physician review or rehearse the types of questions that will be asked and consider the response he or she will give to less typical answers (e.g., responses concerning homosexuality or less common sex-

ual practices). This will help prevent the physician from demonstrating surprise and thus transmitting an attitude of disapproval.

Finally, the patient's contraceptive history should be investigated, including methods used, length of time they have been used, and any complications that may have arisen.

Past General Health History

The patient should be asked to list any significant health problems that she has had during her lifetime. These should include all hospitalizations and operative procedures. It is reasonable for the physician to ask about specific illnesses such as diabetes, hepatitis, tuberculosis, or rheumatic fever that seem likely, based on what is known about the patient or about the patient's situation. Some physicians use a history checklist of the most common conditions, but a careful physician who questions appropriately can be equally effective.

Medications taken and reasons for doing so should be noted, as should allergic responses to medications.

The patient should be questioned for evidence of a bleeding or clotting problem, such as a history of hemorrhage with minor procedures, easy bruisability, or bleeding from mucous membranes.

A smoking history should be obtained in detail, including amount and time she has smoked. She should be questioned about the use of illicit drugs, including marijuana and cocaine. Any affirmative answers should be followed by specific questions concerning length of use, types of drugs used, and side effects that may have been noticed. Her use of alcohol should be detailed carefully, including the number of drinks per day and any history of binge drinking or previous therapy for alcoholism.

Family History

A detailed family history of first-order relatives (mother, father, sisters, brothers, children, and grandparents) should be taken and a family tree constructed (Fig. 5-1). Serious illnesses or causes of death for each individual should be noted. Also, an inquiry should be made about any congenital malformations,

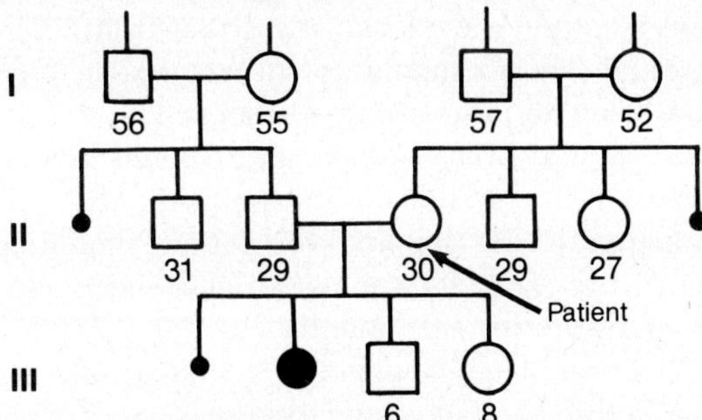

● Spontaneous miscarriage

◯ Living females

□ Living males

● Female who died neonatally because
of prematurity (30 weeks)

FIGURE 5-1
Family tree of typical gynecologic patient.

mental retardation, or pregnancy wastage in either the patient's or her husband's family. Such information may offer clues to hereditarily determined causes of reproductive problems.

Occupational and Social History

The patient should be asked to detail her and her husband's occupational histories, including jobs held and work performed. It is also useful to elicit a history of hobbies and other avocations that might affect health or reproductive capacity.

A social history should be obtained. This involves where and with whom the patient lives, other individuals in the household, areas of the world where the patient and her husband have lived or traveled, and unusual experiences that either may have had.

Review of Systems

A complete review of systems is necessary to uncover symptoms from other areas that relate to reproduction and gynecologic problems (e.g., serious headaches, epileptic seizures, dizziness, or fainting spells). Such a history also may indicate exposure to medications that may be injurious should a pregnancy occur in the future.

It is important to obtain a good cardiovascular-respiratory history as well as a history of hypertension, heart disease, or chest problems such as asthma. Each of these may have an immediate effect on the patient and may also influence a future pregnancy.

Gastrointestinal areas of importance to the gynecologist would be a history of functional bowel problems or hepatitis. Affirmative answers should be investigated more fully with respect to specific illnesses and potential residuals that may affect the patient's current health.

Genitourinary questions are important both from the standpoint of bladder function and as an indication of whether renal function has been or is impaired.

Neurologic or neuromuscular impairment may be important from the standpoint of the ability of the patient to carry and deliver a child without difficulty.

A history of vascular disease, including thrombophlebitis with or without pulmonary embolism, varicose veins, or other vascular problems, should be sought.

The psychiatric history should be detailed carefully for any history of emotional or mental disease processes. In addition, the patient should be asked specifically whether she has ever been sexually abused in adult life, in childhood, by a stranger, or incestuously, or raped. This will be further discussed in Chapter 12.

ESSENCE OF COMPLETE PHYSICAL EXAMINATION

The gynecologist should perform a complete physical examination on every patient at the first visit and at each annual checkup, particularly if the gynecologist is the primary physician caring for the patient. Physical examination is a time to both gather information about the patient and teach the patient information she should know about herself and her body.

The patient should disrobe completely and be covered by a hospital gown that ensures warmth and modesty. During each step of the examination she should be allowed to maintain personal control by being offered options whenever possible. These options begin with the presence or absence of a chaperone. The chaperone, a third party, usually a woman, serves a variety of purposes. She may offer warmth, compassion, and support to the patient during uncomfortable or potentially embarrassing portions of the examination. She may help the physician to carry out procedures such as the Papanicolaou (Pap) smear, and in some cases she offers the physician protection from having his intentions misunderstood by a naive or suspicious individual. While the presence of a chaperone is not absolutely imperative in every doctor/patient relationship, the availability of one for the specific instance where it is deemed advisable should be ensured. Many clinics insist on the presence of a chaperone, and it is wise for the physician to follow local custom.

The examination should begin with a general evaluation of the patient's appearance and posture. Her weight and her blood pressure should be taken initially, and postmenopausal women should have their height measured routinely to document evidence of osteoporosis, which causes vertebral compression fractures.

The patient's eyes, ears, nose, and throat should be examined. Fundoscopic examination should be performed at least annually to inspect the blood vessels of the retina and to observe the lens for evidence of early cataract formation. The gynecologist should either measure intraocular pressures in women over age 40 or suggest that they be seen by an ophthalmologist for this purpose. The patient should be inspected for evidence of upper lip or chin hair, which may indicate increased androgen activity.

The thyroid gland should be palpated for irregularities or increase in size (goiter). Discrete areas of enlargement, hardness, and tenderness should be described. The patient's neck should be palpated for evidence of adenopathy along the supraclavicular and posterior auricular chains.

The chest should be inspected for symmetry of movement of the diaphragms, percussed for areas of consolidation, and auscultated bilaterally for breath and adventitious sounds.

The heart should be examined by palpation for points of maximum impulse, percussed for size, and auscultated for irregularities of rate and evidence of murmurs and other adventitious sounds. An older woman's neck should be auscultated for evidence of vascular bruits. The patient's heart should be auscultated in both the lying and the sitting positions.

A careful breast examination should be carried out in a systematic fashion as described in Chapter 13. At this time the patient should be taught breast self-examination and encouraged to perform this each month.

The abdomen should be systematically examined in the following fashion.

Inspection: the abdomen should be inspected for symmetry; scars, protuberance, or discoloration of the skin; and striations, which may suggest previous pregnancies or adrenal gland hyperactivity. The hair pattern should be noted. The typical female pattern is that of an inverted triangle over the mons pubis. A male pattern involves hair growth between the area of the mons pubis and the umbilicus, also known as a diamond pattern. This may indicate excessive androgen activity (Fig. 5-2).

Palpation: the abdomen should be palpated for organomegaly (enlarged organs), particularly involving the liver, spleen, kidneys, and uterus, and for adnexal masses, which may be palpated abdominally. Palpation also affords the possibility of noting a fluid wave, which would suggest either ascites or hemoperitoneum. Palpation will also yield evidence for rigidity of the abdomen, which would imply spasm in the rectus muscles secondary to intra-abdominal irritation. Where the irritation is caused by intra-abdominal hemorrhage or infection, this rigidity is often evidence of an acute abdomen. During the palpation of the abdomen the physician should elicit the phenomenon of *rebound*, which also signifies intra-abdominal irritation. This is elicited by gently pressing the abdomen and then releasing. The release may cause pain either under the spot (direct rebound) or in a different portion of the abdomen (referred rebound). It should be noted, however, that sudden rough pressure may cause pain even in a normal patient.

Percussion: percussion affords the ability to differentiate fluid waves and to outline solid organs and masses.

Auscultation: the physician should listen for bowel sounds. Hypoactive or absent bowel sounds may imply an ileus caused by peritoneal irritation of the bowel. Hyperactive bowel sounds may imply intrinsic irritation of the

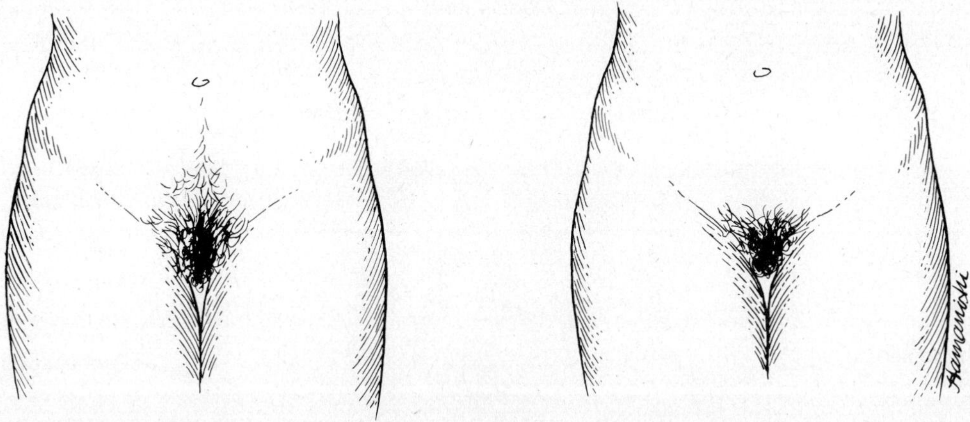

FIGURE 5-2
Normal female pubic hair pattern *(right)* and hair pattern of female showing male (androgenized) pattern.

bowel or partial or complete bowel obstruction.

The area of the groins should be palpated for adenopathy and inguinal hernias. The physician should also elicit the femoral pulses beneath the groin in the femoral triangles, and when these are present, they should be noted from the standpoint of differences that may exist between the two femoral areas.

Legs should be examined for evidence of varicose veins, edema, and other lesions. In addition, it is reasonable to judge arterial circulation to the extremities by palpating pedal pulses on the dorsum of the foot.

PELVIC EXAMINATION

The pelvic examination is conducted with the patient lying supine on the examining table with the legs in stirrups. The patient may or may not desire to be draped with a sheet. Since the physician should be pointing out aspects of the patient's pelvic anatomy where possible, many patients prefer to have the head of the table elevated and to use a small hand mirror to follow the examination with the physician. In such instances, a sheet may be cumbersome. The physician should be sure the patient is as relaxed as possible and should take a few minutes to describe the procedure and allow the shy or nervous patient to prepare herself. Suggesting that the patient allow her legs to fall wide apart and to concentrate on relaxing her abdominal muscles may be helpful.

Inspection

The perineum should be carefully inspected beginning with the mons pubis. The quality and pattern of the hair on the mons and the labia majora should be noted. Areas of alopecia should be noted, as they may imply a skin abnormality. In general, as a woman ages, the pubic hair becomes less dense and may turn grey. During the inspection of the pubic hair the physician should look for evidence of body lice (pediculosis). Next, the skin of the perineum is inspected for redness, excoriation, discoloration, or loss of pigment and for the presence of vesicles, ulcerations, pustules, warty growths, or neoplastic growths. In addition, pigmented nevi or other pigmented lesions should be noted, as should varicose veins. Skin scars denoting previous episiotomy or other obstetrical lacerations should be noted.

Inspection should then systematically evaluate the specific structures of the perineum. The clitoris should be noted and its size and shape described. Normally it is 1 to 1.5 cm in length. Any irregularities or abnormalities of the labia majora or minora should be noted and carefully described. At times these areas are injured by trauma related to coitus, accidental injury, or birth. The patient should be questioned about evidence for trauma when appropriate.

The introitus should be observed closely. Whether the hymen is intact, imperforate, or marital and whether the perineum gapes or re-

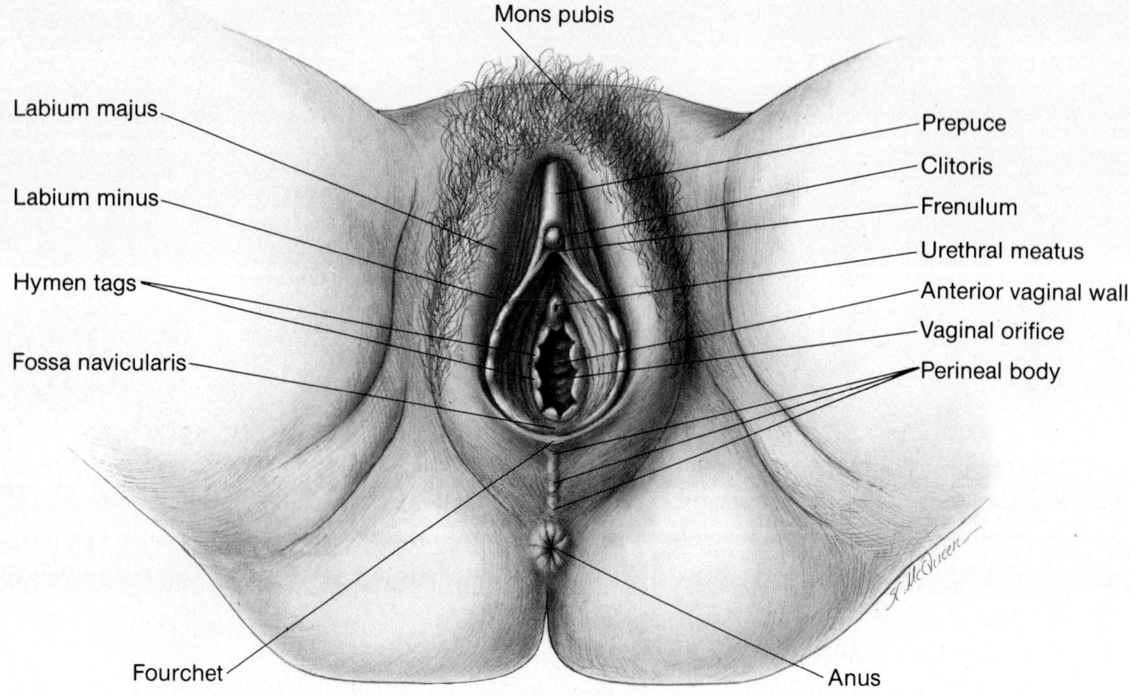

FIGURE 5-3
Normal female perineum. (Redrawn from Krantz KE: Anatomy of the female reproductive system. In Benson RC, ed: Current obstetric and gynecologic diagnosis and treatment, 5th ed. Los Altos, Calif., Lange Medical Publications, 1984.)

mains closed in the usual lithotomy position should be noted.

The perineal body should be inspected. This is the area at the posterior aspect of the labia where the muscles of the superficial perineal compartment come together. It represents the focal point of support for the perineum and is between the vagina and the rectum. The perianal area is then inspected for evidence of hemorrhoids, sphincter continence, and other lesions (Fig. 5-3).

Palpation

The next step in the examination of the perineum involves palpation. With the second and fourth fingers of the gloved hand separating the labia minora, the urethra is inspected and the length of the urethra is palpated and "milked" with the middle finger. In this way, irregularities and inflammation of Skene's glands (periurethral glands), pus or mucus expressed, or a suburethral diverticulum can be noted. Any

pus expressed from the urethra should be submitted to Gram stain and cultured, because it is frequently found to contain gonococcus. The gloved hand then palpates the area of the posterior third of the labia majora, placing the index finger inside the introitus and the thumb on the outside of the labium. In this way, enlargements or cysts of Bartholin glands are noted. This exercise should be performed on each side.

With the gloved hand holding the labia apart, the opening of the vagina should be inspected. The presence of a cystocele or a cystourethrocele should be noted. This would be seen as a bulging of vaginal mucosa downward from the anterior wall of the vagina. The presence of this abnormality may be noted either by simply observing or by asking the patient to bear down (Fig. 5-4). Likewise, the posterior wall should be noted for a bulging upward, which would represent a rectocele (Fig. 5-5). Also, with the patient bearing down, the cervix may become visible, indicating prolapse of the

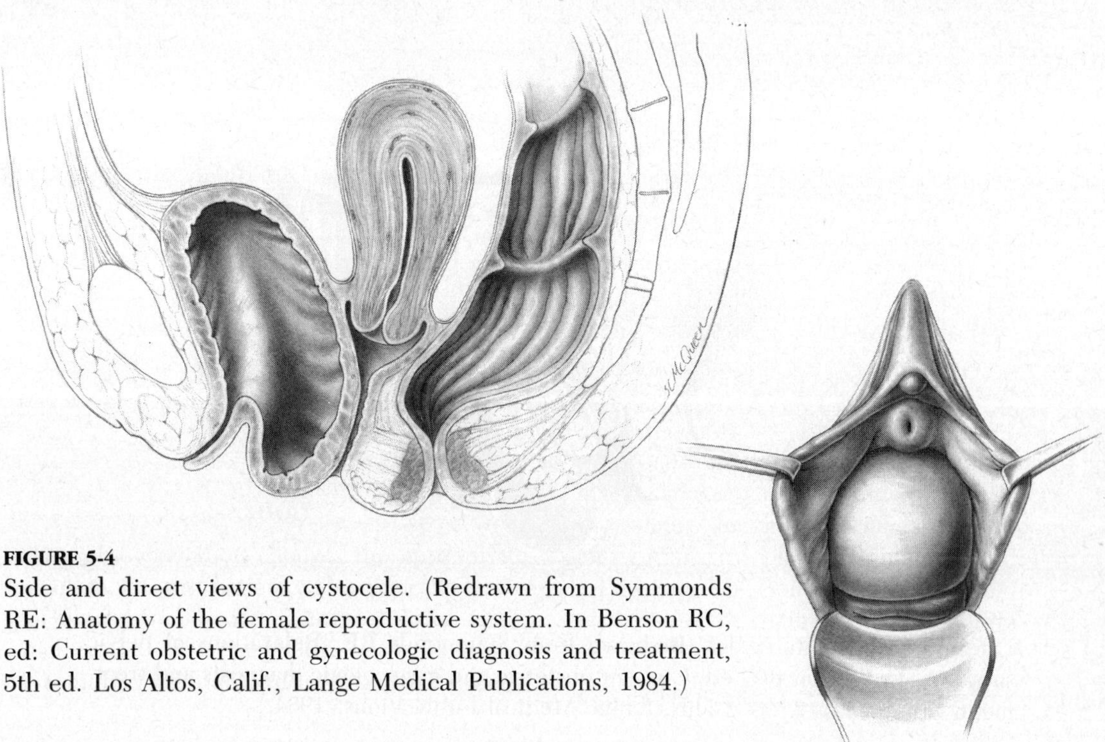

FIGURE 5-4

Side and direct views of cystocele. (Redrawn from Symmonds RE: Anatomy of the female reproductive system. In Benson RC, ed: Current obstetric and gynecologic diagnosis and treatment, 5th ed. Los Altos, Calif., Lange Medical Publications, 1984.)

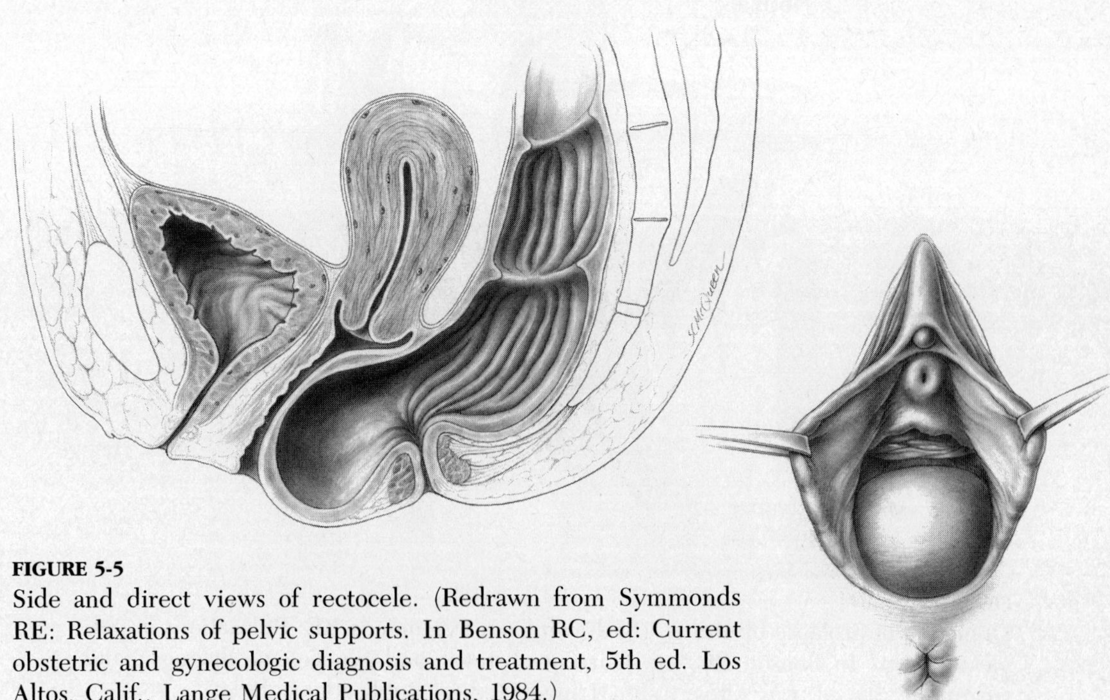

FIGURE 5-5

Side and direct views of rectocele. (Redrawn from Symmonds RE: Relaxations of pelvic supports. In Benson RC, ed: Current obstetric and gynecologic diagnosis and treatment, 5th ed. Los Altos, Calif., Lange Medical Publications, 1984.)

itated by placing two fingers into the introitus and pressing down.

Once the blades are inserted, the speculum should be turned so that the transverse axis of the blades is in the transverse axis of the vagina. The blades should be inserted to their full length and then opened so that the physician may inspect for the position of the cervix. The cervix generally fits into the open blades with ease. If this does not occur, the physician should inspect for the position of the cervix with his or her finger and then reinsert the speculum accordingly. Once the blades are inserted and the cervix visualized, the speculum should be opened and the introitus widened so that the cervix can be adequately inspected and a Pap smear taken. This can be done by using the screw adjustment on the base of the speculum. When inserted properly the speculum will generally stay in place without falling out.

The physician then inspects the vagina and cervix. The vaginal canal is inspected during the insertion of the speculum or on its removal. The mucosa should be noted for evidence of erythema or lesions. Fluid discharge should be evaluated on slides prepared in the following fashion. One drop of vaginal secretion is placed in one drop of sodium chloride solution, coverslipped, and inspected for unicellular flagulated protozoa, *Trichomonas vaginalis*. The vaginal epithelium should also be inspected. The cells should have sharp borders and normal-appearing nuclei. Any variation from the normal may imply infection (see Chapter 21). A drop of potassium hydroxide is placed on another slide and a drop of vaginal secretion is placed within this. The potassium hydroxide will cause lysis of the epithelial cells and trichomonads but leave intact the mycelium of *Monilia*. Thus the presence of mycelium is helpful in diagnosing

vaginal moniliasis. Vaginal lesions such as areas of adenosis (see DES Chapter 14), clear cystic structures (Gartner's cysts), or inclusion cysts on the lines of scars or episiotomy incisions should be noted.

The cervix is inspected next. It should be pink, shiny, and clear. In a nulliparous individual, the external os should be round. When a woman is parous, the external os will take on a fishmouth appearance, and if there have been cervical lacerations, healed stellate lacerations may be noted (Fig. 5-9). Normally the transformation zone (i.e., the junction of squamous and columnar epithelium) is just barely visible inside the external os. Occasionally glandular epithelium may be present on the portio vaginalis, moving the transformation zone onto the portio. This is common in teenage women, women who have been exposed to diethylstilbestrol in utero, some women with vaginitis, or women immediately postpartum or postabortion. Generally, this is cleared by a process of metaplasia in which squamous epithelium covers the columnar epithelium. This process, however, may leave small areas of irregularities and inclusion cysts. These are called nabothian cysts and may be seen in various sizes and shapes. They are of no clinical significance. Often after a women has delivered a baby there is lateral scarring at the 3 and 9 o'clock positions, causing an eversion of the external os so that the reddened columnar epithelium is visible on the anterior and posterior lips of the cervix. If the observer looks closely, the transitional zone can be seen along the edges of this area of eversion and may be perfectly healthy. This is called an *ectropion* and is not evidence of a pathologic condition.

Any lesions of the cervix should be noted and, where appropriate, biopsied. In a patient

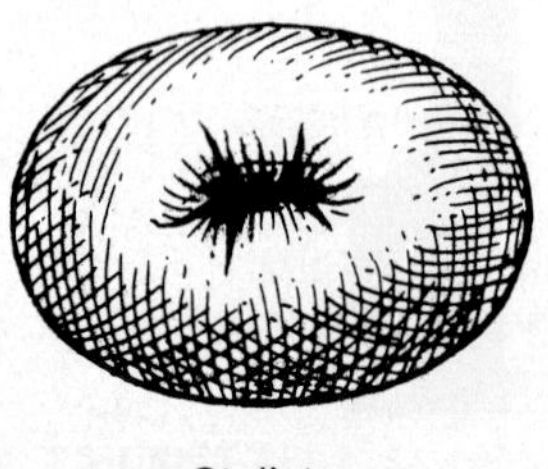
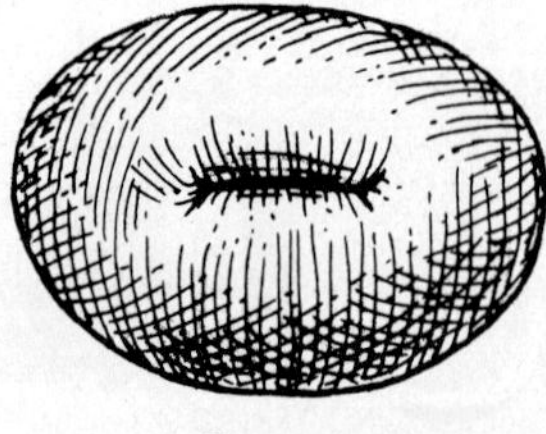
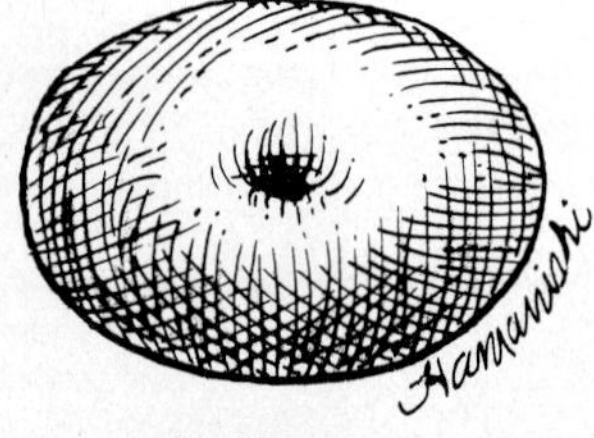

FIGURE 5-9
Nulliparous, parous, and stellate lacerations of cervix.

with acute herpes progenitalis, vesicles or ulcers may be noted. In a patient infected with human papillomavirus, warts (condyloma acuminata) on the cervix may also be observed.

Papanicolaou Smear

At this point in the examination a Pap smear is usually taken. In 1943 Papanicolaou and Trout published their now classic monograph demonstrating the value of vaginal and cervical cytology as a screening tool for cervical neoplasm. With the use of the Pap smear in screening programs, the incidence of invasive cervical cancer has been reduced 50%. Recently, programs focusing on cost-effectiveness have suggested that the screening interval may be extended from the usual 1 year to 3 years in certain low-risk individuals. Since low risk is often difficult to define, the American College of Obstetricians and Gynecologists suggested in 1984 that annual screening was appropriate for most American women. Initial screening should begin at age 18 or when the individual becomes sexually active. High-risk women, those with a history of early sexual activity and multiple partners, should be screened annually. Those patients with later exposure to coitus who have only one sexual partner and who have had two successive negative annual smears may be considered low-risk and should be screened every 1 to 3 years at the discretion of the physician.

There are a number of ways of carrying out this examination. The major objective is to sample secretions from the endocervical canal and to scrape the transitional zone. It is also useful to sample the vaginal pool, although this does not usually yield as high an incidence of cervical disease as does sampling of the canal and the transitional zone. One way of performing the Pap smear is presented:

1. After excess mucus is gently removed, a cotton-tipped swab is placed into the endocervical canal and rotated. The mucus is smeared thinly on a slide by rotation of the swab on the glass. This is labelled *endocervix* and fixed immediately either by a spray fix or by immersing the slide into a fixative solution (Fig. 5-10).
2. Using an Ayers' spatula or some variation thereof, the entire transformation zone is scraped and smeared thinly on a second slide, which is immediately fixed. If the physician wishes a sample of the vaginal pool, this may be taken with the reverse side of the Ayers spatula and smeared on a third slide or on a second portion of the slide containing the transformation zone material (Fig. 5-11).

A number of fixatives are available but it is important that they be applied immediately before drying and distortion of the cells takes place. Pap smears are currently reported using the following descriptive system:

Normal
Atypical
  Inflammation
  Possible dysplasia
Metaplasia
Mild dysplasia
Moderate dysplasia
Severe dysplasia—carcinoma in situ
Invasive cancer

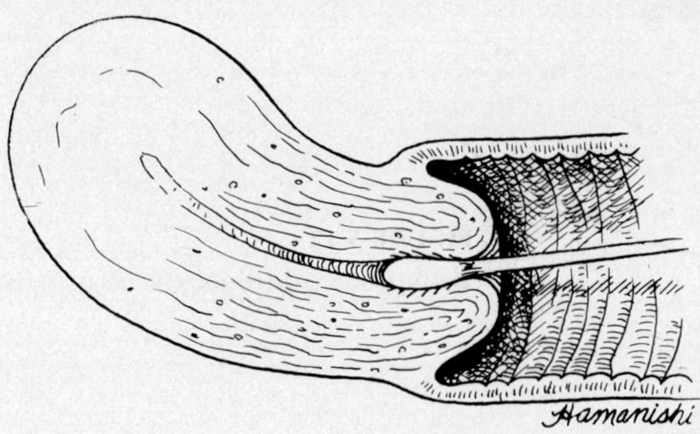

FIGURE 5-10
Obtaining cells from endocervix.

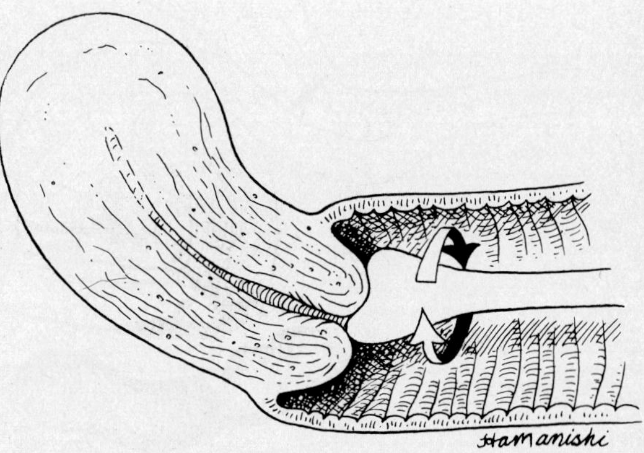

FIGURE 5-11
Obtaining cells from transformation zone using Ayers' spatula.

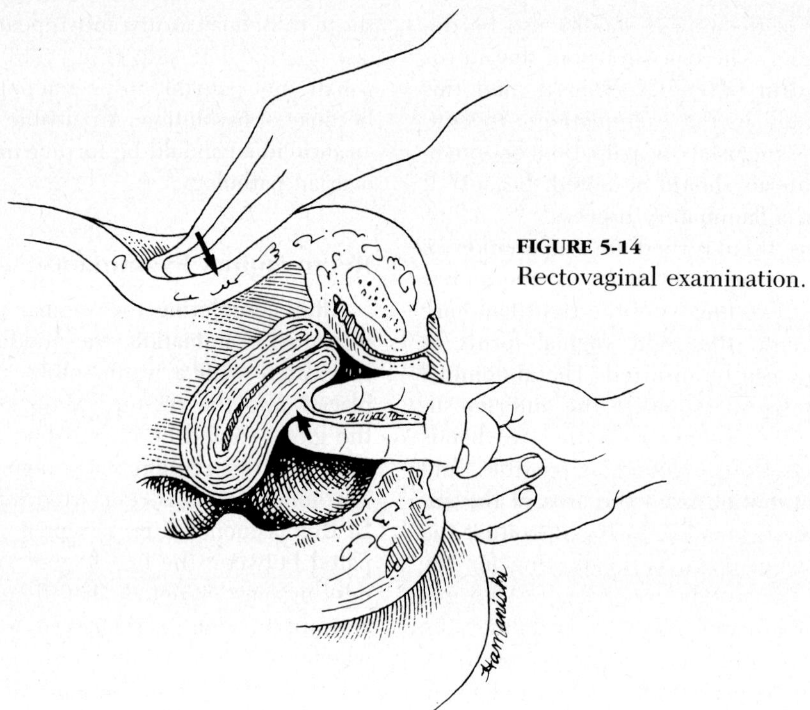

FIGURE 5-14
Rectovaginal examination.

Rectal Examination

The rectum is then palpated in all dimensions with the rectal examining finger. It should be possible to palpate up to 70% of bowel lesions with the rectal finger. Since bowel cancer is common in women, particularly after the age of 35, this part of the examination should not be overlooked. The physician should also note the tone of the anal sphincter and any other anal pathology such as hemorrhoids, fissures, or masses. Finally, a stool sample is taken on the examining finger and tested for occult blood. This is particularly important in women past the age of 35 who may be at risk for bowel cancer.

At the end of the examination the physician should give the patient some tissue so that she may remove the lubricating jelly from her perineum before she dresses.

It is important that each step of the examination be explained to the patient and that she be reassured about all normal findings. Wherever possible, abnormal findings should be pointed out to the patient either by allowing her to palpate the pathologic condition or by demonstrating it to her using a hand mirror. It is also appropriate to demonstrate normal structures to the patient, such as the cervix and portions of the vagina that she may be able to see with her hand mirror. The physician should use the examination as a vehicle for teaching the patient about her body.

KEY POINTS

- Five general impressions of patients may be gleaned nonverbally (by observation). They are happiness, apathy, fear, anger, and sadness.

- Menstrual history includes age of menarche, number of days of cycle, number of days of flow, presence of bleeding between menstrual periods, the date of the last menstrual period, and the date of the previous menstrual period.

- Menstrual cycles occurring just after puberty and just before menopause are frequently anovulatory and may be irregular in frequency.

- Pregnancy history should include the details of term and premature labors, spontaneous abortion, ectopic pregnancies, molar pregnancies, and terminations.

- A complete gynecologic evaluation should always include a sexual history, contraceptive history, and history of physical or sexual abuse.

- A detailed family history includes inquiry about congenital malformations, mental retardations, or pregnancy wastage in the families of the patient and her husband.

- Occupational and avocational activity should be investigated for the presence of potential hazards to the patient's health.

- Pap smears should be performed every 1 to 3 years, depending on the patient's risk level.

- Sexually active women should be evaluated at appropriate intervals for sexually transmitted diseases.

- The physician should use the occasion of the history and physical examination to teach the patient important aspects of self-evaluation.

BIBLIOGRAPHY

American College of Obstetricians and Gynecologists: Cervical Cytology: Evaluation and Management of Abnormalities. Tech Bull 81, 1984.

Papanicolaou GN, Trout HF: Diagnosis of uterine cancer by vaginal smears. New York, The Commonwealth Fund, 1943.

Significant Symptoms and Signs in Different Age Groups

KEY TERMS AND DEFINITIONS

Hematocolpos. Distension of an obstructed vagina (caused by imperforate hymen or transverse septum) with blood and blood products.

Hematometria. A uterus distended with blood, secondary to partial or complete obstruction of any portion of the lower genital tract.

Levator Spasm. Spasm of the levator ani muscles frequently associated with chronic pelvic pain or vaginismus.

Pain. An unpleasant sensory or emotional experience associated with actual or potential tissue damage or described in terms of such damage.

Pelvic Congestion Syndrome. Vascular engorgement of the uterus and the vessels of the broad ligament and lateral pelvic walls, which may lead to chronic pelvic pain.

Trigger Points. Painful spasm of local muscle bundles or areas of scar tissue within the abdominal wall, at times associated with chronic pelvic and lower abdominal pain.

The gynecologist will evaluate a variety of women at different periods of life for relatively few specific symptoms and signs. Perhaps the three most common of these are unusual vaginal bleeding, pelvic pain, and pelvic or abdominal mass. While each of these complaints will be of concern to the individual patient, their diagnostic implications may vary greatly depending on the patient's age. This chapter considers unusual vaginal bleeding, pelvic pain, and pelvic or abdominal mass from the standpoint of differential diagnosis, emphasizing the differences seen at different periods of a woman's life, and includes a detailed consideration of the problem of chronic pelvic pain.

VAGINAL BLEEDING

Abnormal vaginal bleeding includes prepubertal bleeding, menorrhagia, metrorrhagia or postcoital bleeding, and postmenopausal bleeding. Although the cause of the bleeding will frequently determine the characteristics that it exhibits, the physician should develop a systematic approach to the differential diagnosis of abnormal vaginal bleeding. The box on p. 149 offers an outline that can be followed in considering a patient with abnormal vaginal bleeding. In addition, Chapter 35 considers this topic in detail.

Pregnancy

The presence of a pregnancy must be considered in any woman in the reproductive years. This possibility can be rapidly ruled out using a sensitive serum pregnancy test. If the patient is found to be pregnant and vaginal bleeding is noted, the diagnostic possibilities include implantation bleeding; threatened, inevitable, complete, or incomplete abortion; ectopic pregnancy; and molar pregnancy.

Implantation bleeding is quite common. It usually consists of minimal bleeding at about

ETIOLOGY OF ABNORMAL VAGINAL BLEEDING

Pregnancy
  Abortion
    Threatened
    Inevitable
    Complete
    Incomplete
  Ectopic
  Molar—trophoblastic disease
Dysfunctional uterine bleeding
  Postpuberty
  During reproductive years
  Perimenopausal
Neoplastic
  Vulva and vagina
  Cervix
  Uterine corpus
  Fallopian tube
  Ovary
  Other
Inflammatory
  Vulvitis and vaginitis
  Cervicitis
  Endometritis
  Pelvic inflammatory disease
Traumatic
  Foreign body
  Direct trauma
Systemic diseases
  Coagulopathies
  Blood dyscrasias
  Endocrinopathy
  Drug effects
  Others

the time of the first missed menstrual period and generally lasts a very short time. Occasionally it may be present for 1 to 2 days with a flow similar to that of a menstrual period. Often implantation bleeding is not perceptible to the patient but can be seen by the physician as a brownish-tinged cervical mucus if a pelvic examination is performed. Bleeding in excess of a normal menstrual flow is quite rare, and prolonged bleeding does not usually occur.

Bleeding in the first trimester of pregnancy is not uncommon. About 20% to 25% of all pregnant women will spot or bleed in the first trimester. If the bleeding can be observed to be coming from the cervix and the cervix is closed, a diagnosis of threatened abortion can be made (Chapter 15). The uterus should be consistent in size with what is normal for the dates of the pregnancy and may or may not be contracting and tender to the touch. A threatened abortion becomes inevitable when the cervix dilates and products of conception pass through the internal os or when the bleeding is profuse. A complete abortion is noted when the uterus has expelled its contents, the internal os is closed, the bleeding is minimal, and the uterus has returned to near normal size. It is unusual for a patient who has a complete abortion to experience significant pelvic cramping or to cramp when an uterotonic agent such as ergonovine maleate (Ergotrate) or methylergonovine maleate (Methergine) is administered. Incomplete abortion occurs when part of the products of conception have been expelled but others remain within the uterus. The cervix is generally dilated, and there is usually bleeding, which may be profuse. The uterus is generally enlarged, and the patient may experience cramping pain. Most gestations of 6 weeks or less from the time of the last menstrual period will abort completely. Incomplete abortions become more common after 6 weeks of gestation.

A missed abortion occurs when the embryo dies but the products of conception are not expelled from the uterus. Generally the uterus involutes so that it is smaller than expected by dates. There may be dark red or brownish vaginal bleeding, often minimal in amount. Pregnancy tests may remain positive for quite some time in the face of a missed abortion. Such conditions are more common when progestational agents have been given in the hopes of supporting the pregnancy.

Ectopic pregnancies are quite common and seem to be becoming more prevalent (Chapter 16). Currently about 1% of all pregnancies end as ectopic pregnancies but these figures vary from group to group. An ectopic pregnancy is defined as one that is implanted outside of the endometrial cavity. Thus an ectopic pregnancy may exist in the cervix, within various portions of a fallopian tube, in the ovary, in the peritoneal cavity, and, in some rare instances, within the myometrium or a distant organ such as the spleen. A primary ectopic pregnancy in a specific organ implies that the pregnancy was implanted directly within that organ. A secondary ectopic pregnancy implies that the pregnancy ruptured from the fallopian tube and reimplanted completely or partially on another organ.

Ectopic pregnancies cause vaginal bleeding because of the separation of the decidua from the endometrium as the ectopic pregnancy dies or because of direct bleeding from the site of the ectopic pregnancy, with the blood being transported to the uterus and through the cervix. In most but not all cases the patient misses at least one menstrual period, begins to bleed from scant to significant amounts, and generally experiences pelvic pain. The pain may be limited to one side, in the case of a fallopian tube pregnancy, or may present as a more generalized pelvic pain. The pain may be similar to that experienced with pelvic inflammatory disease, but the patient with an ectopic pregnancy has a low-grade temperature or is afebrile.

If the ectopic pregnancy is ruptured, intraperitoneal hemorrhage may occur and the patient may exhibit signs and symptoms of hypovolemia. Such an acute situation requires rapid intervention.

Ectopic pregnancies become a diagnostic problem when they are unruptured. Vaginal bleeding occurs in about 90% of early ectopic pregnancies that are unruptured, and almost all such patients experience pain. The uterus may be slightly enlarged or seem to be normal in size. If the ectopic pregnancy is tubal or ovarian, an adnexal mass may be noted. However, adnexal masses are not uncommon in normal pregnancies, representing the corpus luteum of pregnancy, and this may make the differential diagnosis somewhat more difficult.

With the availability of serum pregnancy tests, rapidly ascertaining the fact that the patient is pregnant is possible. When a pregnancy is diagnosed it becomes necessary to establish whether it is intrauterine or ectopic. An ultrasound examination may be of help. If the pregnancy has progressed beyond 6 weeks' gestation it is frequently possible to see a pregnancy sac within the uterine cavity. Occasionally such a sac may be seen outside the uterine cavity in an adnexa.

Several authors have attempted to compare the levels of human chorionic gonadotrophin (HCG) with the gestational age of the pregnancy and determine from this whether or not a normal pregnancy is developing. However, it is not yet possible to differentiate with certainty between an intrauterine and an ectopic pregnancy by relating levels of HCG to the presence or absence of a sac. This is discussed more completely in Chapter 16.

In a patient experiencing vaginal bleeding and pelvic pain who has a positive pregnancy test and who does not exhibit a gestational sac within the uterus on ultrasound, the physician should consider laparoscopy for a definitive diagnosis. A gestational sac appearing outside the uterine cavity may be suggestive of an ectopic pregnancy, but frequent error has been noted in such diagnoses and often the gestational sac does turn out to be intrauterine. Nonetheless, when there is an element of doubt the physician may wish to consider laparoscopy for definitive diagnosis.

If the patient appears to have intraperitoneal bleeding, a culdocentesis may help. The presence of unclotted blood within the peritoneal cavity is evidence for intraperitoneal hemorrhage. Either a laparotomy or laparoscopy should be undertaken. This procedure may be preceded by dilation and curettage (D&C) with evaluation of the curetting for evidence of products of conception. If these are not noted by visualizing fetal parts, by seeing villi when tissue is floated on water, or by frozen section and microscopic evaluation, then further operative intervention is required.

Several types of patients are at high risk for ectopic pregnancy. These include women who have had previous ectopic pregnancies, those who have undergone tubal reparative procedures, and those who have had previous pelvic infections. Ectopic pregnancy should also be considered in users of intrauterine devices (IUDs), since IUDs only partially protect from tubular implantation.

Another cause of abnormal vaginal bleeding associated with pregnancy is trophoblastic disease (Chapter 33). Most trophoblastic tumors are hydatidiform moles, which occur about once in every 1000 gestations. Although they may present in a variety of ways, the classic molar pregnancy may include vaginal bleeding and a uterus enlarged beyond the size expected for gestational age. These findings may be associated with the passage of grapelike structures per vaginum, representing hydropic villi. At times hypertension, edema, and proteinuria occur. Some molar pregnancies are associated with uteri that are small or normal for gestational age. In these cases the diagnosis may be suspected by an elevation of quantitative chorionic gonadotrophin greater than 100,000 mIU/ml. Molar pregnancy must be differentiated from normal gestation, multiple gestation, and uterine enlargements caused by other factors such as uterine myoma. Bleeding that occurs in the second trimester and is associated with hydatidiform mole may also be associated with a uterus that is large for gestational age; this will also need to be differentiated from hydramnios. An ultrasound examination in the late first trimester or early second trimester will generally detect hydatidiform mole and help in the differential diagnosis of other conditions such as multiple gestation, hydramnios, and other uterine disorders.

Dysfunctional Uterine Bleeding

The endocrinology of this problem is covered in Chapter 35. The frequency with which dysfunctional uterine bleeding occurs, however, is such that it is an important consideration in the differential diagnosis of abnormal vaginal bleeding. The common denominator in most patients with dysfunctional uterine bleeding is anovulation or short ovulatory cycle. It is most commonly seen in the postpubertal period when normal hypothalamic function is not well established. In most instances, menstrual periods occur irregularly, often with long gaps between menses. When menses occurs it may vary from very heavy flow to scanty flow and may continue for a number of days. The bleeding in most instances is from a nonsecretory endometrium. Occasionally the bleeding is profuse with associated signs and symptoms of hypovolemia, requiring emergency care. Endometrial sampling will generally yield scanty nonsecretory endometrium. Rarely is any other pathologic condition noted.

Women in the perimenopausal period who are undergoing some early evidence of ovarian failure may also experience dysfunctional uterine bleeding. Again the pattern may be one of irregularity, and the flow may vary from one that is increased in amount with clots to a scant flow with prolonged spotting. Endometrial biopsy or D&C may yield a pathologic diagnosis of nonsecretory endometrium, but hyperplasia of the endometrium may also be noted. In perimenopausal women it is important to differentiate dysfunctional uterine bleeding from other intrauterine disease, and endometrial sampling is indicated. An endometrial biopsy is generally sufficient to establish the appropriate diagnosis and rule out more serious conditions.

Dysfunctional uterine bleeding may also occur during the reproductive years. It may be associated with polycystic ovarian disease or as a secondary symptom to stress, excessive weight change, or increased exercise performance. In such instances amenorrhea, oligomenorrhea, menorrhagia, or metrorrhagia may all be seen. Endometrial sampling generally produces nonsecretory endometrium; rarely is specific disease seen. In patients with polycystic ovarian disease, hyperplastic endometrium may be present. This is discussed more fully in Chapter 35.

Neoplastic Conditions

Although vaginal bleeding can be caused by a wide variety of neoplastic lesions, both benign and malignant and affecting the various organs of the female reproductive tract, there are specific patterns that are typical of many of these (Table 6-1). In addition, knowledge of occurrence rates of specific neoplasms in various age groups may help the physician in developing a differential diagnosis.

Cancers of the vulva and vagina may present with vaginal bleeding and usually occur in women who are in the latter reproductive years or in the postmenopausal period. Should they occur in women during the reproductive years, the bleeding is generally intermittent and therefore presents as metrorrhagia or postcoital bleeding rather than with any specific relationship to the menstrual cycle. The bleeding is generally minimal, although in advanced cases it can become profuse. An unusual vaginal tumor that may occur in teenage or young women is clear-cell cancer of the vagina, which is most often seen in women who have been exposed in utero to diethylstilbestrol (DES).

TABLE 6-1
Bleeding Pattern Seen in Tumors of the Reproductive Tract

Condition	Menorrhagia	Metrorrhagia	Postmenopausal Bleeding
Vulvar cancer	−	+ +	+ +
Vaginal cancer	−	+ +	+ +
Cervical cancer	−	+ +	+ +
Cervical polyp	−	+ +	+
Uterine myoma	+ +	+	−
Carcinoma of endometrium	−	−	+ +
Fallopian tube cancer	−	−	+
Ovarian cancer	−	±	±

Since this condition was first described by Herbst et al in 1971, the actual incidence has been found to be quite low in such women (Chapter 14). In addition, rare cases of clear-cell cancer of the vagina have been found in women who were not exposed to DES.

Tumors of the cervix are most often squamous cell carcinomas, although as many as 10% are adenocarcinomas and may be present within the endocervical canal (Chapter 27). Such lesions will generally bleed sooner or later, and the bleeding pattern will be one of metrorrhagia or postcoital staining. With larger lesions the bleeding may be quite profuse. Other cervical lesions such as endocervical polyps may also cause metrorrhagia.

The most common lesions of the uterine corpus that cause abnormal bleeding during the reproductive years are leiomyomas (fibroids). Although these are generally benign, they may become quite large and may cause menorrhagia or menometrorrhagia (Chapter 17). Submucous myomata are generally associated with severe menorrhagia. Leiomyomas rarely cause vaginal bleeding in postmenopausal women. Endometrial carcinoma, generally an adenocarcinoma but occasionally a sarcoma, carcinosarcoma, or some intermediate variety, will cause vaginal bleeding (Chapter 28). Most of these occur in postmenopausal women and therefore would present as postmenopausal bleeding. The bleeding may be scant or profuse. Approximately 5% of endometrial adenocarcinomas occur in premenopausal women. These women most often are exposed to continuous endoge-

nous estrogen stimulation and are often found to have polycystic ovarian disease or a functioning ovarian tumor such as a granulosal cell tumor or a thecoma. When adenocarcinoma occurs in premenopausal women, these diagnostic possibilities should be considered.

Vaginal bleeding in association with fallopian tube cancer is quite rare and generally occurs in the postmenopausal woman. Nonetheless, scant vaginal bleeding associated frequently with a watery discharge and occasionally with an adnexal mass should alert the physician to the possibility of this condition (Chapter 32).

Ovarian cancers may present with vaginal bleeding, which is most often the result of intraperitoneal blood finding its way through the fallopian tube and through the uterus into the vagina. In the case of functioning ovarian tumors such as granulosal cell tumor or thecoma, the bleeding may be due to either an hyperplastic endometrium or an endometrial cancer secondary to the estrogen stimulation.

Rarely, other intraperitoneal tumors may cause intraperitoneal bleeding with eventual vaginal bleeding from secondary passage of the blood through the reproductive tract. This is an unusual occurrence but should be considered in the differential diagnosis of unexplained vaginal bleeding.

Inflammatory Conditions

Although bleeding is not common as a symptom in inflammatory conditions, severe inflammation in tissue will often lead to capillary oozing or a small blood vessel erosion. Thus, vulvitis, vaginitis, cervicitis, and endometritis may all be associated with vaginal bleeding or spotting, generally without relationship to menses. At times patients with acute salpingitis or tubo-ovarian abscess may also experience vaginal bleeding. This most likely comes from endometrial inflammation or abnormal uterine bleeding secondary to ovarian dysfunction. The symptoms and signs of inflammation, including discharge, pain and tenderness, and generalized signs and symptoms of infection, will help in the differential diagnosis.

Traumatic Conditions

Direct trauma to the female external genitalia and internal reproductive tract may occur secondary to accidental injury, the placement of foreign bodies within the vagina, and traumatic coitus. Direct lacerations secondary to one of these causes may lead to scant or profuse bleeding, depending on the extent of the injury. Often the bleeding is arterial and requires suture ligations. In children the insertion of foreign bodies into the vagina may lead to vaginal discharge with or without bleeding. Pencils, crayons, pieces of chalk, wads of paper, hairpins, and other items may be found. This is discussed more fully in Chapter 10.

Coital lacerations may occur because of rape or as part of normal sexual function. Tears of the hymen or lacerations of the vagina when tissue is rigid may lead to severe vaginal bleeding. Occasionally, bleeding occurs from the vaginal vault after a hysterectomy. While this often occurs shortly after the operation, there are reports of dehiscence of the upper vault years later.

Systemic Diseases

A number of systemic diseases are associated with clotting defects and therefore may present with vaginal bleeding or have vaginal bleeding associated with the natural history of the disease. These include various coagulopathies, blood dyscrasias, and endocrinopathies. In addition, patients who take medications that interfere with the normal clotting mechanism may suffer vaginal bleeding. Examples of such medications are heparin and sodium warfarin (Coumadin), which may affect the clotting mechanism directly, or agents that interfere with normal platelet function, such as salicylates and other prostaglandin synthetase inhibitors. Many such conditions can be suspected or diagnosed by history and physical examination. General laboratory studies such as complete blood count, cell smear, and assessment of the clotting mechanism will usually help discover such problems if they exist.

Postmenopausal Bleeding

Although postmenopausal bleeding may be associated with a number of different conditions, it must always be investigated because many causes are premalignant or malignant. The most common premalignant and malignant causes are atypical adenomatous hyperplasia and carcinoma of the endometrium. These account for as much as one third of the patients evaluated for postmenopausal bleeding in many series. While many other lesions of the reproductive tract, both benign and malignant, may be discovered, one fourth to one third of the patients evaluated may demonstrate no obvious pathologic condition other than an atrophic endometrium.

PELVIC AND ABDOMINAL PAIN

In 1979 the Taxonomy Committee of the International Association for the Study of Pain defined pain as "an unpleasant sensory and emotional experience associated with actual or potential tissue damage or described in terms of such damage." The committee further stated that pain is always subjective, with each individual learning the application of the word through experience related to injury in early life. It is always unpleasant and is, therefore, an emotional experience. They recognize that people may report pain in the absence of tissue damage or any likely pathophysiologic cause and that this may be secondary to psychological reasons. Blendis points out the most children and adults have experienced abdominal pain that is often short-lived and rarely associated with physical or organic cause. In many cases, both physical and psychogenic elements exist, making it impossible to tell which was the precipitating cause.

TABLE 6-2

Conditions That May Cause Signs and Symptoms of Acute Abdomen and Abdominal Quadrants in Which They Most Often Occur

	Quadrant			
Condition	**Right Upper**	**Right Lower**	**Left Upper**	**Left Lower**
Salpingitis	−	+	−	+
Tubo-ovarian abscess	±	+	±	+
Ectopic pregnancy	−	+	−	+
Torsive adnexa	−	+	−	+
Ruptured ovarian cyst	−	+	−	+
Acute appendicitis	−	+	−	−
Mesenteric lymphadenitis	−	+	−	−
Crohn's disease	−	+	−	−
Acute cholecystitis	+	±	−	−
Perforated peptic ulcer	+	±	+	±
Acute pancreatitis	+	−	+	−
Acute pyelitis	+	±	+	±
Renal calculus	+	+	+	+
Splenic infarct	−	−	+	−
Splenic rupture	−	−	+	−
Acute diverticulitis	−	−	−	+

Acute Abdomen

A number of intra-abdominal conditions can lead to the findings of an acute abdomen. These findings include acute pain, generally of sudden onset, tenderness to palpation, rebound tenderness, and diminished or absent bowel sounds. The pain may be caused by infection, hemorrhage, infarction of tissue, or obstruction of bowel. In the case of bowel obstruction, bowel sounds may be hyperactive. It is important to construct a differential diagnosis when signs and symptoms of acute abdomen are noted. Table 6-2 lists the more common causes of an acute abdomen and identifies the quadrant of the abdomen where findings are more likely to be positive. It should be remembered, however, that the abdominal cavity is a continuum and overlap of signs is extremely common. Disease within a tubular viscus such as the bowel, fallopian tube, or ureter may cause crampy pain. Frequently patients complain of paroxysms of sharp, crampy pain interspaced with no pain at all or with periods of dull ache. Inflammatory conditions involving the ovary are frequently associated with continuous pain often described as sharp and throbbing.

Acute appendicitis, mesenteric lymphadenitis, and occasionally torsion of an adnexa may be found in preadolescent and adolescent girls. Appendicitis is, of course, a possible differential diagnosis in all age groups. It often presents initially as periumbilical pain which localizes to the right lower quadrant and is accompanied by anorexia or nausea and vomiting. Salpingitis, tubo-ovarian abscess, ectopic pregnancy, and ruptured ovarian cysts are common findings in those patients of reproductive age who have an acute abdomen. Patients with salpingitis tend to have a higher fever than those with appendicitis. Although their pain may be severe, they tend to be less ill than those with appendicitis. However, these women may have Crohn's disease, acute cholecystitis, perforated peptic ulcer, acute pyelitis, renal calculi, splenic infarct, and splenic rupture. Occasionally, they may also suffer from acute pancreatitis, which usually presents as epigastric pain often radiating to the back.

Acute abdomen in older women suggests torsion or rupture of an adnexa, acute cholecystitis, perforated ulcer, or acute diverticulitis. Pelvic inflammatory disease is less common in older women, and acute exacerbations are rare in those who have had tubal ligation.

Acute Pelvic Pain

Acute pain of gynecologic origin presents as both pelvic and lower abdominal pain. Diseases and dysfunction of the genitourinary tract, gastrointestinal tract, and musculoskeletal system may also cause pain in these regions. The box at right lists a number of gynecologic and nongynecologic conditions that can cause acute onset of pelvic or lower abdominal pain.

Threatened, inevitable, or incomplete abortion are generally accompanied by midline or bilateral lower abdominal pain, usually of a crampy, intermittent nature. In such instances, vaginal bleeding is generally present. When infection occurs concurrently (septic abortion) there is generally temperature elevation, systemic symptoms of chills and malaise, and often an elevated white cell count and erythrocyte sedimentation rate (ESR). Rapid serum pregnancy tests are generally positive.

Ectopic pregnancy generally is associated with unilateral, continuous crampy pain, although there may be some bilaterality to the presentation. Most ectopic pregnancies are associated with vaginal bleeding. Temperature elevation, if present, is usually minimal, and white cell count and ESR are generally normal but may be slightly elevated, particularly if there is intraperitoneal hemorrhage. Serum β-HCG is positive, and ultrasound examination may help in the diagnosis either by revealing a gestational sac in an adnexa or by ruling out the diagnosis through demonstration of a gestational sac within the uterus. Physical examination frequently demonstrates the presence of a mass in the adnexal region. Intraperitoneal bleeding may be diagnosed by culdocentesis and definitive diagnosis made by laparoscopy.

Acute cervicitis, often caused by *Neisseria gonorrhoeae* or *Chlamydia trachomatis*, may frequently be associated with lower abdominal and pelvic pain. The pain is often of a dull, aching nature and may radiate to the low back or to the upper thighs. There is generally a cervical and vaginal discharge, and there may be a low-grade temperature, slight leukocytosis, and slight increase in ESR. Definitive diagnosis is made by specific culture for the organism.

POSSIBLE CAUSES OF ACUTE PELVIC AND LOWER ABDOMINAL PAIN

Pregnancy-related
  Abortion
  Ectopic
Disorders of the uterus and cervix
  Cervicitis
  Endometritis
  Degenerating myoma
Disorders of the adnexa
  Salpingitis
  Tubo-ovarian abscess
  Endometriosis (endometrioma)
  Torsion of adnexa
  Torsion of hydatid of Morgagni
  Rupture of follicle or corpus luteum cyst
  Ovarian hyperstimulation syndrome
  Degenerating ovarian tumor
Nongynecologic disorders
  Appendicitis
  Mesenteric lymphadenitis
  Diverticulitis
  Functional bowel syndrome
  Cystitis
  Trigonitis
  Renal calculus
  Musculoskeletal disorders

Endometritis is generally transient and occurs in *Neisseria* or *Chlamydia* infections as part of their natural history. Occasionally, vigorous chemical douching will lead to a chemical endometritis. The pain is generally midline, pelvic, or lower abdominal and often aching in type.

Degenerating myoma will frequently cause acute, sharp, or aching pain in the region of the myoma. Diagnosis is aided by the fact that the uterus is irregular and enlarged and that there is tenderness to palpation. There may be a mild leukocytosis, but generally laboratory parameters are normal.

Salpingitis and tubo-ovarian abscess have been discussed under acute abdomen. Endometriosis is discussed in detail in Chapter 18. The pain pattern depends on the location of the endometrial implants and varies from dysmenorrhea and dyspareunia to continuous generalized pelvic discomfort.

TABLE 7-2
Recommended Therapy in Obesity

Degree of Obesity	Percent Above Normal Weight	Therapy
Mild	20-40	Diet and lay supervision
Moderate	41-100	Low-calorie diet and medical supervision
Severe	>100	Gastric reduction operation

common in patients who undergo gastric restriction operations. Seventy-five percent of these individuals report elation and a feeling of well-being. Ninety-one percent of these patients state that before operation they had required a good deal of willpower to keep from overeating and, indeed, 33% stated that they could eat another full meal after eating most of their meals. Only 14% ever felt satisfied after eating. Following the operation 10% state that they require willpower to keep from eating more and only 1% state that they could eat another full meal after eating. Ninety-four percent feel that they could eat no more after completing the usual meal.

Moderately obese patients will lose weight on diets of 1200 to 1500 calories and generally find this approach comfortable. However, weight loss under these circumstances takes a long time. On very low-calorie diets (400 to 700 calories), which consist mostly of protein (fish, fowl, or lean meat), dramatic change in weight can usually be accomplished in 3 months. The patient will lose 1.5 to 2.3 kg per week depending on the amount of body fat at the beginning of dieting. The major problem with such individuals is maintaining weight loss. Craighead et al. point out that unless behavior modification is accomplished, maintenance of weight loss is usually not successful. These workers studied 145 patients who were approximately 60% overweight and divided them into three groups. Treatment continued for 6 months, and there was at least 1 year of follow-up in 99% of those who completed the therapy. Group 1 underwent behavior modification using Ferguson's *Learning to Eat* manual. They lost an average of 11.4 kg and regained only 1.8 kg during the follow-up year. Group 2 received medication therapy with an appetite suppressant, fenfluramine hydrochloride (Pondimin). They lost an average of 14.5 kg but regained 8.6 kg during the follow-up period. The third group was treated with a combination of behavior modification and medication and lost an average of 15.0 kg but regained 9.5 kg during the follow-up period. The authors concluded that behavior modification without medication was the most appropriate therapy for moderate obesity.

Mild obesity seems to respond best to dieting and behavior modification under lay supervision. Such individuals will generally embrace fad diets and look for magic cures. However, if placed on a nutritionally appropriate modified caloric diet, they will generally do well if their attitudes toward eating and response to various stimuli are modified. Lay groups, such as Weight Watchers or Take Off Pounds Sensibly (TOPS), are usually quite successful for motivated individuals.

Obesity in adolescence is a variant of the problem in the general population. Since the risk for progression with increasing morbidity and mortality is great, prompt support and behavior modification are most important. School and parental involvement are important aspects of controlling the problem. Where an obese parent is also present, best results seem to be achieved when both the parent and the child undergo therapy but in separate counselling sessions. In a study by Brownell et al. using 16 weeks of treatment of 42 obese adolescents ages 12 through 16, three groups were studied. When the child alone attended group therapy, there was an average 3.3 kg weight loss; when the child and mother were treated together there was an average 5.3 kg weight loss; and when the child and mother were both treated but separately, there was an 8.4 kg weight loss. After 1 year of follow-up the group in which the mother and child were treated separately maintained their weight loss at a mean of 7.7 kg, whereas the other two groups had regained their previous baseline levels.

Obviously, counselling and behavior modification are important in the management of both the adolescent and adult obese patient, but the means for optimizing such care is yet to be completely defined.

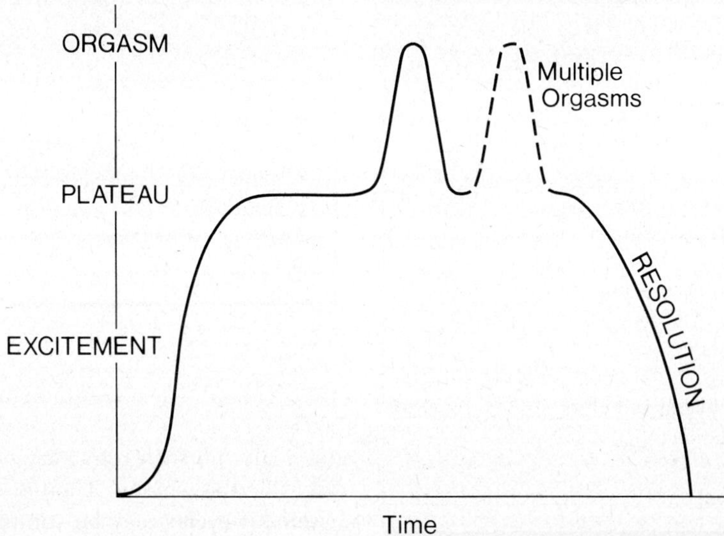

FIGURE 7-1
Sexual response cycle defined by Masters and Johnson. (From Masters WH, Johnson VE: Human sexual response. Boston, Little, Brown & Co., 1966.)

Sexual Function and Dysfunction

Sexual satisfaction is one of the more important human experiences yet it has been estimated that as many as 50% of all married couples experience some sexual dissatisfaction or dysfunction. While there is a strong physiologic basis for sexual function, it is not possible to separate sexual response from the many emotional and other contributing factors that may influence a relationship.

In 1966 Masters and Johnson published their now famous book, *Human Sexual Response,* which was a discussion of observations made on the sexual cycles of 700 subjects. It is on this important work that our current understanding of the female sexual response is based. Masters and Johnson described four phases of the sexual response: excitement, plateau, orgasm, and resolution (Fig. 7-1).

The excitement or seduction phase may be initiated by a number of internal or external stimuli. Physiologically it is associated with deep breathing, increase in heart rate and blood pressure, a total body feeling of warmth associated often with erotic feelings, and an increase in sexual tension. There is generalized vasocongestion which leads to breast engorgement and the development of a maculopapular erythematous rash on the breasts, the chest,

and the epigastrium, which is referred to as the "sex flush." There is also engorgement of the labia majora (seen particularly in multiparous women) and of the labia minora. The clitoris generally swells and becomes erect, causing it to be tightly applied to the clitoral hood. The vagina "sweats" a transudative lubricant, and the Bartholin glands may secrete small amounts of liquid. With the increasing deep breathing the uterus may tent up into the pelvis, perhaps as a result of the Valsalva maneuver. There is also a myotonic effect, which is most notable in nipple erection. Much of the response in the excitement phase is due to stimulation of the parasympathetic fibers of the autonomic nervous system. In some cases anticholinergic drugs may interfere with a full response in this stage.

Next is the plateau stage, which is the culmination of the excitement phase and is associated with a marked degree of vasocongestion throughout the body. Breasts and their areolae are markedly engorged, as are the labia and the lower third of the vagina. The vasocongestion in the lower third of the vagina is such that it forms what has been called the orgasmic platform, causing a decrease in the diameter of the vagina by as much as 50% and thus allowing for greater friction against the penis. At this should identify the quantity and type of drug used by history and should make the appropriate referral to a health care agency. For instance, individuals habituated to cocaine are often treated in a similar fashion to alcoholics, utilizing such help groups as Cocaine Anonymous.

Depression

Depression is a common symptom in a variety of conditions. Patients suffering loss or grief are often depressed. However, depression as a symptom is quite common in the general population. In a recent review, Ripley offered evidence from the world literature to indicate that as many as 10% of all individuals are depressed. Depression associated with psychoses such as is seen in manic-depressive (bipolar) psychosis may occur as often as 3 to 4 per 1000 population. Dorpat and Ripley noted that 9.3% of patients suffering from personality disorders, 26.9% of patients suffering from alcoholism, and 12.0% of schizophrenics had depression as a major symptom. Unfortunately, patients who suffer from depression are more prone to suicide, and psychiatric patients who commit suicide are more likely to have a depressive component to their illness.

Depression in infants and young children is frequently due to deprivation, particularly maternal deprivation. It is frequently characterized by crying and behavior disorders and later by despair and withdrawal. The child may fail to eat and may eventually starve to death. If the child does not die, strong depressive symptomatology may continue into adulthood. Ripley cites the work of several authors who have shown a significantly higher rate of bereavement or broken homes in childhood among adult depressive patients.

It is useful for a gynecologist to understand the way in which depression may present in patients. Early symptoms include chronic fatigue, anxiety and irritability, anhedonia (loss of feelings of joy and pleasure), decreased interest in usual pursuits including sexual activity and personal appearance, and mental changes, including poor concentration and lack of decisiveness. The individual may complain of loss of recent memory; insomnia, especially occurring shortly after falling asleep; a pessimistic outlook about the future, often associated with feelings of guilt; and a number of physical complaints including loss of appetite or a great increase in appetite; change in bowel habits, including constipation or diarrhea; headache; various aches and pains; and general lability. Late in the disease the patient may experience deep feelings of hopelessness with difficulty in presenting ideas. The patient may also complain of generalized weakness, fear of impending doom from a serious illness or fear that serious problems will befall a close family member, suicidal thoughts, and occasionally, delusions.

The physician should be alert to patients who have suffered personal loss or grief but who are still deeply depressed after 6 to 18 months of grieving. While depression is normal in a grief situation, it should not last for a prolonged period.

The diagnosis is often suspected by simply assessing the patient's appearance and asking the usual questions concerning the patient's mood and health. Several psychological tests have been developed to assess depression and can be used in subtle cases. The physician should assess the degree to which the patient is depressed and whether the reason for the depression is appropriate. If the patient is grieving because of a real life situation, the physician should demonstrate concern and offer appropriate assurance that the problem will be relieved with time. If the degree of depression is inappropriate for the life situation, the physician should determine whether the individual has suicidal thoughts and assess whether these thoughts are likely to be put into practice. Such questions as, "Have you considered harming yourself or taking your own life?" are appropriate in this situation. If the patient states that she has had such thoughts, the degree to which she is contemplating them may be assessed by asking if she has considered how she would carry out the suicide or what circumstances deterred her from attempting this act. If the patient seems to be seriously considering suicide, prompt referral to a mental health worker or facility should be made.

Patients who are depressed but give no evidence for psychoses may be helped by medication. Currently the tricyclic drugs are the most useful in usual clinical practice. Table 7-3

TABLE 7-3
Tricyclic Antidepressants

Generic Name	Trade Names
Amitriptyline	Amitril, Elavil, Amitid, Amitriptyline, Endep, SK-Amitriptyline
Amoxapine	Asendin
Desipramine	Norpramin, Pertofrane
Doxepin	Sinequan, Adapin
Imipramine	Tofranil, Antipress, Imavate, Imipramine, Janimine, SK-pramine, Presamine
Protriptyline	Vivactil
Trimipramine	Surmontil

lists a group of these drugs by generic and trade names. Most of the tricyclic drugs have a parasympathomimetic affect. Therefore, dryness of the mouth, blurred vision, hesitancy of urination or dribbling, some menstrual disorders (i.e., amenorrhea or irregularities), and a decrease in sexual arousal are complaints often associated with their use. Each of the tricyclics acts slightly differently, and undesirable side effects in a specific patient may be alleviated by switching to a different medication. Although patients may note reduction of symptoms of depression after 1 to 2 weeks of drug use, real improvement may take as long as 1 month. Dosage of these medications will need to be varied depending on the patient's response.

Lithium salts have been used to treat depression and are most useful in the treatment of manic-depressive psychosis. Monamine oxidase inhibitors are also in common clinical use but frequently have serious side effects and should be administered only by individuals well experienced in their use.

Many patients will have complete relief of symptoms in 1 to 3 months of tricyclic therapy. However, some patients will require counseling to work out serious emotional and social problems as an adjunct to the therapy. Frequently drug therapy is necessary in order to bring the patient's depression under control to

an extent that allows psychotherapy to be useful. Many patients can use tricyclic drugs intermittently when symptomatology warrants.

Loss and Grief

Loss is a common human experience and may affect women of all ages. The loss of a child, a spouse, or a close relative should and probably will precipitate an acute grief reaction. However, the physician must remember that a similar reaction will be precipitated by a spontaneous abortion, by the loss of a body part or organ, or by the realization that infertility and childlessness face the couple. It may also be part of a syndrome in women undergoing separation or divorce.

Lindemann points out that acute grief is a definite syndrome with both psychological and somatic components. In his vast experience with grieving patients he has observed that the syndrome may appear immediately after the loss or be delayed. If it is delayed, grief may appear to be absent only to occur at a future time, often in a more exaggerated fashion. At times the syndrome may occur in a distorted fashion. For successful resolution of grief, the individual must be helped to transform these distorted reactions into normal grief in order to bring about resolution.

Lindemann points out that the symptomatology of normal grief is quite uniform. The individual often complains of tightness in the throat and chest, a choking sensation, a feeling of shortness of breath, and frequent sighing. There is often reported an empty feeling in the abdomen, muscle weakness, and a feeling of tension and mental pain. These symptoms frequently come in waves lasting from minutes to an hour and are often dreaded by the sufferer.

Lindemann further points out that the bereaved experience disorders of the sensorium often involving a sense of unreality, a tendency to place emotional distance between themselves and other people, and a preoccupation with imagery of the deceased. At times the bereaved will assume the mannerisms of the deceased or even attempt to perform the work of the lost loved one. If the mother has died, the bereaved daughter may see the mother's face when she looks at herself in the mirror and may assume the mother's mannerisms in her speech and gestures. There is often the perception that the deceased is nearby and can communicate.

In the immediate grief period the bereaved often feels guilt. This may directly involve the events of the death or of tasks left unfinished before the individual died. The bereaved often feels a lack of warmth and may demonstrate feelings of hostility towards others.

The burden of the grief is often so great that the individual can barely handle the maintenance activities of living, and has little energy left over for social contact or growth and development.

Most authorities feel that a normal grief reaction takes 6 to 18 months and ends when the individual has appropriately experienced the pain and suffering, placed the memory of the deceased in a proper place within the bereaved's life, and established new relationships and new life directions.

Lindemann notes, however, that abnormal grief reactions are possible and divides these into several categories. The first is the delay of reaction which essentially involves a postponement of grieving. This may be seen in an individual who is injured in an accident that kills the person to be grieved. The individual may be preoccupied with personal survival and recuperation and may not have the opportunity to grieve until this has passed. In other instances the individual may delay grieving for a long period of time, often years. There are often psychological reasons why this occurs, but when the grieving is finally precipitated, it may appear quite pathological and out of context for current life situations.

A second variant is a distorted reaction. In this situation the bereaved may take on the characteristics of the deceased without evidencing a sense of loss. The bereaved may actually take on the symptoms of the lost person if that individual had experienced a prolonged illness prior to death.

A third abnormal reaction to grieving may be the development of a psychosomatic condition. Ulcerative colitis, rheumatoid arthritis, and asthma have all been noted to occur in close approximation to bereavement. Lindemann points out that some patients suffering from these problems may improve when the grief reaction is resolved.

Other types of abnormal grief reactions include pathological alterations in relationships with friends and relatives, inappropriate hostility towards others, behavior patterns resembling psychoses, continuing inability to make decisions or to take initiative, and performance of activities which have destructive social and economic outcomes. Finally, Lindemann notes that in the reaction of agitated depression the bereaved develops tension, agitation, insomnia, feelings of worthlessness, and fantasies of a need for punishment. In such situations suicide may be a danger. Fortunately, agitated depression is quite unusual. Lindemann feels that it may be more common in individuals who have experienced a previous depression or in those who have been intensely involved with the deceased, such as mothers who have lost young children.

Loss of a Child by Abortion, Stillbirth, or Neonatal or Infant Death

Obstetricians and gynecologists may need to counsel patients experiencing grief related to several areas of reproduction. Leppert and Pahlka counseled 22 women who had experienced spontaneous abortion. The study format was to hold a counselling session immediately after abortion and again in 4 to 6 weeks. These authors report that all women demonstrated the classic stages of grief, but that guilt was the stage that appeared the most difficult for them and their spouses to resolve. The authors felt that the unexpressed emotions relating to pregnancy loss might affect the relationship of the couple unless they are explored and defused. They suggested that the obstetrician and gynecologist should make it a point to add such counseling to their practice routines. Bruhn and Bruhn point out that a predictable pattern of grief follows every stillbirth and perinatal death and urges physicians to work with their patients in resolving these feelings.

In addition to the physician's offering understanding and counseling, there are many self-help groups that offer aid to parents who have lost children either in the perinatal period or in infancy. The physician should become aware of the agencies or groups within the community that offer group and self-help therapy in neonatal and infant loss. It is reasonable for the physician to learn the techniques used by these groups and to assess whether or not their approach fits the needs of the patient before making referrals.

The physician should also be aware of the fact that each member of the couple may grieve differently and, indeed, the style of grieving that one may exhibit may be in conflict with that of the other. Pointing out these differences and helping the couple to express their true feelings to each other may be very beneficial during this process.

An important issue in understanding the management of grief in couples who have lost infants was brought out in an evaluation of a group of patients by Estok and Lehman. They found that such individuals wished health care providers to acknowledge the couple's feelings of shock, guilt, and grief and to recognize the importance of their memories of the birth and of the baby. In essence, they wished the health care providers to help them sharpen the reality of the death of the child and provide support through the postloss period rather than focus on other life events such as the next pregnancy.

Certain aspects of bereavement should be understood by the physician in dealing with patients who are suffering grief. The loss of a child is always a serious problem. Even the loss of an adult child can have long-term sequelae. Shanfield and Swain noted that parents who have lost adult children in traffic accidents continued to grieve intensely for a prolonged period and had a higher than expected level of psychiatric symptoms and health complaints. Families that were unstable and in which problems had existed with these children suffered more guilt and more psychiatric symptoms. In addition, factors that intensified the bereavement experience were a mother losing a daughter, parents losing children who lived at home, the loss of children born early in the birth order, and the loss of multiple children in a single-car, single-driver accident. A protecting factor seemed to be a prior bereavement experience. These observations were supported by Lundin who used the Texas Inventory of Grief to study first-degree relatives 8 years after bereavement. He noted that relatives of persons who had died suddenly or unexpectedly suffered a more pronounced grief reaction than those who had lost someone in a death that was expected. He also noted that bereavement was greater in parents after the loss of a child than in widows or widowers who lost a spouse.

Unplanned Pregnancy

A special counseling challenge involves the care of a woman with an unplanned pregnancy. Such individuals often suffer conflicting feelings, which may include shame and guilt for their predicament, a genuine desire to have a child, fear of social consequences, and fear for their own future and physical well-being. In addition, they may also suffer from guilt about the destruction of the pregnancy if abortion is considered. While many such women have good support groups (e.g., family, significant other, friends, and religious counselors), others will rely on the physician entirely for advice and direction. The physician should discuss all possible options with the patient, including having and raising the child, offering it for adoption, or terminating the pregnancy. Issues involving the role of the baby's father, the impact of any decision on the future life of the patient, and the risks of the procedure should be considered. The patient should be aided in reaching the most appropriate decision for her needs and then should be supported in carrying out her plan. Where necessary, appropriate referrals to social agencies (i.e., adoption, abortion counseling, or welfare services) should be made.

Infertility

The inability to reproduce leads to a major life frustration and often generates a series of symptoms similar to the grief reaction. Many sequelae may occur that stress the couple's relationship. Guilt, anger, and shame may be components, depending upon the social forces at play in the relationship. Sexual dysfunction may result because of the stresses imposed by the requirements of a treatment regimen or because of general dysfunction within the relationship brought about by the infertility. At times the problems associated with the infertility (e.g., endometrial implants in the cul-de-sac) may cause dyspareunia and lead to sexual dysfunction. External stresses from family and friends who continuously refer to the couple's childlessness may contribute to the tension as well.

The physician must be complete in the medical evaluation of the couple as well as supportive of their emotional needs. The physician should discuss fully all treatment options and the chances for success. He or she should also continuously help the couple to accentuate the positives of their relationship and to consider referring them to self-help groups for infertile couples or to health care counselors who can help with the maintenance of their relationship and self-image.

Death of a Spouse

Holmes and Rahe rate the death of a spouse as one of the major life stresses among survivors independent of age and cultural background, and state that it may be related to a decline in physical and mental well-being of the survivor. Gallagher et al. recently reported the effects of acute bereavement on the indicators of mental health in widows and widowers beyond the age of 55. These workers evaluated a group from the standpoint of past grief, present grief, depression, somatic symptomatology, and self-rating of mental health status. They noted that these individuals in the early stages of their bereavement were suffering from considerable psychological distress as compared to individuals of similar age who were not bereaved. They demonstrated that the degree of effect of bereavement on the patient's mental health did not vary by sex. Those conditions that were more likely to occur in one sex rather than the other occurred with incidence equal to those individuals of the same sex in the study group. Thus findings in women, who tend to have a higher incidence of depression in the general population than do men, demonstrated this to be the case in the same proportions among the study group.

CROSS-CULTURAL DIFFERENCES. Eisenbruch has pointed out that there are significant cross-cultural differences in bereavement while there are great similarities in the grief reaction between different ethnic and cultural groups. Individuals from different backgrounds tend to experience difficulty with their grief when they attempt to respond in a fashion specific for the majority within the culture in which they now reside. Specific rituals, attitudes toward widowhood, mores with respect to length and type of grieving, the way in which the deceased is remembered, and the appropriate period of time for grieving and mourning may be quite different in various minority groups when compared to the general white majority of the United States. Physicians dealing with minority groups are urged to consider the points raised by Eisenbruch in his review in order to have a better ability to help the minority patients through their grieving period.

Separation and Divorce

Currently the number of divorces occurring annually in the United States is about 40% of the number of marriages. There are many reasons for this increase, including the emerging of women to a level of self-support, changing attitudes toward a desire to remain married, and an increased public awareness of family dysfunction such as spouse and child abuse. Often one or both members of a divorcing couple will demonstrate evidence of grief as well as anger, shame, and guilt. Counselling can be very useful in restoration of self-esteem and in helping the individual to emerge from the experience with the ability to survive in new relationships. While physicians should recognize these needs in their patients who are going through separation and divorce, their primary role should be to make appropriate referrals to counsellors who have the time and the skills to deal with the patient in this area.

Loss of an Organ or Body Part

Loss of a body part can be expected to bring about a grief reaction with accompanying symptoms of an emotional and somatic nature. Depression is frequently a strong component. Workers who have investigated the loss of limbs have noted this, and it is reasonable to expect that the loss of organs such as the breast or the uterus would evoke a similar reaction.

Several workers have reported depression among posthysterectomy patients with an incidence ranging from 4% to as high as 70%. In a recent review, Drummond and Field point out that the stages of the process of incorporating the loss of a uterus into the individual's self-image is similar to that of the loss of other body parts. They refer to the four stages of incorporation listed by Roberts, which are defined as impact, retreat, acknowledgement, and reconstruction. The impact stage occurs when the individual becomes aware that she has a problem with her uterus. If she is symptomatic this may be obvious. If she has been told she must lose her uterus because it is diseased, such as with cancer, she will need to make a mental adjustment to this fact. Steiner and Aleksandiewicz have pointed out that when the disease that requires operation is life-threatening or serious, the likelihood of depression is minimized. Richards has pointed out that when disease of the uterus is absent, depression is more likely to occur.

The second stage of organ loss is retreat. This is the period in which the patient accepts the need for the loss of an organ and depersonalizes it in her thinking. If denial occurs at this period, the depression that she notes later may be quite severe.

The third stage is that of acknowledgement. The physician will recognize this stage because it involves the woman's repeated discussion of the procedure, the need for the procedure, and the meaning of the loss of the uterus postoperatively. It is the woman's attempt to place the procedure and the need for the procedure within the appropriate context of her life and her self-image.

The final phase is reconstruction. This involves the redefinition of her self-image without the organ. It will require acceptance by her spouse or significant other and by other members of her community of importance in this event. The physician should attempt to discuss the need for and the likely sequelae of the hysterectomy before it is performed. This discussion should include the significant other in the woman's life so that any fantasies or fears that may arise can be discussed at this point. Some men have difficulty continuing an active sexual experience with a woman who has lost her uterus. These points should be discussed ahead of time so that each realizes the implication of the operation. On the other hand, some women feel that sex is for procreation and after the removal of the uterus may respond quite differently from what the significant other has

been accustomed to in the past. These points, too, should be discussed before the fact.

If the individual is unable to successfully work through the four stages of loss of an organ, disruption of relationships and depression may be sequelae. Newton and Baron have noted that between 20% and 40% of couples have stopped having sexual intercourse after hysterectomy. They do not state whether this is a direct effect of the hysterectomy and the inability to work out feelings related to this procedure or whether other problems may have been in existence, allowing for the hysterectomy to be an excuse to stop experiencing intercourse. Physicians should consider these points, however, and discuss them with the patient and her significant other before embarking on an operative procedure, particularly if it is elective and the time is available for discussion.

Loss of a Pet

A final bereavement situation often overlooked by physicians but frequently important to patients is the grief associated with the death of a pet. Quackenbush recently reviewed the subject and concluded that animals play an important role in the human social system and may contribute greatly to the quality of life of many pet owners. In some cases where the individual lives alone and may be elderly, the animal may be the only living thing in close daily contact with the individual. It is, therefore, not unusual that when the pet dies the owner suffers grief. Quackenbush states that understanding and sensitivity to the feelings and sense of loss that the pet owner experiences will help to facilitate the resolution of the grief.

Counseling the Dying

Elizabeth Kubler-Ross revolutionized our understanding of the death process with her classic book on the subject in 1969. An important paragraph taken from the first chapter describing the fear of death is quite revealing:

When we look back in time and study old cultures and people, we are impressed that death has always been distasteful to man and will probably always be. From the psychiatrist's point of view this is very understandable and can perhaps best be explained by our basic knowledge that, in our unconscious, death is never possible in regard to ourselves. It is inconceivable for our unconscious to imagine an actual ending of our own life here on earth and if the life of ours has to end the ending is always attributed to a malicious intervention from the outside by someone else. In simple terms, in our unconscious mind we can only be killed; it is inconceivable to die of a natural cause or of old age. Therefore, death in itself is associated with a bad act, a frightening happening, something that in itself calls for retribution and punishment.*

Kubler-Ross describes five stages an individual progresses through in the acceptance of the inevitability of death. They are denial, anger, bargaining, depression, and acceptance. Denial and isolation is a temporary state brought about by the shock of learning that the individual suffers from a problem from which he or she cannot recover. The transition from denial to partial acceptance will depend upon the nature of the patient's illness, how long he or she has left before death will occur, and the way in which he or she has prepared throughout life to cope with such serious situations. Kubler-Ross notes that when confronted with multiple health care providers who are likely to express the inevitable in a variety of ways, the dying person often chooses to accept the individual style of presentation that most fits their need. During this period of adjustment, therefore, a number of different opinions may be sought and specific interpretations questioned. Inevitably the individual may be depressed and may isolate herself from those with whom she would normally associate. Frequently the individual may appear confused and in some cases may deny that any information about the impending death has ever been given. Most patients, according to Kubler-Ross, will go through this period long before death occurs. However, in 3 of 200 patients that she studied, acceptance of the inevitable did not occur until the very time of death.

Hospital personnel must guard against avoiding patients after having given the initial information. They must not interpret the period of the patient's denial as a distasteful circumstance with which they cannot cope. Instead

they should help the patient work through this period by patiently repeating information, answering questions, and offering comfort. Terms that remove all hope such as "terminal" or "hopeless" should be avoided.

The second stage described by Kubler-Ross is that of anger. Staff and family members find this the most difficult one with which to cope, since the anger felt by the patient may be inappropriately displaced to everyone and everything in the environment. The physician or nurse caring for the patient falls into the unenviable position of the messenger who is hated because of the bad news he or she has brought. The health care worker who tries to make the patient comfortable may be accused of being overly solicitous, whereas, in contrast, the health care worker who attempts to give the patient the privacy that it is believed she seeks may be accused of being uncaring. Likewise, family members who attempt to be cheerful in visiting the patient may be accused of being glib and uncaring, whereas, if they are more somber they may be accused of being depressing. In such cases the health care worker or family member will probably experience guilt, possibly shame, and may adjust to the problem by avoiding the dying person altogether. During the anger period the dying individual will be irritated by all stimuli. Happiness depicted on television may upset her because she feels that she is not included in it. Discussion of future plans of friends or family members will be equally depressing because the dying individual realizes that she will not be around to participate. The anger period ends when the individual can reconcile the fact that she is different from every healthy person but is still capable of being loved and accepted.

The third stage is that of bargaining. This is an attempt to postpone the inevitable by offering concessions presumably to God. It is essentially the hope of getting more time for good behavior. In this period the individual may do charitable acts, correct past misdeeds, or reconcile damaged relationships. It is a time for relieving guilt and defusing the feeling of required punishment. It may, in many ways, be an opportunity to "put one's house in order."

The fourth stage described by Kubler-Ross is that of depression. While symptoms of depression may occur in the earlier stages, depression

---

*From Kubler-Ross, E: On death and dying. New York, Macmillan Co, 1969.

BIBLIOGRAPHY

Agres WS, Kraemer HC: The treatment of anorexia nervosa: do different treatments have different outcomes? In Stunkard AJ, Stellar E, eds: Eating and its disorders. New York, Raven Press, 1984.

Anderson RE: Where's Dad? parental deprivation in delinquency. Arch Gen Psychiatry 18:641, 1968.

Barker MG: Psychiatric illness after hysterectomy. Br Med J 2:91, 1968.

Barnes GE, Prosen H: Parental death and depression. J Abnorm Psychol 94: 64, 1985.

Birtchnell J: Early parent death in relation to size and constitution of sibship. Acta Psychiatr Scand 47:250, 1971.

Birtchnell J: Early parent death in psychiatric diagnosis. Soc Psychiatry 7:202, 1972.

Brown GW, Harris T, Copeland JR: Depression and loss. Br J Psychiatry 130:1, 1977.

Brownell KD: New developments in the treatment of obese children in adolescence. In Stunkard AJ, Stellar E, eds: Eating and its Disorders. New York, Raven Press, 1984.

Brownell KD, Kelman JH, Stunkard AJ: Treatment of obese children with and without their mothers. Changes in weight and blood pressure. Pediatrics 71:515, 1983.

Bruhn DF, Bruhn P: Stillbirth: A humanistic response. J Reprod Med 29:107, 1984.

Casper RC, Eckert ED, Halmi KA, et al. Bulimia: Its incidence and clinical importance in patients with anorexia nervosa. Br J Psychiatry 27:1030, 1980.

Craighead LW, Stunkard AJ, O'Brien R: Behavior therapy and pharmacotherapy of obesity. Arch Gen Psychiatry 38:763, 1981.

DeGraaf R: New treatise concerning the generative organs of women. In Ladas AK, Whipple B, Perry JD, eds: The G-spot and other recent discoveries about human sexuality. New York, Holt, Rinehart & Winston, 1983.

Dietrich DR: Psychological health of young adults who experienced early parent death: MMPI trends. J Clin Psychol 40:901, 1984.

Dorpat TL, Ripley HS: A study of suicide in the Seattle area. Compr Psychiatry 1:349, 1960.

Drummond J, Field PA: Emotional and sexual sequelae following hysterectomy. Health Care Women Int 5:261, 1984.

Earls F: The fathers (not the mothers): Their importance and influence with infants and young children. In Chess S, Thomas A, eds: Annual progress in child psychiatry and child development 1977, vol. 10. New York, Brunner/Mazel, Publishers, 1977.

Eisenbruch M: Cross cultural aspects of bereavement. II. Ethnic and cultural variations in the development of bereavement practices. Cult Med Psychiatry 8:315, 1984.

Estok P, Lehman A: Perinatal death: Grief support for families. Birth 10:17, 1983.

Ferguson JM: Learning to eat: Leader's manual and patient manual. Palo Alto, Calif., Bull Publishing, 1975.

Frank E, Anderson C, Rubinstein D: Frequency of sexual dysfunction in "normal" couples. N Engl J Med 299:111, 1978.

Gallagher DE, Breckenridge JN, Thompson LW, Peterson JA: Effects of bereavement on indicators of mental health in elderly widows and widowers. J Gerontol 38:565, 1983.

Garrow JS: Treat obesity seriously: A clinical manual. New York, Churchill Livingstone, 1982.

Godkin MA, Krant MJ, Doster NJ: The impact of hospice care on families. Int J Psychiatry Med 13:153, 1983-84.

Grafenberg E: The role of the urethra in female orgasm. Int J Sexol 3:145, 1950.

Green ... field, ...

Gregory ... a par ... amon ... 1965.

Halmi ... to we ... bypas ...

Hammo ... stet ...

Holmes ... J Psy ...

Homek ... fluenc ... dance ...

Hsu LK ... nervo ...

Isager T ... lapse ... J Psyc ...

Johnson ... lates ... lation ...

Johnson ... and t ...

Kaluey ... and p ... 11:35 ...

Kaplan ... zel, 1 ...

Kendell ... miolo ...

Kline N ... Sons, ...

Kubler- ... Co., ...

Laajus ...

LaFerla ... tion i ...

Lamont ... 1978.

Leppert ... spont ... Gynec ...

Lindema ... grief, ...

Lundin ... chiatr ...

Masters ... ton, 1 ...

Masters ... Bosto ...

Melody ... Am J ...

Munro ... childl ...

Nahas ... Press, ...

Newton ... fiction ...

Oppenh ... Adver ... ing di ... 19:35 ...

Parker ... depre ... marit ...

Quacker ...

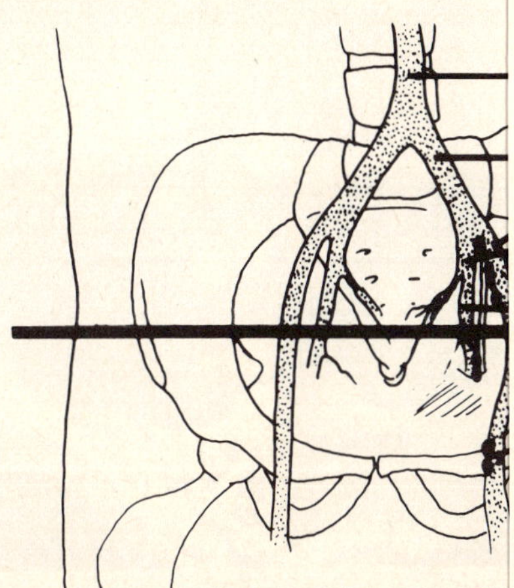

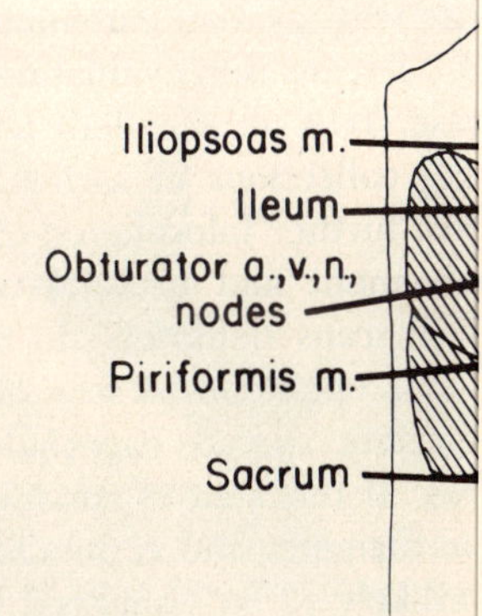

FIGURE 8-7

Illustrations and correspond[ing] normal anatomic features of [...] JW, Amendola MA, Konerd[...] vic and inguinal lymph-node [...] nant disease. Radiology 137:[...]

at this stage may occur because the patient has had to cope with a number of factors associated with the illness. For instance, she may be concerned about the expenses of her care, loss of wages, and the simple fact that she feels poorly, added to the fact that she now realizes she is going to die. In addition, fears that her death will adversely affect other members of her family who depend on her may also add to her depression. Health care workers should be comfortable in allowing the patient to know that they understand the reasons for the depression. They should do everything possible to eliminate the feelings of guilt that the patient may have because of the conditions in which she finds herself. She should be made to realize that the financial burdens that may be developing or the effect that her death may have on family members and their lives are not a result of specific actions that she may have taken. In other words, she is not responsible for the condition she is in and the resulting circumstances are not legitimate reasons for her to feel guilt. Family members can be helpful by accentuating the positive aspects of the patient's life, the love they feel for her, and the happiness they have experienced with her. They should downplay the burdens that the patient's illness and death will create for them. Essentially the patient is working through a period of grief, in this case, grief for herself.

The fifth and final stage is that of acceptance. At this point the individual has worked through the anger that she has felt for her misfortune and for those healthy individuals who do not have to die at this time and has also passed the period of depression and into a period of accepting her fate. This step will most often be achieved if there is a long enough period for the individual to work through the previous stages. Unfortunately, many die before all of these stages have been reconciled. In a very ill patient acceptance is frequently a giving in to the symptoms she has had to bear and a looking forward to peace from these symptoms that the death will bring. However, Kubler-Ross points out that the acceptance stage is not necessarily this alone, as patients who are not physically suffering also will go through this stage. This is often a time when the individual takes comfort in having quality visits with family members in which positive experiences are remembered. She may also obtain comfort from interacting with representatives of her religious faith.

A new innovation in the care of the terminally ill and their families was introduced with the hospice concept during the past decade. There are currently more than 800 hospice organizations in the United States, offering psychosocial support to both patients and families. The service includes postdeath follow-up of the families in order to help them through the grieving period. Hospice organizations include free-standing institutions that offer inpatient services; communituy-based home programs that include both professional and volunteer services; hospital-based hospice teams which may include physicians, nurses, social workers, chaplains, and volunteers who are in a position to minister to any patient in any bed; and hospital-based hospice units that are geographically separate from other patients and often are coordinated with a home care program.

Godkin et al. recently studied 58 bereaved spouses and their families whose loved ones had recently died of late-stage cancer after care in a hospital-based hospice service. These families in general rated hospice care significantly better than that received in prior experiences, stating that the hospice services contributed to an improved family function, greater individual well-being, and the ability of family members to cope with the situation. Over three quarters of the families reported that they were emotionally prepared and prepared in a practical sense for the death of the victim. Health problems were reported by these family members in about the same proportion as was experienced in other bereaved groups, but when these problems occurred they were dealt with within the framework of the program.

Physicians who care for chronically ill and terminal patients, particularly those suffering from cancer, should consider availing themselves of the services of such organizations within their geographic area.

KEY POINTS, cont'd

- Inhibited sexual desire is the most comm

- Heavy drinking of alcohol among pregnar
  that stated in patient histories. Eleven p
  heavy drinkers of alcohol.

- Roughly 7% to 20% of college students u

- Smoking more than 10 cigarettes per day

- High-volume alcohol use is defined as
  drinks or more on specific occasions.

- Ten percent of all individuals suffer depre

- Manic depressive (bipolar) psychoses occu
  1000 population.

- Acute grief reaction lasts 6 to 18 months.

- Currently the number of divorces occur
  about 40% of the number of marriages.

- Posthysterectomy depression occurs in 4
  the indication for the operation and the p

- Roberts's four stages of incorporation as a
  part loss are impact, retreat, acknowledge

- Kubler-Ross defines the stages of individ
  itability of death as denial, anger, bargain

- Hospice programs are support groups for

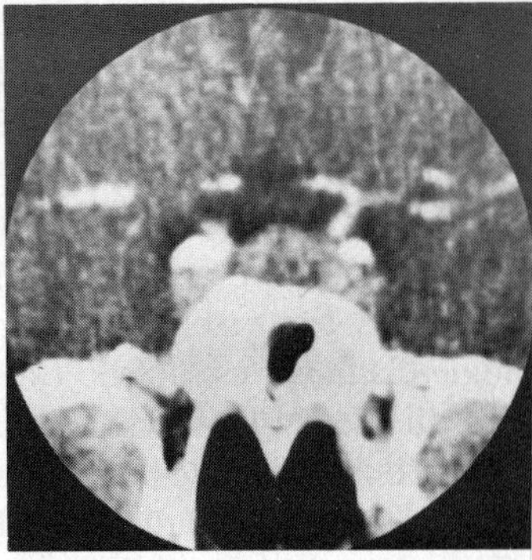

A

FIGURE 8-5
A 17-year-old woman w
Coronal CT scan after i
neous enhancement of p
sellar floor. **B,** Six mon
ovulatory cycles, disappe
shows decrease in size
defect in enhancement,
criptine treatment, sella
less than 4 mm in dian
Computed tomography
microadenoma size. Rad

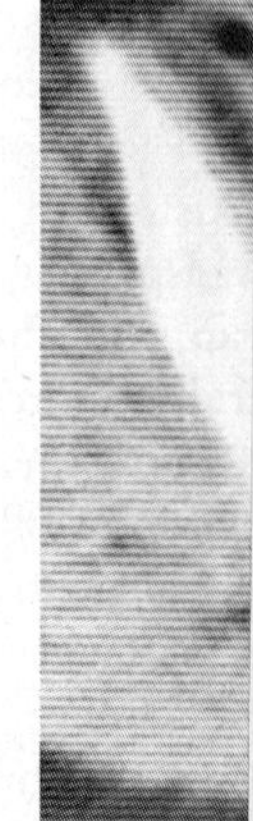

FIGURE 8-6
Stage IIB cervical carci
Right obturator lymph
trioma (E) confirmed a
comparison between c
137:1000, 1981. Copyr

sue is cervical stenosis or spasm. When this is encountered, a paracervical block with 1% xylocaine should be performed. Subsequently, the cervix can be dilated painlessly, with narrow metal dilators, and the biopsy completed.

There are many modifications of the original Novak and Randall endometrial biopsy instruments. Most cannulas are 2 to 4 mm in diameter and are either metal or plastic. Aspiration of the endometrium is accomplished by a syringe or a portable pump. The Vabra aspirator has a reservoir similar to a sputum collection trap. The suction pump with the Vabra aspirator facilitates collection of an adequate sampling of the endometrium in approximately 1 minute. Optimal pressure is 500 to 600 mm Hg. The pressure used determines the depth of the cleavage plane in the endometrium (Fig. 8-18).

Complications following endometrial biopsy are exceedingly rare. The major complication is uterine perforation, with an incidence of 1 or 2 cases per 1000. Infection and postoperative bleeding are very rare. Some women develop a severe vasovagal reflex from instrumentation of the uterine cavity. This reflex can be diminished by either giving the patient intravenous atropine or performing a paracervical block. Some clinicians pretreat women with prostaglandin synthetase inhibitors to decrease the pain associated with this procedure.

Cancer of the endometrium is the most common pelvic malignancy. Statistically 2 to 3 women out of 100 will develop endometrial carcinoma. The increasing incidence of endometrial carcinoma and the increasing popularity of hormonal treatment of menopause have focused research on innovative means of mass screening for endometrial hyperplasia and carcinoma. Several different instruments, including the Endocyte brush, Mimark Helix, and the Isaac's sampler, have been developed. These instruments are designed to obtain cells for cytologic screening. The cellular material obtained should be put into Bouin's solution rather than formalin. Bouin's solution preserves cytonuclear characteristics, while nuclear detail may be distorted by formalin. Examples of tissues obtained by endometrial sampling may be seen in Figs. 8-19 and 8-20.

Direct cytologic material from the endometrial cavity has a false negative rate between 5% and 15% when compared to material from dilation and curettage (D&C) or hysterectomy. Although this false negative rate is substantial, it is virtually identical to the false negative rate of cytologic screening associated with invasive carcinoma of the cervix. Cytologic sampling obtained only from the vaginal pool and endocervical canal is able to diagnose approximately 25% of endometrial carcinomas.

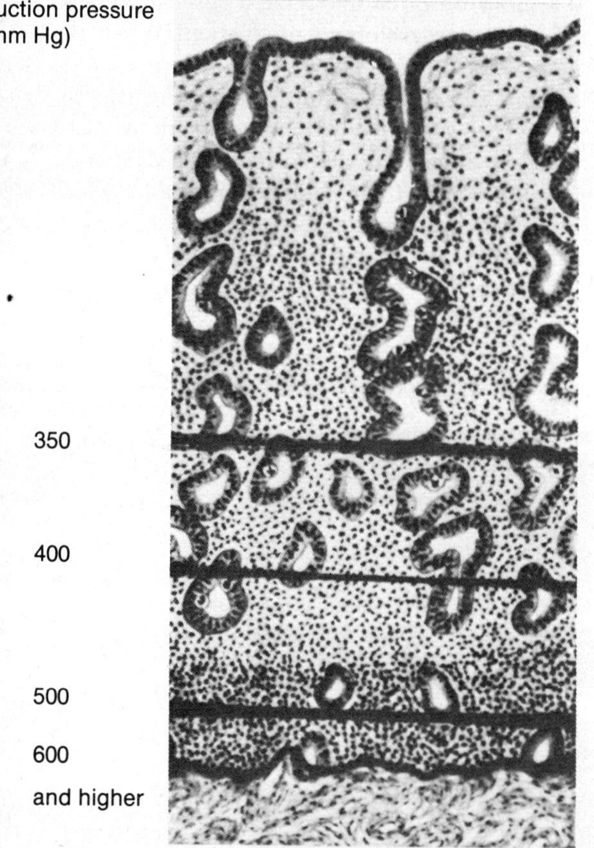

FIGURE 8-18
Schematic interpretation of effects of negative pressures used for vacuum aspiration and depth of cleavage planes in endometrium. (From Marik JJ, Tataryn IV: Dilatation, fractional curretage, and nonpregnant vacuum aspiration. In Symonds EM, Zuspan FP, eds: Clinical and diagnostic procedures in obstetrics and gynecology, Part B, Gynecology. New York, Marcel Dekker, 1984. Reprinted from Gynecology, p. 206, by courtesy of Marcel Dekker, Inc.)

FIGURE 8-19
Cyclic proliferative endometrium. **A,** Endocyte cytology containing sheets of epithelial cells in which nuclei have uniform size and regular contour. Cellular cohesion and orientation are regular (Papanicolaou; ×500). **B,** Kevorkian biopsy of normal proliferative endometrium (H&E; ×250). (From Ferenczy A, Gelfand MM: Obstet Gynecol 63:298, 1984. Reprinted with permission from The American College of Obstetricians and Gynecologists.)

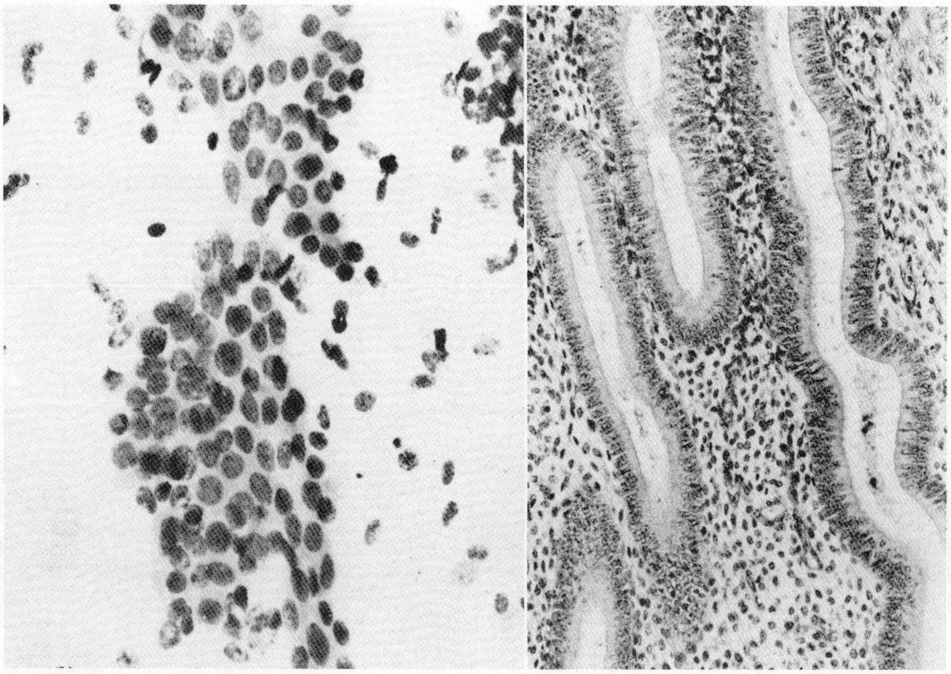

Recommendations and Cost Information

For mass screening, endometrial cytologic sampling has several advantages over endometrial biopsy. The various instruments designed for obtaining endometrial cells for cytology are of a smaller diameter and generally a softer material than biopsy instruments. The majority of procedures performed with the narrow plastic cytologic devices do not require the use of a tenaculum. The foundation of the success or failure of any screening program is patient acceptance, and cytologic screening causes less discomfort than endometrial biopsy. In one comparison study, Ferenczy and Gelfand reported that 100% of the women returned who had undergone sampling of the endometrium with a brush, while only 40% of the women who had endometrial biopsies would consent to a subsequent biopsy procedure. The disadvantages of endometrial cytology as compared to endometrial biopsy are common to most screening procedures. They include decreased accuracy and decreased sensitivity in identifying endometrial hyperplasia.

The major advantages to the patient of the endometrial biopsy over D&C are convenience and cost saving. The financial saving is estimated to be $500 to $750 between an endometrial biopsy and short-stay hospitalization for D&C.

Endometrial biopsy costs between $75 and $150. Cytologic aspiration of cells from the endometrial cavity costs between $20 and $50. The interpretation of a cytologic smear from the endometrium is more complex and takes three to four times longer than interpretation of a cervical cytology smear.

Although multiple instruments are designed for both endometrial biopsy and cytologic sampling, none is superior. The clinical results obtained depend on two factors, the patient's ac-

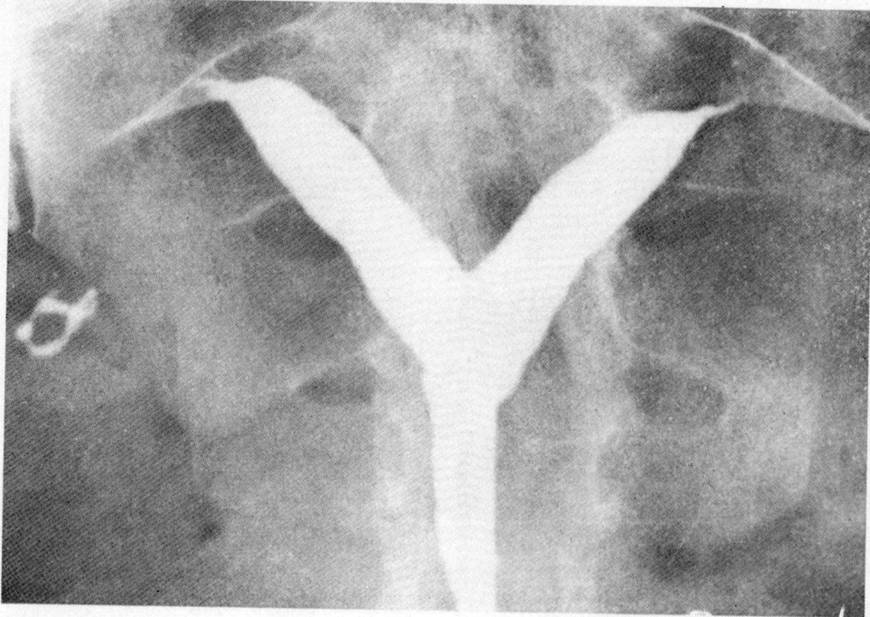

FIGURE 8-23
Hysterosalpingogram from 34-year-old, nulliparous woman who had regular menses and no dysmenorrhea. V-shaped fundal defect with single cervix proved to be bicornuate uterus. (From Siegler AM: Hysterosalpingography. New York, Harper & Row, Publishers, 1967.)

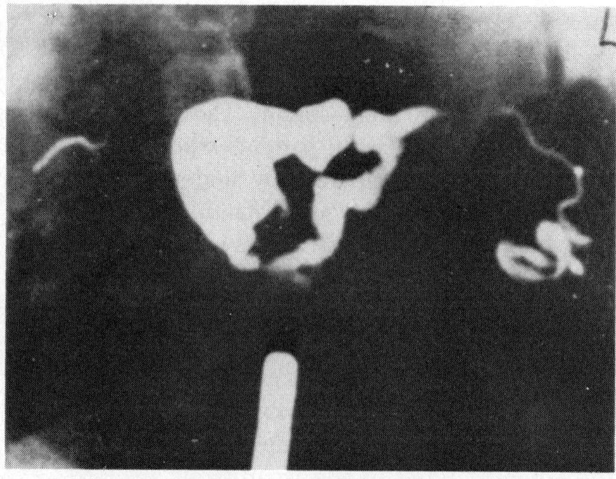

FIGURE 8-24
Hysterosalpingogram demonstrating intrauterine adhesions, grade 3, after repeated curettage for missed abortion. (From Schenker JG, Margalioth EJ: Intrauterine adhesions: an updated appraisal. Fertil Steril 37:593, 1982. Reproduced with permission of the publisher, The American Fertility Society.)

dometrial cavity may also be discovered (Fig. 8-24). HSG is a basic and essential tool in the evaluation of patients with poor reproductive histories. It is specifically applicable for women with repetitive second trimester losses. The technique is frequently performed preoperatively and postoperatively in patients undergoing tubal or plastic surgery to correct tubal obstruction or uterine anomalies or to remove myomas.

HSG is one way of diagnosing an incompetent internal cervical os by measuring its diameter (Fig. 8-25). The maximum normal diameter of the isthmus and internal cervical os is reported to be between 0.7 and 1.0 cm. The anatomic changes in the diameter of the internal os in the nonpregnant state may have little predictive value for future competency in pregnancy because of the dynamic changes during pregnancy that affect cross-linking of collagen and water content of the ground substance in the cervical stroma.

Women with amenorrhea and a history of curettage who do not respond to a progesterone challenge test should have an HSG or hysteroscopy or both. Uterine synechiae are identi-

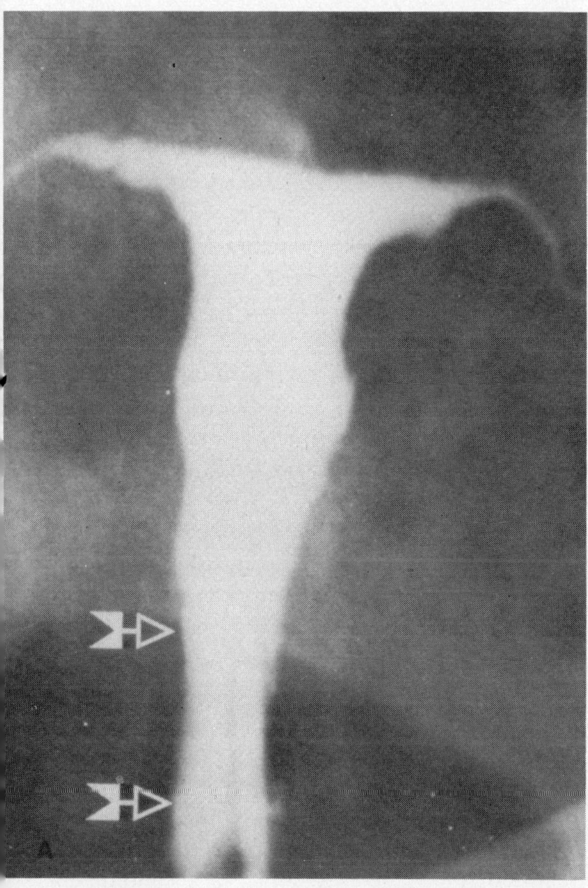

FIGURE 8-25
Hysterosalpingogram demonstrating dilated lower uterine segment (arrows) associated with previous second-trimester abortion suggesting incompetent cervix. (From Siegler AM: Hysterosalpingography. Fertil Steril 40:139, 1983. Reproduced with permission of the publisher, The American Fertility Society.)

fied by slowly injecting a water-soluble medium. If the patient has synechiae, tubal obstruction, and pelvic calcifications, a diagnosis of pelvic tuberculosis should be strongly suspected. HSG will also discover polyps or small submucous myomas in refractory cases of abnormal uterine bleeding.

Contraindications to HSG include the obvious: acute pelvic infection, active uterine bleeding, pregnancy, and allergy to iodine.

The choice of using a small Foley catheter or an adjustable rubber or plastic acorn and cannula for injection depends on physician preference. This decision does not seem to bias re-

sults as long as all air in the system is replaced by the liquid contrast medium. The choice of water-soluble versus oil-based contrast medium depends on the primary indication for the test and physician preference. The advantages and disadvantages of various contrast media have been reviewed by Soules. Water-soluble iodine is preferred for documenting intrauterine filling defects and identifying the severity of mucosal damage in chronic tubal infection. Lipid-based material provides a more distinct and clearer radiographic image. Periodically the opinion has been expressed that the pregnancy rate after HSG is two to three times greater with oil-soluble media. It is difficult to control the multiple variables associated with this finding. However, DeCherney et al. have suggested instillation of 5 ml of oil-based material for its therapeutic effect immediately following a normal diagnostic study with water-based material.

The end point of an x-ray examination for tubal patency is either tubal filling with intraperitoneal spilling or increasing pelvic pain secondary to uterine distension associated with tubal obstruction. Tubal spasm may sometimes be overcome by glucagon (2 mg intravenously), which produces atony of smooth muscle. Glucagon is effective in about one of three women with tubal spasm.

Complications of HSG are rare, but serious when they happen. Acute pelvic infection serious enough to require hospitalization develops in 0.3% to 3.1% of patients. This incidence of pelvic infection is directly related to the population studied, that is, more common in women with dilated tubes. The use of prophylactic antibiotics (tetracycline) may reduce the incidence of acute infection following instrumentation of the uterus. As with surgical procedures that invade the uterus, pelvic pain, uterine perforation, and vasovagal vasomotor reactions do occur. Allergic reactions, particularly to the iodine dye, are a possibility. Intravasation of the dye into the vascular system occurs with high injection pressures, partial perforation of the cannula, and endometrial defects associated with synechiae (Fig. 8-26). Embolic phenomena have been observed with oil-based contrast material. Pelvic peritonitis and granuloma formation with oil-based dye is a very rare complication.

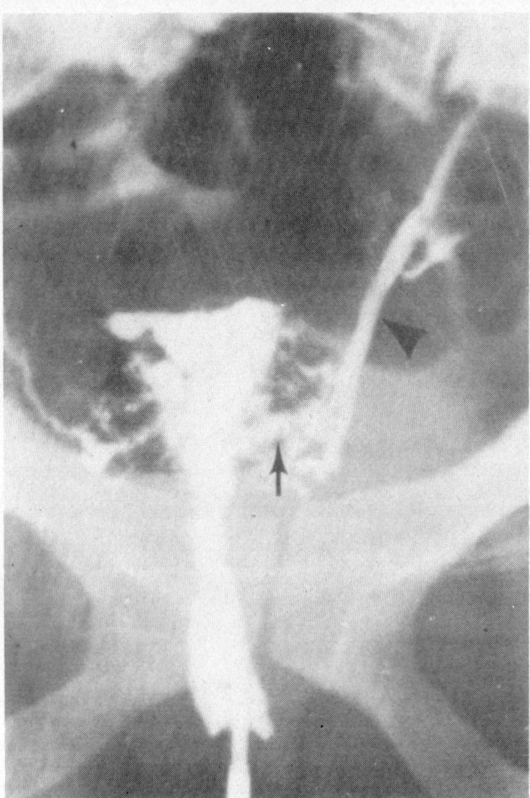

FIGURE 8-26
Hysterosalpingogram showing both lymphatic *(small arrow)* and venous *(large arrow)* intravasation. (From Soules MR, Spadoni LR: Oil versus aqueous media for hysterosalpingography: a continuing debate based on many opinions and few facts. Fertil Steril 38:1, 1982. Reproduced with permission of the publisher, The American Fertility Society.)

Recommendations and Cost Information

In summary, hysterosalpingography is a rapid and relatively safe imaging technique. Its major uses are in the evaluation of patients with infertility or poor pregnancy outcomes. The procedure can diagnose uterine and tubal abnormalities with success. Both oil- and water-based dyes are used.

With a TV screen image intensifier, the average HSG takes 10 minutes to perform. This procedure involves approximately 90 seconds of fluoroscopic time and an average radiation exposure to the ovaries of 1 to 2 rad. The average cost of this outpatient test is between $125 and $175.

HYSTEROSCOPY

Hysteroscopy, the oldest gynecologic endoscopic procedure, is the direct visualization of the endometrial cavity using an endoscope and a light source. The earliest hysteroscope was nothing more than a hollow tube with a kerosene lamp and mirror for a light source. Modern hysteroscopes are modifications of cystoscopes with a channel for a fiberoptic light, a channel to introduce surgical instruments, and a channel to introduce various media to distend the uterus.

Over the past 10 years there has been a renewed interest in hysteroscopy as a result of both improved instrumentation and the use of dextran (Hyskon) as a distending medium. The popularity of hysteroscopy has also been enhanced by the fact that it is a simple technique, much easier to master than laparoscopy. The diagnostic and therapeutic indications for hysteroscopy are also rapidly expanding. Women with recurrent abnormal bleeding, repetitive abortion, uterine synechiae, abnormal hysterosalpingograms, and infertility are candidates for hysteroscopy. Surgical procedures performed under hysteroscopic guidance include location and removal of intact or fragmented IUDs, resection of submucous myomas, lysis of synechiae, incision of uterine septa, removal of endometrial polyps, laser ablation of the endometrium, and placement of silicone plugs into the tubes for sterilization.

The standard hysteroscope is 6 mm in diameter (Fig. 8-27). The angle of view is 30 degrees. Similar to that of a cystoscope, the outer sleeve contains several channels that extend the full length of the instrument, as described earlier.

The cavity of the uterus is a potential space. The success of hysteroscopy depends on the medium used to expand this space. Currently there are three choices: 32% dextran, 5% dextrose and water, and carbon dioxide gas. High molecular weight dextran (average molecular weight 70,000 in 10% glucose) is preferred by the majority of investigators, especially if a surgical procedure is contemplated. This extremely viscous fluid is biodegradable, non-

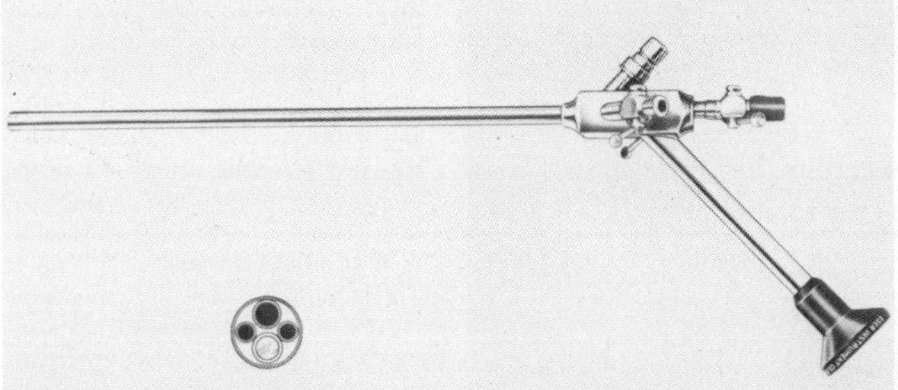

FIGURE 8-27

Hysteroscope (Eder Instrument Co, 8 mm in diameter). Note two side channels for in/out flow of expanding media and middle channel for ancillary instrumentation. (From Schmidt G, Kim MH: Hysteroscopy. In Symonds EM, Zuspan FP, eds: Clinical and diagnostic procedures in obstetrics and gynecology, Part B, Gynecology. New York, Marcel Dekker, 1984. Reprinted from Gynecology, p. 371, by courtesy of Marcel Dekker, Inc.)

toxic, and nonconductive and has good optical qualities. Most importantly, dextran is immiscible with blood; this helps to keep the field clear during intrauterine surgery. Dextran has two drawbacks: it is antigenic, and anaphylaxis has been reported. It also rapidly crystallizes; thus endoscopic instruments must be cleaned shortly after the procedure. Carbon dioxide must be infused with special equipment that carefully limits flow to less than 100 ml per minute and maintains the pressure at approximately 60 to 70 mm Hg. The major precaution with 5% dextrose and water is the monitoring of total fluid intake so as not to produce fluid overload.

Hysteroscopy is ideal to directly visualize and remove partially perforated or broken intrauterine devices. Women with repetitive abortions should have a diagnostic hysteroscopic procedure. Congenital abnormalities that interfere with the success of early pregnancies, such as septa of the uterus, may be seen (Fig. 8-28). Women with recurrent abnormal uterine bleeding may also benefit from this procedure. Often endometrial polyps or small submucous myomas are discovered and may be removed. The extent and location of the uterine synechiae are best described by hysteroscopic examination.

In Europe, endometrial carcinoma is staged by hysteroscopy. In one series, 26% of stage I carcinomas of the endometrium were upgraded to stage II by direct visualization of spread from the fundus to the cervix. Hysteroscopy is helpful in differentiating between adenocarci-

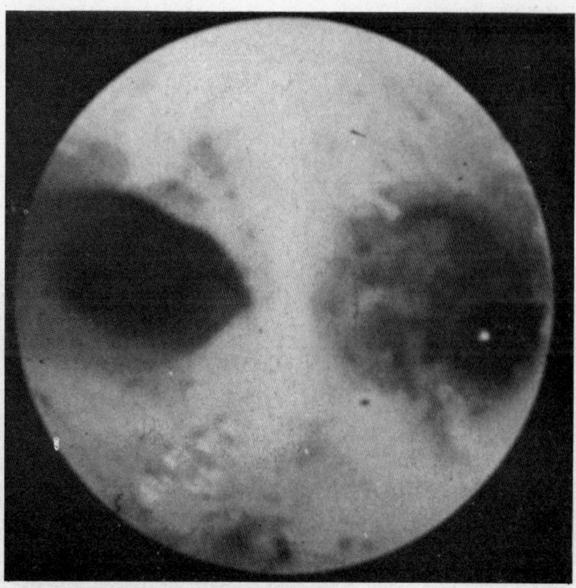

FIGURE 8-28

Intraoperative hysteroscopic view of septate uterus showing inferior point of septum and each uterine horn. (From Israel R, March CM: Am J Obstet Gynecol 149:67, 1984.)

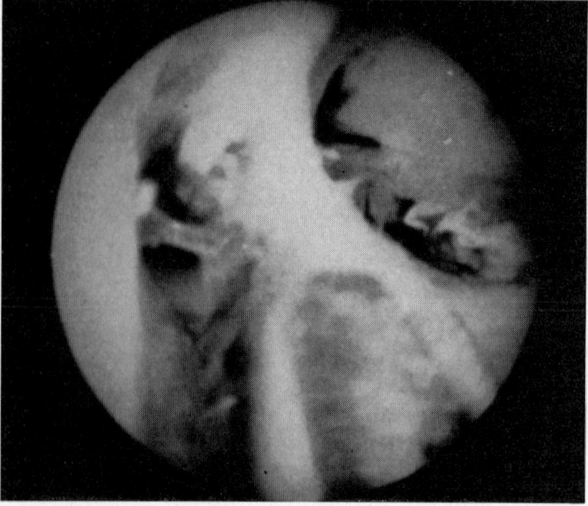

FIGURE 8-29
Hysteroscopic view of intrauterine adhesion in right lateral upper portion of uterus, partially occluding uterotubal junction. (From Valle RF, Sciarra JJ: Hysteroscopic treatment of intrauterine adhesions. In Siegler AM, Lindemann HJ, eds: Hysteroscopy, principles and practice. Philadelphia, J.B. Lippincott Co., 1984.)

noma of the endometrium and endocervix. The theoretical concerns of washing viable malignant cells from the endometrial cavity into the peritoneal cavity and increasing pelvic metastatic disease has not been demonstrated. In the future, hysteroscopy may replace many diagnostic D&C procedures. No matter how meticulous the surgeon is, he or she may miss a focal lesion. D&C is a blind hit-or-miss procedure. With the hysteroscope the gynecologist may visually direct the biopsy forceps to the suspicious area.

Hysteroscopy is superior to hysterosalpingography in discovering intrauterine disease. In comparative studies, the use of hysteroscopy revealed synechiae, polyps, or myomas in 40% of patients with normal hysterosalpingograms (Fig. 8-29). These abnormalities were undetected and unsuspected using x-ray techniques. The false positive rate of hysterosalpingography is 33% when compared to hysteroscopy. One in three women diagnosed as having an intrauterine filling defect by x-ray imaging will have a normal cavity directly visualized with the hysteroscope.

Recently contact hysteroscopy has become more popular because of its simplicity, since a distending medium is not needed (Fig. 8-30). The contact hysteroscope touches the surface to be viewed, and blood and debris are pushed away from the field of vision by gentle tissue contact. The interpretation of endometrial pathology is similar to colposcopy in that it depends on color, contour, and vascular pattern. The contact hysteroscope is the instrument of choice to examine the vagina of an infant or prepubertal child. Hamou developed a microhysteroscope that does not require cervical dilation. This instrument has interchangeable lenses that produce magnifications of $\times 1$, $\times 20$, $\times 60$, and $\times 150$. He uses the higher magnifications to perform contact microcolposcopy of the endocervical canal. This necessitates staining with a vital stain, such as Waterman's blue ink.

The variety and extent of surgery performed

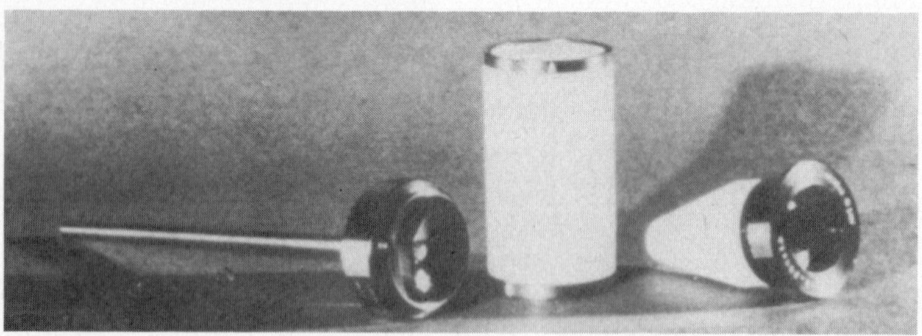

FIGURE 8-30
Contact hysteroscope consisting of three parts: optical guide, cylindric light-collecting chamber, and magnifying eyepiece. (From Baggish MS, Barbot J: Clin Obstet Gynecol 26:221, 1983.)

transcervically with the hysteroscope have expanded significantly during the past 10 years. Endoscopic procedures have progressed from snaring a small polyp to ablating the entire endometrial lining with a laser. The uterine synechiae of a woman with Asherman's syndrome can be cut with microscissors, gradually reestablishing the endometrial cavity. Following the operation a large plastic IUD is placed in the cavity as a stent. For the next 2 months the patient should receive 7.5 mg of conjugated estrogen per day to facilitate regeneration and reepithelialization of the endometrium. An oral progestogen should be given during the last 10 days of estrogen therapy. By performing this operation on an outpatient basis and transcervically, major morbidity and expense can be avoided. The alternative transabdominal metroplasty involves a uterine incision, necessitating that future pregnancies be delivered by cesarean section.

Neuwirth has pioneered a method of removing submucous myomas with a modified urologic resectoscope. He uses a cutting electric current and shaves the myoma until it is flat with the surrounding endometrial lining. An inflatable balloon is inserted into the uterine cavity and left for 24 hours, facilitating hemostasis. After the procedure endometrial regeneration is stimulated with oral estrogen.

Many groups have attempted to develop a method of outpatient transcervical sterilization. The most sophisticated technique uses a hysteroscope to inject liquid silicone into the tubal ostia (Figs. 8-31 and 8-32). A special catalyzer causes the liquid to form a plug within a few minutes. The silicone contains radiopaque silver powder so it may be visualized by a pelvic radiograph. Though the procedure is still in the experimental stages, it is promising. Approximately 85% of women have plugs successfully placed. In the preliminary studies, failure rates have been similar to those in other methods of female sterilization.

Goldrath has discovered that it is possible to ablate the endometrial lining using a hysteroscopic directed laser. The laser photovaporizes the epithelium. This procedure is performed in women with severe dysfunctional uterine bleeding, who for some reason are not candidates for hysterectomy. Hysterograms following laser treatment have demonstrated contraction, scarring, and dense adhesion formation.

There are few contraindications to hystero-

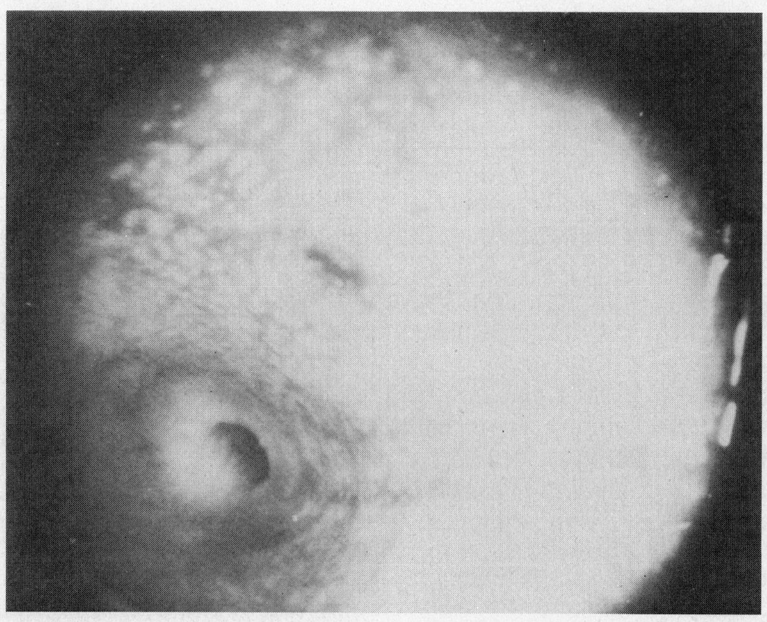

FIGURE 8-31
Hysteroscopic view of tubal ostium. (From Hamou JE: Clin Obstet Gynecol 26:290, 1983.)

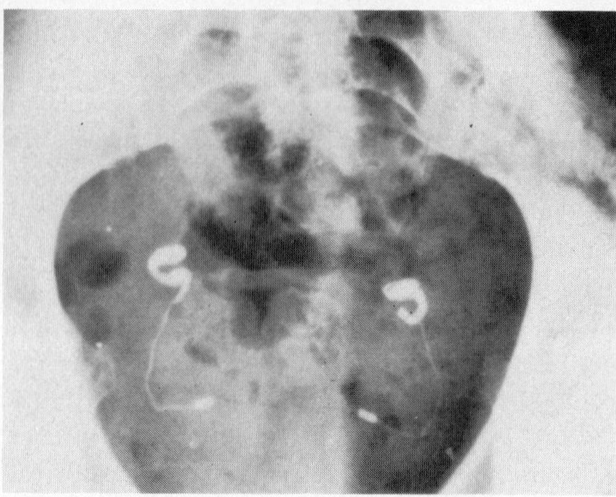

FIGURE 8-32
Normal silicon plugs on pelvic flat-plate radiograph (From Houck RM, Cooper JM, Rigberg HS: Obstet Gynecol 62:588, 1983. Reproduced with permission from The American College of Obstetricians and Gynecologists.)

scopy. Acute pelvic infection is the leading one because of the potential of spreading the disease by the media used for uterine distention. Active bleeding is a relative contraindication. If the bleeding is brisk, the hysteroscopic procedure will be unsatisfactory. Pregnancy is a contraindication.

Complications of hysteroscopy are noted in less than 2% of the procedures. These complications include uterine perforation, pelvic infection, and bleeding. The potential complications of the distending media include anaphylaxis to dextran, circulatory overload with 5% dextrose and water, and the potential of gas embolism with carbon dioxide.

Recommendations and Cost Information

In summary, hysteroscopy is a simple technique for the evaluation of intrauterine pathology. The use of the hysteroscope for intrauterine surgery is rapidly expanding. The cost of a diagnostic hysteroscopic procedure is between $200 and $350.

LAPAROSCOPY

Laparoscopy has radically changed the clinical practice of gynecology over the past 15 to

20 years. This outpatient surgical technique provides a window to directly visualize pelvic anatomy (Fig. 8-33). Today laparoscopy has replaced D&C as the most frequently performed operation by the gynecologic service of university hospitals.

Laparoscopy was first performed in the early 1900s. Two events of the early 1960s renewed interest in this surgical technique, the first being the development of fiberoptic cables and the second the change in society's attitude toward overpopulation and sterilization. Patrick Steptoe is considered the "father" of modern laparoscopy for his work in the mid-1960s with laparoscopic sterilization. By the mid-1970s laparoscopy had been adopted as the method of choice for female sterilization.

The advantages of low cost, convenience, and shorter stay are obvious when laparoscopy is compared to celiotomy. Minilaparotomy in a thin woman may be competitive in time and cost to laparoscopy. However, if a woman is moderately obese there is no comparison.

There are several indications for laparoscopy, both diagnostic and therapeutic. The most common indication is female sterilization. Laparoscopy is an essential step in the diagnostic work-up of a couple with infertility or a woman with chronic pelvic pain. Adventurous gynecologists have progressed from using the laparo-

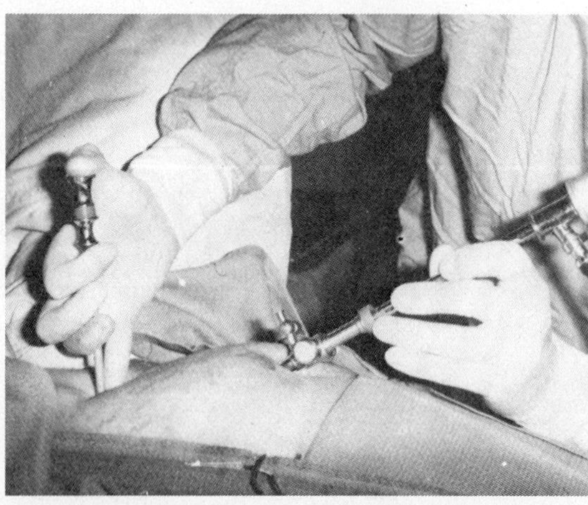

FIGURE 8-33
Insertion of accessory trocar for laparoscopy is made under direct visual control of operator. (From Cibils LA: Gynecologic laparoscopy. Philadelphia, Lea & Febiger, 1975.)

scope to perform such simple surgical tasks as removal of a perforated IUD to more complicated surgery such as evacuating unruptured ectopic pregnancies.

Laparoscopy has made outpatient sterilization available to women throughout the world. The failure rate is approximately 1 in 250 to 1 in 500 cases. Sterilization is accomplished with electric cauterization, Silastic bands, or spring-loaded clips. Because of the serious complications with unipolar cautery, most cautery sterilization procedures are performed with bipolar coagulation of approximately 2 cm of the tube without division (Fig. 8-34). Of the nonelectric alternatives, the Silastic bands have a lower failure rate than the clips (Fig. 8-35). However, with the bands 2 to 3 procedures per 100 result in acute transection of the tube with bleeding from the tube or mesosalpinx. Hemostasis can be obtained by applying another band or with cautery. The spring-loaded clip causes necrosis of less than 1 cm of tube and is the easiest sterilization procedure to successfully reverse (Fig. 8-36). The clip or the band should be placed on the narrow isthmus so the size of the appliance conforms to the diameter of the fallopian tube.

There are several indications for laparoscopy in infertile women. Tubal patency and mobility can be directly observed via the laparoscope (Fig. 8-37). Laparoscopy is able to confirm or rule out intrinsic pelvic disorders such as endometriosis or chronic pelvic inflammatory dis-

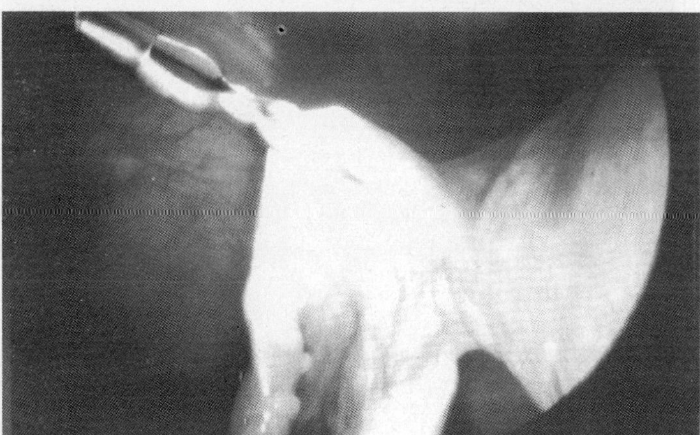

FIGURE 8-34
Laparoscopic view of bipolar coagulation. A Kleppinger bipolar forceps has been used to coagulate isthmic-ampullary junction of this tube in three contiguous places. (From Hulka JF: Textbook of laparoscopy. Orlando, Fla., Grune & Stratton, 1985.)

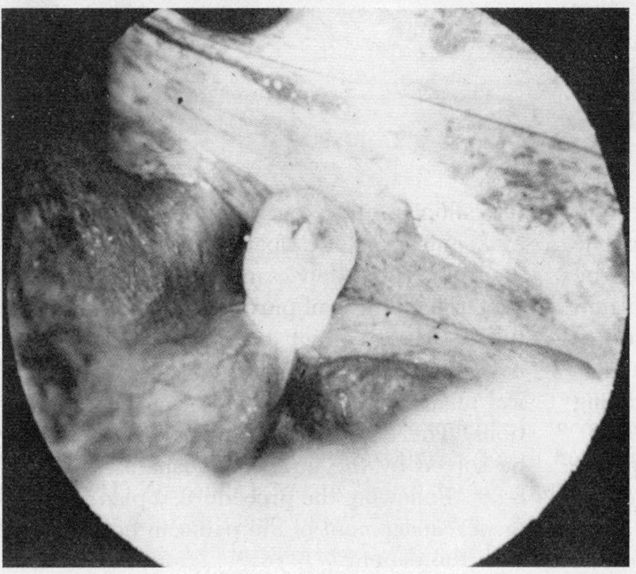

FIGURE 8-35
Laparoscopic view of a Falope-Ring applied to fallopian tube. (From Yoon I: Silicone ring. In Phillips JM, ed: Laparoscopy. Copyright © 1977 by The Williams & Wilkins Co., Baltimore.)

malignancy, large abdominal masses, severe cardiovascular disease, and tuberculous peritonitis. Relative contraindications, in which each case must be individualized, include extensive obesity, hiatal hernia, advanced pregnancy, generalized peritonitis, and extensive intraabdominal scarring.

Laparoscopy may be performed under local or general anesthesia. Many prefer local anesthesia for its safety. The risks associated with general anesthesia are one of the major hazards of laparoscopy. The most frequent complication

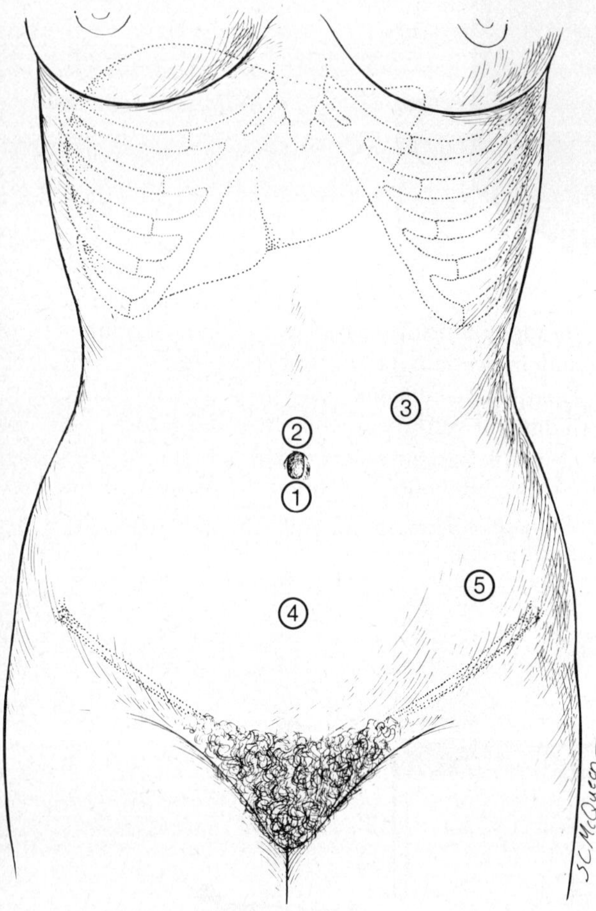

FIGURE 8-40
Usual sites for insertion of insufflating needle: (1) infraumbilical fold; (2) supraumbilical fold; (3) left costal margin; (4) midway between umbilicus and pubis; and (5) left McBurney's point. (From Corson SL: Operating room preparation and basic techniques. In Phillips JM: Laparoscopy. Copyright © 1977 by the Williams & Wilkins Co., Baltimore.)

of laparoscopy is hypercarbia associated with hypoventilation. The standard diagnostic laparoscope is 10 mm in diameter. Secondary puncture trochars vary from 5 mm (bipolar forceps) to 7 or 8 mm in width (spring-loaded clip and Silastic band). A laparoscope is 30 cm long and provides a field of vision of 60 to 75 degrees. The inferior margin of the umbilicus is the preferred site of entry, as this is the thinnest area of the abdominal wall. Alternative sites are detailed in Fig. 8-40. The choice of gas to develop the pneumoperitoneum depends on the choice of anesthesia. Nitrous oxide is preferable with local anesthesia, while carbon dioxide is the choice with general anesthesia. Nitrous oxide is nonflammable but does support combustion. Carbon dioxide quickly forms carbonic acid on the moist parietal peritoneal surface, which results in considerable discomfort to a patient without regional or general anesthesia.

The three major categories of complications with laparoscopy are laceration of vessels, intestinal injuries, and cardiorespiratory problems arising from the pneumoperitoneum. Since abdominal wall hematomas are usually subfascial in location, care must be taken to avoid the epigastric vessels. Laceration of the aorta, inferior vena cava, or iliac vessels is a surgical emergency. Intestinal injuries may be produced by the Veress needle or the trochar.

Hasson has advocated open laparoscopy to avoid intestinal injury (Fig. 8-41). Instead of blind entry into the peritoneal cavity, a small incision is made in the fascia and parietal peritoneum. The cone is placed in the abdominal cavity under direct visual control. The fascia is secured to the sleeve of the cone to obtain an airtight seal. Open laparoscopy reduces the incidence of both bowel and vascular trauma. It is the procedure of choice if the patient has a history of multiple abdominal operations.

Complications directly related to the pneumoperitoneum include pneumothorax, diminished venous return, gas embolism, and cardiac arrhythymias. It is important not to develop pressures greater than 20 mm Hg in establishing the pneumoperitoneum. High pressures impede venous return and limit excursion of the diaphragm. A rare but life-threatening complication of laparoscopy is gas embolism, which produces hypotension and the classical

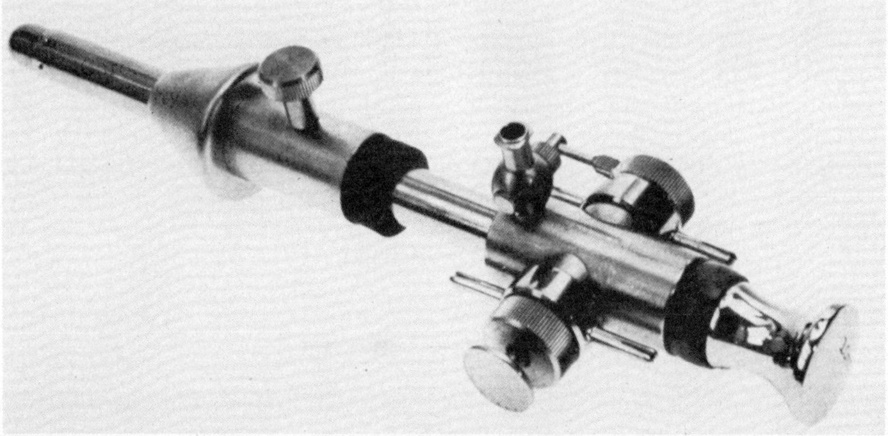

FIGURE 8-41
Open laparoscopy cannula. (From Hasson HM: Open laparoscopy. In Symonds EM, Zuspan FP, eds: Clinical and diagnostic procedures in obstetrics and gynecology, Part B, Gynecology. New York, Marcel Dekker, 1984. Reprinted from Gynecology, p. 312, by courtesy of Marcel Dekker, Inc.)

"mill wheel" murmur, which can be heard over the entire precordium. The patient with this complication should be turned on her left side and the frothy blood aspirated by a central venous catheter directed into the right side of the heart.

Recommendations and Cost Information

In summary, laparoscopy, more than any other advance, has changed the clinical practice of gynecology over the past two decades. Today's residents have a difficult time contem-

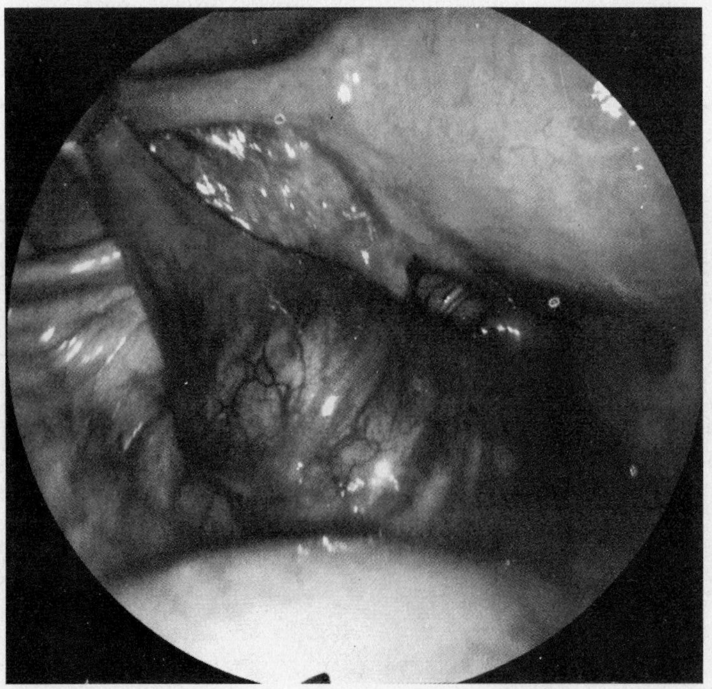

FIGURE 8-42
Laparoscopic view of unruptured ectopic pregnancy. (From Hulka JF: Textbook of laparoscopy. Orlando, Fla., Grune & Stratton, 1985.)

plating the practice of the specialty prior to the introduction of the "silver tube." Laparoscopy provides a window for the diagnosis of infertility, pelvic pain, ectopic pregnancy, abdominal and pelvic trauma, staging the extent of pelvic disease, and the visual diagnosis of abnormal anatomy. Therapeutically the primary use of the laparoscope is female sterilization. However, one can biopsy abnormal tissue, lyse adhesions, aspirate oocytes, retrieve lost IUDs, and treat endometriosis and early ectopic pregnancies with this technique (Fig. 8-42). The total cost of a laparoscopic procedure is between $600 and $1000, which is approximately 25% of the cost of a celiotomy.

KEY POINTS

- A sector scanner is preferable for gynecologic ultrasound exams as it provides greater visualization of the pelvis than a linear array.

- Sonography has not been found to cause adverse clinical effects in humans with the energy levels used in diagnostic studies.

- Computed tomography is useful in discovering extension of pelvic cancer into the fat of the retroperitoneal space and the detection of enlarged lymph nodes.

- For computed tomography the surface radiation dose is between 2 and 10 rads. This radiation exposure is similar to that of a barium enema.

- The major use of computed tomography scans in gynecology has been in evaluating women with pituitary tumors and in identifying retroperitoneal disease during the initial evaluation of pelvic carcinoma.

- Magnetic resonance imaging penetrates bone and air without attenuation. Therefore, this technique allows identification of soft tissue disease inaccessible to other imaging techniques.

- Magnetic resonance imaging uses radio frequency radiation, which is nonionizing radiation.

- Magnetic resonance imaging has the capacity to differentiate normal from malignant tissue and also may identify areas of abnormal tissue metabolism.

- The hematocrit of unclotted blood obtained during culdocentesis will be over 15% when bleeding emanates from an ectopic pregnancy.

- The incidence of false positive culdocentesis in the diagnosis of ectopic pregnancy is less than 2%.

- The diagnostic accuracy of endometrial biopsy is 90% to 98% when compared to subsequent findings at D&C or hysterectomy.

- The evaluation of direct cytological material from the endometrial cavity has a false negative rate for malignancy between 5% and 15%.

- Fifteen percent of women who have obstructed fallopian tubes as determined by hysterosalpingography subsequently become pregnant without further treatment.

- Pain relief does not invariably alleviate tubal spasm during hysterosalpingography.

- Acute pelvic infection develops in 0.3% to 3.1% of patients following a hysterosalpingogram.

- The major indications for hysteroscopy are abnormal uterine bleeding, infertility, or recurrent abortion.

- Hysteroscopy is superior to hysterosalpingography in discovering and diagnosing intrauterine pathology.

- Dextran is an extremely viscous fluid used to distend the uterus during hysteroscopy. Dextran is nontoxic, nonconductive, and immiscible with blood.

- The failure rate with laparoscopic sterilization is between 1 in 250 and 1 in 500 cases.

- Absolute contraindications to laparoscopy include significant hemoperitoneum, anticoagulation therapy, advanced malignancy, large abdominal masses, severe cardiovascular disease, and tuberculous peritonitis.

- Three major complications of laparoscopy are laceration of vessels, intestinal injuries, and cardiorespiratory problems arising from the pneumoperitoneum. The incidence of major complications is less than 1 in 1000 cases.

BIBLIOGRAPHY

Angel JL, Knuppel RA: Computed tomography in diagnosis of puerperal ovarian vein thrombosis. Obstet Gynecol 63:61, 1984.

Baggish MS, Barbot J: Contact hysteroscopy. Clin Obstet Gynecol 26:219, 1983.

Bamford DS, Hall EW, Newman MR: The Isaacs endometrial cell sampler, an evaluation in 100 patients with postmenopausal bleeding. Acta Cytol 28:101, 1984.

Bhiwandiwala PP, Mumford SD, Feldblum PJ: A comparison of different laparoscopic sterilization occlusion techniques in 24,439 procedures. Am J Obstet Gynecol 144:319, 1982.

Bonneville JF, Poulignot D, Cattin F, et al: Computed tomographic demonstration of the effects of bromocriptine on pituitary microadenoma size. Radiology 143:451, 1982.

Cibils LA: Gynecologic Laparoscopy. Philadelphia, Lea & Febiger, 1974.

Copenhaver EH, Malone PD, Steckel FE, et al: Surgery of the vulva and vagina, a practical guide. Philadelphia, WB Saunders Co., 1981.

Crooks LE, Hoenninger J, Arakawa M, et al: High-resolution magnetic resonance imaging. Radiology 150:163, 1984.

DeCherney AH, Romero R, Polan ML: Ultrasound in reproductive endocrinology. Fertil Steril 37:323, 1982.

Dietemann JL, Portha C, Cattin F, et al: CT follow-up of microprolactinomas during bromocriptine-induced pregnancy. Neuroradiology 25:133, 1983.

Einerth Y: Vacuum curettage by the Vabra® method. Acta Obstet Gynecol Scand 61:373, 1982.

Federle MP: Computed tomography in obstetrics and gynecology. Female Patient 9:39, 1984.

Ferenczy A, Gelfand MM: Outpatient endometrial sampling with endocyte: comparative study of its effectiveness with endometrial biopsy. Obstet Gynecol 63:295, 1984.

Goldrath MH, Fuller TA, Segal S: Laser photovaporization of endometrium for the treatment of menorrhagia. Am J Obstet Gynecol 140:14, 1981.

Grimes DA: Diagnostic dilation and curettage: a reappraisal. Am J Obstet Gynecol 142:1, 1982.

Gross BH, Moss AA, Mihara K, et al: Computed tomography of gynecologic diseases. AJR 141:765, 1983.

Hamou JE: Microhysteroscopy. Clin Obstet Gynecol 26:285, 1983.

Hasson HM: The optimum method of abdominal entry for laparoscopy. In Phillips JM, ed: Endoscopy in gynecology. Downey, Calif, The American Association of Gynecologic Laparoscopists, 1978.

Hill GJ: Outpatient surgery. Philadelphia, WB Saunders Co., 1973.

Houck RM, Cooper JM, Rigberg HS: Hysteroscopic tubal occlusion with formed-in-place silicone plugs: a clinical review. Obstet Gynecol 62:587, 1983.

Hulka JF: Textbook of Laparoscopy. Orlando, Fla, Grune & Stratton, 1985.

Hutchins CJ: Laparoscopy and hysterosalpingography in the assessment of tubal patency. Obstet Gynecol 49:325, 1977.

Israel R, March CM: Hysteroscopic incision of the septate uterus. Am J Obstet Gynecol 149:66, 1984.

Iversen OE, Segadal E: The value of endometrial cytology. A comparative study of the Gravlee Jet-Washer, Isaacs cell sampler, and endoscan versus curettage in 600 patients. Obstet Gynecol Surv 40:14, 1985.

Johnson IR, Symonds EM, Kean DM, et al: Imaging the pregnant human uterus with nuclear magnetic resonance. Am J Obstet Gynecol 148:1136, 1985.

Johnson IR, Symonds EM, Worthington BS, et al: Imaging ovarian tumors by nuclear magnetic resonance. Br J Obstet Gynaecol 91:260, 1984.

Lewis BV: Hysteroscopy in gynaecological practice: a review. J R Soc Med 77:235, 1984.

Mann WJ, Mendonca-Dias MH, Lauterbur PC, et al: Preliminary in vitro studies of nuclear magnetic resonance spin-lattice relaxation times and three-dimensional nuclear magnetic resonance imaging in gynecologic oncology. Am J Obstet Gynecol 148:91, 1984.

Mendonca-Dias MH, Mann WJ, Chumas J, et al: Three-dimensional nuclear-magnetic-resonance zeugmatographic imaging of surgical specimens. Biosci Rep 2:713, 1982.

Moldofsky PJ, Sears HF, Mulhern CB, et al: Detection of metastatic tumor in normal-sized retroperitoneal lymph nodes by monoclonal-antibody imaging. N Engl J Med 311:106, 1984.

Neuwirth RS: Hysteroscopic management of symptomatic submucous fibroids. Obstet Gynecol 62:509, 1983.

O'Brien WF, Buck DR, Nash JD: Evaluation of sonography in the initial assessment of the gynecologic patient. Am J Obstet Gynecol 149:598, 1984.

Oldendorf WH: NMR imaging: its potential clinical impact. Hosp Pract 17:114, 1982.

Partain CL, James AE Jr, Rollo FD, et al: Nuclear magnetic resonance imaging. Philadelphia, WB Saunders Co., 1983.

Peterson HB, DeStefano F, Rubin GL, et al: Deaths attributable to tubal sterilization in the United States 1977-1981. Am J Obstet Gynecol 146:131, 1983.

Phillips JM: Laparoscopy. Baltimore, Williams & Wilkins, 1977.

Pittaway DE, Winfield AC, Maxson W, et al: Prevention of acute pelvic inflammatory disease after hysterosalpingography: efficacy of doxycycline prophylaxis. Am J Obstet Gynecol 147:623, 1983.

Sanders RC, James AE Jr: The principles and practice of ultrasonography in obstetrics and gynecology, ed 2. New York, Appleton-Century-Crofts, 1980.

Schenker JG, Margalioth EJ: Intrauterine adhesions: an updated appraisal. Fertil Steril 37:593, 1982.

Siegler AM: Hysterosalpingography. New York, Harper & Row, Publishers, 1967.

Siegler AM: Hysterosalpingography. Fertil Steril 40:139, 1983.

Siegler AM, Lindemann HJ: Hysteroscopy, principles and practice. Philadelphia, JB Lippincott Co., 1984.

Sommer FG, Walsh JW, Schwartz PE, et al: Evaluation of gynecologic pelvic masses by ultrasound and computed tomography. J Reprod Med 27:45, 1982.

Soules MR, Spadoni LR: Oil versus aqueous media for hysterosalpingography: a continuing debate based on many opinions and few facts. Fertil Steril 38:1, 1982.

Swayne LC, Love MB, Karasick SR: Pelvic inflammatory disease: sonographic-pathologic correlation. Radiology 151:751, 1984.

Symonds EM, Zuspan FP: Clinical and diagnostic procedures in obstetrics and gynecology. New York, Marcel Dekker, 1984.

Taylor PJ, Hamou JE: Hysteroscopy. J Reprod Med 28:359, 1983.

Thickman D, Kressel H, Gussman D, et al: Nuclear magnetic resonance imaging in gynecology. Am J Obstet Gynecol 149:835, 1984.

Voss SC, Lacey CG, Pupkin M, et al: Ultrasound and the pelvic mass. J Reprod Med 28:833, 1983.

Walsh JW, Amendola MA, Konerding KF, et al: Computed tomographic detection of pelvic and inguinal lymph-node metastases from primary and recurrent pelvic malignant disease. Radiology 137:157, 1980.

Walsh JW, Goplerud DR: Prospective comparison between clinical and CT staging in primary cervical carcinoma. AJR 137:997, 1981.

Wentz AC: Endometrial biopsy in the evaluation of infertility. Fertil Steril 33:121, 1980.

Wittenberg J: Computed tomography of the body. I. N Engl J Med 309:1160, 1983.

Wittenberg J: Computed tomography of the body. II. N Engl J Med 309:1224, 1983.

Worthington BS: Clinical prospects for nuclear magnetic resonance. Clin Radiol 34:3, 1983.

GENERAL
GYNECOLOGY

CHAPTER 9

Congenital Abnormalities

KEY TERMS AND DEFINITIONS

Accessory Ovary. Excess ovarian tissue near a normally placed ovary and connected to it.

Ambiguous Genitalia. Anatomic modification of the external genitalia, which makes specific determination of gender difficult.

Androgen Insensitivity Syndrome. An X-linked condition of a testosterone receptor defect in a 46, XY individual with testes and normal male testosterone levels. These individuals have absent uterus, normal female phenotype, and scanty body hair.

Arcuate Uterus. A minimum septate uterus; probably of no clinical importance.

Bicornuate Uterus. A partial lack of fusion of two uterine corpora to varying degree. A single cervix is present.

Didelphic Uterus. Complete duplication of the uterus and cervix without fusion of the two cavities. One fallopian tube joins each fundal cavity. This condition may be associated with a septate vagina.

Hematocolpos. Distension of an obstructed vagina (caused by imperforate hymen or transverse septum) with blood and blood products.

Hydrocolpos. Distension of an obstructed vagina (caused by imperforate hymen or transverse septum) with fluid.

Labial Fusion. Fusion of the labia minora in the midline, closing the introitus.

Mucocolpos. A vagina blocked by an imperforate hymen or transverse septum and filled with mucus.

Ovotestes. A gonad that contains both ovarian and testicular remnants.

Repetitive Spontaneous Abortion. The loss of three or more pregnancies before 20 weeks' gestation. Functionally, however, many physicians will do a workup for repetitive spontaneous abortion after two or more pregnancy losses.

Rokitansky-Küster-Hauser Syndrome. A 46,XX female with müllerian failure, usually showing absence of all or most of vagina, cervix, uterus, and fallopian tubes.

Rudimentary Uterine Horn. A structure that develops from one müllerian duct and does not communicate with the uterine cavity. The contralateral fallopian tube communicates with the uterine cavity. The ipsilateral fallopian tube communicates with that horn.

Septate Uterus. The presence of a septum that separates the uterine cavity either partially or completely into two separate cavities.

Supernumerary Ovary. The presence of a third ovary separated from the normally situated ovaries.

Unicolic (Unicornuate) Uterus. A uterus and cervix that develop from a single müllerian duct joined at the top of the fundus by only one fallopian tube. It represents complete arrest of one müllerian duct.

Vaginal Agenesis. Absence of the vagina.

Congenital abnormalities of the female reproductive tract can be caused by a genetic error or by a teratologic event during embryonic development. Minor abnormalities may be of little consequence, but major abnormalities may lead to severe impairment of menstrual and reproductive functions. This chapter categorizes a number of such abnormalities and discusses diagnosis and treatment. For discussion of the etiology of these problems, the reader is referred to Chapter 1, Embryology.

EXAMINATION OF THE NEWBORN FOR SEXUAL AMBIGUITIES

The first major diagnostic decision of the obstetrician or neonatal physician with respect to the newborn is gender assignment. In most cases the designation is clear. However, in newborns with ambiguous genitalia there is a potentially serious problem for both physician and parents. The female who has been androgenized may appear similar to the male pseudohermaphrodite suffering from incomplete androgen insensitivity syndrome. Also, some vulvar abnormalities may resemble partial androgenization. It is therefore appropriate to systematically evaluate the newborn's genitalia to define appropriate sex assessment.

The first, and probably most important, aspect of the examination is inspection. The physician should systematically observe the newborn's perineum, beginning with the mons pubis. The clitoris should be noted for any obvious enlargement, the opening of the urethra should be identified, and the labia should be separated to see if the introitus can be visualized. If the labia are fused, this maneuver will be impossible. At times the labia are joined by flimsy adhesions; these generally separate in later childhood or respond to the application of estrogen cream. If it is possible to separate the labia, the hymen may be observed. Generally it is partially perforate, revealing the entrance into the vagina. Posteriorly the labia fuse in the midline at the posterior fourchette of the perineum. Posterior to the perineal body the rectum can be visualized, and it should be tested to be sure that it is perforate. Meconium staining about the rectum is evidence for perfora-

tion. If there is doubt, the rectum may be penetrated with a cotton-tipped swab or, if necessary, with the little finger encased in a well-lubricated finger cot.

If the labia are fused and the clitoris is not enlarged, other abnormalities may also be present. For instance, defects of the anterior abdominal wall may exist as well. The infant should be carefully examined for other defects. An enlarged clitoris and fused labia are evidence of androgen effect and may imply congenital adrenal hyperplasia, maternal ingestion of androgens, or increased natural androgen production.

In most instances, inspection is all that is necessary. If for any reason, however, the physician wishes to examine the vagina or see the cervix of the newborn, an endoscope, such as a cystoscope, may be used, since the hymen is generally perforate and will accept this instrument.

If labial fusion is noted, the physician should palpate the groins and labial folds for evidence of gonads. Gonads palpable in the inguinal canal, labioinguinal region, or labioscrotal folds are almost always testes. Thus such a finding implies a male with ambiguous genitalia rather than a virilized female. Conversely, an infant with ambiguous genitalia but without palpable testes in the scrotum is likely to be a virilized female, most often the result of congenital adrenal hyperplasia. Rectal examination may make it possible to palpate a cervix and uterus, thus helping in the differential diagnosis.

Where ambiguous genitalia are noted, further testing, such as chromosome analysis or buccal smear and blood or urinary studies for androgens and related enzymes, may be required. It is important to order these studies immediately, as gender assignment is an important event that should take place as soon after birth as possible.

SPECIFIC DEFECTS OF THE EXTERNAL AND INTERNAL GENITALIA

In the remaining sections of this chapter, specific defects of each level of the external and internal female genitalia will be discussed.

Perineal and Vaginal Defects

Defects of the Clitoris

The clitoris is generally 1 to 1.5 cm long and 0.5 cm wide in the nonerect state. The glans is partially covered by a hood of skin. The urethra opens near the base of the clitoris. Abnormalities are unusual, although the clitoris may be enlarged because of androgen stimulation. In such circumstances the shaft of the clitoris may be quite enlarged, and partial development of a penile urethra may have occurred. Extreme cases of androgen stimulation are generally associated with fusion of the labia. These findings occur in infants with congenital adrenal hyperplasia and in those exposed in utero to androgens of natural origin (Fig. 9-1).

Labial Fusion

Although labial fusion may result from exposure to exogenous androgens or be associated with defects of the anterior abdominal wall, the most common cause is congenital adrenal hyperplasia. The most common form is due to an inborn error of metabolism involving the enzyme 21-hydroxylase. This condition is transmitted as an autosomal recessive gene coded on chromosome 6, and because of the error in 21-hydroxylase metabolism, the major biosynthesis pathway to cortisol is diminished. Homozygous individuals occur at a rate of 1 per 490 to 1 per 67,000 of the population, depending on the community. Heterozygotic carriers are present in the population in a frequency ranging from 1 per 20 to 1 per 250.

The genetically mutated 21-hydroxylase enzyme interferes with cortisol production in such a fashion that plasma 17-hydroxyprogesterone levels are elevated. Two other enzyme defects also transmittable as autosomal recessive traits that may give similar abnormal findings are 11-hydroxylase deficiency and 3-β-hydroxysteroid dehydrogenase deficiency.

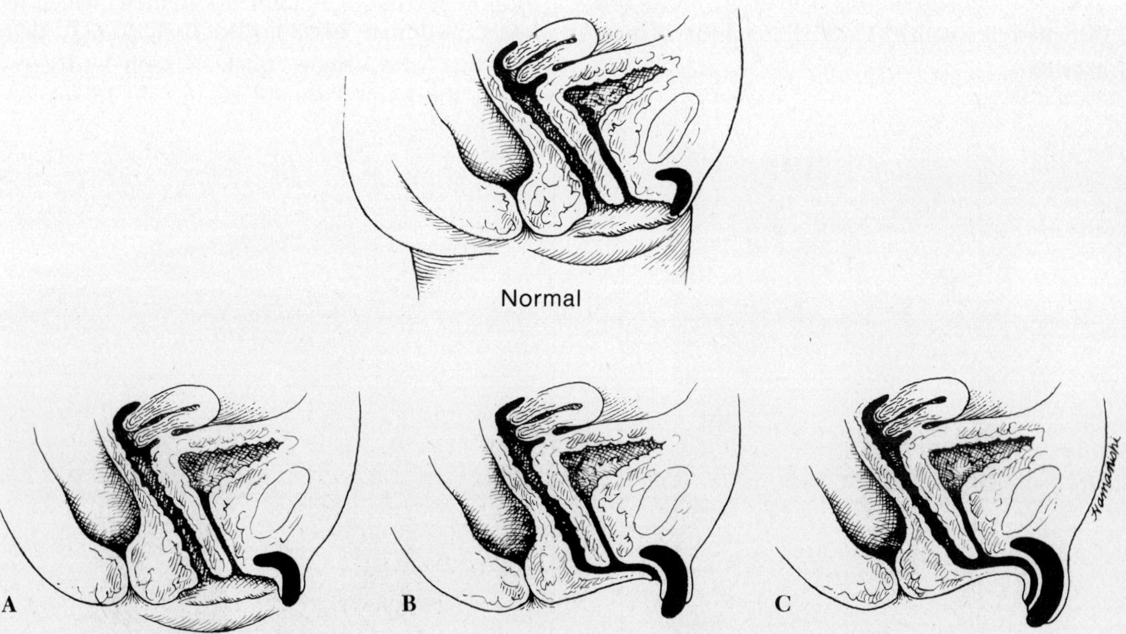

FIGURE 9-1
Sagittal views of genital deformities seen in female infants who are masculinized. **A,** Minimal masculinization with slight enlargement of the clitoris. **B,** Labial fusion and more marked enlargement of the clitoris. **C,** Complete labial fusion, enlargement of the clitoris, and formation of a partial penial urethra. (Modified from Verkauf BS, Jones HW, Jr: Reprinted by permission from the South. Med. J. 63:634, 1970.)

Congenital adrenal hyperplasia may be demonstrated at birth by the presence of ambiguous genitalia in genetic females (Fig. 9-2). However, a significant proportion of newborns with this condition may develop a life-threatening adrenal crisis as a result of salt loss. Delayed diagnosis may result in accelerated bone maturation, leading ultimately to short stature. The development of premature secondary sexual characteristics in males and further virilization in females may also occur.

In 1977 Pang et al. described a reliable and valid screening test employing capillary blood obtained by heel prick of infants that allowed for the radioimmunoassay determination of 17-hydroxyprogesterone in the serum. This test has been used in screening newborns for 21-hydroxylase deficiency, particularly in known high-risk populations such as Alaskan Eskimos. Using a 3 mm filter paper disk elution technique to study the presence of 17-hydroxyprogesterone in capillary blood of these day-old newborns, these authors determined levels in normal infants to be less than 40 pg/3 mm disk. Affected infants had 17-OHP levels of 57 to 980 pg/disk.

Treatment of congenital adrenal hyperplasia involves replacement cortisol. This suppresses adrenocorticotropic hormone (ACTH) output and therefore decreases the stimulation of the cortisol-producing pathways of the adrenal cortex.

Imperforate Hymen

The hymen represents the junction of the sinovaginal bulbs with the urogenital sinus and therefore is composed of endoderm from the urogenital sinus epithelium. Ordinarily the hymen is perforated during embryonic life to establish a connection between the lumen of the vaginal canal and the vestibule. If this perforation does not take place, the hymen is imperforate (Fig. 9-3).

It is rare to make the diagnosis of imperforate hymen before puberty, at which point primary amenorrhea is the major symptom. Occasionally in childhood a hydrocolpos or mucocolpos may occur. This is due to a collection of secretions behind the hymen, which in rare cases may build up to form a mass that obstructs the urinary tract. If such is discovered, the hymen should be incised to release the build-up.

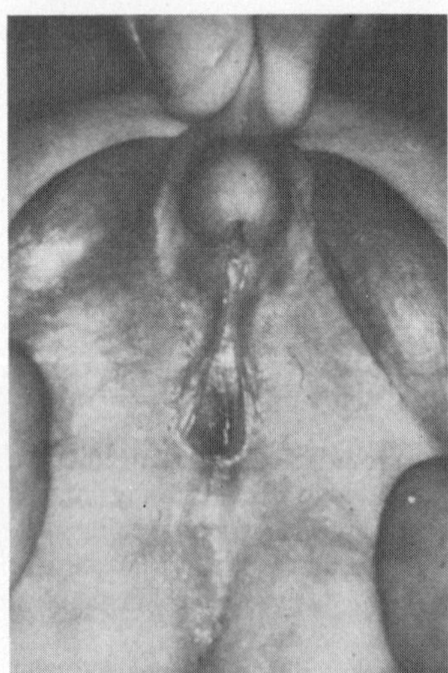

FIGURE 9-2
External genitalia of female with congenital adrenal hyperplasia showing clitoral enlargement and labial fusion. (From Jones HW Jr, Scott WW: Hermaphroditism, genital anomalies and related endocrine disorders, 2nd ed. Baltimore, Williams & Wilkins, 1971.)

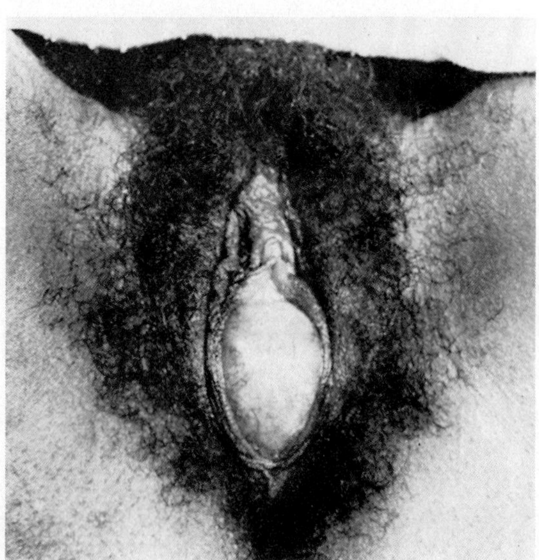

FIGURE 9-3
Imperforate hymen distended by hematocolpos. (From Baramki TA: J Reprod Med 29:376, 1984.)

At puberty the patient may experience cyclic cramping but no menstrual flow. Over time the patient may develop a hematocolpos and a hematometrium. In more advanced cases the fallopian tubes may be distended with menstrual flow, and the flow may back up through the tubes and form endometrial implants in the peritoneal cavity. Quite surprisingly, many patients are free of symptoms.

The diagnosis can be determined by history and by the presence of a bulging membrane at the introitus. Therapy consists of a cruciate incision into the hymen extending to the 10, 2, and 6 o'clock positions. In dense hymens a triangular section may be excised, although this is rarely necessary. Hemostasis is secured by fine suture, and evolution to normal usually occurs rapidly.

Vaginal Agenesis

Vaginal agenesis is usually associated with the Rokitansky-Küster-Hauser syndrome (Fig. 9-4). This syndrome is characterized by congenital absence of the vagina and uterus, although small masses of smooth muscular material resembling a rudimentary bicornuate uterus may be noted. These masses rarely have an epithelial lining and rarely menstruate, although occasionally this does occur, giving rise to monthly cyclic cramping. The ovaries are normal, and the fallopian tubes are usually present. Complete vaginal agenesis is discovered in 75% of patients with Rokitansky-Küster-Hauser syndrome. Approximately 25% of patients have a short vaginal pouch. These individuals have a 46,XX karyotype. The disorder seems to be an accident of development and not an inherited condition.

The androgen insensitivity syndrome (testicular feminization syndrome) demonstrates a 46,XY karyotype. While vaginal agenesis or the presence of a short pouch vagina is usually found, these patients have undescended testicles and male sex ducts. They usually exhibit minimal pubic hair after puberty. The testes should be removed after puberty to prevent the development of seminomas. The ovaries of the patient with Rokitansky-Küster-Hauser syndrome are normal and should not be removed.

Phelan reported that of 72 patients with vaginal agenesis, 25% had urologic abnormalities noted on intravenous pyelography. A later study by Baramki demonstrated that 40% of 92 patients had urologic abnormalities. Further, Turunen and Unnerus found that 25 of 200 such patients had skeletal anomalies, usually involving congenital fusion or absence of vertebrae.

Diagnosis of Rokitansky-Küster-Hauser syndrome is demonstrated by the presence of primary amenorrhea at the time of puberty, physical examination that demonstrates the absence of a vaginal opening or the presence of a short vaginal pouch, and failure to palpate a uterus on rectal examination, coupled with the finding of a normal karyotype. Laparoscopic examination may be performed in cases where the diagnosis is not clear or where there is some concern over the presence of a functioning uterus.

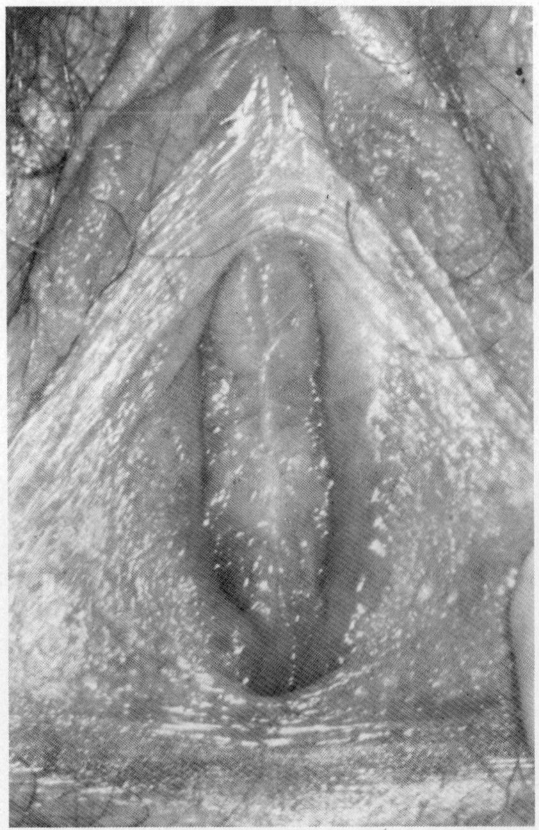

FIGURE 9-4
External genitalia of patient with congenital absence of vagina. (From Baramki TA: J Reprod Med 29:376, 1984.)

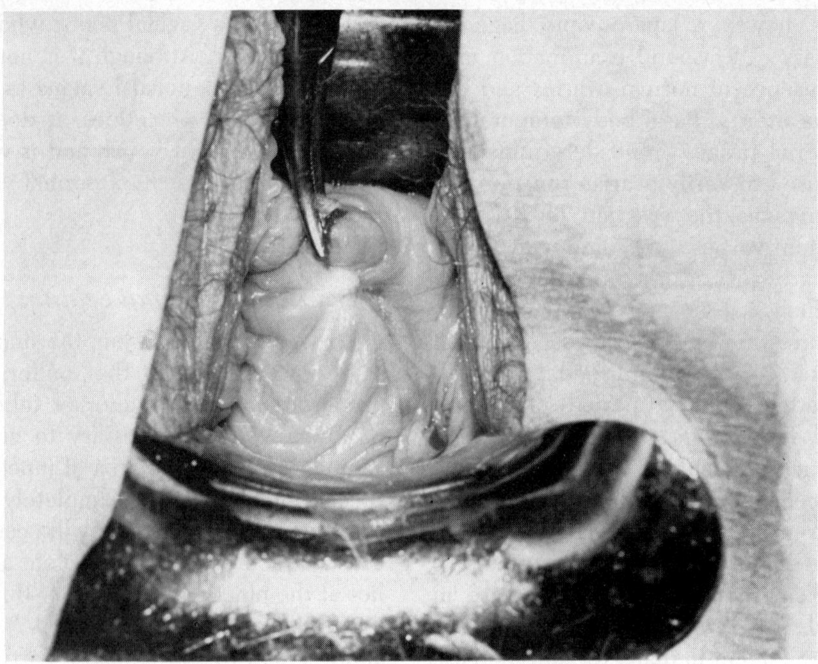

FIGURE 9-7
Patient with complete transverse vaginal septum.

the imperforate hymen, except that there is no bulging at the introitus. The patient complains of primary amenorrhea with cyclic cramping. The patient with a transverse septum may bleed somewhat but will still develop hematocolpos and hematometrium over time and may also complain of foul-smelling vaginal discharge.

The septum is usually thin, generally less than 1 cm thick. If an opening is noted, it may be expanded by manual dilation or simple incision, with suturing of the edges of the vagina on either side. Occasionally the septum is thick, and the two areas of the vagina are quite distantly separated. In such a case excision may require the implantation of a split-thickness skin graft in a fashion similar to the McIndoe procedure.

Longitudinal septa of the vagina will be discussed with duplication of the uterus and cervix.

Vaginal Adenosis

In the female exposed to DES in utero the junction between the müllerian ducts and the sinovaginal bulb may not be sharply demonstrated. If müllerian elements invade the sinovaginal bulb, remnants may remain as areas of adenosis in the adult vagina. They are generally palpated submucosally, although they may be observable at the surface. These anomalies are discussed more fully in Chapter 14.

Abnormalities of the Cervix and Uterus

Embryologic Considerations

Between the third and fifth weeks of gestation the metanephric ducts develop and join the cloaca. By the fifth week two ureteric buds develop from the mesonephric ducts close to the distal ends. These grow cephalad toward the mesonephric mass. The müllerian or paramesonephric duct forms from a cleft between the mesonephros and the forming gonad. These ducts are bilateral and grow caudally just lateral to and intimately associated with the mesonephric ducts. The fate of these various elements is therefore closely entwined. Damage to one usually affects the others. The paramesonephric ducts grow caudally, meet in the midline, and descend into the pelvis, reaching the urogenital sinus at an elevation known as the müllerian tubercle.

Musset analyzed 133 cases of genital urinary malformation and described a three-stage process for fusion of the two müllerian ducts into the uterus and cervix. The first stage is described as short, taking place at the beginning of the tenth week. The medial aspect of the more caudal portions of the two ducts fuse, starting in the middle and proceeding simultaneously in both directions. In this way a median septum is formed. The second stage continues from the tenth to the thirteenth week and occurs because of a rapid cell proliferation and the filling in of the triangular space between the two uterine cornua. In this way a thick upper median septum is formed. This is wedgelike and gives rise to the usual external contour of the fundus. At the same time the lower portion of the median septum is resorbed, unifying the cervical canal first and then the upper vagina. The third stage lasts from the thirteenth to about the twentieth week. In this stage the degeneration of the upper uterine septum occurs, starting at the isthmic region and proceeding cranially up to the top of the fundus. In this way a unified uterine cavity is formed.

The vagina develops from a combination of the müllerian tubercles and the urogenital sinus. Cells proliferate from the upper portion of the urogenital sinus to form solid aggregates known as the sinovaginal bulbs. These cell masses develop into a cord, the vaginal plate, which extends from the müllerian ducts to the urogenital sinus. This plate canalizes starting at the hymen, which is where the sinovaginal bulb attaches to the urogenital sinus, and proceeding cranially to the developing cervix, which has by this time already canalized. The process is completed at about the twenty-first week of intrauterine life.

Toaff et al. have pointed out from their review of the literature that the type of communicating abnormality of the uterus depends on a teratogenic process active at different stages in the embryonic development. Most symmetric communicating uteri have a normal urinary system, indicating that normal growth of the two mesonephric ducts had taken place before the fusion problem occurred. They point out,

however, that all patients with communicating uteri with atretic hemivagina who were studied had ipsilateral renal agenesis. Likewise, in patients with anomalies wherein a hemicervix was absent, ipsilateral renal agenesis occurred. They implied from these findings that an early teratogenic process active during the fourth week of gestation resulted in arrested growth of one mesonephric duct, agenesis of the ureteric bud, and therefore renal agenesis.

Genetic Studies of Müllerian Fusion Difficulties

Elias et al. recently reviewed the cases of sisters, mothers, and aunts of 24 women with known müllerian fusion abnormalities. Only 1 sister out of 37 (2.7%) was found to have a similar abnormality. No such abnormalities were found among 24 mothers, 45 maternal aunts, or 50 paternal aunts. However, the data in this study were accumulated by history and medical records and not by direct uterine examination. Nonetheless, Elias et al. concluded that the major genetic transmission mechanism could only be polygenic or multifactorial.

Incidence

It is difficult to estimate the incidence of uterine fusion anomalies because the data in most reports are derived from study groups rather than from the general population. The incidence is reported as 0.1% in retrospective studies and from 2% to 3% in observations of uteri at the time of delivery. Most uteri in the latter study, however, fit into the category of arcuate uterus or subseptate uterus.

Symptoms and Signs

Complete duplication of the vagina, uterus, and cervix may be asymptomatic until the woman begins to menstruate. Frequently the earliest symptom brought to the attention of the gynecologist is the fact that tampons do not obstruct menstrual flow. What occurs is that the patient puts a tampon into one vagina but the other vagina is still open. The second most common way the diagnosis is made is by observation at the time of the first pelvic examination.

TABLE 9-1

Results of Studies Evaluating Reproductive Success in Women Who Have Had Repair of Septate Uterus

Author(s) (Year)	No.	Live Births	Abortions	Ectopic Pregnancy
Musich and Behrman (1978)	21	9	2	0
Buttram (1979)	46	23	1	1
Palmer (1981)	100	67	4	0
Rochet and Dargert (1981) (per Audebert, Cittadini, and Cognat [1983])	38	29	2	0
Cardiani and Fedele (1981)	68	31	2	0
Audebert, Cittadini, and Cognat (1983)	54	19	3	0
Total	327	178	14	1

Obstructive vaginal lesions often lead to cyclic pain at the time of menstruation or to the presence of a mucus-filled or blood-filled mass present in the vagina. This may be mistaken for a paravaginal tumor.

A noncommunicating uterine horn may be indicated in one of two fashions. The first may be pain or a mass exacerbated cyclically at the time of menses, which occasionally is associated with symptoms and signs of endometriosis in a teenage woman. The early onset of signs and symptoms of endometriosis should alert the physician to this possibility. A mass is often noted on physical examination. The second way such a problem may present is as an ectopic pregnancy. Since sperm may migrate through the patent horn and since the rudimentary horn may have a normal tube attached to it, pregnancy can occur in the rudimentary horn. But since such horns are frequently small, rupture or pain caused by the obstruction may point to the diagnosis.

One of the major presenting symptoms is reproductive wastage. Didelphic uteri are usually not associated with this complaint. Musset estimated that abnormalities of the uterus may occur in as many as 15% to 25% of women with a history of repetitive abortion. Most patients with pregnancy wastage, however, had a variation of septate uterus. Whereas pretherapy pregnancy wastage rates were as high as 85% to 90%, improvement of pregnancy efficiency to as much as 80% occurred after metroplasty. Table 9-1 summarizes the results of a number of such reports. It is important to thoroughly evaluate such patients before exposing them to an operative procedure, since other problems may cause pregnancy wastage.

Uterine dysfunction and incoordinate uterine action are complicating problems seen in labor in women with septate and bicornuate uteri. Likewise, breech presentations and transverse lies occur more commonly in women with such abnormal uteri.

Diagnosis

Diagnosis of a uterine anomaly may be indicated by history of spontaneous abortion, especially in the second trimester, but is best proven by hysterosalpingography, hysteroscopy, and at times, laparoscopy. Valdes et al. recently reviewed the use of ultrasound for diagnosing female genital tract anomalies. Sixty-four patients with an ultrasound diagnosis of an anomaly were studied retrospectively to determine the accuracy and usefulness of the sonographic examination in such cases. Sixty-four percent of the patients were pregnant; 36% were not. Of 46 patients who had ultrasound diagnoses, 21 cases were diagnosed as bicornuate/septate uterus, 18 cases as didelphia, 3 cases as vaginal and cervical atresia, 2 cases as obstructed lower but normal upper genital

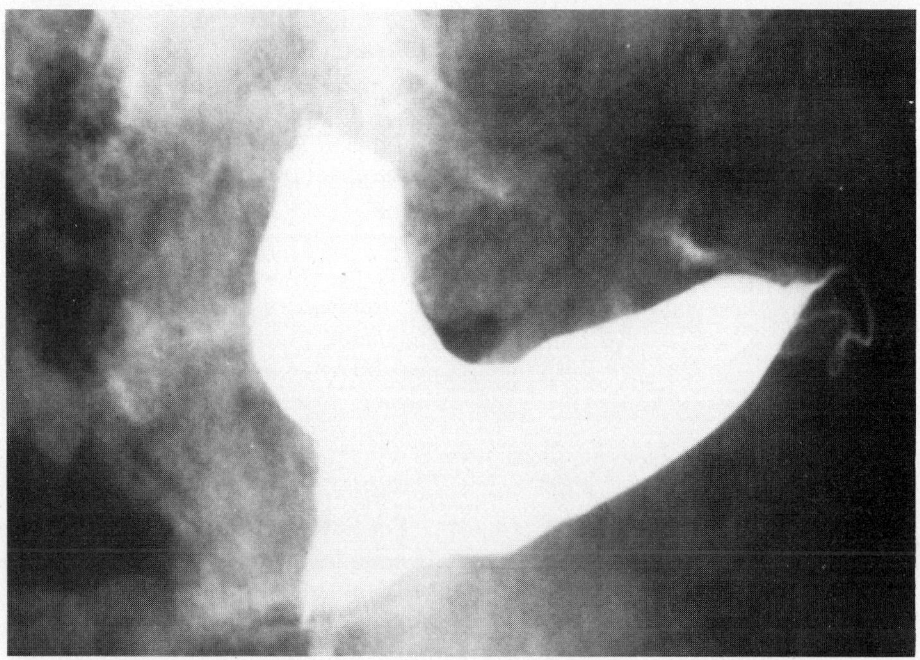

FIGURE 9-8
Hysterosalpingogram of bicornuate uterus seen in patient with repetitive abortions.

tract, and 2 cases as abnormal-appearing uterus. Ultrasound diagnosis was compared with hysterosalpingographic and operative findings in 43 patients and with physical examination in three patients. Scan results were classified as diagnostic in 26%, confirmatory in 63%, and incorrect in 11%. Ultrasound is a reasonable diagnostic procedure in such cases but should not be considered diagnostic until supplementary studies are performed. Hysterosalpingography and direct observation via hysteroscopy are the perferred methods of diagnosis. Laparoscopy and laparotomy may be useful in unusual cases (Fig. 9-8).

Specific Anomalies

ABSENCE OF CERVIX AND UTERUS. As discussed under Rokitansky-Küster-Hauser syndrome, the cervix and uterus are often not completely absent; the fallopian tubes and possibly some fibrous tissue are usually present. Absence is frequently associated with urinary tract anomalies.

UNICORNUATE UTERUS. Destruction of one müllerian duct may occur for various embryonic reasons. It is often related to lack of development of the mesonephric system on one side associated with lack of the appropriate development of the müllerian system. When this is the case, there is almost always a missing kidney and ureter on the same side. A single cervix and a single horn of the uterus with the fallopian tube of the side entering it are seen. The ovary may be present on the opposite side. Such a uterus usually supports a pregnancy. Unicornuate uterus may not be diagnosed unless the patient is evaluated with a hysterosalpingogram or is subjected to an operative procedure.

In a review of the literature consisting of 31 patients, Buttram found a 48% spontaneous abortion rate, a 17% prematurity rate, and a 40% live birth rate in patients with this anomaly.

ANOMALIES OF LATERAL FUSION OF MÜLLERIAN DUCTS. Partial or complete duplication of the vagina, cervix, and uterus may be seen clinically. These may be classified as didelphic, which may involve a complete duplication of vagina, uterus, and cervix; bicornuate, which consists of a single-chamber vagina

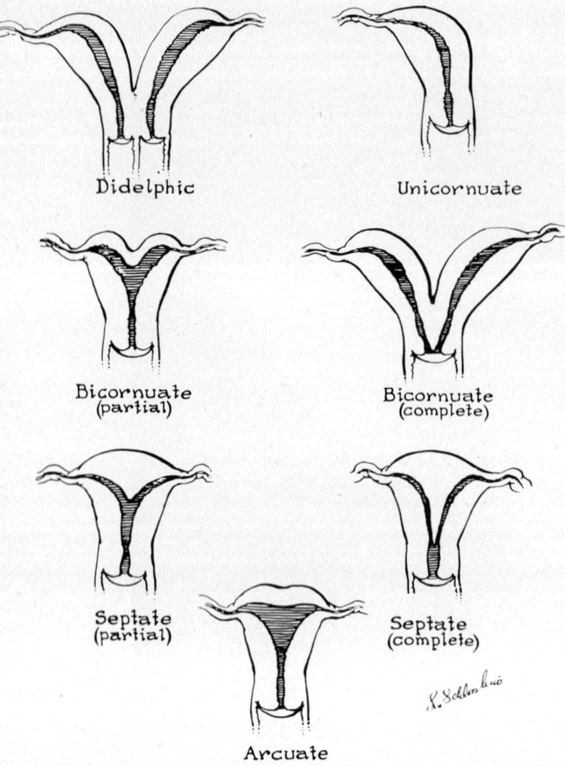

FIGURE 9-9
Nonobstructive maldevelopment of the Müllerian system. (From Baramki TA: J Reprod Med 29:376, 1984.)

and cervix with a complete or partial septate uterus and two uterine bodies (Fig. 9-8); septate, in which the uterus appears as a single organ but contains a midline septum that is either partial or complete; or arcuate, which demonstrates a small septate indentation at the upper end of the fundus. Fig. 9-9 graphically depicts these.

Recently Toaff et al. reviewed the subgroup of malformed uteri that includes duplication of the vagina, cervix, and uterus with communication between the horns. Nine subcategories have been described and are depicted in Fig. 9-10. Some involve septate uteri and others didelphic uteri. Some involve obstructive areas of the vagina. Because of the structural differences the clinical findings may be quite different from case to case.

Finally, obstructive varieties of duplication may be noted, again involving the uterus or the vagina.

Management

For patients with nonobstructed abnormalities, no therapy may be indicated. This is particularly true for women with unicornuate and didelphic uteri. On the other hand, septate uteri are frequently associated with reproductive wastage problems, and correction may be necessary to relieve these situations. A number of metroplasty procedures are available. The first was described by Strassman and involved the removal of the septum by a wedge incision and the reunification of the two cavities. However, a number of other means have been devised to eliminate the septum. Table 9-2 summarizes some of these and outlines their differences.

Recently septate uteri have been treated by division of the septum through the hysteroscope.

To perform this procedure, a laparoscope should first be introduced into the peritoneal cavity so that the uterus can be directly visualized during the procedure. This will also allow differentiation of a septate uterus from a bi-

TABLE 9-2
Procedures for Performing Metroplasty on Uteri with Müllerian Fusion Anomalies

Procedure	Technique
Strassman	Wedge excision of septum—reunification of cavity
Jones	Cone resection of septum
Tompkins Bret Palmer	Sagittal incision with severance of septum
Chervenak, Neuwirth	Hysteroscopically controlled severance of septum

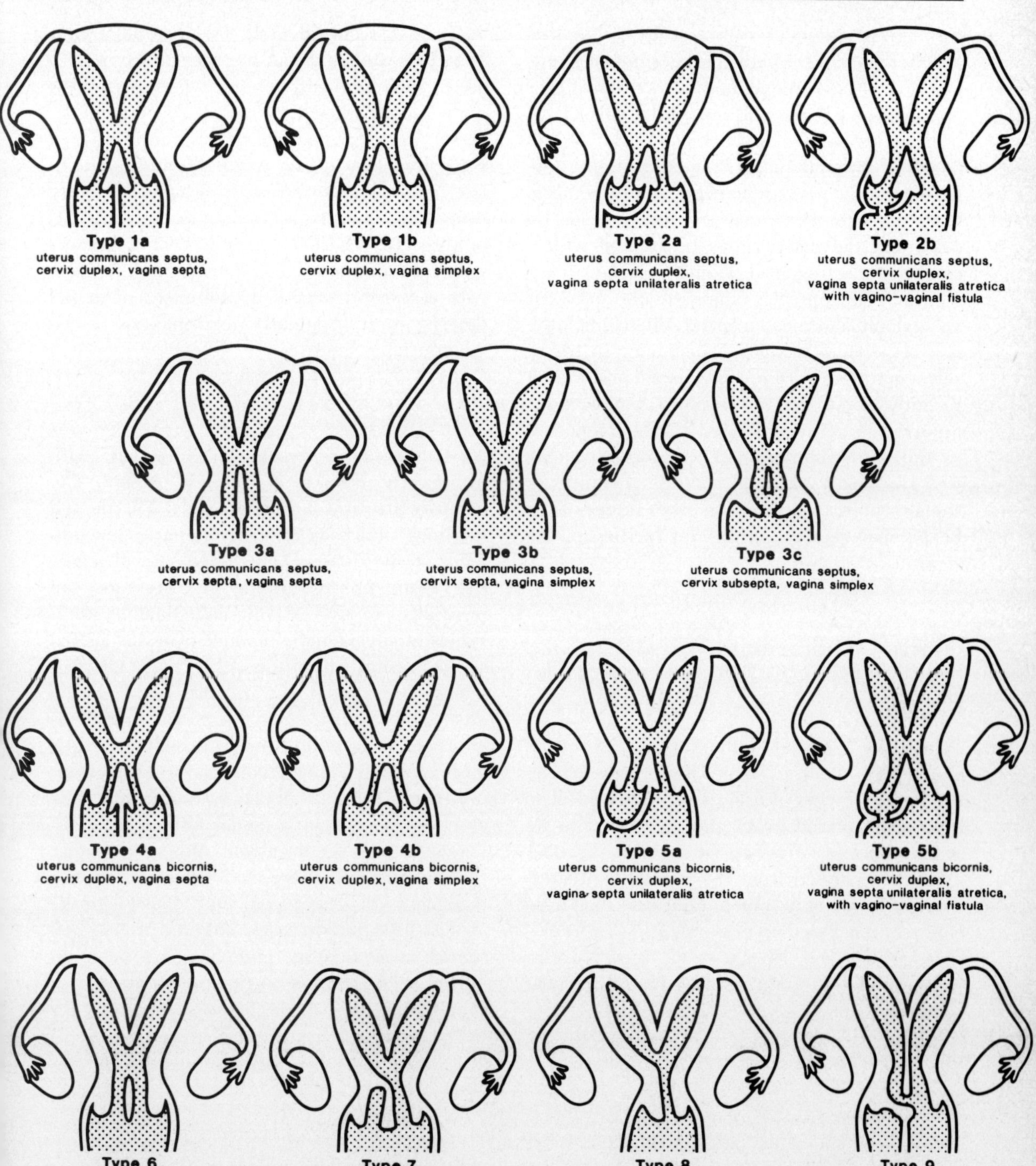

FIGURE 9-10

Morphologic classification of communicating uteri. All have an isthmic communication except type 9, which has a low cervical communication. (From Toaff ME, Lev-Toaff AS, Toaff R: Communicating uteri: review and classification with introduction of two previously unreported types. Fertil Steril 41:661, 1984. Reproduced with permission of the publisher, The American Fertility Society.)

cornuate or didelphic uterus. Flexible scissors are then passed through the instrument chamber of the hysteroscope, and the septum is progressively cut in the midline until a normal-appearing cavity is developed. Little or no bleeding generally occurs, since the septum is fibrous and poorly vascularized. After operation a Lippes-type IUD may be inserted for 30 days, and the patient may be treated with a conjugated estrogen (1.25 mg per day) for 1 month. This approach eliminates the need for an abdominal procedure and thus limits the risk of pelvic adhesions, which may in themselves interfere with fertility. Israel and March recently noted that no serious complications occurred in 72 such treated patients reported in the world literature. This procedure may well eventually make all abdominal repairs of septate uteri obsolete. In the future laser beams may replace scissors for incision of the septum.

Ovarian Abnormalities

Accessory Ovary and Supernumerary Ovary

In 1959 Wharton defined accessory ovary and supernumerary ovary. The former term is used when excess ovarian tissue is noted near a normally placed ovary and connected to it. Supernumerary ovary occurs when a third ovary is separated from the normally situated ovaries. Printz et al. pointed out that such ovaries may be found in the omentum or retroperitoneally, and Hogan et al. reported the presence of a dermoid cyst in a supernumerary

ovary that occurred in the greater omentum. Wharton estimated that the occurrence of both accessory ovary and supernumerary ovary was quite rare, finding approximately 1 case of accessory ovary per 93,000 patients and 1 case of supernumerary ovary in 29,000 autopsies. In fact, only 13 reported cases of supernumerary ovary have been found to date in the world literature. In Wharton's review, 3 of 4 patients with supernumerary ovary and 5 of 19 patients with accessory ovary had additional congenital defects, most frequently abnormalities of the genitourinary tract.

Ovotestes

Ovotestes are present in individuals with ovaries who have an HY antigen present. The majority are true hermaphrodites. The degree to which müllerian and mesonephric development occurs depends on the amount of testicular tissue present in the ovotestes and the proximity to the developing duct system. Where a considerable amount of testicular tissue is present within the organ, there is a tendency for descent toward the labial scrotal area. Thus palpation of the gonad in the inguinal canal or within the labial scrotal area is fairly common. Ovulation and menstruation may occur if the müllerian system is appropriately developed. In a similar fashion, spermatogenesis may occur as well. Where testicular tissue is present, there is an increased risk for malignant degeneration, and these gonads should be removed after puberty. Germ cell tumors such as dysgerminomas have been reported in the ovarian portion of ovotestes.

KEY POINTS

- Gender identification in a newborn infant has such emotional impact that it should be considered an emergency procedure.

- Congenital adrenal hyperplasia is an autosomal recessive condition most commonly due to an inborn error of metabolism involving the enzyme 21-hydroxylase. Homozygous individuals occur in 1 out of every 490 to 67,000 births. Heterozygote carriers are present in 1 in 20 to 1 in 250 individuals. Differences depend on ethnic background of people tested.

- The hymen is the junction of the sinovaginal bulb with the urogenital sinuses and is derived from endoderm.

- Vaginal agenesis is most often associated with Rokitansky-Küster-Hauser syndrome. From 25% to 40% of these will have urologic abnormalities. Approximately one eighth will have skeletal abnormalities as well.

- Abnormalities of the uterus and cervix may be transmitted as a polygenic or multifactorial pattern of inheritance. They occur in about 2% to 3% of the female population.

- From 15% to 20% of women with repetitive abortion histories may be found to have anomalies of the uterus.

- Pretherapy pregnancy wastage rates in women with anomalies of the uterus may be as high as 85% to 90%. After surgical repair the pregnancy efficiency rate may be as high as 80%.

- Accessory ovaries occur in approximately 1 per 93,000 patients. Supernumerary ovaries occur in approximately 1 out of every 29,000 women.

BIBLIOGRAPHY

Abrego D, Ibrahim AA: Mesenteric supernumerary ovary. Obstet Gynecol 45:352, 1975.

Audebert AJM, Cittadini E, Cognat M: Habitual abortion in uterine malformations. Acta Eur Fertil 14:273, 1983.

Baramki TA: The treatment of congenital anomalies in girls and women. J Reprod Med 29:376, 1984.

Beheshti M, Hardy BE, Churchill BM, et al: Gender assignment in male pseudo hermaphrodite children. Urology 22:604, 1983.

Blair RG: Pregnancy associated with congenital malformations of the reproductive tract. J Obstet Gynaecol Br Emp 67:36, 1960.

Buttram VC: Müllerian anomalies and their management, Fertil Steril 40:159, 1983.

Buttram VC, Zanotti L, Acosta AA, et al: Surgical correction of septate uterus. Fertil Steril 25:373, 1974.

Cardiani GB, Fedele L: Clinical management of uterine anomalies. Acta Eur Fertil 12:83, 1981.

Cruikshank SH, VanDrie DM: Supernumerary ovaries. Update and Review. Obstet Gynecol 60:126, 1982.

Daly DC, Walters CA, Soto-Albers CE, et al: Hysteroscopic metroplasty: surgical technique and obstetric outcome. Fertil Steril 39:623, 1983.

Dillon WP, Dewey M: A case of accessory ovary. Obstet Gynecol 58:660, 1981.

Elias S, Simpson JL, Carson SA, et al: Genetic studies in incomplete müllerian fusion. Obstet Gynecol 63:276, 1984.

Emans SJ, Grace E, Fleischnick E, et al: Detection of late onset 21-hydroxylase deficiency congenital adrenal hyperplasia in adolescents. Pediatrics 72:690, 1983.

Fleischnick E, Rum D, Alosco SM, et al: Extended MHC haplotypes in 21-hydroxylase deficiency congenital adrenal hyperplasia: shared genotypes in unrelated patients. Lancet 1:152, 1983.

Greiss FC, Mauzy CH: Congenital anomalies in women. An evaluation of diagnosis, incidence and obstetric performance. Am J Obstet Gynecol 82: 330, 1961.

Hahn-Pedersen J, Larsen PM: Supernumerary ovary. Acta Obstet Gynecol Scand 63:365, 1984.

Hauser GA, Schreiner WE: Das Mayer-Rokitansky-Küster-Syndrom. Schweiz Med Wochenschr 91:381, 1961.

Hay D: Uterus unicornis and its relationship to pregnancy. J Obstet Gynaecol Br Emp 68:371, 1961.

Hogan ML, Barber DD, Kaufmann RH: Dermoid cyst in supernumerary ovary. The greater omentum. Report of a case. Obstet Gynecol 29:405, 1967.

Israel R, March CM: Hysteroscopic incision of the septate uterus. Am J Obstet Gynecol 149:66, 1984.

Kaufman RH, Noller K, Adam E, et al: Upper genital tract abnormalities and pregnancy outcome in diethylstilbestrol-exposed progeny. Am J Obstet Gynecol 148:973, 1984.

McIndoe, A: Treatment of congenital absence and obliterative conditions of vagina. Br J Plast Surg 2:254, 1950.

Muller U, Mayerova A, Debus B, et al: Correlation between testicular tissue and HY phenotype in intersex patients. Clin Genet 23:49, 1983.

Musich JR, Behrman SJ: Obstetric outcome before and after metroplasty in women with uterine anomalies. Obstet Gynecol 52:63, 1978.

Musset R: Classification globale des malformations uterines. Gynécol Obstét 66:145, 1967.

Palmer R: Anomalies uterines congenitales. In Boury-Heyler C, Maulbeon P, Rochet Y, et al: Uterus et fécondité, vol. 1. Paris, Masson, 1981.

Pang S, Hotchkiss J, Drash AL, et al: Microfilter paper method for 17-hydroxyprogesterone radioimmunoassay—its application for rapid screening for congenital adrenal hyperplasia. J Clin Endocrinol Metab 45:1003, 1977.

Pang S, Murphey W, Levine LS, et al: A pilot newborn screening for congenital adrenal hyperplasia in Alaska. J Clin Endocrinol Metab 55:413, 1982.

Phelan JT, Counseller VS, Greene LF: Deformities of the urinary tract with congenital absence of the vagina. Surg Gynecol Obstet 97:1, 1953.

Printz JL, Choate JW, Townes PL, et al: The embryology of supernumerary ovaries. Obstet Gynecol 41:246, 1973.

Semens JP: Congenital anomalies of the female genital tract. Functional classification based on a review of 56 personal cases and 5 unreported cases. Obstet Gynecol 19:328, 1962.

Toaff ME, Lev-Toaff AS, Toaff R: Communicating uteri: review and classification with introduction of two previously unrecorded types. Fertil Steril 41:661, 1984.

Turunen A, Unnerus CE: Spinal changes in patients with congenital aplasia of the vagina. Acta Obstet Gynecol Scand 46:99, 1967.

Valdes C, Malini S, Malinak LR: Ultrasound evaluation of female genital tract anomalies: a review of 64 cases. Am J Obstet Gynecol 149:285, 1984.

Wharton LR: Two cases of supernumerary ovary and one of accessory ovary within an analysis of previously reported cases. Am J Obstet Gynecol 78:1101, 1959.

Pediatric Gynecology

KEY TERMS AND DEFINITIONS

Adhesive Vulvitis. A self-limiting consequence of chronic vulvitis in which denuded epithelium of adjacent labia minora agglutinate and fuse the two labia together.

Factitious Precocious Puberty. The result when a young girl has used or has been given hormonal creams or has ingested adult medications such as oral estrogens or birth control pills.

Gelastic Seizures. An unusual neurologic symptom that is sometimes associated with precocious puberty. It involves seizures with inappropriate laughter.

Heterosexual Precocious Puberty. Premature virilization in a female child, including development of secondary sexual characteristics.

Incomplete or Pseudoprecocious Puberty. Premature female sexual maturation and uterine bleeding without associated ovulation.

McCune-Albright Syndrome (Polyostotic Fibrous Dysplasia). A rare triad of cafe-au-lait spots, fibrous dysplasia, and cysts of the skull and long bones.

Precocious Puberty. The appearance of signs of secondary sexual maturation at an age more than 2.5 standard deviations below the mean for the population to which the child belongs. In girls in North America, precocious puberty is defined as initiation of signs of sexual maturation occurring before 8 years of age.

Premature Adrenarche. Isolated early development of axillary hair without other signs of secondary sexual maturation.

Premature Pubarche. Isolated early development of pubic hair without other signs of secondary sexual maturation.

Premature Thelarche. Isolated early unilateral or bilateral breast development without other signs of secondary sexual maturation.

Puberty. The process of biologic and physical development after which sexual reproduction first becomes possible.

Gynecologic diseases are uncommon in children, especially in comparison with the incidence of diseases in women of reproductive age. This chapter considers gynecologic diseases of children from infancy until the completion of puberty. Congenital anomalies and neoplasia of infants are covered in other chapters. The evaluation of children's gynecologic problems involves considerations of physiology, psychology, and treatments that are different from those of adult gynecology.

An outpatient visit by a prepubertal or pubertal child to a gynecologist should be structured differently from a gynecologic visit by a woman of reproductive age. Considerable time must be devoted to gaining the child's confidence and establishing rapport. If the interaction is poor during the first visit, the negative experience will detract from future physician-patient interactions. In addition, a child's visit to a gynecologist usually focuses on a perceived problem rather than on preventive medicine,

cystectomy with preservation of ovarian tissue. Again, cystic teratoma was the most common benign tumor in these children.

The most common differential diagnosis of an abdominopelvic mass in children, which is not an ovarian mass, is a benign cyst of the mesentery or omentum. Benign uterine tumors are rare in children. However, functional luteal cysts of the ovary are not uncommon in neonates secondary to maternal gonadotrophins. These cysts do not need operative intervention, as they will regress spontaneously.

In summary, approximately 75% of ovarian neoplasms in premenarcheal females are benign teratomas, and approximately 25% are malignant tumors. Abdominal pain is the most common symptom, and an abdominopelvic mass is the most frequent sign of an ovarian tumor in childhood. Even though ovarian neoplasia is rare in children, this diagnosis must be considered in a young girl with abdominal pain and a palpable mass.

PRECOCIOUS PUBERTY

Puberty in the female is the process of biologic change and physical development after which sexual reproduction becomes possible. This is a time of accelerated linear skeletal growth and development of secondary sexual characteristics, such as breast development and the appearance of axillary and pubic hair. Normal puberty occurs over a wide range of ages (Chapter 36). Precocious puberty is arbitrarily defined as the appearance of any signs of secondary sexual maturation at an age more than 2.5 standard deviations below the mean. Thus in females in North America, precocious puberty is initiation of sexual maturation occurring before 8 years of age. Precocious puberty is associated with a wide range of disorders (see box at right). When it is diagnosed, the physician should undertake a detailed investigation of the etiology of the condition in order not to overlook a potentially correctable anatomic lesion. The two primary concerns of parents of children with precocious puberty are the social stigma associated with the child's being physically different from her peers and the diminished ultimate height caused by the premature closure of epiphyseal growth centers.

Puberty is a time of accelerated growth, skel-

DIFFERENTIAL DIAGNOSIS OF PRECOCIOUS PUBERTY

I. Complete true precocious puberty
  A. Idiopathic or constitutional causes
  B. Neurogenic, cerebral lesions
    1. Tumors of hypothalamus, pineal gland, or cortex including hamartoma, craniopharyngioma, glioma
    2. Infections, including toxoplasmosis, encephalitis, and meningitis
    3. Neurocutaneous syndromes, neurofibromatosis
    4. Developmental defects, including microcephaly, tuberous sclerosis, aqueductal stenosis, craniostenosis
    5. Trauma
    6. Miscellaneous causes: Sturge-Weber syndrome, diffuse encephalopathy, idiopathic epilepsy
  C. McCune-Albright syndrome
  D. Juvenile primary hypothyroidism
  E. Silver's syndrome (craniofacial disproportion, small stature, retarded bone age, increased gonadotrophin levels)
II. Incomplete or pseudoprecocious puberty
  A. Premature pubarche
  B. Premature thelarche
  C. Adrenal lesions: congenital adrenal hyperplasia, Cushing syndrome, tumors
  D. Ovarian tumors: estrogen-producing, granulosa-theca cell, luteoma
  E. Iatrogenic causes: androgen or estrogen administration, vitamins, oral contraceptives
III. Extrapituitary gonadotrophin production
  A. Gonadotrophin-secreting tumors: choriocarcinoma, teratoma, hepatoblastoma, dysgerminoma
  B. Exogenous gonadotrophin administration

Adapted from Goldfarb AF: Endocrine disturbance of puberty. In Lavery JP, Sanfilippo JS, eds.: Pediatric and adolescent obstetrics and gynecology. New York, Springer-Verlag, 1985, p. 176.

---

etal maturation, and resulting epiphyseal closure. Although precocious puberty occurs early in a child's life, it usually develops in this normal sequence. This produces the paradox of precocious puberty. Early in the course of the disease the girls are taller and heavier than

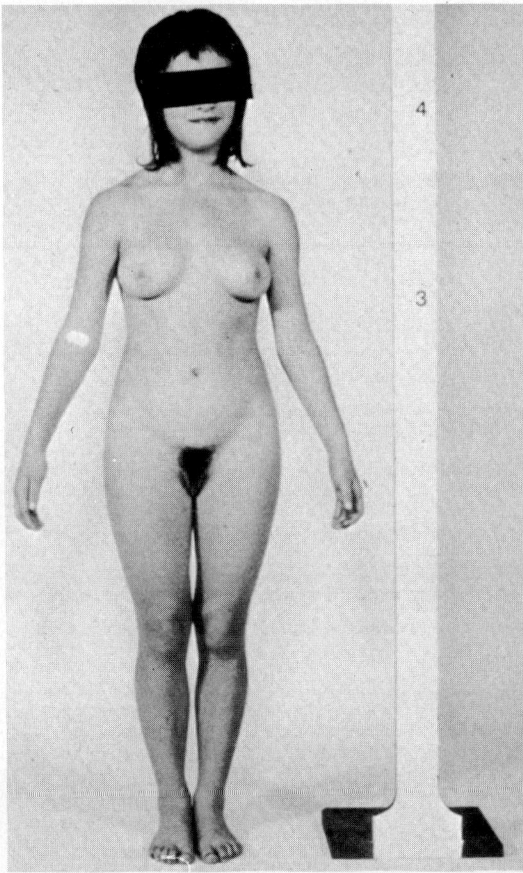

FIGURE 10-8
Child aged 7 years with constitutional precocious puberty. Note increased height for age. (From Dewhurst CJ: Practical pediatric and adolescent gynecology. New York, Marcel Dekker, 1980. Reprinted courtesy of Marcel Dekker, Inc.)

their chronologic peers who have not experienced the growth spurt (Fig. 10-8). However, although the patient is tall as a child, her eventual adult height will be shorter than normal. Without therapy, approximately 50% of females with precocious puberty will not reach a height of 5 feet.

The syndrome of precocious puberty is subdivided into complete (true) or incomplete (pseudo) and isosexual and heterosexual disorders. These definitions are only of clinical value after the eventual diagnosis has been established. Complete or true precocious puberty involves premature maturation of the hypotha-

lamic pituitary-ovarian axis and includes normal menses, ovulation, and the possibility of pregnancy. Incomplete or pseudoprecocious puberty involves premature female sexual maturation and uterine bleeding but without associated ovulation. In the latter syndrome, secretion of estrogens is independent of hypothalamic-pituitary control. Obviously, depending on when the patient is first seen in relationship to the natural history of her disease, it may be necessary to observe patients at regular intervals for 2 to 3 years to distinguish one syndrome from another (Tables 10-3 and 10-4). Prolonged follow-up is sometimes necessary to rule out subtle, slow-growing lesions of the brain, ovary, or adrenal gland. The exact etiology of the majority of cases of true precocious puberty is unknown (constitutional); however, approximately 10% are secondary to life-threatening central nervous system disease. A definitive diagnosis is established more often for pseudoprecocious puberty, and it is usually related to an ovarian or adrenal disorder. Both true precocious puberty and pseudoprecocious puberty are rare; however, true precocious puberty is five to six times more frequent than pseudoprecocious puberty. Heterosexual precocious puberty is premature virilization in a female child and includes development of masculine secondary sexual characteristics. The androgens that cause heterosexual precocious puberty usually come from the adrenal gland.

Premature Thelarche

Premature thelarche is defined as isolated unilateral or bilateral breast development as the only sign of secondary sexual maturation. It is not accompanied by other associated evidence of pubertal development, such as axillary or pubic hair or changes in vaginal epithelium. Premature thelarche usually occurs between 2 and 4 years of age. Nipple development is absent. This is a benign, self-limiting condition that does not require treatment. Often the breast enlargement spontaneously regresses. The etiology of premature thelarche is not understood. However, it is postulated to be related either to a slight increase in circulating estrogen levels or an increased end organ sensitivity of breast tissue to endogenous estrogens.

TABLE 10-3

Physical Findings Among Patients with Various Syndromes of True Precocious Puberty

| | | | True Precocious Puberty | | | |
Findings	Premature Thelarche	Premature Adrenarche	Idiopathic	Central Nervous System Tumor	McCune-Albright Syndrome	Hypothyroid
Breast enlargement	Yes	No	Yes	Yes	Yes	Yes
Pubic hair	No	Yes	Yes	Yes	Yes	Unusual
Vaginal bleeding	No	No	Yes	Yes	Yes	Yes
Virilizing signs	No	No	No	No	No	No
Bone age	Normal	Normal to minimally advanced	Advanced	Advanced	Advanced	Normal or retarded
Neurological deficit	No	No	No	Yes	Yes	No
Abdominopelvic mass	No	No	Occ'l	No	No	Occ'l

From Ross GT: Disorders of the ovary and female reproductive tract. In Wilson JD, Foster DW, eds: Williams textbook of endocrinology,7th ed. Philadelphia, WB Saunders Co., 1985, p. 230.

Premature Pubarche or Adrenarche

Premature pubarche is early isolated development of pubic hair without other signs of secondary sexual maturation. Premature adrenarche is isolated early development of axillary hair. Neither of these conditions is progressive, and the girls do not have clitoral hypertrophy. However, it is important to differentiate premature pubarche from the adrenogenital syndrome. Some children with premature pubarche have abnormal electroencephalographs without significant neurologic disease. The bone age should not be advanced. The etiology is poorly understood but believed to be related to increased androgen production by the adrenal glands.

Etiology

Idiopathic (constitutional) development is responsible for approximately 85% of the cases of true precocious puberty. Some of these children are simply at the earliest limits of the normal distribution of the biologic curve. Most idiopathic cases are sporadic in distribution; however, a few are familial. The mode of inheritance is believed to be autosomal recessive.

These girls have no genital abnormality except early development. Occasionally they develop follicular cysts of the ovaries secondary to increased levels of pituitary gonadotrophins (Fig. 10-9). In these cases the cysts are a result, not the cause, of precocious puberty. Gonadotrophin levels, sex steroid levels, and response of luteinizing hormone (LH) after administration of gonadotrophin-releasing hormone (GnRH) are similar to those in normal puberty. The cause of premature maturation of the hypothalamic-pituitary-ovarian axis is unknown. The syndrome may appear as early as age 3 to 4 years. When observed for several decades, these women have normal menopausal ages. Emotional problems are a concern, because the young girls suffer with extreme social pressures. The intellectual and psychological development of girls with precocious puberty is appropriate for their chronologic age. Most are shy and withdrawn from their peers. The diagnosis of idiopathic or constitutional precocious puberty is made by exclusion. A recent report by Cacciari et al. has stimulated the hypothesis that many cases of idiopathic puberty may be related to small hamartomas of the hypothalamus. They studied 15 children who underwent

TABLE 10-4
Physical Findings Among Patients with Various Syndromes of Pseudoprecocious Puberty

	Isosexual			Heterosexual		
Findings	**Ovarian Tumors**	**Adrenal Tumors**	**Factitious**	**Ovarian Tumors**	**Adrenal Tumors**	**Adrenal Hyperplasia**
Breast enlargement	Yes	Yes	Yes	Yes	Yes	Yes
Pubic hair	Yes	Yes	Yes	Yes	Yes	Yes
Vaginal bleeding	Yes	Yes	Yes	Yes	Yes	Yes
Virilizing signs	No	Yes	No	Yes	Yes	Yes
Bone age	Advanced	Advanced	Advanced	Advanced	Advanced	Advanced
Neurological deficit	No	No	No	No	No	No
Abdominopelvic mass	Usually	No	No	Occ'l	No	No

From Ross GT: Disorders of the ovary and female reproductive tract. In Wilson JD, Foster DW, eds: Williams textbook of endocrinology, 7th ed. Philadelphia, WB Saunders Co., 1985, p. 230.

cranial computed tomography, and six had subsequent pneumoencephalography. In their series, 33% of the children were found to have small hamartomas of the tuber cinereum. This series selected children with early onset of precocious puberty and high levels of follicle-stimulating hormone (FSH) and LH.

A wide range of inflammatory, degenerative, or neoplastic diseases that involve the central nervous system may produce true precocious puberty. Usually, symptoms of a neurologic disease, especially headaches and visual disturbances, precede the manifestations of precocious puberty. A most unusual neurologic symptom that may be associated with precocious puberty is seizures with inappropriate

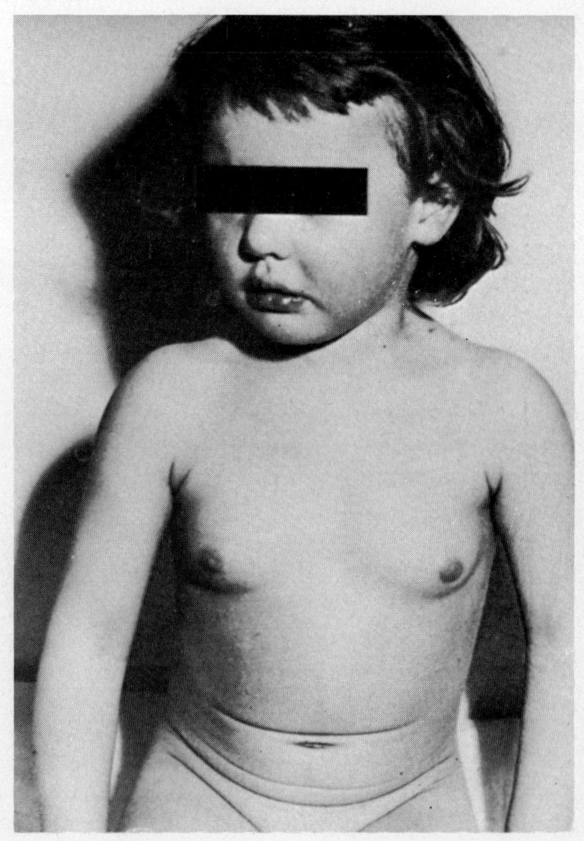

FIGURE 10-9
Precocious puberty in young girl. Child had large lower abdominal swelling, which at operation was shown to be bilateral follicular cysts (result of premature ovarian stimulation and not cause of condition). (From Dewhurst CJ: Practical pediatric and adolescent gynecology. New York, Marcel Dekker, 1980. Reprinted courtesy of Marcel Dekker, Inc.)

laughter (gelastic seizures). Anatomically, most central nervous system lesions are located near the hypothalamus in the region of the third ventricle, tuber cinereum, or mamillary bodies. Among the central nervous system diseases associated with true precocious puberty are tuberculosis, encephalitis, trauma, hydrocephalus, neurofibromatosis, granulomas, hamartomas, and teratomas. These space-occupying masses are most difficult to successfully treat surgically.

McCune-Albright syndrome (polyostotic fibrous dysplasia) is a rare triad of cafe-au-lait spots, fibrous dysplasia, and cysts of the skull and long bones (Fig. 10-10). These patients also have definite facial asymmetry. Approximately 40% of girls with McCune-Albright syndrome have associated isosexual true precocious puberty.

Hypothyroidism most commonly is associated with delayed pubertal development. However, in rare instances, untreated hypothyroidism results in isosexual true precocious puberty. The hypothyroidism associated with precocious puberty is due to primary thyroid insufficiency, not a deficiency in pituitary thyroid-stimulating hormone (TSH). This syndrome is seen in girls between the ages of 6 and 8 years.

Silver's syndrome is a rare congenital disease with multiple anomalies including low birth weight, asymmetry of the body, abnormal jaw, cafe-au-lait spots, abnormal and short little fingers, and a tendency for the corner of the mouth to turn down. Silver's syndrome is another rare cause of precocious puberty.

The relationship between congenital adrenal hyperplasia and puberty depends on the time of initial diagnosis and therapy. If the disease is diagnosed in the neonatal period and treated, normal puberty ensues. If the disease is untreated, the girl usually develops heterosexual precocious puberty from the adrenal androgens. However, if congenital adrenal hyperplasia is diagnosed late in childhood, isosexual precocious puberty may follow initial treatment of the adrenal disease.

The most common cause of pseudoprecocious puberty is a functioning ovarian tumor. Granulosa cell tumors are the most common type, accounting for approximately 60%. These tumors are usually greater than 8 cm when as-

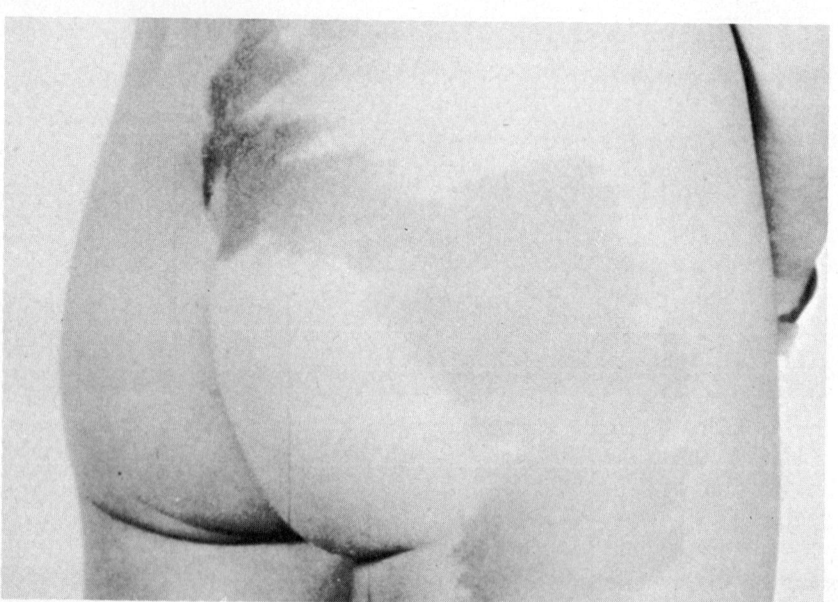

FIGURE 10-10
Large cafe-au-lait spot in child with precocious puberty as result of McCune-Albright syndrome. (From Dewhurst CJ: Practical pediatric and adolescent gynecology. New York, Marcel Dekker, 1980. Reprinted courtesy of Marcel Dekker, Inc.)

sociated with precocious puberty; 80% can be palpated abdominally. Other ovarian tumors that may be associated with precocious puberty include thecomas, luteomas, teratomas, Sertoli-Leydig tumors, choriocarcinomas, and benign follicular cysts. Thecomas and luteomas are much smaller than granulosa tumors and usually cannot be palpated abdominally. Overall, these tumors are rare during childhood; only 5% of granulosa cell tumors and 1% of thecomas occur before puberty. On rare occasions follicular cysts of the ovary enlarge and secrete enough estrogen to be the cause rather than the result of precocious puberty. It is speculated that the benign cysts function in an autonomous fashion. The ability of many tumors to secrete human chorionic gonadotrophin (HCG) or estrogen, including teratomas, choriocarcinomas, and dysgerminomas, has been established by radioimmunoassay. Rarely do these tumors produce precocious puberty. Adrenocortical neoplasms usually produce heterosexual precocious puberty, although isosexual precocity is occasionally seen. Congenital adrenal hyperplasia usually produces virilization and heterosexual precocious puberty.

Iatrogenic or factitious precocious puberty results when a young female has used hormonal cream or ingested adult medication such as oral estrogen or birth control pills. The secondary sexual characteristics regress after discontinuation of the medication.

Recently, Wierman et al. identified a new subset of children with precocious puberty. They have found a small number of children with gonadotrophin-independent precocity. Gametogenesis and steroidogenesis may occur in these individuals despite the absence of pubertal patterns of gonadotrophin release. When the children were tested with an analogue of GnRH, there was no effect on the pattern or mean levels of gonadotrophins or circulating sex steroids.

Diagnosis

A battery of tests including brain scan, estradiol, and FSH levels and thyroid function tests may be needed to establish the diagnosis. Initial emphasis in diagnosis is placed on the exclusion of serious neoplasms of the central nervous system, ovaries, or adrenal glands.

Acceleration of growth is one of the earliest clinical features of precocious puberty. Thus bone age should be determined by hand-wrist films and compared with standards for a patient's age (Fig. 10-11). Usually these films are repeated at 6-month intervals to evaluate the rate of skeletal maturation and correspondingly the necessity of active treatment of the disease. Advancement of bone age more than 95% of the norm for the child's chronologic age documents a peripheral estrogen effect.

Recent improved radiologic diagnosis of subtle central nervous system abnormalities with use of cranial computed axial tomography, pneumoencephalography, and magnetic resonance imaging has increased the sensitivity and frequency of discovery of the underlying cause of true precocious puberty. Ultrasound and computed axial tomography of the abdomen should be performed to discover enlargement of the ovaries and uterus.

Serum levels of FSH, LH, prolactin, TSH, estradiol, testosterone, dehydroepiandrosterone (DHEA) or DHEA-S, HCG, triiodothyronine, and thyroxine all may be of value in establishing the differential diagnosis. Sometimes a GnRH stimulation test is diagnostic in differentiating incomplete from true precocious puberty, but this test does not specifically identify children with central nervous system lesions. The LH responses to gonadotrophin stimulation after reaching a basal level are similar in cases of true precocious puberty to the responses of a mature adult. In contrast a child with precocious puberty secondary to a feminizing ovarian neoplasm does not have a significant elevation in LH response to gonadotrophins.

Management

The treatment of precocious puberty depends on the cause, the extent and progression of precocious symptoms, and whether the cause may be removed operatively. For example, extirpation of a granulosa cell tumor and subtotal removal of a hypothalamic hamartoma are rapid solutions. Because most cases involve premature maturation of the hypothalamic-pituitary-ovarian axis without a lesion, this discussion will focus on medical management of these cases. Girls with menarche before age 8

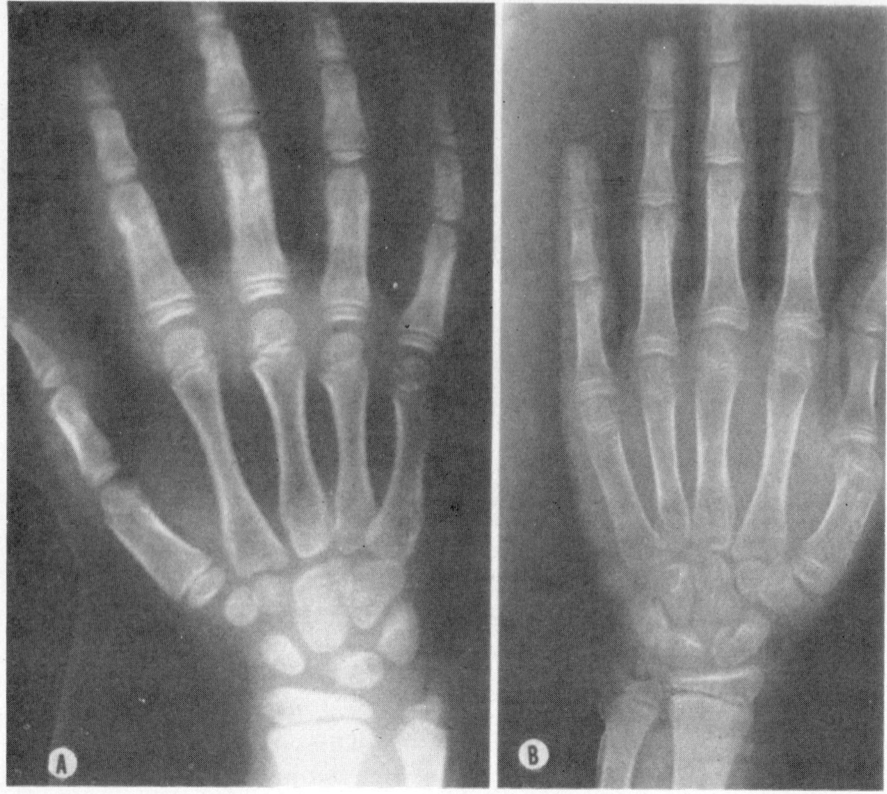

FIGURE 10-11

X-ray films demonstrating bone age. **A,** Normal for 7 years of age. **B,** Advanced bone age in girl 7 years of age who also shows other signs of isosexual precocity. (From Huffman JW: The gynecology of childhood and adolescence, 2nd ed. Philadelphia, W.B. Saunders Co., 1981.)

years, progressive thelarche and pubarche, and bone age more than 2 years greater than their chronologic ages definitely should be treated. The goals of therapy are to reduce gonadotrophin secretions and reduce or counteract the peripheral actions of the sex steroids, decrease growth rate to normal, and slow skeletal maturation.

The present drug of choice for true precocious puberty is one of the potent agonists or analogues of GnRH (Table 10-5). These drugs may be given either subcutaneously or by the intranasal route. They are rapid, safe, and effective treatments for children with the disease secondary to disturbances in the hypothalamic-pituitary-ovarian axis. Wierman et al., using daily injections of the agonist, observed involution of secondary sexual characteristics, with menstruation ceasing and breast development

and pubic hair regressing. In their series of nine children, spontaneous LH and FSH pulsations were abolished. Most importantly the drug not only reversed the ovarian cycle but changed the growth pattern. Growth velocity was decreased approximately 50% (Fig. 10-12). In their series the predicted adult height increased a mean of 3.3 cm. The potent agonist inhibits gonadotrophin secretion by increasing the down regulation of GnRH receptors.

Styne et al. have reported results of a similar series. They discovered that the agonist decreased gonadotrophins within 1 week and decreased sex steroids to prepubertal range within the first 2 weeks of therapy. These investigators performed serial ultrasonic examinations to document the sizes of the uterus and ovaries. Both organs slowly regressed in size. The only observed side effect to the drug was

TABLE 10-5

Gonadotrophin and Estradiol Levels in Girls with Precocious Puberty Before and After Administration of 100 µg GnRH

	No.	LH (IU/L, mean ± SD)		FSH (IU/L, mean ± SD)		Estradiol (pmol/L)	
		Basal	Peak	Basal	Peak	Mean	Range
Idiopathic precocious puberty	18	2.4 ± 2.0	36.9 ± 20.0	3.0 ± 1.8	16.3 ± 7.9	91.2	22-318
Intracranial lesion	9	2.6 ± 2.0	30.7 ± 17.3	4.4 ± 3.0	24.6 ± 5.1	107	22-240

From Lyon AJ, De Bruyn R, Grant DB: Isosexual precocious puberty in girls. Acta Pediatr Scand 74:953, 1985.

cutaneous reaction at the site of injection. Stanhope et al. have recently reported the use of an intranasal GnRH analogue. One hundred micrograms is administered two to three times per day. Once again these authors report decreasing growth rate to normal and the ability to slow the process of skeletal maturation. Pescovitz et al. from the National Institutes of Health have recently reported the largest series. Ninety-five girls were treated for at least 6 months with a long-acting GnRH analog. Their positive findings were similar; however, they found the analogue ineffective in patients with McCune-Albright syndrome. The effects of these new drugs are quickly reversible when the drugs are discontinued after normal adult height is achieved.

Before the introduction of agonists or analogues to GnRH, most children with true precocious puberty were treated with medroxyprogesterone acetate (Depo-Provera) at a dosage of 100 to 200 mg weekly. High levels of this progestin did suppress menstruation and produce regression of breast development. However, medroxyprogesterone did not change skeletal growth rates. Danazol has also been used in selected cases. It produced amenorrhea and inhibited further breast development; however, once again, there was no effect on growth rate or skeletal maturation. Cyproterone acetate is an antiandrogen that has been prescribed for precocious puberty in doses of 70 and 150 mg/m² per day in Europe. The results are similar to results obtained with medroxyprogesterone and danazol.

Both the child with precocious puberty and her family need intensive counseling. The child may be exposed to ridicule by her peers and to sexual exploitation. Thus the child needs extensive sex education and help in anticipating and confronting various social experiences. Often it is possible to dress the child in clothes that diminish the appearance of her advanced sexual maturation until the effects of her disease are reversed by drug therapy.

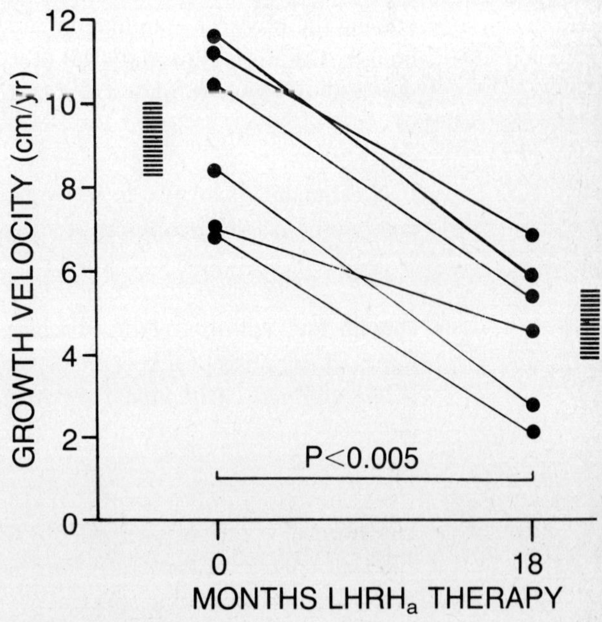

FIGURE 10-12

Effect of luteinizing hormone–releasing hormone therapy on growth velocities of six previously untreated girls. Data on growth before and during 18 months of therapy were available for six subjects. Hatched bars indicate mean values ±SEM. (From Mansfield MJ, Beardsworth ED, Loughlin JS, et al: N Engl J Med 309:1288, 1983. Reprinted by permission of The New England Journal of Medicine.)

───────────── **KEY POINTS** ─────────────

- The most frequent gynecologic problem of children is vulvovaginitis.

- In the field of pediatric gynecology, most diagnostic errors result from errors of omission during the examination rather than errors of commission.

- If a child is anxious about the physical examination, mild sedation may be helpful: the combination of 50 mg meperidine, 12.5 mg chlorpromazine hydrochloride, and 12.5 mg promethazine hydrochloride given in a dose of 1 ml intramuscularly for every 20 pounds, up to a maximum of 2 ml.

- The vaginal epithelium of the prepubertal child appears redder and thinner than the vaginal epithelium of a woman in her reproductive years. The prepubertal vagina is also narrower, thinner, and lacking in the distensibility of the vagina of a woman in her reproductive years.

- During the physical examination and rectal examination, no pelvic masses should be felt. The normal prepubertal uterus and ovaries are nonpalpable. The relative size ratio of cervix to uterus is 2 to 1 in a child.

- It is estimated that 80% to 90% of outpatient visits of children to gynecologists involve the classic symptoms of vulvovaginitis: introital irritation and discharge.

- One in four cultures of the discharge from vulvovaginitis identifies mycotic or bacterial vaginosis or a specific organism, such as *Neisseria gonorrhoeae, Trichomonas vaginalis, Chlamydia trachomatis,* herpes simplex virus, or *Shigella boydii.*

- The normal vagina of the prepubertal child is colonized by an average of nine different species of bacteria—four aerobic and facultative anaerobic species and five obligatory anaerobic species.

- In the period from 6 to 12 months before menarche, children often develop a physiologic discharge secondary to the increase in circulating estrogen levels.

- A discharge that is both bloody and foul smelling strongly suggests the presence of a foreign body.

- The vast majority of cases of nonspecific vulvovaginitis respond to a combination of topical estrogen cream and oral antibiotics given for 10 to 14 days.

- The classic symptom of pinworms *(Enterobius vermicularis)* is nocturnal vulvar and perianal itching, the treatment for which is the anthelmintic agent mebendazole (Vermox).

- The usual cause of genital trauma during childhood is an accidental fall. The majority of such traumas involve straddle injuries.

- The treatment of nonexpanding vulvar hematomas consists of an ice pack or ice sitz bath.

- Ovarian tumors constitute approximately 1% of all neoplasms in premenarcheal children. Approximately 75% of ovarian tumors are benign, with cystic teratomas being the most common.

- Precocious puberty is the appearance of signs of sexual maturation before 8 years of age. It usually develops in a normal sequence.

- Without therapy, approximately 50% of females with true precocious puberty will not reach a height of 5 feet.

- The exact etiology of the majority of cases of true precocious puberty is unknown; however, approximately 10% of cases are secondary to life-threatening central nervous system disease.

- Idiopathic (constitutional) development is responsible for approximately 85% of the cases of true precocious puberty.

- The most common cause of pseudoprecocious puberty is a functioning ovarian tumor. Granulosa cell tumors are the most common type, accounting for approximately 60%.

- The goals of therapy of precocious puberty are to reduce gonadotrophin secretions and reduce or counteract the peripheral actions of sex steroids, decreasing growth rate to normal, and slowing skeletal maturation. This is best accomplished by agonists or analogues to GnRH.

BIBLIOGRAPHY

Altchek A: Pediatric vulvovaginitis. J Reprod Med 29:359, 1984.

Altchek A: Vulvovaginitis in adolescents and younger girls. Contemp OB/GYN, p. 85, June 1986.

Bump RC: *Chlamydia trachomatis* as a cause of prepubertal vaginitis. Obstet Gynecol 65:384, 1985.

Cacciari E, Frejaville E, Cicongnani A, et al: How many cases of true precocious puberty in girls are idiopathic? J Pediatr 102:357, 1983.

Capraro VJ: Pediatric gynecology. In Danforth DN, ed.: Obstetrics and gynecology, 4th ed. Philadelphia, Harper & Row, Publishers, 1982.

Comite F, Cassorln F, Barnes KM: Luteinizing hormone releasing hormone analogue therapy for central precocious puberty. JAMA 255:243, 1986.

Danforth DN: Obstetrics and gynecology, 4th ed. Philadelphia, Harper & Row, Publishers, 1982.

De Jong AR: Sexually transmitted diseases in children. Am Fam Physician 30:185, 1984.

Dewhurst CJ: Gynaecological disorders of infants and children. Philadelphia, FA Davis Co., 1963.

Dewhurst CJ: Practical pediatric and adolescent gynecology. New York, Marcel Dekker, 1980.

Duffy TJ: Torsion of the fallopian tube in a premenarchal girl. Postgrad Med J 56:267, 1981.

Ehren IM, Mahour GH, Isaacs H: Benign and malignant ovarian tumors in children and adolescents. Am J Surg 147:339, 1984.

Emans SJ, Goldstein DP: The gynecologic examination of the prepubertal child with vulvovaginitis: Use of the knee-chest position. Pediatrics 65:758, 1980.

Emans SJH, Goldstein DP: Pediatric and adolescent gynecology, 2nd ed. Boston, Little, Brown & Co., 1982.

Golladay ES, Mollitt DL: Ovarian masses in the child and adolescent. South Med J 76:954, 1983.

Haney PJ, Whitley NO: CT of benign cystic abdominal masses in children. AJR 142:1279, 1984.

Huffman JW: Premenarchal vulvovaginitis. Clin Obstet Gynecol 20:581, 1977.

Huffman JW: The Gynecology of childhood and adolescence 2nd ed. Philadelphia, WB Saunders Co., 1981.

Jenkinson SD, Mackinnon AE: Spontaneous separation of fused labia minora in prepubertal girls. Br Med J 289:160, 1984.

Jones JG, Yamauchi T, Lambert B: *Trichomonas vaginalis* infestation in sexually abused girls. Am J Dis Child 139:846, 1985.

Kennedy LA, Pinckney LE, Currarino G, et al: Amputated calcified ovaries in children. Radiology 141:83, 1981.

Kingsbury A: The clinical importance of vaginal discharge in childhood. Aust NZ J Obstet Gynaecol 24:135, 1984.

Kosloske AM, Goldthorn JF, Kaufman E, et al: Treatment of precocious pseudopuberty associated with follicular cysts of the ovary. Am J Dis Child 138:147, 1984.

Lavery JP, Sanfilippo JS: Pediatric and adolescent obstetrics and gynecology. New York, Springer-Verlag. 1985.

Levine MD, Rappaport LA: Recurrent abdominal pain in school children: the loneliness of the long-distance physician. Pediatr Clin North Am 31:969, 1984.

Lyon AJ, De Bruyn R, Grant DB: Isosexual precocious puberty in girls. Acta Paediatr Scand 74:950, 1985.

Mansfield MJ, Beardsworth DE, Loughlin JS, et al: Long-term treatment of central precocious puberty with a long-acting analogue of luteinizing hormone–releasing hormone. N Engl J Med 309:1286, 1983.

McCrea RS: Uterine adnexal torsion with subsequent contralateral recurrence. J Reprod Med 25:123, 1980.

Mishell DR, Davajan V: Infertility, reproductive endocrinology and contraception, 2nd ed. Oradell, NJ, Medical Economics Books, 1986.

Paradise JE, Campos JM, Friedman HM, et al: Vulvovaginitis in premenarcheal girls: clinical features and diagnostic evaluation. Pediatrics 70:193, 1982.

Paradise JE, Willis ED: Probability of vaginal foreign body in girls with genital complaints. Am J Dis Child 139:472, 1985.

Pescovitz OH, Comite F, Hench K, et al: The NIH experience with precocious puberty: diagnostic subgroups and response to short-term luteinizing hormone releasing hormone analogue therapy. J Pediatr 108:47, 1986.

Root AW, Shulman I: Isosexual precocity: Current concepts and recent advances. Fertil Steril 45:749, 1986.

Shawis RN, El Gohary AE, Cook RCM: Ovarian cysts and tumours in infancy and childhood. Ann R Coll Surg Engl 67:17, 1985.

Singleton AF: Vaginal discharge in children and adolescents. Clin Pediatr 19:799, 1980.

Stanhope R, Adams J, Brook CGD: The treatment of central precocious puberty using an intranasal LHRH analogue (Buserelin). Clin Endocrinol 22:795, 1985.

Styne DM, Harris DA, Egli CA, et al: Treatment of true precocious puberty with a potent luteinizing hormone–releasing factor agonist: effect on growth, sexual maturation, pelvic sonography, and the hypothalamic-pituitary-gonadal axis. J Clin Endocrinol Metab 61:142, 1985.

Swischuk LE, Hayden CK: Abdominal masses in children. Pediatr Clin North Am 32:1281, 1985.

Takeuchi J, Hajime H: Pubertas praecox and hypothalamic hamartoma. Neurosurg Rev 8:225, 1985.

Widholm O: Genital bleeding during childhood. Pediatr Ann 10:170, 1981.

Wierman ME, Beardsworth DE, Mansfield MJ, et al: Puberty without gonadotropins. N Engl J Med 312:65, 1985.

Wilson JD, Foster DW: Williams textbook of endocrinology, 7th ed. Philadelphia, WB Saunders Co., 1985.

Contraception, Sterilization, and Pregnancy Termination

KEY TERMS AND DEFINITIONS

Contraception. The temporary avoidance of pregnancy.

Contraceptive Failure Rate. Pregnancy rates with various types of contraceptives at different intervals, usually yearly. This is frequently expressed as a failure per 100 women at 1 year or per 100 woman-years.

Family Planning. The birth of each child is planned and desired by the parents.

Gestagen. A class of sex steroids having progestational activity. The terms *progestagen* and *progestin* are synonymous.

Induced Abortion. Intentional medical or surgical termination of pregnancy prior to 20 weeks gestation. Also called elective pregnancy termination if performed for woman's desires or therapeutic abortion if performed for reasons of maintaining health of the mother.

Intrauterine Device (IUD). A small foreign body, usually made of plastic with or without copper, which when placed into the endometrial cavity provides an effective method of contraception.

IUD Event Rates. Incidence of adverse effects such as expulsion, removal for medical reasons, and pregnancy at various times after insertion of an IUD.

Life Table Method. An actuarial technique for determining rates of occurrence of events such as pregnancy and discontinuation at various intervals after the starting of any type of contraceptive.

Method Effectiveness. The rate of effectiveness when the contraceptive method is always used correctly.

Oral Contraceptive Steroids (OCs). Formulations of synthetic gestagens and usually estrogens that are ingested orally to prevent conception.

Pearl Index. A nonactuarial method used for determining the pregnancy (failure) rate of any contraceptive technique:

$$\text{Pregnancy rate} = \frac{\text{No of pregnancies} \times 1200}{\text{Woman-months of use}}$$

Rhythm. Periodic abstinence from intercourse during the periovulatory time of the cycle.

Spermicide. A local contraceptive containing the agent nonoxyl 9, which is toxic to sperm.

Sterilization. The permanent prevention of pregnancy.

Use Effectiveness. Overall effectiveness rate in actual use for a specific contraceptive method.

An ideal method of contraception has not yet been developed. All existing contraceptive techniques have advantages and disadvantages. Therefore the physician's advice about contraception should include an explanation of the advantages and disadvantages of each method so that the patient is fully informed and can rationally choose the method most suitable for her. If there are medical reasons for not using certain methods, the physician should inform the patient and offer her alternatives.

Except for the condom, no acceptable

method has been developed for use by the male. A great deal of research effort is currently being expended to develop one or more methods of contraception for the male, but there are several problems that will be difficult to overcome. These include (1) difficulty in separating suppression of the major testicular functions, spermatogenesis and androgen production, (2) the long lag period from initiation of treatment until the elimination of sperm from the ejaculate, usually about 3 months, (3) the problems of reversibility, including a variable delay in the time required for restoration of fertility as well as the possibility that abnormal sperm may be produced initially, and (4) the lack of motivation of most men to use a contraceptive, as the male is not the member of the couple who becomes pregnant. For these reasons, even if a contraceptive for males such as a combination progestin-androgen agent is developed, its use will be limited.

CONTRACEPTIVE USE

The use of contraceptives has steadily increased in the United States since 1960. By 1982, of the 55 million U.S. women aged 15 to 44, about one third were not exposed to pregnancy, and of the remaining 36 million women all but 3 million were using a method of contraception. The most frequently used method to prevent conception was male and female sterilization. Of the nonsurgical methods of contraception, oral contraceptives were most popular, being used by 18% of all women in this age group, followed by the condom, IUD, spermicides, diaphragm, withdrawal, and rhythm (Table 11-1). Of all women practicing contraception, 27% used oral contraception, with this method's greatest popularity being among women under 30 (Table 11-2). Of women under 25 using contraception in 1982, almost half (48%) used oral contraception. For women over 35 the condom was the most popular method of nonsurgical contraception. Overall, 8% of women exposed to the risk of unwanted pregnancy, more than 3 million women in the United States, did not practice any form of contraception.

The use of sterilization increased from 7.8% in 1965 to 18.6% in 1976 among married U.S. women and by 1982 to 21% of all U.S. women aged 15 to 44. Oral contraceptive use among all married couples in the United States aged 15

TABLE 11-1

Estimated Number and Percentage Distribution of U.S. Women Aged 15 to 44, by Exposure to the Risk of Unintended Pregnancy and Method of Contraception Currently Used

Exposure to Risk/Method	No. (in thousands)	%
Exposed and using a contraceptive	33,425	61
Sterilization	11,643	21
Tubal ligation	(6,783)	(12)
Vasectomy	(4,860)	(9)
Oral contraceptive	9,996	18
IUD	2,307	4
Condom	4,475	8
Spermicide	1,463	3
Diaphragm	1,908	3
Withdrawal	930	2
Rhythm	553	1
Douche and other method	150	*
Exposed and not using a contraceptive	3,053	6
Not exposed	18,137	33
Total	54,615	100

From Forrest JD, Henshaw SK: What U.S. women think and do about contraception. Reprinted with permission from *Family Planning Perspectives*, 15:162, 1983.
*<0.5%.

TABLE 11-2

Percentage Distribution of U.S. Women Aged 15 to 44 Who are Exposed to the Risk of Unintended Pregnancy, by Contraceptive Method Currently Used, According to Age Group

| | | Age Group | | | | | |
Method	Total	15-19	20-24	25-29	30-34	35-39	40-44
Sterilization	32	0	6	25	43	62	61
Tubal	(19)	(*)	(4)	(15)	(25)	(36)	(35)
Vasectomy	(13)	(*)	(2)	(10)	(17)	(26)	(26)
Oral contraceptive	27	44	50	34	17	8	5
IUD	6	3	6	8	9	6	4
Condom	12	21	13	12	12	8	11
Spermicides	4	7	3	3	4	3	5
Diaphragm	5	1	7	7	7	3	3
Withdrawal	3	5	3	3	2	2	2
Rhythm	2	*	1	1	1	3	2
Other	*	2	*	*	1	*	*
None	8	18	11	6	5	6	8
TOTAL	100	100	100	100	100	100	100

From Forrest JD, Henshaw SK: What U.S. women think and do about contraception. Reprinted with permission from *Family Planning Perspectives* 15:157, 1983.
*<0.5%.

to 44 increased from 15.3% in 1965 to a high of 25.1% in 1973 and then declined to 22.5% in 1976. In 1975, pharmacy purchases of oral contraceptives began declining in the United States, and by 1982, oral contraceptives were used by only 18% of all U.S. women in this age group. Likewise, use of the IUD increased from 0.7% in 1965 to 6.7% in 1973; it then declined to 6.3% in 1976 among married women and by 1982 to 4% of all U.S. women aged 15 to 44. Thus since 1976 although use of sterilization has increased, use of the two most effective nonsurgical methods of contraception has declined with a concomitant increase in use of the less effective barrier methods of contraception.

CONTRACEPTIVE EFFECTIVENESS

It is difficult to determine the actual effectiveness of various methods of contraception because of a large number of factors that affect contraceptive failure. The terms *method effectiveness* and *use effectiveness* (or *method failure* and *patient failure*) have been used to differentiate whether conception occurred while the contraceptive method was being used correctly or incorrectly. In general, methods used at the time of coitus, such as the diaphragm, condom, spermicidal jelly or foam, rhythm, and withdrawal, have a much greater method effectiveness than use effectiveness. With use of the methods in which coitus-related activities are not needed, such as the oral contraceptives and IUD, there is less difference between method and use effectiveness, and thus their overall effectiveness is greater than that of the coitus-related methods.

The overall value of a contraceptive method as used by a couple (correctly or incorrectly) is determined by calculation of actual effectiveness as well as the continuation rate. To determine these rates, actuarial methods such as the log-rank life table method should be used instead of the less accurate Pearl index.

Even with the use of these excellent statistical techniques, it is difficult to determine the effectiveness of the various methods in actual practice. Most studies undertaken to determine effectiveness of a contraceptive method are performed under carefully controlled clinical trials during which frequent contact with supportive clinical personnel results in lower failure rates and higher continuation rates than occur in normal use. Furthermore, these clinical trials are infrequently performed in a comparative randomized manner, so clinicians cannot compare results of a trial of one type of contraceptive method with the results of a trial of another type.

Several other factors influence contraceptive failure rates. One of the most important is motivation of the couple. Contraceptive failure is more likely to occur in couples seeking to delay a wanted birth than in couples seeking to prevent any more births, especially for coitus-related methods. The woman's age has a strong negative correlation with the failure of a contraceptive method, as does the socioeconomic class and level of education. Thus one must consider many variables when evaluating the effectiveness of any method of contraception for an individual patient. In addition, failure rates of prospective studies are consistently lower than those of retrospective interview studies.

According to data obtained from questionnaires used in the 1973 and 1976 National Surveys of Family Growth, first-year failure rates were lowest for oral contraceptives (2.5%) and highest for rhythm (18.8%) (Table 11-3). For all methods, failure rates were lower for women wishing to prevent any pregnancy than for women wishing to delay a pregnancy, lower among women aged 35 to 44 (1.4%) than among women aged 15 to 24 (10.7%), and inversely related to education and income (socioeconomic class). The least variation among failure rates occurred with oral contraceptives and the greatest with rhythm. Theoretically the method failure rates could be estimated by the lowest failure rate found in the subgroup of women who wished to prevent a pregnancy, had the highest income, and were over 30. In this group the first-year failure rates were 0.8% for the oral contraceptives and 1.5% for the IUD (Table 11-3). Further data from these surveys indicate that 1-year continuation rates for the various contraceptive methods were highest for the IUD and oral contraceptives and lowest for the diaphragm, condom, and spermicides (Table 11-4).

TABLE 11-3

Percentage of Married Women Aged 15 to 44 Who Experienced a Contraceptive Failure During the First Year of Use, by Contraceptive Method (United States, 1970-1975)

Contraceptive Method	All Women*	Women over 30 with at Least High School Education Wishing to Prevent Pregnancy with Annual Income >$15,000†
Sterilization	0.0	0.0
Oral contraceptive	2.5	0.8
IUD	4.8	1.5
Condom	9.6	0.9
Diaphragm	14.4	6.4
Spermicidal foam, cream, jelly, suppository	17.7	6.1
Rhythm	18.8	8.3
Other	11.5	4.0

*Data from Grady WR, Hirsch MB, Keen N, et al: Contraceptive failure and continuation among married women in the U.S., 1970-75. Stud Fam Plann 14(1):12, 1983.
†Data from Schirm AL, Trussell J, Menken J, et al: Contraceptive failure in the United States: The impact of social, economic and demographic factors. Fam Plann Perspect 14:68, 1982.

TABLE 11-4

Percentage of Married Women Aged 15 to 44 Who Continued to Use the Same Contraceptive Method for 1 Year if Only Method-Related Reasons for Discontinuation (Excluding Unintended Pregnancy) are Considered (United States, 1970-1975)

Contraceptive Method	All Women
All methods except sterilization	69.3
Oral contraceptives	74.1
IUD	78.6
Condom	61.9
Diaphragm	64.3
Spermicidal foam, cream, jelly, suppository	53.8
Rhythm	71.4
Other (excluding sterilization)	66.5

From Grady WR, Hirsch MB, Keen N, Vaughan B: Contraceptive failure and continuation among married women in the U.S., 1970-75. Stud Fam Plann 14(1):16, 1983.

SPERMICIDES—VAGINAL FOAMS, CREAMS, JELLIES, AND SUPPOSITORIES

All spermicides contain an ingredient (usually nonoxyl 9) that immobilizes or kills sperm on contact. They also provide a mechanical barrier and must be placed into the vagina before each coital act. There are no available data comparing the efficiency of the various types of vaginal spermicides, but as noted earlier, their effectiveness increases with increasing age of the woman and is similar to that of the diaphragm in all age and income groups. The increased effectiveness of vaginal spermicides in older women is probably due to increased motivation. Also, acts of coitus are more likely to be less spontaneous and to occur less frequently than in younger women. A spermicide incorporated into a vaginal sponge that can be left in place for 24 hours avoids the need for use before each coital act. However, the vaginal sponge had significantly higher failure rates than the diaphragm in clinical trials comparing these two methods. It has been suggested that contraceptive failures with spermicides may be associated with an increased incidence of congenital malformations, but this finding has not been confirmed by several large studies and is not believed to be valid.

DIAPHRAGM

The diaphragm must be carefully fitted by the physician or nursing personnel. The largest diaphragm that does not cause discomfort or undue pressure on the vaginal epithelium should be used. After the fitting the patient should remove the diaphragm and reinsert it herself. The patient should then be examined to make sure the diaphragm is covering the cervix. When the woman is wearing the diaphragm, she should not be aware of its presence or have any discomfort. The diaphragm should be used with spermicidal cream or jelly and should be left in place for at least 8 hours after the last coital act.

Data from the Oxford Family Planning Association Study indicate that women who have been using a diaphragm successfully should be informed that it is very effective, and they need not switch to another method. In this study of married women over 25 who had been using the diaphragm for at least 5 months, the failure rate was only 2.4 per 100 woman-years. Therefore prospective new users should be informed that the diaphragm is an effective method of contraception after the first few months of use.

CERVICAL CAP

Various types of plastic and rubber cup-shaped devices that fit around the cervix have been used as barrier contraceptives for decades, mainly in Britain and Europe. Each type of device is manufactured in different sizes and should be fitted to the cervix by a clinician. The cervical cap should not be left in place more than 72 hours because of possible problems of ulceration, odor, and infection. Although these devices are not currently approved for general use in the United States, they are a popular method of contraception among a segment of the population. Clinical trials with cervical caps among motivated women report first year failure rates of about 9%.

CONDOM

The use of the condom by individuals with multiple sexual partners should be encouraged, as it is the method of contraception that is most effective in preventing transmission of sexually transmitted disease. The condom should not be applied tightly. The tip should extend beyond the end of the penis by about ½ inch to collect the ejaculate. Care must be taken on withdrawal not to spill the ejaculate. In the Oxford Family Planning Association Study all condom users had previously used another method, mainly oral contraception. During 12,497 woman-years of exposure, 449 unplanned pregnancies occurred, for a use-pregnancy rate of 3.6 per 100 woman-years. The pregnancy rate increased linearly over time, from 0.7 per 100 woman-years at 3 months to 8.4 per 100 woman-years at 24 months. Accidental pregnancy rates were slightly lower among women over 35 years of age and among women who had completed their families, even when these factors were standardized for the other characteristics. This study is one of the largest for which findings have been published, and the results are consistent with those of several older studies that show a similar high level of effectiveness for the condom when used by couples with enough motivation for the wife to attend a family planning clinic. In the United States survey discussed previously the first-year condom failure rate was only 0.9% among women over 30 who wanted to prevent further pregnancies and had an annual income of more than $15,000.

RHYTHM

The Roman Catholic church officially proscribes all methods of contraception other than rhythm, or periodic abstinence. The rationale for the rhythm method is based on three assumptions: first, the ovum is capable of being fertilized for only about 24 hours after ovulation; second, sperm can retain their fertilizing ability for only about 48 hours after coitus; and third, ovulation usually occurs 12 to 16 days (14 ± 2 days) before the onset of the subsequent menses. According to these assumptions, after the woman records the length of her cycles for several months, she determines her fertile period by subtracting 18 days from the total days of her shortest cycle and 11 days from the total days of her previous longest cycle. Then in each subsequent cycle the couple abstains from coitus during this calculated fertile period. The use-effectiveness of this calendar method of periodic abstinence is poor. Failure rates have been reported to vary between 21 and 47 per 100 woman-years. In the United States survey the first-year failure rate of the rhythm method was 18.8%. As summarized by Mastroianni, the reasons for this lack of success are numerous, despite advances in knowledge of human reproductive physiology. First, there is no good evidence to indicate that the three assumptions on which the rhythm method is based have scientific validity. Second, there is great irregularity in menstrual cycle length, so that women with previously regular cycles not infrequently have occasional marked variation in cycle length. Cycle irregularity is common in perimenarcheal and perimenopausal women, a time of life when most pregnancies are unwanted. Third, because a woman is menstruating during several of the nonfertile days and

most couples do not have coitus during this time, the period of abstinence is frequently greater than the time during which sexual relations may be practiced.

To increase the effectiveness of the rhythm method, instead of relying solely on the calendar method previously described, it is advisable to also measure the basal body temperature every day. Because progesterone causes an increase in basal body temperature, if the couple abstains from intercourse from the start of menses until at least 48 hours after the rise in basal body temperature (2 days after ovulation), sexual relations will take place only after the ovum is no longer capable of being fertilized. Data from several sources indicate that the use of daily basal body temperature for determining the days of periodic abstinence increases the effectiveness of the rhythm method. One British study reported a failure rate of only 6.6 per 100 woman-years for women practicing the temperature method for determining the time of periodic abstinence.

Recently there have been reports that women could detect changes in the quality and quantity of their own cervical mucus and could be taught to predict the time when ovulation was going to occur. Although reports of extraordinary success with this method have been made by some enthusiasts, careful analysis of their results suggests that the actual effectiveness of this modification is substantially less than claimed.

Thus periodic abstinence, or the rhythm method, requires a high degree of motivation, communication, and sophistication. Even with these qualities the rhythm method of family planning is associated with a high failure rate, and all couples who choose this method should be aware of this.

ORAL STEROIDS

There were originally three major types of oral steroid contraceptive formulations: combination, sequential, and daily gestagen. The combination is the most widely used and most effective type. It consists of tablets containing both an estrogen and a gestagen given continuously for 3 weeks. The original sequential type, which is no longer marketed, consisted of a regimen of estrogen alone given for about 2 weeks followed by 1 week of a combination estrogen and gestagen. Recently combination formulations have been marketed that contain two or three different amounts of the same estrogen and gestagen. Each of the tablets containing one of these various dosages is given for intervals varying from 7 to 11 days during the 21-day medication period. These formulations have been given the description of biphasic or triphasic and are generally known as multiphasic. The rationale for this type of formulation is that a lower total dose of steroid is administered without increasing the incidence of breakthrough bleeding. When combination oral contraceptives are prescribed, usually no medication is given for 1 week out of 4 to allow withdrawal bleeding to occur. The third type of contraceptive formulation consists of a tablet of gestagen without any estrogen. This formulation is ingested daily without a steroid-free interval.

Pharmacology

Oral contraceptives presently being used are formulated from synthetic steroids and do not contain natural estrogens or gestagens. There are two major types of synthetic gestagens: derivatives of 19-nortestosterone and derivatives of 17-alpha-acetoxyprogesterone. The latter group are C_{21} gestagens, consisting of steroids such as medroxyprogesterone acetate and megestrol acetate. They are not utilized in present contraceptive formulations. In contrast to the 19-nortestosterone derivatives, when the C_{21} gestagens were given in high dosages to female beagle dogs, the animals developed an increased incidence of mammary cancer. Because of this carcinogenic effect, contraceptives with these gestagens are not marketed. All oral contraceptive formulations now available in the United States consist of varying dosages of one of the following five 19-nortestosterone gestagens: norethynodrel, norethindrone, norethindrone acetate, ethynodiol diacetate, or norgestrel (or its active isomer, levonorgestrel) (Fig. 11-1). With the exception of two daily gestagen formulations the gestagens are combined with varying dosages of two estrogens, ethinyl estradiol and ethinyl estradiol-3-methyl ether (also known as mestranol) (Fig. 11-2). All the synthetic estrogens and gestagens in oral contraceptives have an ethinyl group on the 17 position. The presence of this ethinyl group enhances the oral activity of these agents, as their essential functional groups are not rapidly hydroxylated and then conjugated as they initially pass through the liver via the portal sys-

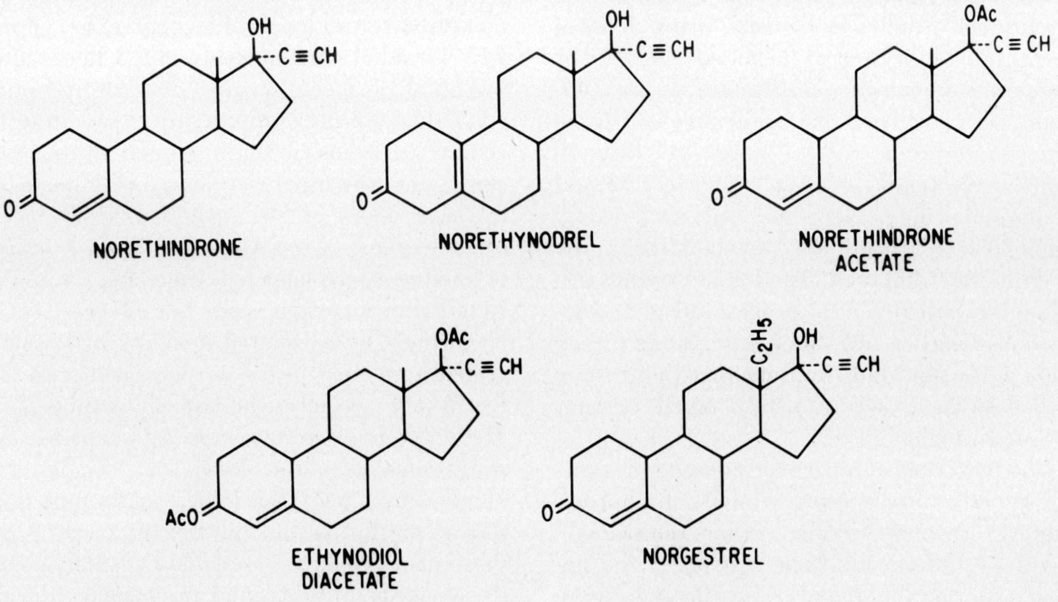

FIGURE 11-1
Structural formulas of the five gestagens used in combination oral contraceptives.

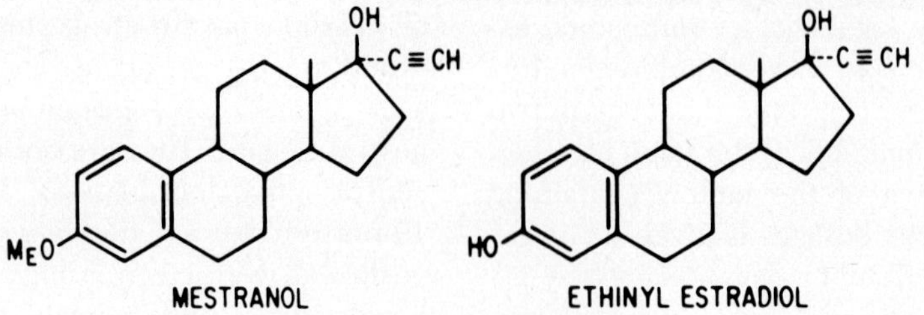

FIGURE 11-2
Structural formulas of the two estrogens used in combination oral contraceptives in the United States.

tem, in contrast to what occurs with the natural sex steroids when they are ingested orally. The synthetic steroids thus have greater potency per unit weight than the natural steroids when both are ingested orally.

The various modifications in chemical structure of the different synthetic gestagens and estrogens also alter their biologic activity. For these reasons, one cannot compare the pharmacologic activity of the various gestagens or estrogens present in the particular contraceptive steroid only on the basis of the amount of steroid present in the formulation. The biologic activity of each steroid must be considered also. Based on established tests for progestational activity in animals, it has been found that a given weight of norgestrel is several times more potent than the equivalent weight of norethindrone. Studies in humans, using delay of menses or endometrial histologic alterations such as subnuclear vacuolization as an endpoint, also conclude that norgestrel is 5 to 10 times more potent and levonorgestrel 10 to 20 times more potent than an equivalent weight of norethindrone. Norethindrone acetate and ethinyldiol diacetate are metabolized in the body to norethindrone. The human studies utilizing the parameters of progestational activity described earlier and studies comparing the effects on serum lipids indicate that these three gestagens have approximately equal potency per unit weight.

The two types of estrogenic compounds present in oral contraceptives, ethinyl estradiol and ethinyl estradiol-3-methyl ether (mestranol), also have different biologic activity in the human. To become biologically effective, mestranol must be demethylated to ethinyl estra-

diol, because mestranol does not bind to the estrogen cytosol receptors. The degree of conversion of mestranol to ethinyl estradiol varies among individuals; some are able to convert it completely; others convert only a portion of it. Thus in some individuals a given weight of mestranol is as potent as the equivalent weight of ethinyl estradiol, whereas in others it is only about half as potent. Overall it has been estimated that ethinyl estradiol is about 1.7 times as potent as an equivalent weight of mestranol, using human endometrial response and effect on liver corticosteroid-binding globulin (CBG) production as end points. Thus it is necessary to evaluate the biologic activity as well as the quantity of both steroid components when comparing potency of the various formulations.

Using radioimmunoassay, Brenner et al. measured serum levels of levonorgestrel, FSH, LH, estradiol, and progesterone 3 hours after ingestion of a combination oral contraceptive containing 0.5 mg of *dl*-norgestrel and 50 μg of ethinyl estradiol in three women during two consecutive treatment cycles as well as during the intervening pill-free interval. Daily levels of levonorgestrel rose during the first few days of medication, plateaued thereafter, and declined after ingestion of the last pill (Fig. 11-3). Nevertheless, substantial amounts of levonorgestrel remained in the serum for at least the first 3 to 4 days after the last pill was ingested. These levels of steroid were sufficient to suppress gonadotrophin release, and estradiol levels remained low. Thus follicle maturation does not occur during the pill-free interval. From these data it seems reasonable to conclude that the majority of accidental pregnancies during oral contraceptive therapy probably do not re-

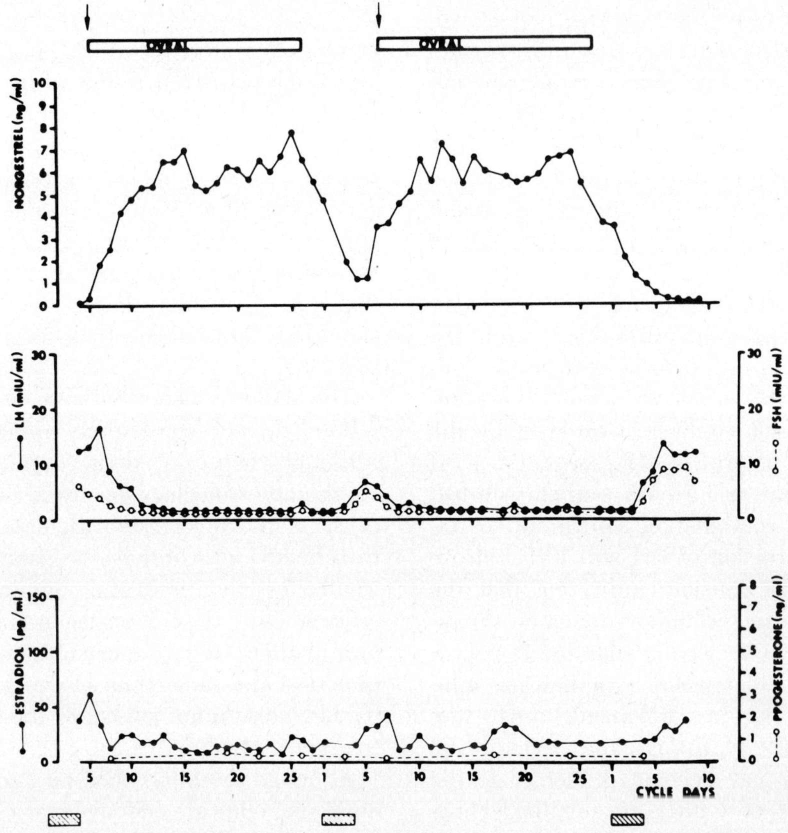

FIGURE 11-3
Serum *d*-norgestrel, FSH, LH, estradiol, and progesterone levels in patient during and after oral administration of 500 μg of dl-norgestrel and 50 μg of ethinyl estradiol (Ovral) for two subsequent 21-day periods interrupted by a pill-free interval of 6 days. (From Brenner PF, Mishell DR Jr, Stanczyk FZ, et al: Am J Obstet Gynecol 129:133, 1977.)

sult from failure to ingest one or two pills more than a few days after treatment is initiated but rather because initiation of the next cycle of medication is delayed for a few days. Therefore it is important that the pill-free interval be limited to no more than 7 days. This is best accomplished by administering either a placebo or an iron pill daily during the steroid-free interval (the so-called 28-day package). Alternatively, treatment may be started on the first Sunday after menses begins instead of the fifth day of the cycle. It is easier to remember to start the next cycle on a Sunday. Patients should be warned that the most important pill to remember to ingest is the first pill of the cycle.

Physiology

The combination of estrogen and gestagen is the most effective type of oral contraceptive formulation because these preparations consistently inhibit the midcycle gonadotrophin surge and thus prevent ovulation. In addition these drugs act on other aspects of the reproductive process. They alter the cervical mucus, making it consistently thick, viscid, and scanty in amount, which thus retards sperm penetration. They alter motility of the uterus and oviduct, thus altering transport of both ova and sperm. Furthermore they alter the endometrium so that its glandular production of glycogen is diminished and less energy is available for the blastocyst to survive in the uterine cavity. Finally they may alter ovarian responsiveness to gonadotrophin stimulation. Nevertheless, neither gonadotrophin production nor ovarian steroidogenesis is completely abolished, and levels of those endogenous hormones in the peripheral blood during ingestion of combination oral contraceptives are similar to those found in the early follicular phase of the normal cycle.

Contraceptive steroids mainly prevent ovulation by interfering with GnRH release from the hypothalamus. In rats, as well as in a few studies in humans, this inhibitory action of the contraceptive steroids could be overcome by the administration of GnRH. However, in most other studies, the majority of women who had been ingesting combination contraceptive steroids had suppression of LH and FSH release following GnRH infusion, indicating that the steroids had a direct inhibitory effect on the pituitary as well as the hypothalamus. It is possible, however, that when hypothalamic inhibition occurs for a prolonged time, the mechanism for synthesis and release of gonadotrophins may become refractory to the normal amount of GnRH stimulation. However, in a few oral contraceptive users studied, after serial daily administration of GnRH, there was still a refractory response to a GnRH infusion. It is thus probable that the combination contraceptive steroids do have a direct inhibitory effect on the gonadotrophin-producing cells of the pituitary in addition to their effect on the hypothalamus. This direct pituitary effect occurs in about 80% of women ingesting combination steroids and is related not to the age of the patient or the duration of steroid use but to potency of the preparations, being more frequent with use of formulations containing 50 μg of estrogen or more than with use of those containing 30 to 35 μg. It is not known if the amount of pituitary suppression is related to the occurrence of postpill amenorrhea, but if there is a relation, lower dose formulations should be associated with a lower frequency of this entity.

The daily gestagen without estrogen preparations do not consistently inhibit ovulation. Although they exert their contraceptive action via the other mechanisms listed previously, because of the inconsistent ovulation inhibition, the effectiveness of these preparations is significantly less than with the combined type. Because a lower dose of gestagen is used in these formulations, it is important that they be ingested at the same time of day to ensure that blood levels do not fall below the effective contraceptive level.

Although there has been no significant difference in clinical effectiveness demonstrated among the various combination formulations currently available in the United States, listed in Table 11-5, the formulations containing only 20 μg of ethinyl estradiol may be slightly less effective. Provided no tablets are omitted, the pregnancy rate is about 0.2% per year with all combination formulations.

TABLE 11-5

Composition of Oral Contraceptives Currently Marketed in the United States

Manufacturer/Product	Type	Progestin	Estrogen
Mead Johnson & Co.			
Ovcon-50	Comb.	1.0 mg Norethindrone	50 μg Ethinyl estradiol
Ovcon-35	Comb.	0.4 mg Norethindrone	35 μg Ethinyl estradiol
Ortho Pharmaceuticals, Inc.			
Modicon	Comb.	0.5 mg Norethindrone	35 μg Ethinyl estradiol
Ortho-Novum 1/35	Comb.	1.0 mg Norethindrone	35 μg Ethinyl estradiol
Ortho-Novum 1/50	Comb.	1.0 mg Norethindrone	50 μg Mestranol
Ortho-Novum 1/80	Comb.	1.0 mg Norethindrone	80 μg Mestranol
Ortho-Novum 2	Comb.	2.0 mg Norethindrone	100 μg Mestranol

TABLE 11-5, cont'd
Composition of Oral Contraceptives Currently Marketed in the United States

Manufacturer/ Product	Type	Progestin	Estrogen
Ortho Pharmaceuticals, Inc., cont'd			
Ortho-Novum 10/	Comb.-biphasic	0.5 mg Norethindrone	35 μg Ethinyl estradiol
11		1.0 mg Norethindrone	35 μg Ethinyl estradiol
Micronor	Prog.	0.35 mg Norethindrone	
Ortho-Novum 7/	Comb.-triphasic	0.5 mg Norethindrone	35 μg Ethinyl estradiol
7/		0.75 mg Norethindrone	35 μg Ethinyl estradiol
7		1.0 mg Norethindrone	35 μg Ethinyl estradiol
Parke-Davis			
Loestrin 1/20	Comb.	1.0 mg Norethindrone acetate	20 μg Ethinyl estradiol
Loestrin 1.5/30	Comb.	1.5 mg Norethindrone acetate	30 μg Ethinyl estradiol
Norlestrin 2.5/50	Comb.	2.5 mg Norethindrone acetate	50 μg Ethinyl estradiol
Norlestrin 1/50	Comb.	1.0 mg Norethindrone acetate	50 μg Ethinyl estradiol
Searle Laboratories			
Demulen 1/35	Comb.	1.0 mg Ethynodiol di-acetate	35 μg Ethinyl estradiol
Demulen 1/50	Comb.	1.0 mg Ethynodiol di acetate	50 μg Ethinyl estradiol
Ovulen	Comb.	1.0 mg Ethynodiol di-acetate	100 μg Mestranol
Enovid-E21	Comb.	2.5 mg Norethynodrel	100 μg Mestranol
Enovid-5	Comb.	5.0 mg Norethynodrel	75 μg Mestranol
Enovid-10	Comb.	9.85 mg Norethynodrel	150 μg Mestranol
Syntex Laboratories			
Brevicon	Comb.	0.5 mg Norethindrone	35 μg Ethinyl estradiol
Norinyl 1 + 35	Comb.	1.0 mg Norethindrone	35 μg Ethinyl estradiol
Norinyl 1 + 50	Comb.	1.0 mg Norethindrone	50 μg Mestranol
Norinyl 1 + 80	Comb.	1.0 mg Norethindrone	80 μg Mestranol
Norinyl 2	Comb.	2.0 mg Norethindrone	100 μg Mestranol
NOR-QD	Prog.	0.35 mg Norethindrone	
Tri-Norinyl 2/	Comb.-triphasic	0.5 mg Norethindrone	35 μg Ethinyl estradiol
9/		1.0 mg Norethindrone	35 μg Ethinyl estradiol
5		0.5 mg Norethindrone	35 μg Ethinyl estradiol
Wyeth Laboratories			
Lo/Ovral	Comb.	0.3 mg Norgestrel	30 μg Ethinyl estradiol
Nordette	Comb.	0.15 mg Levonorgestrel	30 μg Ethinyl estradiol
Ovral	Comb.	0.5 mg Norgestrel	50 μg Ethinyl estradiol
Ovrette	Prog.	75 μg Norgestrel	
Triphasil 6/	Comb.-triphasic	50 μg Levonorgestrel	30 μg Ethinylestradiol
5/		75 μg Levonorgestrel	40 μg Ethinylestradiol
10		125 μg Levonorgestrel	30 μg Ethinylestradiol

Metabolic Effects

It is important to realize that oral contraceptives have metabolic effects in addition to the effects on the reproductive axis (Table 11-6). Some of these produce adverse clinical effects. The incidence of these effects has been exaggerated in the lay press and has steadily decreased as the dosage of steroids in the formulation has decreased. Fortunately, in most instances the more common adverse effects are relatively mild. Some are produced by the estrogenic component of the formulation, while the others are produced by the progestin component alone or by a combination of the two. The most frequent symptoms produced by the estrogenic component include nausea, breast tenderness, and fluid retention, which usually does not exceed 3 to 4 pounds of body weight.

Estrogen can also produce changes in mood and depression brought about by diversion of tryptophan metabolism from its minor pathway in the brain to its major pathway in the liver. The end product of tryptophan metabolism, serotonin, is thus decreased in the central ner-

TABLE 11-6
Metabolic Effects of Contraceptive Steroids

	Effects	
	Chemical	Clinical
Estrogen—Ethinyl Estradiol		
Proteins		
Albumin	↓	None
Amino acids	↓	None
Globulins	↑	
Angiotensinogen		↑ Blood pressure
Factors VII and X		Hypercoagulability
Carrier proteins (CBG, TBG, transferrin, ceruloplasmin)		None
Carbohydrate		
Plasma insulin	None	None
Glucose tolerance	None	None
Lipids		
Cholesterol	None	None
Triglyceride	↑	None
HDL-Cholesterol	↑	None
LDL-Cholesterol	↓	None
Electrolytes		
Sodium excretion	↓	Fluid retention Edema
Tryptophan metabolism	↓	Depression Mood changes Sleep disturbance
Vitamins		
B complex	↓	None
Ascorbic acid	↓	None
Vitamin A	↑	None
Skin		
Sebum production	↓	Less acne
Pigmentation	↑	Chloasma
Target tissues		
Breast	↑	Breast tenderness
Endometrial receptors	↑	Hyperplasia

vous system, and the resultant lowering of serotonin can produce depression in some women and sleepiness and mood changes in others. This state is reversible and fortunately not too common; it disappears when oral contraceptives are discontinued. The incidence of all these estrogenic side effects is much lower now than a decade ago because the formulations in use today contain only one fifth as much estrogen as the formulations used in the 1960s.

The gestagens, because they are structurally related to testosterone, produce certain adverse androgenic effects. These include weight gain, acne, and a symptom perceived by some women as nervousness. Some women gain a considerable amount of weight when they take oral contraceptives, and this weight gain is produced by the anabolic effect of the progestin component. Although estrogens decrease sebum production, gestagens increase sebum production and can cause acne to develop or worsen. Thus patients who have acne should be given a formulation with a low gestagen/estrogen ratio. The final symptom produced by the gestogenic component is failure of with-

drawal bleeding or amenorrhea. Because the progestins decrease the synthesis of estrogen receptors in the endometrium, endometrial growth is decreased, and some women have failure of withdrawal bleeding. Although this symptom is not important medically, since bleeding serves as a signal that the patient is not pregnant, it is desirable to have some amount of periodic withdrawal bleeding during the days the woman is not taking these steroids. Although gestagens may produce a temporary slight decrease of glucose tolerance, high doses of certain oral contraceptives do not cause the development of diabetes mellitus. Both steroid components can act together to produce irregular bleeding or chloasma or both. Breakthrough bleeding (which is usually produced by insufficient estrogen, too much gestagen, or a combination of both, as well as failure of withdrawal bleeding) can be alleviated by increasing the amount of estrogen in the formulation or by switching to a more estrogenic formulation. The symptom of chloasma, pigmentation of the malar eminences, is accentuated by sunlight and usually takes a

---

TABLE 11-6, cont'd
Metabolic Effects of Contraceptive Steroids

	Effects	
	Chemical	**Clinical**
Gestagens—19-Nortestosterone Derivatives		
Proteins	None	None
Carbohydrate		
Plasma insulin	↑	None
Glucose tolerance	↓	None
Lipids		
Cholesterol	↓	None
Triglyceride	↓	None
HDL-Cholesterol	↓ ⎫	
LDL-Cholesterol	↑ ⎭	? ↑ Cardiovascular disease
Nitrogen retention	↑	↑ Body weight
Skin—sebum production	↑	↑ Acne
Androgenic effect	↑	Nervousness
Endometrial receptors	↓	Amenorrhea

From Mishell DR Jr: Oral steroid contraceptives. Reproduced with permission from Infertility, contraception and reproductive endocrinology, 2nd ed., by Daniel R. Mishell, Jr., M.D., and Val Davajan, M.D. Copyright © 1986 Medical Economics Books, Oradell, N.J. 07649. All rights reserved.
CBG, Corticosteroid-binding globulin; *TBG*, thyroxine-binding globulin.

long time to disappear after oral contraceptives are discontinued.

In addition to these more common adverse effects, there is an increased risk of developing more serious problems that can lead to death or severe morbidity. The synthetic estrogen, ethinyl estradiol, used in oral contraceptives causes an increase in hepatic production of several globulins. The amount of increase is directly related to the dosage of estrogen in the formulation and thus is less with formulations containing a lower dose of estrogen. Some of these globulins are involved in the blood-clotting process, and their increase may cause a hypercoagulable state and the development of thrombosis in certain oral contraceptive users. Increased levels of one of the globulins, angiotensinogen, may cause increased angiotensin II, which may produce an increase in blood pressure in certain individuals. The elevated globulin levels return to normal shortly after stopping ingestion of the drug. The blood hypercoagulability and elevated blood pressure, if present, also disappear. There is no evidence that oral contraceptive use produces permanent hypertension.

Although the incidence of cholelithiasis is increased about twofold compared to its incidence in controls in the first few years of oral contraceptive use, data from the Royal College study in Britain indicate that after 4 years of oral contraceptive use the incidence of cholelithiasis is decreased as compared with controls. Thus oral contraceptives appear to accelerate the process of cholelithiasis but do not increase its overall incidence. The risk of developing deep vein thrombophlebitis is also increased about three or four times, as is the risk of developing thromboembolism. However, the absolute incidence of these disorders, which are not necessarily related (i.e., patients with thromboembolism do not have to have clinical symptoms of thrombophlebitis), has been estimated by Vessey in women using the older, higher estrogen formulations to be about 1 per 10,000 users annually for thrombophlebitis and about 1 per 30,000 users annually for thromboembolism. Oral contraceptives appear to increase the incidence of hemorrhagic and possibly thrombotic stroke, although the epidemiologic data relating oral contraceptive use to stroke are conflicting and indicate that the increased risk of stroke in oral contraceptive

users, if it does occur, is mainly limited to women ingesting formulations with 50 mg of estrogen or more and who have underlying vascular disorders such as hypertension or who are older and smoke. Although the relative risk of developing stroke is possibly increased about three times, the actual incidence remains quite low, estimated in women using the higher estrogen dose formulations to be about 1 per 20,000 to 1 per 30,000 users per year. Benign liver adenomas occur rarely in oral contraceptive users, with an estimated frequency of about 1 per 30,000 to 1 per 50,000 users per year. The incidence is increased in women who have used the formulations for more than 5 years. Also, as discussed later, although there is epidemiologic evidence that women over 35 years who smoke or have other associated risk factors, such as hypertension or hypercholesterolemia, have an increased risk of developing myocardial infarction with oral contraceptive use, the actual incidence of developing myocardial infarction in this group is also low, about 1 per 5000 users annually.

Major Concerns

Women have three major concerns about oral contraceptives: an increased risk of developing cancer, problems with future childbearing, and an increased chance of developing heart attacks and stroke. These concerns are mostly unwarranted, as the following discussion indicates.

Cancer

A thorough review of the literature reveals that in the 26 years of widespread use of oral contraceptives only scant evidence exists that their use increases the risk of any type of cancer, including breast cancer, cancer of the uterus, cancer of the cervix, and cancer of the liver. Three large prospective studies were started in 1968, two in Great Britain (the Royal College of General Practitioners Study [RCGP] and the Oxford Family Planning Study) and one in the United States (the National Institutes of Health [NIH]-sponsored Walnut Creek Study). Each study compared large groups of women using oral contraceptives with a similar number of control women using other methods of contraception. To date, none of these studies has found an increased risk of any type of cancer except for cervical cancer in the Oxford study, which may have been due to confounding factors. Although data from the Walnut Creek study indicate that women using oral contraceptives and exposed to large amounts of sunlight may have an increased risk of melanoma, this association has not been found in other studies.

BREAST CANCER. At the present time the women using oral contraceptives in these prospective as well as other retrospective epidemiologic studies do not have a higher incidence of cancer of the breast than a control group of women of similar age who are using other methods of contraception. Furthermore, oral contraceptives contain a gestagen in addition to the estrogen, and the gestagen counteracts the stimulatory action of the estrogen on target tissues. For this reason, women ingesting oral contraceptives have a lower incidence of nonmalignant cystic disease of the breast than do controls.

A large multicenter epidemiologic study performed by the Centers for Disease Control in the United States (the Cancer and Steroid Hormone study [CASH]) has shown there is no increased risk of breast cancer in oral contraceptive users overall as well as various high-risk subgroup users, such as those with a family history of breast cancer, those with and without benign breast disease, and those using oral contraceptives for many years before their first pregnancy. Furthermore, there was no change in risk of breast cancer with increasing duration of oral contraceptive use, age at first use, or time since last use (Table 11-7). Data from this and other studies indicate no increased risk of breast cancer with any specific type of oral contraceptive formulation or with long-term use at an early age.

ENDOMETRIAL CANCER. There is no evidence that an increased incidence of carcinoma of the endometrium occurs in oral contraceptive users. Data from several epidemiologic studies including the CASH study indicate that women who are using combination oral contraceptives are less likely to develop cancer of the endometrium than are a control group of women who do not use oral contraceptives, probably because the formulations contain a gestagen as well as an estrogen. Gestagens inhibit the synthesis of estrogen receptors and thus, when given with an estrogen, prevent the growth-promoting action of the estrogen.

CERVICAL CANCER. Evidence from one epidemiologic study (the Oxford study) suggests that users of oral contraceptives have an increased incidence of cancer of the cervix. In this and other studies, oral contraceptive users have been found to have an increased incidence of dysplasia of the cervix (including carcinoma in situ), as compared with controls using other methods of contraception. Dysplasia and epidermoid cancer of the cervix have also been linked with onset of sexual intercourse at a young age and with multiple sexual partners. In other studies in which oral contraceptive users were found to have a higher incidence of

TABLE 11-7
Relative Risk* of Breast Cancer† with Oral Contraceptive Use

Time Since First Use (Years)	Duration of Use (Years)					All Who Have Ever Used
	<2	2-5	6-7	8-10	≥11	
<10	0.7	2.0	2.8	0.8	—	1.4
10-12	1.2	2.0	0.3	0.9	1.2	1.2
13-15	0.9	1.0	1.2	0.8	1.1	1.0
≥16	0.9	1.0	0.8	0.7	0.8	0.9
All	0.9	1.2	1.0	0.7	0.9	0.9

Adapted from Centers for Disease Control Cancer and Steroid Hormone Study: Long-term oral contraceptive use and the risk of breast cancer. JAMA 249:1591, 1983. Copyright 1983, American Medical Association.
*Relative to persons who have never used oral contraceptives. None of the figures are statistically significant.
†By time since first oral contraceptive use and duration of use. Excludes 53 women with unknown duration of use.

dysplasia than the controls, it was also found that oral contraceptive users had more sexual partners and had intercourse at a younger age than did the controls who used other methods of contraception. These studies indicated that the increased incidence of dysplasia was most likely due to other factors, including more sexual partners, more frequent cytologic screening, and increased protection by those in the control group who used diaphragms or condoms. A similar problem of confounding factors may have occurred in the Oxford study noted earlier. The individuals using oral contraceptives may have begun sexual activity earlier than the control group, which used IUDs. Thus although oral contraceptive users are a high-risk group for cervical neoplasia and require annual screening with cervical cytology, there is no evidence that the oral contraceptives are the causative factor.

LIVER CANCER. Cancer of the liver is very uncommon in young women, and women using oral contraceptives do not have a greater chance of developing this rare cancer, as the incidence of this cancer in women of reproductive age in the United States has not changed since oral contraceptives became widely used. Women using oral contraceptives for more than 5 years appear to have a greater chance of developing benign liver adenomas. Although these benign liver tumors can spontaneously rupture and cause serious hemorrhage, they gradually decrease in size and eventually disappear after oral contraceptives are discontinued. Thus these adenomas, which occur in only about 1 in 30,000 oral contraceptive users, are temporary and do not become malignant.

OTHER CANCERS. The incidence of ovarian cancer is diminished by about 50% in oral contraceptive users (see later discussion). Although some studies show an increased incidence of malignant melanoma related to oral contraceptive use, they did not control for the confounding effect of exposure to sunlight, which is increased in oral contraceptive users.

Pregnancy After Discontinuation of Oral Contraceptives

Although the rate of return of fertility after discontinuation of oral contraceptives in both nulligravid and nulliparous women may be delayed a few months as compared with women who stop using other methods of contraception, such as the diaphragm or IUD, eventually the percentage of women who conceive after stopping all methods is the same. Thus although oral contraceptives produce a period of temporary infertility in some women after their discontinuation, this infertility is usually not permanent, as reported by Vessey in the Oxford Family Planning Study. After 2 or 3 years fertility rates were the same among groups of former oral contraceptive users and former users of other methods of contraception (Fig. 11-4).

Since the return of ovulation is delayed for variable periods of time after discontinuation of oral contraceptives, it is difficult to estimate the expected date of delivery if conception takes place before spontaneous menstruation resumes. For these reasons, if women stop oral contraceptives in order to conceive it is probably best that they continue to use barrier methods for 1 or 2 months until they resume regular cycles. If they do conceive before the resumption of spontaneous menses, gestational age should be estimated by serial sonography.

The spontaneous abortion rate in women who conceive in the first or subsequent months after stopping oral contraceptives is the same as the spontaneous abortion rate in the general population or that in women who stop using other contraceptive methods. One study reported a high incidence of lethal chromosomal abnormalities in abortuses of women who conceived within a few months after stopping oral contraceptives. However, more recent studies have shown that abortuses of women who did not use oral contraceptives had the same incidence of these chromosomal abnormalities as abortuses of women who did use them.

Several studies of large numbers of babies born to women who stopped using oral contraceptives have been undertaken. These studies show that these infants have no greater chance of being born with any type of birth defect even if conception occurred in the first month after stopping the medication. The incidence of congenital anomalies was the same in babies born to women who had previously used oral contraceptives as in babies born to women who had previously used other methods of contraception or women who had not used any method of contraception. The largest of these studies contained data from the Walnut Creek Study. The rate of major malformation in

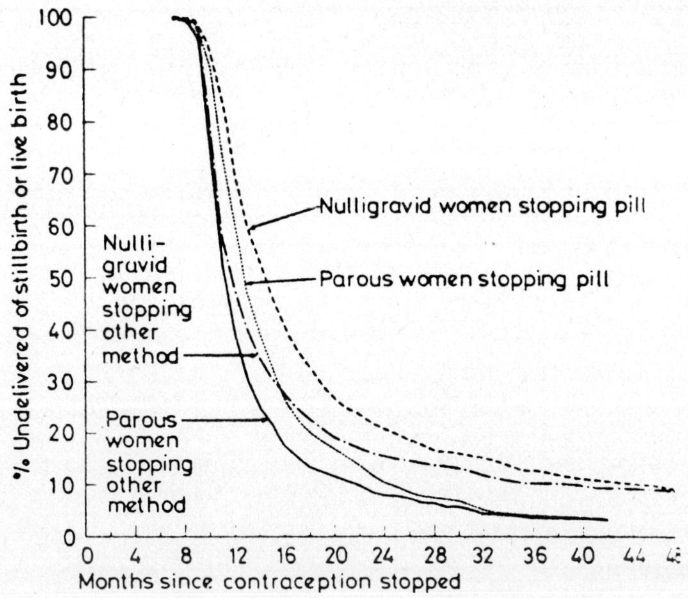

FIGURE 11-4
Fertility after discontinuation of different methods of contraception in order to conceive. (From Vessey MP, Wright NH, McPherson K, et al: Br Med J 1:265, 1978.)

women who had used oral contraceptives before conception was 173 in 10,000, compared with the rate of 150 and 201 in 100,000 in the groups who had used other methods or no method before conception. These differences are not significant. In this study, women conceiving within 1 month of stopping oral contraceptives had fewer malformed babies than those conceiving 1 to 5 months later.

Cardiovascular Disease

One of the problems with the retrospective case control epidemiologic studies performed to determine risks of drugs producing disease is that they provide a figure called a *relative risk* or *times rate*. For example, in studies of oral contraceptives it has been stated that myocardial infarction occurs three times more frequently in oral contraceptive users than nonusers. Nevertheless, because young women rarely develop myocardial infarction, in terms of absolute risk the chance that any one woman will develop the disease is extremely low. Although the relative risk figure may frighten an individual, the absolute risk figure is more important. As an example, the relative risk of dying in an automobile accident is much higher if one drives frequently. Nevertheless, most people drive frequently because the absolute risk is so low. The three prospective studies of oral contraceptive users mentioned before, which have been ongoing for more than 10 years, indicate that the absolute risk that an individual oral contraceptive user will develop cardiovascular disease is very low. In the United States and Britain death rates for persons who have had heart attacks have decreased in women aged 20 to 45 years during the past 15 years, years in which oral contraceptive use increased dramatically. Furthermore, the decrease in heart attack death rates in these countries has been similar for men and women. Results from the three prospective oral contraceptive studies indicate that a significantly increased risk of developing cardiovascular disease occurs only in current oral contraceptive users over 35 years of age who smoke or those of any age who use oral contraceptives and also have some type of preexisting vascular disease, such as hypertension, diabetes, or hypercholesterolemia (Tables 11-8 and 11-9). There is no reliable evidence that nonsmokers under age 45 and smokers under 35 who use oral contraceptives have an increased chance of dying from a heart attack provided they do not have preexisting vascular diseases. Thus, if a woman is under 35 and is a cigarette smoker,

TABLE 11-8

Circulatory Disease Mortality Rates per 100,000 Woman-Years by Age, Smoking Status, and Oral Contraceptive Use

| | Mortality Rate (No. Deaths) | | % Relative Risk: Ever-Users vs. Controls |
Age	Ever-Users	Controls	
15-25			
Nonsmokers	0.0 (0)	0.0 (0)	—
Smokers	10.5 (1)	0.0 (0)	—
25-34			
Nonsmokers	4.4 (2)	2.7 (1)	1.6
Smokers	14.2 (6)	4.2 (1)	3.4
35-44			
Nonsmokers	21.5 (7)	6.4 (2)	3.3
Smokers	63.4 (18)	15.2 (3)	4.2*
45-			
Nonsmokers	52.4 (4)	11.4 (1)	4.6
Smokers	206.7 (17)	27.9 (2)	7.4*

Adapted from Royal College of General Practitioners' Oral Contraception Study: Further analysis of mortality in oral contraceptive users. Lancet 1:541, 1981.
*Significantly different.

TABLE 11-9

Walnut Creek Study: Diseases of the Circulatory System

| | Standard Rates | | | RR | |
Disease	Never	Current	Past	Current	Past
Acute myocardial infarction	0.23	0.27	0.20	1.1	0.8
Ischemic heart disease	0.79	1.09	0.90	1.4	1.1
Subarachnoid hemorrhage	0.04	0.43	0.10	10.1*	2.3*
Cerebral thrombosis	0.24	0.53	0.29	2.2*	1.2
Arterial thrombosis	0.24	0.76	0.24	3.2*	1.0
Pulmonary embolism	0.38	0.22	0.29	0.6	0.0
Thrombophlebitis	0.51	0.42	0.48	0.8	1.8

Adapted from Ramcharan S, Pellegrin FA, Ray RM, et al: The Walnut Creek Contraceptive Drug Study: A prospective study of the side effects of oral contraceptives, vol. 3, NIH Publ. No. 81-564. Washington, DC, US Government Printing Office, 1981.
*Not significantly different overall. Significantly different only in smokers over 40 years of age.

she may still use oral contraceptives. Likewise, a woman between 35 and 45 years can continue to use oral contraceptives provided she does not smoke cigarettes or have any other type of vascular disease such as hypertension, diabetes, or hypercholesterolemia.

A few years ago there was concern that women should not use oral contraceptives for more than 5 years, because a 1978 analysis of mortality data from women enrolled in the RCGP Study suggested an increased risk of dying from cardiovascular disease in women who had used oral contraceptives for more than 5 years. Data published in 1981 from the same study indicate that this concern is not valid, as the incidence of deaths from cardiovascular disease did not increase with increased duration of oral contraceptive use. This information, together with data from many other epidemiologic studies that show no increased deaths from myocardial infarction in former users of oral contraceptives, indicates that the cause of myocardial infarction or stroke in oral contraceptive users is due to arterial thrombosis, not atherosclerosis. Thus, despite data indicating that certain oral contraceptive formulations lower HDL-cholesterol (high-density lipoprotein) and raise LDL-cholesterol (low-density lipoprotein) (changes which theoretically could be atherogenic), there is no evidence that long-term use of oral contraceptives produces a permanent harmful effect on the blood vessels such as development of atherosclerosis. Furthermore the adverse lipid alterations produced by some formulations, especially those with high gestagen potency, are small and usually within the normal range. No data show that these small alterations in lipids increase the incidence of atherosclerosis in humans. Thus women can take oral contraceptives for an unlimited time period no matter how old they are when they start taking it. In addition, there is no evidence that there is need for a rest period after a few years of oral contraceptive use. A rest period does not serve any value.

Other Concerns

Included among other concerns about taking oral contraceptives that have proven to be untrue is the belief that women need to take vitamin supplements because oral contraceptives produce vitamin deficiency. Although oral contraceptives do lower the blood levels of the B-complex vitamins and vitamin C, these low vitamin levels are not accompanied by any clinical evidence of vitamin deficiency, and vitamin supplementation is not necessary. There has also been concern that oral contraceptives should not be prescribed for young teenagers because their use might cause permanent changes in their hypothalamic-pituitary-ovarian axis as well as produce premature epiphyseal closure and cause the individuals to stop growing. Both these concerns have proven to be unfounded, and oral contraceptives can be used

by women of any age who have started to have regular menstrual cycles. Finally, there has been concern that oral contraceptives should not be taken by women who developed morphologic alterations in their vagina and uterus as a result of exposure to diethylstilbestrol during fetal life. There is no evidence that when oral contraceptives are ingested by women with adenosis or other genital tract changes caused by antenatal diethylstilbestrol exposure that there is an increase in cancer or other harmful alterations. Therefore oral contraceptives can be used safely by these women.

Contraindications to Oral Contraceptive Use

Oral contraceptives can be prescribed for the majority of women in the reproductive age group because they are young and healthy; however, there are certain absolute contraindications for their use. These include a present and past history of vascular disease, including thromboembolism, thrombophlebitis, atherosclerosis, stroke, and systemic vascular disease, such as lupus erythematosus or hemoglobin SS disease. In addition, hypertension, diabetes mellitus with vascular disease, and hyperlipidemia, as well as women over 35 who smoke, are contraindications to oral contraceptives because use of these agents in women with these disorders can increase the risk for stroke or myocardial infarction. One of the contraindications for oral contraceptive use listed by the United States Food and Drug Administration is cancer of the breast or endometrium, although no data indicate that oral contraceptives are harmful in women with these diseases. In addition, patients who are pregnant should not ingest oral contraceptives because of the masculinizing effect of the gestagens on the external genitalia of the female fetus.

Concerns that ingestion of oral contraceptives during pregnancy produces other deleterious effects on the fetus such as limb reduction defects and heart defects have not been proven by epidemiologic studies. These concerns were raised by articles linking ingestion of all progestational agents in pregnancy to an increased incidence of congenital abnormalities and were flawed by probable recall bias. As shown by Wilson and Brent the major use of gestagens in pregnancy was for women having a threatened abortion. Bleeding in pregnancy by itself is associated with an increased number of anomalies. In addition, the incidence of anomalies has not decreased since gestagens are no longer being used for treatment of threatened abortion. There is therefore no conclusive evidence showing that oral contraceptive usage per se in pregnancy increases the incidence of any anomalies other than masculinization of the female external genitalia. This effect will not occur before 8 weeks of gestation.

Patients with heart disease should not use oral contraceptives, since the fluid retention produced by these agents could produce congestive heart failure. Nor should patients with active liver disease use oral contraceptives, since steroids are metabolized in this organ. However, patients who have had liver disease (e.g., viral hepatitis) in the past but whose liver function tests have returned to normal can receive these agents.

Relative contraindications to oral contraceptive use include heavy cigarette smoking under the age of 35, migraine headaches, amenorrhea, and depression. Migraine headaches can be made worse by oral contraceptive use, and patients who develop a stroke while taking oral contraceptives frequently have an increased incidence of headaches of the migraine type, fainting, loss of vision or speech, or paresthesias before development of the cardiovascular accident. If any of these symptoms develop in oral contraceptive users, the patient should stop ingesting these agents. Patients who are amenorrheic for a cause other than polycystic ovarian syndrome should probably not receive oral contraceptives, because they may have a pituitary microadenoma. Oral contraceptive use will mask the symptoms of both amenorrhea and galactorrhea, which are the symptoms produced by enlargement of the adenoma. Thus patients with amenorrhea should not receive oral contraceptives until the diagnosis for this symptom is established.

Anyone who develops galactorrhea while taking oral contraceptives should discontinue these agents, and after 2 weeks, a serum prolactin level should be measured. If the prolactin level is elevated, further diagnostic evaluation, such as x-ray examination of the sella turcica, is indicated. A recent NIH study reported by the Pituitary Adenoma Study Group confirmed findings of other studies that showed that oral contraceptives do not produce prolactin secretory pituitary adenomas, because the incidence of these tumors was the same in oral contraceptive users and controls.

Beginning Oral Contraceptives

Adolescents

In deciding whether the pubertal, sexually active girl should use oral contraceptives for contraception, the clinician should be more concerned about compliance than possible physiologic harm. Provided the postmenarcheal girl has demonstrated maturity of the hypothalamic-pituitary-ovarian axis by having at least three regular, presumably ovulatory, cycles, it is safe to prescribe oral contraceptives without being concerned about causing permanent damage to the reproductive process. It is probably best not to prescribe oral contraceptives for women of any age with oligomenorrhea, except those with polycystic ovarian syndrome, because of the increased likelihood of their developing postpill amenorrhea, and oligomenorrhea is more frequent in adolescence than later in life. One need not be concerned about accelerating epiphyseal closure in postmenarcheal females. Their endogenous estrogens have already initiated the process a few years before menarche, and the contraceptive steroids will not hasten it.

Following Pregnancy

There is a difference in the relationship of the return of ovulation and bleeding in the postabortal woman and one who has had a term delivery. The first episode of menstrual bleeding in the postabortal woman is usually preceded by ovulation. Following a term delivery, the first episode of bleeding is usually, but not always, anovulatory. Ovulation occurs sooner after an abortion, usually between 2 and 4 weeks, than after a term delivery, when ovulation is usually delayed beyond 6 weeks but may occur as early as 4 weeks in a woman who is not breastfeeding.

Thus after spontaneous or induced abortion of a fetus of less than 12 weeks' gestation, oral contraceptives should be started immediately to prevent conception following the first ovulation. For patients who deliver after 28 weeks and are not nursing, the combination pills should be initiated 2 to 3 weeks after delivery. If the termination of pregnancy occurs between 21 and 28 weeks, contraceptive steroids should be started 1 week later. The reason for delay in the latter instances is that the normally increased risk of thromboembolism occurring postpartum may be further enhanced by the hypercoagulable state associated with contraceptive steroid ingestion. Because the first ovulation is delayed for at least 4 weeks after a term delivery, there is no need to expose the patient to this increased risk.

It is probably best for women who are nursing not to use combination oral contraceptives, as their use has been shown to diminish the amount of milk produced, as estrogen inhibits prolactin's action on the breast. Women who are breastfeeding every 4 hours, including at nighttime, will not ovulate until at least 10 weeks after delivery and thus do not need contraception before that time. Once supplemental feeding is introduced, ovulation can resume promptly. Since only a small percentage of full breastfeeding women will ovulate as long as they continue full nursing and remain amenorrheic, either a barrier method or gestagen-only oral contraceptive can be used. The latter does not diminish the amount of breast milk and is effective in this group of women.

All Patients

At the initial visit, after a history and physical examination have determined that there are no medical contraindications for oral contraceptives, the patient should be informed about the benefits and risks. For medicolegal reasons it is best to use a written informed consent signed by the patient as well as noting on the patient's medical record that the benefits and risk have been explained to her.

Type of Formulation

In determining which formulation to use, it is best to initially prescribe a formulation with 30 or 35 µg of ethinyl estradiol. A study from Great Britain by Meade et al. reported that the rates of total deaths as well as deaths from ar-

TABLE 11-10

Ratio of Observed/Expected Events by Estrogen Dose (United Kingdom, 1974-1977)

	Ethinyl Estradiol	
	50 µg	30 µg
Venous deaths	1.40	0.65
Nonvenous deaths	1.52	0.53*
Ischemic heart disease	1.48	0.54*
Stroke	1.20	0.80
Pregnancy	0.62	1.33*

Adapted from Meade TW, Greenberg G, Thompson SG: Progestogens and cardiovascular reactions associated with oral contraceptives and a comparison of the safety of 50- and 30-µg estrogen preparations. Br Med J 1:1157, 1980. *Significant difference.

terial causes alone were significantly lower in patients using formulations with 30 µg of ethinyl estradiol than in those using formulations of 50 µg of ethinyl estradiol (Table 11-10). Furthermore, the rates of ischemic heart disease and stroke were also significantly decreased in women using the lower dose estrogen formulations. As stated earlier, the increase in amounts of serum globulins, including angiotensinogen as well as those involved with coagulation, is related to the dose of estrogen administered. Thus, it would appear reasonable that lower doses of estrogen formulations should not cause as great or frequent an increase in blood pressure or venous thrombosis. There is some indication from the Royal College Study that the incidence of total arterial disease in oral contraceptive users is related to the dose of gestagen when the estrogen dosage is unchanged. For this reason, it would appear reasonable to use formulations with the lowest dosage of a particular gestagen. The development of multiphasic formulations has allowed the total dose of gestagen to be reduced compared with the monophasic formulations without increasing the incidence of breakthrough bleeding.

The FDA has stated that the product prescribed should be one that contains the least amount of estrogen and progestin that is compatible with a low failure rate and the needs of the individual patient. Because few randomized studies have been performed comparing the different marketed formulations, until large-scale comparative studies are performed, the clinician must decide which formulation to use based on which formulations have the least adverse effects among patients in his or her practice. Unless acne is present there is no evidence that some patients do better with formulations that are more estrogenic while other patients do better with formulations that are more gestagenic.

The contraceptive formulations containing gestagens without estrogen have a lower incidence of adverse metabolic effects. Since the factors that predispose to thromboembolism are caused by the estrogen component, the incidence of thromboembolism in women ingesting these compounds is probably not increased. Furthermore, blood pressure is not affected, nausea and breast tenderness are eliminated, and milk production and quality are unchanged. Despite these advantages, these agents have the disadvantages of a high frequency of intermenstrual and other abnormal bleeding patterns, including amenorrhea, and a lower rate of effectiveness. The actual use failure rate of these preparations has been reported to vary between 2% and 8% per year, and a relatively high percentage of these pregnancies are ectopic. Since nursing mothers have reduced fertility and are amenorrheic, the major disadvantages of these preparations are minimized for these patients. Furthermore, since milk production and quality are unaffected in contrast to the changes produced by combination pills, the formulations with gestagens alone may be offered to these women while they are nursing. However, a small portion of these synthetic steroids have been detected in breast milk. The long-term effects (if any) of these gestagens on the infant are not known, but none have been detected to date.

Follow-Up

If the patient has no contraindications to oral contraceptive use, the only routine laboratory tests indicated are a complex blood count, urinalysis, and Pap smear. At the end of 3 months, the patient should be seen again; at this time a nondirected history should be obtained and the blood pressure measured. After this visit the patient should be seen annually, at which time a nondirected history should

again be taken, blood pressure and body weight measured, and a physical examination (including breast, abdominal, and pelvic examination with Pap smear) performed. It is important to perform annual Pap smears on oral contraceptive users, as they are a relatively high risk group for development of cervical neoplasia. The routine use of other laboratory tests is not indicated unless the patient is over 35 years or has a family history of diabetes or vascular disease. For patients over 35 who wish to continue taking oral contraceptives, it is advisable to obtain a lipid panel, including HDL- and LDL-cholesterol, total cholesterol, and triglycerides. If the lipid levels are abnormal, another method of contraception may be safer. In addition, because of the increased incidence of diabetes after age 35, a 2-hour postprandial blood glucose level should be obtained; if this is elevated, a full glucose tolerance test should be performed. If results of this test are abnormal, the oral contraceptives should probably be stopped. Routine use of these tests in women under 35 is not indicated because the incidence of positive results is extremely low. However, if the patient has a family history of vascular disease, such as myocardial infarction occurring in family members under the age of 50, it would be advisable to obtain a lipid panel before and after oral contraceptive use is started; if the patient has a family history of diabetes or evidence of diabetes during pregnancy, a 2-hour postprandial blood glucose test should be performed before and after oral contraceptives are started. If the patient has a past history of liver disease, a liver panel should be obtained to make certain that liver function is normal before oral contraceptives are started.

Drug Interactions

Although synthetic sex steroids can retard the biotransformation of certain drugs (e.g., phenazone and meperidine) as a result of substrate competition, such interference is not important clinically. Oral contraceptive use has not been shown to inhibit the action of other drugs. However, some drugs can clinically interfere with the action of oral contraceptives by inducing liver enzymes that convert the steroids to more polar and less biologically active metabolites. Certain drugs have been shown to accelerate the biotransformation of steroids in the human. These include barbiturates, sulfonamides, cyclophosphamide, and rifampicin. Several investigators have reported a relatively high incidence of oral contraceptive failure in women ingesting rifampicin, and these two agents should not be given concurrently. The clinical data concerning oral contraceptive failure in users of other antibiotics (e.g., penicillin, ampicillin, and sulfonamides), analgesics (e.g., phenytoin), and barbiturates are less clear. A few anecdotal studies have appeared in the literature, but reliable evidence for a clinical inhibitory effect of these drugs, such as occurs with rifampicin, is not available. Until controlled studies are performed, it would appear prudent when both agents are given simultaneously to suggest use of a barrier method in addition to the oral contraceptives because of possible interference with oral contraceptive action by the action of the antibiotic or the gut flora. In addition, women with epilepsy requiring medication are best treated with 50 μg estrogen formulations because a higher incidence of abnormal bleeding has been reported in these women with the use of lower dose estrogen formulations.

Noncontraceptive Health Benefits

In addition to being the most effective method of contraception, oral contraceptives provide several other health benefits. Some are due to the fact that the combination oral contraceptives contain a potent, orally active gestagen as well as an orally active estrogen and there is no time when the estrogenic target tissues are stimulated by estrogens without a gestagen (unopposed estrogen).

Both natural progesterone and the synthetic gestagens inhibit the proliferative effect of estrogen, the so-called antiestrogenic effect. Estrogens increase the synthesis of both estrogen and progesterone receptors, while progesterone decreases their synthesis. Thus one mechanism whereby progesterone exerts its antiestrogenic effects is by decreasing the synthesis of estrogen receptors. Relatively little gestagen is needed to do this, and the amount present in oral contraceptives is sufficient. Another way progesterone produces its antiestrogenic action is by stimulating the activity of the enzyme, es-

tradiol-17-beta-dehydrogenase, within the endometrial cell. This enzyme converts the more potent estradiol to the less potent estrone, reducing estrogenic action within the cell.

Benefits from Antiestrogenic Action of Progestins

As a result of the antiestrogenic action of the progestins in oral contraceptives, the height of the endometrium is less than in an ovulatory cycle, and there is less proliferation of the glandular epithelium. These changes produce several substantial benefits for the oral contraceptive user. One is a reduction in the amount of blood loss at the time of endometrial shedding. In an ovulatory cycle the mean blood loss during menstruation is about 35 ml, compared with 20 ml for women ingesting oral contraceptives. This decreased blood loss makes the development of iron deficiency anemia less likely. Data from the RCGP study showed that oral contraceptive users were about half as likely to develop iron deficiency anemia as were the controls. Moreover, the beneficial effect persisted to a similar degree in women who had previously used oral contraceptives and then stopped them, probably because of an increase in the iron stores that remained for several years after the drug was discontinued.

Since the oral contraceptives produce regular withdrawal bleeding, it would be expected that oral contraceptive users would have fewer menstrual disorders than controls. The results of the RCGP study confirmed the fact that oral contraceptive users were significantly less likely to develop menorrhagia, irregular menstruation, or intermenstrual bleeding. Since these disorders are frequently treated by curettage, oral contraceptive users require this procedure less frequently.

Because gestagens inhibit the proliferative effect of estrogens on the endometrium, it is not surprising that women who use oral contraceptives have been found to be significantly less likely to develop adenocarcinoma of the endometrium. Data from several retrospective case comparison studies, including the CASH study, indicate that the relative risk of developing endometrial cancer among combination oral contraceptive users was only half that among controls. The protective effect increased the longer these agents were used, and the reduced risk of endometrial cancer persisted for at least 5 years after treatment was discontinued.

Estrogen exerts a proliferative effect on breast tissue, which also contains estrogen receptors. Gestagens probably inhibit the synthesis of estrogen receptors in this organ as well, exerting an antiestrogenic action on the breast. Several studies have shown that oral contraceptives reduce the incidence of benign breast disease, and two prospective studies have indicated that this reduction is directly related to the amount of gestagen in the compounds.

Data from the Oxford Study indicate that current users of oral contraceptives have an 85% reduction in the incidence of fibroadenomas and 50% reductions in chronic cystic disease and nonbiopsied breast lumps, as compared with controls using IUDs or diaphragms. The risk of developing these three diseases decreased with increased duration of oral contraceptive use and persisted for about 1 year following discontinuation of oral contraceptives, after which no reduction in risk was observed.

Benefits from Inhibition of Ovulation

Other noncontraceptive medical benefits of oral contraceptives result from their main action, inhibition of ovulation. Some disorders, such as dysmenorrhea and premenstrual tension, occur much more frequently in ovulatory than anovulatory cycles. In fact, inhibition of ovulation by exogenous steroids has been used as therapy for severe dysmenorrhea for decades. The 1974 report of the RCGP study showed that oral contraceptive users had 63% less dysmenorrhea and 29% less premenstrual tension than controls.

Another serious adverse effect of ovulatory menstrual cycles is the development of functional ovarian cysts—specifically, follicular and luteal cysts—that frequently require laparotomy because of enlargement, rupture, or hemorrhage. When ovulation is inhibited, functional cysts do not usually develop. In a survey performed by the Boston Collaborative Drug Surveillance Program, less than 2% of women with a discharge diagnosis of functional ovarian cysts were taking oral contraceptives, in contrast to 20% of controls. However, 20% of women with nonfunctional cysts were taking oral contraceptives, an incidence similar to that observed in the controls.

Another disorder linked to incessant ovulation is ovarian cancer. Several case control studies have shown that the risk of developing ovarian cancer decreases as the number of pregnancies increases, and it has been reported that the incidence of ovarian cancer correlated inversely with the number of children born. The trauma to the ovarian surface epithelium produced by incessant ovulation may in some way contribute to the development of ovarian cancer. Casagrande et al. reported data from a case control study that indicated that the relative risk of ovarian cancer decreased as the numbers of live births and incomplete pregnancies as well as oral contraceptive use increased. When the anovulatory years from all three factors were added, the decreased relative risk was statistically significant. These investigators found that the protective effect of oral contraceptives was about the same as pregnancy with 12 months of oral contraceptive use, protecting to about the same degree as one live birth. Several recent case control studies, including the CASH study, reported that oral contraceptive users had only about one-half the risk of developing ovarian cancer, and this protection persisted for at least 10 years after the oral contraceptive was stopped.

Other Benefits

The RCGP study showed that the risk of developing rheumatoid arthritis in oral contraceptive users was only about half that in controls. Another benefit is protection against salpingitis, commonly referred to as pelvic inflammatory disease (PID). There have been at least 11 published epidemiologic studies estimating the relative risk of developing PID among oral contraceptive users. Seven of these studies compared oral contraceptive use to nonuse of any other contraception. The relative risk of developing PID among oral contraceptive users in most of these studies was about 0.5%. It has been estimated that between 15% and 20% of women with cervical gonorrheal infection will develop salpingitis. In a study from Sweden by Ryden et al., all cases of suspected salpingitis were confirmed by laparoscopic visualization 1

TABLE 11-11

Rate and Estimated Number of Hospitalizations Prevented Annually by Use of Oral Contraceptives (United States)*

Disease	Rate/100,000 Users	Estimated Number
Benign breast disease	235	20,000
Ovarian retention cysts	35	3,000
Iron deficiency anemia†	320	27,200
Pelvic inflammatory disease (first episodes)		
Total episodes†	600	51,000
Hospitalizations	156	13,300
Ectopic pregnancy	117	9,900
Rheumatoid arthritis†	32	2,700
Endometrial cancer‡	5	2,000
Ovarian cancer‡	4	1,700

From Ory HW: The noncontraceptive health benefits from oral contraceptive use. Reprinted with permission from *Family Planning Perspectives*, 14:182, 1982.

*Except where noted, figures refer to hospitalizations prevented among the estimated 8.5 million current users of oral contraceptives.

†Episodes prevented regardless of whether hospitalizations occurred.

‡Based on an estimated 39 million U.S. women who have ever used oral contraceptives.

day after hospital admission. Of those who used contraception other than the IUD and oral steroids, 15% developed salpingitis; only about half as many, 8.8%, of those who used oral contraceptives developed salpingitis. The results of this study indicate that oral contraceptives reduce the clinical development of salpingitis in women infected with gonorrhea. Although the incidence of cervical infection with *Chlamydia trachomatis* is increased in oral contraceptive users compared with controls, Wølner-Hanssen et al. reported that the incidence of chlamydial salpingitis in oral contraceptive users was only half that of controls. This protection may be related to the decreased duration of menstrual flow, which permits a smaller number of gonococcal organisms to ascend to the upper genital tract and allows the body's defenses to eliminate them more easily. One sequela of PID is ectopic pregnancy, an entity that has tripled in incidence in the last decade. Oral contraceptives reduce the risk of ectopic pregnancy by more than 90% in current users and may reduce the incidence in former users by decreasing their chance of developing salpingitis.

Ory has estimated that of 100,000 women in the United States using oral contraceptives each year, this use will prevent 320 from developing iron deficiency anemia, 32 from developing rheumatoid arthritis, and 450 from developing PID that does not require hospitalization. In addition, there will be 150 fewer women hospitalized for PID, 235 fewer hospitalized for breast disease, 35 fewer hospitalized for ovarian tumors, and 117 fewer hospitalized for tubal pregnancies (Table 11-11). Ory estimated that each year about 1 out of every 750 women taking oral contraceptives will not require hospitalization for a serious disease she would have developed if she had not taken this drug. He estimated that use of oral contraceptives prevents 50,000 women from being hospitalized in the United States each year. It is unfortunate that the infrequent adverse effects of oral contraceptives have received widespread publicity, while the more common noncontraceptive health benefits have attracted little attention.

INJECTABLE STEROIDS

Four injectable steroid contraceptive formulations have undergone extensive clinical trials. Depomedroxyprogesterone acetate (DMPA), a microcrystalline suspension of the gestagen, administered in a dosage of 150 mg every 3 months, is marketed in many countries, including Sweden and the United Kingdom, but it has not been approved for use as a contraceptive in the United States. Studies have also been undertaken with 300 mg of DMPA administered every 6 months; norethindrone enanthate (NET-EN), 200 mg every 2 months and every 12 weeks; combinations of dihydroxyprogesterone acetofenide and estradiol enanthate; and medroxyprogesterone acetate (MPA) and estradiol cypionate, administered monthly. NET-EN is formulated in an oily suspension, and its duration of action is shorter than that of DMPA. It is marketed as a contraceptive in some European countries.

Effectiveness

DMPA is given by deep gluteal intramuscular injection without manual massage in a dosage of 150 mg every 3 months. More than 500 scientific articles have been written about DMPA since it was made available for use as a contraceptive 25 years ago. More than 11 million women have used DMPA, and currently there are more than 2 million users in the world. It is an effective method of contraception. Pregnancy rates from individual clinics with substantial numbers of patients vary from 0.0 to 0.5 per 100 woman-years. Because the contraceptive action of 150 mg of DMPA usually lasts longer than 3 months, patients who delay receiving their next scheduled injection for a few weeks are still protected against accidental pregnancy. This enhances the effectiveness of this preparation.

NET-EN in a dosage of 200 mg every 12 weeks is slightly less effective than DMPA. Because most pregnancies occurred in the last 4 weeks of the first injection interval, NET-EN is now being administered every 2 months for the first 6 months and every 3 months thereafter, or every 2 months for the duration of usage. With this method of administration the pregnancy rate with NET-EN was less than 1% at the end of 1 year and approached the 0.1% failure rate of DMPA, according to a 1983 WHO randomized study (Table 11-12).

Mechanism of Action

The large dose of gestagens alone is effective because of the multiple mechanisms of action, similar to those of the combination oral steroids. They inhibit secretion of gonadotrophins, including the midcycle release of LH, and thus prevent ovulation. DMPA and the combination oral steroids are the only steroid contraceptive formulations developed to date that consistently inhibit ovulation, a quality that appears to be essential for optimal effectiveness of steroid contraceptives. Estradiol levels measured daily during treatment with DMPA show only slight fluctuation and usually approximate those found in the early follicular phase of the normal menstrual cycle, which are significantly higher than the levels in postmenopausal women. Uterine size is slightly decreased in patients who receive the drug for several years, but there are no other signs or

TABLE 11-12

Net Termination Rates per 100 Women in WHO Study of DMPA and NET-EN

Reason for Termination	1-Year Net Cumulative Event Rates			2-Year Net Cumulative Event Rates		
	DMPA	NET-EN 60	NET-EN 60-84	DMPA	NET-EN 60	NET-EN 60-84
Pregnancy	0.1	0.4	0.6	0.4	0.4	1.4
Amenorrhea	11.9	6.8	8.4	24.2	14.7	14.6
Bleeding	15.0	13.6	13.7	18.8	18.4	21.8
Medical	11.8	13.7	12.7	15.0	16.0	16.7
Personal	20.7	24.5	22.8	38.8	42.6	40.2
TOTAL	51.4	49.7	50.3	73.5	70.7	72.4

From World Health Organization Expanded Programme of Research, Development and Research Training in Human Reproduction Task Force on Long-Acting System Agents for the Regulation of Fertility. Contraception 28:1, 1983. *DMPA*, Depomedroxyprogesterone acetate; *NET-EN*, norethindrone enanthate.

symptoms of deestrogenization. There is no subjective decrease in breast size, and vaginas remain moist and well rugated.

The delay in resumption of ovulation after DMPA administration is due to the slow release from the injection site and the prolonged presence of effective MPA levels in the serum. In clinical studies, resumption of ovulation and fertility occurs in most women within 1 year after treatment is discontinued. Because of the unpredictable length of this delay in resumption of ovulation in the individual patient, this method of contraception is usually restricted to women whose childbearing is completed.

Metabolic Effects

In contrast to the metabolic effects noted with combination estrogen-gestagen oral contraceptives, no changes in liver function, lipid metabolism, or blood pressure have been noted during DMPA treatment. There is some evidence, however, that DMPA at a dosage of 150 mg every 3 months (but not NET-EN) may cause a clinically insignificant deterioration of glucose tolerance and an increase in plasma insulin levels. Also, there is some evidence that DMPA has a clinically insignificant glucocorticoid effect at this dose. Nearly all clinical studies with DMPA indicate that an increase in body weight occurs during therapy, according to the duration of use. In the WHO comparative study, the average weight gain after 1 year of DMPA was 2 kg; with NET-EN, it was 1.5 kg.

Beagle dogs treated with high doses of DMPA have an increased incidence of mammary cancer. Similar tumors in dogs have also been noted following administration of high doses of other related C-21 gestagens, but not with the 19-nortestosterone gestagens such as NET-EN. Studies with DMPA in monkeys, as well as in humans, have shown no increased incidence of mammary carcinoma, although two monkeys treated with DMPA for more than 10 years developed endometrial cancer. The relevance of the carcinogenic effect of DMPA in the beagle to the development of breast cancer in humans is not known. Because of these findings, the FDA has not approved the use of DMPA as a contraceptive, despite its availability in the United States for treatment of other disorders. NET-EN is not available for any use in the United States.

Bleeding Pattern

Patients who receive DMPA have complete disruption of the normal menstrual cycle and a totally irregular bleeding pattern. During the 3 months after the first injection of DMPA, most patients bleed from 8 to 30 days of each 30-day

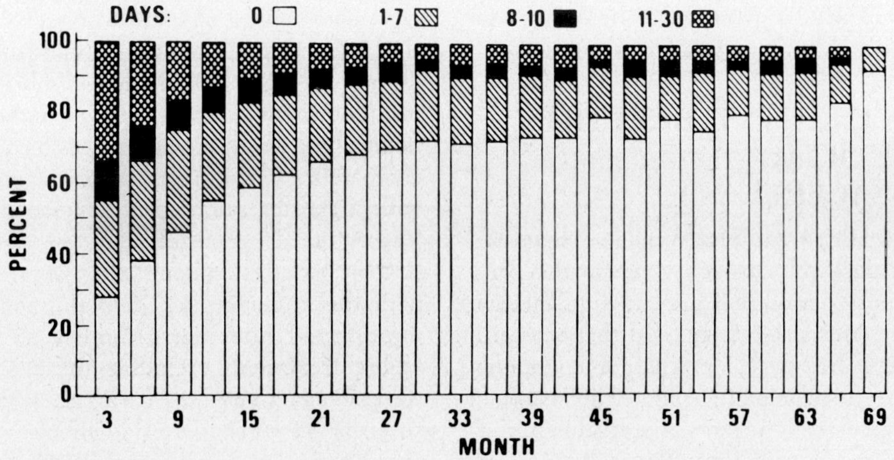

FIGURE 11-5
Percent of patients with bleeding or spotting on days 0, 1 to 7, 8 to 10, or 11 to 30 per 30-day cycle while receiving injectable DMPA, 150 mg, every 3 months. (From Schwallie PC, Assenzo JR: Fertil Steril 24:331, 1973. Reproduced with permission of the publisher, The American Fertility Society.)

period. Thereafter the incidence of amenorrhea gradually increases in direct proportion to the amount of time the patient has received the drug, while the incidence of increased bleeding steadily diminishes (Fig. 11-5). In the WHO comparative study, bleeding with DMPA tended to be somewhat more irregular than that with NET-EN. DMPA was associated with more frequent days of spotting and fewer normal cycles. Nevertheless the 1-year rates of discontinuation for bleeding problems for both drugs were similar, 10.0 in 100 women for DMPA and 12.0 in 100 women for NET-EN. When bleeding does occur, it is usually not excessive and is frequently characterized as spotting. Periodic bleeding can be regulated by the cyclic administration of oral estrogen, and some researchers have advocated that it be used in conjunction with DMPA for this purpose.

Amenorrhea is more common among DMPA users than NET-EN users, yet at the end of 1 and 2 years, continuation rates with both drugs are similar. After discontinuing DMPA treatment, about 50% of the patients resume a regular cyclic menstrual pattern within 6 months; about 75% have regular menses within 1 year. When bleeding does resume after the effect of the last injection is dissipated, it is initially regular in about half the patients. In one study, some of the women with irregular bleeding after discontinuation of therapy had to be treated with hormonal steroids for a short period. Resumption of regular menses may be delayed for more than 1 year in about 25% of women.

PREGNANCY INTERCEPTION (POSTCOITAL CONTRACEPTION)

In 1966 Morris and van Waganen suggested that high doses of estrogen given in the early postovulatory period will prevent implantation in women. Morris has suggested that the term *interception* be used for what is commonly called the "morning-after pill." The estrogen compounds used by various investigators for interception include diethylstilbestrol, 25 to 50 mg/day; diethylstilbestrol diphosphate, 50 μg/day; ethinyl estradiol, 1 to 5 mg/day; and conjugated estrogens, 20 to 30 mg/day. Treatment is continued for 5 days, and if it is begun within 72 hours after an isolated midcycle act of coitus, it is effective. If more than one episode of coitus has occurred or if treatment is initiated more than 72 hours after coitus, effectiveness is markedly reduced. Morris and van Waganen reported that 29 pregnancies occurred in 9000 patients with midcycle exposures treated with estrogen—that is, a pregnancy rate of approximately 0.3%. Only 3 of the pregnancies appeared to be due to method failure, a Pearl index of 0.4 per 100 woman-years. Of the 29 pregnancies, 3 were ectopic, an incidence of approximately 10%. Garcia et al. reported a failure rate of 0.7% in 4595 treatment cycles.

Side effects associated with this therapy are, as expected, nausea and vomiting, breast soreness, and menstrual irregularities. The United States Centers for Disease Control performed a five-center study comparing use of ethinyl estradiol (5 mg per day) for 5 days with conjugated equine estrogen (30 mg per day). Treatment with ethinyl estradiol resulted in a slightly lower pregnancy rate (0.7%) as compared with conjugated equine estrogen (1.6%). However, patients treated with ethinyl estradiol also had greater incidences of nausea and vomiting, indicating the potency of this dose of estrogen may have been greater. If treatment was begun 2 days after coitus, the pregnancy rate was 1.7 times greater than if it was begun the day after coitus. Thus it is best to start treatment within 24 hours of coitus.

Because the side effects of high-dose estrogen cause failure of some women to complete the 5-day course, a regimen of two tablets of ethinyl estradiol 0.05 mg and *dl*-norgestrel 0.5 mg (Ovral) given twice with an interval of 12 hours has been advocated. Effectiveness is comparable to the high-dose estrogen regimen with a shorter duration of adverse symptoms. Yuzpe et al. reported that 11 pregnancies (1.6%) occurred among 692 women treated with this regimen, but 4 of the subjects had unprotected intercourse more than 72 hours before treatment; excluding those 4 subjects, the pregnancy rate was 1.0%. About half of the subjects (42.4%) had no side effects, while nausea or vomiting occurred in 51.7%. Other side effects such as mastalgia and menorrhagia were infrequent, occurring in less than 1% of the women. Thus the effectiveness of this method is similar to that of higher dosages of estrogen alone and results in a lower incidence of abnormal and delayed menses. Side effects appear to be less and, because of the 1-day treatment regimen, patient compliance should be greater. If the patient has a continuing need for contraception, after the cycle in which interception is used, she should be advised to use one of the conventional contraceptive methods.

INTRAUTERINE DEVICES

The main benefits of IUDs are (1) a high level of effectiveness, (2) a lack of associated systemic metabolic effects, and (3) a single act of motivation required for long-term use. In contrast to other types of contraception, there is no need to ingest a pill daily or to regularly use a coitus-related method. These characteristics, as well as the fact that a visit to a health care facility is required for discontinuing the method, account for the fact that IUDs have the highest continuation rate of all currently available reversible methods of contraception. Of course it is desirable for all women to have annual pelvic examinations, but in some areas of the world this is not possible.

Unlike barrier techniques that rely on use by the acceptor and have higher use failure rates than method failure rates, the method effectiveness and use effectiveness rates for IUDs are similar. First-year failure rates are generally reported to range from 2% to 3%; however, following IUD insertion by experienced clinicians the pregnancy rates are lower. Pregnancy rates are related to the skill of the inserting clinician. With experience, correct high fundal insertion occurs more frequently, and there is a lower incidence of partial or complete expulsion with resultant lower pregnancy rates. Furthermore, the annual incidence of accidental pregnancy decreases steadily after the first year of IUD use. After 6 years of use of the loop and 5 years of the copper-bearing IUD, the cumulative failure rate is 5% to 6%, about 1% per year.

The incidence of all major adverse events with IUDs, including pregnancy as well as expulsion or removal for bleeding or pain, steadily decreases with increasing age, and women over 35 have pregnancy rates less than 2% in the first 2 years of use of the loop (Table 11-13). Thus the IUD is especially suited for older parous women who wish to prevent further pregnancies.

Mechanism of Action

It is generally accepted that the mechanism of contraceptive action of the IUD is via production of a local sterile inflammatory reaction caused by the presence of the foreign body in the uterus. Nearly a 1000% increase in the number of leukocytes is present in uterine washings of the human endometrial cavity 18 weeks after the insertion of an IUD, as compared with washings obtained before insertion. Tissue breakdown products of these leukocytes are toxic to all cells, including the sperm and blastocyst. Small IUDs do not produce as great an inflammatory reaction as larger devices do. Therefore smaller IUDs have higher pregnancy

TABLE 11-13
Two-Year Net Cumulative Event Rates with the Loop IUD per 100 Women

	Age at Insertion (Years)			
	15-24	**25-29**	**30-34**	**35-49**
Pregnancies	5.8	4.7	2.8	1.5
Expulsions	17.4	9.8	7.1	5.4
Removals for bleeding or pain	18.0	17.7	16.8	16.2
Continuation rate	58.0	66.7	72.0	75.4
First insertions	2,753	2,082	1,397	1,187
Woman-months of use	41,758	34,574	23,874	19,912

From Tietze C, Lewit S: Evaluation of intrauterine devices: Ninth progress report of the Cooperative Statistical Program. Stud Fam Plann 1:55, 1970.

TABLE 11-14

Fertility Rates (mean % ±SE) of Parous Women Remaining Undelivered of Live Birth or Stillbirth at Given Intervals After Stopping Contraception to Plan Pregnancy

Method of Contraception Stopped	Mean Age (Years)	% Women Remaining Undelivered by Months Since Discontinuation					
		12	18	24	30	36	42
IUD	31.4	48.8 ± 2.4	18.1 ± 1.9	10.6 ± 1.6	9.3 ± 1.5	6.7 ± 1.4	6.3 ± 1.4
Oral contraceptive	30.6	60.7 ± 1.2	20.4 ± 1.0	10.8 ± 0.8	7.6 ± 0.7	5.4 ± 0.6	4.5 ± 0.6
Diaphragm	30.9	36.8 ± 1.5	13.8 ± 1.1	8.2 ± 0.9	6.2 ± 0.9	4.6 ± 0.8	4.2 ± 0.8
Other method	31.8	39.4 ± 1.5	16.2 ± 1.3	10.6 ± 1.1	7.8 ± 1.0	6.2 ± 0.9	5.0 ± 0.9
IUD users in past, stopped for medical reasons	32.7	49.3 ± 4.7	19.1 ± 4.1	13.6 ± 3.8			

From Vessey MP, Lawless M, McPherson K, Yeates D: Fertility after stopping use of intrauterine contraceptive device. Br Med J 286:106, 1983.

rates than larger devices of the same design. The addition of copper also increases the inflammatory reaction.

IUDs mainly act as a spermicide. Tredway et al. reported that the short phase of sperm transport from the cervix to the oviduct is markedly impaired in women wearing an IUD. Thus very few (if any) sperm reach the oviducts, and the ovum usually does not become fertilized. Further evidence for this action of IUDs on sperm transport was found by a group of Chilean investigators. They performed oviductal flushings in 54 women with and without IUDs who were sterilized by salpingectomy soon after ovulation and also had unprotected sexual intercourse shortly before ovulation. They found that in about half of the women not wearing an IUD, normally cleaving ova were found in the tubal flushings, whereas no normally cleaving ova were found in the oviducts of the women wearing IUDs. If fertilization does occur, copper ions, as well as the locally released prostaglandins, probably alter the normal process of implantation, increasing contraceptive effectiveness. Upon removal of both copper-bearing and non-copper-bearing IUDs the inflammatory reaction rapidly disappears and resumption of fertility occurs at the same rate following discontinuation of use of barrier methods of contraception.

Vessey et al. reported that pregnancy rates of women who discontinued using an IUD were similar to those of women discontinuing barrier methods at 1 and 2 years. However, women discontinuing IUDs for medical problems, including infection, had a slightly lower pregnancy rate at 2 years (Table 11-14).

Types of IUDs

In the past 15 years, numerous models of IUDs have been designed and used clinically. Many of these devices are available for use in Europe, Canada, and other countries. In the United States four types of IUDs, all of which have a monofilament tail, are approved for use by the FDA (Fig. 11-6). The FDA-approved types of IUDs are the copper-bearing copper 7, the copper T 200B, the copper T 380A and the progesterone-releasing T-shaped device. Only the last device is currently being marketed in the United States. The others are not being sold because of corporate decisions regarding their profitability.

There is no need to ever change the non-copper-bearing plastic IUDs unless the patient develops increased bleeding after the IUD has been in place for more than 1 year. Calcium salts are deposited on the plastic in time, and their roughness can cause ulceration and bleeding of the endometrium. If increased bleeding develops after a non-copper-bearing plastic IUD has been in the uterus for 1 year or more, the old IUD should be removed and a new one inserted.

Because of the constant dissolution of cop-

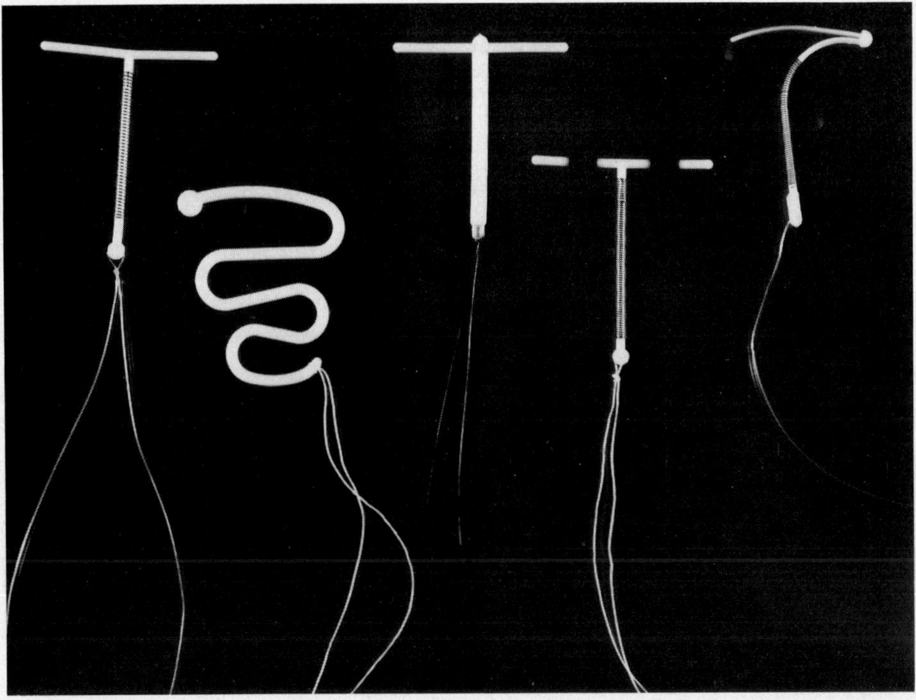

FIGURE 11-6
IUDs currently approved for use in the United States: copper T 200, loop, progesterone-releasing IUD, copper T 380 A, and copper 7.

per, of which the daily amount is less than that ingested in the normal diet, the copper IUDs must be replaced at periodic intervals. The necessary interval was originally estimated to be 2 to 3 years but is now believed to be 4 to 5 years. Five published studies have indicated that the annual pregnancy rates with the copper 7 and copper T 200 IUDs do not increase in the fourth and fifth years after insertion; the World Health Organization stated in 1982 that the copper 7 is safe and effective for at least 4 years of use; and the copper T 200B is now approved for use in the United States for 4 years. At the time of scheduled removal one device can be removed and a new one inserted at the same visit.

Adding a reservoir of progesterone to the vertical arm also increases the effectiveness of the T device. The presently marketed progesterone IUD releases 65 μg of progesterone daily. This amount is sufficient to prevent pregnancy by local action in the endometrial cavity but is not enough to cause a measurable increase in peripheral serum progesterone levels.

The currently approved model of the progesterone-releasing IUD must be replaced annually, because the reservoir of progesterone becomes depleted after about 18 months of use.

Time of Insertion

Although it is widely believed that the optimal time for insertion of an IUD is during the menses, there are data indicating that if a woman is not pregnant, the IUD can be safely inserted on any day of the cycle. White et al. analyzed 2-month event rates of about 10,000 women who had a copper T 200 inserted on various days of the cycle. Rates of expulsion were lowest with devices inserted the week after menses stopped, while rates of removal for bleeding and pain as well as pregnancy were higher with insertions performed after cycle day 18. However, the differences were small and of little clinical relevance. It has also been recommended that IUDs not be inserted until more than 2 or 3 months have elapsed following a pregnancy. However, event rates of copper IUDs inserted between 4 and 8 weeks postpartum and more than 8 weeks postpartum are similar, indicating that copper IUDs can be safely inserted at the time of the routine postpartum visit. A withdrawal technique of insertion should be used to avoid perforation, as in one study the perforation rate has been reported to be higher if the IUD is inserted when a woman is lactating.

Adverse Effects

Incidence

In general, in the first year of use, IUDs have about a 2% pregnancy rate, a 10% expulsion rate, and a 15% rate of removal for medical reasons, mainly bleeding and pain. The incidence of each of these events, especially expulsions, diminishes steadily in subsequent years.

At the end of 6 years the continuation rate of the loop was 42.4% (Table 11-15). A total of 5.4% of the terminations during 6 years were due to pregnancy, a little less than 1% per year. Thus, although the pregnancy rate in the first year is greater with the IUD than with oral contraceptives, within the framework of longer periods, the use-pregnancy rate with the IUD is similar to that of the combination oral contraceptives. About one half of all women discontinuing use of the loop IUD after 6 years do so because of bleeding, pain, or other medical reasons or a combination of these factors.

The results of 5 years of experience with the copper T 200 showed a net pregnancy rate of 5.8% (about 1% per year), a discontinuation rate for expulsion of 7.2%, and a removal rate for bleeding and pain of 23.7%, similar to event rates with the loop (Table 11-16). Another copper T device—the copper T 380A, which has copper on both the horizontal and vertical arms and was recently approved for use in the United States—also has a low pregnancy rate. Sivin and Tatum reported that the net cumulative pregnancy rate with this device at the end of 4 years was only 1.9%. Thus the addition of copper on the horizontal arm appears to lower the pregnancy rate as well as increase the estimated duration of action to 8 years or more.

Type

UTERINE BLEEDING. Nearly all medical reasons accounting for IUD removal involve one or more types of abnormal bleeding: heavy or prolonged menses or intermenstrual bleeding. The IUD does not influence follicular maturation, the time or incidence of ovulation, or corpus luteum function; however, it does exert a local effect on the endometrium, causing the onset of menses to take place about 2 days earlier than the normal onset, when steroid levels are higher than in control cycles. It is possible that this early onset of menses may be produced by a premature and increased rate of release of prostaglandins, brought about by the

---

TABLE 11-15

Net Annual and Cumulative Rates of Closures per 100 Women Using the Loop in 6 Years of Use

| | | Expulsion | | | Removals | | | | |
| | | | | | | | | | |
Year	Pregnancy	Initial	Later	Bleeding and Pain	Medical	Planned Pregnancy	Personal	Total Closures	Active
First	2.4	2.9	1.9	10.4	2.5	0.6	1.9	22.6	77.4
Second	1.6	0.9	0.7	6.3	2.2	1.5	2.1	15.3	65.6
Third	1.0	0.5	0.6	6.4	1.3	1.9	1.9	13.6	56.6
Fourth	1.1	0.3	0.2	5.0	1.2	1.9	2.2	11.9	49.9
Fifth	0.4	0.1	0.0	2.2	2.1	2.2	1.6	8.6	45.4
Sixth	0.6	0.0	0.0	2.2	0.3	1.1	2.1	6.3	42.6
TOTAL	5.4	7.1		31.3		13.6		57.4	42.6

Adapted from Tietze C, Lewit S: Evaluation of intrauterine devices: Ninth progress report of the Cooperative Statistical Program. Stud Fam Plann 1:55, 1970.

TABLE 11-16

IUD Cumulative Net Rates per 100 Acceptors by Device and Year

	First Year		Second Year		Third Year		Fourth Year		Fifth Year	
	Nova-T	Copper T	Nova-T	Copper T	Nova-T	Copper T	Nova-T	Copper T	Nova-T	Copper T
Pregnancy	0.7	1.9	1.4	3.8	1.9	4.9	2.0	5.1	2.2	5.8
Expulsion	5.5	4.2	6.9	5.2	8.1	5.7	8.7	6.8	9.3	7.2
Removals										
Bleeding or pain	11.1	11.4	17.0	14.9	21.1	19.7	24.1	22.8	26.7	23.7
Infection	2.3	1.8	2.9	2.3	3.7	3.6	4.2	4.2	4.8	4.3
Other medical reasons	0.8	1.4	1.6	2.7	2.0	3.4	2.3	5.0	2.9	5.2
Planning pregnancy	2.5	1.9	6.1	5.3	10.5	8.7	12.9	10.8	14.5	12.3
Other personal reasons	1.0	0.5	2.2	1.1	4.7	2.9	5.1	4.8	6.4	5.5
Continuation	76.1	77.0	62.0	64.7	48.2	51.1	39.8	40.5	33.2	36.0

From Luukkainen T, Allonen II, Nielsen N-C, et al: Five years' experience of intrauterine contraception with Nova-T and the Copper-T-200. Am J Obstet Gynecol 147:885, 1983.

presence of the intrauterine foreign body. The stimulation of uterine contractions by excessive prostaglandin levels may prolong the duration of the menstrual flow, which is significantly longer in women wearing IUDs.

The amount of blood lost in each menstrual cycle is also significantly greater in women wearing inert as well as copper-bearing IUDs than in nonwearers. In a normal cycle, the mean amount of menstrual blood loss is about 35 ml. After insertion of a loop IUD, the mean loss increases to 70 to 80 ml. The increase is less with copper-bearing devices. With a copper 7 the mean menstrual blood loss has been found to vary from 50 to 55 ml, whereas with the copper T 200 the mean loss varies from 50 to 60 ml. In contrast, with the progesterone-releasing IUD the amount of blood loss is actually reduced to about 25 ml per cycle.

Some investigators report that the increase in menstrual blood loss with copper-bearing IUDs is greatest in the first cycle after IUD insertion, after which it declines steadily, whereas others report that the increase in blood loss is similar during each menses for 1 year after copper IUD insertion. Guillebaud has shown that after insertion of copper-bearing as well as inert IUDs, a greater percentage of women have menstrual blood loss in excess of 80 ml, which has been shown to produce severe iron deficiency. In this British study a group of women were inserted with either the loop or copper 7 IUD. One year after insertion of either device, there were significant decreases in mean hemoglobin levels as well as in the percentage of women with hemoglobin levels of less than 12 g/dl. As expected, because the mean blood loss increases and the percentage of women losing more than 80 ml was greater with the loop than with the copper 7, the decrease in mean hemoglobin level and incidence of anemia were less with the group inserted with the copper 7 than with the loop. In a study of Swedish women inserted with the copper 7 and copper T 200, there was no significant change in mean values of hemoglobin concentration, serum iron, and total iron-binding capacity determined 6 and 12 months after IUD insertion when compared with mean values measured before insertion. A sensitive noninvasive indicator for measuring tissue iron stores is measurement of serum ferritin. Several studies have shown that among women wearing either a copper-bearing or inert IUD there is a significant decrease in serum ferritin levels overall as well as an increase in percentage of women with extremely low ferritin levels (less than 16 μg/L), indicating an absence of iron in bone marrow. Low serum ferritin levels are a good predictor of development of anemia. Therefore it is best that both ferritin and hemoglobin be measured annually in all wearers of non-steroid-releasing IUDs. If either parameter decreases significantly, supplemental iron should be administered to the patient.

The exact mechanism whereby IUDs increase menstrual blood loss is not completely understood, despite extensive investigation. Histologic studies of endometrium obtained by biopsy and hysterectomy have demonstrated two types of lesions in association with IUDs. Vascular erosions have been seen in areas of direct contact with the IUD, and evidence of increased vascular permeability has been found in areas not in direct contact with the IUD. Both types of lesion could cause increased menstrual blood loss as well as intermenstrual bleeding. It has been shown that in the endometrial tissue adjacent to the device there is an increased concentration of proteolytic enzymes and plasminogenic activators, which may lead to increased fibrinolytic activity. This increase in fibrinolytic activity adversely affects hemostasis and increases menstrual blood loss.

Patients who experience excessive bleeding in the first few months after IUD insertion should be treated with reassurance and supplemental oral iron. The bleeding may diminish with time as the uterus adjusts to the presence of the foreign body. Patients with excessive bleeding that continues or develops several months or more after IUD insertion may be treated by systemic administration of one of the prostaglandin synthetase inhibitors such as mefenamic acid in a dosage of 500 mg three times daily, which was shown by Anderson et al. to significantly reduce menstrual blood loss in IUD users. If bleeding continues despite this treatment, the device should be removed. After a 1-month interval another device may be inserted if the patient still wishes to use an IUD for contraception. If the original device was nonmedicated, the new device should be a copper- or a progesterone-releasing IUD, because these smaller devices are associated with less blood loss than the larger plastic devices.

PERFORATION. Although it is uncommon, one of the potentially serious complications associated with use of the IUD is perforation of the uterine fundus. Perforation initially occurs at insertion and can best be prevented by straightening of the uterine axis with a tenaculum and then probing of the cavity with a uterine sound before IUD insertion, which is best performed by the withdrawal technique. Sometimes only the distal portion of the IUD penetrates the uterine muscle at insertion, and then the uterine contractions over the next few months force the IUD into the peritoneal cavity. IUDs correctly inserted entirely within the endometrial cavity do not wander through the uterine muscle into the peritoneal cavity. The incidence of perforation is generally related to the shape of the device or the amount of force used during its insertion as well as the experience of the clinician. Perforation rates with the loop and the copper IUDs have been reported to be about 1 in 1000 insertions. The clinician should always suspect that perforation has occurred if a patient states she cannot feel the appendage but did not notice the device was expelled. One should not assume that an unnoticed expulsion has occurred. Frequently, the device has rotated 180 degrees and the appendage has been withdrawn into the cavity. In this situation, after pelvic examination is performed, and the possibility of pregnancy excluded, the uterine cavity should be probed. Millen and Bernstein conducted a study of 100 patients with IUDs who had no IUD appendages visible at the time of a routine examination, it was found that 69 had the IUD in utero with the strings drawn up into the endometrial cavity, 17 had an unnoticed expulsion, and 10 had a uterine perforation. If the device cannot be felt with a uterine sound or biopsy instrument, an x-ray film or sonogram should be ordered. It is best to obtain x-ray films with both anteroposterior and lateral views with contrast medium or a uterine sound inside the uterine cavity. The IUD may be located in the cul de sac and the diagnosis may be missed with only an anteroposterior film.

If the IUD is found to be outside the uterus, it should be electively removed, because complications such as adhesions and bowel obstruction have been reported with intraperitoneal IUDs. Both the copper IUDs and shields have been found to produce severe peritoneal reactions. Therefore, it is best to remove these devices as soon as possible after the diagnosis of perforation is made. Unless severe adhesions have developed most intraperitoneal IUDs can be removed by means of laparoscopy, avoiding the necessity of laparotomy.

Perforation of the cervix has also been reported to occur with devices having a straight vertical arm such as the copper T or 7. The incidence of downward perforation of these devices into the cervix has been reported to range from about 1 in 600 to 1 in 1000 insertions. When follow-up examinations are performed on patients with these devices, the cervix should be carefully inspected and palpated, as frequently the perforation does not extend completely through the ectocervical epithelium. Cervical perforation is not a major problem, but devices that have perforated downward should be removed through the endocervical canal with uterine packing forceps in the clinic, because their downward displacement is associated with a reduced contraceptive effectiveness.

Complications Related to Pregnancy

Congenital Anomalies

When pregnancy occurs with an IUD in place, implantation occurs away from the device itself, so the device is always extra-amniotic. Although there is a paucity of published data, to date there is no evidence of an increased incidence of congenital anomalies in infants born with an IUD in utero. In Poland's study of aborted tissue from women having a spontaneous abortion, 21% who conceived with an IUD in situ had evidence of embryonic abnormalities. This incidence was considerably less than the 44% incidence of abnormalities occurring in abortuses from women using no contraception and was similar to the incidence of embryonic abnormalities occurring in abortuses of women who had induced abortions. This study suggests that the presence of the IUD has no influence on embryonic development and that the increased incidence of spontaneous abortion in IUD users is not due to an increased incidence of embryo abnormalities.

Tatum and associates reported that of 166 conceptions occurring with a copper T IUD in place which progressed to a size that permitted adequate examination for anomalies, only one infant had a congenital anomaly, a fibroma of the vocal cords. Guillebaud reported that of 167 pregnancies with the copper 7 in place that reached viability, 159 normal babies were born. No details were given regarding three infants, and the other five had a variety of anomalies. The incidence of congenital defects, 3%, was similar to the expected rate. Thus there is no evidence from these studies to indicate that the presence of copper in the uterus exerts a deleterious effect on fetal development. Although relatively few infants have been born with a progesterone-releasing IUD in the uterus, careful examination of these infants has also revealed no increased incidence of cardiac or other anomalies.

Spontaneous Abortion

In all series of pregnancies with any type of IUD in situ, the incidence of fetal death was not significantly increased; however, a significant increase in the incidence of spontaneous abortion has been consistently observed. In the first 7 years of the prospective Oxford Family Planning Association contraceptive study, there were a total of 494 unplanned pregnancies among women using IUDs, oral contraceptives, and diaphragms. After the pregnancies that were electively terminated were excluded, the spontaneous abortion rates among the remaining pregnancies were 55.7% for women wearing IUDs, 13.6% for women using oral contraceptives, and 18.1% for women using the diaphragm. This and other studies with the loop and copper IUDs indicate that if a patient conceives with an IUD in place and the IUD is not removed, the incidence of spontaneous abortion is about 55%, approximately three times greater than would occur if the patient conceives without an IUD.

If after conception the IUD is spontaneously expelled or if the appendage is visible and the IUD is removed by traction, the incidence of spontaneous abortion is significantly reduced to about 20%. Thus if a woman conceives with an IUD in situ and she wishes to continue the pregnancy, the IUD should be removed if the appendage is visible in order to significantly reduce the chance of spontaneous abortion. If the appendage is not visible, the uterine cavity should not be probed in an attempt to locate the IUD, as the probing may increase the risk of abortion as well as sepsis.

Septic Abortion

If the IUD cannot be easily removed or the appendage is not visible, evidence suggests that the risk of septic abortion may be increased if the IUD remains in place. Most of the evidence indicating an increased risk of sepsis is based on data from women who conceived with the shield-type of IUD that had a multifilament tail. The design of this tail string allowed bacteria to enter the spaces between the filaments of the tail underneath the sheath, in contrast to the inability of bacteria to enter the monofilament tails of other devices. When the shield device was drawn upward into the uterus as gestation advanced, the bacteria within the tail had the potential for causing a severe and sometimes fatal uterine infection. Currently, there is no conclusive evidence that a patient conceiving with an IUD with a monofilament tail has an increased risk of septic abortion, except for the fact that the spontaneous abortion rate is increased, and about 2% of all abortions become septic.

Thus if a patient who conceives with an IUD in utero wishes to continue the pregnancy and the device cannot be removed without entering the uterine cavity, she should be informed of the possibility of an increased incidence of sepsis and, if she wishes to continue the pregnancy, of the need to report symptoms of infection promptly. If intrauterine infection does occur with an IUD in the pregnant uterus, the endometrial cavity should be evacuated after a short interval of appropriate antibiotic treatment, similar to the treatment of uterine sepsis without an IUD in place.

Ectopic Pregnancy

The IUD prevents intrauterine pregnancy more effectively than it prevents ectopic pregnancy, but it does reduce the overall incidence of ectopic pregnancy. Nevertheless, if pregnancy occurs with an IUD in place, there is a greater chance it is ectopic than if no IUD were used. If a patient conceives with an IUD in place, her chances of having an ectopic pregnancy range from 3% to 9%. This incidence is about 10 times greater than the reported ectopic pregnancy frequency of 0.3% to 0.7% of total births in similar populations.

Thus if a patient conceives with an IUD in place, there should be a high index of suspicion of ectopic pregnancy. There is a higher frequency of ectopic pregnancies with use of the progesterone-releasing IUD, and patients conceiving while wearing this device should have sonography performed early in gestation. Also, the possibility of ovarian pregnancy should always be considered. Patients wearing an IUD who have a clinical diagnosis of ruptured corpus luteum may in fact have an unrecognized ovarian pregnancy. If any patient with an IUD has an elective termination of pregnancy, the evacuated tissue should be examined histologically to be certain that the gestation was intrauterine.

Nevertheless, it should be remembered that the IUD does not cause ectopic pregnancy. A Centers for Disease Control study indicates that patients using an IUD are 60% less likely to develop an ectopic pregnancy than women using no method of contraception, similar to the protection against ectopic pregnancy provided by barrier methods but not as effective as that provided by oral contraceptives.

Prematurity

Several studies indicate that the rate of preterm delivery is higher if an IUD remains in the uterus throughout gestation. If it is not possible to remove the IUD and the patient wishes to continue her pregnancy, she should be warned of the possible increased risk of prematurity in addition to the increased risk of spontaneous abortion. She should also be informed about an increased risk of ectopic pregnancy and possibly septic abortion and should be instructed to report the first signs of pelvic pain or fever. There is no evidence that pregnant women with an IUD in utero have an increased incidence of other obstetrical complications. In addition, there is no evidence that prior use of an IUD results in a greater incidence of complications in subsequent pregnancies.

Infection in the Nonpregnant Woman

In the 1960s, despite great concern among gynecologists that use of the IUD would markedly increase the incidence of salpingitis, there was little evidence that such an increase did oc-

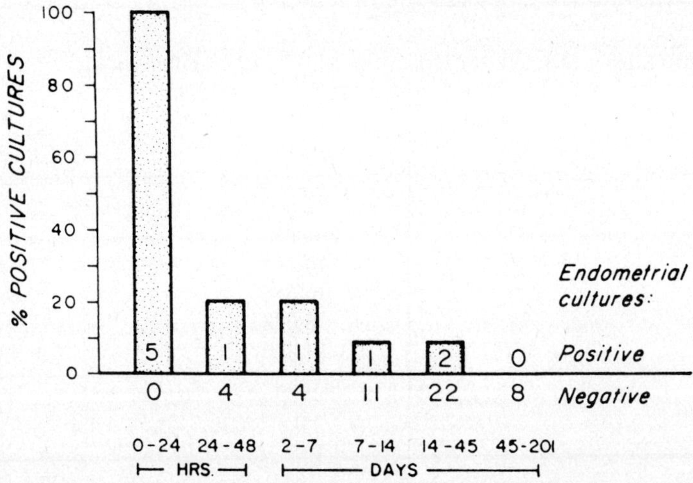

FIGURE 11-7
Relationship of incidence of positive endometrial cultures to duration of use of IUD before hysterectomy. (From Mishell DR Jr, Bell JH, Good RG, et al: Am J Obstet Gynecol 96:119, 1966.)

cur. In this decade the IUD was mainly inserted into parous women, and the incidence of sexually transmitted disease was not as high as it is currently. Mishell et al. prepared aerobic and anaerobic cultures of endometrial homogenates obtained transfundally at varying intervals after insertion of a loop. In the first 24 hours following insertion of a loop, the normally sterile endometrial cavity was consistently infected with bacteria. Nevertheless, the natural defenses destroyed these bacteria within 24 hours in 80% of instances. In this study the endometrial cavity, the IUD, and the portion of the thread within the cavity were found to be consistently sterile when transfundal cultures were obtained more than 30 days after insertion (Fig. 11-7). These findings indicated that development of salpingitis more than 1 month after insertion of the loop type of IUD is of venereal origin and unrelated to the presence of the IUD.

These findings agree with the incidence of a clinical diagnosis of pelvic inflammatory disease (PID) found in a group of 23,977 mainly parous women wearing IUDs analyzed by Tietze and Lewit in 1970. When PID rates were computed according to length of time the IUD was in place, the rates were highest in the first 2 weeks after insertion and then steadily diminished. Rates after the first month were in the range of 1 to 2.5 per 100 woman-years (Table 11-17). The results of both these studies provide evidence that one should not insert an IUD into a patient who may have been recently infected with a pathogen such as gonococcus, as insertion of the device will transport these pathogens into the upper genital tract. If there is clinical suspicion that a gonococcal or chlamydial endocervicitis exists, cultures should be obtained and the IUD should not be inserted until negative results are obtained. It does not appear to be cost effective to administer systemic antibiotics routinely during the period of IUD insertion, but the insertion technique should be performed as aseptically as possible.

Following introduction and widespread use of the shield, particularly among nulliparous women in whom IUDs were previously inserted only occasionally, several studies appeared which suggested that use of IUDs increased the relative risk of developing salpingitis or PID severalfold.

There are several problems with all these studies. One problem is that uniform guidelines for the diagnosis of salpingitis or PID were not used. Differences in the criteria used to establish the diagnosis of salpingitis may increase the frequency of the diagnosis among IUD wearers. Patients with lower abdominal

TABLE 11-17

Rate of Pelvic Inflammatory Disease by Duration of IUD Use at Diagnosis

Period	Cases	Woman-Years	Rate Per 100 Woman-Years (95% Confidence Limits)
1-25 days	75	969	7.7 (6.0-9.5)
16-30 days	34	913	3.7 (2.5-5.0)
2-12 months	421	16,144	2.6 (2.4-2.9)
13-24 months	236	10,588	2.2 (1.9-2.5)
25-36 months	94	6,068	1.5 (1.2-1.9)
27-72 months	40	4,420	0.9 (0.6-1.2)

From Tietze C, Lewit S: Evaluation of intrauterine devices: Ninth progress report of the Cooperative Statistical Program. Stud Fam Plann 1:55, 1970.

pain who have only minimal or no elevation in temperature may have the diagnosis of salpingitis made more often if an IUD is in the uterus. A second problem is the evidence that use of oral contraceptives, condoms, and diaphragms provides protection against development of salpingitis. The data from numerous studies indicate that the incidence of both febrile and nonfebrile PID is about half as great in women using oral contraceptives and barrier methods as in women using no method of contraception. In the Oxford Family Planning Study, the incidence of hospitalized cases of PID with these two methods of contraception was similar. Sexually active women usually use a method of contraception, mainly oral contraceptives, barriers, or the IUD. The increased risk of infection with the IUD is due in a large part to the protective effect of the other contraceptives. In many of the studies performed in the 1970s, a high percentage of IUD patients were using the shield. This device is more likely to have a causal relationship with salpingitis than other devices. Tatum et al. carefully examined the sheaths of the appendages of new shields, in their sterile packages, and those removed from patients. They found that 34% of the former and 9% of the latter had breaks in the sheath around the knot attaching it to the device. These breaks would allow bacteria continuous access from the vagina into the endometrial cavity and thus increase the risk of upper genital tract infection. Finally, in all of these studies there was no differentiation between episodes of salpingitis developing in the

first few months after IUD insertion, which has previously been shown to be related to insertion of the IUD, and episodes developing a few months after insertion. Lee et al. reported results from a multicenter case control study of the relationship of the IUD and PID. They found the overall risk of PID in IUD users as compared with noncontraceptives users to be 1.9%. Shield users had a risk of 8.3%, and other IUD users only 1.6%. When the PID risk of IUD users (other than the shield) was correlated with duration of use, it was found that a significantly increased risk of PID for the loop and copper 7 was present only during the first 4 months after insertion (Table 11-18). After that period there was no significantly increased risk of PID in users of IUDs other than the shield. Thus the findings of this more recent study agree with those of earlier studies mentioned previously which indicate that salpingitis occurring more than a few months after insertion of the loop or copper device is most likely due to a sexually transmitted disease and not related to the IUD.

The populations at high risk for developing PID include those who have a prior history of PID, nulliparous women under 25 years of age, and women with multiple sexual partners. The FDA has recommended that women with these characteristics be especially advised about the risks of developing salpingitis with use of an IUD and the possibility of subsequent loss of fertility. They should be told to be alert for the early symptoms of PID, so treatment can be started before complications occur. These data,

TABLE 11-18

Duration of Current IUD Use (Excluding Dalkon Shield) for Women with PID and Controls

Duration of Use of Current IUD (months)*	Women with PID†	Controls†	Relative Risk‡ (95% Confidence Limits)
≤1	27	17	3.8 (2.1-6.8)
2-4	22	32	1.7 (1.1-3.1)
5-12	33	90	1.1 (0.7-1.7)
13-24	32	81	1.2 (0.7-1.8)
25-60	23	62	1.2 (0.7-2.0)
>60	13	40	1.4 (0.7-2.7)
No method	250	763	1 (Referrent)

From Lee NC, Rubin GL, Ory HW, Burkman RT: Type of intrauterine device and the risk of pelvic inflammatory disease. Obstet Gynecol 62:1, 1983. Reprinted with permission from The American College of Obstetricians and Gynecologists.
PID, Pelvic inflammatory disease.
*IUD used in the 3 months before interview.
†Limited to women who reported no past history of PID.
‡Relative risk adjusted for age, marital status, and number of sexual partners within the previous 6 months.

as well as those of two recent studies showing an increased risk of tubal causes of infertility in nulliparous women who had used an IUD, indicate that the clinician should avoid using IUDs in nulliparous women who may want to conceive in the future. The risk of impairing future fertility because of the increased possibility of developing salpingitis in the first few months after IUD insertion as well as the possibility of developing an ectopic pregnancy must be considered when deciding on use of an IUD in a nulliparous woman.

Symptomatic salpingitis may be successfully treated by antibiotics without removal of the IUD until the patient becomes free of symptoms. In patients who have clinical evidence of a tuboovarian abscess or who have a shield in place, the IUD should be removed after a therapeutic serum level of appropriate parenteral antibiotics has been reached and preferably after a clinical response has been observed. An alternate method of contraception should be used in patients who develop salpingitis with an IUD in place or in those with a past history of salpingitis. There is evidence that IUD users are at increased risk of colonizing actinomycoses organisms in the upper genital tract. The relationship of actinomycosis to salpingitis is unclear, but at present it appears best to try to identify these organisms on the routine annual cytologic smear, and if they are present, the IUD should be removed and left out until the organisms disappear, at which time a new device can be safely inserted. The use of antibiotics in women with actinomycosis who are free of symptoms is unnecessary.

Overall Safety

Several long-term studies have indicated that the IUD is not associated with an increased incidence of carcinoma of the cervix or endometrium. Jain estimated that IUD users have an annual mortality of 3 to 5 deaths per million women, mainly due to infection. He calculated, however, that as far as mortality is concerned the IUD is as safe or safer than other methods of contraception, including sterilization, and safer than no contraception at all at any age. However, the IUD does produce morbidity that may result in hospitalization. The main causes of hospitalization among IUD users are complications of pregnancy, uterine perforation, and hemorrhage, as well as pelvic infection. Despite the increased morbidity with IUDs, the actual incidence of these problems is low and is probably decreased now that the shield is no longer being used and physicians are aware of the potential complications associated with IUDs in pregnancy. The IUD is a particularly useful method of contraception for women who have completed their families and do not wish to undergo sterilization as well as for older women, in whom the risk of taking steroid contraceptives may be increased. Unfortunately its availability in the United States is now limited.

STERILIZATION

In 1982 one partner had been sterilized in about one-third of all married couples in the United States who were using a method of contraception. Sterilization was the most popular method of preventing pregnancy (1) if the wife was over 30 years, (2) if the couple had been married more than 10 years, and (3) if the couple desired no further children. In contrast to the other methods of contraception, which are reversible or temporary, sterilization should be considered permanent. Although reanastomosis following vasectomy or tubal ligation is possible, the reconstructive operation is much more

difficult than the original sterilizing procedure, and the results are variable. Pregnancy rates following reanastomosis of the vas range from 45% to 60%, while those following oviduct reanastomosis range from 50% to 80%, depending on the amount of tissue damage associated with the original procedure, as well as technical competency.

Voluntary sterilization is legal in all 50 states, and the decision to be sterilized should be made solely by the patient in consultation with the physician. Since all currently available sterilization procedures require surgical techniques, patients who request sterilization should be counseled regarding both the risks and the irreversibility of the procedures. It is advisable to fully inform the patient, and the spouse if possible, of the benefits and risks of these surgical procedures. In addition, it has been useful to have more than one counsellor when sterilization is requested by a woman less

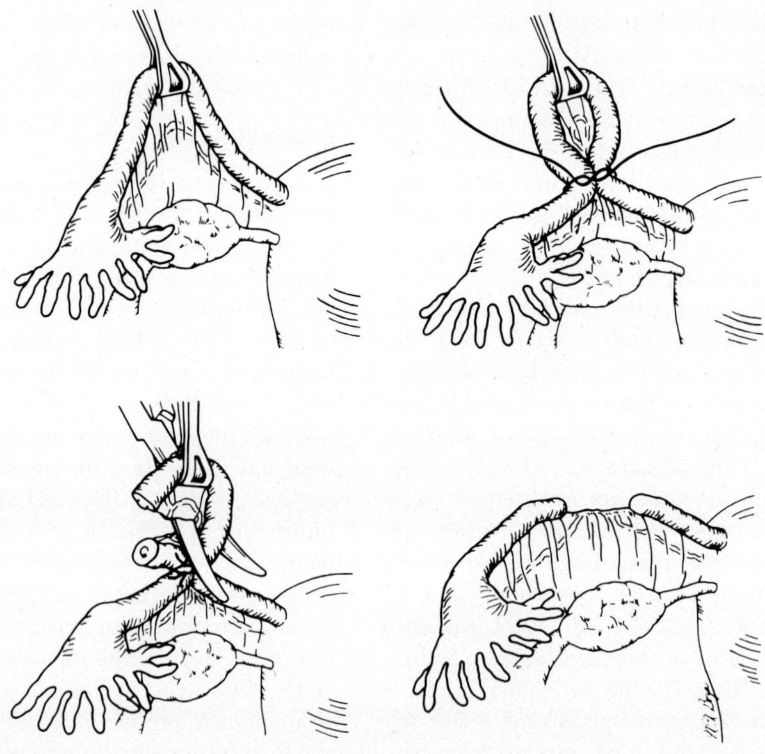

FIGURE 11-8
Modified Pomeroy technique of female sterilization. (From Sciarra JJ: Surgical procedures for tubal sterilization. In Sciarra JJ, Zatuchni GI, Daly MJ: Gynecology and Obstetrics, vol. 6. Philadelphia, Harper & Row Publishers, 1984.)

than 25 years of age, as well as a woman under 40 years of age without any children.

The rationale for such careful scrutiny of younger candidates for sterilization is that they tend to change their minds more often, their attitudes may be less fixed, and they face a longer period of reproductive life during which divorce, remarriage, or death among their children can occur. About 1% of sterilized women subsequently request reversal. In the United States approximately 7000 women request reversal each year.

The most effective, least destructive method of tubal occlusion is the most desirable in younger patients, since ovarian dysfunction and adhesion formation are diminished, while the incidence of successful reversal procedures is increased. The effective laparoscopic band techniques or the modified Pomeroy technique (Fig. 11-8) should be used in patients who are less than 25 years of age. Reversal after this method of sterilization is followed by pregnancy in about 75% of cases, a rate that is higher than that reported following most laparoscopic fulgurations, where more tube is destroyed.

Male Sterilization

Sterilization in the male is performed by vasectomy, an outpatient procedure that takes about 20 minutes and requires only local anesthesia. The vas deferens is isolated and cut. The ends of the vas are closed, either by ligation or by fulguration; they are then replaced in the scrotal sac, and the incision is closed. Complications of vasectomy include hematoma (in up to 5% of subjects), sperm granulomas (inflammatory responses to sperm leakage), and spontaneous reanastomosis (if this is to occur, it usually does so within a short time after the procedure). Hematoma is best prevented by ligating all small vessels in the scrotal wall. The occurrence of sperm granuloma is minimized by cauterizing or fulgurating the ends of the vas instead of ligating them. After the procedure the man is not considered sterile until two sperm-free ejaculates have been produced. Semen analysis should be performed 1 and 2 months after the procedure. It usually requires about 15 to 20 ejaculations after the operation before the man is sterile. Although in the

United States requests for reversal range from 6% to 7%, vas reanastomosis is a difficult and meticulous procedure that has a success rate of about 50%.

Female Sterilization

Sterilization of the female is more complicated, requiring a transperitoneal incision and, usually, general anesthesia. Postpartum sterilization is performed by making a small infraumbilical incision and performing either a Pomeroy or modified Irving-type of tubal ligation. These simple and rapid procedures can be performed either in the delivery room immediately after delivery or in the operating room the following day without prolonging the patient's hospital stay. The same operative techniques can be used for female sterilization at times other than the puerperium, but additional techniques are also used for what has been termed *interval sterilization*. Ligation of the oviducts by the Pomeroy technique can be easily and rapidly performed through a small abdominal incision. The latter has been termed *minilaparotomy*. On occasion a colpotomy incision may also be used, but this incision is associated with a higher incidence of postoperative infection.

The development of fiberoptic light sources has made laparoscopy a popular gynecologic operative technique. By utilizing various accessories, in addition to the laparoscope, the operator can fulgurate and cut the oviducts without making an intraperitoneal incision other than one or two small punctures. Most gynecologists find the two-puncture technique for laparoscopy sterilization easier to learn and perform than the single-puncture technique. General anesthesia is usually utilized for laparoscopic sterilization, but overnight hospitalization is unnecessary. The failure rate following this technique is about 1 per 1000 procedures. Because the pregnancy rate following fulguration and transection is similar to that following fulguration alone, it is now recommended that the oviducts not be cut following fulguration. The incidence of complications following laparoscopic fulguration ranges from 1% to 6%; major complications (hemorrhage, puncture, or cautery of bowel) occur in about 0.6% of cases.

In an attempt to eliminate the problem of

bowel injury, bipolar forceps were developed to replace the unipolar apparatus, which has a grounding plate attached to the patient through which the current passes. In the bipolar system, the current passes from one prong of the forceps, through the tissue, to the other prong, thus producing a limited coagulation with destruction of a small segment of the oviduct. After coagulation, if division is to be performed, scissors are introduced to cut the oviduct. If division is not to be performed, some operators perform a coagulation of two or three contiguous burns on each oviduct to ensure adequate obliteration of the lumen. When the unipolar apparatus is used, a single 1 cm burn on each oviduct is sufficient. However, even with this small amount of coagulation, local tissue damage following unipolar coagulation is extensive and attempts at reanastomosis have a very low rate of success. Because bipolar coagulation not only is safer but also is associated with a higher success rate following a reanastomosis procedure, this technique is now preferred.

Because of the problems of electrocoagulation, efforts have been made to develop safer methods that destroy less tissue. Nonelectrical tubal occlusion techniques that may be performed through the laparoscope are those using the tantalum, plastic, and spring-loaded clips; the Silastic band (Falope ring). All of these techniques require a modification of the conventional laparoscope, as well as specialized training in their use. The failure rate for the clip and band techniques averages about 2 per 1000 procedures, with a range of 1 to 6 per 1000.

INDUCED ABORTION

When contraception or sterilization is not used or fails, abortion may now be legally performed in the United States and many other countries. After the first trimester of pregnancy, each state, in promoting its interest in the health of the mother, may regulate the abortion procedure in ways that are reasonably related to maternal health.

From 1973 to 1980 the number of legal abortions performed in the United States steadily increased, but since then the abortion rate has remained stable. In 1982 there were an estimated 1.6 million legal abortions; in the same year 26% of all pregnancies were terminated by induced abortion, a rate of 29 per 1000 women between the ages of 15 and 44 years, and 300 abortions were performed for every 1000 live births plus abortions. In 1982 about 3% of all women of childbearing age in the United States had an abortion performed. About one third of the abortions were in women under age 20 years, another third in women aged 20 to 24. One fourth of these abortions were obtained by married women. About 90% of abortions were performed at 8 weeks' gestation or less. About 85% of abortions were performed by suction curettage, 10% by surgical curettage, and 5% by saline infusion. Less than 2% were terminated by means of prostaglandins.

Methods

There are three major methods for termination of pregnancy: instrumental evacuation by the vaginal route, stimulation of uterine contractions, and major surgical procedures.

Vaginal Evacuation

Vaginal evacuation by either dilation and curettage or vacuum aspiration (suction) is mainly limited to abortion in the first trimester. In the first few weeks of gestation, endometrial aspiration, sometimes misnamed "menstrual extraction," can be done with a small, flexible plastic cannula without dilation or anesthesia. Abortions 8 or more weeks after the onset of the last menses require dilation of the cervix and general or local paracervical anesthesia. Mechanical dilation of the cervix can be facilitated or avoided entirely by insertion of *Laminaria* tents or other osmotic dilators, for several hours before evacuation of the uterus. Their use is particularly helpful in the nulliparous woman, and their routine use allows the majority of first trimester abortions to be performed without anesthesia. Beyond 12 to 13 weeks it is advisable to evacuate the uterus in the operating suite, but overnight hospitalization is usually not necessary.

Formerly, suction curettage was primarily restricted to those individuals in whom gestation was less than 13 weeks. Recent studies have shown that dilation and evacuation (D &

E) can be performed in the second trimester by means of either graduated dilators or preinsertion of several *Laminaria,* a larger suction cannula, and forceps. At 12 to 16 weeks' gestation, it is safer, more rapid, and less expensive than the infusion technique or major surgical procedure. Between 16 and 20 weeks the incidence of minor complications is probably similar to the incidence after saline or prostaglandin infusion, but the incidence of major complications, such as uterine and bowel perforation, is probably greater. Disadvantages include the greater technical expertise that is required, the emotional trauma to participating physicians and paramedical personnel, and the possible long-term effects of cervical trauma.

Stimulation of Uterine Contractions

Second trimester abortion is usually initiated by the stimulation of uterine contractions. The most commonly used method is infusion of 200 ml of 20% saline solution. Labor usually starts within 12 to 24 hours after the instillation, and evacuation of the uterine contents usually follows 12 to 24 hours later. The delay can usually be shortened by the concomitant use of oxytocin; however, the addition of oxytocin increases the incidence of complications, especially consumption coagulopathy and cervical rupture, which may result in cervicovaginal fistula.

Intraamniotic administration of 40 mg of prostaglandin $F_{2\alpha}$ is also used to stimulate uterine contractions in the second trimester. This technique has a slightly higher success rate (90% to 95%) than saline instillation (85% to 90%), and the interval between infusion and abortion is somewhat shorter.

Other solutions that have been injected into the amniotic fluid to induce abortion include urea and hypertonic glucose. The former is frequently used in Great Britain, but the latter is associated with a high incidence of infection and is not recommended.

Transvaginal extraamniotic administration of Rivanol or prostaglandin $F_{2\alpha}$ and placement of a metreurynter into the lower uterine segment have also been used to initiate uterine contractions in the early second trimester.

Two additional prostaglandins have been approved for abortion. These are vaginal suppositories of prostaglandin E_2 (20 mg) and intra-muscular 15-methyl prostaglandin $F_{2\alpha}$. Both are noninvasive techniques with a decreased morbidity, primarily infection, and ease of administration. They should not be used in patients with asthma or those with prior uterine surgery, but otherwise they have a success rate greater than 95% with a rapid abortion time of 8 to 12 hours. Repeated administration is necessary for both substances. Also, both have a high incidence of gastrointestinal side effects, primarily nausea, vomiting, and diarrhea, which can usually be controlled by appropriate premedication. The prostaglandin E_2 suppositories also cause a chilly sensation and temperature elevation.

Major Surgical Procedures

Hysterectomy or hysterotomy can be performed in both the first and second trimesters. Hysterotomy has a high incidence of morbidity and should be avoided if possible. Despite the increased morbidity of the procedure, however, hysterectomy has the advantage of sterilizing the patient without problems of subsequent menstrual disorders. Abortion hysterectomy has been performed both abdominally and vaginally in both the first and early second trimesters in relatively large numbers of patients with a low incidence of morbidity.

Currently the following procedures are recommended for elective or induced abortion. Ideally every patient should have ultrasound scanning, and unless fetal heart activity is seen, a qualitative human chorionic gonadotrophin (HCG) assay should also be performed before pregnancy termination. Ultrasound examination is helpful in determining if a gestational sac or fetus is present in the uterus and if so, gestational age. Thus it is important to perform this procedure before EPT in all individuals with a gestation greater than 12 weeks. It is best not to attempt EPT in an individual who has missed a menstrual cycle and has a negative HCG assay or in one who has a positive assay but in whom less than 6 weeks has elapsed since the onset of the last menses. Failure to terminate the pregnancy occurs more frequently when the procedure is done 6 weeks or less after the last menstrual period. From 6 to 8 weeks of gestation the uterus is best evacuated by means of a small, flexible cannula attached to a hand or machine suction device. From 8 to 12 weeks, abortion is best performed by vacuum aspiration. For the nulligravid individual a single *Laminaria* or other osmotic dilator should be placed in the cervical canal 4 to 24 hours before the aspiration procedure to decrease the incidence of cervical trauma resulting from mechanical dilation. *Laminaria* should also be inserted in all patients with a gestational period greater than 12 weeks before all abortion techniques.

From 12 to 16 weeks' gestation the best methods for pregnancy termination are intramuscular 15-methyl-$F_{2\alpha}$-prostaglandin, vaginal prostaglandin E_2, and dilation and evacuation by an individual with training and experience with this technique.

From 16 to 18 weeks these same techniques as well as intraamniotic infusion with saline are the most acceptable procedures. Beyond 18 weeks vaginal prostaglandin E_2 suppositories, intraamniotic infusion with saline, and dilation and evacuation are the procedures of choice.

Complications

The possible immediate complications of evacuation of the uterus include perforation of the uterus, hemorrhage, and cervical laceration. Hypertonic saline may cause consumption coagulopathy with severe hemorrhage, as well as adverse central nervous system effects. Complications of prostaglandins include hypertension, tachycardia, bronchoconstriction, nausea, vomiting, diarrhea, and development of slow-healing cervicovaginal fistulas. The possible delayed complications of all therapeutic abortions include retention of a portion of the placenta, which causes bleeding problems; infection; thrombophlebitis; a possible increased incidence of preterm labor in subsequent pregnancies; sensitization of Rh-negative women; and a possible increased incidence of sterility, especially in patients who develop infection and perhaps in others who develop intrauterine synechiae.

Complication rates are three to four times higher for second trimester abortions than for first trimester abortions. By technique, complication rates are lowest for vacuum aspiration, followed in order by dilation and curettage, hypertonic saline infusion, hysterotomy, and hysterectomy. The complication rate for abortion by hysterotomy is two to three times higher than the usual high rates for second trimester abortion by other methods.

In young women the incidence of serious complications and death is higher for abortion than for any method of contraception. For this reason, contraception or sterilization should be used to prevent unwanted pregnancy, and therapeutic abortion should be reserved for failure of these safer techniques.

———————————— KEY POINTS ————————————

- In 1982, of the 55 million women in the United States aged 15 to 44 years, about one third were not exposed to pregnancy, and of the remaining 36 million women all but 3 million were using a method of contraception.

- The most frequently used method to prevent conception in the United States is male and female sterilization. Of the nonsurgical methods of contraception, oral contraceptives are most popular, being used by 18% of all women in this age group, followed by the condom (8%), IUD (4%), spermicides (3%), diaphragm (3%), withdrawal (2%), and rhythm (1%).

- First-year use failure rates are lowest for oral contraceptives (2.5%); higher for the IUD (4.8%), condom (9.6%), diaphragm (14.4%), and spermicides (17.7%); and highest for rhythm (18.8%).

- Contraceptive failure rates are increased in inverse relation to the user's age, level of education, and socioeconomic class.

- First-year method failure rates were 0.8% for oral contraceptives, 0.9% for the condom, 1.5% for the IUD, 6.1% for spermicides, 6.4% for the diaphragm, and 8.3% for rhythm.

- Oral contraceptive formulations in the United States consist of varying dosages of one of the following five 19-nortestosterone gestagens: norethynodrel, norethindrone, norethindrone acetate, ethynodiol diacetate, or norgestrel; and either of two estrogens: ethinyl estradiol or ethinyl estradiol-3-methyl ether.

- A given weight of norgestrel is 5 to 10 times more potent than the equivalent weight of norethindrone, whereas norethindrone acetate and ethinyl estradiol are similar in potency to norethindrone.

- Ethinyl estradiol is about 1.7 times as potent as an equivalent weight of mestranol.

- There is no significantly increased risk of breast cancer in oral contraceptive users, nor in various high-risk subgroups of oral contraceptive users.

- The rate of return of fertility after stopping oral contraceptives is delayed, but eventually the percentage of women who conceive after stopping all methods of contraception including oral contraceptives is the same.

- Babies born to women who discontinue oral contraceptives have no greater incidence of any type of birth defect.

- A significantly increased risk of developing cardiovascular disease occurs only in current oral contraceptive users over 35 years of age who smoke or those of any age who use oral contraceptives and also have some type of preexisting vascular disease.

- Adverse effects produced by the estrogenic component of oral contraceptives include nausea, breast tenderness, fluid retention, temporary increase in blood pressure, thrombosis, changes in mood, and depression. Gestagens produce certain androgenic adverse effects including weight gain, nervousness, and acne, as well as failure of withdrawal bleeding or amenorrhea.

________________ **KEY POINTS, cont'd** ________________

- Absolute contraindications for oral contraceptive use include presence or history of vascular disease (e.g., thromboembolism or thrombophlebitis), hypertension, diabetes mellitus with vascular disease, smoking after age 35, cancer of the breast or endometrium, pregnancy, and active liver disease. Relative contraindications to oral contraceptive use include heavy cigarette smoking, migraine headaches, amenorrhea, and depression.

- In an ovulatory cycle the mean blood loss during menstruation is about 35 ml, as compared with 20 ml for women ingesting oral contraceptives.

- Oral contraceptive users are about half as likely to develop iron deficiency anemia as are controls.

- Oral contraceptive users are significantly less likely to develop menorrhagia, irregular menstruation, or intermenstrual bleeding than nonusers.

- The risk of developing endometrial cancer as well as ovarian cancer in oral contraceptive users is only half that in controls. Oral contraceptive users also have a 50% reduction in the incidence of benign breast disease.

- Oral contraceptive users have about 60% less dysmenorrhea and 39% less premenstrual tension than controls.

- Functional ovarian cysts rarely occur in oral contraceptive users.

- Oral contraceptives reduce the clinical development of salpingitis in women infected with gonorrhea or chlamydia by 50%, and the overall incidence of salpingitis in oral contraceptive users is reduced 50%.

- Oral contraceptives reduce the risk of ectopic pregnancy by more than 60% in women currently using them.

- Oral contraceptives prevent 50,000 women from being hospitalized in the United States each year as a result of their noncontraceptive health benefits.

- The annual incidence of accidental pregnancy decreases steadily after the first year of IUD use. After 6 years of use of the loop or copper IUD, the cumulative failure rate is about 1% per year.

- The incidence of adverse events with IUDs steadily decreases with increasing age of the patient.

- The main mechanism of contraceptive action of IUDs (other than the progesterone-releasing IUD) is production of a local sterile inflammatory reaction of leukocytes, which destroys sperm and prevents fertilization.

- Resumption of fertility following IUD removal is not delayed and occurs at the same rate as resumption following discontinuation of use of mechanical methods of contraception.

- Several types of IUDs are approved for use in the United States: the plastic loop, the copper-bearing copper 7, the copper T 200, the copper T 380A, and the progesterone-releasing T-shaped device, but only the last is currently marketed.

- At the time of scheduled removal of copper or progesterone-releasing IUDs the device can be removed and reinserted at the same clinic visit. The IUD can be safely inserted on any day of the cycle.

- In the first year of use, IUDs have about a 2% pregnancy rate, a 10% expulsion rate, and a 15% rate of removal for medical reasons, and the incidence of each of these events diminishes steadily in subsequent years.

- In women wearing a loop IUD, about 70 to 80 ml of blood is lost; in those wearing a copper T IUD, 50 to 60 ml is lost per cycle; with the progesterone-releasing IUD the amount of blood loss is 25 ml per cycle.

- Mefenamic acid in a dosage of 500 mg twice daily significantly reduces menstrual blood loss in IUD users.

- IUD fundal perforation rates are about 1 in 1000 insertions. The incidence of cervical perforation by copper IUDs ranges from about 1 in 600 to 1 in 1000 insertions.

- There is no evidence of an increased incidence of congenital anomalies in infants born with any type of IUD in utero.

_____________ **KEY POINTS, cont'd** _____________

- If a patient conceives with an IUD in place and the IUD is not removed, the incidence of spontaneous abortion is about 55%, approximately three times greater than would occur without an IUD. If after conception the IUD appendage is visible and the IUD is removed by traction, the incidence of spontaneous abortion is reduced to about 20%.

- If a patient conceives with an IUD in place, her chances of having an ectopic pregnancy range from 3% to 9%, about 10 times greater than occurs in conception without an IUD.

- Patients using an IUD have about a 60% lower risk of having an ectopic pregnancy than women using no method of contraception.

- The rate of prematurity among live births occurring with an IUD in situ is increased two to four times.

- The overall risk of salpingitis in users of IUDs, excluding the shield type, is about 1.5 times that in controls, and a significantly increased risk of PID for the loop and copper 7 IUDs is present only during the first 4 months after insertion.

- Injectable DMPA (150 mg every 3 months) has a first-year pregnancy rate of 0.1%.

- Patients treated with injectable gestagens for contraception have complete disruption of the normal menstrual cycle and a totally irregular bleeding pattern.

- In 1982 one partner had been sterilized in about one-third of all married couples in the United States who were using a method of contraception.

- Pregnancy rates following reanastomosis of the vas range from 45% to 60%, whereas those following oviduct reanastomosis range from 50% to 80%.

- About 1% of sterilized women request reversal. In the United States approximately 7000 women request reversal each year.

- It usually requires about 15 to 20 ejaculations after vasectomy before a man is sterile.

- Following vasectomy two aspermic ejaculates are required before the male is considered sterile.

- The failure rate following laparoscopic fulguration of the oviducts is about 1 in 1000 procedures; with the clip and band techniques it is about 2 in 1000 procedures.

- In 1982 there were an estimated 1.6 million legal abortions in the United States, and 26% of all pregnancies were terminated by induced abortion.

- About 90% of elective abortions in the United States were performed at 8 weeks' gestation or less.

- Complication rates are three to four times higher for second trimester abortions than for first trimester abortions.

BIBLIOGRAPHY

Alvior GTI Jr: Pregnancy outcome with removal of intrauterine device. Obstet Gynecol 41:894, 1973.

Anderson ABM, Haynes PJ, Guillebaud J, et al: Reduction of menstrual blood loss by prostaglandin synthetase inhibitors. Lancet 1:774, 1976.

Brenner PF, Mishell DR Jr, Stanczyk FZ: Serum levels of *d*-norgestrel, luteinizing hormone, follicle-stimulating hormone, estradiol, and progesterone in women during and following ingestion of combination oral contraceptives containing *dl*-norgestrel. Am J Obstet Gynecol 129:133, 1977.

Casagrande JT, Louie EW, Pike MD, et al: "Incessant ovulation" and ovarian cancer. Lancet 2:170, 1979.

Centers for Disease Control Cancer and Steroid Hormone Study: Long-term oral contraceptive use and the risk of breast cancer. JAMA 249:1591, 1983.

Dixon GW, Schlesselman JJ, Ory HW, Blye RP: Ethinyl estradiol and conjugated estrogens as postcoital contraceptives. JAMA 244:1336, 1980.

Forrest JD, Henshaw SK: What U.S. women think and do about contraception. Fam Plann Perspect 15:162, 1983.

Garcia C-R, Huggins GR, Rosenfeld DL, et al: Postcoital contraception: Medical and social factors of the morning after pill. Contraception 15:445, 1977.

Grady WR, Hirsch MB, Keen N, Vaughan B: Contraceptive failure and continuation among married women in the U.S., 1970-75. Stud Fam Plann 14:9, 1983.

Guillebaud J: Copper IUCDs and pregnancy. (letter) Br J Fam Plann 7(3):88, 1981.

Jain AK: Safety and effectiveness of intrauterine devices. Contraception 11:243, 1975.

Klein TA, and Mishell DR Jr: Gonadotropin, prolactin and steroid hormone levels after discontinuation of oral contraceptives. Am J Obstet Gynecol 127:585, 1977.

Layde PM, Beral V, Kar CR: Further analyses of mortality in oral contraceptive users. Royal College of General Practitioners' Oral Contraceptive Study. Lancet 1:541, 1981.

Lee NC, Rubin GL, Ory HW, Burkman RT: Type of intrauterine device and the risk of pelvic inflammatory disease. Obstet Gynecol 62:1, 1983.

Lehfeldt H, Tietze C, Gorstein F: Ovarian pregnancy and the intrauterine device. Am J Obstet Gynecol 108:1005, 1970.

Lewit SL: Outcome of pregnancies with intrauterine devices. Contraception 2:47, 1970.

Liedholm P, Sjöberg N-O, Astedt B: Increased bleeding and increased fibrinolytic activity in the endometrium in women using the copper T. In Hefnawi F, Segal SJ, eds: Analysis of intrauterine contraception. Amsterdam, Elsevier-North Holland. 1975, p. 391.

Luukkainen T, Allonen H, Nielsen N-C, et al: Five years experience of intrauterine contraception with Nova-T and the Copper-T-200. Am J Obstet Gynecol 147:885, 1983.

Mastroianni L Jr: Rhythm: Systematized chance-taking. Fam Plann Perspect 6:209, 1974.

Meade TW, Greenberg G, Thompson SG: Progestogens and cardiovascular reactions associated with oral contraceptives and a comparison of the safety of 50- and 30-μg estrogen preparations, Br Med J 1:1157, 1980.

Millen A, Austin FJ, Bernstein GS: Analysis of 100 cases of missing IUD strings. Contraception 8:485, 1978.

Mishell DR Jr: The effects of contraceptive steroids on hypothalamic-pituitary function. Am J Obstet Gynecol 128:60, 1977.

Mishell DR Jr: Oral steroid contraceptives. In Mishell DR Jr, Davajan V, eds.: Infertility, contraception and reproductive endocrinology, 2nd ed. Oradell, NJ, Medical Economics Books, 1986.

Mishell DR Jr, Roy S: Copper intrauterine contraceptive device event rates following insertion 4 to 8 weeks postpartum. Am J Obstet Gynecol 143:29, 1982.

Mishell DR Jr, Bell JH, Good RG, et al: The intrauterine device: A bacteriologic study of the endometrial cavity. Am J Obstet Gynecol 96:119, 1966.

Morehead JE, Matthews A, Guillebaud J, Bonnar J: Menstrual blood loss in users of an IUD. In Hefnawi F, Segal SJ, eds: Analysis of intrauterine contraception. Amsterdam, Elsevier-North Holland. 1975, p. 381.

Morris JM, van Waganen G: Interception: The use of postovulatory estrogens to prevent implantation. Am J Obstet Gynecol 115:101, 1973.

Nash HA: Depo-provera: A review. Contraception 12:377, 1975.

Oral contraceptives and health: An interim report from the Oral Contraceptive Study of the Royal College of General Practitioners. New York, Pitman Publishing, 1974.

Oral contraceptives and venous thromboembolic disease, surgically confirmed gall-bladder disease, and breast tumors. Report from the Boston Collaborative Drug Surveillance Program. Lancet 1:1399, 1973.

Ory HW: The noncontraceptive health benefits from oral contraceptive use. Fam Plann Perspect 14:182, 1982.

Pike MC, Henderson BE, Krailo MD, et al: Breast cancer in young women and use of oral contraceptives: Possible modifying effect of formulation and age at use. Lancet 2:926, 1983.

Pituitary Adenoma Study Group: Pituitary adenomas and oral contraceptives: A multi-center case-control study. Fertil Steril 39:753, 1983.

Poland B: Conception control and embryonic development. Am J Obstet Gynecol 106:365, 1970.

Porter JB, Hunter JR, Danielson DA, et al: Oral contraceptive and nonfatal vascular disease—recent experience. Obstet Gynecol 59:299, 1982.

Porter JB, Hunter JR, Jick H, et al: Oral contraceptives and nonfatal vascular disease, Obstet Gynecol 66:1, 1985.

Ramcharan S, Pellegrin FA, Ray RM, Hsu J-P: The Walnut Creek Contraceptive Drug Study: A prospective study of the side effects of oral contraceptives, vol. 3, NIH Pub. No. 81-564. Washington, DC, US Government Printing Office, 1981.

Royal College of General Practitioners: Oral contraceptives and health. An interim report from the Oral Contraceptive Study of the Royal College of General Practitioners. New York, Pitman Medical Publishing, 1974.

Royal College of General Practitioners' Oral Contraceptive Study: Mortality among oral contraceptive users. Lancet 2:727, 1977.

Royal College of General Practitioners' Oral Contraceptive Study: Further analysis of mortality in oral contraceptive users. Lancet 1:541, 1981.

Ryden G, Fahraeus L, Molin L, et al: Do contraceptives influence the incidence of acute pelvic inflammatory disease in women with gonorrhea? Contraception 20:149, 1979.

Schirm AL, Trussell J, Menken J, Grady WR: Contraceptive failure in the United States: The impact of social, economic and demographic factors. Fam Plann Perspect 14:68, 1982.

Schwallie PC, Assenzo JR: Contraceptive use—efficacy study utilizing medroxyprogesterone acetate administered as an intramuscular injection once every 90 days. Fertil Steril 24:331, 1973.

Schwallie PC, Assenzo JR: The effect of depomedroxyprogesterone acetate on pituitary and ovarian function, and the return of fertility following its discontinuation: A review. Contraception 10:181, 1974.

Sciarra, J.J: Surgical procedures for tubal sterilization. In Sciarra JJ, Zatuchni GI, Daly MJ: Gynecology and obstetrics, vol. 6, Philadelphia, Harper & Row, Publishers, 1984.

Scott JA, Kletzky OA, Brenner PF: Comparison of the effects of contraceptive steroid formulations containing two doses of estrogen on pituitary function. Fertil Steril 30:141, 1978.

Sivin I, Tatum HJ: Four years of experience with the T Cu 380A intrauterine contraceptive device. Fertil Steril 36:159, 1981.

Stadel BV, Rubin GL, Webster LA, et al: Oral contraceptives and breast cancer in young women. Lancet 2:970, 1985.

Swyer GIM: Potency of progestins in oral contraceptives—further delay of menses data. Contraception 26:23, 1982.

Tatum HJ, Schmidt FH, Jain AK: Management and outcome of pregnancies associated with the copper T intrauterine contraceptive device. Am J Obstet Gynecol 7:869, 1976.

Tatum HJ, Schmidt FH, Phillips DM: Morphological studies of Dalkon Shield tails removed from patients. Contraception 11:465, 1975.

Tietze C, Lewit S: Evaluation of intrauterine devices: Ninth progress report of the Cooperative Statistical Program. Stud Fam Plann 1:55, 1970.

Tredway DR, Umezaki CU, Mishell DR Jr: Effect of intrauterine devices on sperm transport in the human being: Preliminary report. Am J Obstet Gynecol 123:734, 1975.

Vessey MP, Lawless M, McPherson K, Yeates D: Fertility after stopping use of intrauterine contraceptive device. Br Med J 286:106, 1983.

Vessey MP, Wright NH, McPherson K, et al: Fertility after stopping different methods of contraception. Br Med J 1:265, 1978.

Vessey MP, Doll R, Peto R: A long-term follow-up study of women using different methods of contraception—an interim report. J Biosoc Sci 8:373, 1976.

Weström L: Incidence, prevalence and trends of acute pelvic inflammatory disease and its consequences in industrialized countries. Am J Obstet Gynecol 138:880, 1980.

White MK, Ory HW, Rooks JB, Rochat RW: Intrauterine device termination rates and the menstrual cycle day of insertion. Obstet Gynecol 55:220, 1980.

Williams P, Johnson B, Vessey MP: Septic abortion in women using intrauterine devices. Br Med J 4:263, 1975.

Wilson JG, Brent RL: Are female sex hormones teratogenic? Am J Obstet Gynecol 141:567, 1981.

Wølner-Hanssen P, Svensson L, Märdh P-A, et al: Laparoscopic findings and contraceptive use in women with signs and symptoms of acute salpingitis. Obstet Gynecol 66:233, 1985.

World Health Organization Expanded Programme of Research Development and Research Training in Human Reproduction: Task force on long-acting systemic agents for the regulation of fertility. Contraception 15:513, 1977.

Yuzpe AA, Smith RP, Rademaker AW: A multicenter clinical investigation employing ethinyl estradiol combined with *dl*-norgestrel as a postcoital contraceptive agent. Fertil Steril 37:508, 1982.

Rape, Incest, and Abuse

KEY TERMS AND DEFINITIONS

Rape. Any act of sexual intimacy performed by one person on another without mutual consent by force, by threat of force, or by the inability of the victim to give appropriate consent.

Incest. Sexual intimacy with or without coitus involving a close family member. The act may include fondling, exposure, or the penetration of an orifice by the phallus.

Abuse. This may be defined as aggressive behavior including acts of a sexual or physical nature, verbal belittling, or intimidation. The act may be premeditated, as when one individual wishes to gain control over another, or spontaneous, as a spontaneous response to anger or frustration.

Rape, incest, and other forms of physical and sexual abuse are very common. Physicians in general, and obstetricians and gynecologists in particular, are in a position to detect these problems and offer treatment and counsel when their patients have been found to be victims. In the acute state, a careful history using a compassionate and nonjudgmental approach will often allow an accurate story to be obtained. When the patient seeks medical advice at a time remote from the experience, or when the experience is ongoing, the presenting chief complaint may have little to do with the actual problem. For the physician to elicit a clear picture, it is necessary to resort to open-ended questions and interviewing techniques that allow the patient to comfortably discuss truthfully the actual problem.

These patients are at risk for severe physical and emotional distress, and as victims they may suffer psychological damage to their self-image, which in turn may lead to many long-term poor choices in important life situations. While rape, incest, and abuse will be dealt with separately, there is frequently a relationship in the social pathology involved as well as in the long-term effects that the patient must endure. In each instance appropriate physician response and physician responsibility will be discussed.

RAPE

Rape, or the sexual assault of children, women, and men, is a common act. Only recently has society identified the real scope of this problem. In 1978 an FBI report indicated that close to 200,000 rapes were reported nationwide each year and that this could likely represent no more than 50% of the actual rapes committed. Victims, even today, are reluctant to report rapes to authorities because of embarrassment, fear of retribution, feelings of guilt, or simply lack of knowledge of their rights.

In the past, society has held many misconceptions about the rape victim, particularly a female. These included the notion that the individual encouraged the rape by specific behavior or dress and that no person who did not wish to be could be raped. Further, the feeling that rape was an indication of basic promiscuity was widely held. In many instances sexual assault victims were accused of lying to cause

strating that such events are extremely common.

Marriages involving spouse abuse are often complex. Women who marry men who abuse them frequently stay in the marriage for a number of reasons, including psychological need, fear of being unable to support themselves or their children, and ignorance with respect to the abnormal nature of this behavior.

The physician's suspicion may be raised by the nature of the patient's complaint. As with child abuse victims, bizarre or recurrent injuries should stimulate the physician's suspicion. Most patients are not so accident prone that they are bruised all the time. It is reasonable for a physician to ask the patient how she acquired specific injuries that may be obvious, such as bruises, burns, or lacerations. In most cases, with sympathetic questioning the patient will discuss the problem. Such patients require time and understanding so that they may tell their stories. The physician should seek specific details of the type of abuse, circumstances under which it was perpetrated, and the conception of the patient about the motives of the spouse in performing the abuse.

Many communities have sexual assault crisis intervention centers, usually associated with major hospitals. Domestic violence cases are frequently handled by shelters for battered women, community mental health agencies, or counseling through the domestic court system. Several communities have developed hot lines specializing in the care of abuse victims. Physicians should acquaint themselves with the resources in their community. A number of private health care workers of various disciplines such as psychiatry, psychology, and medical social work are available for referral. When making such referrals the physician should identify individuals who can help with such problems and develop an understanding of how these workers will manage the patient. In most families where abuse is a routine matter, the entire family is usually involved. Counseling resources that address the problems of both the abuser and the abusee as well as the children in the family who have observed the abuse or been victims of it themselves are the most useful. Caseworkers may be assigned to one or more family members, and in some cases multiple therapists may work with the entire family. The physician should take the responsibility of making the appropriate referral and of following up with the family from time to time to see that members are continuing in therapy.

The Elderly

The Select Committee on Aging to consider domestic violence against the elderly heard hearings before the Subcommittee of Human Services of the House of Representatives in 1980. They noted that approximately 500,000 to 2.5 million cases involving abuse of the elderly occur per year in the United States. The committee documented the fact that abuse of the elderly may be as large a nationwide problem as child abuse. Usually the abused person is a woman past the age of 75, often with a physical impairment. She is generally white, widowed, and living with relatives. The abuser is generally an adult child living within the family. Counseling issues involve the entire family but particularly the individual causing the abuse. Physicians who care for geriatric patients need to be alert for signs and symptoms of this type of domestic abuse; when it is found, community resources should be activated.

______ KEY POINTS ______

- About 200,000 rapes are reported nationwide each year. This figure may represent many fewer rapes than actually occur.

- Sexual assault happens to people of all ages, races, and socioeconomic groups, but the very young, the mentally and physically handicapped, and the very old are particularly susceptible.

- Two phases of the rape trauma syndrome occur. The first is the immediate or acute phase and lasts hours to days. The second, the reorganization stage, lasts months to years.

- In caring for rape trauma victims, the physician's responsibilities are medical, medical-legal, and supportive.

- From 12% to 40% of victims who are sexually assaulted have injuries.

- Rape trauma victims should always be treated as victims. At no time should guilt be implied.

- About 10% of all child abuse cases involve sexual abuse.

- Roughly 336,000 children are sexually abused each year in the United States.

- Incestual activity may be experienced by as many as 15% to 25% of all women and approximately 12% of all men.

- Approximately 80% of all sexual abuse cases of children involve a family member.

- Father-daughter incest accounts for about 75% of reported cases; however, although brother-sister incest may be the commonest type, it may not be reported often.

- As many as 25% of women treated for injuries in an emergency room are likely to be victims of wife battering. Diagnosis of this by a physician is rare.

- Between 500,000 and 2.5 million cases of abuse of the elderly reportedly occur in the United States each year.

BIBLIOGRAPHY

Batten DA: Incest: A review of the literature. Med Sci Law 23:245, 1983.

Benward J, Densen-Gerber J: Incest as a causative factor in antisocial behavior: An exploratory study. Contemp Drug Probl 4:322, 1975.

Browning DH, Boatman B: Incest: Children at risk. Am J Psychiat 134:69, 1977.

Burgess AW, Holmstrom LL: Rape: Victims of crisis. In Bowie, Md., R.J. Brady Co., 1974.

Davis LD: Beliefs of service providers about abused women and abusing men. Soc Work 29:2, 1984.

Finkelhor D: Sex among siblings. Arch Sex Behav 9:195, 1981.

Flugel J: Psychoanalytic study of the family. London, Hogarth Press, 1926.

Galleno H, Oppenheim W: The battered child syndrome revisited. Clin Ortho Rel Res 162:11, 1982.

Gentry CE: Incestuous abuse of children: The need for an objective view. Child Welfare 58:355, 1978.

Giordano NH, Giordano JA: Elder abuse: A review of the literature. Soc Work 29:232, 1984.

Hilberman E, Monson K: Sixty battered women. Victimatology 2:460, 1977.

Jones JG: Sexual abuse of children. Am J Dis Child 136:142, 1982.

Kahn M, Sexton M: Sexual abuse of young children. Clin Pediatr 22:369, 1983.

Kaplan HS: The evaluation of sexual disorders. New York, Brunner/Mazel, 1983.

Kempe CH: Sexual abuse: Another hidden pediatric problem. The 1977 C. Anderson Aldrich lecture. Pediatrics 62:382, 1978.

Kerns DL: Child abuse and neglect: The pediatrician's role. J Cont Educ Pediatr 21:11, 1979.

Lukianowicz N: Incest. I. Paternal. II. Other types. Br J Psychiat 120:301, 1972.

Meiselman KC: Incest: A psychological study of cases and effects with treatment recommendations. London, Jossey-Bass, 1978.

Nadelson CC, Notman MT, Zackson H, et al: Follow-up study of rape victims. Am J Psychiat 139:1267, 1982.

Nakashima II, Zakus GE: Incest: Review and clinical experience. Pediatrics 60:696, 1977.

Pedrick-Cornell C, Gelles RJ: Elderly abuse: The status of current knowledge. Fam Rela 31:457, 1982.

Rimsza ME, Niggemann EH: Medical evaluation of sexually abused children: A review of 311 cases. Pediatrics 69:8, 1982.

Sarafino EP: An estimate of nationwide incidence of sexual offenses against children. Child Welfare 58:127, 1979.

Sarles RM: Incest. Pediatrics 2:51, 1980.

Select Committee on Aging: Domestic violence against the elderly. Hearings before the Subcommittee of Human Services, House of Representatives, April 21, 1980, Washington, D.C., U.S. Government Printing Office, 1980.

Sgroi SM: Sexual molestation of children: The last frontier of child abuse. Child Today 4:18, 1975.

Star B: Patterns of family violence. Social Case Work 60:339, 1980.

Breast Diseases

—————————— KEY TERMS AND DEFINITIONS ——————————

Axillary Tail of Spence. A lateral projection of glandular tissue that extends from the upper outer portion of the breast toward the axilla.

Cluster. A mammographic finding of five or more calcifications within a volume of a cubic centimeter.

Cooper's Ligaments. Fibrous septa that extend from the skin over the breast to the underlying pectoralis fascia.

Cystosarcoma Phyllodes. Fibroepithelial breast tumors that are rare and usually arise from fibroadenomas.

Diaphanography. The technique of transillumination of the breast by which a camera measures the light transmitted through breast tissue.

Digital Radiography. The technique by which x-ray photons are detected after passing through the breast tissue.

Fibroadenomas. Firm, freely mobile, solitary, solid breast masses usually present in adolescents and teenagers.

Fibrocystic Changes. An exaggerated response of breast tissue to the cyclic changes of ovarian hormones.

Intraductal Papilloma. Benign breast mass that is usually microscopic but may grow to 2 to 3 mm in diameter. The predominant symptom of an intraductal papilloma is spontaneous discharge from one nipple.

Lumpectomy. Conservative surgical procedure for breast carcinoma that involves removal of a wide margin of normal breast tissue surrounding a breast carcinoma less than 2 cm.

Modified Radical Mastectomy. An operation that includes removal of the breast and only the fascia over the pectoralis major muscle.

Paget's Disease. Rare breast carcinoma that has an innocent appearance and looks like eczema or dermatitis of the nipple.

Polymastia. More than two breasts.

Polythelia. More than two nipples.

Radical Mastectomy. An operation that includes en bloc removal of the breast as well as underlying pectoralis major and pectoralis minor muscles.

Simple Mastectomy. An operation that includes removal of the breast without underlying muscle or fascial tissue.

Thermography. Technique to potentially diagnose breast disease by directly measuring either cutaneous temperatures of the breast or infrared radiation from the breast by electronic detectors.

Virginal Hypertrophy of the Breasts. Rare condition in which there is massive hypertrophy of the breasts at puberty.

Xeromammography. Mammographic technique in which the image is produced by a photoelectric process on aluminum plates coated with selenium.

The importance of early detection and diagnosis of breast carcinoma cannot be overemphasized. Breast carcinoma is the most common malignancy of women and is one of the two leading causes of cancer deaths. It is the number one cause of death in women in their 40s. One out of ten women, 10% of American females, develop carcinoma of the breast during their lifetime.

It is noteworthy that mortality from breast carcinoma has not changed significantly over the past 40 years. However, recent improvements in mammography and meticulous physical examination have facilitated earlier detection of breast carcinoma and may improve survival rates.

The prognosis and survival of a woman with breast carcinoma is improved by early discovery. Thus every gynecologist has an obligation to educate patients concerning self-examination of the breast and to develop a routine for carefully screening patients for breast disease. Detailed physical examination of the breast must be an important and integral step in evaluating every female patient.

Our culture attaches great significance to the female breast. An individual patient may react to the tremendous anxiety of suspected breast disease with behavior that varies from frequent visits to the physician for breast pain to denial of the presence of an obvious mass. The patient's description of her problem and her reactions to diagnoses, benign or malignant, must never be taken out of the context of this anxiety.

The major emphasis of this chapter is the epidemiology, detection, and diagnosis of breast carcinoma. The chapter also includes a brief discussion of benign breast diseases, since the symptoms of benign breast disease present fre-

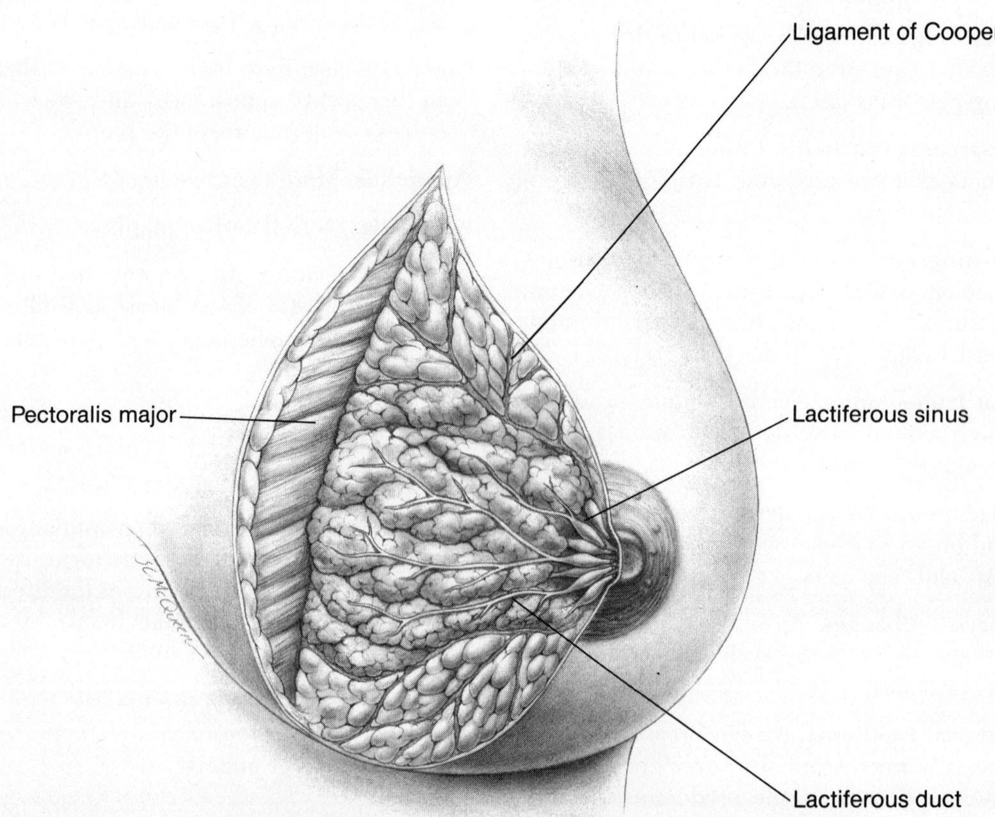

FIGURE 13-1
Anatomy of breast. (From Rehman I: Embryology and anatomy of the breast. In Gallager HS, Leis HP, Synderman RK, et al, eds: The breast. St. Louis, The C.V. Mosby Co., 1978, p. 6.)

quently. Galactorrhea is presented in Chapter 37.

ANATOMY

The breasts are large, modified sebaceous glands contained within the superficial fascia of the anterior chest wall. A lateral projection of glandular tissue extends from the upper outer portion of the breast toward the axilla and is called the axillary tail of Spence. The average weight of the adult breast is 200 to 300 g during the menstruating years. The periphery of breast tissue is predominantly fat, while the central area consists primarily of glandular tissue.

The breast is composed of 12 to 20 lobes arranged in radial fashion from the nipple. Each lobe is triangular and has one central excretory duct that opens to the exterior at the nipple.

Milk originates in the secretory cells of the alveoli. It is subsequently transported by the branching collecting ducts of the lobules into the lactiferous sinuses and terminally into the excretory ducts of each respective lobe of the breast. Fibrous septa, Cooper's ligaments, extend from the skin to the underlying pectoralis fascia (Fig. 13-1). Invasion of these ligaments by malignant cells produces skin retraction, which is a sign of advanced breast carcinoma.

The lymphatic distribution of the breast is complex. Approximately 75% of the lymphatic drainage goes to the axilla. Other metastatic routes include lymphatics adjacent to the internal mammary vessels and direct lymphatic spread into the mediastinum and subpectoral and subdiaphragmatic areas (Fig. 13-2). Metastases from one breast across the midline to the other breast or chest wall occur occasionally.

Breast tissue is sensitive to the cyclic

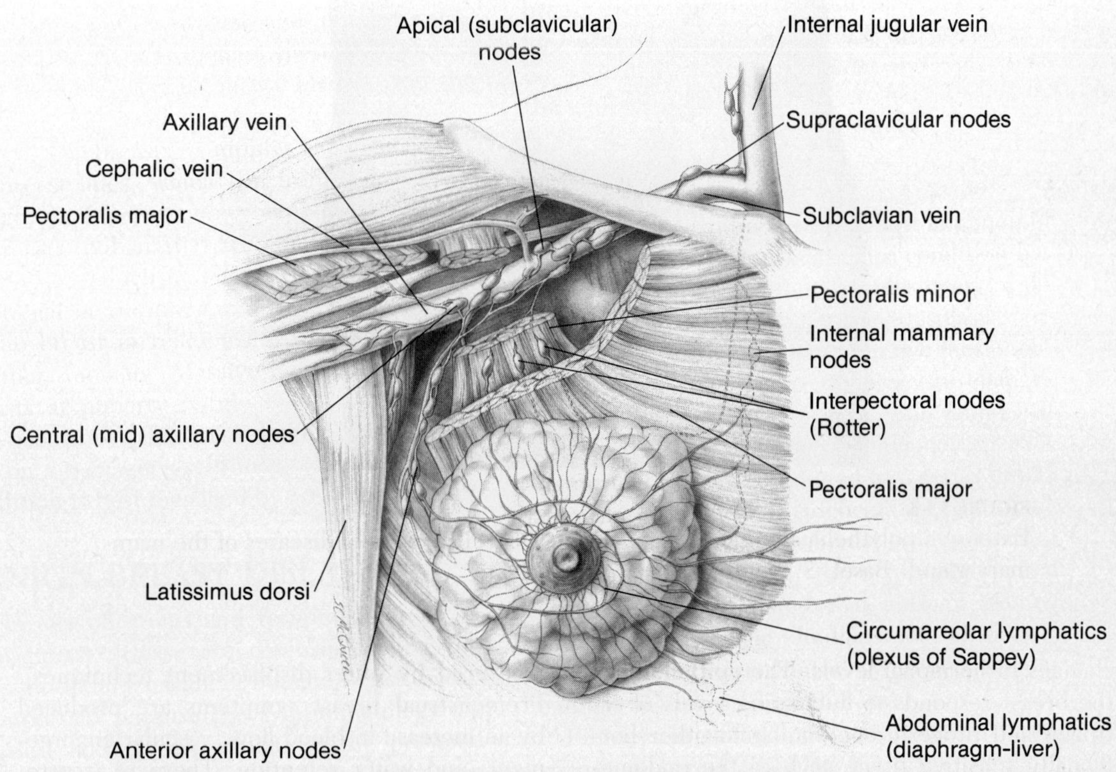

FIGURE 13-2
Lymphatics of breast. (From Rehman, I: Embryology and anatomy of the breast. In Gallager HS, Leis HP, Synderman RK, et al eds: The breast. St. Louis, C.V. Mosby Co., 1978, p. 17.)

ogy is believed to be an imbalance of the ratio of estrogen to progesterone with a relative lack of progesterone. However, Peters and others have postulated that fibrocystic changes are secondary to increased daily prolactin production.

The classic symptom of fibrocystic changes is cyclic bilateral breast pain. The signs of fibrocystic change include increased engorgement and density of the breasts, excessive nodularity, rapid change and fluctuation in the size of cystic areas, increased tenderness, and occasionally spontaneous nipple discharge. Both signs and symptoms are most disturbing during the premenstrual phase of the cycle. The breast pain is bilateral, and it is difficult for the patient to localize. Often the pain radiates to the shoulders and upper arms. Severe localized pain may occur when a simple cyst undergoes rapid expansion. The differential diagnosis of breast pain includes referred pain from a dorsal radiculitis or inflammation of the costal chondral junction (Tietze's syndrome). The latter two conditions have symptoms that are not cyclic and are unrelated to the menstrual cycle.

On physical examination the findings of excessive nodularity of fibrocystic changes have been described as similar to palpating the surface of a plateful of peas. Multiple solid areas are rubbery and may seem more two dimensional than the three-dimensional mass associated with a carcinoma. The larger cysts have a consistency during palpation similar to a balloon filled with water.

There are three clinical stages of the condition, with each stage having associated predominant histologic findings. Clinically these stages have considerable overlap. They are described to develop an understanding of the natural history of the condition.

The first stage occurs in women in their twenties and is termed *mazoplasia*. Breast pain is noted primarily in the upper outer quadrants of the breast. The indurated axillary tail is in the most tender area of the breast. During this phase there is intense proliferation of the stroma.

The second clinical stage of *adenosis* occurs generally in women in their thirties. The breast pain and tenderness are premenstrual but less severe. Multiple small breast nodules vary from 2 to 10 mm in diameter. The histologic picture of adenosis demonstrates marked proliferation and hyperplasia of ducts, ductules, and alveolar cells.

The last stage is termed the *cystic* phase and usually occurs in women in their forties. There is no severe breast pain unless a cyst increases rapidly in size. In this situation a woman experiences a sudden pain with point tenderness and discovers a lump. Cysts are tender to palpation and vary from microscopic to 5 cm in diameter. The cysts in fibrocystic changes often regress in size. The fluid aspirated from a large cyst is straw colored, dark brown, or green, depending on the chronicity of the cyst.

The histology of fibrocystic changes is characterized by proliferation and hyperplasia of the lobular, ductal, and acinar epithelium. Usually proliferation of fibrous tissue occurs and accompanies epithelial hyperplasia. Many histologic variants of fibrocystic change have been described, including cysts (from microscopic to large blue domed cysts), adenosis (florid, blunt duct, and sclerosing), fibrosis (periductal and stromal), duct ectasia, apocrine metaplasia, intraductal epithelial hyperplasia, and papillomatosis. Ductal hyperplasia and atypia and apocrine metaplasia with atypia are the most prominent histologic findings directly associated with the subsequent development of breast carcinoma. If these two conditions are discovered on breast biopsy, the chance of breast carcinoma in the future is fivefold greater than in controls.

The treatment of fibrocystic disease depends on the severity of symptoms and varies from mechanical support of the breast to surgical therapy for intractable pain. The vast majority of symptoms can be controlled by medical therapy. If a persistent dominant three-dimensional mass develops during the course of the disease, a tissue biopsy is mandatory. Initial therapy of fibrocystic disease consists of the patient wearing a "support" bra, which provides adequate support for the breasts both night and day. Diuretics during the premenstrual phase occasionally relieve breast discomfort. Minton has been an advocate of advising patients to reduce their consumption of methylxanthines and tobacco. Methylxanthines are commonly found in coffee, tea, cola drinks, chocolate, and many nonprescription medications. Minton studied 106 women with fibrocystic changes and found that in 68% the condition resolved and in another 24% the clinical symptoms improved by decreasing consumption of methylxanthines and nicotine. However, a recent case-control study by Lubin and associates found no association between caffeine or methylxanthine consumption and benign breast disease.

Oral contraceptives or supplemental progestogens during the secretory phase of the cycle have both been used to treat fibrocystic change but the drug of choice for severe symptoms is danazol. Dosages of 100, 200, and 400 mg daily continuously for 4 to 6 months have been employed. Danazol relieves breast symptoms and decreases nodularity of the breast in approximately 90% of patients. This effect lasts for several months after discontinuation of danazol.

Patients who do not respond to danazol should receive a trial of bromocriptine or tamoxifen. Bromocriptine, an inhibitor of prolactin, is given continuously in a dosage of 5 mg daily. Tamoxifen is a synthetic antiestrogen commonly used as a chemotherapeutic agent for breast carcinoma. Tamoxifen competes with estradiol for estrogen receptors in the breast. Small clinical studies have documented a 70% relief of breast symptoms when tamoxifen is prescribed for fibrocystic changes.

On rare occasions a woman with severe fibrocystic changes is treated surgically by simple mastectomy. Indications for surgery include intractable pain not relieved by medical therapy, a history of multiple breast biopsies, or biopsy evidence of a precancerous lesion.

Fibroadenomas

Fibroadenomas are firm, freely mobile, solid, solitary breast masses (Fig. 13-5). They are the second most common type of benign breast disease. Fibroadenomas usually present in adolescents and teenagers. Typically the young woman discovers the painless mass accidentally while bathing. Growth of the mass is usually slow but may be quite rapid. Fibroadenomas do not change in size with the menstrual cycle, and they do not produce breast pain or tenderness.

The average fibroadenoma is 2.5 cm in diameter. Multiple fibroadenomas are discovered in 15% to 20% of patients. After surgical removal fibroadenomas recur in approximately 20% of women.

Sometimes it is difficult to distinguish a fibroadenoma from a cyst. If the mass cannot be aspirated with a needle, surgical removal is indicated. Only histologic examination will differentiate this lesion from a medullary or papillary carcinoma. Fibroadenomas can be removed without difficulty under local anesthesia. They are rubbery in consistency, well circumscribed, and easily delineated from surrounding breast tissue.

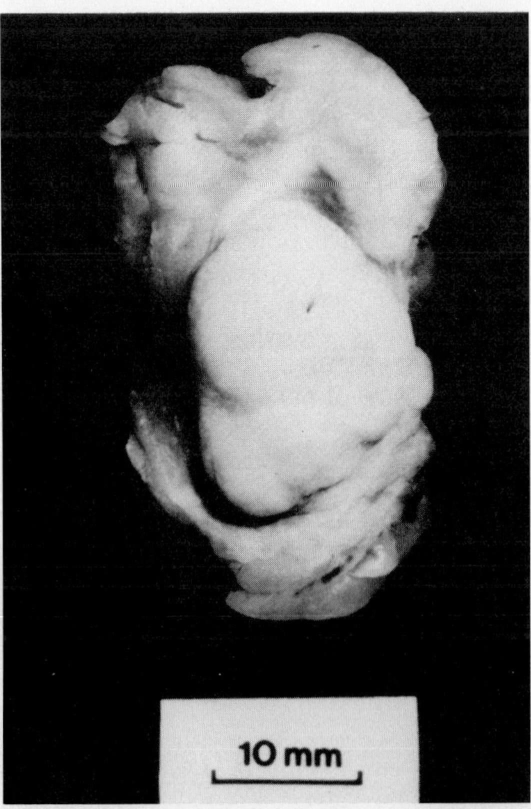

FIGURE 13-5
Surface of fibroadenoma adjacent to normal fibrous and fatty tissue of the breast. (From Millis, R: Principles of breast pathology. In Parsons CA, ed: Diagnosis of breast disease: Imaging, clinical features, and pathology. London, Chapman & Hall Ltd, © 1983, p. 5.)

Cystosarcoma Phyllodes

Cystosarcoma phyllodes are fibroepithelial breast tumors that usually arise from fibroadenomas. Cystosarcoma phyllodes are rare in that they represent only 2.5% of fibroepithelial tumors and 1% of breast malignancies. They are the most frequent breast sarcoma. These rapidly growing tumors are most common in the fifth decade of life. One in four of these tumors is malignant, yet only one out of ten metastasizes. If metastatic disease is discovered, it is the stromal tissue that predominates. Treatment of benign cystosarcoma phyllodes is local excision with a wide margin of normal breast tissue.

Intraductal Papilloma

The predominant symptom of an intraductal papilloma is spontaneous discharge from one nipple. This symptom usually appears in a woman in the perimenopausal age group. The discharge from the nipple is *spontaneous* and intermittent. The consistency of the discharge associated with an intraductal papilloma can be watery, serous, or serosanguineous. The amount of discharge varies from a few drops to several milliliters of fluid. During examination of the breast, it is important to circumferentially put pressure on different areas of the areola. This technique will help to identify whether the discharge emanates from a single duct or multiple openings. When the discharge comes from a single duct, the differential diagnosis involves both intraductal papilloma and carcinoma. If multiple ducts are involved, the diagnosis of

carcinoma is more likely. Intraductal papillomas are usually microscopic but may grow to 2 to 3 mm in diameter extending radially from the alveolar margin.

Nipple Discharge

Nipple discharge is a common complaint of women with both benign and malignant breast disease. Leis reported a series of 7588 breast operations; 85% had a mass, and 7% had a chief complaint of discharge from the nipple. Of the 560 patients operated on for nipple discharge, 493 findings were benign and 67 malignant.

To be medically significant, discharge from the breast should be spontaneous and persistent in a nonlactating woman. Many normal women can express a few drops of sticky gray, green, or black viscous fluid. The importance of diagnosing the etiology of *spontaneous* discharge from the nipple is to rule out carcinoma. The color of the discharge does not differentiate a benign from a malignant process. Malignancies have been associated with clear, serous, or serosanguineous or bloody nipple discharges. Cytology of the discharge is important but not invariably diagnostic. Most series document a false negative rate of approximately 20%. Therefore a negative cytology should not deter surgical biopsy.

Before surgical biopsy a patient with a per-

TABLE 13-1

Relation Between Nipple Discharge and Diagnosis in 432 Operations from New York Medical College 1960-1975

Discharge	Galactorrhea	Duct Ectasia	Infection	Intraductal Papilloma	Fibrocystic Disease	Cancer	Total
Milky	2	0	0	0	0	0	2
Multicolored and sticky	0	46	0	0	0	0	46
Purulent	0	0	14	0	0	0	14
Watery	0	0	0	3	1	5	9
Serous	0	5	0	79	52	11	147
Serosanguineous	0	8	0	59	34	14	115
Sanguineous	0	6	0	45	28	20	99
TOTAL	2	65	14	186	115	50	432

Reprinted with permission from Pilnik S: Clinical diagnosis of benign breast diseases. J Repro Med 22:286, 1979.

sistent discharge of any type should have mammography. In a young woman with a suspected intraductal papilloma the involved duct, which is usually blue, and a small area of surrounding breast tissue can be removed. Table 13-1 documents that intraductal papillomas and fibrocystic disease are the two most common etiologies of spontaneous nipple discharge. In this series 50 out of 432 patients had a carcinoma diagnosed by breast biopsy.

Fat Necrosis

Fat necrosis is rare but important because it is often confused with carcinoma. The patient presents with a tender, ill-defined breast mass that may have an area of surrounding ecchymosis. Occasionally there is skin retraction, which further confuses the prebiopsy diagnosis. The usual etiology of fat necrosis is trauma. However, the majority of women do not remember the event that injured the breast. Treatment of fat necrosis is excisional biopsy.

BREAST CARCINOMA

Epidemiology

The etiology of breast carcinoma is poorly understood despite extensive investigation. Epidemiologists, hoping to identify the etiology, have documented risk factors that predispose to or promote the induction of breast cancer. The risk factors can be divided into several categories: heredity, age, hormones, nutrition-demography, radiation, and previous breast disease. Generalizations concerning etiology follow similar categories: genetic predisposition, environmental carcinogens, viral agents, and radiation exposure.

Two problems obscure a clear understanding of the risk factors of breast cancer. One is the long latent period, 15 to 25 years, before the development of clinically recognizable carcinoma. The other is the consideration both of the duration and the intensity of factors that may induce or promote cancer. For example, the peak incidence of breast carcinoma in Japanese women after the bombing of Hiroshima and Nagasaki occurred in women who were in the premenarcheal age group at the time of the atomic explosions. Subsequently these teenagers developed breast carcinoma in their mid-

thirties after the characteristic prolonged latent period. Korenman's estrogen window hypothesis suggests that the radiation (cancer inducer) acted with the background of the unopposed estrogen of adolescents (cancer promoter).

Although there are limits in the clinical applicability of risk factors, women at increased risk should be screened at more frequent intervals. Many risk factors are additive. Risk factors are estimates developed by epidemiologists that allow patients and physicians to consider the probability of developing the disease. They have been widely publicized in the lay press. The fact that has not been emphasized is that risk factors identify *only* 25% of women who will eventually develop breast carcinoma.

The United States has one of the highest rates of breast carcinoma in the world. Presently in the United States approximately 130,000 new cases are diagnosed, and approximately 41,000 deaths occur yearly from breast carcinoma. The specific risk to an American woman of developing a breast carcinoma is 1 in 10 (10%) during her lifetime. The risk for an American woman without a single risk factor is 1 in 17 (6%). Therefore the message concerning risk should be that every woman in the United States is at risk for breast carcinoma.

Berg has made an interesting comparison contrasting breast cancer with another common gynecologic neoplasm, carcinoma of the cervix. In women ages 35 to 39 the rate of breast carcinoma is 55/100,000 women per year. This rate is three times greater than the rate for cervical carcinoma in the same age group. The risk of breast carcinoma during a woman's lifetime is similar to the risk of lung cancer in a heavy smoker during his or her lifetime.

A genetic predisposition to develop breast carcinoma has been recognized in some families. This tendency is not strong enough to develop a specific genetic pattern of inheritance. The basic hypothesis is that women in susceptible families have a genetic predisposition to develop breast carcinoma when exposed to environmental carcinogens. The two to four times increased risk extends from the mother to first-degree relatives, that is, daughters and sisters. The highest genetic risk (sixfold to ninefold) occurs in first-degree relatives of a premenopausal woman who develops bilateral breast carcinoma.

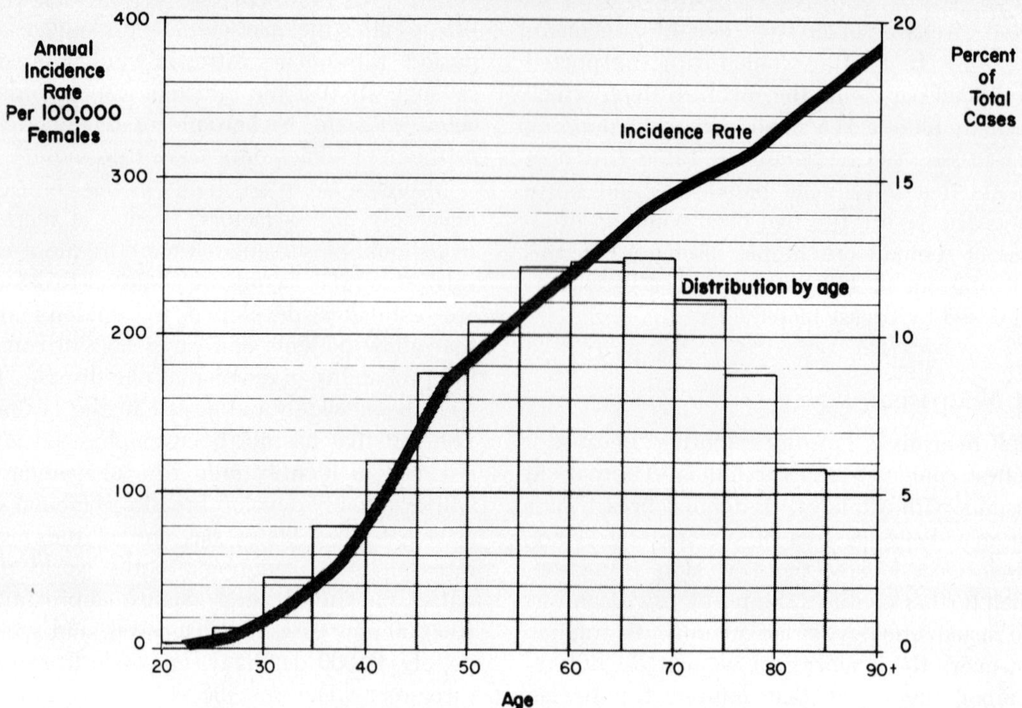

FIGURE 13-6

Incidence in the United States, by age, of female breast cancer. (From Seidman H, Mushinski MH: Breast cancer incidence, mortality, survival, and prognosis. In Feig SA, McLelland R, eds: Breast carcinoma: Current diagnosis and treatment. New York, Masson Publishing, 1983. Copyright by American College of Radiology.)

The frequency of breast carcinoma increases directly with the patient's age (Fig. 13-6). Breast carcinoma is almost nonexistent before puberty, and the incidence gradually increases during the reproductive years. Eighty-five percent of breast carcinoma occurs after the age of 40. During the perimenopausal years there is a brief plateau in the number of newly discovered cases. After menopause the incidence of breast carcinoma increases directly with a woman's age.

The relationship between endogenous ovarian hormones and breast carcinoma has been studied extensively. Several clinical observations support the hypothesis that the risk of breast carcinoma is related to the intensity and duration of exposure to unopposed endogenous estrogen. Cancer of the breast is most unusual in the prepubertal female. Bilateral oophorectomy before age 35, without hormonal replacement, reduces the risk of breast carcinoma by 70%. Women have an incidence of breast carcinoma 100 times greater than that of men. Coulam et al. have followed 1270 women with chronic anovulation. They discovered a relative risk of 1.45 for the postmenopausal development of breast carcinoma in women with a history of many years of premenopausal unopposed estrogen. Their study is another example of the prolonged latent period between exposure and development of clinical disease.

Obese women are at a higher risk for developing breast carcinoma during the postmenopausal years. The pathophysiology of this tendency is believed to be an increased amount of peripheral conversion of androstenedione to estrone and decreased levels of sex hormone binding globulin. Marchant described the increased risk associated with prolonged menstrual function. Women with spontaneous menopause before age 45 experience one half the risk of developing breast carcinoma as do women who are still menstruating at age 54. A similar study documented a twofold increased risk for women who menstruated for 40 years or longer contrasted with that for women who menstruated for 30 years or less.

Demographic data describe significant variations in the incidence of breast carcinoma from country to country. De Waard in a descriptive review of the epidemiology of breast carcinoma points out that women living in the United States have a much higher rate of breast carcinoma than women living in Africa, Asia, or the Middle East. The age-specific incidence of breast carcinoma in American women is six times greater than among women in Japan. Interestingly, studies of Japanese families who moved to the United States demonstrate that their rate of breast carcinoma becomes similar to that of American women after two generations. The demographic data are believed to be due to differences in total dietary fat and obesity. Epidemiologic studies performed within the same culture have demonstrated differences in incidences of breast cancer directly related to the amount of fat in the diet.

Ionizing radiation is a definite risk factor because of the long-accepted relationship between radiation and malignant transformation. The experience of Japanese women who survived the atomic bomb has been discussed. There are small groups of women who received either multiple radiation treatments for postpartum mastitis or multiple fluoroscopic examinations for respiratory disease who have subsequently developed breast carcinoma at an increased rate. Women with immunologic deficiencies are at a slightly greater risk of breast carcinoma.

Previous history of breast disease is an important risk factor. Once the patient has developed carcinoma of one breast, her risk is approximately 1% per year of developing cancer in the other breast. As stated previously, the extent of epithelial hyperplasia and atypia in women with benign breast disease determines the magnitude of risk for developing carcinoma.

The age at which a woman delivers her first child is more important as a risk factor than parity. If a woman's first term birth occurs before age 20, she has 50% less risk than a nulliparous woman. If the first term pregnancy occurs after 35, the risk is 1.5 times greater than that for women who have their first baby before age 26. For many years it was believed that nursing an infant offered a protective effect for the future development of breast neoplasia. Subsequent studies have documented that nursing is neither a positive nor a negative risk factor. Reserpine, which elevates prolactin levels, has been shown not to be a risk factor. Rosenberg et al. could find no relationship between cigarette smoking and the incidence of breast cancer.

The vast majority of studies involving exogenous estrogen either in oral contraceptives or given to postmenopausal women have not reported an increased incidence of subsequent breast carcinoma.

Detection and Diagnosis

Detection of breast carcinoma is defined as the use of tests in asymptomatic women at periodic intervals to discover breast neoplasms. The advantage of early detection and diagnosis is reduced mortality because of smaller-sized cancers, more localized lesions, and a lower percentage of positive nodes. Established methods of detection include self-examination of the breasts, periodic examination by physicians, and mammography.

Physical examination and mammography are complementary procedures that must be considered together. Self-examination has the major advantages of no cost to the patient and convenience. Thermography and ultrasound are unproven as methods to detect early breast carcinoma and should be considered experimental. Diagnosis can be established only by biopsy. A negative mammogram does not rule out breast carcinoma.

The kinetics of growth in breast carcinoma are important for understanding screening and detection. The average breast mass doubles in volume every 100 days and doubles in diameter every 300 days. A breast carcinoma grows for 6 to 8 years before reaching a diameter of 1 cm. In slightly less than another year the carcinoma will reach 2 cm in diameter. The mean diameter of a breast mass discovered by women who perform breast self-examination at monthly intervals is 2 cm.

Greenwald et al. studied the results of breast self-examination and of physician examination on the stage of breast carcinoma at initial diagnosis. Of 293 women with breast carcinoma, cancer was detected in clinical stage 1 in 54% when the detection method was routine physical examination, in 38% when the detection method was self–breast examination, and in only 27% when the detection of the mass was accidental. In their study, only 50% of women who performed breast self-examination did so on a monthly basis. These authors estimated that the breast cancer mortality might be reduced 19% by self-examination and 24% by annual examination of the breasts by physicians.

In a more recent study, Foster and Costanza determined the relationship between breast self-examination and survival of breast cancer patients. Their study group included 1004 newly diagnosed invasive breast carcinomas in Vermont from July 1975 to December 1982. During this time there was not widespread use of screening mammography in their state. The survival rate at 5 years was 75% for women who examined their own breasts versus 57% for women who did not examine their breasts. The authors concluded that in their population, breast self-examination was responsible for earlier detection, improved survival, smaller tumor size, and fewer axillary node metastases. Their findings persisted after controlling the analysis for the potential bias of confounding variables such as age, length-biased sampling, and lead-time bias.

Self-Examination of the Breasts

The majority of breast masses are initially discovered by the patient, either accidentally or during breast self-examinations (BSE). In a group of women having annual mammography and physical examinations by physicians, one out of three carcinomas was discovered by the patients in the interval between professional detection methods. Even with widespread national publicity, approximately 50% of women do not perform monthly BSE. However, over 90% of women who regularly practice BSE were instructed in the techniques by their physicians. It is ironic that the group of women who are most eager to perform BSE are women between the ages of 18 and 34. This age group has the greatest anxiety concerning breast cancer, yet because of their young age they are at the lowest risk. In Foster's study of newly di-

agnosed carcinomas, 424 women performed BSE and 411 did not. The average size of the breast mass in women who performed BSE monthly was 2.1 cm. For those who performed BSE less than monthly it was 2.4 cm; for the nonexaminers, 3.2 cm

The most effective teaching of BSE occurs in a one-to-one relationship. It is ideal to test the patient's ability to palpate masses in manufactured breast models. These models should contain masses with diameters as small as 0.3 to 0.5 cm.

Instructions for the patient concerning the techniques of breast self-palpation should emphasize timing, inspection, and palpation. The few days immediately after a menstrual period are the best time to detect changes in normal lumps or texture of the breasts. Postmenopausal women or women who have had a hysterectomy should be instructed to perform self-examination on the same calendar days each month. The patient should inspect her breasts in the mirror, looking for changes in shape and contour of the breasts and changes in the skin or nipples.

Palpation should begin in the shower, as many women have increased tactile sensitivity by using a "wet" technique. After the shower, the patient should lie down on the bed with one arm underneath her head. Using the pads of her fingers in a massaging motion with firm pressure, she should examine the entire breast and surrounding chest wall in a systematic fashion. One of the easier techniques to follow is to palpate the breasts in a clockwise fashion.

Physical Examination

The ability to detect breast lumps varies widely from physician to physician. Fletcher et al. recently tested the physical examination techniques of 80 different physicians using manufactured breast models. The simulated breasts of the mannequins had a volume of 250 ml and the consistency of the breast tissue of a 50-year-old woman. The ability to detect the mass was directly related to the size of the mass; 87% of 1 cm, 33% of 0.5 cm, and 14% of 0.3 cm masses were discovered. The most disturbing finding was the wide range of detection rates among physicians, ranging from 17% to 83%. In general, physicians with higher discovery rates spent more time performing the examination.

A thorough breast examination by the physician should take 3 to 5 minutes to complete. This time is also an ideal opportunity to instruct the patient in the technique of self-examination. A complete breast examination involves inspecting and palpating the breasts with the patient in the sitting as well as the supine position.

Initially, with a woman sitting on the examining table, the physician inspects the contour, symmetry, and vascular pattern of the breasts and skin for irritation, retraction, or edema. It is important to have the patient place her arms above her head and subsequently place her hands on her hips. This sequence will contract the pectoralis muscles, which may allow the physician to visualize an abnormality. The patient in the sitting position is in the optimal position for the physician to determine the presence of adenopathy in the axilla (Fig. 13-7).

The patient's breasts should be subsequently examined with the woman in the supine position. It is important to examine both nipples looking for retraction, skin irritation, or a discharge. The normal breast has a small depression directly below the nipple. The skin of the breast is again carefully inspected, looking for unusual vascular patterns, edema, erythema, or retraction.

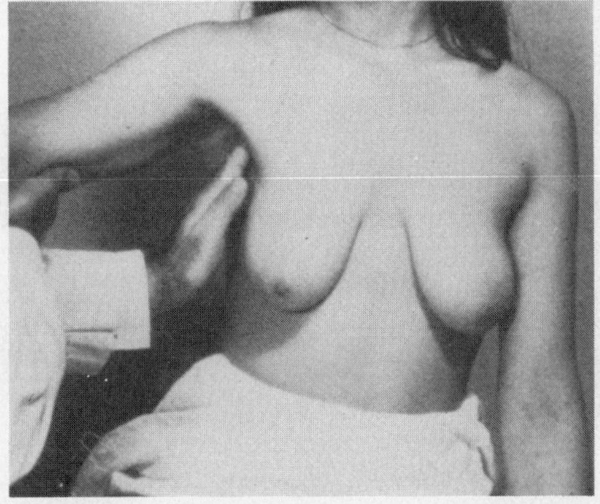

FIGURE 13-7
Examination of axilla in sitting position during breast examination. (From Marchant DJ: Clin. Obstet. Gynecol. 25:361, 1982.)

Palpation is performed with the patient's arms at her side and raised above the head and should not be limited to the breast tissue alone. The examiner should palpate the axilla, the supraclavicular areas, and the adjacent chest wall. Palpation should use the pads of the first three fingers places together, exerting firm but gentle pressure. Each physician determines his or her own systematic fashion, the majority preferring concentric circles. It is very important that the physician draw a descriptive picture of any positive finding. This picture should include notations concerning the site, shape, size, consistency, and mobility of the mass. Special notation should be made as to whether the mass is tender and whether it is attached to skin or deep structures (Fig. 13-8).

Mammography

Mammography is the only nonexperimental method of detecting breast carcinoma at an early and highly curable stage. Mammography is also the most accurate method of detecting breast carcinoma. The clinical advantages of discovering breast carcinoma during its earliest stage include higher percentage of localized disease, lower incidence of positive regional nodes, and reduced mortality. The 5-year survival of women whose breast cancer is believed to be localized to the breast with negative axillary nodes is 85%. In contrast, the 5-year survival is only 53% when axillary nodes are positive.

Most physicians are able to consistently palpate breast masses when they are 1 cm in diameter or greater. Mammography may discover fine calcifications in breast neoplasms months to years before the carcinoma enlarges to a size that may be palpated on physical examination. Studying the kinetics of growth of breast cancer helps the clinician to appreciate why breast carcinoma is so often a systemic disease. Breast carcinoma must develop neovascularization to grow beyond 1 to 2 mm in diameter. Neovascularization provides the breast carcinoma the capability of metastasizing via the vascular system. The average breast carcinoma grows for 3 years to enlarge from 1 mm to 1 cm.

There have been major improvements in image quality in mammography during the past

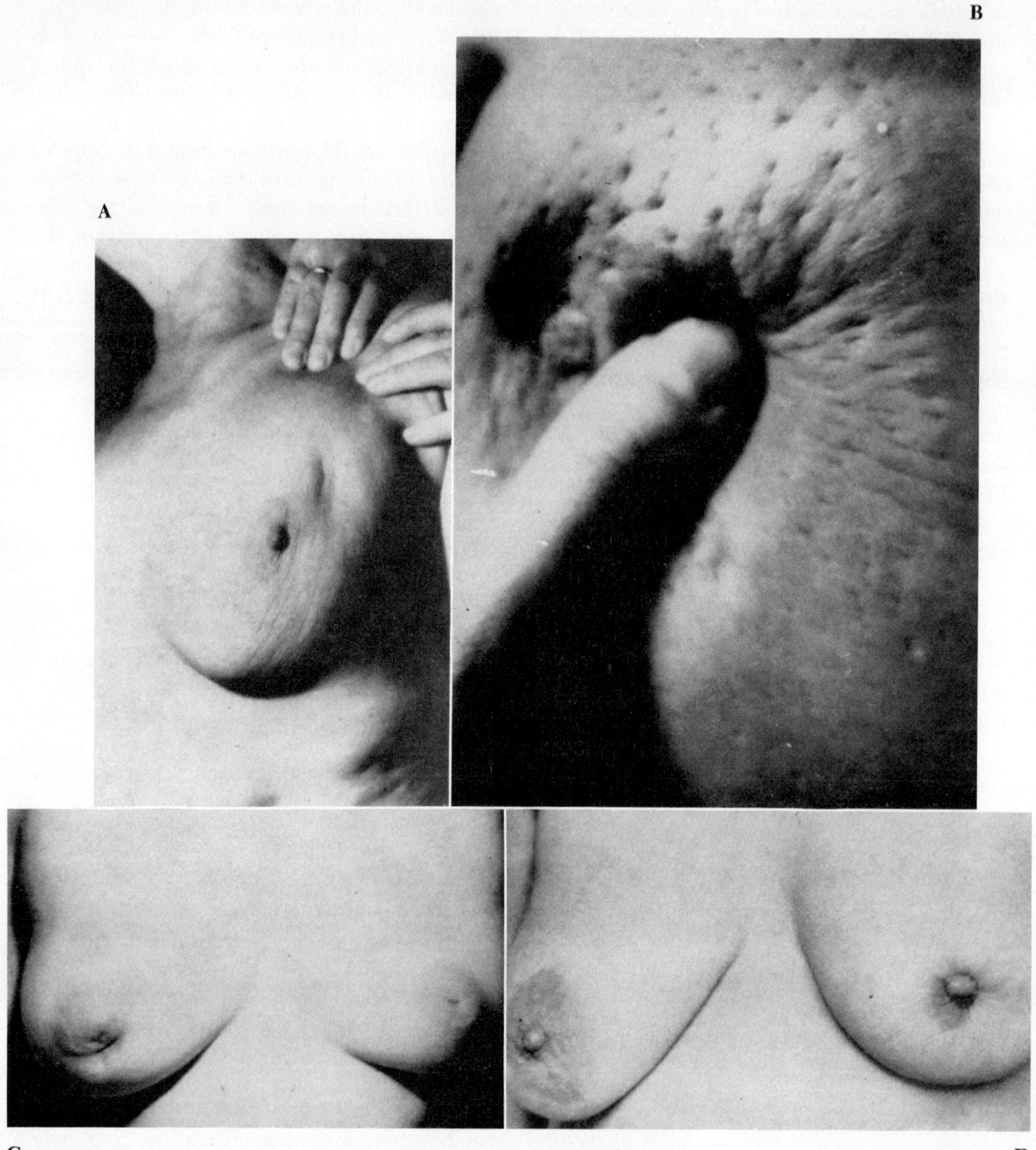

FIGURE 13-8

Signs of breast carcinoma. **A,** Retraction found during physical examination. **B,** Peau d'orange from underlying carcinoma. **C,** Retraction of right nipple. **D,** Retraction of left nipple from carcinoma. (From Degrell I: Atlas of diseases of the mammary gland. Basel, S. Karger AG, 1976, p. 20.)

10 years. New equipment has decreased the radiation exposure associated with mammography approximately tenfold. Because of these two changes, the guidelines regarding the use of mammography for detection of early breast carcinoma have been expanded. Conservative estimates are that 50 million American women should be screened by mammography each year. This challenge to radiologists has been summarized by McLelland. He believes there are two definite restraints on the optimal use of mammography to identify early breast carcinoma: a lack of properly trained and committed radiologists and the cost of the test. McLelland emphasizes that mammography is a technically demanding procedure that requires an experienced and meticulous interpretation of the films as well as correlation of the images with a thorough clinical examination.

Historically two landmark studies are the foundation of the scientific credibility of mammography as a screening procedure. Screening by definition is the search for breast disease in a large population, not all of whose members will be asymptomatic. The first large randomized control study was undertaken in the early 1960s by the Health Insurance Plan of New York (HIP). The HIP investigation involved yearly screening by both mammography and physical examination for 5 years. The women were followed for 10 to 14 years, and the study demonstrated a 30% reduction in mortality from breast carcinoma in the women who had yearly mammography compared to the control group.

The second pivotal study was performed in 29 centers throughout the United States during the late 1970s. This immense undertaking was sponsored by the National Institutes of Health and was named the Breast Cancer Detection Demonstration Project (BCDDP). The BCDDP involved screening 275,000 women, and during the 5 years of the project, 3557 breast carcinomas were found, 42% discovered only by mammography. The definite improvements in mammographic diagnosis over the 12-year time interval between the two studies is documented by comparing their results. Cancer detection was approximately two times more frequent in the BCDDP study. In women aged 40 to 49, mammography found 39% of carcinomas in the HIP investigation compared to 85% identified in the BCDDP project. Most important in the detection of early carcinoma less than 1 cm, the results were 36% in the BCDDP versus 8% in the HIP.

In the mid-1970s there was an intense controversy over the risks versus benefits of mammography in women under the age of 50. At that time the benefits of screening premenopausal women were questioned, and the higher sensitivity of the breasts of younger women to the harmful effect of radiation was stressed. However, improved diagnostic techniques and equipment have eliminated the controversy, and the American Cancer Society expanded its recommendations for mammography in 1983 (Table 13-2).

Nemoto et al. surveyed 12,315 new breast carcinomas diagnosed in 1977. Patients initially discovered 73%, physicians found 23%, and only 4% were initially identified by mammography. It is speculated that these percentages will be reversed by the increased use of mammography during the mid-1980s.

Present recommendations to detect early breast cancer include encouraging all women to perform BSE annually after age 21. For women between ages 35 and 40, it is important to emphasize annual physical examination of the breast for the rest of their lives and to obtain a baseline mammogram. Between ages 40 to 49 a mammogram is obtained approximately every 1 to 2 years. After age 50, every asymptomatic woman should have a mammogram at least at

---

TABLE 13-2

American Cancer Society Guidelines for Mammographic Screening of Asymptomatic Women

---

1. Base-line mammogram for all women at age 35 to 40 years.
2. Mammography at 1- to 2-year intervals from 40 to 49 years.
3. Annual mammogram for women 50 years or older.

From Kopans DB, Meyer JE, Sadowsky N: Breast imaging. N Engl J Med 310:966, 1984. Reprinted by permission of The New England Journal of Medicine.

yearly intervals. Obviously, more frequent physical examinations and mammograms may be indicated depending on individual risk factors and the finding of precursors of breast carcinoma.

Mammography is established as part of the diagnostic work-up of women with breast symptoms. Often significant occult disease is identified in another quadrant of the same breast or in the contralateral breast. All patients with breast masses or persistent spontaneous nipple discharge should have mammograms of both breasts before biopsy. Mammography is also indicated in evaluating a breast mass the patient has found but that the physician cannot confirm by palpation. This technique is helpful in difficult clinical problems such as the evaluation of large breasts or following augmentation mammoplasty. It is important to stress once again that mammography and physical examination are complementary procedures. One procedure does not replace the necessity of carefully performing the other.

There are two major types of radiologic equipment to obtain mammography: xeromammography and screen film mammography. Although there are minor advantages and disadvantages of each technique, the sensitivity and specificity of mammography depend primarily on the skill of the technician and radiologist and not on the equipment used.

In xeromammography the image is produced by a photoelectric process on aluminum plates coated with selenium. The two definite advantages of xeromammograms are wide recording latitude and edge enhancement. Wide recording latitude emphasizes subtle differences in density of breast tissues. The edge-enhancement phenomenon improves the visualization of microcalcifications and spiculations, especially in dense breasts.

Screen film mammography was developed initially to reduce the radiation exposure from mammography by the use of specialized x-ray equipment. This technique is excellent to delineate soft tissue masses from surrounding tissue. Reduced exposure time causes less distortion of the image by motion. This technique requires vigorous breast compression to obtain optimal results, including uniform tissue thickness, maximal geometric detail, and increased image contrast.

Optimal identification of early breast carcinoma by mammography depends on a competent technician's obtaining excellent images and the radiologist's searching for subtle changes. Breast cancer may be detected by visualizing clusters of fine calcifications or spiculations or ill-defined multinodular masses with irregular contours, all characteristic of malignancy.

Calcifications are often smaller than 0.5 mm in diameter and thus must be identified by a magnifying lens. The presence of five or more calcifications within a volume of 1 cm^3 is termed a cluster. Subsequent breast biopsies will find 25% of clusters associated with cancer and 75% with benign disease.

Sickles emphasized the importance of vigorous breast compression to spread apart areas of dense tissue within the breast and possibly identify "hidden" carcinoma (Fig. 13-9). He further advocated the importance of side-by-side comparison of both breasts and evaluating current films with previous ones. This facilitates identification of the less classic, indirect signs of breast carcinoma, such as a single dilated duct with intraductal carcinoma, asymptomatic architectural distortion in dense breasts, and a developing density.

The relationship between high levels of radiation and increased risk for breast carcinoma raises questions concerning the relative risk of the carcinogenic effect of diagnostic mammography. Long-term studies of fluoroscopy patients and survivors of the atomic explosion who were exposed to less than 100 rads (1 Gy) do not show an increased rate of breast carcinoma.

Feig has measured the radiation dose to the breast by state-of-the-art mammography equipment as 0.1 to 0.8 rad (1 to 8 mGy) for a two-view examination. A special committee of the National Research Council estimated that the low dose of radiation exposure involved in mammography might produce one excess breast carcinoma per year per 1 million women. Wilson has compared this radiation risk to other risks of life. This risk of death is similar to driving 300 miles by car, riding a bike for 10 miles, or a 60-year-old woman living for 20 minutes.

The national incidence of breast carcinoma is 1000 cases per million women per year for women in their early 40s. There is no evidence

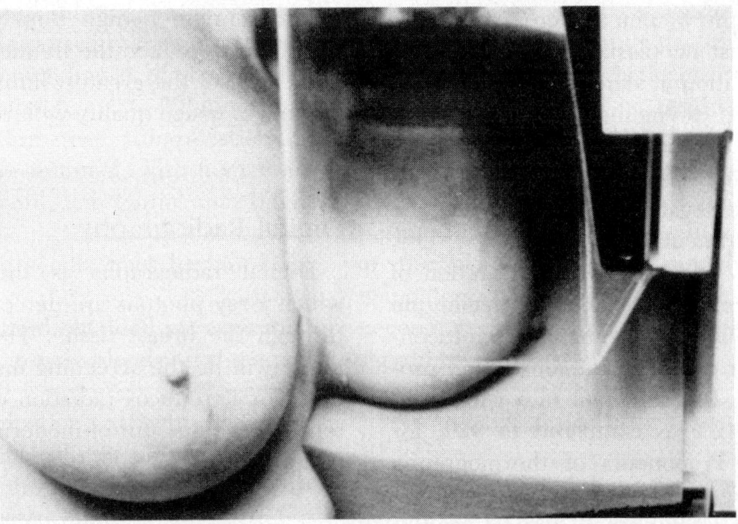

FIGURE 13-9
Photograph of mammography being performed with oblique technique with appropriate compression applied. (From Wilson OL: Mammographic technique. In Parsons CA, ed: Diagnosis of breast disease: Imaging, clinical features, and pathology. London, Chapman & Hall Ltd, © 1983, p. 67.)

of synergism between radiation risk and other risks such as genetic and nutritional factors. In summary, the risk of radiation from mammography is negligible compared to the benefits of the discovery of early and potentially curable breast carcinoma.

Ultrasound

Ultrasound has a definite role as a complementary procedure to other imaging techniques in the diagnosis of breast disease. The primary advantage of ultrasound is the ability to produce images of breast tissue on multiple occasions without harmful effects. The greatest limitation of ultrasonography of the breast is the limited spatial resolution. Microcalcifications are not visualized because resolution of less than 2 mm is difficult with ultrasound. Sonography cannot differentiate benign from malignant masses.

Ultrasonography of the breast can be performed by a hand-held transducer, the water tank immersion, or water bag techniques. Breast cancer is usually hypoechoic, and early cancers are difficult to distinguish from surrounding normal hypoechoic breast tissue. Ultrasound is helpful in differentiating a cystic breast mass from a solid mass when the mass cannot be aspirated. This imaging technique is also useful in diagnosing women with augmentation mammoplasty and in the differential diagnosis of breast masses in teenagers.

Sickles et al. recently reported a comparison study using state-of-the-art equipment. Mammography detected 62 of 64 (97%) carcinomas, while ultrasound diagnosed only 37 of 64 (58%). Only 8% of carcinomas smaller than 1 cm in diameter were discovered by ultrasound. The majority of breast carcinomas visualized by ultrasound can be palpated clinically. In a small series of 31 proven carcinomas, Egan and Egan found 68% diagnosed by ultrasound versus 77% by mammography.

In summary, ultrasound should never be used as a sole imaging technique for breast disease. It is more time consuming and expensive than mammography. Because of its lack of sensitivity and specificity for early breast carcinoma, it should not be used in an attempt to detect subclinical disease.

Thermography

Thermography is unreliable as a screening technique for breast carcinoma or as a tech-

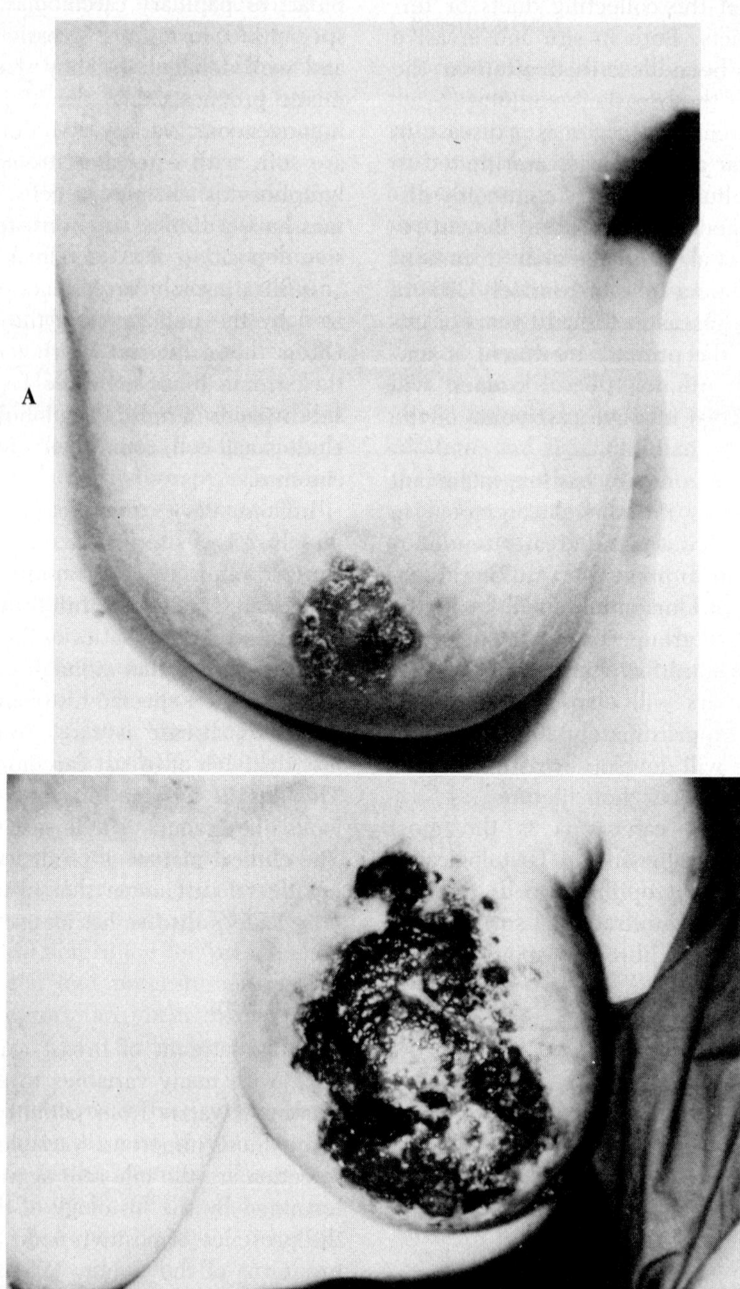

FIGURE 13-12
A, Paget's disease of left nipple. **B,** Extensive Paget's disease involving skin of breast. (From McKinna JA: Clinical features of breast disease. In Parsons CA, ed: Diagnosis of breast disease: Imaging, clinical features, and pathology. London, Chapman & Hall Ltd, © 1983, p. 38.)

static disease occurs early via both hematogenous and lymphatic routes. For example, 30% to 40% of women without gross adenopathy in the axilla will have positive nodes discovered during histologic examination. Two thirds of all women with breast carcinoma eventually develop distant metastatic disease regardless of the type of initial therapy. Fifty percent of women diagnosed eventually die of the disease (Table 13-4). The major changes in management of breast carcinoma over the past 10 to 20 years have resulted from changing concepts regarding the biology of the disease, with the understanding that many women with breast carcinoma have systemic disease at the time the diagnosis is initially established. It is beyond the scope of this book to present the details of treatment of breast carcinoma.

Veronesi et al. have listed the three major objectives of treating breast carcinoma: control of local disease, treatment of distant metastasis, and improved quality of life for women treated for the disease. There are several methods of controlling local disease. However, no difference in long-term survival rates has been documented, regardless of the extent of surgical therapy or aggressiveness of local radiotherapy. Chemotherapy is used not only for patients with proven metastatic disease but also for women at high risk for recurrent disease. Recent emphasis on conservative surgery (lumpectomy) plus radiation therapy to control mul-

TABLE 13-4
Stages and Survival of Women with Breast Cancer

Clinical Staging (American Joint Committee)	Crude 5-Year Survival (%)	Range of Survival (%)
Stage 1	85	82-94
Tumor <2 cm in diameter		
Nodes, if present, not felt to contain metastases		
Without distant metastases		
State II	66	47-74
Tumors <5 cm in diameter		
Nodes, if palpable, not fixed		
Without distant metastases		
Stage III	41	7-80
Tumor >5 cm or,		
Tumor any size with invasion of skin or attached to chest wall		
Nodes in supraclavicular area		
Without distant metastases		
State IV	10	—
With distant metastases		

Histologic Staging (NSABP*)	Crude Survival (%)		5-Year Disease-Free Survival (%)
	5-Year	10-Year	
All patients	63.5	45.9	60.3
Negative axillary lymph nodes	78.1	64.9	82.3
Positive axillary lymph nodes	46.5	24.9	34.9
1-3 positive axillary lymph nodes	62.2	37.5	50.0
>4 positive axillary lymph nodes	32.0	13.4	21.1

From Henderson IC, Canellos GP: Cancer of the breast. N Engl J Med 302:18, 1980. Reprinted by permission of The New England Journal of Medicine.
*NSABP denotes National Surgical Adjuvant Breast Project.

TABLE 13-5
Ten-year Disease-free Survival Rates

	Conservation Surgery and Radiation	Radical or Modified Radical Mastectomy Alone
Minimal breast cancer	92%	95%
Stage I	78%	80%
Stage II	73%	65%

Reprinted with permission from Montague ED: Conservation surgery and radiation therapy in the treatment of operable breast cancer. Cancer 53:702, 1984.

ticentric foci of cancer within the same breast and on reconstructive surgery after simple mastectomy have improved the quality of life of women with breast carcinoma (Table 13-5).

Surgical Therapy

The decision concerning appropriate therapy and extent of the surgical operation to treat breast carcinoma should be made by the patient in consultation with the surgeon, radiotherapist, and medical oncologist who will treat her. As emphasized previously, the initial extent of disease, virulence of the neoplasms, and presence of estrogen and progesterone receptors are the key medical factors in the decision. Intensive discussions concerning breast reconstruction or external prostheses are important to help the patient and family contemplate the effects of surgery on body image. Morris et al. have studied the psychological and social adjustments to mastectomy in 160 women. These patients were followed at intervals of 3, 12, and 24 months after surgery. One in four women was still having problems with depression and associated marital and sexual problems 2 years after initial therapy.

Until 20 years ago radical mastectomy was the standard operation for carcinoma of the breast. Radical mastectomy was designed to control local disease by an extensive en bloc removal of the breast and underlying pectoralis major and pectoralis minor muscles and complete axillary dissection. It is a cosmetically mutilating operation, leaving a significant deformity of the chest wall. Recently, less radical operations have grown in popularity. The modified radical operation removes the breast and only the fascia over the pectoralis major muscle. The pectoralis minor muscle may be removed to facilitate a complete axillary dissection. Simple mastectomy includes removal of the breast without underlying muscle tissue.

The place of radical or modified radical mastectomy in early breast cancer has been challenged. Veronesi et al. published a controlled study of 701 women with carcinomas measuring less than 2 cm in diameter without palpable axillary lymph nodes. The women were randomized preoperatively into two treatment groups. One group of 349 patients had radical mastectomy. The other group included 352 women who had excision of a quadrant of the breast to control the primary lesion, axillary dissection, and radiotherapy involving both external and interstitial sources. Five-year survival rates were virtually identical—90% in both groups. Five-year disease-free survival rates were similar, 83% and 84%. Fisher and colleagues in the National Surgical Adjuvant Breast Project have recently reported similar findings.

It is important to offer every woman alternatives in treatment for early breast carcinoma. The cosmetic result obtained by lumpectomy and radiation therapy depends on the size and shape of the breast and the size of the initial tumor. For some women mastectomy followed by reconstructive surgery may give a superior cosmetic result. Postoperative adjuvant radiation is not indicated after simple mastectomy if the axillary nodes are negative.

Medical Therapy

Estrogen receptors and progesterone receptors are important predictors of extended disease-free survival in women with a breast carcinoma. The presence and concentration of receptors should be obtained at the time of the initial diagnostic surgery, as receptor status may change after radiotherapy or chemotherapy. In general, receptor-positive tumors are well differentiated and exhibit a less aggressive clinical behavior, including a lower risk of recurrence and lower capacity to proliferate. When estrogen receptors are positive, approximately 60% of breast cancers will respond to hormonal therapy; 80% response is noted when both estrogen and progesterone receptors are present. If estrogen receptors are negative, less than 10% of tumors respond to hormonal manipulation. Thus chemotherapy is the treatment of choice when receptors are absent.

Hormonal therapy includes ablative surgery and the addition of drugs that change endocrine function by blocking receptor sites or blocking synthesis of hormones. The most commonly used ablative surgery is bilateral oophorectomy in a premenopausal woman with breast carcinoma. Hormonal therapy is effective in producing a response in advanced metastatic carcinoma for approximately 1 year. Metastatic disease in soft tissue and bone is the most sensitive to hormonal manipulation. Tamoxifen, an oral antiestrogen, is an alternative to surgical castration. Adrenalectomy or hypophysectomy has largely been replaced by medical adrenalectomy using aminoglutethimide. Oral estrogens, depo-medroxyprogesterone, androgens, and danazol have also been used to treat breast carcinoma. Two endocrine agents used simultaneously do not produce better results than a single agent. However, Levine and Lippman have combined hormonal therapy and chemotherapy. They believe "synchronization" of the cancer with hormonal therapy improves the cytotoxicity of chemotherapy.

Adjuvant chemotherapy has produced positive responses and an increase in disease-free survival in several clinical studies. Initially, chemotherapy was selected to treat women with positive axillary nodes or remote disease. Recently chemotherapy has been given in hopes of eradicating occult metastatic disease.

It is now firmly established that combinations of cytotoxic drugs are superior to a single agent. The chemotherapeutic agents most frequently chosen for breast carcinoma include cyclophosphamide, methotrexate, adriamycin, 5-fluoroucil, and vinblastine. The average total response rate to combined chemotherapy is 55%. Approximately 10% to 20% of women treated with combination chemotherapy experience a complete remission for about 18 months.

KEY POINTS

- One out of ten women, 10% of American females, develop carcinoma of the breast during their lifetime.

- The classic symptom of fibrocystic changes is cyclic bilateral breast pain. The signs of fibrocystic changes include increased engorgement and density of the breasts, excessive nodularity, rapid change and fluctuation in the size of cystic areas, increased tenderness, and occasionally spontaneous nipple discharge.

- The importance of diagnosing the etiology of a *spontaneous* discharge from the nipple is to rule out carcinoma. The color of the discharge does not differentiate a benign from a malignant process.

- Intraductal papilloma and fibrocystic changes are the two most common etiologies of spontaneous nipple discharge.

- Risk factors identify only 25% of women who will eventually develop breast carcinoma.

———————— KEY POINTS, cont'd ————————

- In the United States there are approximately 130,000 new cases diagnosed and approximately 41,000 deaths yearly from breast carcinoma.

- The frequency of breast carcinoma increases directly with the patient's age; 85% occur after 40 years of age.

- Once a woman has developed carcinoma of one breast, her risk is approximately 1% per year of developing cancer in the other breast.

- Thermography and ultrasound are unproven as methods to detect early breast carcinoma.

- Mammography is the only nonexperimental method of detecting breast carcinoma at an early and highly curable stage.

- The 5-year survival of a woman whose breast carcinoma is believed to be localized to the breast with negative axillary nodes is 85%. In contrast, the 5-year survival is only 53% when axillary nodes are positive.

- For women between ages 35 and 40, it is important to emphasize annual physical examination of the breasts and to obtain a baseline mammography. For women aged 40 to 49, mammography should be obtained approximately every 1 to 2 years, depending on the patient's risk factors. After age 50, every asymptomatic woman should have mammography at least at yearly intervals.

- The radiation dose to the breast by state-of-the-art mammography equipment is 0.1 to 0.8 rad (1 to 8 mGy) for a two-view examination.

- If the fluid aspirated from a cystic mass in the breast is bloody or the mass remains, a biopsy should be performed. Cysts that recur within 2 weeks or necessitate more than one repeat aspiration should be biopsied.

- The incidence of carcinoma in biopsies corresponds directly with the patient's age. Approximately 20% of breast biopsies in women aged 50 are positive, and this figure increases to 33% in women aged 70 or older.

- Regardless of the diagnostic accuracy of imaging techniques and needle aspiration, open breast biopsy is the definitive step to establish that a breast mass is not carcinoma.

- The classic sign of a breast carcinoma is a solitary, solid, three-dimensional breast mass. The borders of the mass are usually indistinct.

- Infiltrating ductal carcinoma is the most common breast malignancy.

- Two thirds of all women with breast carcinoma eventually develop distant metastatic disease regardless of the type of initial therapy. Fifty percent of women will eventually die of the disease.

- Three major objectives of treating breast carcinoma are control of local disease, treatment of distant metastasis, and improved quality of life for women treated for the disease.

- The initial extent of disease, virulence of the neoplasms, and presence of estrogen and progesterone receptors are the key medical factors in deciding on the appropriate therapy for breast carcinoma.

- In general, receptor-positive tumors are well differentiated and exhibit a less aggressive clinical behavior, including a lower risk of recurrence and lower capacity to proliferate.

- When estrogen receptors are positive, approximately 60% of breast cancers will respond to hormonal therapy. If estrogen receptors are negative, less than 10% of tumors respond to a hormonal manipulation. Therefore chemotherapy is the treatment of choice when receptors are absent.

- Approximately 10% to 20% of women treated with combination chemotherapy experience a complete remission for about 18 months.

BIBLIOGRAPHY

Anderson I, Andren L, Hildell J, et al: Breast cancer screening with mammography. Radiology 132:273, 1979.

Bassett LW, Gold RH: Mammography, thermography, and ultrasound in breast cancer detection. New York, Grune & Stratton, 1982.

Beljan JR, Bohigian GM, Dolan WD, et al: Early detection of breast cancer: A council report from the Council on Scientific Affairs. JAMA 252:3008, 1984.

Berg JW: Clinical implications of risk factors for breast cancer. Cancer 53:589, 1984.

Betsill WL, Rosen PP, Lieberman PH, et al: Intraductal carcinoma: Long-term follow-up after treatment by biopsy alone. JAMA 239:1863, 1978.

Carlile T: Breast cancer detection. Cancer 47:1164, 1981.

Carlile T, Kopecky KJ, Donovan JT, et al: Breast cancer prediction and the Wolfe classification of mammograms. JAMA 254:1050, 1985.

Clark GM, McGuire WL, Hubay CA, et al: Progesterone receptors as a prognostic factor in stage II breast cancer. N Engl J Med 309:1343, 1983.

Coulam CB, Annegers JR, Kranz JS: Chronic anovulation syndrome and associated neoplasia. Obstet Gynecol 61:403, 1983.

Crile G, Cooperman A, Esselstyn CB: Results of partial mastectomy in 173 patients followed for from five to ten years. Surg Gynecol Obstet 150:563, 1980.

Degrell I: Atlas of the diseases of the mammary gland. New York, S. Karger, 1976.

De Waard F: Epidemiology of breast cancer; a review. Eur J Cancer Clin Oncol 19:1671, 1983.

Dodd GD: Mammography: State of the art. Cancer 53:652, 1984.

Egan RL, Egan KL: Detection of breast carcinoma: Comparison of automated water-path whole-breast sonography, mammography, and physical examination. AJR 143:493, 1984.

El Yousef SJ, Duchesneau RH, Alfidi FJ, et al: Magnetic resonance imaging of the breast. Radiology 150:761, 1984.

Feig SA: Radiation risk from mammography: Is it clinically significant? AJR 143:469, 1984.

Feller WF: Evaluating a solitary breast lump. Contemp OB/GYN (special issue):107, 1983.

Fentiman IS, Cuzick J, Millis RR, et al: Which patients are cured of breast cancer? Br Med J 289:1108, 1984.

Fisher B, Bauer M, Margolese R, et al: Five-year results of a randomized clinical trial comparing total mastectomy and segmental mastectomy with or without radiation in the treatment of breast cancer. N Engl J Med 312:665, 1985.

Fisher B, Redmond C, Fisher ER, et al: Ten-year results of a randomized clinical trial comparing radical mastectomy and total mastectomy with or without radiation. N Engl J Med 312:674, 1985.

Fletcher SW, O'Malley MS, Bunce LA: Physicians' abilities to detect lumps in silicone breast models. JAMA 253:2224, 1985.

Foster RS, Costanza MC: Breast self-examination practices and breast cancer survival. Cancer 53:999, 1984.

Frable WJ: Fine-needle aspiration biopsy: A review. Hum Pathol 14:9, 1983.

Frantz VK, Pickren JW, Melcher GW, et al: Incidence of chronic cystic disease in so-called "normal breasts." Cancer 4:762, 1951.

Gambrell RD: Proposal to decrease the risk and improve the prognosis of breast cancer. Am J Obstet Gynecol 150:119, 1984.

Gautherie M: Thermobiological assessment of benign and malignant breast disease. Am J Obstet Gynecol 147:861, 1983.

Goldhirsch A, Stjernsward J, Zava D, et al: Randomized trial of chemo-endocrine therapy, endocrine therapy, and mastectomy alone in postmenopausal patients with operable breast cancer and axillary node metastasis. Lancet 1:1256, 1984.

Golinger RC: Hormones and the pathophysiology of fibrocystic mastopathy. Surg Gynecol Obstet 146:273, 1978.

Greenwald P, Nasca PC, Lawrence CE, et al: Estimated effect of breast self-examination and routine physician examinations on breast-cancer mortality. N Engl J Med 299:271, 1978.

Henderson IC, Canellos GP: Cancer of the breast, the past decade. New Engl J Med 302:17, 1980.

Hicks MJ, Davis JR, Layton JM, et al: Sensitivity of mammography and physical examination of the breast for detecting breast cancer. JAMA 242:2080, 1979.

Howe HL: Proficiency in performing breast self-examination. Patient Counselling and Health Education Fourth Quarter 151, 1980.

Kaufman DW, Miller DR, Rosenberg L, et al: Noncontraceptive estrogen use and the risk of breast cancer. JAMA 252:63, 1984.

Kopans DB: "Early" breast cancer detection using techniques other than mammography. AJR 143:465, 1984.

Kopans DB, Meyer JE, Sadowsky N: Breast imaging. New Engl J Med 310:960, 1984.

Korenman SG: Estrogen window hypothesis of the etiology of breast cancer. Lancet 1:700, 1980.

Korenman SG: The endocrinology of breast cancer. Cancer 46:874, 1980.

Lamas AM, Horwitz RI, Peck D: Usefulness of mammography in the diagnosis and management of breast disease in postmenopausal women. JAMA 252:2999, 1984.

Leis HP, Kwon CS: Fibrocystic disease of the breast. J Reprod Med 22:291, 1979.

Leis HP Jr: The significance of nipple discharge. In Schwartz GF, Marchant D, eds: Breast disease, diagnosis and treatment. New York, Symposia Specialists, 1980, p. 111.

Lester RG: The contributions of radiology to the diagnosis, management, and cure of breast cancer. Radiology 151:1, 1984.

Levine RM, Lippman ME: Breast cancer management: Recent advances and recommendations. Adv Intern Med 29:215, 1984.

Levitt SH, Mandel J: Benefits versus risks in conservation surgery with irradiation for breast cancer. Am J Med 77:93, 1984.

London RS, Sundaram GS, Goldstein PJ: Medical management of mammary dysplasia. Obstet Gynecol 59:519, 1982.

Love SM, Gelman RS, Silen W: Fibrocystic "disease" of the breast—non-disease? N Engl J Med 307:1010, 1982.

Lubin F, Ron E, Wax Y, et al: A case-control study of caffeine and methylxanthines in benign breast disease. JAMA 253:2388, 1985.

Lundgren B, Jakobsson S: Single view mammography: a simple and efficient approach to breast cancer screening. Cancer 38:1124, 1976.

Lundy J: What treatment alternatives for minimal breast cancer? Contemp OB/GYN p. 107, October 1983.

Marchant DJ: Epidemiology of breast cancer. Clin Obstet Gynecol 25:387, 1982.

McLelland R: Mamography 1984: Challenge to radiology. AJR 143:1, 1984.

Minton JP: Methylxanthines in breast disease. In Schwartz GF, Marchant D, eds: Breast disease, diagnosis and treatment. New York, Symposia Specialists, 1980, p. 143.

Montague ED: Conservation surgery and radiation therapy in the treatment of operable breast cancer. Cancer 53:700, 1984.

Morris T: Psychological adjustment to mastectomy. Cancer Treat Rev 6:41, 1979.

Morris T, Greer HS, White P: Psychological and social adjustments to mastectomy. Cancer 40:2381, 1977.

Moskowitz M: Mammography to screen asymptomatic women for breast cancer: AJR 143:457, 1984.

Nemoto T, Natarajan N, Smart CR, et al: Patterns of breast cancer detection in the United States. J Surg Oncol 21:183, 1982.

Nyirjesy I, Billingsley FS: Detection of breast carcinoma in a gynecologic practice. Obstet Gynecol 64:747, 1984.

Page DL, Dupont WD, Rogers LW, et al: Intraductal carcinoma of the breast: Follow-up after biopsy only. Cancer 49:751, 1982.

Parsons CA: Diagnosis of breast disease imaging, clinical features and pathology. Baltimore, University Park Press, 1983.

Paulus DD: Conservative treatment of breast cancer: Mammography in patient selection and follow-up. AJR 143:483, 1984.

Peters F, Schuth W, Scheurich B, et al: Serum prolactin levels in patients with fibrocystic breast disease. Obstet Gynecol 64:381, 1984.

Pilnik S: Clinical diagnosis of benign breast disease. J Reprod Med 22:277, 1979.

Redding WH, Monaghan P, Imrie SF, et al: Detection of micrometastases in patients with primary breast cancer. Lancet 2:1271, December 1983.

Rehman I: Embryology and anatomy of the breast. In Gallager HS, Leis HP, Synderman RK, et al, eds: The breast. St. Louis, The C.V. Mosby Co., 1978, p. 3.

Roberts MM, Jones V, Elton RA, et al: Risk of breast cancer in women with history of benign disease of the breast. Br Med J 288:275, 1984.

Rosen PP, Braun DW, Kinne DE: The clinical significance of preinvasive breast cancer. Cancer 46:919, 1980.

Rosenberg L, Schwingl PJ, Kaufman DW, et al: Breast cancer and cigarette smoking. N Engl J Med 310:92, 1984.

Rosenberg L, Miller DR, Kaufman DW, et al: Breast cancer and oral contraceptive use. Am J Epidemiol 119:167, 1984.

Senie RT, Rosen PP, Lesser ML, et al: Breast self-examination and medical examination related to breast cancer stage. Am J Pub Health 71:583, 1981.

Sickles EA, Filly RA, Callen PW: Breast cancer detection with sonography and mammography: Comparison using state-of-the-art equipment. AJR 140:843, 1983.

Sickles EA: Mammographic features of "early" breast cancer. AJR 143:461, 1984.

Strawbridge HTG, Bassett AA, Foldes I: Role of cytology in management of lesions of the breast. Surg Gynecol Obstet 152:1, 1981.

Sundaram GS, Manimekalai S, Wenk RE, et al: Estrogen and progesterone receptor assays in human breast cancer. A brief review of the relevant terms, methods, and clinical usefulness. Obstet Gynecol Survey 39:719, 1984.

Tabar L, Gad A, Akerlund E, et al: Screening for breast cancer in Sweden. In Feig AS, McLelland R, eds: Breast carcinoma: current diagnosis and treatment. New York, American College of Radiology and Masson, 1983, p. 315.

Verbeek ALM, Holland R, Sturmans F, et al: Reduction of breast cancer mortality through mass screening with modern mammography. Lancet 1:1222, 1984.

Veronesi V, Sacozzi R, Del Vecchio M, et al: Comparing radical mastectomy with quadrantectomy, axillary dissection, and radiotherapy in patients with small cancers of the breast. New Engl J Med 305:6, 1981.

Vorherr H: Breast aspiration biopsy. Am J Obstet Gynecol 148:127, 1984.

Problems of Prenatal DES Exposure

KEY TERMS AND DEFINITIONS

Abnormal Transformation Zone. Area in the vagina or on the cervix that may contain columnar epithelium and squamous metaplasia and that often contains intraepithelial neoplasia that has an abnormal colposcopic pattern.

Adenosis. The presence of glandular (columnar) epithelium in the vagina.

Cervicovaginal Ridge. A structural change in the cervix or upper vagina of DES-exposed females (hood, cockscomb, pseudopolyp, and collar).

Clear Cell Adenocarcinoma of the Vagina and Cervix. Rare genital tract malignancies that occur with increased frequency in DES females.

Colposcope. An instrument used to magnify and examine the epithelium of the transformation zone to identify abnormal areas in the lower genital tract that warrant biopsy.

Diethylstilbestrol (DES). An orally active synthetic nonsteroidal estrogen.

Ectropion. The presence of glandular (columnar) epithelium on the ectocervix (portio of the cervix).

Intraepithelial Neoplasia. Premalignant changes in the surface epithelium. This may also be termed dysplasia or carcinoma in situ, depending on its severity.

Müllerian Ducts. Paired structures in the embryo that in part lead to the formation of the female reproductive tract (primarily upper vagina, cervix, uterus, and fallopian tubes).

Normal Transformation Zone. Area of columnar epithelium and squamous metaplasia in the vagina or on the cervix that has normal colposcopic patterns.

Squamous Metaplasia. Physiologic process by which squamous epithelium replaces the columnar epithelium of adenosis and ectropion.

Uterine Constriction Ring and T-Shaped Uterus. Types of abnormal shapes of the endometrial cavity diagnosed by hysterosalpingogram in DES females.

Vaginal Epithelial Changes (VEC). Epithelial changes in the vagina of DES-exposed women that consist of adenosis or squamous metaplasia or both.

Diethylstilbestrol (DES) was initially synthesized in 1938 and was the first commercially available orally active estrogen. It is derived from the stilbene molecule and biologically acts in a fashion similar to steroidal estrogens such as estradiol (Fig. 14-1). Because it was relatively inexpensive and is orally active, its use for human therapy became widespread. In the late 1940s, DES treatment was used during pregnancy to prevent complications such as threatened abortion and prematurity. Many initial studies reported beneficial effects for DES pregnancy therapy, but some investigations in the early 1950s did not confirm these initial claims. The popularity of the drug for pregnancy support subsequently waned but continued into the 1960s. Finally, in 1971 it was noted that young women whose mothers took DES during pregnancy were at increased risk to develop a rare malignancy, clear cell adenocarcinoma of the vagina. Soon after this association was established, the use of estrogens for treatment of pregnancy complications in the United States was proscribed by the Food and Drug Administration.

The size of the DES-exposed population is unknown, but it is estimated that in the United States there have been approximately 3 million pregnant women treated with nonsteroidal synthetic estrogens, primarily DES. Soon after the initial association with clear cell adenocarcinoma of the vagina, intrauterine exposure to DES was also associated with clear cell adenocarcinoma of the cervix. Subsequently, a number of nonmalignant epithelial structural abnormalities of the female genital tract were also discovered in this population.

This chapter reviews the various malignant and nonmalignant alterations of the genital tract in DES females including changes that have been observed in their reproductive functions. The histogenesis of DES-associated genital changes is reviewed. In addition, a brief summary is provided of psychological studies of DES females and the current health status of DES-exposed males and mothers.

LOWER GENITAL TRACT (VAGINA AND CERVIX) ABNORMALITIES

Several nonneoplastic abnormalities of the cervix and vagina are found frequently in the genital tract of females exposed to DES in utero. These changes include vaginal adenosis, cervical ectropion, structural abnormalities of the cervix and upper vagina, and alterations in the shape of the endometrial cavity.

Vaginal adenosis (Fig. 14-2) consists of glandular (columnar) epithelium or its mucinous products in the vagina; cervical ectropion refers to similar changes on the ectocervix. The columnar epithelium of vaginal adenosis usually contains various cell types. One resembles the epithelium of the endocervix (Fig. 14-2, *A*), and the other contains cells that are similar to the epithelium of the endometrium and fallopian tube (so-called tuboendometrial cells [Fig. 14-2, *B*]). It appears that the clear cell adenocarcinomas arise from the tuboendometrial cell.

Squamous metaplasia is frequently seen with adenosis and ectropion and is the physiologic process by which columnar epithelium is re-

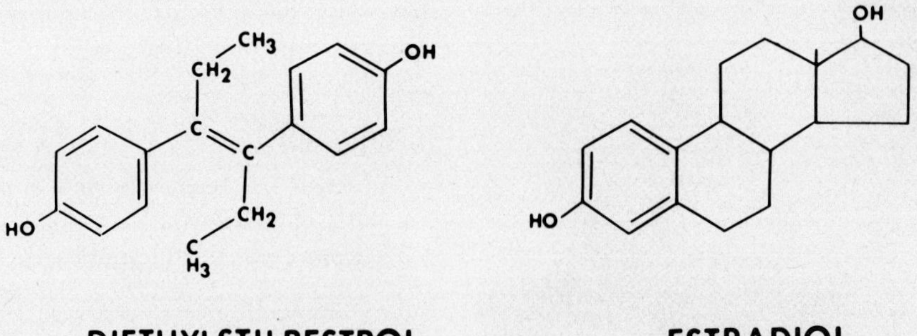

DIETHYLSTILBESTROL

ESTRADIOL

FIGURE 14-1
Structures of diethylstilbestrol and estradiol.

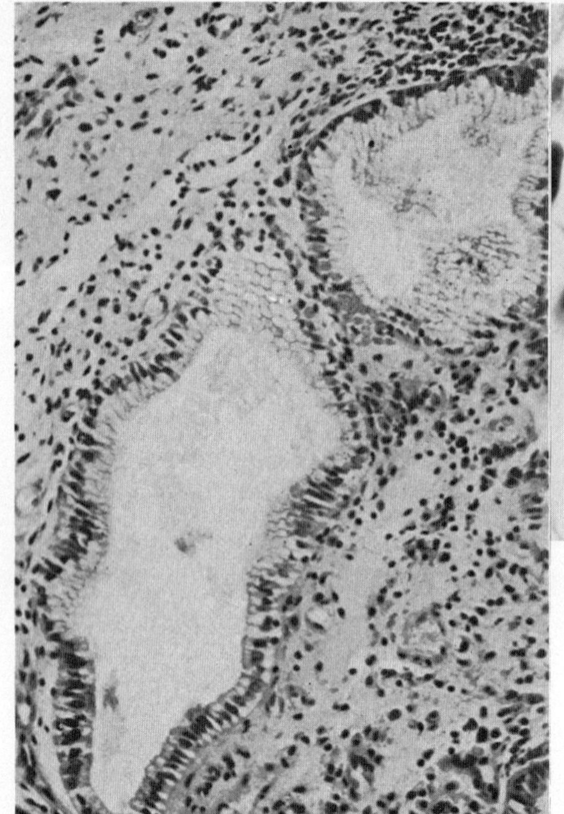

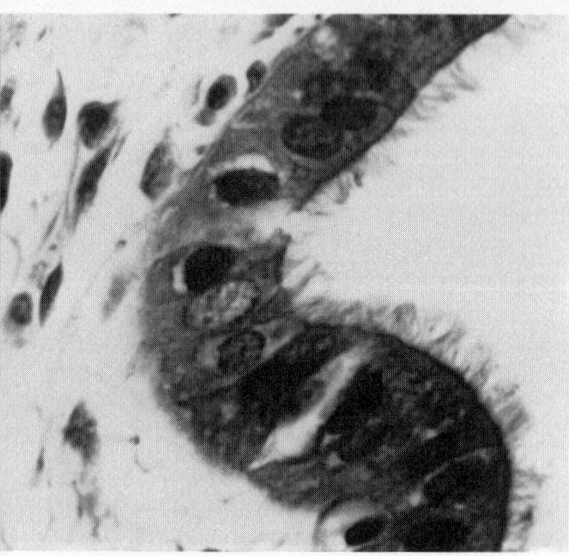

FIGURE 14-2
Vaginal adenosis. **A,** Glands are lined by endocervical-type epithelium (×200). **B,** Glands are lined by ciliated tuboendometrial cells (×890). (**A** from Herbst AL, Scully RE: Cancer 25:745, 1970. **B** from Herbst AL, ed: Intrauterine exposure to diethylstilbestrol in the human. Washington, DC, American College of Obstetricians and Gynecologists, 1978.)

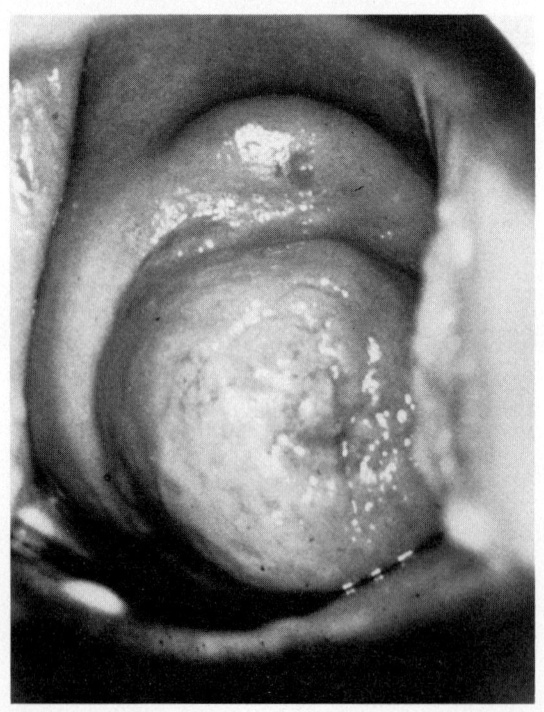

placed by squamous epithelium. This process occurs normally in both DES-exposed and unexposed females.

Structural malformations of the lower genital tract including transverse ridges, cervical collars, hoods, cockscombs, hypoplasia of the cervix, and pseudopolyps have been described (Fig. 14-3). Upper genital tract abnormalities (changes in the shape of the endometrial cavity) have also been identified on hysterosalpingogram examinations (Fig. 14-4).

Frequency

Adenosis has been reported to occur in 30% to 90% of DES-exposed subjects. However, data from case-control studies that are not in-

FIGURE 14-3
Vaginal hood. (From Robboy SJ, Scully RE, Herbst AL: J Reprod Med 15:13, 1975.)

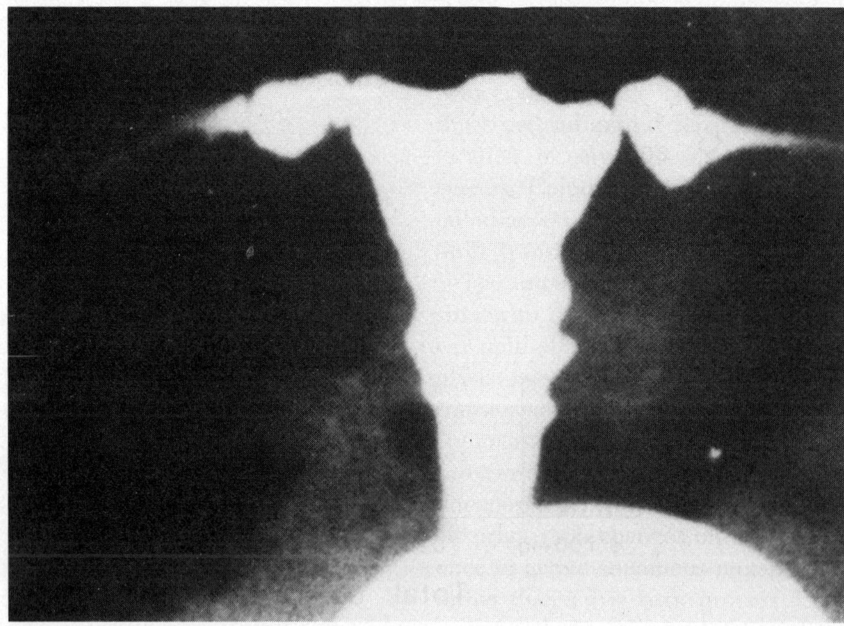

FIGURE 14-4

Hysterosalpingogram. Constrictions are noted in proximal portion of hornlike extension from uterine cavity. Uterine cavity is somewhat irregular. (From Am J Obstet Gynecol 137:299, 1980.)

fluenced by the potential bias of self-selection or physician referral suggest the overall prevalence is of the order of 30% to 40%. Specific risk factors affect the occurrence of vaginal adenosis in the exposed, including the age of the patient, the total dosage of the drug ingested by the mother, and the time during pregnancy the treatment was begun. The term vaginal epithelial changes (VECs) has been used by some investigators to indicate the changes of vaginal adenosis and squamous metaplasia in the vagina. Biopsy studies have indicated the highest rate of adenosis occurs among those whose mothers began DES in early pregnancy, and changes are rarely observed in subjects whose mothers started treatment after the eighteenth week. As shown in Fig. 14-5, dosage of DES and time started during pregnancy are important interrelated factors. A larger dosage of the drug or initiation of treatment early in pregnancy leads to a greater risk of adenosis. As subjects grow older, the columnar epithelium is replaced in many instances by squamous metaplasia (Fig. 14-6). Over a period of years the healing process appears to proceed in a high proportion of the DES-exposed subjects,

but in some the decrease in the size of the areas of columnar epithelium does not appear to have occurred (Table 14-1). The factors that seem to promote the changes of squamous metaplasia are not clearly identified, although some have theorized that a more acid pH of the vagina may accelerate the process. The highest rates of adenosis are seen in young subjects and those whose mothers ingested larger doses of DES and started treatment in early pregnancy. Cervicovaginal structural abnormalities (ridges, hoods, collars, etc.) occur in approximately 25% of DES-exposed subjects. The presence of these changes, like those of vaginal adenosis, is more common with higher dosages of maternal medication and an initiation of DES treatment early in pregnancy. These structural abnormalities also undergo modification over a period of years and in some subjects disappear entirely. As shown in Table 14-1 the epithelial changes of cervical ectropion decreased or disappeared in about three fourths of the subjects observed for up to 5 years, while ridges decreased or disappeared in one half and appeared to be stable in the remaining. Other factors that appear to decrease the frequency of structural changes of

a solid core of squamous epithelium that arises from the vaginal plate (Fig. 14-9). The vaginal plate grows cephalad from the urogenital sinus, and the solid core of squamous epithelium ultimately canalizes to form the permanent lining of the vagina, which consists primarily of squamous epithelium.

The laboratory mouse has been used frequently to study the effects of hormones on the developing genital tract. In the newborn mouse the vagina is immature, and the reproductive tract continues to develop neonatally, similar to the changes that occur in humans during the latter part of intrauterine life. By administering estrogens such as estradiol or DES to neonatal mice, it has been found that the squamous transformation of columnar epithelium is arrested, resulting in the persistence of müllerian-type columnar epithelium in the upper vagina and cervix.

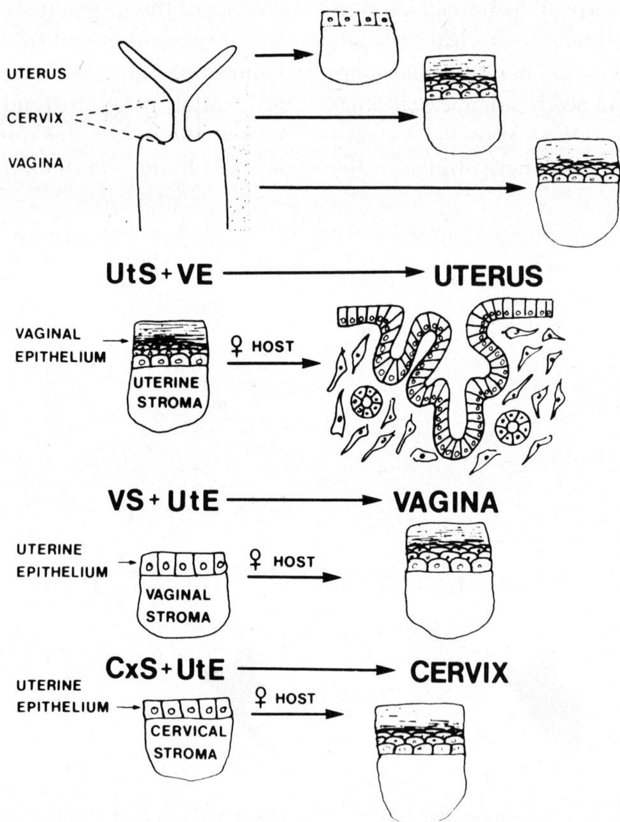

FIGURE 14-10

Summary of recombination experiments between epithelium and stroma from uterus, cervix, and vagina from neonatal mice (1 to 5 days old). Upper portion of figure depicts morphologic organization of epithelium in these organs: Uterine epithelium is a simple columnar glandular epithelium, whereas vaginal and cervical epithelium is stratified squamous. Uterine stroma *(UtS)* induces uterine morphogenesis and cytodifferentiation from vaginal epithelium *(VE)*. In reciprocal recombination composed of vaginal stroma *(VS)* plus uterine epithelium *(UtE)*, normally simple columnar epithelium is induced to differentiate as vaginal epithelium. Similarly, cervical stroma *(CxS)* induces development of stratified epithelium from *UtE*. (From Cunha GR, Fujii H: Stromal parenchymal interactions in normal and abnormal development of the genital tract. In Herbst AL, Bern HA, eds: Developmental effects of diethylstilbestrol [DES] in pregnancy. New York, Thieme-Stratton, 1981.)

In utero exposure to DES in humans may have a similar effect, that is, a DES-induced persistence of glandular epithelium in the vagina leading to adenosis. The increased risk of clear cell adenocarcinoma in subjects whose mothers began DES treatment in early pregnancy may in part be due to the larger area of ectopic glandular epithelium in the vagina of these patients. Insofar as clear cell adenocarcinomas are related to the tuboendometrial cell of adenosis, increased areas of tuboendometrial-type epithelium in patients exposed to DES in early gestation may provide a greater area for interaction with an unidentified carcinogen. Endogenous estrogens could act as such a promoter insofar as the adenocarcinomas primarily occur after the onset of menstruation. However, not all the factors that lead to the appearance of these tumors are understood at present.

The structural abnormalities of the uterus and cervicovaginal areas may also be associated with anomalous development of the müllerian ducts. Although the mechanism is not clear, some unfavorable pregnancy outcomes observed in DES-exposed women may be related to the configuration of the endometrial cavity or to anomalies of the cervix. A defect in the development of the myometrium or in cervical-uterine connective tissue is also possible. Recently it has been shown experimentally that the stroma of different parts of the embryonic female genital tract can have inductive effects that determine the histology of the overlying epithelium (Fig. 14-10). For example, combining cervical stroma with uterine epithelium leads to cervical differentiation, while combining vaginal stroma with cervical epithelium leads to vaginal epithelial development. These observations suggest a primarily stromal action of DES that could account for both the epithelial and the connective tissue abnormalities often observed. Presumably, DES ingested by the mother crosses the uteroplacental barrier and enters the fetal circulation. It is known that estrogen receptors develop in the fetal genital tract in early intrauterine life. Insofar as DES is a nonsteroidal estrogen, it appears that it may not be handled in the fetal tissues in the same manner as steroidal estrogens. This would allow it to have the developmental effects noted in exposed offspring.

The genital abnormalities associated with DES in humans pertain to the ingestion of any stilbene-type (see Fig. 14-1) estrogen. Ingestion of steroidal estrogens during pregnancy has not been reported to be associated with such changes.

PSYCHOLOGICAL STUDIES

There have not been extensive psychological studies of DES-exposed females compared to those of unexposed females. As might be anticipated, increased anxiety and concern have existed among the exposed population in regard to health risks they encounter as a consequence of intrauterine exposure to DES. A major problem has also been the guilt and anxiety felt by the mothers of these patients because of concern about damage to their daughters. The guilt is present despite the fact that the medication was prescribed in an effort to help them achieve a better outcome for the pregnancy with their daughters. A number of self-help and consumer groups have been formed to deal with some of these issues.

DES-EXPOSED MALES

Abnormalities have been described in DES-exposed males, including cryptorchidism, hypoplasia of the testis, and more frequent epididymal cysts as well as abnormalities in semen analyses. It should be remembered that the effect of DES on the female genital tract appears to occur primarily on the müllerian ducts. In the male genital tract the müllerian remnants are found in the epididymis of the testis and the utricle of the prostate. An increased risk in the development of malignancy in DES-exposed males has not been demonstrated. The testicular and semen changes observed with increasing frequency among DES-exposed males in some studies have not been verified in others. If cryptorchidism is confirmed to be more common among those exposed, an increased risk of testicular cancer would be expected, insofar as cryptorchidism is a known risk factor for the development of this malignancy in men. Because of the delay in childbearing among men in their twenties and thirties, analysis of fertility rates among DES-exposed men is not sufficient to evaluate adequately the risk of infertility in this group.

DES-EXPOSED MOTHERS

Because of the high doses of estrogen taken during pregnancy by DES mothers, there have been concerns of an increased risk of estrogen-sensitive tumors in this group. In particular, breast cancer and endometrial cancer, as well as other genital tract cancers, have been evaluated in case-control studies. Currently increased risk has not been conclusively demonstrated. Table 14-6 summarizes the occurrence of breast cancer, citing studies that have evaluated this in DES-exposed women. Two of the studies indicate no significant difference in breast cancer risk. The third study shows a slightly increased risk of breast cancer among

those exposed who are now over the age of 60 years. Currently the guidelines for breast cancer screening and examination in DES-exposed mothers is the same as for other women (see Chapter 13).

TABLE 14-6
Breast Cancer Occurrence

	DES-Exposed	Unexposed
Herbst, 1981	34/655	28/645
Brian, 1980	8/408	9.4*
Greenberg, 1984	118/3033	80/3033

*Expected number derived from general population statistics.

____________ **KEY POINTS** ____________

- Vaginal adenosis occurs in about one third of DES-exposed females.

- Cervicovaginal ridges occur in about one fourth of DES-exposed females.

- Vaginal adenosis is more frequent among those whose mothers took DES in early pregnancy, those whose mothers took DES at a higher dose, and in exposed females who are younger at the time of examination.

- Adenosis and ectropion usually heal by the physiologic process of squamous metaplasia.

- Adenosis, ectropion, and cervicovaginal ridges heal spontaneously in many but *not* all DES-exposed females.

- Unfavorable pregnancy outcomes, particularly premature birth, midtrimester loss, and ectopic pregnancy, occur in about one half of DES-exposed females.

- Over 80% of DES daughters have a liveborn child.

- Routine hysterosalpingogram studies are not indicated for DES-exposed females.

- Analysis of nuclear DNA content is useful to help distinguish intraepithelial neoplasia from squamous metaplasia.

- The risk of development of clear cell adenocarcinoma of the vagina and cervix is increased in DES-exposed females, but these tumors occur in less than 1 per 1000 exposed.

- Abnormal development of the müllerian ducts in utero results in reproductive tract alterations in the DES-exposed female.

- Factors that appear to increase the risk of development of clear cell adenocarcinoma in addition to intrauterine DES exposure include history of miscarriage in the mother and prematurity and fall season of birth of the daughter.

BIBLIOGRAPHY

Antonioli DA, Burke L, Friedman EA: Natural history of diethylstilbestrol-associated genital tract lesions: Cervical ectopy and cervicovaginal hood. Am J Obstet Gynecol 137:847, 1980.

Barnes AB: Menstrual history of young women exposed in utero to diethylstilbestrol. Fertil Steril 32:148, 1979.

Barnes AB, Colton T, Gundersen J, et al: Fertility and outcome of pregnancy in women exposed in utero to diethylstilbestrol. N Engl J Med 302:609, 1980.

Bibbo M, Gill WB, Azizi F, et al: Follow-up study of male and female offspring of DES-exposed mothers. Obstet Gynecol 49:1, 1977.

Brian DD, Tilley BC, Labarthe DR, et al: Breast cancer in DES-exposed mothers. Absence of association. Mayo Clin Proc 55:89, 1980.

Cousins L, Karp W, Lacey C, et al: Reproductive outcome of women exposed to diethylstilbestrol in utero. Obstet Gynecol 56:70, 1980.

Cunha G, Fujii H: Stromal-parenchymal interactions in normal and abnormal development of the genital tract. In Herbst AL, Bern HA, eds: Developmental effects of diethylstilbestrol (DES) in pregnancy. New York, Thieme-Stratton, 1981.

DeCherney AH, Cholst I, Naftolin A: Structure and function of the fallopian tubes following exposure to diethylstilbestrol (DES) during gestation. Fertil Steril 36:741, 1981.

Dieckmann WE, Davis ME, Rynkiewicz SM, et al: Does the administration of diethylstilbestrol during pregnancy have therapeutic value? Am J Obstet Gynecol 66:1062, 1953.

Dodds EC, Goldberg L, Larson W, et al: Oestrogenic activity of certain synthetic compounds. Nature 141:247, 1938.

Forsberg MD, Kalland T: Embryology of the genital tract in humans and in rodents. In Herbst AL, Bern HA, eds: Developmental effects of diethylstilbestrol (DES) in pregnancy. New York, Thieme-Stratton, 1981.

Fu Y, Robboy SJ, Prat J: Nuclear DNA study of vaginal and cervical squamous cell abnormalities in DES-exposed progeny. Obstet Gynecol 52:129, 1978.

Greenberg ER, Barnes AB, Resseguie L, et al: Follow-up study of mothers exposed to diethylstilbestrol in pregnancy. N Engl J Med 311:1393, 1984.

Herbst AL, Scully RE: Adenocarcinoma of the vagina in adolescence: A report of 7 cases including 6 clear cell carcinomas (so-called mesonephromas). Cancer 25:745, 1970.

Herbst AL, Ulfelder H, Poskanzer DC: Adenocarcinoma of the vagina: Association of maternal stilbestrol therapy with tumor appearance in young women. N Engl J Med 284:878, 1971.

Herbst AL, Scully RE, Robboy SJ: Effects of maternal DES ingestion on the female genital tract. Hosp Pract 10:51, 1975.

Herbst AL, Cole P, Colton T, et al: Age-incidence and risk of diethylstilbestrol-related clear cell adenocarcinoma of the vagina and cervix. Am J Obstet Gynecol 128:43, 1977.

Herbst AL, ed: Intrauterine exposure to diethylstilbestrol in the human. Chicago, American College of Obstetricians and Gynecologists, monograph, 1978.

Herbst AL, Hubby MM, Blough RR, et al: A comparison of pregnancy experience in DES-exposed and DES-unexposed daughters. J Reprod Med 24:62, 1980.

Herbst AL, Bern HA, eds: Developmental effects of diethylstilbestrol (DES) in pregnancy. New York, Thieme-Stratton, 1981.

Herbst AL, Hubby MM, Azizi F, et al: Reproductive and

gynecologic surgical experience in diethylstilbestrol-exposed daughters. Am J Obstet Gynecol 141:1019, 1981.

Herbst AL, Anderson S, Hubby M, et al: Risk factors for the development of DES associated clear cell adenocarcinoma: A case control study. Am J Obstet Gynecol 154:814, 1986.

Jeffries JA, Robboy SJ, O'Brien PC, et al: Structural anomalies of the cervix and vagina in women enrolled in the Diethylstilbestrol Adenosis (DESAD) Project. Am J Obstet Gynecol 148:59, 1984.

Kaufman RH, Adam H, Binder GL, et al: Upper genital tract changes and pregnancy outcome in offspring exposed in utero to diethylstilbestrol. Am J Obstet Gynecol 137:299, 1980.

Kaufman RH, Noller KL, Adam E, et al: Upper genital tract abnormalities and pregnancy outcome in diethylstilbestrol exposed progeny. Am J Obstet Gynecol 148:973, 1984.

Noller KL, Townsend DE, Kaufman RH, et al: Maturation of vaginal and cervical epithelium in women exposed in utero to diethylstilbestrol (DESAD Project). Am J Obstet Gynecol 146:279, 1983.

O'Brien PC, Noller KL, Robboy SJ, et al: Vaginal epithelial changes in young women enrolled in the National Cooperative Diethylstilbestrol Adenosis (DESAD) Project. Obstet Gynecol 53:300, 1979.

Robboy SJ, Scully RE, Herbst AL: Pathology of vaginal and cervical abnormalities associated with prenatal exposure to diethylstilbestrol (DES). J Reprod Med 15:5, 1975.

Robboy SJ, Szyfelbein WM, Goellner JR, et al: Dysplasia and cytologic findings in 4589 young women enrolled in Diethylstilbestrol Adenosis (DESAD) Project. Am J Obstet Gynecol 140:579, 1981.

Robboy SJ, Welch WR, Young RH, et al: Topographic relation of cervical ectropion and vaginal adenosis to clear cell adenocarcinoma. Obstet Gynecol 60:546, 1982.

Robboy SJ, Noller KL, O'Brien, P, et al: Increased incidence of cervical and vaginal dysplasia in 3980 DES-exposed young women. JAMA 252:2979, 1984.

Abortion

KEY TERMS AND DEFINITIONS

Abortion. Termination of pregnancy before 20 weeks' gestation calculated from date of onset of last menses. An alternative definition is delivery of a fetus with a weight of less than 500 g. If abortion occurs before 12 weeks' gestation, it is called early; from 12 to 20 weeks it is called late.

Aneuploid Abortus. An abortus with the number of chromosomes less or greater than the normal 46.

Cerclage. A circular ligature used to treat the incompetent cervix. The suture is placed beneath the epithelium of the cervix at the level of the internal cervical os.

Complete Abortion. Spontaneous expulsion of all fetal and placental tissue from the uterine cavity before 20 weeks' gestation.

Euploid Abortus. An abortus in which the chromosome complement is normal, 46X or 46XY.

Incompetent Cervix (Cervical Incompetence). Condition whereby the internal cervical canal dilates at 16 weeks of gestation or later resulting in recurrent premature pregnancy loss.

Incomplete Abortion. Passage of some but not all fetal or placental tissue through the cervix before 20 weeks' gestation.

Induced Abortion. Intentional medical or surgical termination of pregnancy before 20 weeks' gestation. Also called elective pregnancy termination if performed for woman's desires or therapeutic abortion if performed for reasons of maintaining health of the mother.

Inevitable Abortion. Uterine bleeding from a gestation of less than 20 weeks accompanied by cervical dilation but without expulsion of any placental or fetal tissue through the cervix.

Lupus Anticoagulant. An IgG or IgM immunoglobulin found in the serum of women with lupus erythematosus and other connective tissue disease as well as in women without systemic disease. The presence of this antibody is associated with recurrent pregnancy loss due to thrombosis in the placental circulation.

Metroplasty. A surgical procedure to unify the endometrial cavity of a bicornuate uterus or remove the septum of a septate uterus.

Missed Abortion. Fetal death before 20 weeks' gestation without expulsion of any fetal or maternal tissue for at least 8 weeks thereafter.

Recurrent Spontaneous Abortion. The loss of three or more pregnancies before 20 weeks' gestation. Functionally, however, many physicians will do a work up for recurrent spontaneous abortion after two or more pregnancy losses.

Septic Abortion. Any type of abortion that is accompanied by uterine infection.

Threatened Abortion. Any uterine bleeding from a gestation of less than 20 weeks without any cervical dilation or effacement.

Uterine Adhesions. Tissue within the uterine cavity that obliterates part or all of the endometrium.

About 15% to 20% of all known human pregnancies terminate in clinically recognized abortion. However, the incidence of total human embryonic loss is estimated to be much higher. In 1952 Hertig and Rock, using morphologic techniques, reported that about 40% of all human embryos either fail to implant or are aborted before the time of the expected menses. Edmonds et al., utilizing a specific assay for β-HCG in a group of normal women wishing to become pregnant, found that the fecundity rate in an ovulatory cycle was about 60%. However, these investigators reported that the total embryonic loss before 12 weeks' gestation was about 60%, yielding a clinical fecundity rate of 25% per cycle, similar to that found in several demographic studies. The majority of abortions in Edmonds' study were not recognized clinically. Since some fertilized ova do not implant and thus do not secrete detectable HCG, the rate of human pregnancy loss is probably even higher; it has been estimated by Léridon to be as high as 70% (Table 15-1). Therefore the process of human reproduction is inefficient. However, since most early pregnancy losses are due to chromosomal or genetic abnormalities, the high frequency of abortion, as stated by Austin, is "an important and valuable provision of Nature . . . and . . . is in the best interests of the race," as "disadvantageous features from gene mutation are prevented from being incorporated into the overall hereditary pattern."

About 80% of abortions occur in the first trimester, with the incidence decreasing with increasing gestational age. Harlap et al. reported that the incidence of clinical abortion is relatively stable during each week of gestation before 12 weeks and declines steadily thereafter (Fig. 15-1). These investigators also reported that if conception occurs within 3 months after a prior live birth, the incidence of abortion is increased compared to the relatively stable rate if conception occurs later than 3 months (Fig. 15-2).

Warburton and Fraser studied the incidence of abortion over a 10-year period in a group of more than 2000 women who had had at least one pregnancy of at least 20 weeks' gestation. The overall incidence of clinical abortion was 14.7%, and the risk of a pregnancy terminating in spontaneous abortion increased with increasing parity, maternal age, and paternal age (Table 15-2). Each of these parameters was an independent risk factor for abortion, and this

---

TABLE 15-1

Life Table for Intrauterine Mortality in the Human (Per 100 Ova Exposed to Risk of Fertilization)

Week After Ovulation	Death (Expulsion of Dead Embryos)	Survivors
—	16 (not fertilized)	100
0	15 (failed to cleave)	84 (fertile)
1	27	69 (implanted)
2	5.0	42
6	2.9	37
10	1.7	34.1
14	0.5	32.4
18	0.3	31.9
22	0.1	31.6
26	0.1	31.5
30	0.1	31.4
34	0.1	31.3
38	0.2	31.32
Live births (including birth defects)		31
Natural wastage		69

From Léridon H: Intrauterine mortality. In Human fertility. Chicago, The University of Chicago Press, 1977.

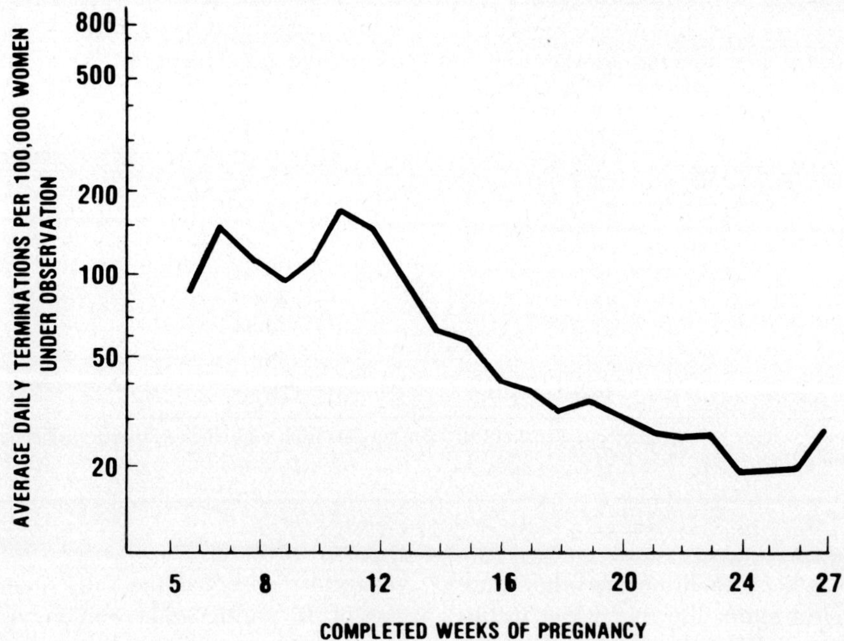

FIGURE 15-1

Spontaneous abortion by week of pregnancy. (From Harlap S, Shiono PH, Ramcharan S: A life table of spontaneous abortions and the effects of age, parity, and other variables. In Porter IH, Hook, EB, eds: Human embryonic and fetal death. New York, Academic Press, 1980.)

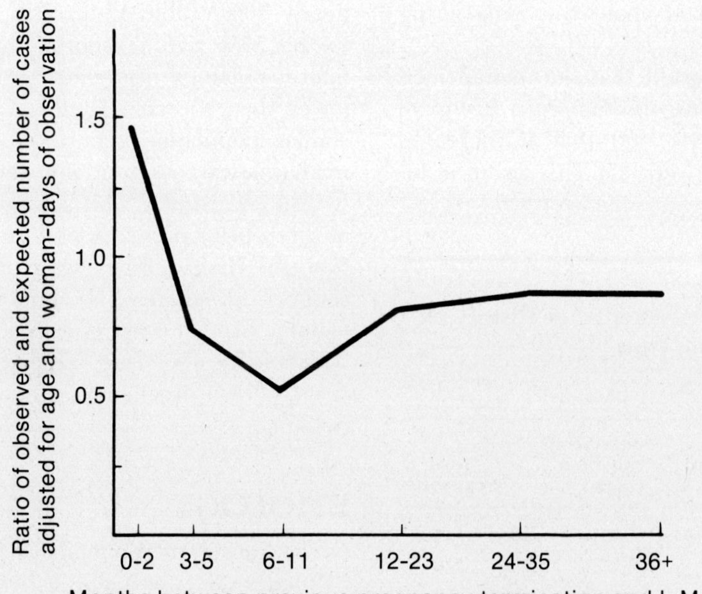

FIGURE 15-2

Spontaneous abortions by pregnancy spacing and outcome of previous pregnancy. (Modified from Harlap S, Shiono PH, Ramcharan S: A life table of spontaneous abortions and the effects of age, parity, and other variables. In Porter IH, Hook, EB, eds: Human embryonic and fetal death. New York, Academic Press, 1980.)

TABLE 15-2
Relation of Abortion Frequency to Maternal and Paternal Age at Conception

Maternal Age	% Abortion Frequency	Paternal Age	% Abortion Frequency
< 20	12.2	< 20	12.0
20-24	14.3	20-24	11.8
25-29	13.7	25-29	15.7
30-34	15.5	30-34	13.1
35-39	18.7	35-39	15.8
40-44	25.5	40-44	19.5
		44 +	23.1
TOTAL	14.7	TOTAL	14.7

From Warburton D, Fraser FC: Spontaneous abortion risks in man: Data from reproductive histories collected in a medical genetics unit. Am J Hum Genet 16:1, 1964.

information has been confirmed in other studies. These investigators also found that in this group of women who prior to this had delivered at least one live-born infant, the incidence of clinical abortion was 12.3% if they had no prior abortion. After having one or more abortions, there was a 24% to 32% risk of abortion in each successive pregnancy. They also recognized that a woman with multiple abortions has a tendency to abort at about the same gestational length.

Poland et al. reported that the overall incidence of spontaneous abortion in a group of 472 women was 14% and that it increased markedly after they were 35. This group of investigators observed the subsequent pregnancies of 46 multigravida women, all of whose prior pregnancies had ended in abortion. If the woman had had only one prior abortion, the rate of spontaneous abortion in a subsequent pregnancy was 20%, similar to the overall rate in the general population, but after a woman experienced three consecutive abortions, her chance of having a subsequent abortion was nearly 50% (Table 15-3). This figure is similar to the 55% figure reported by James. These figures obtained from clinical studies are much lower than the calculated value of 84% for a similar population reported by Malpas using mathematical assumptions. Thus for women with no live births and a reproductive history of three prior pregnancies terminating in abortion, the chance of having an abortion in a subsequent pregnancy is about 50%, whereas women with at least one live birth and three spontaneous abortions only have a 30% chance that the next pregnancy will terminate in abortion.

TABLE 15-3
Outcome of First Pregnancy After History of Spontaneous Abortion Only

| No. of Consecutive Spontaneous Abortions | Outcome | | Total Pregnancies |
	Live Birth (%)	Spontaneous Abortion (%)	
1*	79	19	145
2	65	35	26
3*	50	47	30
TOTAL			201

From Poland BJ, Miller JR, Jones DC, et al: Reproductive counseling in patients who have had a spontaneous abortion. Am J Obstet Gynecol 127:685, 1977.
*0.005 < P < 0.006 (47% versus 19%).

ETIOLOGY

The causes of spontaneous abortion can be divided into two major categories, fetal and maternal, also called genetic and environmental. By far the major causes of abortion are genetic. There have been several large cytogenetic studies of spontaneous abortion, including the survey of 1500 abortuses by Boué, Boué, and Lazar and the more recent study by

TABLE 15-4
Chromosome Abnormalities by State at Which Error Occurred

| | | Chromosomal Abnormalities (% of All Recognizable Fetal Loss) | | | | |
| | | Polyploidy | | Structural | | |
Stage	Trisomy	Triploid	Tetraploid	Familial	De Novo	Total
Maternal gametogenesis	23.0	1.6	-	0.67	0.75*	26
Paternal gametogenesis	2.0	2.4	-	0.33	0.25*	5
Fertilization	-	4.0	-	-	-	4
Zygote	-	-	4.0	-	-	4
TOTAL	25.0	8.0	4.0	1.0	1.0	39

From Jacobs PA, Hassold TJ: The origin of chromosome abnormalities in spontaneous abortion. In Porter IH, Hook EB: Human embryonic and fetal death. New York, Academic Press, 1980.
*Based on only four cases.

Kajii et al. of 565 abortuses utilizing chromosomal banding techniques. These and other large studies indicate that the incidence of chromosomal anomalies in abortuses is about 50%. Only about 5% of the abnormal karyotypes are abnormalities in the structure of individual chromosomes, such as translocation. The vast majority are numerical abnormalities due to errors occurring during gonadogenesis (chromosomal nondisjunction during meiosis), fertilization (triploidy due to digyny or dispermy), or the first division of the fertilized ovum (tetraploidy or mosaicism). Except for monosomy, it is possible to determine the parental origin of the chromosome abnormality. Jacobs and Hassold reported that 26% of all fetal loss is due to errors of maternal gametogenesis, 5% to errors of paternal gametogenesis, 4% to errors of fertilization, and 4% to errors of zygote division (Table 15-4).

In most surveys of chromosomal anomalies of abortuses the relative frequency of the different types of anomalies is similar. The most frequent type of anomaly is autosomal trisomy, which accounts for about half the abnormal karyotypes (Table 15-5). Trisomies of all autosomes except for autosome 1 have been reported after karyotyping of abortions, with tri-

TABLE 15-5
Chromosome Results of 447 Abortuses

	Karyotyped (Banded)	% of All Known Karyotype
Chromosomally Normal		
46.XY	111	24.8
46.XX	95	21.3
TOTAL	206	46.1
Chromosomally Abnormal		
45.X	44	9.8
Primary autosomal trisomy	138	30.9
Double trisomy	7	1.7
Triple trisomy	1	0.4
Triploidy	29	6.5
Tetraploidy	8	1.8
Mosaicism	1	0.4
Structural rearrangement	11	2.5
Others (XXY, Monosomy 21)	2	0.8
TOTAL	241	53.9

From Kajii T, Ferrier A: Anatomic and chromosomal anomalies in 639 spontaneous abortuses. Hum Genet 55:87, 1980.

somy 16 being the most frequent. About one third of all autosomal trisomies in abortuses are trisomy 16, with trisomy 13, 15, 21, and 22 being next most frequent. Many trisomies occurring in abortions have not been reported in live births, probably because the phenotype is incompatible with fetal development.

The second most common chromosome abnormality is monosomy 45X, which occurs in 15% to 20% of abortuses with abnormal karyotypes. It is estimated that the survival rate of 45X conceptions is about 1 in 300. About 15% of chromosomal anomalies in abortuses are triploidy, with tetraploidy being less frequent, about 5% to 10%. To summarize, autosomal trisomy is the most common abnormal karyotype (~50%) followed in decreasing frequency by monosomy 45X (~20%), triploidy (15%), tetraploidy (10%), and structural abnormalities (5%). The most common single chromosomal abnormality is monosomy 45X. Karyotypes of abortuses of women who have had more than one abortion tend to be similar if the first abortus had either a normal karyotype or an autosomal trisomy (Table 15-6).

The various surveys have revealed no seasonal variability in the incidence of any type of chromosomal abnormality in abortions. There is also no effect of paternal age. Maternal age, however, is directly related to the incidence of trisomies, mainly those in the D and G group.

Maternal age has no effect on the incidence of the other chromosomal anomalies in abortions, although there is evidence that monosomy 45X is associated with a younger maternal age than other aneuploid or euploid abortions. Chromosome abnormalities in the parents are an infrequent cause of abortions, as more than 90% of couples who have two or more spontaneous abortions are chromosomally normal. In a review of the literature, Simpson reported that in only 3.2% of cases did either parent have a balanced rearrangement of chromosome structure. A large recent study by Sachs et al. of 500 couples with two or more abortions found that 4.4% of the parents had a balanced translocation. In both these studies the translocations were more commonly maternal than paternal. Sachs et al. also reported that an additional 5% of the couples had mosaicism in one parent (nearly all X chromosome mosaicism of the mother, which could account for the high frequency of monosomy X conceptions).

Using a definition of gestational age as time from onset of the last menstrual period to time of abortion, Kajii et al. reported that the greatest prevalence of chromosomally abnormal abortions (74%) occurred at 9 weeks of gestation, and gradually decreased thereafter. The lower prevalence of abnormal karyotypes occurring in gestations terminating at less than 9 weeks may be artifactual, as the success of karyo-

---

TABLE 15-6

Karyotypes of Abortions in Women with Two Karyotyped Abortions—Combined Series

| | Second Abortion | | | | | | | | | | | |
| | Normal | | Monosomy | | Trisomy | | Triploidy | | Tetraploidy | | Structural Rearrangements | | |
First Abortion	No.	%	No.	%	No.	%	No.	%	No.	%	No.	%	Total
Normal	69	84.1	2	2.4	6	6.3	5	6.1	0	0	0	0	82
Monosomy	7	58.3	1	8.3	3	25.0	1	8.3	0	0	0	0	12
Trisomy	10	25.0	1	0.3	27	67.5	2	5.0	0	0	0	0	40
Triploidy	6	50.0	1	8.3	3	25.0	2	16.7	0	0	0	0	12
Tetraploidy	1	100.0	0	0	0	0	0	0	0	0	0	0	1
Structural rearrangement	0	0	1	14.7	0	0	0	0	0	0	6	85.7	7

From Warburton D, Stein Z, Kline J, et al: Chromosome abnormalities in spontaneous abortion: data from the New York City study. In Porter IH, Hook EB, eds: Human embryonic and fetal death. New York, Academic Press, 1980.

typing by culture is less likely if an embryo is not present, and the frequency of empty gestational sacs is greatest in abortions of 8 weeks or less. However, the lower rate may also be due to the fact that chromosomally abnormal conceptuses may be retained in utero longer than ones destined to abort that are chromosomally normal.

Abortion of chromosomally normal conceptuses is found to occur later in gestation than abortion of chromosomally abnormal ones. The peak incidence of euploid abortion is about 12 to 13 weeks of gestation; the peak incidence of aneuploid abortions is about 11 weeks. Stein et al. reported that the incidence of chromosomally normal abortions increased markedly after a maternal age of 35, rising to more than 30% of clinically recognized conceptions after age 40 (Fig. 15-3). Whether this increase in risk of abortion of euploid conceptions is due to an increase in genetic abnormalities or abnormalities in the maternal environment has not yet been elucidated, but there is an increased incidence of both first- and second-trimester abortions after age 35, and uterine abnormalities generally are a cause of second-trimester abortion (Fig. 15-4).

There are many possible causes for abortion of chromosomally normal conceptions. Simpson has postulated that a frequent, but yet unproven, cause is a genetic abnormality, most probably a mutation, or polygenic factors. He based this assumption on the fact that about 2% of live births have a disorder involving a single gene mutation or polygenic inheritance, whereas only 0.5% of live births have a chromosomal abnormality. Thus, in humans, genetic abnormalities are more common than chromosomal abnormalities. These genetic disorders could produce abortion by interfering with fetal metabolism or embryonic structural differentiation.

Two reports published in 1985 support the concept that genetic abnormalities may be a cause of spontaneous abortion in humans. Thomas et al. performed histocompatibility locus antigen (HLA) typing in couples with repeated abortion and showed that these couples had a greater frequency of sharing more than one antigen at the A, B, and DR locus than a

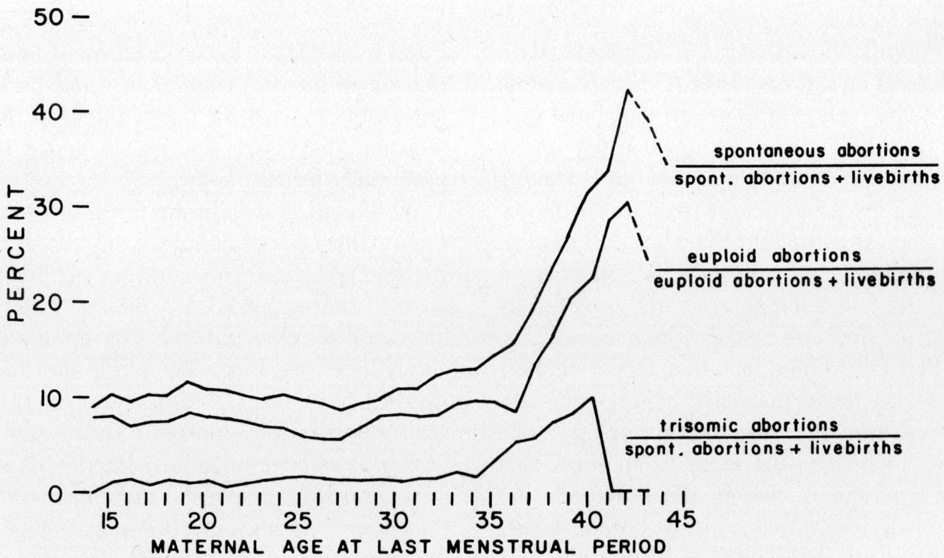

FIGURE 15-3
Estimated rates (%) of spontaneous abortion, euploid abortion, and trisomic abortion by maternal age for private and public patients combined. Broken line, denominator less than 25. (From Stein Z, Kline J, Susser E, et al: Maternal age and spontaneous abortion. In Porter IH, Hook EB, eds: Human embryonic and fetal death. New York, Academic Press, 1980.)

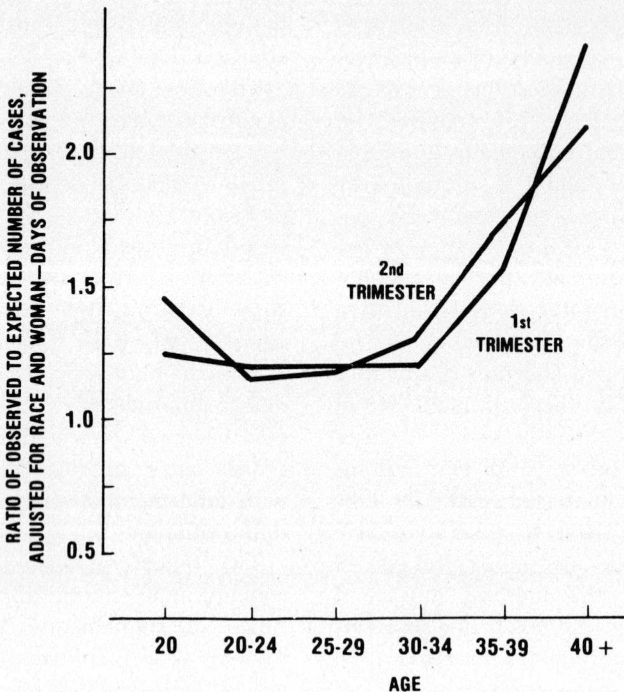

FIGURE 15-4

Spontaneous abortions by age. (From Harlap S, Shiono PH, Ramcharan S: A life table of spontaneous abortions and the effects of age, parity, and other variables. In Porter IH, Hook EB, eds: Human embryonic and fetal death. New York, Academic Press, 1980.)

control population. Other investigators have also reported an increased HLA sharing among couples with recurrent abortion and have postulated that the abortion occurs because of the absence of a maternal immunologic blocking factor normally produced in response to paternal antigens. It is thought that the blocking factor, a circulating IgG antibody, is important in allowing the fetal allograft not to be rejected by the maternal immune system. Thomas et al. reported that the women who had repeated abortions had a normal maternal lymphocytic immune response to stimulation by paternal lymphocytes. They therefore concluded that the cause of the recurrent abortions was not immunologic but genetic due to homozygosity for recessive major histocompatibility complex genes that could be the responsible factor for the abortion. In several animal species, genes contributing to spontaneous abortion are located in the region of the chromosome that controls the major histocompatibility complex. In humans the histocompatibility complex is located in the HLA locus on chromosome 6. The sharing of the HLA antigens could be just the detectable marker for the segment of the chromosome that carries recessive genes that are potentially lethal.

Weitkamp and Schacter reported that chromosomally normal couples who experience recurrent abortion, in addition to having increased sharing of HLA-A alleles, also have an increased incidence of the transferrin C3 allele and a decreased frequency of the most common transferrin allele, C1. These transferrin alleles are located on chromosome 3. Although transferrin genes have been associated with abortion in several animal species, the effect of transferrin on spontaneous abortion may not be necessarily direct but, as with HLA antigens, could be an effect of genes closely located to the transferrin locus.

Thus these two reports support the concept that the presence of certain recessive genes located on chromosomes 3 and 6 could interfere with normal fetal development and increase the possibility of spontaneous abortion of euploid embryo. Further evidence for a genetic mechanism is the fact that in the gestation after a spontaneous abortion in a primigravida there is an increased frequency of congenital malformations and perinatal deaths.

Environmental Causes

In contrast to the frequent genetic causes of abortion, maternal or environmental causes are less frequent. Uterine abnormalities, either congenital or acquired, may not provide the optimal environment for nourishment and survival of the embryo and thus may cause abortion of a genetically normal embryo. Congenital uterine abnormalities can be divided into those brought about by abnormal uterine fusion, those produced by maternal diethylstilbestrol (DES) ingestion, and those due to abnormal cervical function. The latter condition, the incompetent cervix, can also be acquired after mechanical cervical dilation.

Anomalies of Uterine Development

Anomalies of uterine development are relatively frequent, with the incidence reported in the literature ranging from about 1:200 to 1:600 women. Overall about 20% to 25% of women with anomalies of uterine fusion have severe problems with reproduction, recurrent abortion being the most serious. Although it has been stated that the bicornuate and septate uterus are the anomalies most frequently associated with abortion, this belief has arisen from the fact that these anomalies can be corrected surgically and thus are more frequently reported as a cause of abortion before surgical correction. In a study of all 182 women with uterine anomalies detected during an 18-year period at a large Finnish hospital, Heinonen et al. reported that the least frequent uterine anomaly, the unicornuate uterus, was associated with the greatest incidence of spontaneous abortion, about 50%. This incidence was higher than the 25% to 30% incidence of abortion that occurred in women with either a septate or bicornuate uterus. Buttram and Gibbons also reported that a unicornuate uterus was the uterine developmental anomaly associated with the highest incidence of abortion.

Surgical correction of bicornuate and septate uteri is possible by utilizing one of the transfundal metroplasty techniques described by Strassman, Jones, or Tompkins (Fig. 15-5) or by transcervical hysteroscopic resection of the uterine septum. The Strassman technique of metroplasty is usually utilized for a bicornuate uterus, whereas the other techniques are used for resection of a uterine septum. In the series of Heinonen et al., about one fifth of the women with bicornuate and septate uteri had a metroplasty performed, and the abortion rate declined from 84% to 12%. Similar results were reported in the series of 43 patients of Rock and Jones and the 21 patients of Musich and Behrman. In both these reports the live birth rate increased from 7% to 8% before metroplasty to 75% to 77% after unification of the uterine cavity. DeCherney et al. reported that of 103 patients with recurrent abortion and a uterine septum, it was possible to perform a hysteroscopic resection in about 70%. Of these patients, 80% had a subsequent successful delivery. In the 30% of patients with a septum greater than 1 cm thick, a metroplasty was not performed.

March and Israel reported that it was possible to incise the septum, even those thicker than 1 cm, of all 82 women with recurrent abortion with flexible scissors placed transcervically through the hysteroscope. After this treatment the abortion rate declined from 95% to 13%. Because these results are as good as or better than those for an abdominal metroplasty without the need to perform a laparotomy or subsequent cesarean section, hysteroscopic incision should now be the treatment of choice for the septate uterus.

Uterine Anomalies After Diethylstilbestrol (DES)

Comparative studies have shown that women exposed to DES during their fetal life have impaired reproductive function compared with controls. Numerous studies, including the comparative ones of Barnes et al. and Herbst et al., indicate that women exposed to DES who subsequently conceived have a significantly greater incidence of spontaneous abortion than controls (Table 15-7). In 1980 Kaufman et al. reported that women exposed to

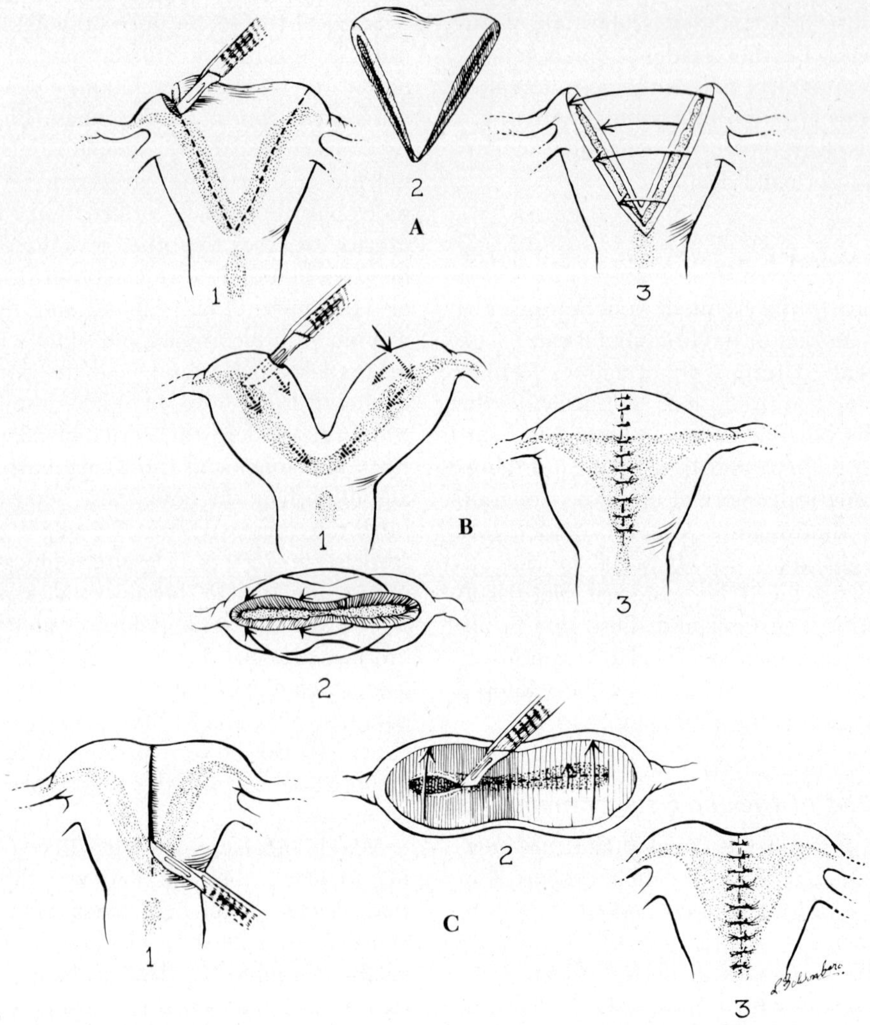

FIGURE 15-5
A, Wedge technique of Jones and Jones. **B,** Transverse fundal incision of Strassmann. **C,** Median bivalving technique of Tompkins. (From Rock JA, Jones, HW: The clinical management of the double uterus. Fertil Steril 28:798, 1977. Reproduced with permission of the publisher, The American Fertility Society.)

DES who had an abnormal hysterosalpingogram (HSG), mainly a small T-shaped uterine cavity, had a greater chance of having a spontaneous abortion with a subsequent pregnancy than did DES-exposed women with a normal HSG. However, in a larger series published in 1984 these same investigators reported that the percentage of first or all pregnancies in women exposed to DES that ended in spontaneous abortion was similar regardless of whether their HSG revealed abnormalities in the shape of the cavity or intrauterine defects. Haney et al. reported that the endometrial cavity of women exposed to DES in utero had a significantly smaller surface area than normal, which could perhaps contribute to the increased spontaneous abortion rate in women exposed to DES in utero. No therapy, including routine uterine cerclage, has been shown to be beneficial in lowering the abortion rate in women exposed to DES who have abnormalities of the uterine cavity and recurrent abortion.

Acquired Uterine Defects

LEIOMYOMAS. Leiomyomas are common benign uterine tumors that are present in

TABLE 15-7
Numbers and Percentages of Women Exposed to DES and of Control Subjects
Who Had Unfavorable Outcomes of Pregnancy, and Relative Risks of Unfavorable Outcomes
with DES Exposure

Outcome	Exposed to DES (220)*	Controls (224)*	Relative Risk	P Value	95% Confidence Limits on Relative Risk
Any unfavorable outcome	83 (37.7)	50 (22.3)	1.69	0.001	1.20-2.18
Miscarriage	57 (25.9)	36 (16.1)	1.61	0.008	1.11-2.34
Ectopic pregnancy	8 (3.6)	3 (1.3)	2.77	ns†	0.73-10.46
Premature birth	17 (7.7)	10 (4.5)	1.71	ns	0.80-3.65
Stillbirth	8 (3.6)	3 (1.3)	2.77	ns	0.80-3.65
Never had a full-term live birth	42 (19.1)	11 (4.9)	3.90	0.001	2.06-7.37

From Barnes AB, Colton T, Gundersen J, et al: Fertility and outcome of pregnancy in women exposed in utero to diethylstilbestrol. N Engl J Med 302:609, 1980. Reprinted by permission of The New England Journal of Medicine.
*Figures in parenthesis denote percentages.
†Not significant ($P > 0.10$).

about one fourth of women of reproductive age. Uterine leiomyomas, especially if they are submucosal, can be associated with repetitive abortion. Although a causal relationship is difficult to establish, in a review of the literature, Buttram and Reiter reported that when myomectomy was performed for recurrent abortion in a total of 1941 women, the spontaneous abortion rate was reduced from 41% to 19%. These data indicate that on occasion uterine leiomyomas are a cause of abortion.

INCOMPETENT CERVIX. Cervical incompetence is characterized by an asymptomatic dilation of the internal cervical os leading to dilation of the cervical canal and external os during the second trimester of pregnancy. The consequent lack of support of the fetal membranes leads to their spontaneous rupture, which is usually followed by expulsion of the fetus and placenta. The incidence of this problem, which was originally described in 1948, has been estimated to vary from 1 in 57 to 1 in 1730 pregnancies. Mann estimated that about 20% of midtrimester pregnancy losses are due to cervical incompetence. Although excessive mechanical cervical dilation at the time of dilation and curettage was formerly the most com-

mon cause of this problem, since recognition of this syndrome, the use of excessive mechanical cervical dilation is less common. Consequently, as stated in the review by Cousins, the most common cause of cervical incompetence is now due to a congenital defect in the cervical tissue. The diagnosis of cervical incompetence is best made by a history of second-trimester pregnancy loss accompanied by spontaneous rupture of the fetal membranes without preceding uterine contractions. Cervical incompetence has been found to be associated with uterine anomalies, particularly uterus didelphys, as well as with anomalies produced by fetal DES exposure.

The best treatment of cervical incompetence is placement of a concentric nonabsorbable silk or Mersilene suture at the level of the internal os (cerclage), utilizing either the technique described by Shirodkar or McDonald (Fig. 15-6). Since, as reported by Harger, these techniques yield a similar rate of success, with the rate of fetal survival increasing from about 20% before suture placement to 80% after the cerclage procedure, the McDonald procedure is preferable, as this procedure is technically easier and is associated with less morbidity than the Shirodkar technique is. It is recommended that

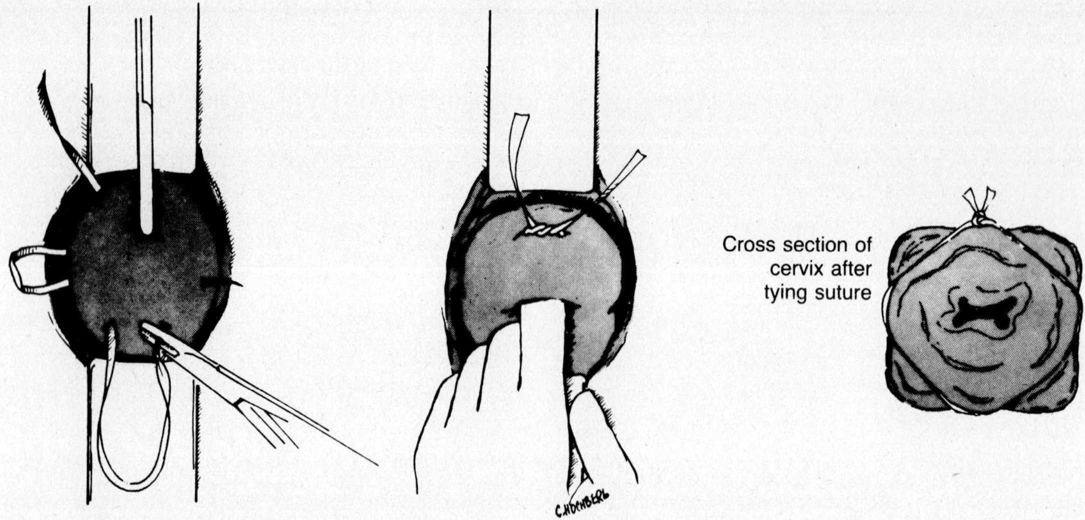

FIGURE 15-6

Steps in performing McDonald cerclage using Mersilene suture. Index finger is used to ensure closure of internal os. (From March CM: Recurrent abortion. Reproduced with permission from Infertility, contraception, and reproductive endocrinology, 2nd ed, edited by Daniel R. Mishell, Jr., M.D., and Val Davajan, M.D. Copyright © 1986. Medical Economics Books, Oradell, N.J. 07649. All rights reserved.)

the suture be placed electively between 12 to 14 weeks of gestation after major embryogenesis has been completed and the incidence of spontaneous abortion due to genetic abnormality has markedly lessened. An ultrasound examination should be performed before cerclage to document a normal gestation. Occasionally if there is a markedly shortened cervix or placement of the McDonald cerclage has failed to maintain the pregnancy, a transabdominal cerclage, as described by Benson and Durfee, should be performed. If the suture is placed externally, it is usually removed at 38 weeks' gestation, and vaginal delivery allowed. However, because of cervical scarring, cesarean section is required in about 15% of pregnancies.

INTRAUTERINE ADHESIONS. Adhesions in the uterine cavity can cause partial or complete obliteration of the endometrium, leading to menstrual abnormalities and amenorrhea as well as being a cause of abortion. The latter is thought to be due to insufficient endometrium to support adequate fetal growth. The major cause of adhesions is curettage of the endometrial cavity in association with a pregnancy or in the early puerperium (Table 15-8). In the series of March and Israel the most common antecedent factor was curettage for incomplete abortion. Curettage after a missed abortion or following postpartum hemorrhage had a high incidence of subsequent intrauterine adhesion (IUA) formation. On occasion IUAs develop after a diagnostic curettage as well as in women with genital tuberculosis. The diagnosis of IUA is usually made by the finding of filling defects seen at the time of hysterosalpingogram. The defects are typically irregular with sharp contours and homogeneous opacity that persist in a series of films (Fig. 15-7). The diagnosis is best confirmed by hysteroscopy.

The recommended treatment for IUA is lysis of the adhesions by miniature scissors during hysteroscopy. After adhesion lysis, either an IUD or small Foley catheter is usually placed in the cavity, and high-dose estrogen (conjugated equine estrogen 2.5 mg bid) is administered for 60 days. Medroxyprogesterone acetate 10 mg per day is added for the last 5 to 10 days, and then the foreign body is removed. March and Israel reported that the abortion rate decreased from 83% to 13% after hysterographic lysis of adhesions. To minimize the chances of development of IUA, curettage of the pregnant or recently pregnant uteri should

TABLE 15-8
Definite Causes of IUA in 1856 Cases

	No. of Cases	%
Trauma associated with pregnancy		
Curettage after abortion	1237	66.7
Spontaneous	544	
Induced	557	
Unknown	136	
Postpartum curettage	400	21.5
Cesarean section	38	2.0
Evacuation of hydatidiform mole	11	0.6
Trauma without pregnancy		
Myomectomy	24	1.3
Diagnostic curettage	22	1.2
Cervical manipulation (biopsy, polypectomy, etc.)	10	0.5
Curettage because of menometrorrhagia	8	0.4
Insertion of IUD	3	0.3
Insertion of radium	1	
Without known trauma		
Postpartum; after abortion; others	28	1.5
Genital tuberculosis	74	4.0
TOTAL	1856	100.00

From Schenker JG, Margalioth EJ: Intrauterine adhesions: An updated appraisal. Fertil Steril 37:593, 1982. Reproduced with permission of the publisher, The American Fertility Society.

be gentle and superficial and not extend deep into the mucosa. After curettage for missed abortion or postpartum hemorrhage, consideration should be given to prophylactic high oral dose estrogen treatment for 1 to 2 months to enhance endometrial growth.

Endocrine Causes

Progesterone Deficiency

Maintenance of the endometrium for the first 7 weeks of gestation depends on progesterone produced by the corpus luteum. The function of the latter depends on HCG produced by the trophoblast. When progesterone secretion from the corpus luteum is lower than normal or the endometrium has an inadequate response to normal circulating levels of progesterone, endometrial development may be inadequate to support the implanted blastocyst and may lead to spontaneous abortion. Several investigators have reported that in conception cycles, midluteal peak progesterone levels in the circulation are always greater than 9 ng/ml. Horta et al. measured daily plasma progesterone levels during the luteal phase of a group of normal fertile women as well as in a group of women whose previous three gestations terminated in spontaneous abortion. In the former group the lowest midluteal peak progesterone level was 9 ng/ml, while in the latter group mean progesterone levels reached a peak of 6 mg/ml, significantly lower than the normal fertile group. Hensleigh and Fainstat also reported that five of nine women with recurrent spontaneous abortion had maximum midluteal serum progesterone levels less than 10 ng/ml.

Diagnosis of luteal insufficiency as a cause of infertility has also been made by performing histologic examination of the endometrium and finding a discrepancy of three days or more between the expected and actual endometrial dating pattern in at least two menstrual cycles. Several investigators using this method of diagnosis have reported luteal deficiency to occur in as many as one-third of women with recurrent abortion, whereas others have reported it to be an infrequent cause of abortion. This discrepancy may have occurred because the precision of endometrial dating by histologic examination varies among different observers.

Several investigators have treated women with recurrent abortion and evidence of luteal deficiency with progesterone vaginal suppositories 25 mg twice daily or intramuscular progesterone 12.5 mg/day beginning 3 days after ovulation and continuing throughout the first trimester. With this treatment, term pregnancy rates have been reported to range from 80% to 90%. However, no randomized placebo studies have been reported to verify the effectiveness of progesterone in preventing abortion in women with luteal insufficiency.

There is no evidence that administration of synthetic progestins, which themselves may be luteolytic, are of benefit in reducing the incidence of abortion. There is also no benefit to

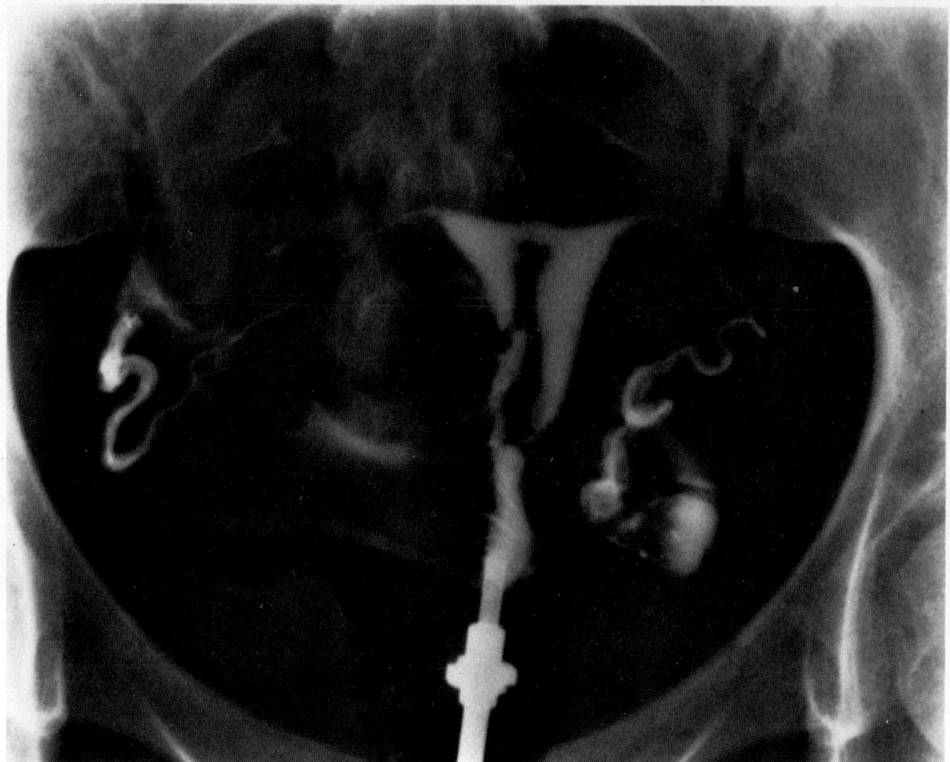

FIGURE 15-7
Endometrial adhesions. The patient was a 23-year-old gravida 5, para 0, spontaneous abortus 4, ectopic 1 (G5 P0 SAB4 ECT), with previous left linear salpingostomy, being evaluated for recurrent abortion. Irregular, linear filling defect represents adhesions between anterior and posterior walls of endometrial cavity, extending from internal os to level near fundus. (From Richmond JA: Hysterosalpingography. Reprinted with permission from Infertility, contraception, and reproductive endocrinology, 2nd ed, edited by Daniel R. Mishell, Jr., M.D., and Val Davajan, M.D. Copyright © 1986. Medical Economics Books, Oradell, N.J. 07649. All rights reserved.)

be derived by initiating progesterone therapy after the expected menstrual period is missed, especially if the women develop symptoms of threatened abortion. Low progesterone levels at this time are a result, not the cause, of the abortion.

Thyroid Disease

Although older studies indicate that hypothyroidism may be a cause of abortion, a recent study by Montoro et al. reported that no abortions occurred in 11 pregnancies of nine markedly hypothyroid women. In three recent studies of large numbers of women with recurrent abortion, only a few women in one of the stud-

ies were found to have abnormal thyroid function. Thus there is no definitive evidence that hypothyroidism is a cause of abortion in humans.

Diabetes Mellitus

Although uncontrolled diabetes mellitus has been associated with an increased abortion rate, Crane and Wahl found the incidence of spontaneous abortion was similar in a group of women with either gestational diabetes (12.3%) or frank diabetes (12.2%) and matched control groups (10.9% and 14.5%). In this study the diabetes was controlled with insulin. They also reported that the number of women with multiple spontaneous abortions were similar in the diabetic and control groups. Other studies of pregnancy in diabetics in the past 25 years reported a spontaneous abortion rate varying from 6% to 11.5%. Thus it appears that diabetes, if controlled by diet or insulin, is not a cause of abortion.

Immunologic Factors

As mentioned previously, the foreign antigens produced by the fetus should cause it to be rejected by the mother's immune system. Although some protection from this immunologic effect is offered by progesterone, it has been hypothesized by Rocklin et al. and others that a maternal blocking factor, an IgG antibody, coats the foreign fetal antigens and prevents the fetus from being rejected. These investigators reported that women with recurrent abortion lacked this blocking factor.

The sharing of major histocompatibility locus antigens (HLA) (which may cause the maternal immune system to fail to produce blocking antibodies, as discussed earlier) as a cause of abortion has been refuted by Caudle et al., who found no difference in the degree of HLA antigen sharing in couples with recurrent abortion and a control group. However, Mowbray et al. performed a randomized treatment trial in a group of women with recurrent abortion and no detectable antibody against paternal lymphocytes. Women injected with paternal white cells had a significantly greater chance of a subsequent successful pregnancy (78%) than those injected with their own white cells (37%). Thus the data regarding an immunologic cause of abortion are conflicting, and at present the evidence for such an etiology cannot be considered definitive.

Lupus Anticoagulant

Although an association between several systemic medical diseases and an increased rate of abortion has been postulated, a relation has been definitely established for lupus erythematosus. Since 1980 several reports, as summarized by Lubbe and Liggins, have appeared indicating that the cause of frequent abortion in some women with systemic lupus erythematosus is associated with the presence of an autoantibody, called lupus anticoagulant, in the maternal circulation. This antibody, which is an IgG or IgM immunoglobulin, has been found in about 5% to 15% of women with systemic lupus as well as in those with other connective tissue diseases. In addition, it has been found in women with a history of recurrent thrombotic episodes as well as in women with no other disease process.

The presence of this antibody in the circulation is associated with arterial and venous thrombosis as well as with recurrent pregnancy loss. It is thought that one mechanism for this effect is that the antibody interferes with prostacyclin formation, leading to a relative excess of thromboxane A_2, thus causing a thrombotic tendency. It has been postulated that abortion occurs because of thrombosis in the placental blood supply and resultant embryonic or fetal death. About 50% of pregnant women with the lupus anticoagulant have a false positive serologic test for syphilis, and many, but not all, have antinuclear antibodies. Thus the absence of an antinuclear antibody in a patient with a suggestive history for the lupus anticoagulant should not prevent specific testing for the lupus anticoagulant. Only about 40% of pregnant women with the antibody have lupus erythematosus. Screening for the antibody can be undertaken by performing a kaolin clotting time or the platelet neutralization procedure. If either of these tests is prolonged, there is a high likelihood the antibody is present. Other tests such as the tissue thromboplastin inhibition test or the activated partial thromboplastin time have been proposed for screening but have been criticized for being nonspecific or insensitive, respectively.

Lubbe and Liggins recommend that women who have had one or more abortions and who have lupus anticoagulant be treated throughout their pregnancy with immunosuppressive doses of prednisone (40 to 60 mg per day) combined with low-dose aspirin (75 mg per day). This regimen suppresses the antibody as measured by in vitro procedures and has been reported to improve the chances of fetal survival. With this therapy several women with a history of recurrent abortions and no live-born infants have carried pregnancies to term. The antibody against cardiolipin has also been associated with fetal demise in a small study of patients with systemic lupus erythematosus. Although there is currently no specific treatment to offer when this antibody is detected, vigilant fetal surveillance is recommended.

Infections

Numerous infectious agents present in the cervix, uterine cavity, or seminal fluid have been postulated to be etiologic factors for abortion. Although there is evidence that clinical endometritis due to any infectious agent can produce an abortion, the evidence is unclear as to whether subclinical infections with certain microorganisms or viruses are a cause of spontaneous abortion. The parasite *Toxoplasma gondii* may infect the embryo and cause an abortion. However, it is difficult to document the presence of this organism before abortion because there is a lack of correlation between serologic immunoassays for this organism and its detection in the endometrium by immunofluorescence. Furthermore, Kimball et al. reported that there is a similar incidence of positive immunologic screening tests for this organism in women with a history of none, one, or more than one abortion.

Although *Listeria monocytogenes* produces abortion in several animal species, there is no evidence that it is an abortifacient in women. Rabau and David found no bacteriologic or serologic evidence of *Listeria* infection in 554 women who had aborted, including 74 with recurrent abortions, and Stray-Pedersen et al. were unable to isolate this organism from a group of 48 women with recurrent abortion. *Chlamydia trachomatis* is a common sexually transmitted pathogen, but there is no evidence that it causes abortion in asymptomatic women.

Infection with herpes simplex virus in the genital tract has been reported to cause abortion. If genital herpes initially occurs in the first half of pregnancy, Nahmias et al. reported that the abortion rate is about 34%. Naib et al. reported that if pregnancy occurs within 18 months after initial detection of herpes infection, the abortion rate was 55%. Both these rates were significantly higher than the 11.5% abortion rate in the control population.

Several authors have suggested that T strain mycoplasma, both *Ureaplasma urealyticum* and *Mycoplasma hominis,* can cause abortion. Data indicating the first organism as a cause of abortion are stronger than for the latter. Stray-Pedersen et al. found that although the incidence of cervical colonization of *U. urealyticum* was similar in a group of women with recurrent abortion and controls, the incidence of endometrial colonization was significantly more frequent (28%) in the group with recurrent abortions than in the control group (7%). In this study the cultures were obtained at least 6 months after the last abortion, and there were no clinical or laboratory signs of infection in any of the women. These investigators could not correlate the presence of *M. hominis* in the uterus with an increased frequency of abortion.

Stray-Pedersen and Stray-Pedersen reported that eradication of *U. urealyticum* in the endometrium by tetracyline treatment for 10 days resulted in a significantly lower subsequent abortion rate (19%). However, there are no randomized placebo controlled treatment studies to prove that these organisms cause abortion and that treatment is effective.

Environmental Factors

Smoking

In a retrospective study Kline et al. reported that women who smoked during pregnancy had a significantly greater chance of having a spontaneous abortion than did a control group (Table 15-9). For women who smoked more than 14 cigarettes per day the risk of having an abortion was 1.7 times greater than for women who did not smoke, but smoking less than this did not result in a significantly greater incidence of abortion. These investigators found that heavy smokers had an increased risk of aborting chromosomally normal embryos only. There was no increased risk of an aneuploid abortion in smokers. These data indicate that smoking acts as a toxic agent to destroy chromosomally normal fetuses.

Alcohol

Kline et al. also reported that alcohol, acting independently from smoking, was a risk factor for abortion (Table 15-10). Women who drank alcohol at least 2 days a week had about a twofold greater risk of having an abortion than women who did not drink during pregnancy, with the risk increasing to threefold with daily

TABLE 15-9

Frequency (%) of Smoking among Women Experiencing Spontaneous Abortions (Cases) and Women Delivering at 28 Weeks' Gestation or Later (Controls)

No. of Cigarettes per Day	% Distribution		Adjusted Odds Ratio	95% Confidence Interval
	Cases	Controls		
None	62.0	69.8	1.00	--
1-13	20.5 ⎫ 37.9	20.0 ⎫ 30.2	1.07 ⎫ 1.28	.80-1.42
14-80	17.4 ⎭	10.2 ⎭	1.73 ⎭	1.23-2.43
TOTAL	648	645		

From Kline J, Stein Z, Susser M, et al: Environmental influences on early reproductive loss in a current New York City study. In Porter IH, Hook EB, eds: Human embryonic and fetal death. New York, Academic Press, 1980.

TABLE 15-10

Frequency (%) of Alcohol Consumption among Women Experiencing Spontaneous Abortions (Cases) and Women Delivering at 28 Weeks' Gestation or Later (Controls)

Frequency of Alcohol Consumption During Pregnancy	% Distribution		Adjusted Odds Ratio	95% Confidence Interval
	Cases	Controls		
Never	42.6	43.7	1.00	
Twice a month and less	28.9	38.0	.77	.59 - .99
Less than twice a month	10.8	10.4	1.04	.71 - 1.52
2 to 6 days a week	13.3 ⎫ 17.9	6.5 ⎫ 7.9	1.96 ⎫ 2.36	1.30 - 2.95
Daily	4.5 ⎭	1.4 ⎭	3.00 ⎭	1.39 - 6.49
TOTAL	648	645		

From Kline J, Stein Z, Susser M, et al: Environmental influences on early reproductive loss in a current New York City study. In Porter IH, Hook EB, eds: Human embryonic and fetal death. New York, Academic Press, 1980.

ingestions of alcohol. As with smoking, an increased risk of abortion was confined to chromosomally normal embryos, indicating that alcohol, like smoking, can act as a toxic agent on the normal embryo to cause its death.

Irradiation

Animal studies have shown that ionizing radiation can produce congenital malformation, growth retardation, and embryonic death. These effects are dose related, and there is a threshold dose below which an adverse effect does not occur. Although there is evidence in the human that high-energy radiation exposure is associated with teratogenic effects and growth retardation, there is no conclusive evidence that similar exposure increases the risk of spontaneous abortion.

Extrapolation from animal data indicates that the embryo is most sensitive to the lethal effect of irradiation during the day of implantation and a few days later (Table 15-11). The sensitivity decreases during the period of early embryogenesis, after which the minimum lethal dose (MLD) remains constant to term gestation. Brent reported that the MLD of irradiation to rats is 5 rads on the day of implantation. These data thus indicate that there is little likelihood that irradiation of less than 5 rads (severalfold greater than the amount used in nearly all diagnostic procedures) will cause an abortion in the human, even if it is administered during the time of implantation.

TABLE 15-11
Estimation of Abortigenic Hazards of
X-Irradiation to Human Embryo from Animal
Experiments

Stage of Human Gestation (Days)	Lethal Dose/50 (Rads)	MLD (Rads)
1	70-100	10
14	140	25
18	150	25
28	220	50
50	260	50
Late fetus to term	300-400	50

From Brent RL: Radiation-induced embryonic and fetal loss from conception to birth. In Porter IH, Hook EB, eds: Human embryonic and fetal death. New York, Academic Press, 1980.

Environmental Toxins

Little valid information exists concerning the effect of environmental toxins on human abortion. Although some studies have shown an increased risk of abortion among female anesthesiologists, other studies have not found such an effect. Most studies reporting such a relation are retrospective questionnaire studies of marginal validity. A well-done recent case control study by Axelsson et al. indicated that the incidence of abortion in women exposed to anesthetic gases was not significantly increased.

Information concerning a possible abortifacient effect after increased exposure to other environmental toxins is even less clear. Vianna reported that the entire population of women exposed to toxic chemical wastes in the Love Canal area had no significant excess of spontaneous abortions, although groups of women living in certain areas with a higher exposure may have had an increased risk of abortion.

DIAGNOSIS

Threatened Abortion

It has been estimated that bleeding occurs during the first 20 weeks of pregnancy in about 30% to 40% of human gestations, with about half of these pregnancies ending in spontaneous abortion. There is no evidence that women with gestational bleeding who do not abort have an increased incidence of complications of pregnancy, but they may have a slightly increased incidence of fetal anomalies and preterm birth. To determine the prognosis of the pregnancy in a woman with threatened abortion, endocrinologic studies, ultrasonography, and a combination of both techniques have been used.

Nygren et al. measured HCG, progesterone, and estradiol in the serum of a group of women with threatened abortion and found that a low level of HCG correlated best with a poor outcome of the pregnancy. Of 46 women who subsequently aborted, 44 had HCG levels less than 10,600 mIU/ml, while all 23 women who did not abort had levels greater than 18,600 mIU/ml (Fig. 15-8). Unlike HCG there was a considerable overlap in levels of progesterone and estradiol between the women who aborted and those who did not. Mishell and Davajan reported that if the urinary HCG level was less than 10,000 mIU/ml in a group of women with threatened abortion with a gestational age between 55 and 110 days (measured from onset of the last menstrual period), spontaneous abortion consistently occurred. Thus a low level of HCG during this time of gestation is a poor prognostic sign. Because progesterone levels normally fall to a nadir 9 to 11 weeks after the last menstrual period, the finding of a low progesterone level is of little prognostic significance. Many women bleed at this stage of gestation because this is the time when luteal production of progesterone ceases and trophoblastic production has not yet begun to increase sufficiently to consistently maintain the endometrium.

Kadar et al. reported that in normal gestation the presence of a gestational sac should be seen with an ultrasound examination when the serum HCG level is greater than 6500 mIU/ml, about 5 to 6 weeks of gestation (Table 15-12). Fetal heart activity and fetal motion should become detectable using real-time ultrasound by at least the end of 7 weeks of gestation (measured from onset of last menstrual period). Anderson reported that the presence or absence of fetal heart motion and spontaneous fetal extremity motion between 8 and 13 weeks' gestation in a group of 158 women with threatened

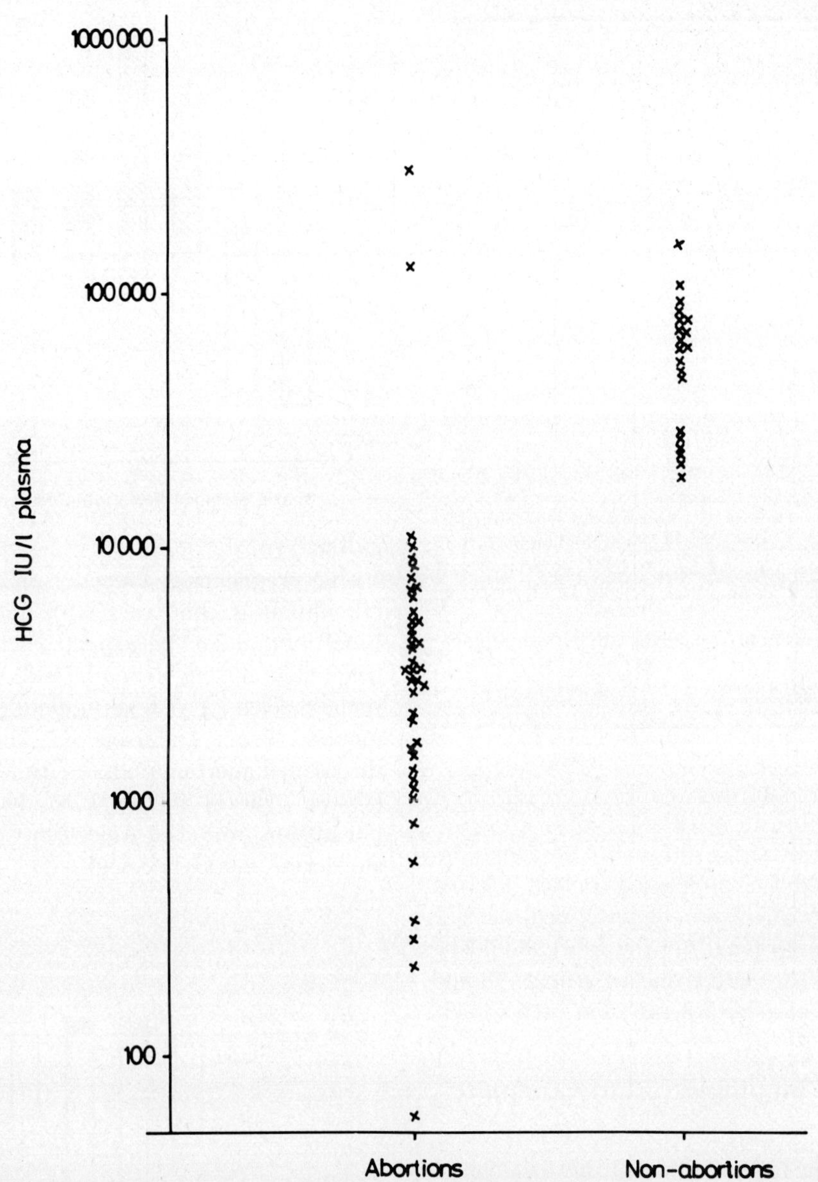

FIGURE 15-8

Peripheral plasma levels of HCG when diagnosis of TA was made. (From Nygren K-G, Johansson EDB, Wide L: Am J Obstet Gynecol 116:916, 1973.)

abortion correlated well with the subsequent pregnancy outcome (Figs. 15-9 and 15-10). Between 6 and 8 weeks' gestation the presence of a fetal heart beat correlated well with the continuation of the pregnancy, but failure to detect fetal heart activity occurred in both those who had a good and those who had a poor outcome. Beyond 8 weeks of gestation the absence of fetal cardiac activity and absence of fetal movements in a 10-minute period is diagnostic of fetal death, especially if the fetus sinks slowly toward the posterior inferior uterine wall when the uterus is touched. Because of the possible discrepancy between the actual day of conception and estimated date based on calculation from time of onset of last menses, confirmation

TABLE 15-12
Correlation Between Sonar Findings and
Serum HCG Values on Day of Scan*

Serum HCG Levels (mIU/ml)	No. of Scans	
	No Sac	Sac
>15,500	1	28
8500-15,500	2	10
6500-8500	0	5
6000-6500	†	†
4000-6000	4	0
2000-4000	8	0
<2000	8	0

From Kadar N, DeVore G, Romero R: Discriminatory
hCG zone: Its use in the sonographic evaluation for ectopic
pregnancy. Obstet Gynecol 58:156, 1981. Reprinted with
permission from The American College of Obstetricians
and Gynecologists.
*Based on 66 scans from 53 patients with normal intrauter-
ine pregnancies.
†Discriminatory HCG zone.

of fetal death by serial ultrasound at weekly intervals should be performed before uterine
evacuation. A correlation of gestational sac size
and crown-rump length of the fetus should be
performed. The latter measurement should
normally increase by at least 1 cm each week.

Inevitable, Incomplete, and Complete Abortions

In a patient bleeding during the first half of
pregnancy the diagnosis of inevitable abortion
is strengthened if the bleeding is profuse and
associated with uterine cramping pains.
Women with threatened abortion who do not
abort usually do not have cramps. When bleeding or pain in the first half of pregnancy is severe enough to require hospitalization, the
most likely diagnosis is inevitable or incomplete abortion, occurring in more than 60% of
women who are hospitalized for vaginal bleeding in the first half of pregnancy (Table 15-13).
The diagnosis can be confirmed by examination
of the cervical os. If cervical dilation has occurred with or without rupture of membranes,
the abortion is inevitable. If only a portion of

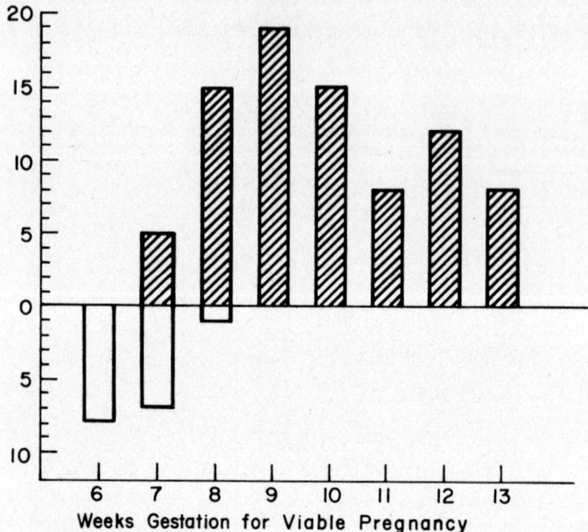

FIGURE 15-9
Viable pregnancies. Presence or absence of fetal motion is compared with gestational age.
Fetal motion can be expected with increasing
frequency during seventh and eighth gestational weeks. ▨ = fetal motion; ☐ = no fetal
motion. (From Anderson SG: Management of
threatened abortion with real-time sonography.
Obstet Gynecol 55:259, 1980. Reprinted with
permission from The American College of Obstetricians and Gynecologists.)

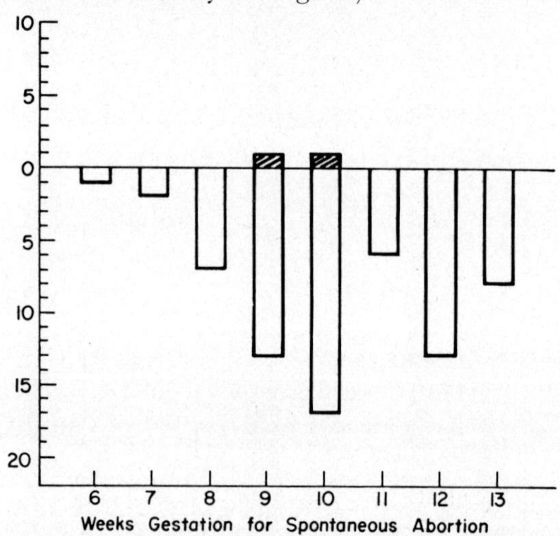

FIGURE 15-10
Spontaneous abortion. Fetal motion was rarely
observed regardless of gestational age. ▨ = fetal motion; ☐ = no fetal motion. (From Anderson SG: Management of threatened abortion
with real-time sonography. Obstet Gynecol
55:259, 1980. Reprinted with permission from
The American College of Obstetricians and
Gynecologists.)

TABLE 15-13
Causes of Vaginal Bleeding Before Twentieth Week of Pregnancy

Final Diagnosis	No. of Patients	%
Threatened abortion	211	13.6
Inevitable and incomplete abortion	951	61.4
Complete abortion	203	13.1
Septic abortion	67	4.3
Missed abortion	27	1.7
Benign hydatidiform mole	12	0.8
Tubal pregnancy	78	5.1
TOTAL	1549	

From Cavanagh D, Fleisher A, Ferguson JH: Inevitable and incomplete abortion. Am J Obstet Gynecol 90:216, 1964.

the products of conception have been expelled and the cervix remains dilated, a diagnosis of incomplete abortion is made. However, if all fetal and placental tissue has been expelled, the cervix is closed, bleeding from the canal is minimal or decreasing, and uterine cramps have ceased, a diagnosis of complete abortion can be made. A complete abortion usually occurs before 6 weeks' and after 14 weeks' gestation. Abortions occurring within this time frame are usually incomplete and may be accompanied by profuse uterine bleeding.

Missed Abortion

The diagnosis of missed abortion is suspected when the uterus fails to continue to enlarge with or without uterine bleeding or spotting. Typically after an episode of bleeding subsides, a continuous brown vaginal discharge is noted. The diagnosis can be confirmed by a continuous fall in HCG levels until they become undetectable or there is absence of fetal heart rate and absence of movement of the fetal extremities during an ultrasound examination. When a dead fetus is retained in the uterus beyond 5 weeks after fetal death, consumptive coagulability with resultant hypofibrogenemia may occur. The incidence of this condition is correlated with both the length of gestation and the duration of fetal death, being uncommon in gestations of less than 14 weeks' duration or duration of fetal death less than 6 weeks.

Septic Abortion

Infection occurs in about 1% to 2% of all spontaneous abortions, with the incidence increasing if the abortion has been induced by a nonsterilized instrument. Any patient with uterine bleeding or spotting during the first half of pregnancy accompanied by clinical signs of infection must be considered to have a septic abortion if no obvious source of infection outside the genital tract is evident.

Septic abortions can be threatened, inevitable, or incomplete. The infection frequently spreads from the endometrium through the myometrium to the parametrium and sometimes to the peritoneum. Thus in addition to endometritis, parametritis and peritonitis frequently occur in women with septic abortions. In addition to an elevated temperature and leukocytosis, lower abdominal tenderness, cervical motion tenderness, and a foul uterine discharge are signs of septic abortion. The cause of the infection is usually polymicrobal, with *Escherichia coli* and other aerobic gram-negative rods frequently involved. Group B beta-hemolytic streptococci, anaerobic streptococci, *Bacteroides* species, and on occasion *Clostridium perfringens* are other organisms that can cause septic abortion. Since endotoxins can be released from the gram-negative bacilli, endotoxic shock may accompany septic abortion, particularly if it is caused by insertion of nonsterile agents into the uterine cavity.

TREATMENT
Threatened Abortion

Although some physicians recommend that patients with threatened abortion restrict their physical activities or stay at bed rest, there is no evidence that these measures or any active medical therapy improves the prognosis of threatened abortion. Treatment with natural progesterone or synthetic progestins was previously advocated, but there is no evidence that such therapy improves the prognosis. Since such treatment may increase the probability of having a missed abortion, the use of this or any type of hormonal therapy is contraindicated. Nevertheless, staying at home with restriction of physical activities and avoidance of coitus is usually advised until the bleeding ceases. If bleeding increases, especially if it is accompanied by uterine cramps, it is likely that the abortion is becoming inevitable and the patient should be examined in a medical facility. Serial HCG measurements and uterine sonography aid in predicting the outcome. If fetal activity ceases or HCG levels steadily decline to less than 10,000 mIU/ml, then it is probably best to evacuate the uterine contents medically with an oxytocic agent or surgically with curettage, depending on the stage of gestation.

Inevitable and Incomplete Abortion

Most abortions that occur between 8 and 14 weeks of pregnancy are incomplete and require surgical evacuation. This procedure can usually be accomplished on an outpatient basis in a hospital or surgical outpatient facility, as bleeding may be profuse and it may be necessary to administer a blood transfusion. Women with an incomplete abortion who do not develop sepsis or hypotension can usually be treated in the emergency room. After measurement of vital signs and placement of an intravenous line with an 18-gauge needle, blood is drawn for a complete blood count as well as typing and cross matching for possible transfusion. An infusion of 10 to 30 units of oxytocin in 1000 ml of 5% Ringer's lactate is advocated, and an intramuscular analgesic (meperidine 75 mg and diazepam [Valium] 5 mg) is given, followed by placement of a paracervical block at 3 and 9 o'-clock with 10 ml of 1% lidocaine (Xylocaine). Approximately 5 to 10 minutes later the uterine contents are evacuated with sponge forceps, and the cavity curetted gently with a sharp curette. Deep curettage should be avoided to prevent the subsequent development of uterine synechiae. Following the procedure the patient's vital signs and amount of vaginal bleeding should be monitored for 4 to 8 hours, after which the patient may be discharged home to remain at bed rest for 24 hours and avoid intercourse for 2 weeks. Oral ergonovine maleate 0.2 mg is administered every 4 to 6 hours for 1 to 2 days. In addition, iron sulfate 200 mg should be administered orally three times a day until hemoglobin levels return to normal and tissue iron stores are replenished. If the mother is Rh negative and the father Rh positive, 50 μg anti-D gamma globulin should be administered intramuscularly. Numerous investigations, including the large series reported by Decenzo and Cavanagh, have shown this management approach to have good results.

Women with a complete abortion, usually before 8 weeks' gestation, need not be hospitalized but can be treated as outpatients with administration of ergonovine maleate as described. However, if patients are already in the hospital and are thought to spontaneously pass all the products of conception, a curettage should be performed as described to be certain that the abortion is not incomplete.

Septic Abortion

Septic abortion is a potentially fatal disease process with an estimated fatality rate of 0.4 to 0.6/100,000 spontaneous abortions. In the United States between 1975 and 1977, Grimes reported that 41 women died after having a spontaneous abortion; 15 (37%) of these deaths were due to sepsis. All patients with the diagnosis of septic abortion should have a complete blood count, urinalysis, chemistry, and electrolyte panel obtained. In addition, a specimen of the uterine discharge should be sent to the laboratory for culture and sensitivity. A Gram stain of the discharge should be performed in the admitting area. If the patient is seriously ill, blood cultures, a chest x-ray examination, and tests of blood coagulability should be obtained. Antibiotics should be administered intravenously and the uterine contents evacuated. It is best to use combination antibiotic therapy including an agent that will be effective against anaerobic bacteria. After adequate blood levels of antibiotics are obtained, usually within 2 hours, the uterus should be evacuated as described previously.

If the uterus is larger than 14 weeks gestation and the cervix is closed (threatened septic abortion), management is more difficult. The uterine cavity needs to be evacuated to provide drainage of the infected material. This can be performed either by curettage, dilation and evacuation, oxytocics, or prostaglandins. Sometimes it is necessary to perform a hysterectomy if the sepsis is severe and the uterus cannot be evacuated through the cervical canal. All patients with septic abortions need to have close monitoring of vital signs and urinary output. If signs of septic shock should develop, a central venous pressure catheter should be placed and additional intravenous fluids administered. Additional therapeutic agents such as nasal oxygen, vasopressor agents, digitalis, and corticosteriods may also be used.

Recurrent Abortion

The expected probability of a woman's having three consecutive spontaneous abortions is about 0.3% to 0.4%, but the actual incidence is reported to range from 0.4% to 0.8%, indicating that there is a specific cause for recurrent pregnancy loss in some women.

The abortuses of women who have three or more abortions are more likely to be chromosomally normal (80% to 90%) than those of women with a spontaneous abortion. Women with recurrent abortions also have a tendency to abort later in gestation, with two thirds of such abortions occurring beyond 12 weeks' gestation, indicating that maternal or environmental factors are a more likely cause of repeated pregnancy loss. Recurrent abortion is also called habitual abortion, but this term implies that every pregnancy will end in an abortion. As stated, if a woman has had no live births and three abortions, she has about a 50% chance of having a term gestation in her next pregnancy, and if she has had one live birth this chance is increased to about 70%. Thus the term habitual abortion should not be used.

Couples with recurrent abortion require careful sympathetic management by the practitioner, as an abortion is an emotionally traumatic experience that can result in as much grief as intrauterine fetal death in late pregnancy or a neonatal death. With recurrent abortion this emotional trauma is magnified, and the practitioner needs to express sympathy and understanding as counseling is performed and a diagnostic regimen is outlined.

Because the etiology of a second-trimester loss is more likely to be uterine in origin and thus more likely to be able to be determined, a diagnostic evaluation should be performed after a woman has had only one second-trimester spontaneous abortion. There is no need to wait for a woman to have three first-trimester abortions with their accompanying emotional trauma before beginning a diagnostic evaluation. Because one early abortion is relatively common, it is recommended that diagnostic evaluation be initiated only after a woman has two first-trimester abortions.

After a history and physical examination are performed with pertinent questions regarding cervical incompetence, a complete blood count, a serum TSH, and a midluteal serum progesterone measurement should be ob-

TABLE 15-14

Identification of Etiologic Factors in 195 Couples According to Prior Obstetric History

	Total	
Etiologic Factor	**No.**	**%**
Uterine body abnormalities	30	15.4
Müllerian fusion anomaly	19	
Fixed retroversion	5	
Uterine fibroids	4	
Synechiae	2	
Cervical incompetence	25	12.8
Endocrine dysfunction	10	5.1
Luteal insufficiency	6	
Thyroid dysfunction	4	
Endometrial infection	29	14.9
U. urealyticum	22	
T. gondii	7	
Chromosomal abnormalities	5	2.6
Systemic disorders (ulcerative colitis)	2	1.0
Sperm factors	8	4.1
Excessive smoking	1	0.5
Total "known etiology"	110	56.4
"Unknown etiology"	85	43.6
Total	195	100

From Stray-Pedersen B, Stray-Pedersen S: Etiologic factors and subsequent reproductive performance in 195 couples with a prior history of habitual abortion. Am J Obstet Gynecol 148:140, 1984.

tained. A hysterogram should be performed to rule out congenital uterine anomalies, submucous leiomyomas, and intrauterine adhesions. If no abnormalities are found, a karyotype of the husband and wife should be performed to determine if some chromosomal anomaly such as balanced translocation or 45X mosaicism exists. The value of obtaining endometrial bacteriologic cultures and HLA typing of husband and wife is controversial; however, tests to detect the lupus anticoagulant antibody should be performed.

If any of these tests reveals an abnormality that can be corrected with appropriate surgical or medical therapy as described, such therapy should be initiated. If a chromosomal abnormality is found, then genetic counseling is in-

dicated. There have been three recent series of large numbers of couples with recurrent abortion who have undergone a comprehensive diagnostic evaluation (Table 15-14). Although different criteria for abnormal diagnostic tests were used by each group of investigators, no specific etiology for the recurrent abortion (all tests normal) was found in 35% to 44% of the couples studied.

If no diagnosis can be obtained, the couple should be counseled regarding the probability of abortion in a subsequent pregnancy. After conception, measurement of HCG levels twice weekly will allow early prognosis of the outcome of the pregnancy. In normal gestations the levels of HCG double about every 2 days, and the rate of increase in a particular patient

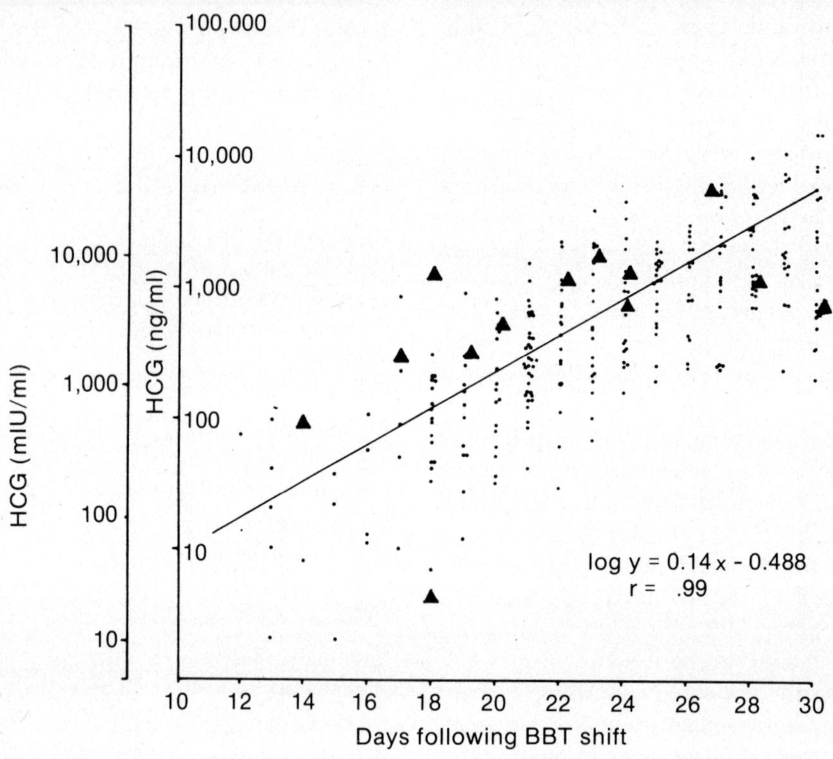

FIGURE 15-11

β-HCG RIA values during first 30 days of successful pregnancies. Each point represents concentration of HCG on specific day from 189 successful pregnancies. ▲, twin gestation. Line represents linear regression of means of data taken by days (5.7 mIU; 1 ng). (From Batzer FR, Schlaff S, Goldfarb AF, et al: Serial β-subunit human chorionic gonadotropin doubling time as a prognosticator of pregnancy outcome in an infertile population. Fertil Steril 35:307, 1981. Reproduced with permission of the publisher, The American Fertility Society.)

can be compared with the expected normal rate of increase (Fig. 15-11). In most individuals with an early abortion, levels of HCG will rise at a slower rate than normal, plateau, and then decline (Fig. 15-12). Batzer et al. found that when β-HCG doubling time in the first month of gestation was normal, it predicted a good outcome 88% of the time, and when abnormal, predicted a poor outcome 76% of the time. If HCG levels are increasing normally, an ultrasound examination should be performed after they reach 6500 mIU/ml, at which time a gestational sac should be found. A re-peat ultrasound 2 weeks later should demonstrate a normal fetal heart rate. These findings are reassuring, both to the mother and to the clinician.

Some individuals recommend that prophylactic antibiotic treatment be given to the husband and wife in the conception cycle or that progesterone supplementation be given to all women with recent abortion in the first trimester of pregnancy. Neither of these modalities has been demonstrated to improve the outcome of the pregnancy.

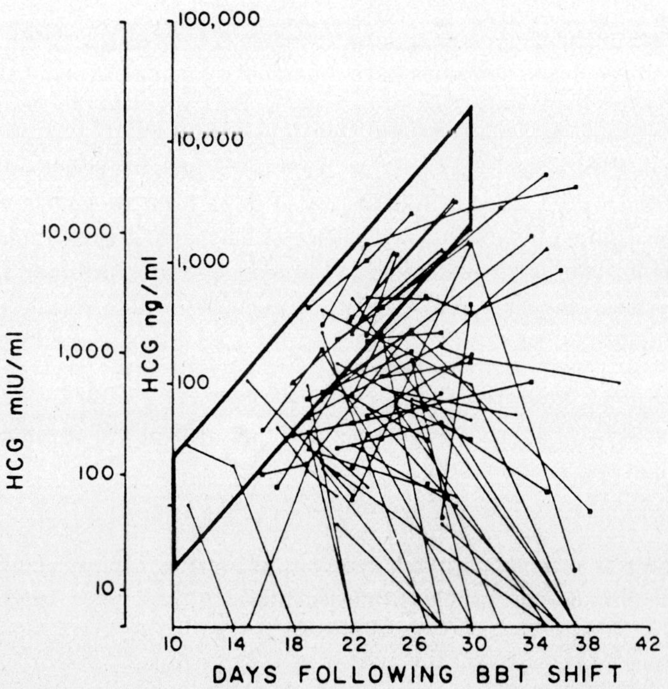

FIGURE 15-12
Serial β-HCG RIA values in 53 patients who aborted spontaneously. Twenty-six patients had a negative slope. Five patients with a normal slope aborted in second trimester. Solid line encloses 95% confidence limits in successful pregnancies. (From Batzer FR, Schlaff S, Goldfarb AF, et al: Serial β-subunit human chorionic gonadotropin doubling time as a prognosticator of pregnancy outcome in an infertile population. Fertil Steril 35:307, 1981. Reproduced with permission of the publisher, The American Fertility Society.)

_______________ **KEY POINTS** _______________

- About 15% to 20% of all human pregnancies terminate in clinically recognized abortion.

- In the human the total embryonic loss before 12 weeks' gestation is about 60%.

- About 80% of abortions occur in the first trimester, with the incidence decreasing with increasing gestational age.

- If conception occurs within 3 months after a live birth, the incidence of abortion is increased compared to the relatively stable rate if conception occurs later than 3 months.

- The risk of a pregnancy terminating in spontaneous abortion increases independently with increasing parity, maternal age, and paternal age.

- Women with multiple abortions have a tendency to abort at about the same gestational age.

- For a woman with a reproductive history of three prior pregnancies terminating in abortion with no live births, her chance of having an abortion in a subsequent pregnancy is about 50%; if she has had at least one live birth and three spontaneous abortions, the chance that her next pregnancy will terminate in abortion is only about 30%.

- The major cause of abortion is genetic, and the incidence of chromosomal anomalies in abortuses is about 50%.

- Only about 5% of the abnormal karyotypes of abortuses are structural abnormalities of the chromosomes such as translocation.

- Autosomal trisomy is the most common abnormal karyotype (50%), followed in decreasing frequency by monosomy 45X (20%), triploidy (15%), tetraploidy (10%), and structural abnormalities (5%).

- The most common single chromosomal abnormality is monosomy 45X.

- Karyotypes of abortuses of women who have had more than one abortion tend to be similar if the first abortus had either a normal karyotype or an autosomal trisomy.

- Maternal age is directly related to the incidence of trisomic abortions.

- Monosomy 45X abortion is associated with a younger maternal age than other aneuploid or euploid abortions.

- Abortion of chromosomally normal conceptuses is found to occur later in gestation than abortions of chromosomally abnormal conceptuses does, with the peak incidence of euploid abortion being about 12 to 13 weeks of gestation; the peak incidence of aneuploid abortions is about 11 weeks.

- The incidence of chromosomally normal abortions increases markedly after a maternal age of 35, rising to more than 30% of clinically recognized conceptions after age 40.

- About 20% to 25% of women with anomalies of uterine fusion have severe problems with reproduction, recurrent abortion being the most serious.

- The least frequent uterine anomaly, the unicornuate uterus, is associated with the greatest incidence of spontaneous abortion, about 50%.

- Women with either a septate or bicornuate uterus have a 25% to 30% incidence of spontaneous abortion.

- Women with recurrent abortion due to bicornuate and septate uteri have a decline in the abortion rate from about 88% to 15% after surgical correction.

- Women exposed to DES who subsequently conceive have a significantly greater incidence of spontaneous abortion than controls do.

- In women with an incompetent cervix the rate of fetal survival increases from about 20% to 80% after cerclage.

KEY POINTS, cont'd

- Spontaneous and induced abortion is the cause of about two thirds of intrauterine adhesions.

- Diabetes, if controlled by diet or insulin, is not a cause of abortion.

- In women who smoke more than 14 cigarettes per day the risk of having an abortion is 1.7 times greater than in women who do not smoke.

- Smoking and alcohol are both toxic agents that can destroy chromosomally normal fetuses.

- Women who drink alcohol at least 2 days a week have about a twofold greater risk of having an abortion.

- Irradiation of less than 5 rads will not cause an abortion in the human.

- Threatened abortion occurs in about 30% to 40% of human gestations, with only about half of these pregnancies ending in spontaneous abortion.

- A poor prognosis for pregnancy is associated with a serum HCG level less than 10,000 mIU/ml in a woman with threatened abortion in the first trimester of pregnancy.

- The presence or absence of fetal heart motion or of spontaneous fetal extremity motion beyond 8 weeks' gestation in women with threatened abortion correlates well with a poor pregnancy outcome.

- Complete abortion usually occurs before 6 weeks' and after 14 weeks' gestation. Abortions occurring within this time frame are usually incomplete.

- When a dead fetus is retained in the uterus beyond 5 weeks after fetal death, consumptive coagulability with resultant hypofibrogenemia may occur.

- About 1% to 2% of all spontaneous abortions become infected.

- The expected probability of a woman's having three consecutive abortions is about 0.3% to 0.4%, but the actual incidence is reported to range from 0.4% to 0.8%.

- The abortuses of women who have three or more abortions are more likely to be chromosomally normal (80% to 90%) than those of women with a spontaneous abortion.

- Women with recurrent abortions also have a tendency to abort later in gestation, with two thirds of such abortions occurring beyond 12 weeks' gestation, indicating that maternal or environmental factors are a more likely cause of repeated pregnancy loss.

- A diagnostic evaluation should be performed after a woman has had only one second-trimester spontaneous abortion or two first-trimester abortions.

- In most individuals with an early abortion, levels of HCG will rise at a slower rate than normal, plateau, and then decline.

BIBLIOGRAPHY

Anderson SG: Management of threatened abortion with real-time sonography. Obstet Gynecol 55:259, 1980.

Austin CR: Pregnancy losses and birth defects. In Austin CR, Short RV, eds: Reproduction in mammals, vol. 2. London, Cambridge University Press, 1972.

Axelsson G, Rylander R: Exposure to anaesthetic gases and spontaneous abortion: Response bias in a postal questionnaire study. Int J Epidemiol 11:250, 1982.

Barnes AB, Colton T, Gundersen J, et al: Fertility and outcome of pregnancy in women exposed in utero to diethylstilbestrol. N Engl J Med 302:609, 1980.

Batzer FR, Schlaff S, Goldfarb AF, et al: Serial β-subunit human chorionic gonadotropin doubling time as a prognosticator of pregnancy outcome in an infertile population. Fertil Steril 35:307, 1981.

Beer AE, Quebbeman JF, Ayers JWT, et al: Major histocompatibility complex antigens, maternal and paternal immune responses, and chronic habitual abortions in humans. Am J Obstet Gynecol 141:987, 1981.

Benson RC, Durfee RB: Transabdominal cervicouterine cerclage during pregnancy for the treatment of cervical incompetency. Obstet Gynecol 25:145, 1965.

Boué J, Boué A, Lazar P: Retrospective and prospective epidemiological studies of 1500 karyotyped spontaneous human abortions. Teratology 12:11, 1975.

Brent RL: Radiation-induced embryonic and fetal loss from conception to birth. In Porter IH, Hook EB, eds: Human embryonic and fetal death. New York, Academic Press, 1980.

Buttram VC, Gibbons WE: Müllerian anomalies: A proposed classification (an analysis of 144 cases). Fertil Steril 32:40, 1979.

Buttram VC Jr, Reiter RC: Uterine leiomyomata: Etiology, symptomatology, and management. Fertil Steril 36:433, 1981.

Carr DH: Cytogenetic aspects of induced and spontaneous abortions. Clin Obstet Gynecol 15:203, 1972.

Caudle MR, Rote NS, Scott JR, et al: Histocompatibility in couples with recurrent spontaneous abortion and normal fertility. Fertil Steril 39:793, 1983.

Cavanagh D, Fleisher A, Ferguson JH: Inevitable and incomplete abortion. Am J Obstet Gynecol 90:216, 1964.

Chartier M, Roger M, Barrat J, et al: Measurement of plasma human chorionic gonadotropin (hCH) and β-hCG activities in the late luteal phase: Evidence of the occurrence of spontaneous menstrual abortions in infertile women. Fertil Steril 31:134, 1979.

Cousins L: Cervical incompetence, 1980: A time for reappraisal. Clin Obstet Gynecol 23:467, 1980.

Crane JP, Wahl N: The role of maternal diabetes in repetitive spontaneous abortion. Fertil Steril 36:477, 1981.

Creasy MR, Crolla JA, Alberman ED: A cytogenetic study of human spontaneous abortions using banding techniques. Hum Genet 31:177, 1976.

Decenzo JA, Cavanagh D: Management of incomplete abortion on an outpatient basis. Am J Obstet Gynecol 97:17, 1967.

DeCherney AH, Russell JB, Graebe RA, et al: Resectoscopic management of müllerian fusion defects. Fertil Steril 45:726, 1986.

Edmonds DK, Lindsay KS, Miller JF, et al: Early embryonic mortality in women. Fertil Steril 38:447, 1982.

Glass RH, Golbus MS: Habitual abortion. Fertil Steril 29:257, 1978.

Gottesfeld KR: The use of ultrasound in the first trimester of pregnancy. Semin Ultrasound 1:254, 1980.

Grimes DA, Cates W Jr, Selik RM: Fatal septic abortion in the United States, 1975-1977. Obstet Gynecol 57:739, 1981.

Haney AF, Hammond CB, Soules MR, et al: Diethylstilbestrol-induced upper genital tract abnormalities. Fertil Steril 31:142, 1979.

Harger JH: Comparison of success and morbidity in cervical cerclage procedures. Obstet Gynecol 56:543, 1980.

Harger JH, Archer DF, Marchese SG, et al: Etiology of recurrent pregnancy losses and outcome of subsequent pregnancies. Obstet Gynecol 62:574, 1983.

Harlap S, Shiono PH, Ramcharan S: A life table of spontaneous abortions and the effects of age, parity, and other variables. In Porter IH, Hook EB, eds: Human embryonic and fetal death. New York, Academic Press, 1980.

Heinonen PK, Saarikoski S, Pystynen P: Reproductive performance of women with uterine anomalies. Acta Obstet Gynecol Scand 61:157, 1982.

Hensleigh PA, Fainstat T: Corpus luteum dysfunction: Serum progesterone levels in diagnosis and assessment of therapy for recurrent and threatened abortion. Fertil Steril 32:396, 1979.

Herbst AL, Hubby MM, Azizi F, et al: Reproductive and gynecologic surgical experience in diethylstilbestrol-exposed daughters. Am J Obstet Gynecol 141:1019, 1981

Herbst AL, Hubby MM, Blough RR, et al: A comparison of pregnancy experience in DES-exposed and DES-unexposed daughters. J Reprod Med 24:62, 1980.

Hertig AT, Rock J, Adams EC, et al: Thirty-four fertilized human ova, good, bad and indifferent, recovered from 210 women of known fertility. Pediatrics 23:202, 1959.

Horta JLH, Fernandez JG, Soto de Leon B, et al: Direct evidence of luteal insufficiency in women with habitual abortion. Obstet Gynecol 49:705, 1977.

Jacobs PA, Hassold TJ: The origin of chromosome abnormalities in spontaneous abortion. In Porter IH, Hook EB, eds: Human embryonic and fetal death. New York, Academic Press, 1980.

James WH: On the possibility of segregation in the propensity to spontaneous abortion in the human female. Ann Hum Genet 25:207, 1961.

Kadar N, DeVore G, Romero R: Discriminatory hCG zone: Its use in the sonographic evaluation for ectopic pregnancy. Obstet Gynecol 58:156, 1981.

Kajii T, Ferrier A, Niikawa N, et al: Anatomic and chromosomal anomalies in 639 spontaneous abortuses. Hum Genet 55:87, 1980.

Kajii T, Ohama K: Inverse maternal age effect on monosomy X. Hum Genet 51:147, 1979.

Kaufman RH, Adam E, Binder GL, et al: Upper genital tract changes and pregnancy outcome in offspring exposed in utero to diethylstilbestrol. Am J Obstet Gynecol 137:299, 1980.

Kaufman RH, Noller K, Adam E, et al: Upper genital tract abnormalities and pregnancy outcome in diethylstilbestrol-exposed progeny. Am J Obstet Gynecol 148:973, 1984.

Kline J, Shrout P, Stein ZA, et al: Drinking during pregnancy and spontaneous abortion. Lancet 2:176, 1980.

Kline J, Stein Z, Susser M, et al: Environmental influences on early reproductive loss in a current New York City study. In Porter IH, Hood EB, eds: Human embryonic and fetal death. New York, Academic Press, 1980.

Kline J, Stein ZA, Susser M, et al: Smoking: A risk factor for spontaneous abortion. N Engl J Med 297:793, 1977.

Lauritsen JG: Aetiology of spontaneous abortion. Acta Obstet Gynecol Scand (Suppl) 52:3, 1976.

Léridon H: Human fertility. Chicago, University of Chicago Press, 1977.

Lubbe WF, Butler WS, Palmer SJ, et al: Fetal survival after prednisone suppression of maternal lupus-anticoagulant. Lancet 1:1361, 1983.

Lubbe WF, Liggins GC: Lupus anticoagulant and pregnancy. Am J Obstet Gynecol 153:322, 1985.

Malpas P: A study of abortion sequences. Br J Obstet Gynaecol 45:932, 1938.

Mann, EC: Habitual abortion. Am J Obstet Gynecol 77:706, 1959.

March CM, Israel R: Gestational outcome following hysteroscopic lysis of adhesions. Fertil Steril 36:455, 1981.

March CM, Israel R: Hysteroscopic management of recurrent abortion secondary to septate uterus. Am J Obstet Gynecol (in press).

Mishell DR Jr, Davajan V: Quantitative immunologic assay of human chorionic gonadotropin in normal and abnormal pregnancies. Am J Obstet Gynecol 96:231, 1966.

Montoro M, Collea JV, Frasier D, et al: Successful outcome of pregnancy in women with hypothyroidism. Ann Intern Med 94:31, 1981.

Mowbray JF, Gibbings C, Liddell H, et al: Controlled trial of treatment of recurrent spontaneous abortion by immunisation with paternal cells. Lancet 1:941, 1985.

Musich Jr, Behrman SJ: Obstetric outcome before and after metroplasty in women with uterine anomalies. Obstet Gynecol 52:63, 1978.

Nahmias AJ, Josey WE, Naib ZM, et al: Perinatal risk associated with maternal genital herpes simplex virus infection. Am J Obstet Gynecol 110:825, 1971.

Naib ZM, Nahmias AJ, Josey WE, et al: Association of maternal genital herpetic infection with spontaneous abortion. Obstet Gynecol 35:260, 1970.

Naylor AF, Warburton D: Sequential analysis of spontaneous abortion. II. Collaborative study data show that gravidity determines a very substantial rise in risk. Fertil Steril 31:282, 1979.

Nygren K-G, Johansson ED, Wide L: Evaluation of the prognosis of threatened abortion from the peripheral plasma levels of progesterone, estradiol, and human chorionic gonadotropin. Am J Obstet Gynecol 116:916, 1973.

Poland BJ, Miller JR, Jones DC, et al: Reproductive counseling in patients who have had a spontaneous abortion. Am J Obstet Gynecol 127:685, 1977.

Rabau E, David A: Listeria monocytogenes in abortion. J Obstet Gynaecol Br Comm 70:481, 1963.

Roberts JM, Laros RK: Hemorrhagic and endotoxic shock: A pathophysiologic approach to diagnosis and management. Am J Obstet Gynecol 110:1041, 1971.

Rock JA, Jones HW: The clinical management of the double uterus. Fertil Steril 28:798, 1977.

Rock JA, Zacur HA: The clinical management of repeated early pregnancy wastage. Fertil Steril 39:123, 1983.

Rocklin RE, Kitzmiller JL, Carpenter CB, et al: Maternal-fetal relation: Absence of an immunologic blocking factor from the serum of women with chronic abortions. N Engl J Med 295:1209, 1976.

Sachs ES, Jahoda MGJ, Van Hemel JO, et al: Chromosome studies of 500 couples with two or more abortions. Obstet Gynecol 65:375, 1985.

Schenker JG, Margalioth EJ: Intrauterine adhesions: An updated appraisal. Fertil Steril 37:593, 1982.

Simpson JL: Genes, chromosomes, and reproductive failure. Fertil Steril 33:107, 1980.

Stein Z, Kline J, Susser E, et al: Maternal age and spontaneous abortion. In Porter IH, Hook EB, eds: Human embryonic and fetal death. New York, Academic Press, 1980.

Stillman RJ: In utero exposure to diethylstilbestrol: Adverse effects on the reproductive tract and reproductive performance in male and female offspring. Am J Obstet Gynecol 142:905, 1982.

Stray-Pedersen B, Eng J, Reikvam TM: Uterine T-mycoplasma colonization in reproductive failure. Am J Obstet Gynecol 130:307, 1978.

Stray-Pedersen B, Stray-Pedersen S: Etiologic factors and subsequent reproductive performance in 195 couples with a prior history of habitual abortion. Am J Obstet Gynecol 148:140, 1984.

Tho PT, Byrd TR, McDonough PG: Etiologies and subsequent reproductive performance of 100 couples with recurrent abortion. Fertil Steril 32:389, 1979.

Thomas ML, Harger JH, Wagener DK, et al: HLA sharing and spontaneous abortion in humans. Am J Obstet Gynecol 151:1053, 1985.

Warburton D, Stein Z, Kline J, et al: Chromosome abnormalities in spontaneous abortion: Data from the New York City study. In Porter IH, Hook EB, eds: Human embryonic and fetal death. New York, Academic Press, 1980.

Warburton D: Monosomy X: A chromosomal anomaly associated with young maternal age. Lancet 1:167, 1980.

Warburton D, Fraser FC: Spontaneous abortion risks in man: Data from reproductive histories collected in a medical genetics unit. Am J Hum Genet 16:1, 1964.

Weitkamp LR, Schacter BZ: Transferrin and HLA: Spontaneous abortion, neural tube defects, and natural selection. N Engl J Med 313:925, 1985.

CHAPTER
16

Ectopic Pregnancy

Abdominal Pregnancy. Pregnancy that develops in any portion of the peritoneal cavity. It usually occurs after a secondary implantation of the trophoblast following tubal abortion (secondary abdominal pregnancy). A primary abdominal pregnancy is one that implants directly into the peritoneal cavity.

Arias-Stella Reaction. Hypersecretory appearance of endometrial glands. The cells demonstrate hyperchromatism, pleomorphism, increased mitotic activity, and hypertrophy.

Cervical Pregnancy. Pregnancy developing in the cervical canal below the level of the internal os.

Chronic Ectopic Pregnancy. Ectopic gestational tissue in the peritoneal cavity following tubal abortion or rupture. It produces chronic symptoms of lower abdominal pain and usually forms adhesions to bowel and peritoneum.

Cornual Pregnancy. Pregnancy developing in one horn of a bicornuate uterus.

Culdocentesis. Aspiration of fluid in cul-de-sac (pouch) of Douglas via a needle placed through the vagina.

Decidual Cast. Sloughing of nearly all of the decidua lining the endometrial cavity.

Ectopic Pregnancy. Pregnancy that develops following implantation of the blastocyst anywhere other than the endometrium lining the uterine cavity.

Hemoperitoneum. Blood in the peritoneal cavity. The blood from a ruptured ectopic pregnancy initially clots and then lyses so that hemoperitoneum is a combination of blood clots and hemorrhagic fluid that will not clot.

Interstitial Pregnancy. Pregnancy developing in the interstitial portion of the oviduct.

Ovarian Pregnancy. Pregnancy developing in the ovary. For the diagnosis to be made, the following four characteristics must be fulfilled: (1) the tube on the affected side should be intact, (2) the gestational site must occupy the normal position of the ovary, (3) the gestational site must be connected to the uterus by the ovarian ligament, and (4) histologically identified ovarian tissue must be present in the sac wall.

Ruptured Ectopic Pregnancy. Ectopic pregnancy that has eroded through the tissue in which it has implanted, producing hemorrhage from exposed vessels.

Salpingitis Isthmica Nodosa. (Tubal Diverticulum). Direct invasion of the tubal muscularis by the tubal epithelium for varying distances between the lumen and the serosa.

Salpingostomy. Operative opening made in the oviduct and used to remove an unruptured tubal pregnancy for the purpose of retaining the oviduct.

Salpingotomy. Operative opening made in the oviduct, followed by removal of an ectopic pregnancy and closure of the incision in the oviduct.

Tubal Abortion. Tubal pregnancy that is extruded out of the fimbrial end of the oviduct.

Tubal Pregnancy. Pregnancy occurring in the oviduct in the ampulla, fimbria, or isthmus. This is the most frequent site of ectopic pregnancy.

Unruptured Tubal Gestation. Tubal pregnancy that has not yet eroded through the wall of the oviduct.

Ectopic pregnancy was probably first described in AD 963 by Albucasis, an Arab writer. In 1876, before the initiation of surgical therapy, the mortality from ectopic pregnancy was estimated to be 60%. The first successful operative treatment of ectopic pregnancy was performed in 1883 by Lawson Tait in England. In 1887 he reported that he had performed salpingectomy on four women with ectopic pregnancy and that they all survived.

EPIDEMIOLOGY

The incidence of ectopic pregnancy is expressed in different ways in the literature, with the most common denominator being number of recognized conceptions (number of ectopic pregnancies per 1000 conceptions). Other denominators include the number of women of reproductive age (number of ectopic pregnancies per 10,000 women aged 14 to 44) and number of total births (number of ectopic pregnancies per 1000 births).

It would be best to be able to calculate the incidence of ectopic pregnancies per 1000 total conceptions; however, since most spontaneous abortions and many elective abortions are not reported, the denominator is always smaller than the actual number, yielding a spuriously increased incidence. Nevertheless, since an unknown number of ectopic pregnancies remain asymptomatic and thus are not reported, the numerator is also lower. Thus the true incidence of ectopic pregnancies per 1000 total conceptions can never be accurately calculated, but the incidences reported are good approximations and, since the same methodology is used, can be validly compared.

The incidence of ectopic pregnancy varies among different countries, with rates as high as 1 in 28 and 1 in 40 deliveries being reported in Jamaica and Vietnam. In the United States the incidence per live births in different series has varied from 1 in 64 to 1 in 241. Using a population base, Sivin reported that the annual ectopic pregnancy rate in the United States in 1976 was 0.72 per 1000 women aged 15 to 44 and 0.95 per 1000 women at risk for pregnancy.

During the past 25 years the incidence of ectopic pregnancy has been steadily increasing in the United States as well as in several Euro-

TABLE 16-1

Increases in Incidence of Ectopic Pregnancy as Reported in Different Regions

Geographic Area	Period	Increase Factor
Czechoslovakia, Prague	1955-1966	1.7
England and Wales	1966-1976	1.6
Finland		
Helsinki	1968-1976	1.9
Turku	1966-1975	1.8
Scotland (unpublished observations)	1964-1974	1.7
Sweden		
Lund	1960-1979	1.9
Uppsala	1960-1975	2.5
United States	1965-1977	2.7

From Weström L, Bengtsson L PH, Mårdh P-A: Incidence, trends and risks of ectopic pregnancy in a population of women. Br Med J 282:15, 1981.

pean countries (Table 16-1). Weström et al. reported that in 20 years the rate of ectopic pregnancy doubled in Sweden, increasing from 5.8 per 1000 diagnosed conceptions between 1960 and 1964 to 11.1 between 1975 and 1979. The Centers for Disease Control reported a similar marked increase in the United States. Between 1970 and 1980 there was nearly a threefold increase in the annual number of women hospitalized for ectopic pregnancies (from 17,800 to 52,200) as well as in the rate per 1000 live births (from 4.8 to 14.5), and there was a doubling of the rate per reported pregnancies (from 4.5 to 10.5) (Table 16-2). Thus in the United States in 1980 more than 1 woman of every 100 who was known to conceive was hospitalized for ectopic gestation. This increased incidence of ectopic pregnancy is thought to be mainly due to an increased incidence of salpingitis, a major risk factor for ectopic pregnancy, as well as improved diagnostic techniques.

In both the Swedish and United States studies there was also a marked increase in the rate of ectopic pregnancy with increasing age when calculated as incidence per 1000 reported conceptions. In the United States the rate increased from 4.5 in women aged 15 to 24 years to 15.2 in those aged 35 to 44 years. However, when the number was calculated per 10,000 women aged 15 to 44, the rate of ectopic preg-

TABLE 16-2
Numbers and Rates of Ectopic Pregnancies by Year (United States, 1970-1980)

		Rates		
Year	No.	Age Group 15-44 Years*	Live Births†	Reported Pregnancies‡
1970	17,800	4.2	4.8	4.5
1971	19,300	4.4	5.4	4.8
1972	24,500	5.5	7.5	6.3
1973	25,600	5.6	8.2	6.8
1974	26,400	5.7	8.4	6.7
1975	30,500	6.5	9.8	7.6
1976	34,600	7.2	11.0	8.3
1977	40,700	8.3	12.3	9.2
1978	42,400	8.5	12.8	9.4
1979	49,900	9.9	14.3	10.4
1980	52,200	9.9	14.5	10.5
TOTAL	363,700	7.0	9.9	7.8

From Centers for Disease Control: Ectopic pregnancies—United States, 1979-1980. MMWR 33(15):201, 1984.
*Rate per 10,000 females.
†Rate per 1000 live births.
‡Rate per 1000 reported pregnancies (live births, legal induced abortions, and ectopic pregnancies).

nancy was lowest in the older group, reflecting the lower total number of pregnancies in this group. These data indicate that the incidence rate of ectopic pregnancy should be calculated using total pregnancies as the denominator to determine the actual risk for a woman exposed to pregnancy. Because of the lower pregnancy rate in older women, overall only about 11% of ectopic pregnancies in the United States occur in women aged 35 to 44, whereas more than half (53%) occur in women aged 25 to 34.

Most ectopic pregnancies occur in multigravid women. Only 10% to 15% of ectopic pregnancies occur in nulligravid women, whereas more than half occur in women who have been pregnant three or more times.

In the United States the rates of ectopic pregnancy were similar in each section of the country, but the rates were about twice as high for nonwhite as for white women (Fig. 16-1). About 2.6% of all reported pregnancies in nonwhite women aged 35 to 44 in the United States are ectopic.

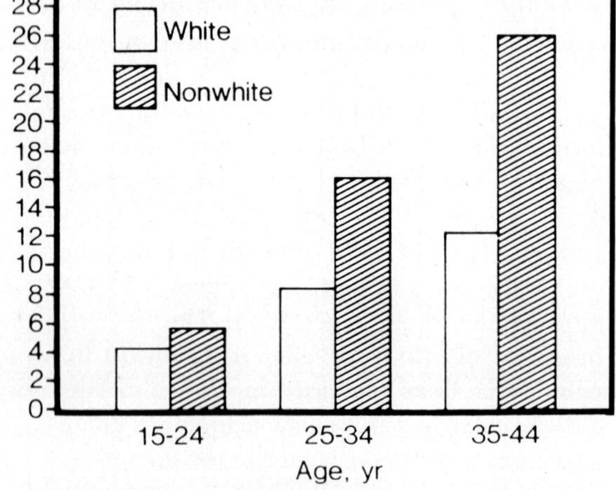

FIGURE 16-1
Ectopic pregnancy rates per 1000 reported pregnancies (including live births, legal induced abortions, and ectopic pregnancies) by age and race (United States, 1970-1978). (From Rubin GL, Peterson HB, Dorfman SF, et al: JAMA 249:1725, 1983. Copyright 1983, American Medical Association.)

MORTALITY

Even with the increased use of surgery and blood transfusions and earlier diagnosis, ectopic pregnancy remains a major cause of maternal death in the United States today. About 40 to 50 deaths from ectopic pregnancy occur annually. Ectopic pregnancy is the most common cause of maternal death in the first half of pregnancy. Although the percentage of all maternal deaths in the United States that are due to ectopic pregnancy increased from 8% in 1970 to 14% in 1980, the percentage of ectopic pregnancies that become fatal has decreased. The overall death-to-case rate of ectopic pregnancy has decreased fourfold from 3.5 per 1000 women with ectopic pregnancy in 1970 to 0.9 in 1980 (Fig. 16-2). The death-to-case rate is similar in all age groups but is about 3 times higher in black women. Because the incidence of ectopic pregnancy is also higher in blacks in the United States, a pregnant black woman is about 6 times more likely to die of ectopic pregnancy than a white woman. Ectopic pregnancy is the most common single cause of all maternal deaths among black women, causing about one fifth of such deaths. Unmarried women of all races have a 1.7 times greater chance of dying of ectopic pregnancy than married women do. Overall risk of death from ectopic pregnancy is about 10 times greater than the risk of childbirth and more than 50 times greater than the risk of legal abortion.

Dorfman et al. studied the clinical aspects of

deaths resulting from ectopic pregnancy in the United States in 1979 and 1980. They found that blood loss was the major cause of death (85%), with infection (5%) and anesthesia complications (2%) much less common. About 80% of these gestations were in the oviduct itself, and the other 20% were interstitial or abdominal gestations. Because the overall incidence of ectopic pregnancy occurring in these latter locations is slightly less than 4%, interstitial and abdominal ectopic pregnancies have about a 5 times greater risk of being fatal than those pregnancies located in the portion of the tube distal to the uterus. About three fourths of the women with fatal ectopic pregnancies initially developed symptoms and died in the first 12 weeks of gestation. Of the remaining one fourth who developed symptoms and died after the first trimester, 70% had interstitial or abdominal pregnancies. Patient delay in consulting a physician after development of symptoms accounted for one third of the deaths, whereas treatment delay resulting from misdiagnosis contributed to the death in one half. More than one half of the patients died of hemorrhage without emergency surgery. The most common

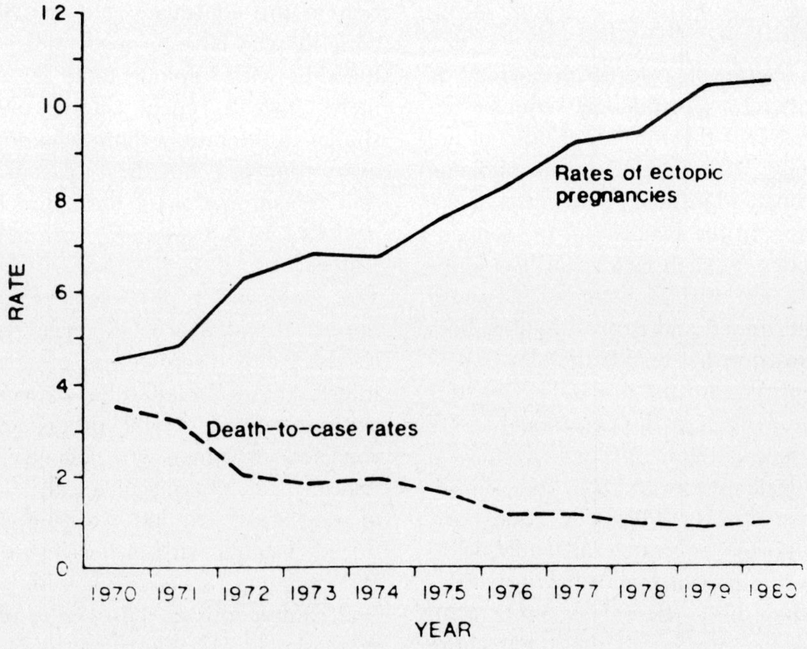

FIGURE 16-2
Rates of ectopic pregnancies and death-to-case ratios by year (United States, 1970-1980). (From Centers for Disease Control: MMWR 33[15]:201, 1984.)

TABLE 16-3
Misdiagnoses for Fatal Ectopic Pregnancies (United States, 1979-1980)

Misdiagnoses	Occurrences*	
	No.	%
Gastrointestinal disorder	14	25
Intrauterine pregnancy	10	18
Pelvic inflammatory disease	8	14
Psychiatric disorder	5	9
Spontaneous abortion	5	9
Sequelae of recent induced abortion	4	7
Urinary tract infection	4	7
Adnexal cyst	2	4
Dysfunctional uterine bleeding	2	4
Fetal death in utero	1	2
Placental abnormality (placenta previa, abruptio placentae)	1	2
Total	56	(100)†

From Dorfman SF, Grimes DA, Cates W Jr, et al: Ectopic pregnancy mortality, United States, 1979 to 1980: Clinical aspects. Obstet Gynecol 64:386, 1984. Reprinted with permission from The American College of Obstetricians and Gynecologists.
*Based on all recorded diagnostic errors. Misdiagnoses did not occur in some cases and occurred more than once in others.
†These percentages do not add up to 100% because of rounding.

misdiagnoses were intestinal disorders and intrauterine pregnancy (Table 16-3).

ETIOLOGY

The major cause of ectopic pregnancy is acute salpingitis. Its morphologic sequelae account for about half the initial episodes of ectopic pregnancy. Although other morphologic factors have been identified as a cause of ectopic pregnancy, in the majority of the remaining first episodes no such factor can be identified. Thus in about 40% of instances the cause cannot be determined and is presumed to be a physiologic disorder that results in delay of passage of the embryo into the uterine cavity so it remains in the oviduct at the gestational age (7 days) when implantation occurs. Ovulation from the contralateral ovary has been implicated as a cause of delay of blastocyst transport, and Breen reported contralateral ovulation to occur in about one third of tubal gestations treated by laparotomy. However, Saito et al. observed that the portion of the tube where implantation occurred in women with ectopic pregnancies was similar whether the corpus luteum was ipsilateral or contralateral to the pregnancy. If transmigration was a factor, they hypothesized that there would be a greater incidence of distal tubal pregnancies with ovulation in the contralateral ovary. Furthermore, patients who have an ipsilateral oophorectomy together with salpingectomy for ectopic pregnancy have a repeat ectopic pregnancy rate similar to the rate in those who do not have the ovary removed. For these reasons it is unlikely that transmigration of the ovum from the opposite ovary is a common cause of ectopic pregnancy.

A more likely physiologic cause would be hormonal imbalance, as excessive circulating levels of either estrogen or progesterone could interfere with normal tubal contractility. An increased rate of ectopic pregnancies has been reported in women who conceive with physiologically and pharmacologically elevated levels of progestins. The latter condition can be produced locally with a progesterone-releasing IUD as well as systemically with progestin-only oral contraceptives. Iatrogenic, physiologically increased levels of estrogen and progesterone occur after ovulation induction with either clomiphene or human menopausal gonadotrophins, and an increased rate of ectopic pregnancies has been reported in women conceiving after either of these treatment modalities.

Another probable etiology is an abnormality of embryonic development. Stratford examined 44 human conceptuses from ectopic gestations by microdissection and histologic sections and found that about two thirds were abnormal and half had gross structural abnormalities. These types of abnormalities could interfere with normal tubal transport. Genetic abnormalities have not been shown to be a cause of ectopic pregnancy, because there is no familial increased incidence, and Elias et al. have shown that the chromosomal complements of ectopic gestations are similar to those of intrauterine gestations.

The causes of ectopic pregnancy will now be discussed in more detail.

Tubal Pathology

The permanent agglutination of the plicae (folds) of the endosalpinx produced by salpingitis can allow normal passage of the smaller sperm while preventing normal transport of the larger blastocyst. The blastocyst can be trapped in blind pockets formed by adhesions of the endosalpinx. In their 20-year longitudinal study, Weström et al. found that nearly half (45.3%) of the women with ectopic pregnancy had a clinical history or histologic findings of a prior episode of acute salpingitis. This figure is in close agreement with the incidence of histologic evidence of prior salpingitis found in the pathologic review of oviducts removed from women with ectopic pregnancy by Bone and Greene as well as Niles and Clark (Fig. 16-3). These and previous investigations found the incidence of histologic evidence of prior salpingitis to be about 40%.

Weström et al. prospectively followed 900 women aged 15 to 34 who had laparoscopically confirmed acute salpingitis and found that the ectopic pregnancy rate was 68.8 per 1000 conceptions, yielding a sixfold increase in the risk of ectopic pregnancy after acute salpingitis as

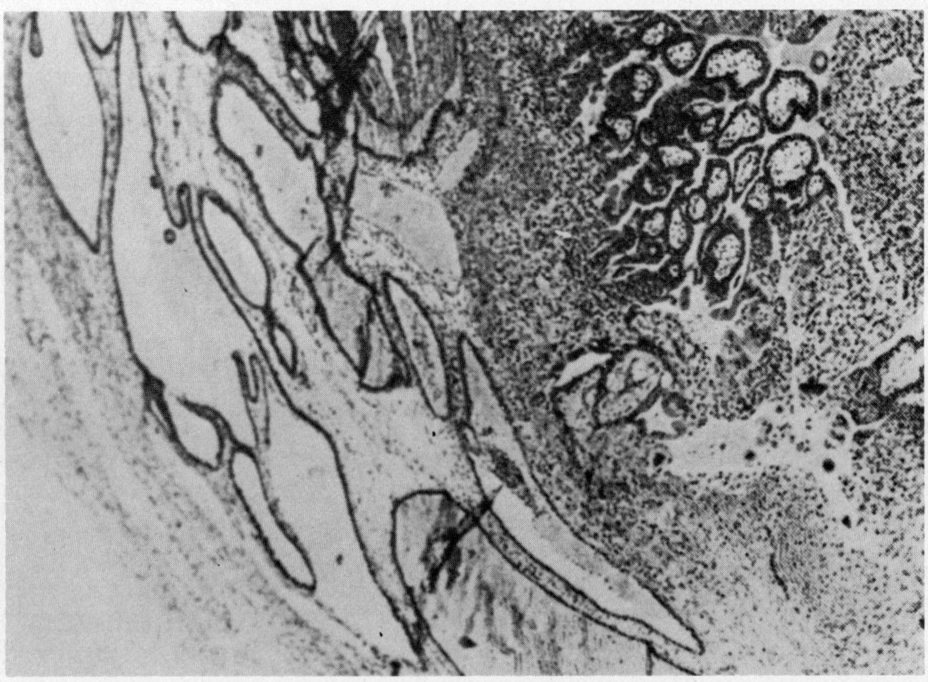

FIGURE 16-3
Tubal pregnancy with placental villi and trophoblastic cells to the right and wall of the tube to the left showing marked degree of follicular salpingitis. (Original magnification, ×70.) (From Bone NL, Greene RR: Am J Obstet Gynecol 82:1166, 1961.)

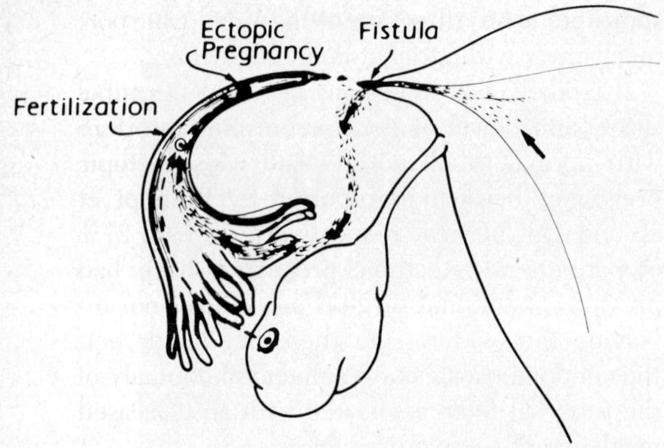

FIGURE 16-6
Mechanism of ectopic pregnancy after sterilization. (From Corson SL, Batzer FR: J Reprod Med 31:78, 1986.)

it was reported that if pregnancy occurred after tubal sterilization by laparoscopic fulguration without concomitant transection, the ectopic pregnancy rate was about 50%. McCausland hypothesized that with the extensive tissue destruction caused by electrocoagulation, a utero-peritoneal fistula could develop that would allow sperm to pass into the distal segment of the oviduct and fertilize the egg (Fig. 16-6). Such fistulas were demonstrated radiographically by Shah et al. in 11% of 150 women following laparoscopic electrocoagulation and demonstrated histologically by McCausland, who called the process endosalpingosis or endosalpingoblastosis. McCann and Kessel also reported a 50% ectopic pregnancy rate following failure of laparoscopic electrocoagulation but only a rare ectopic pregnancy occurred following failure of sterilization with metal clips or silicone rings.

With the marked increase in use of female sterilization techniques, failure of sterilization is becoming a more frequent cause of ectopic pregnancy. In contrast to a large series of ectopic pregnancies in the United States in the 1950s and 1960s reported by Breen, in which only 0.6% of women with ectopic pregnancy had had tubal sterilization, Brenner et al. reported that 3% of 300 ectopic pregnancies occurring in 1976 to 1977 were due to tubal sterilization failure.

Women who have had a prior ectopic pregnancy, even if treated by unilateral salpingectomy, are at increased risk for having a subse-

quent ectopic pregnancy. Of women who conceive after having one ectopic pregnancy, about 15% of subsequent pregnancies are ectopic. In the series of Brenner et al. and Breen, 7% of the women with ectopic pregnancy had a prior ectopic pregnancy.

Contraceptive Failures

As summarized by Tatum and Schmidt, pregnancies occurring as a result of a failure of certain contraceptive methods have a greater chance of being ectopic. Although women who become pregnant while using diaphragms or combination oral contraceptives do not have an increased chance of having an ectopic pregnancy, women who become pregnant while using IUDs or progestin-only oral contraceptives have about a 5% chance of having an ectopic pregnancy. The incidence of ectopic pregnancy in women who become pregnant with the progesterone-releasing IUD is even higher, about 15%. Women using these methods of contraception who elect to have their pregnancies terminated should have a histologic examination of the uterine cavity to be sure the pregnancy was intrauterine.

Women using any type of contraception have a significantly decreased chance of having an ectopic pregnancy as compared with sexually active, noncontraceptive users (Table 16-5). Oral contraceptives prevent ectopic pregnancy to a greater extent than barrier methods or IUDs, but women using the latter methods have less than half the chance of having an ectopic pregnancy than women using no method have. Ory as well as Tatum and Schmidt have reported that the chance of a pregnancy being ectopic in a woman using an IUD is increased if the IUD has been in place for 2 years or more. This increase with longer duration of IUD use is most likely due to the fact that the intrauterine pregnancy rate with IUDs is highest in the first year of use and declines steadily thereafter. Thus the IUD prevents both tubal and uterine pregnancies but is more effective in preventing intrauterine pregnancies. Following discontinuation of any method of contraception, including the IUD, the ectopic pregnancy rate is not increased. An exception is women who were using the shield-type of IUD with its multifilament tailstring, which en-

TABLE 16-5
Percent Distribution of Current Contraceptive Methods and Relationship
with Ectopic Pregnancy

Current Method	Women with Ectopic Pregnancy (No. = 475)	Control Subjects (No. = 2923)	Relative Risk (95% Confidence Interval)
IUD	14.1	17.0	0.4 (0.3-0.6)
Traditional methods	12.0	19.6	0.4 (0.3-0.5)
Oral contraceptives	6.7	26.5	0.1 (0.1-0.2)
None	67.2	36.9	1.0 (Referent)
TOTAL	100.0	100.0	

From Ory HW, The Women's Health Study: Ectopic pregnancy and intrauterine contraceptive devices: New perspectives. Obstet Gynecol 57:137, 1981. Reprinted with permission from The American College of Obstetricians and Gynecologists.

hanced the development of salpingitis. As reported by Chow et al., women discontinuing use of the shield IUD have a 2.4 times increased risk of having an ectopic gestation.

Herbst et al. as well as others have shown that the incidence of ectopic gestation is significantly greater (4 to 5 times) in women who have been exposed to diethylstilbestrol (DES) in utero than in a control group. In various series the ectopic pregnancy rate in such individuals is about 4% to 5%. Kaufman et al. reported that among women exposed to DES whose hysterosalpingograms demonstrated abnormalities in the uterine cavity, the ectopic pregnancy rate was 13%.

Hormonal Alterations

As occurs with exogenous progesterone administration, if increased levels of exogenous or endogenous estrogens are present shortly after the time of ovulation, the incidence of ectopic pregnancy is increased. Morris and Van Wagenen reported that 3 of 30 pregnancies were ectopic in women receiving postovulatory high-dose estrogen to prevent pregnancy. Several investigators have reported that the ectopic pregnancy rate is about 1.5% for conceptions occurring after ovulation has been induced with clomiphene citrate. McBain et al. as well as Gemzell reported the ectopic rate in pregnancies occurring after human menopausal gonadotrophin–induced ovulation to be about 3% to 4%. McBain et al. reported that if the urinary estrogen excretion during human

menopausal gonadotrophin therapy exceeded 200 μg per day, the ectopic rate was 12.5%. These reports indicate that increased levels of estrogen as well as of progesterone interfere with tubal motility and increase the chance of ectopic gestation. Ectopic gestation has also been reported to occur after in vitro fertilization and embryonic transfer. The mechanism remains obscure but may be related to altered sex steroid hormone levels, proximal tubal disease, or both.

Previous Abortion

Although some studies have suggested that a prior induced abortion increases the risk of ec-

TABLE 16-6
Standardized* Relative Risks of Ectopic Pregnancy and 95% Confidence Intervals According to Selected Characteristics

History Characteristic	Relative Risk	95% Confidence Interval
One induced abortion	1.3	0.6-2.7
Two or more induced abortions	2.6	0.9-7.4
Ectopic pregnancy	7.7	1.9-31.5
Pelvic infection	7.5	3.5-16.0
Pelvic operation	2.6	1.4-4.6

From Levin AA, Schoenbaum SC, Stubbfield PG, et al: Ectopic pregnancy and prior induced abortion. Am J Public Health 72:253, 1982.
*Standardized using the multiple logistic regression model.

topic pregnancy, Levin et al. showed that when statistical techniques were used to control the effects of other risk factors, the history of one prior induced abortion did not significantly increase the risk of ectopic pregnancy (Table 16-6). However, the risk for ectopic pregnancy doubled if a woman had had two or more prior induced abortions, which (although not significant) indicates a possible association between multiple induced abortions and subsequent ectopic gestation, probably related to postabortal infection.

PATHOLOGY

Most ectopic pregnancies occur in the oviduct. In Breen's series 97.7% of the ectopic pregnancies were tubal, 1.4% were abdominal, and less than 1% were ovarian or cervical (Fig. 16-7). The majority of tubal gestations, 81%, were located in the ampullary portion of the oviduct, being about equally divided between the distal and middle third of the tube. About 12% of tubal gestations occur in the isthmus and 5% in the fimbrial region. Although Breen considered pregnancies located in the cornual

area of the uterus to be uterine in origin, they are in fact pregnancies implanted in the interstitial portion of the oviduct. About 2% of all ectopic pregnancies are interstitial and are associated with severe morbidity, as they become symptomatic later in gestation than other tubal pregnancies, are difficult to diagnose, and frequently produce massive hemorrhage when they rupture (Fig. 16-8). A true cornual pregnancy is one located in the rudimentary horn of a bicornuate uterus, and this is quite rare. In a review of 240 true cornual pregnancies reported by O'Leary and O'Leary, about 90% of them ruptured with massive hemorrhage.

About 1 in 200 ectopic pregnancies are true ovarian pregnancies that fulfill the four criteria originally described by Spiegelberg. In IUD users the incidence increases to 1 in 15. Many patients with ovarian pregnancies are believed clinically to have a ruptured corpus luteum cyst. In Hallatt's series of 25 primary ovarian pregnancies, correct diagnosis was made during the surgical procedure for only 28%. In his series the hemorrhagic mass was always located adjacent to the corpus luteum, never within it. Ovarian pregnancy is also associated with pro-

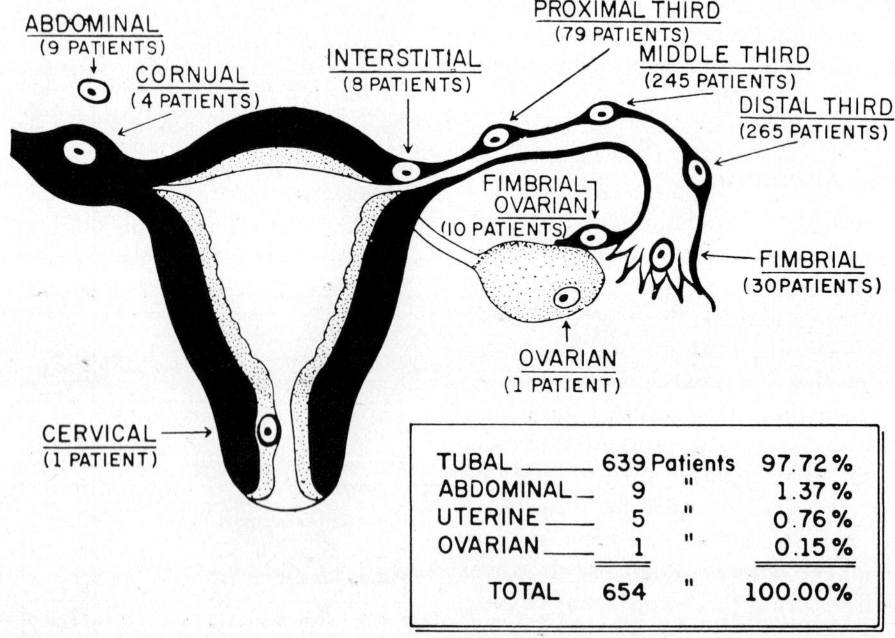

TUBAL	639 Patients	97.72%
ABDOMINAL	9 "	1.37%
UTERINE	5 "	0.76%
OVARIAN	1 "	0.15%
TOTAL	654 "	100.00%

FIGURE 16-7
Anatomic site of ectopic pregnancy. (From Breen JL: Am J Obstet Gynecol 106:1004, 1970.)

fuse hemorrhage, with 81% of Hallatt's cases having a hemoperitoneum greater than 500 ml. Nevertheless, most can be successfully treated by ovarian resection and not oophorectomy.

Most abdominal pregnancies occur secondary to tubal abortion with secondary implantation into the peritoneal cavity (Fig. 16-9). On rare occasions a primary abdominal pregnancy may occur. For the latter diagnosis to be made the following three criteria originally set forth by Studdiford must be present: (1) the tubes and ovaries must be normal with no evidence of recent or past injury, (2) there must be no evidence of a uteroplacental fistula, and (3) the pregnancy must be related only to the peritoneal surface and early enough in gestation to eliminate the possibility of secondary implantation following primary tubal nidation. An unusual type of primary abdominal pregnancy may implant in the spleen or liver and produce massive intraperitoneal hemorrhage.

The prognosis for fetal survival in abdominal pregnancy is poor, found to be 11% by Clark and Guy. Diagnosis is difficult but has become easier with the use of ultrasonography. Once the diagnosis is established, a laparotomy with removal of the fetus should be performed immediately to prevent a possible fatal hemorrhage. On occasion, when the placenta is tightly adherent to bowel and blood vessels, it should be left in the abdominal cavity. In such instances the placental tissue usually resorbs, but symptoms of abdominal pain and intermittent fever may persist for many months as a result of partial bowel obstruction and abscess formation. Thus when it is surgically feasible, the placenta should be entirely removed. Partial removal may result in massive hemorrhage.

The four pathologic criteria for the diagnosis of cervical pregnancy as reported by Rubin et al. are (1) cervical glands must be present opposite the placental attachment, (2) the attachment of the placenta to the cervix must be intimate, (3) the placenta must be below the entrance of the uterine vessels or below the peritoneal reflection of the anteroposterior sur-

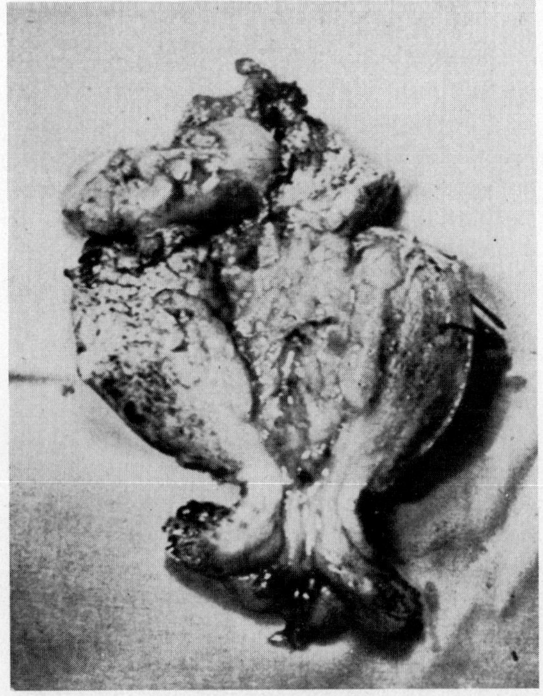

FIGURE 16-8
Anterior view of uterus that has been opened with an anterior Y incision, showing conceptus replaced in site it had formerly occupied in cornual bed. (From Kalchman GG, Meltzer RM: Am J Obstet Gynecol 96:1139, 1966.)

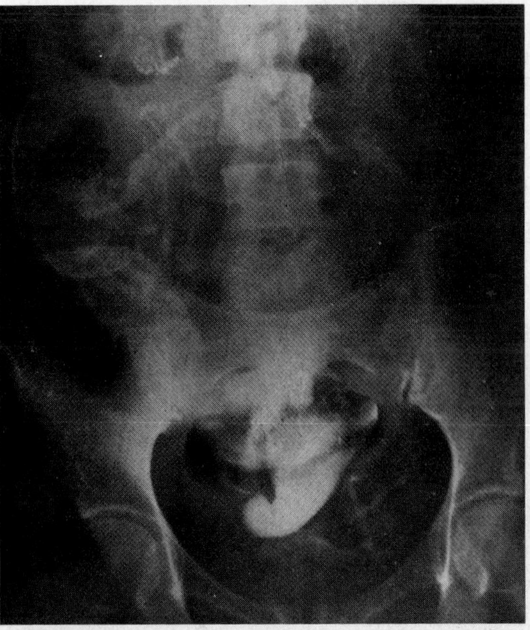

FIGURE 16-9
Hysterosalpingography demonstrating size of uterus and fetus, which is located outside of uterus. (From Clark JF, Guy RS: Am J Obstet Gynecol 96:511, 1966.)

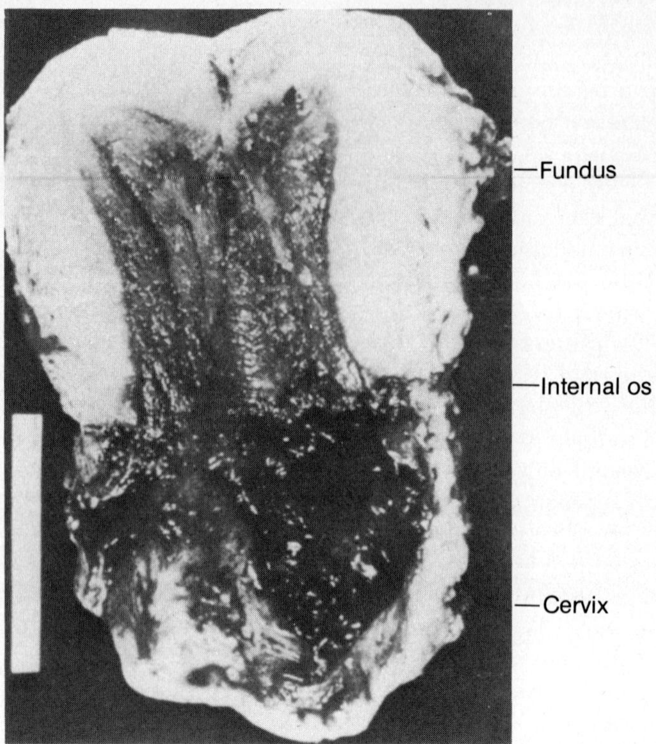

FIGURE 16-10
Cervical pregnancy, 10 weeks' gestation. (From Parente JT, Ou C-S, Levy J: Obstet Gynecol 62:79, 1983. Reprinted with permission from The American College of Obstetricians and Gynecologists.)

face of the uterus, and (4) fetal elements must not be present in the corpus uteri (Fig. 16-10).

The clinical criteria for the diagnosis of cervical pregnancy described by Paalman and McElin are (1) uterine bleeding after amenorrhea without cramping pain, (2) a softened cervix that is disproportionately enlarged to a size equal to or larger than the corpus, (3) complete confinement and firm attachment of the products of conception to the endocervix, and (4) a snug internal os.

Most cervical pregnancies occur after a previous sharp uterine curettage. The differential diagnosis is difficult and includes incomplete abortion, placenta previa, carcinoma of the cervix, and degenerative leiomyoma. Although this entity was primarily associated with a high mortality rate because of massive hemorrhage, currently, with better methods of diagnosis and modern surgical techniques, death is rare. More than half the patients with cervical pregnancy require a hysterectomy for treatment, and it is nearly always necessary if the preg-

nancy has advanced more than 18 weeks in gestational age. Even if a hysterectomy is not performed, the prognosis for future fertility is poor.

An extremely rare location for ectopic pregnancy is between the leaves of the broad ligament, called intraligamentous pregnancy. A single case of vaginal pregnancy presenting as a suburethral cyst has been reported.

Another uncommon form of ectopic gestation is combined intrauterine and extrauterine pregnancy (94% tubal and 6% ovarian). With the use of mathematic calculation the incidence of this entity has previously been estimated to be either 1 in 17,000 or 1 in 30,000 pregnancies. However, a review of the recent experience at one institution by Reece et al. revealed that 1 of 8000 pregnancies was combined intrauterine and extrauterine and 1 of 70 ectopic pregnancies was associated with an intrauterine pregnancy. Combined intrauterine and extrauterine pregnancy may be more common following pharmacologic ovulation induction with fuse hemorrhage, with 81% of Hallatt's cases having a hemoperitoneum greater than 500 ml. Nevertheless, most can be successfully treated by ovarian resection and not oophorectomy.

Most abdominal pregnancies occur secondary to tubal abortion with secondary implantation into the peritoneal cavity (Fig. 16-9). On rare occasions a primary abdominal pregnancy may occur. For the latter diagnosis to be made the following three criteria originally set forth by Studdiford must be present: (1) the tubes and ovaries must be normal with no evidence of recent or past injury, (2) there must be no evidence of a uteroplacental fistula, and (3) the pregnancy must be related only to the peritoneal surface and early enough in gestation to eliminate the possibility of secondary implantation following primary tubal nidation. An unusual type of primary abdominal pregnancy may implant in the spleen or liver and produce massive intraperitoneal hemorrhage.

The prognosis for fetal survival in abdominal pregnancy is poor, found to be 11% by Clark and Guy. Diagnosis is difficult but has become easier with the use of ultrasonography. Once the diagnosis is established, a laparotomy with removal of the fetus should be performed immediately to prevent a possible fatal hemorrhage. On occasion, when the placenta is tightly adherent to bowel and blood vessels, it should be left in the abdominal cavity. In such instances the placental tissue usually resorbs, but symptoms of abdominal pain and intermittent fever may persist for many months as a result of partial bowel obstruction and abscess formation. Thus when it is surgically feasible, the placenta should be entirely removed. Partial removal may result in massive hemorrhage.

The four pathologic criteria for the diagnosis of cervical pregnancy as reported by Rubin et al. are (1) cervical glands must be present opposite the placental attachment, (2) the attachment of the placenta to the cervix must be intimate, (3) the placenta must be below the entrance of the uterine vessels or below the peritoneal reflection of the anteroposterior sur-

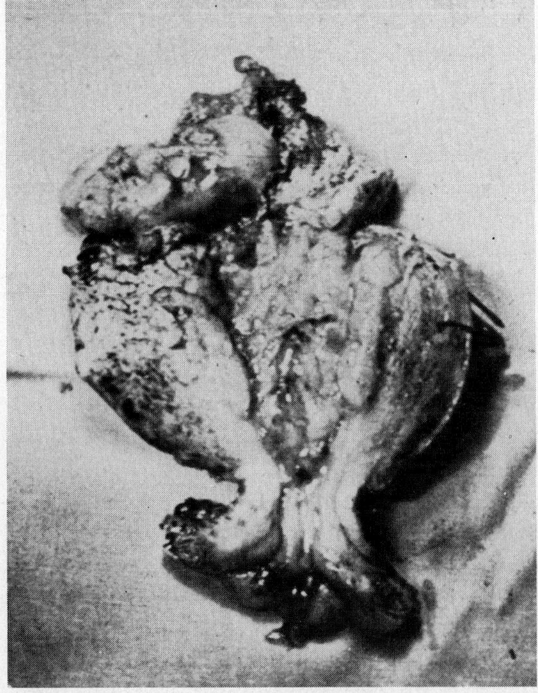

FIGURE 16-8
Anterior view of uterus that has been opened with an anterior Y incision, showing conceptus replaced in site it had formerly occupied in cornual bed. (From Kalchman GG, Meltzer RM: Am J Obstet Gynecol 96:1139, 1966.)

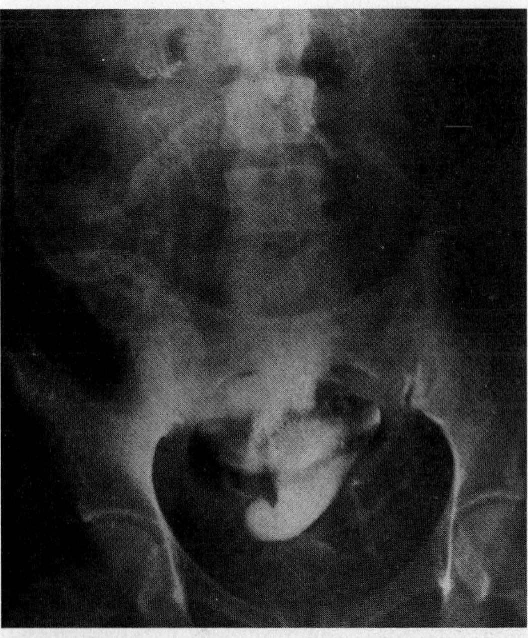

FIGURE 16-9
Hysterosalpingography demonstrating size of uterus and fetus, which is located outside of uterus. (From Clark JF, Guy RS: Am J Obstet Gynecol 96:511, 1966.)

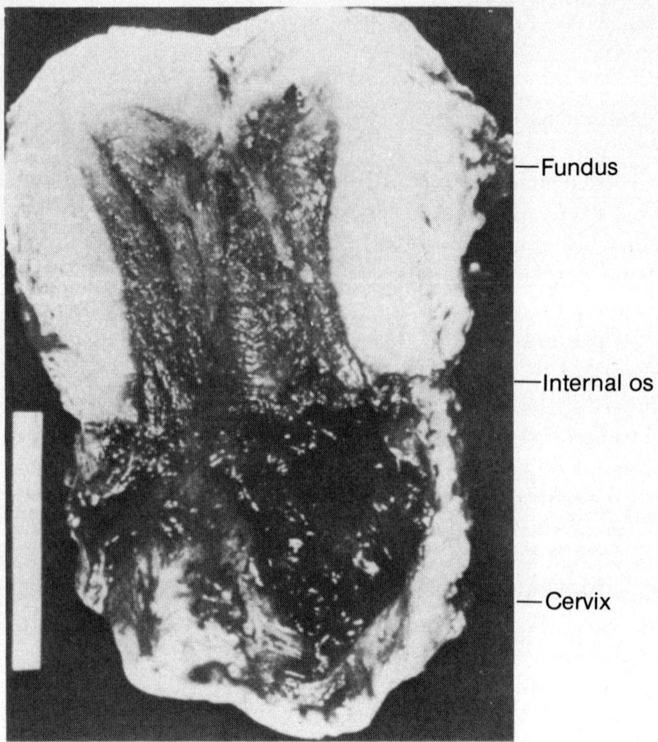

FIGURE 16-10
Cervical pregnancy, 10 weeks' gestation. (From Parente JT, Ou C-S, Levy J: Obstet Gynecol 62:79, 1983. Reprinted with permission from The American College of Obstetricians and Gynecologists.)

face of the uterus, and (4) fetal elements must not be present in the corpus uteri (Fig. 16-10).

The clinical criteria for the diagnosis of cervical pregnancy described by Paalman and McElin are (1) uterine bleeding after amenorrhea without cramping pain, (2) a softened cervix that is disproportionately enlarged to a size equal to or larger than the corpus, (3) complete confinement and firm attachment of the products of conception to the endocervix, and (4) a snug internal os.

Most cervical pregnancies occur after a previous sharp uterine curettage. The differential diagnosis is difficult and includes incomplete abortion, placenta previa, carcinoma of the cervix, and degenerative leiomyoma. Although this entity was primarily associated with a high mortality rate because of massive hemorrhage, currently, with better methods of diagnosis and modern surgical techniques, death is rare. More than half the patients with cervical pregnancy require a hysterectomy for treatment, and it is nearly always necessary if the preg-

nancy has advanced more than 18 weeks in gestational age. Even if a hysterectomy is not performed, the prognosis for future fertility is poor.

An extremely rare location for ectopic pregnancy is between the leaves of the broad ligament, called intraligamentous pregnancy. A single case of vaginal pregnancy presenting as a suburethral cyst has been reported.

Another uncommon form of ectopic gestation is combined intrauterine and extrauterine pregnancy (94% tubal and 6% ovarian). With the use of mathematic calculation the incidence of this entity has previously been estimated to be either 1 in 17,000 or 1 in 30,000 pregnancies. However, a review of the recent experience at one institution by Reece et al. revealed that 1 of 8000 pregnancies was combined intrauterine and extrauterine and 1 of 70 ectopic pregnancies was associated with an intrauterine pregnancy. Combined intrauterine and extrauterine pregnancy may be more common following pharmacologic ovulation induction with the subsequent increase in multiple ovulation. With the increased use of these agents as well as increased incidence of salpingitis, combined intrauterine and extrauterine pregnancy may occur more frequently than previously estimated and should be suspected when any of the following clinical criteria are present: (1) a fundus compatible with gestational age estimated by date of onset of last menses in a patient believed to have an ectopic gestation; (2) two corpora lutea at laparotomy or laparoscopy and an enlarged, soft, and globular uterus; (3) the absence of withdrawal bleeding and the presence of pregnancy symptoms following excision of an ectopic pregnancy; (4) hemoperitoneum following the termination of an intrauterine pregnancy; and (5) the combination of abdominal pain, adnexal mass with pain and tenderness, peritoneal irritation, and a uterus enlarged more than 8 weeks' gestational age.

A chronic ectopic pregnancy occurs when the intraperitoneal hemorrhage associated with tubal abortion or rupture is relatively minor and ceases spontaneously, but the ectopic gestation neither resolves completely or implants and continues to develop as an abdominal pregnancy. The trophoblast continues to secrete human chorionic gonadotrophin (HCG) in small amounts, with half the circulating levels being less than 1000 mIU/ml in 50% and less than 100 mIU/ml in 20%. In the series of Cole and Corlett about 6% of all surgically treated ectopic pregnancies in one institution were classified as chronic. The most common (72%) gross pathologic finding was dense adhesions produced by the inflammatory response to the trophoblast. These adhesions attach omentum and bowel to the site of the ectopic pregnancy. In one third of the cases a collection of clotted blood or old hematoma was present. Cole and Corlett reported that because of the extensive disease it is necessary to perform a hysterectomy in 25% and an oophorectomy in 60% of patients with a chronic ovarian ectopic pregnancy.

HISTOPATHOLOGY

When the blastocyst implants in the tube it does not grow mainly in the tubal lumen as has been assumed for many years. In a recent review of the pathology of tubal gestation, Bu-

dowick et al. found that after implanting on the mucosa of the endosalpinx, the trophoblast invades the lamina propria and then the muscularis of the oviduct and grows mainly between the lumen of the tube and its peritoneal covering (Fig. 16-11). Growth occurs both parallel to the long axis of the tube and circumferentially around it. As the trophoblast invades vessels, retroperitoneal tubal hemorrhage occurs that is mainly extraluminal but may extrude from the fimbriated end and create a hemoperitoneum before tubal rupture (Fig. 16-12).

The stretching of the peritoneum covered by this hemorrhage results in episodic pain before the final perforation into the peritoneal cavity. Rupture occurs when the serosa is maximally stretched, producing necrosis secondary to an inadequate blood supply.

Hemoperitoneum is nearly always found in ectopic pregnancy other than that which is cervical in origin. Usually there is a combination of clotted and unclotted blood in the peritoneal cavity. The unclotted blood has not clotted because it results from lysis of blood that has previously coagulated, similar to what occurs during menstrual bleeding. The hematocrit value of this nonclotting blood is nearly always greater than 15%, such a finding being reported in 98% of specimens obtained by culdocentesis in the series of ectopic pregnancies reported by Brenner et al. At the time of laparotomy for a ruptured ectopic pregnancy about half the patients have less than 500 ml of hemoperitoneum, one quarter between 500 and 1000 ml, and one fifth more than 1000 ml.

When the oviduct is removed and examined histologically, inflammatory cells are nearly always seen. These include plasma cells, lymphocytes, and histiocytes. Chorionic villi, which are frequently degenerated or hyalinized, as well as nucleated red cells are diagnostic of ectopic pregnancy. Decidual reaction in the tube is uncommon.

Because of limited space or inadequate nourishment, the trophoblastic tissue of most ectopic pregnancies does not grow as rapidly as that of pregnancies within the uterine cavity. As a result HCG production does not increase as rapidly as in a normal pregnancy, and although steroid production of the corpus luteum is initiated, elevated progesterone levels cannot be maintained. Thus initially the endome-

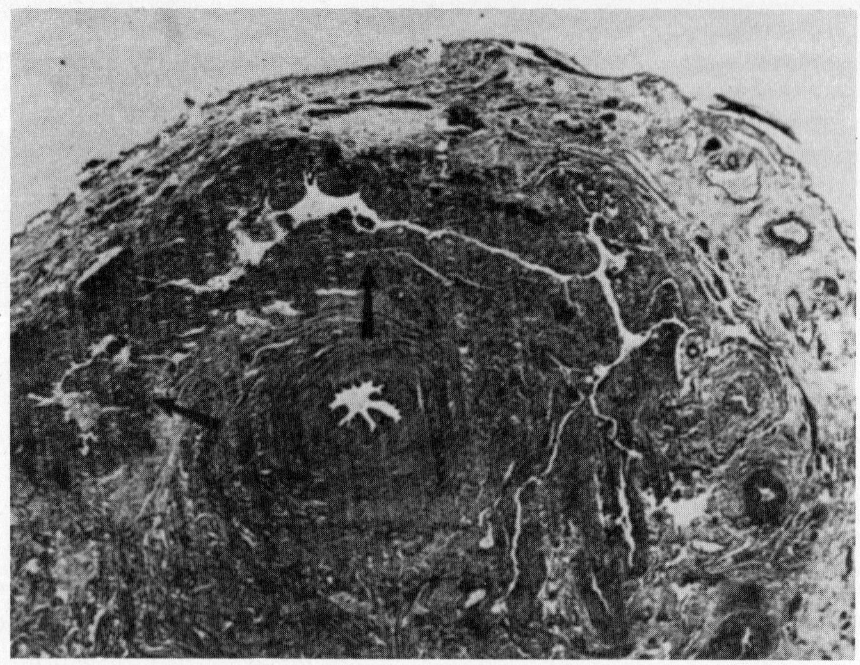

FIGURE 16-11

Low-power photograph showing tube almost completely surrounded by cleftlike space *(arrows)*. Closer inspection revealed that cleft was produced by trophoblast that had implanted elsewhere, perforated wall of tube, and was dissecting along broad ligament between tube and peritoneum. (From Budowick M, Johnson TRB, Genadry R, et al: The histopathology of the developing tubal ectopic pregnancy. Fertil Steril 34:169, 1980. Reproduced with permission of the publisher, The American Fertility Society.)

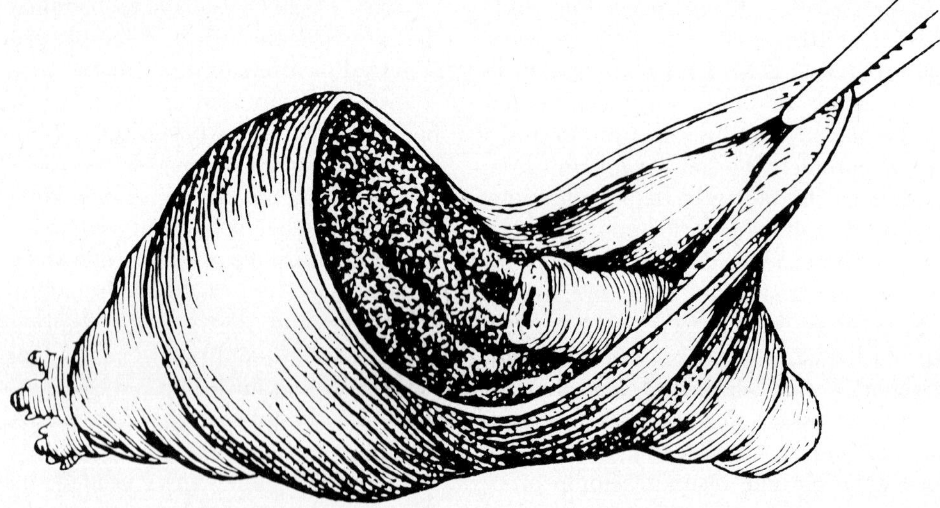

FIGURE 16-12

Artist's rendition of dissected ampullary ectopic pregnancy showing space between tube and peritoneum, revealed when blood clots and placenta were removed. Toward fimbriated end, no dissection was performed and external appearance is that of dilated tube. (From Budowick M, Johnson TRB, Genadry R, et al: The histopathology of the developing tubal ectopic pregnancy. Fertil Steril 34:169, 1980. Reproduced with permission of the publisher, The American Fertility Society.)

trium becomes decidualized because of continued progesterone production by the corpus luteum. Sometimes the secretory cells of the endometrial glands become hypertrophied with hyperchromatism, pleomorphism, and increased mitotic activity, as originally described by Arias-Stella (Fig. 16-13). The Arias-Stella reaction can be confused with neoplasia, but it is not unique for ectopic pregnancy, as it can occur with intrauterine pregnancy as well as fol-

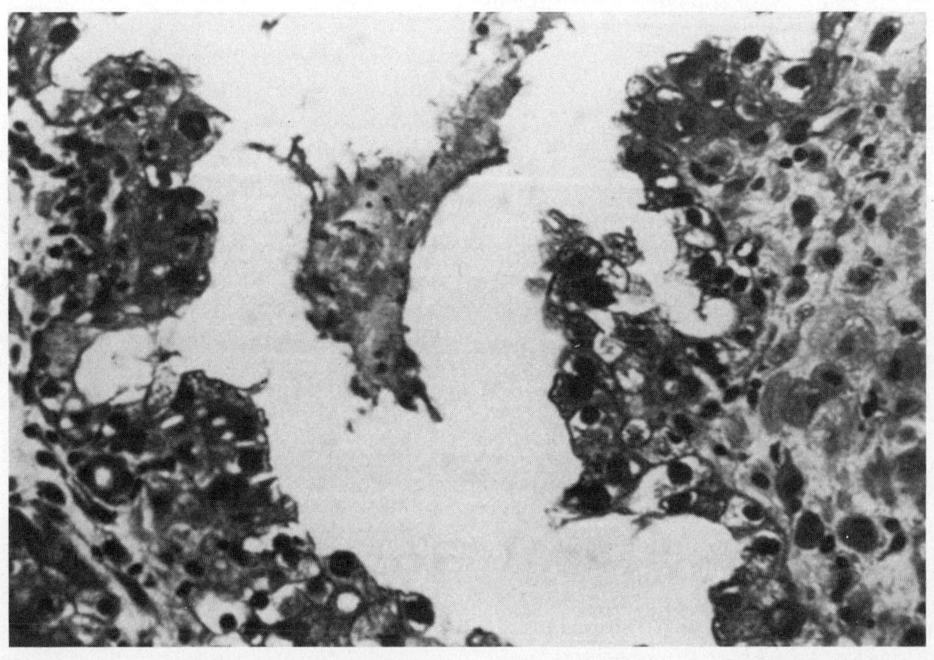

FIGURE 16-13
Arias-Stella reaction. (From DeCherney AH, Maheux R: Curr Probl Obstet Gynecol 6:2, 1983. Reproduced with permission.)

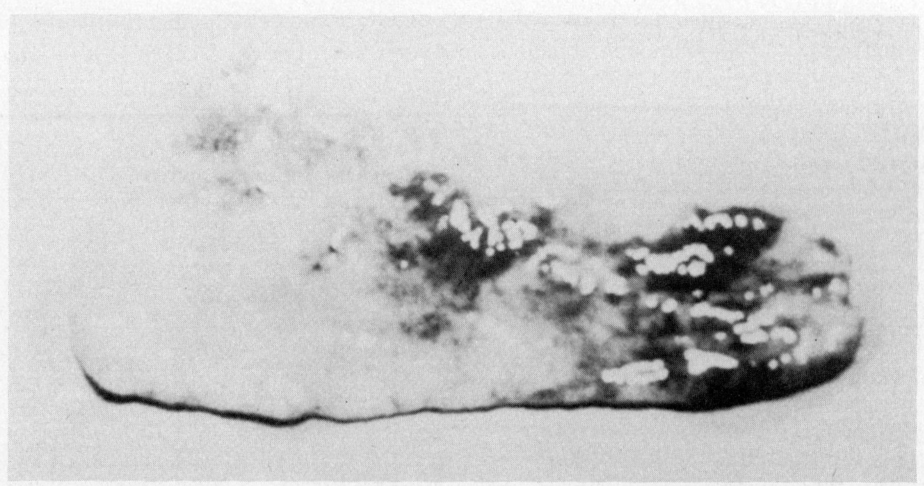

FIGURE 16-14
Decidual cast. (From DeCherney AH, Maheux R: Curr Probl Obstet Gynecol 6:2, 1983. Reproduced with permission.)

lowing stimulation with clomiphene. When progesterone levels fall as a result of insufficient daily increase of HCG, the endometrium is no longer maintained, and it sloughs, producing uterine bleeding. Sometimes nearly all the decidua is passed through the cervix intact, producing a decidual cast that may be clinically confused with a spontaneous abortion (Fig. 16-14).

SYMPTOMS

The most common symptoms of ectopic pregnancy are abdominal pain, absence of menses, and irregular vaginal bleeding (Table 16-7). Pain is nearly a universal symptom but is not type specific. Before rupture the pain may be only a vague soreness or colicky in nature. Its location may be generalized, unilateral, or bilateral. Shoulder pain occurs in about one fourth of patients with ectopic pregnancy as a result of diaphragmatic irritation from the hemoperitoneum. During rupture of the pregnancy the pain usually becomes intense, and syncope occurs in about one third of patients with tubal rupture.

The majority of patients with ectopic pregnancy fail to have menses at the expected time but have one or more episodes of irregular vaginal bleeding when the decidual endometrial tissue is sloughed. The interval of amenorrhea is usually 6 weeks or more. The bleeding is usually characterized as spotting but may simulate menstrual bleeding. It is rarely as heavy as that which occurs in spontaneous abortion.

Other symptoms include dizziness, an urge to defecate, breast tenderness, and nausea. About 5% to 10% of women will note passage of a decidual cast.

SIGNS

The most common presenting sign is abdominal tenderness, which, together with adnexal tenderness elicited at the time of the bimanual pelvic examination, is present in nearly all patients with an ectopic pregnancy (Table 16-8). It is possible to palpate an adnexal mass in half the patients, and about one third have some degree of uterine enlargement that is nearly always smaller than a normal 8-week gestation except when interstitial gestation is present. Tachycardia and hypotension can occur following rupture if blood loss is profuse, but temperature elevation is an uncommon finding, being present in only about 5% to 10% of patients, and is rarely greater than 38° C.

DIAGNOSIS

Laboratory Tests

At the time of rupture a hematocrit of less than 30% is found in about one fourth of patients. About half the patients have a normal leukocyte count, with a mild elevation of 10,000 to 15,000/mm^3 in one third and a greater elevation in one fifth.

HCG is present in the circulation of nearly every patient with an ectopic gestation, but the

TABLE 16-7
Symptoms of Ectopic Pregnancy

Symptoms	% Patients with Symptom
Abdominal pain	90-100
Amenorrhea	75-95
Vaginal bleeding	50-80
Dizziness, fainting	20-35
Urge to defecate	5-15
Pregnancy symptoms	10-25
Passage of tissue	5-10

From Weckstein LN: Current perspective on ectopic pregnancy. Obstet Gynecol Surv 40:259, © by Williams & Wilkins, 1985.

TABLE 16-8
Signs of Ectopic Pregnancy

Sign	% Patients with Sign
Adnexal tenderness	75-90
Abdominal tenderness	80-95
Adnexal mass*	50
Uterine enlargement	20-30
Orthostatic changes	10-15
Fever	5-10

From Weckstein LN: Current perspective on ectopic pregnancy. Obstet Gynecol Surv 40:259, © by Williams & Wilkins, 1985.
*20% present on the side opposite the ectopic pregnancy.

levels are lower than 3000 mIU/ml in about half. As shown by Barnes et al., the incidence of positive qualitative pregnancy tests depends on the sensitivity of the assay (Table 16-9). With use of the sensitive enzyme-linked immunosorbent assays (ELISA), more than 90% of patients with an ectopic pregnancy will have a positive pregnancy test. This incidence increases to nearly 100% if a radioimmunoassay for HCG is utilized.

Differential Diagnosis

The diagnosis is usually obvious for patients with the classic symptoms of ruptured ectopic pregnancy: a history of irregular bleeding followed by sudden onset of pain and syncope accompanied by signs of peritoneal irritation. However, before rupture the symptoms and signs are nonspecific and also occur with other gynecologic disorders. Entities frequently confused with ectopic pregnancy include salpingitis, threatened or incomplete abortion, ruptured corpus luteum, appendicitis, dysfunctional uterine bleeding, adnexal torsion, degenerative uterine leiomyoma, and endometriosis.

In the series of Brenner et al., about 50% of the patients with ruptured ectopic pregnancy had at least one medical consultation without the correct diagnosis having been made before the admission when the diagnosis was established. About 33% were seen once, 11% twice, and the remainder 3 to 5 times before the diagnosis was made. Other studies have confirmed this high frequency of misdiagnosis and physician delay in determining that an ectopic pregnancy is present. Because of the possibility of a fatal outcome from undiagnosed ruptured ectopic pregnancy, it is essential that the diagnosis of ectopic pregnancy be considered in any woman of childbearing age with abdominal pain and irregular menstrual bleeding even if she has had a previous tubal sterilization procedure or is wearing an IUD.

Establishment of Diagnosis

Ectopic pregnancy should be suspected in any patient who develops the symptoms just listed, particularly if she has previously had a pelvic operation, especially tubal operation, whether it was a tubal reconstructive procedure or a sterilization procedure. Other risk factors include one or more episodes of salpingitis, a previous ectopic gestation, current use of an IUD, use of a progestin-only oral contraceptive, or use of pharmacologic methods of ovulation induction. In any patient with the symptoms of ectopic gestation the diagnosis is facilitated by the use of culdocentesis, a sensitive assay for HCG, and pelvic ultrasonography and can be established by laparoscopy or laparotomy.

TABLE 16-9

Comparison of Pregnancy Tests in Detecting Ectopic Pregnancy in 108 Patients

Test	Lower Sensitivity Limit of Serum Assay (mIU/ml)	Positive Test	Negative Test	Sensitivity (%)
β-HCG serum	5	107	1	99.1
Tandem-visual HCG	50	97	11	89.8
Mod El	50	97	11	89.8
Sensi-Tex	250	92	16	85.2
UCG-Beta Stat	200	92	16	85.2
β-Neocept	150	88	20	81.5
Sensi Slide	800	66	42	61.1
UCG-Beta Slide	500	54	52	50.9

From Barnes RB, Roy S, Yee B, et al: Reliability of urinary pregnancy tests in the diagnosis of ectopic pregnancy. J Reprod Med 30:827, 1985.

Culdocentesis

The finding of nonclotting blood, especially if the hematocrit is above 15%, is of great diagnostic assistance in establishing the diagnosis of ectopic pregnancy. In the literature review of Cartwright et al. of nearly 5000 ectopic pregnancies a positive finding at culdocentesis was reported to be present between 70% and 97% of the time, with most series reporting a positive finding at culdocentesis in more than 90% of ectopic pregnancies. A positive finding at culdocentesis indicates hemoperitoneum. This may be due to other pathologic conditions, most frequently a hemorrhagic corpus luteum or upper abdominal pathology. However, about 85% of patients with hemoperitoneum suspected of having an ectopic pregnancy do have one. The finding of nonclotting blood at the time of culdocentesis does not always indicate that rupture of the ectopic pregnancy has occurred, as mentioned previously. Finally, hemoperitoneum can occur without causing symptoms or signs of peritoneal irritation.

Human Chorionic Gonadotrophin

Although a negative qualitative urine test for HCG does not rule out ectopic pregnancy, if a sensitive ELISA assay is negative, the diagnosis is unlikely. If β-HCG is not detected with use of radioimmunoassay of serum, the diagnosis of ectopic pregnancy can, with a rare exception, be ruled out. Although about 85% of women with ectopic pregnancy have serum HCG levels lower than those seen in normal pregnancy at a similar gestational age, a single quantitative HCG assay usually cannot be used to diagnose ectopic pregnancy because the actual dates of ovulation and conception are not known for most women. Even if the date of ovulation is known, 10% of women with normal gestations will have HCG levels lower than the normal 90% confidence limits. Furthermore, low HCG levels are also found in women with various stages of spontaneous abortion, conditions which must be considered in the differential diagnosis.

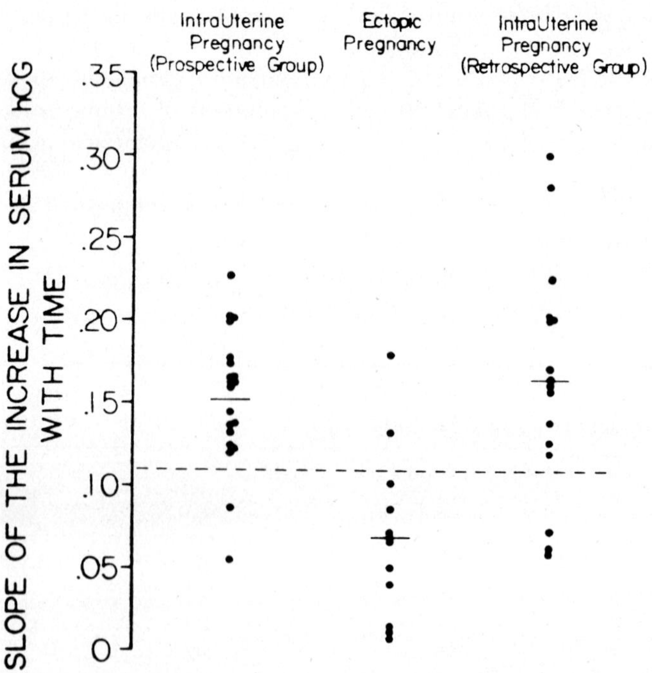

FIGURE 16-15

Slopes (mean ± SD) of human chorionic gonadotrophin (HCG) increase in three groups of patients: prospective, 0.152 ± 0.04 (range, 0.054-0.23); retrospective, 0.17 ± 0.08 (range, 0.06-0.3); and ectopic, 0.069 ± 0.05 (range, 0.01-0.18). Broken line indicates lower limit of rate of increase. (From Kadar N, Caldwell BV, Romero R: Obstet Gynecol 58:162, 1981. Reprinted with permission from The American College of Obstetricians and Gynecologists.)

In normal pregnancies in early gestation the levels of circulating HCG double about every 2 days. Kadar et al. have shown that in abnormal pregnancies (ectopic gestations and those destined to abort) HCG levels usually do not increase at the same rate (Fig. 16-15). These investigators calculated that if the percentage increase in β-HCG during a 2-day period is less than 66%, the chance that the patient has an abnormal pregnancy is high (Table 16-10). In their series only 15% of normal pregnancies failed to have this amount of increase and only

TABLE 16-10

Lower Normal Limits of Percentage Increase of Serum HCG during Early Pregnancy

Sampling Interval (Days)	Increase in HCG (%)
1	29
2	66
3	114
4	175
5	255

From Kadar N, Caldwell BV, Romero R: A method of screening for ectopic pregnancy and its indications. Obstet Gynecol 58:162, 1981. Reprinted with permission from The American College of Obstetricians and Gynecologists.

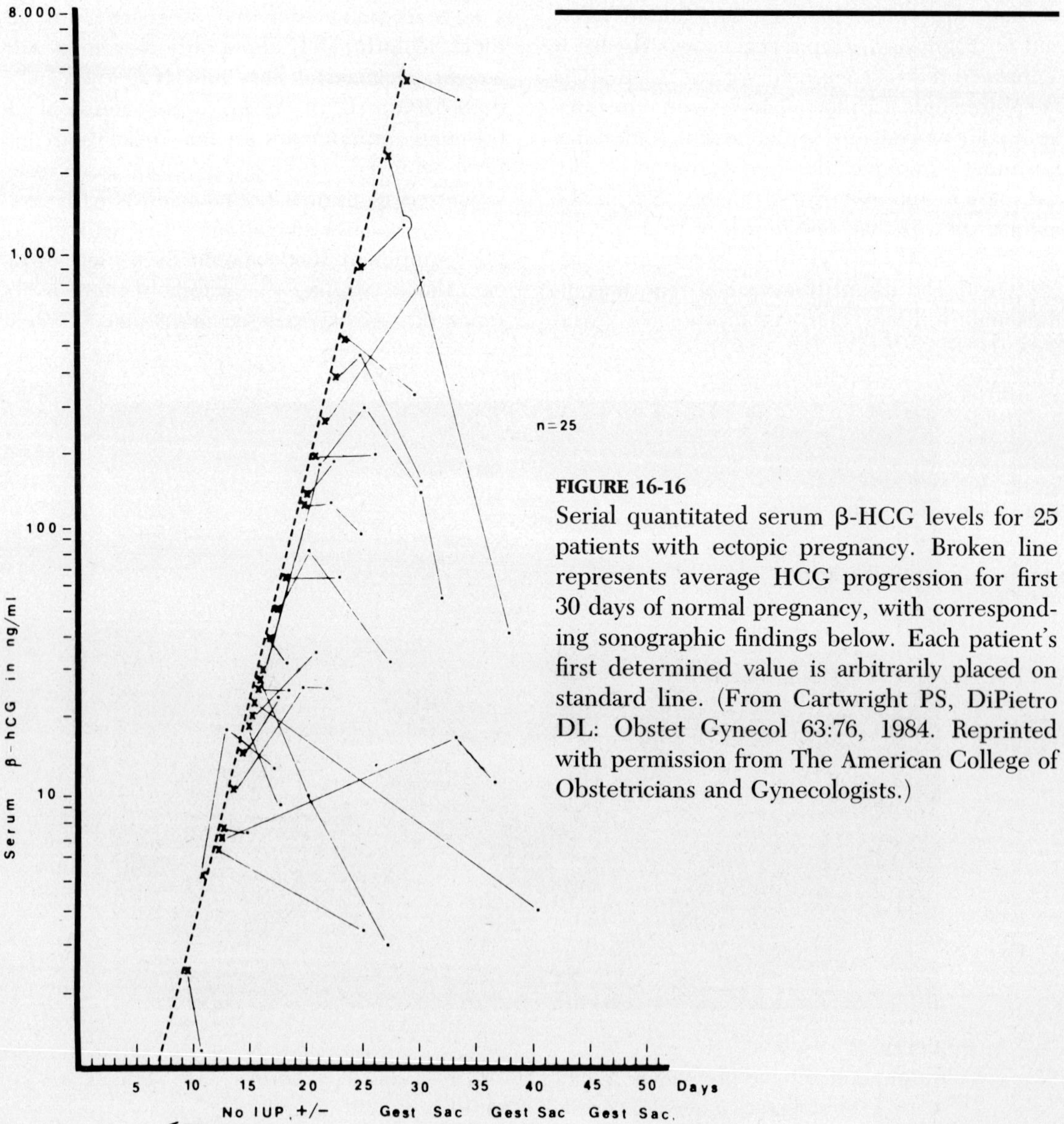

FIGURE 16-16
Serial quantitated serum β-HCG levels for 25 patients with ectopic pregnancy. Broken line represents average HCG progression for first 30 days of normal pregnancy, with corresponding sonographic findings below. Each patient's first determined value is arbitrarily placed on standard line. (From Cartwright PS, DiPietro DL: Obstet Gynecol 63:76, 1984. Reprinted with permission from The American College of Obstetricians and Gynecologists.)

13% of ectopic pregnancies had this normal rate of increase.

When symptoms of pain occur, it is probable that trophoblastic growth is impaired as a result of localized hemorrhage, and a decrease in HCG production occurs. Cartwright and Di-Pietro reported that of 25 patients with ectopic pregnancies and serial HCG levels, 20 showed a plateau or decrease in HCG levels over at least 48 hours (Fig. 16-16). Thus serial HCG measurements are of aid in the early diagnosis of ectopic pregnancy.

Ultrasonography

With present technology, ultrasound offers aid in diagnosing ectopic pregnancy. Its use is enhanced if it is combined with serial β-HCG measurements. Unfortunately with the discrimination available with current abdominal scanning equipment the demonstration of a fetal mass or embryonic sac can be seen in the oviduct of less than one fourth of women with tubal pregnancies (Fig. 16-17). Preliminary results with the use of transvaginal real time ultrasound indicate that visualization of extra-uterine pregnancies can be significantly increased to greater than 50%. Since combined intrauterine and extrauterine pregnancy is so uncommon, if a true gestational sac can be visualized within the uterus, especially if a fetus is present, the diagnosis of ectopic pregnancy is nearly always excluded. Sometimes early in gestation the ultrasonic appearance of the decidual reaction accompanying the ectopic pregnancy may be confused with a gestational sac; the sonographer should be certain that a true gestation sac is present before reporting such a finding. In 1981 Kadar et al. reported that if the β-HCG level was greater than 6500 mIU/ml and no sac was seen in the uterus, there was a high likelihood that the pregnancy was ectopic. Unfortunately about 90% of women with ectopic pregnancies have a β-HCG level lower than 6500 mIU/ml. With improvements in ultrasound equipment greater resolution has been achieved enabling a gestational sac to be visualized in normal pregnancies as early as 3 to 4 weeks after ovulation. Thus with use of this equipment there should be a high suspicion that a pregnancy is ectopic if there is absence of a gestational sac more than 4 weeks

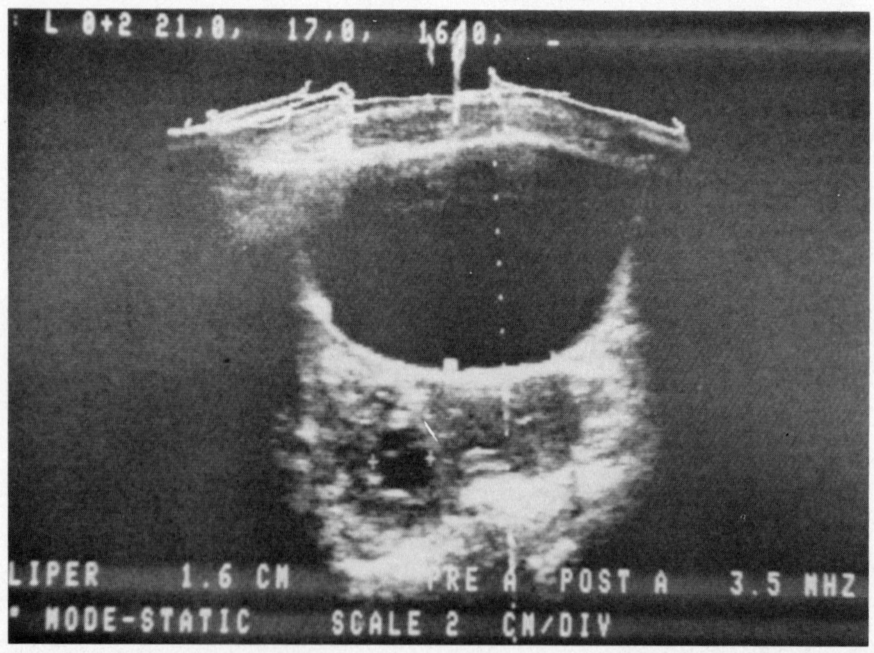

FIGURE 16-17
Ultrasound of ectopic pregnancy in fallopian tube. (From DeCherney AH, Maheux R: Curr Probl Obstet Gynecol 6:2, 1983. Reproduced with permission.)

after ovulation. Nevertheless, absence of a gestational sac in the uterus cannot differentiate among a normal pregnancy with an inaccurate estimate of the true gestational age, a blighted ovum, or an ectopic gestation.

Dilation and Curettage

If the gestational age is known to exceed 5 weeks and no intrauterine gestational sac is seen with ultrasonography, a curettage with histologic examination of the scrapings, by frozen section if desired, can be undertaken to determine if any products of gestation are present in the uterus. If no chorionic villi are visualized in the scrapings, laparoscopy should be performed to establish the diagnosis of ectopic pregnancy. The finding of a decidual reaction or the Arias-Stella reaction in the scrapings cannot establish the diagnosis of ectopic pregnancy, because these findings can also appear with intrauterine gestation and have been reported to occur in only about half the patients with ectopic gestation.

Laparoscopy

A definitive diagnosis of ectopic pregnancy can nearly always be made by direct visualization of the pelvis with laparoscopy. However, sometimes because of hemoperitoneum, adhesions, or obesity, it is difficult to visualize the pelvic organs. In a study by Samuellson and Sjovall, 4 of 166 ectopic pregnancies were not visualized by the laparoscopist, and 6 of 120 patients with an intrauterine pregnancy were thought to have ectopic pregnancies. Thus there is a 2% to 5% chance of a false positive or false negative diagnosis with laparoscopy. If sufficient hemoperitoneum is present to prevent adequate laparoscopic visualization, exploratory laparotomy should be performed.

Clinical Evaluation of Patients with Suspected Ectopic Pregnancy

Flow sheets have been developed by Thorneycroft, by Weckstein, and by DeCherney and Maheux to aid the clinician in the diagnosis of the patient with ectopic pregnancy who is not hypotensive and requires immediate laparotomy. They involve the use of ultrasonography and serial quantitative β-HCG assays. These diagnostic aids are of particular use in observing an asymptomatic patient beginning shortly after conception if the patient is at high risk for ectopic pregnancy, such as when she has had a prior ectopic pregnancy or distal tubal infertility surgery. Performing a quantitative β-HCG assay twice weekly and calculating the rate of increase as well as performing ultrasonography beginning 3 weeks after ovulation will help to establish the diagnosis of ectopic pregnancy before tubal rupture. The combination of these two techniques is particularly applicable to stable patients treated in institutions with adequate facilities for ultrasound and serial quantitative β-HCG assays.

However, for the patient who develops symptoms of an ectopic pregnancy that are of sufficient magnitude to require emergency care, a sensitive qualitative pregnancy test and culdocentesis are usually all the diagnostic aids necessary to establish the diagnosis. If both these tests are positive, it is most likely that an ectopic pregnancy is present, and laparoscopy or laparotomy or both should be performed, depending on the findings of the physical examination. For the patient with a positive finding at culdocentesis and a negative quantitative HCG assay, the diagnosis of ruptured corpus luteum is likely, and the patient should either have a laparoscopy or be studied with radioimmunoassay for β-HCG, depending on her clinical condition.

The patient with a negative finding at culdocentesis and a positive quantitative HCG assay will benefit most from ultrasound and serial β-HCG assays; however, she must be warned that she may have an ectopic pregnancy and be prepared to enter the hospital quickly if her symptoms suddenly worsen.

An algorithm for the use of these modalities has been prepared by Thorneycroft and demonstrates schematically a reasonable method of evaluation for the patient with a history compatible with ectopic pregnancy (Fig. 16-18).

MANAGEMENT

Surgical Therapy

The treatment of ectopic gestations in uncommon locations other than the oviduct was discussed earlier in the chapter (see pathology).

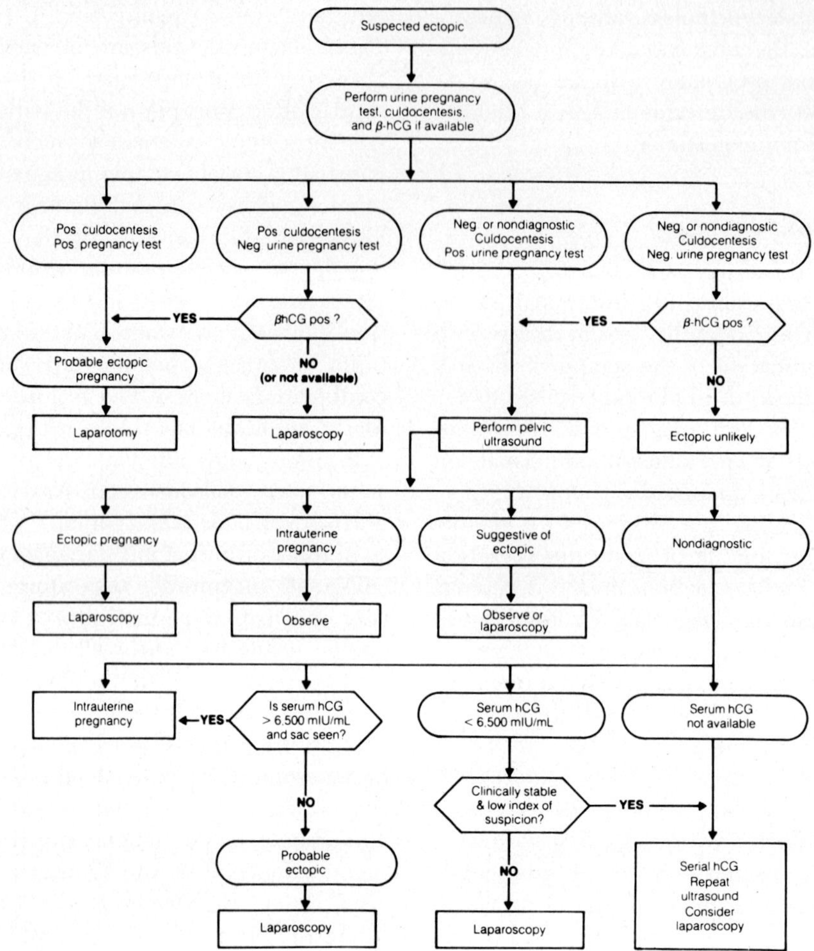

FIGURE 16-18
Ectopic pregnancy workup for patient not in shock. (From Thorneycroft IH: Contemp OB/GYN 22:91, July 1983.)

An interstitial pregnancy, because it usually becomes symptomatic at a late gestational age, is usually large and may require hysterectomy. Otherwise a resection of the cornual region of the uterus may be sufficient. On occasion, tubal gestations abort through the fimbriated end of the oviduct or regress spontaneously without symptoms; however, the vast majority require surgical treatment, which can be either a radical or a conservative procedure. If the pregnancy has produced rupture of the oviduct or has involved the entire oviduct or if no further pregnancies are desired, radical tubal operation is usually performed. Radical operation consists of salpingectomy with or without accompanying oophorectomy or hysterectomy. It was previously advocated that an elective ipsi-lateral oophorectomy be performed in a woman wishing future fertility to theoretically increase the chance of conception and reduce the chance of another ectopic pregnancy by having ovulation occur each month from the ovary proximal to the remaining tube. Results from various studies yield conflicting data. Some studies report similar conception rates in women treated with salpingectomy and salpingo-oophorectomy, whereas others report higher pregnancy rates in women having the ovary removed, and still others report lower subsequent pregnancy rates in women having the ovary removed. Because the subsequent ectopic pregnancy rate in these studies was not decreased when oophorectomy was performed and because the number of eggs available for the in vitro fertilization procedure is greater with two ovaries, it is best not to remove the ipsilateral ovary unless its involvement in the pathologic process technically necessitates its removal.

Removal of the uterus may sometimes be indicated if another disease, such as leiomyoma, is present. On occasion a hysterectomy can be performed if the woman has undergone a prior tubal sterilization and develops a tubal pregnancy. However, because of the increased operating time and morbidity associated with hysterectomy as well as the need for extensive preoperative counseling, elective hysterectomy should usually not be performed at the time of laparotomy for ectopic pregnancy.

Resection of the distal portion of the interstitial oviduct, commonly called a cornual resection, is frequently performed at the time of salpingectomy, but the procedure is unnecessary because it does not prevent a subsequent interstitial pregnancy. Of the 75 cases of interstitial pregnancy following homolateral salpingectomy reported by Kalchman and Meltzer, 20% had been preceded by a cornual resection. In Hallatt's series of repeat ectopic pregnancies, 8 of 10 ruptured homolateral interstitial pregnancies were preceded by deep cornual resection. Thus cornual resection does not prevent a subsequent interstitial pregnancy, and if it is performed, it should be only superficial.

Although a colpotomy incision has been used to perform salpingectomy in an unruptured tubal pregnancy as well as to aid in establishing the diagnosis, because of the extensive use of laparoscopy for diagnosis this incision is used infrequently.

Conservative treatment (not removing the oviduct) for an unruptured ectopic pregnancy is being used with increasing frequency for a woman who desires future fertility. When salpingostomy is correctly performed for an unruptured ectopic pregnancy, the repeat ectopic pregnancy rate is not increased compared with salpingectomy, whereas the subsequent live birth rate is increased. The techniques utilized include salpingotomy, salpingostomy, fimbrial evacuation, and partial salpingectomy, also called segmental resection of the portion of the oviduct containing the ectopic pregnancy. Fimbrial evacuation of the gestational products by digital expression or blunt curettage traumatizes the endosalpinx and has a high rate of recurrent ectopic pregnancy (24%), about twice as high as the rate following salpingectomy. In addition, this procedure may not remove the tubal gestation, and another operative procedure may be required a few days later. The best results of conservative operation occur after salpingotomy or salpingostomy. The latter technique is used more frequently in the U.S.

These techniques can be performed for the vast majority of unruptured tubal pregnancies not located in the isthmic portion of the oviduct. It is best to use microsurgical principles when performing salpingostomy, and when the unruptured pregnancy is small (less than 3 cm), it is possible to perform the salpingostomy with a laparoscopic procedure. After salpingostomy, because persistence of trophoblast tissue has been reported in a small percentage of women treated in this manner, serial quantitative HCG assays should be performed postoperatively. If hemostasis cannot be maintained after a salpingostomy, which frequently occurs for those unruptured pregnancies located in the isthmus, a segmental resection of the oviduct can be performed and a reanastomosis done a few months later. Timonen and Nieminen reported that women who had a segmental resection had a lower subsequent term pregnancy rate (17%) than women who had salpingectomy (29%). Therefore, DeCherney and Maheux recommended that a partial salpingectomy only be performed if salpingostomy is impossible and the contralateral oviduct is absent or irrevocably damaged.

Medical Therapy

In 1982 Tanaka et al. reported the successful use of methotrexate in a patient with an unruptured interstitial pregnancy. In 1983 Miyazaki et al. reported the use of methotrexate in eight patients with unruptured tubal pregnancies. Of the eight, only one required subsequent laparotomy, and tubal patency was observed in four of five who had a subsequent hysterosalpingogram. Recently investigators in the United States have been using this technique with a careful research protocol. The use of methotrexate or other medical therapy such as progesterone receptor blockers is still experimental but offers the possibility of avoiding operation in select patients.

Observation without Treatment

As late as 1955 Lund reported on 119 women with unruptured tubal pregnancy expectantly treated with only bed rest and frequent observation. Of these 119, 68 (57%) were eventually discharged from the hospital without operation, but about 60% of them required hospitalization for more than 1 month. The remainder had a tubal rupture or required operative intervention for other reasons. The subsequent fertility rates were similar in the group treated surgically and those requiring no further operation. In 1982 Mashiach et al. reported that if at the time of the initial laparoscopy a small unruptured tubal pregnancy was found and that if serial HCG levels subsequently fell, it was possible to avoid surgical therapy, although they performed a repeat laparoscopy before discharge. At the present time it is considered better to remove the unruptured ectopic pregnancy at the time of the first laparoscopy to avoid the additional expense of hospitalization, serial HCG assays, and a second laparoscopy.

Rh Factor

It is recommended that all Rh-negative, unsensitized women with ectopic pregnancies receive Rh immunoglobulin at a dosage of 50 μg if the gestation is of less than 12 weeks' duration and 300 μg if it is beyond 12 weeks. However, Grimes et al. have reported that because most of their hospitalizations were unscheduled and not preceded by Rh screening, the majority of women with ectopic pregnancies in the United States who are Rh negative do not receive Rh(D) immunoglobulin. The magnitude of the risk of sensitization is unknown but is estimated to vary from nil at 1 month to about 9% at 3 months' gestation. Because of the potential benefits and lack of risk, this treatment should be undertaken in all Rh-negative, unsensitized women with ectopic pregnancy.

PROGNOSIS

Overall the subsequent conception rate in women with an ectopic pregnancy is about 60%. A little less than half of these pregnancies terminate in another ectopic pregnancy or spontaneous abortion, so only about one third of women with an ectopic pregnancy have a subsequent live birth. However, these general figures are modified by several factors, particularly age, parity, evidence of contralateral tubal disease, and whether the ectopic material is ruptured or not (Table 16-11). The subsequent fertility rate is significantly higher in parous women under the age of 30. However, if the ectopic pregnancy occurs in a woman's first pregnancy, her subsequent conception rate is only about 35%. On the other hand, women with high parity (more than three deliveries) who develop an ectopic pregnancy have a relatively high rate of conception ($\approx$80%). The subsequent conception rate is lower in women who have had a prior history of salpingitis as well as in those who have gross evidence of

TABLE 16-11

Factors Significantly Associated with Postoperative Fertility of 151 Patients with Primary Ectopic Pregnancy

Factor	Fertile Patients b (No. = 114)	Infertile Patients c (No. = 37)	Significant Difference (P)
Mean age (years ± SD)	26.2 ± 4.7	28.0 ± 4.4	<0.05
History of sterility	17 (15%)	15 (41%)	<0.003
Adhesions or tubal disease or both	20 (18%)	19 (51%)	<0.001
Unruptured ectopic pregnancy	77 (68%)	17 (46%)	<0.03

From Sherman D, Langer R, Sadovsky G, et al: Improved fertility following ectopic pregnancy. Fertil Steril 37:497, 1982. Reproduced with permission of the publisher, The American Fertility Society.
b, Subsequent intrauterine pregnancies.
c, Subsequent sterility or repeat ectopic pregnancy only.

TABLE 16-12

Surgical Treatments and Subsequent Fertility Among 151 Patients with Primary Ectopic Pregnancy

| Surgical Treatment | No. of Patients | Subsequent Pregnancies | | |
		Intrauterine	Repeat Ectopic	Sterility
Conservative*	21	16 (76%)	1 (5%)	4 (19%)
Radical*	32	14 (44%)	3 (9%)	15 (47%)
Conservative†	26	23 (88%)	2 (8%)	1 (4%)
Radical†	72	61 (85%)	3 (4%)	8 (11%)
Conservative‡	47	39 (83%)	3 (6.4%)	5 (10.6%)
Radical‡	104	75 (72.1%)	6 (5.8%)	23 (22.1%)

From Sherman D, Langer R, Sadovsky G, et al: Improved fertility following ectopic pregnancy. Fertil Steril 37:497, 1982. Reproduced with permission of the publisher, The American Fertility Society.
*Patients with either history or operative findings suggestive of coexistent sterility factors ($P = .04$, significant difference).
†Patients with otherwise normal reproductive history and organs ($P = .9$, no significant difference).
‡All patients ($P = .2$, no significant difference).

damage in the opposite oviduct due to previous salpingitis. Future fertility is significantly higher in women who have an unruptured tubal pregnancy than in those with a ruptured ectopic pregnancy so that early diagnosis with serial β-HCG and ultrasound is desirable. In the report of Sherman et al., although only 65% of patients with a ruptured ectopic pregnancy subsequently conceived, the conception rate in women with an unruptured tubal pregnancy was 82%. In a group of patients with a high incidence of unruptured ectopic pregnancy (58%) brought about by the liberal use of early laparoscopy in patients with suspected ectopic pregnancy, these authors reported a high incidence of subsequent fertility (81%) and a low incidence of subsequent ectopic pregnancy (8%). The intrauterine pregnancy rates were high ($\approx$85%) in patients with no history of infertility or gross evidence of prior salpingitis, and these rates were similar whether the patients were treated with salpingectomy or salpingostomy. However, in the group of women with evidence of prior pelvic infection or a history of infertility, subsequent intrauterine conception rates were higher when they

TABLE 16-13

Results of Conservative Microsurgery for Tubal Pregnancy in Women with a Single Fallopian Tube

| Author | No. of Women Desiring Pregnancy | Women Who Conceived | | Women with IUP | | Women with Repeat EUP | |
		No.	%	No.	%	No.	%
Henry-Suchet et al.*	14	10	71	8	57	2	15
DeCherney et al.*	12	8	67	6	50	2	17
Valle and Lifchez	11	11	100	11	100	0	--
Oelsner et al.	21	16*	76	10	47	9	43
TOTAL	58	45	77	35	60	13	22

From Oelsner G, Rabinovitch O, Morad J, et al: Reproductive outcome after microsurgical treatment of tubal pregnancy in women with a single fallopian tube. J Reprod Med 31:483, 1986.
IUP, Intrauterine pregnancy; EUP, extrauterine pregnancy.
*Three had had an intrauterine pregnancy before repeat extrauterine pregnancy.

were treated with salpingostomy (76%) than with salpingectomy (44%) (Table 16-12). Most studies in the literature indicate that the overall subsequent ectopic pregnancy rate is similar among women treated radically or conservatively, and this study indicates that conservative surgery is most beneficial in women with evidence of contralateral tubal damage or peritubal adhesions.

The rate of repeat ectopic pregnancies after a single ectopic pregnancy ranges from 8% to 20% with a mean of about 15%. Thus about one of four conceptions after an ectopic pregnancy is a repeat ectopic pregnancy. Only about one of three nulliparous women who have an ectopic pregnancy ever conceives again (35%), and about one third of them have another ectopic pregnancy (13%).

With two ectopic pregnancies the subsequent fertility is decreased even further, with infertility rates as high as 90% being reported.

There have been several reports of the use of conservative microsurgery, either salpingostomy or salpingotomy, on women with an unruptured tubal pregnancy in the only remaining oviduct. In the great majority of the subjects the other oviduct had been previously removed for another ectopic gestation. In the total of 58 patients so treated in four different centers, as reviewed by Oelsner et al., the conception rate was 77% with an intrauterine pregnancy rate of 60% (Table 16-13). A total of 13 (22%) of the women had a subsequent ectopic gestation. Since this intrauterine pregnancy rate is much higher than that achieved by in vitro fertilization and embryo transfer, it is now recommended that all women with an unruptured tubal pregnancy have a salpingostomy performed even if they have had two ectopic pregnancies and have only one oviduct remaining.

KEY POINTS

- The annual ectopic pregnancy rates in the United States are about 0.72 per 1000 women aged 15 to 44 and 0.95 per 1000 women at risk for pregnancy.

- Between 1970 and 1980 there was nearly a threefold increase in the annual number of women hospitalized for ectopic pregnancies in the United States (from 17,800 to 52,200) as well as in the rate per 1000 live births (from 4.8 to 14.5) and a doubling of the rate per reported pregnancies (from 4.5 to 10.5).

- In the United States in 1980 more than 1 woman of every 100 who was known to conceive was hospitalized for ectopic gestation.

- In the United States the rate of ectopic pregnancy increased from 4.5 per 1000 conceptions in women aged 15 to 24 to 15.2 in those aged 35 to 44.

- About 11% of ectopic pregnancies in the United States occur in women aged 35 to 44, and more than half (53%) occur in women aged 25 to 34.

- Only 10% to 15% of ectopic pregnancies occur in nulligravid women, and more than half the ectopic pregnancies occur in women who have been pregnant three or more times.

- In the United States the rates of ectopic pregnancy were similar in each section of the country, but the rates were about twice as high for nonwhite women as for white women.

- About 2.6% of all reported pregnancies in nonwhite women aged 35 to 44 in the United States are ectopic.

- Ectopic pregnancy is the most common cause of maternal death in the first half of pregnancy, and about 40 to 50 deaths from ectopic pregnancy occur in the United States each year.

- The death-to-case ratio of ectopic pregnancy is similar in all age groups but is about 3 times higher in black women.

- A pregnant black woman is about 6 times more likely to die of ectopic pregnancy than a white woman, and ectopic pregnancy is the most common single cause of all maternal deaths among black women, causing about one fifth of such deaths.

- Overall risk of death from ectopic pregnancy is about 10 times greater than with childbirth and more than 50 times greater than with legal abortion.

- Blood loss is the major cause of death (85%) from ectopic pregnancy, with infection (5%) and anesthesia complications (2%) much less common.

- Extratubal pregnancies have about a fivefold greater risk of being fatal than tubal gestations do.

- Patient delay in consulting a physician after development of symptoms accounted for one third of the deaths from ectopic pregnancy, whereas treatment delay due to misdiagnosis contributed to death in one half.

- The major cause of ectopic pregnancy is acute salpingitis. Its morphologic sequelae account for about half the initial episodes of ectopic pregnancy.

- In about 40% of instances the etiology of ectopic pregnancy cannot be determined.

- The ectopic pregnancy rate was 68.8 per 1000 conceptions in women with a prior history of salpingitis, which is a sixfold increase in the risk.

————————— **KEY POINTS, cont'd** —————————

- About half the oviducts removed from patients with tubal pregnancies have evidence of salpingitis isthmica nodosa.

- About one fifth of women with ectopic pregnancy have had previous abdominal surgical procedures not involving the oviduct.

- The incidence of ectopic pregnancy in pregnancies occurring after salpingoplasty or salpingostomy precedures for distal tubal disease ranges from 15% to 25%.

- The rate of ectopic pregnancy in pregnancies following reversal of sterilization procedures is about 4%.

- When women conceive after a tubal sterilization has been performed, the incidence of ectopic pregnancy is about 15%.

- If pregnancy occurs after tubal sterilization by laparoscopic fulguration without concomitant transection, the ectopic pregnancy rate is about 50%.

- About 15% of women who have had one ectopic pregnancy will have a subsequent ectopic pregnancy.

- Women who become pregnant while using IUDs or progestin-only oral contraceptives have about a 5% chance of having an ectopic pregnancy.

- Women discontinuing use of the shield IUD have a 2.5 times greater chance of having an ectopic gestation, but women discontinuing use of other IUDs do not have an increased risk of ectopic pregnancy.

- The incidence of ectopic gestation is significantly greater (4 to 5 times) in women who have been exposed to diethylstilbestrol (DES) in utero than in a control group. The ectopic pregnancy rate in such individuals is about 4% to 5%.

- Approximately 98% of ectopic pregnancies are tubal, 1.5% are abdominal, and less than 1% are ovarian or cervical.

- Most tubal gestations (81%) are located in the ampullary portion of the oviduct, being about equally divided between the distal and middle third of the tube. About 12% of tubal gestations occur in the isthmus and 5% in the fimbrial region. About 2% of all ectopic pregnancies are interstitial and are associated with severe morbidity.

- About 1 of 8000 pregnancies is combined intrauterine and extrauterine pregnancy.

- The hematocrit value of the blood removed by culdocentesis in ectopic pregnancy is nearly always greater than 15%.

- The most common symptoms of ectopic pregnancy are abdominal pain, absence of menses, and irregular vaginal bleeding.

- Shoulder pain occurs in about one fourth of patients with ectopic pregnancy.

- Syncope occurs in about one third of patients with tubal rupture.

- The most common presenting sign of ectopic pregnancy is abdominal tenderness, which together with adnexal tenderness elicited at the time of the bimanual pelvic examination is present in nearly all patients with an ectopic pregnancy.

- It is possible to palpate an adnexal mass in half the patients, and about one third have some degree of uterine enlargement.

- HCG is present in the circulation of nearly every patient with an ectopic gestation, but the levels are lower than 3000 mIU/ml in about half.

- With use of the sensitive ELISA assays, more than 90% of patients with an ectopic pregnancy will have a positive pregnancy test. This incidence increases to nearly 100% if a radioimmunoassay for HCG is utilized.

- It is essential that the diagnosis of ectopic pregnancy be considered for any woman of childbearing age with abdominal pain and irregular menstrual bleeding even if she has had a previous tubal sterilization procedure or is wearing an IUD.

_____________ **KEY POINTS, cont'd** _____________

- Most series report that nonclotting blood is obtained by culdocentesis in more than 90% of ectopic pregnancies.

- About 85% of women with an ectopic pregnancy have serum HCG levels lower than those seen in normal pregnancy at a similar gestational age.

- In women with an ectopic gestation, HCG levels usually do not increase at the same rate as in women with normal pregnancy.

- Laparoscopy has a 2% to 5% misdiagnosis rate (false positive or false negative) for ectopic pregnancy.

- If the pregnancy has produced rupture of the oviduct or has involved the entire oviduct or if no further pregnancies are desired, salpingectomy is the treatment of choice.

- Similar subsequent conception rates and ectopic pregnancy rates occur in women treated with salpingectomy or salpingo-oophorectomy.

- Cornual resection does not prevent a subsequent interstitial pregnancy.

- For an unruptured ectopic pregnancy the repeat ectopic pregnancy rate with salpingostomy is not increased as compared with salpingectomy, whereas the subsequent live birth rate is increased.

- Fimbrial evacuation of the gestational products by digital expression has about twice the rate of recurrent ectopic pregnancy as salpingectomy.

- It is recommended that all Rh-negative unsensitized women with ectopic pregnancies receive Rh immunoglobulin.

- Overall the subsequent conception rate in women with an ectopic pregnancy is about 60%. A little less than half of these pregnancies terminate in another ectopic pregnancy or spontaneous abortion, so only about one third of women with an ectopic pregnancy have a subsequent live birth.

- If the ectopic pregnancy occurs in a woman's first pregnancy, her chance of subsequent conception is only about 35%.

- The subsequent conception rate is lower in women who have had a prior history of salpingitis as well as in those who have gross evidence of damage in the opposite oviduct caused by previous salpingitis.

- Future fertility is significantly higher in women who have an unruptured tubal pregnancy than in those with a ruptured ectopic pregnancy.

- Conservative tubal surgery is most beneficial in women with evidence of contralateral tubal damage or peritubal adhesions.

- About one of four conceptions after an ectopic pregnancy is a repeat ectopic pregnancy.

- About one third of nulliparous women with an ectopic pregnancy have a subsequent ectopic pregnancy.

- In women with one remaining oviduct where unruptured ectopic pregnancy is treated by salpingostomy, the conception rate is 77% with an intrauterine pregnancy rate of 60% and a subsequent ectopic gestation rate of 22%.

BIBLIOGRAPHY

Barnes AB, Grover JW, Sudduth SS: Simultaneous extra- and intrauterine pregnancy. Obstet Gynecol 31:50, 1968.

Barnes AB, Wennberg CN, Barnes BA: Ectopic pregnancy: Incidence and review of determinant factors. Obstet Gynecol Surv 38:345, 1983.

Barnes RB, Roy S, Yee B, et al: Reliability of urinary pregnancy tests in the diagnosis of ectopic pregnancy. J Reprod Med 30:827, 1985.

Batzer FR, Weiner S, Corson SL, et al: Landmarks during the first forty-two days of gestation demonstrated by the β-subunit of human chorionic gonadotropin and ultrasound. Am J Obstet Gynecol 146:973, 1973.

Bone NL, Greene RR: Histologic study of uterine tubes with tubal pregnancy. Am J Obstet Gynecol 82:1166, 1961.

Braunstein GD, Asch RH: Predictive value analysis of measurements of human chorionic gonadotropin, pregnancy specific β_1-glycoprotein, placental lactogen, and cystine aminopeptidase for the diagnosis of ectopic pregnancy. Fertil Steril 39:62, 1983.

Breen JL: A 21 year survey of 654 ectopic pregnancies. Am J Obstet Gynecol 106:1004, 1970.

Brenner PF, Roy S, Mishell DR Jr: Ectopic pregnancy. A study of 300 consecutive surgically treated cases. JAMA 243:673, 1980.

Budowick M, Johnson TRB, Genadry R, et al: The histopathology of the developing tubal ectopic pregnancy. Fertil Steril 34:169, 1980.

Cartwright PS, DiPietro DL: Ectopic pregnancy: Changes in serum human chorionic gonadotropin concentration. Obstet Gynecol 63:76, 1984.

Cartwright PS, Vaughn B, Tuttle D: Culdocentesis and ectopic pregnancy. J Reprod Med 29:88, 1984.

Centers for Disease Control: Ectopic pregnancies—United States, 1979-1980. MMWR 33(15):201, 1984.

Chavkin W: The rise in ectopic pregnancy—exploration of possible reasons. Int J Gynaecol 20:341, 1982.

Chow W-H, Daling JR, Weiss NS, et al: IUD use and subsequent tubal ectopic pregnancy. Am J Public Health 76:536, 1986.

Clark JF, Guy RS: Abdominal pregnancy. Am J Obstet Gynecol 96:511, 1966.

Cole T, Corlett R Jr: Chronic ectopic pregnancy. Obstet Gynecol 59:63, 1982.

Corson SL, Batzer FR: Ectopic pregnancy. A review of the etiologic factors. J Reprod Med 31:78, 1986.

DeCherney AH, Kase N: The conservative surgical management of unruptured ectopic pregnancy. Obstet Gynecol 54:451, 1979.

DeCherney AH, Maheux R: Modern management of tubal pregnancy. Curr Probl Obstet Gynecol 6:2, 1983.

DeCherney AH, Romero R, Naftolin F: Surgical management of unruptured ectopic pregnancy. Fertil Steril 35:21, 1981.

Delke I, Veridiano NP, Tancer ML: Abdominal pregnancy: Review of current management and addition of 10 cases. Obstet Gynecol 60:200, 1982.

Dorfman SF: Deaths from ectopic pregnancy, United States, 1979 to 1980. Obstet Gynecol 62:334, 1983.

Dorfman SF, Grimes DA, Cates W Jr, et al: Ectopic pregnancy mortality, United States, 1979 to 1980: Clinical aspects. Obstet Gynecol 64:386, 1984.

Elias S, LeBeau M, Simpson JL, et al: Chromosome analysis of ectopic human conceptuses. Am J Obstet Gynecol 141:698, 1981.

Franklin EW III, Zeiderman AM, Laemmle P: Tubal ectopic pregnancy: etiology and obstetric and gynecologic sequelae. Am J Obstet Gynecol 117:200, 1973.

Gemzell CA: Experience with the induction of ovulation J Reprod Med 21(suppl):205, 1978.

Grimes DA, Geary FH Jr, Hatcher RA: Rh immunoglobulin utilization after ectopic pregnancy. Am J Obstet Gynecol 140:246, 1981.

Hallatt JG: Primary ovarian pregnancy: A report of twenty-five cases. Am J Obstet Gynecol 143:55, 1982.

Herbst AL, Hubby MM, Azizi F, et al: Reproductive and gynecologic surgical experience in diethylstilbestrol-exposed daughters. Am J Obstet Gynecol 141:1019, 1981.

Kadar N, Caldwell BV, Romero R: A method of screening for ectopic pregnancy and its indications. Obstet Gynecol 58:162, 1981.

Kadar N, DeCherney AH, Romero R: Receiver operating characteristic (ROC) curve analysis of the relative efficacy of single and serial chorionic gonadotropin determinations in the early diagnosis of ectopic pregnancy. Fertil Steril 37:542, 1982.

Kadar N, DeVore G, Romero R: Discriminatory hCG zone: Its use in the sonographic evaluation for ectopic pregnancy. Obstet Gynecol 58:156, 1981.

Kalchman GG, Meltzer RM: Interstitial pregnancy following homolateral salpingectomy. Am J Obstet Gynecol 196:1139, 1966.

Kaufman RH, Noller K, Adam E, et al: Upper genital tract abnormalities and pregnancy outcome in diethylstilbestrol-exposed progeny. Am J Obstet Gynecol 148:973, 1984.

Levin AA, Schoenbaum SC, Stubblefield PG, et al: Ectopic pregnancy and prior induced abortion. Am J Public Health 72:253, 1982.

Lund J: Early ectopic pregnancy. J Obstet Gynaecol Br Emp 62:70, 1955.

Majmudar B, Henderson PH III, Semple E: Salpingitis isthmica nodosa: A high-risk factor for tubal pregnancy. Obstet Gynecol 62:73, 1983.

Mangan CE, Borow L, Burtnett-Rubin MM, et al: Pregnancy outcome in 98 women exposed to diethylstilbestrol in utero, their mothers, and their unexposed siblings. Obstet Gynecol 59:315, 1982.

Mashiach S, Carp HA, Serr DM: Nonoperative management of ectopic pregnancy. A preliminary report. J Reprod Med 2:127, 1982.

McBain JC, Evans JH, Pepperell RJ, et al: An unexpectedly high rate of ectopic pregnancy following the induction of ovulation with human pituitary and chorionic gonadotrophin. Br J Obstet Gynaecol 87:5, 1980.

McCann MF, Kessel E: International experience with laparoscopic sterilization: Follow-up of 8500 women. Adv Planned Parent 12:199, 1978.

McCausland A: High rate of ectopic pregnancy following laparoscopic tubal coagulation failures. Am J Obstet Gynecol 136:97, 1980.

McCausland A: Endosalpingosis ("endosalpingoblastosis") following laparoscopic tubal coagulation as an etiologic factor of ectopic pregnancy. Am J Obstet Gynecol 143:12, 1982.

Miyazaki Y, Shiina Y, Wake N, et al: Studies on nonsurgical therapy of tubal pregnancy. Acta Obstet Gynaecol Jpn 35:489, 1983.

Morris JM, Van Wagenen G: Interception: The use of postovulatory estrogens to prevent implantation. Am J Obstet Gynecol 115:101, 1973.

Nagamani M, London S, St Amand P: Factors influencing fertility after ectopic pregnancy. Am J Obstet Gynecol 149:533, 1984.

Niles JH, Clark JJ: Pathogenesis of tubal pregnancy. Am J Obstet Gynecol 105:1230, 1969.

Oelsner G, Rabinovitch O, Morad J, et al: Reproductive outcome after microsurgical treatment of tubal pregnancy in women with a single fallopian tube. J Reprod Med 31:483, 1986.

O'Leary JL, O'Leary JA: Rudimentary horn pregnancy. Obstet Gynecol 22:371, 1963.

Ory HW, The Women's Health Study: Ectopic pregnancy and intrauterine contraceptive devices: New perspectives. Obstet Gynecol 57:137, 1981.

Paalman RJ, McElin TW: Cervical pregnancy. Am J Obstet Gynecol 77:1261, 1959.

Parente JT, Ou C-S, Levy J: Cervical pregnancy analysis: A review and report of five cases. Obstet Gynecol 62:79, 1983.

Persaud V: Etiology of tubal ectopic pregnancy. Obstet Gynecol 36:257, 1970.

Peterson HB: Extratubal ectopic pregnancies: J Reprod Med 31:108, 1986.

Reece EA, Petrie RH, Sirmans MF, et al: Combined intrauterine and extrauterine gestations: A review. Am J Obstet Gynecol 146:323, 1983.

Rubin GL, Peterson HB, Dorfman SF, et al: Ectopic pregnancy in the United States 1970 through 1978. JAMA 249:1725, 1983.

Saito M, Koyama T, Yaoi Y, et al: Site of ovulation and ectopic pregnancy. Acta Obstet Gynecol Scand 54:227, 1975.

Samuellson S, Sjovall A: Laparoscopy in suspected ectopic pregnancy. Acta Obstet Gynecol Scand 51:31, 1972.

Schenker JG, Evron S: New concepts in the surgical management of tubal pregnancy and the consequent postoperative results. Fertil Steril 40:709, 1983.

Schenker JG, Eyal F, Polishuk WZ: Fertility after tubal pregnancy. Surg Gynecol Obstet 135:74, 1972.

Schoen JA, Nowak RJ: Repeat ectopic pregnancy. A 16-year clinical survey. Obstet Gynecol 45:542, 1975.

Shah A, Courey NG, Cunanan RG: Pregnancy following laparoscopic tubal electrocoagulation and division. Am J Obstet Gynecol 129:459, 1977.

Sherman D, Langer R, Sadovsky G, et al: Improved fertility following ectopic pregnancy. Fertil Steril 37:497, 1982.

Siegler AM, Hulka J, Peretz A: Reversibility of female sterilization. Fertil Steril 43:499, 1985.

Siegler AM, Kontopoulos V: An analysis of macrosurgical and microsurgical techniques in the management of the tuboperitoneal factor in infertility. Fertil Steril 32:377, 1979.

Siegler AM, Wang CF, Westoff C: Management of unruptured tubal pregnancy. Obstet Gynecol Surv 36:599, 1981.

Sivin I: Copper T IUD use and ectopic pregnancy rates in the United States. Contraception 19:151, 1979.

Stratford B: Abnormalities of early human development. Am J Obstet Gynecol 107:1223, 1970.

Tanaka T, Hayashi H, Kutsuzawa T, et al: Treatment of interstitial ectopic pregnancy with methotrexate: Report of a successful case. Fertil Steril 37:851, 1982.

Tatum HJ, Schmidt FH: Contraceptive and sterilization practices and extrauterine pregnancy: A realistic perspective. Fertil Steril 28:407, 1977.

Thorneycroft IH: When you suspect ectopic pregnancy. Contemp OB/GYN 22:91, July 1983.

Timonen S, Nieminen U: Tubal pregnancy, choice of operative method of treatment. Acta Obstet Gynecol Scand 46:327, 1967.

Weckstein LN: Current perspective on ectopic pregnancy. Obstet Gynecol Surv 40:259, 1985.

Weckstein LN, Boucher AR, Tucker H, et al: Accurate diagnosis of early ectopic pregnancy. Obstet Gynecol 65:393, 1985.

Weström L, Bengtsson LPH, Mårdh P-A: Incidence, trends and risks of ectopic pregnancy in a population of women. Br Med J 282:15, 1981.

Benign Gynecologic Lesions

Brenner Tumor. A small, smooth, solid fibro-epithelial tumor of the ovary. It may be benign or malignant.

Degeneration of a Myoma. The process by which a myoma outgrows its blood supply and begins to necrose centrally. Forms of degeneration include hyaline, myxomatous, calcific, cystic, fat, and red degeneration.

Dermoid (Benign Cystic Teratoma). A benign germ cell tumor that may contain elements of all three germ cell layers.

Dysontogenic Cysts. Thin-walled cysts of embryonic origin.

Endometrial Polyp. A localized outgrowth of endometrial glands and stoma projecting beyond the surface of the endometrium and including a vascular stalk.

Follicular Hematoma. Follicular cysts filled with blood, usually from hemorrhage in the vascular theca zone.

Gartner's Duct Cysts. Cysts primarily of mesonephric origin found laterally in the vagina.

Hematometra. A uterus distended with blood, secondary to partial or complete obstruction of any portion of the lower genital tract.

Hidradenoma. A rare, small, benign vulvar tumor originating from apocrine sweat glands.

Hidradenitis Suppurative. A chronic infection involving skin, subcutaneous tissue, and apocrine glands.

Hydatid Cysts of Morgagni. Pedunculated paratubal cysts found near the fimbria of the oviduct.

Hydrometra. A collection of clear fluid in the uterine cavity.

Hyperreactio Luteinalis. Multiple theca lutein cysts causing bilateral ovarian enlargement during pregnancy.

Intravenous Leiomyomatosis. An extremely rare condition in which benign, smooth muscle fibers invade and slowly grow into the venous channels of the pelvis.

Itch-Scratch Cycle. The cycle of itching leading to scratching. The scratching leads to excoriation, irritation, and healing, with subsequent irritation and itching.

Leiomyoma (Myoma or Fibroid). A benign tumor of muscle cell origin found in any tissue that contains smooth muscle.

Leiomyomatosis Peritonealis Disseminata. A benign disease with multiple small nodules over the surface of the pelvis and abdominal peritoneum, grossly mimicking disseminated carcinoma.

Lichenification. Changes in the skin from chronic irritation, characterized by whiteness, thickening, and leathery appearance.

Luteoma of Pregnancy. A rare, specific, benign, hyperplastic reaction of ovarian theca lutein cells during pregnancy.

Meigs' Syndrome. The constellation of symptoms of ascites and hydrothorax associated with a benign ovarian fibroma, resolving after the removal of the tumor.

Nabothian Cysts. Cervical retention cysts lined by endocervical-type columnar cells.

Parasitic Myoma. A myoma that outgrows its uterine blood supply and obtains a secondary blood supply from another organ, such as the omentum.

Prominence or Tubercle of Rokitansky. The protrusion of solid elements of a dermoid into the cyst cavity.

Pruritus. A symptom of intense itching with an associated desire to scratch.

Pyometra. A collection of pus in the uterine cavity.

Struma Ovarii. A specialized ovarian teratoma that consists of thyroid tissue as a major or exclusive component. It may rarely produce sufficient thyroid hormone to induce hyperthyroidism.

Submucosal Myoma. A myoma located immediately below the endometrial lining.

Subserosal Myoma. A myoma found just beneath the serosa of the uterus.

Syringoma. A benign tumor of the eccrine sweat glands.

Vulvodynia. A recently developed term describing chronic vulvar discomfort.

This book is divided primarily into chapters dealing with benign diseases and chapters dealing with malignant ones. For the clinician, however, the difference is not always clear. As in all areas of medicine, gynecologic problems do not fall into definitive categories, and those that include malignant disease often overlap with those that include benign disease. When the diagnosis from the history, physical examination, and laboratory tests is clear, management is usually self-evident. When a specific diagnosis is unclear, tissue biopsy is appropriate. This chapter deals primarily with benign lesions; however, the symptoms and differential diagnoses of these lesions have tremendous overlap with those of malignant disease.

The discussions in this chapter are arranged anatomically, beginning with the vulva and then covering the vagina, cervix, uterus, oviducts, and ovaries. This chapter does not attempt to be encyclopedic; rather, lesions have been selected based on their clinical significance and incidence. Therefore, lesions such as glomus tumors of the vulva or papillomas of the cervix have been omitted. Because several nonneoplastic abnormalities and lesions present in ways similar to those of benign tumors, this chapter also discusses entities that are not specifically abnormal growths. Lesions such as torsion of the ovary, lacerations of the vagina, and hematomas of the vulva are examples of these common clinical problems.

The successful clinician must use deductive as well as inductive reasoning in solving a problem. To have mastered both these techniques, he or she not only must be adept at physical examination and history taking but also must be able to form a complete list of possible lesions that may be involved in the patient's complaint. An understanding of the entities of this chapter will be helpful toward that goal.

VULVA

Urethral Caruncle

A urethral caruncle is a small, fleshy outgrowth of the edge of the urethra. The tissue of the caruncle is soft, smooth, and bright red and initially appears as an eversion of the urethra (Fig. 17-1). Urethral caruncles are generally small, single, and sessile but may be pedunculated and grow to be 1 to 2 cm in diameter. They occur most frequently in postmenopausal women and must be differentiated from urethral carcinomas. Urethral caruncles are believed to arise from an ectropion of the posterior urethral wall secondary to retraction and atrophy of the postmenopausal vagina. The growth of the caruncle is secondary to chronic irritation or infection. Histologically the caruncle is composed of transitional and stratified squamous epithelium with a loose connective tissue (Fig. 17-2). Caruncles are frequently subdivided into papillomatous, granulomatous, and angiomatous varieties. They are often secondarily infected, producing ulceration and bleeding.

The symptoms associated with urethral caruncles are variable. Many women are asymptomatic, whereas others experience dysuria, frequency, and urgency. Sometimes the caruncle produces point tenderness after contact

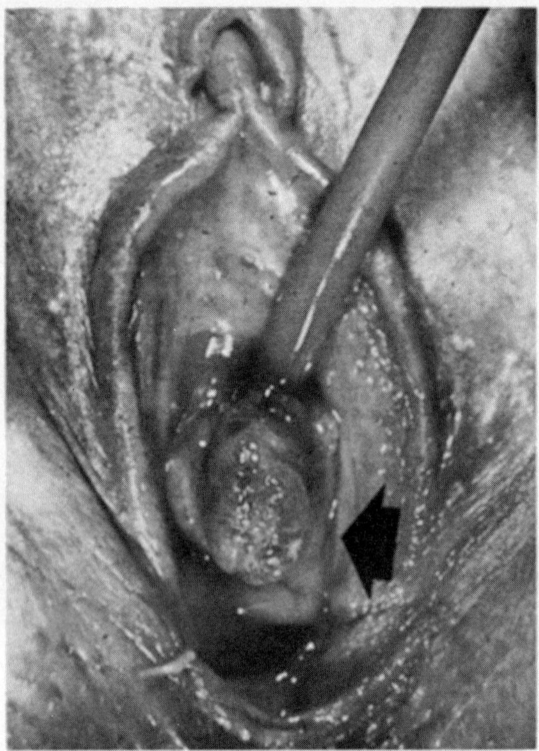

FIGURE 17-1
A large benign urethral caruncle, thought clinically to be a urethral carcinoma because of its size (arrow). (From Marshall FC, Uson AC, Melicow MM: Surg Gynecol Obstet 110:724, 1960. By permission of Surgery, Gynecology & Obstetrics.)

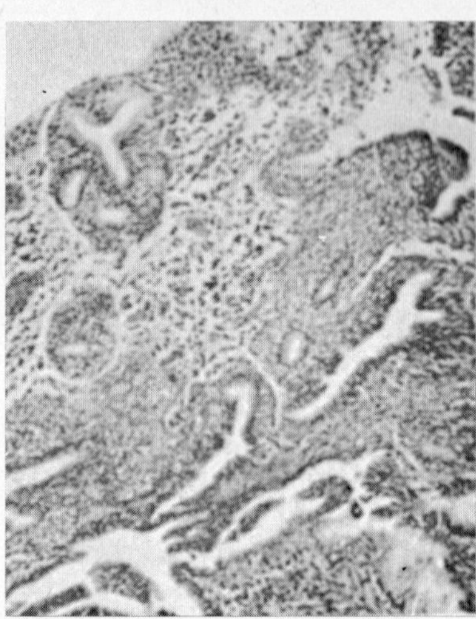

FIGURE 17-2
Urethral caruncle. Hyperemia, inflammation, and some infolding of transitional epithelium (H&E stain). (From Kaufman RH: Solid tumors. In Gardner HL, Kaufman RH, eds: Benign diseases of the vulva and vagina, 2nd ed. Boston, G.K. Hall, 1981, p. 88. Reproduced with permission.)

with undergarments or during intercourse. Ulcerative lesions usually produce spotting on contact more commonly than hematuria.

The differential diagnosis of urethral caruncles includes primary carcinoma of the urethra and prolapse of the urethral mucosa. Although urethral caruncles are not a precursor for urethral carcinoma, grossly the two are often confused. Both diseases are most common in postmenopausal women. Marshall et al. reported a series of 394 urethral tumors. A clinical diagnosis of urethral caruncle was made in 376 of these women. Histologic examination of biopsy material demonstrated urethral carcinoma in nine patients in their series. Thus, approximately 1 out of 40 women with a clinical diagnosis of urethral caruncle has a malignant urethral neoplasm.

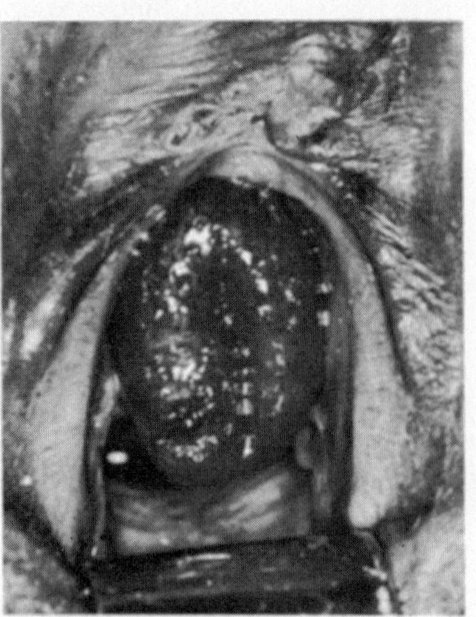

FIGURE 17-3
Prolapse of urethral mucosa in a 7-year-old child. Edematous red collar of tissue surrounds urethral meatus. (From Kaufman RH: Solid tumors. In Gardner HL, Kaufman RH, eds: Benign diseases of the vulva and vagina, 2nd ed. Boston, G.K. Hall, 1981, p. 89. Reproduced with permission.)

The diagnosis of a urethral caruncle is established by biopsy under local anesthesia. Initial therapy is oral or topical estrogen and avoidance of irritation. If the caruncle does not regress or is symptomatic, it may be destroyed by cryosurgery, laser therapy, fulguration, or operative excision. Following operative destruction, a Foley catheter should be left in place for 48 to 72 hours. Follow-up is necessary to ensure that the patient does not develop urethral stenosis.

Urethral prolapse is predominantly a disease of the premenarchal female (Fig. 17-3), although it does occur in postmenopausal women. The rosette of friable, edematous prolapsed mucosa does not have the bright red color of a caruncle and is not as circumscribed in gross configuration. Therapy of a prolapsed urethra is hot sitz baths and antibiotics to reduce inflammation and infection. In rare cases it may be necessary to excise the redundant mucosa.

Cysts

The most common large cyst of the vulva is a cystic dilation of an obstructed Bartholin's duct. Approximately 2% of new gynecologic patients present with an asymptomatic Bartholin's duct cyst. Treatment is not necessary unless the cyst becomes infected or enlarges enough to produce symptoms. A more complete discussion of Bartholin's duct cysts and abscesses is included in Chapter 21. Occasionally the ducts of mucous glands of the vestibule are occluded. The resulting cysts may be clear, yellow, or blue. Similar small mucous cysts occur in the periurethral region. Wolffian duct cysts or mesonephric cysts are rare, but when they do occur, they are found near the clitoris and lateral to the hymen.

The most common small vulvar cysts are epidermal inclusion cysts or sebaceous cysts. Because these cysts cannot be differentiated grossly from those previously mentioned and since a continuing controversy exists with respect to their histogenesis, these two are discussed together in this chapter. These cysts are located immediately beneath the epidermis. Most commonly they are discovered on the anterior half of the labia majora. These cysts are usually multiple, freely movable, round, slow

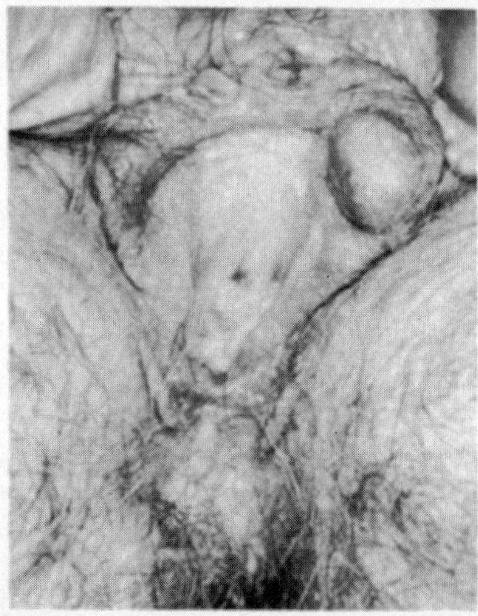

FIGURE 17-4
Epidermal inclusion cyst. Large single cyst of labium minus. (From Kaufman RH: Cystic tumors. In Gardner HL, Kaufman RH, eds: Benign diseases of the vulva and vagina, 2nd ed. Boston, G.K. Hall, 1981, p. 97. Reproduced with permission.)

growing, and nontender. They are firm to shotty in consistency, and their contents are usually under pressure. Grossly, they are white or yellow, and the contents are caseous like a thick cheese.

An inclusion cyst develops following trauma when an infolding of squamous epithelium has occurred beneath the epidermis in the site of an episiotomy or obstetric laceration. Alternative theories of histogenesis include embryonic remnants and occlusion of pilosebaceous ducts of sweat glands. The histology of these cysts is characterized by an epithelial lining of keratinized, stratified squamous epithelium with a center of cellular debris that grossly resembles sebaceous material. Most vulvar epidermal cysts do not have sebaceous cells or sebaceous material identified on microscopic examination (Fig. 17-4). These cysts are asymptomatic unless they are secondarily infected. Large epidermal cysts may be confused with fibromas, lipomas, and hidradenomas.

Most of these cysts require no treatment. If the cyst becomes infected, treatment consists of heat applied locally and incision and drainage. Cysts that become recurrently infected or produce pain should be excised when the acute inflammation has subsided.

Nevus

A nevus, commonly referred to as a *mole*, is a localized nest or cluster of melanocytes. These undifferentiated cells arise from the embryonic neural crest and are present from birth. Many nevi are not recognized until they become pigmented at the time of puberty. Vulvar nevi are one of the most common benign neoplasms in females. As with nevi in other parts of the body, they exhibit a wide range in depth of color, from blue to dark brown to black, and some may be amelanotic. The diameter of most nevi ranges from a few millimeters to 2 cm. Grossly, a benign nevus may be flat, elevated, or pedunculated. Other lesions in the differential diagnosis include hemangiomas and endometriosis of the vulva.

Vulvar nevi are generally asymptomatic. Most women do not closely inspect their vulvar skin and are unaware of biologic changes in gross appearance of these lesions. Histologically, the lesions are subdivided into three major groups: junctional, compound (Fig. 17-5), and intradermal nevi.

Although the vulvar area contains approximately 1% of the skin surface of the body, 5% to 10% of all malignant melanomas in women arise from this region. The biologic reasons for this discrepancy are unknown. Speculation includes the hypothesis that junctional activity is common in vulvar nevi, and the many irritants to which vulvar skin is exposed may lead to malignancy. It is estimated that 30% of malignant melanomas arise from a preexisting nevus.

Ideally, all vulvar nevi should be excised and examined histologically. This may be accomplished with local anesthesia or coincidentally with obstetric delivery or gynecologic surgery. Proper excisional biopsy should be three dimensional and adequate in width and depth. Approximately 5 mm of normal skin surrounding the nevus should be included, and the biopsy should include the underlying dermis as well. Some patients are reluctant to have a "normal"-appearing nevus removed. Recent changes in growth or color, ulceration, bleeding, or the development of satellite lesions mandate biopsy. Friedman et al. listed the characteristic clinical features of an early malignant melanoma, which may be remembered by thinking ABCD: *asymmetry*, *border* irregularity, *color* variegation, and a *diameter* usually greater than 6 mm.

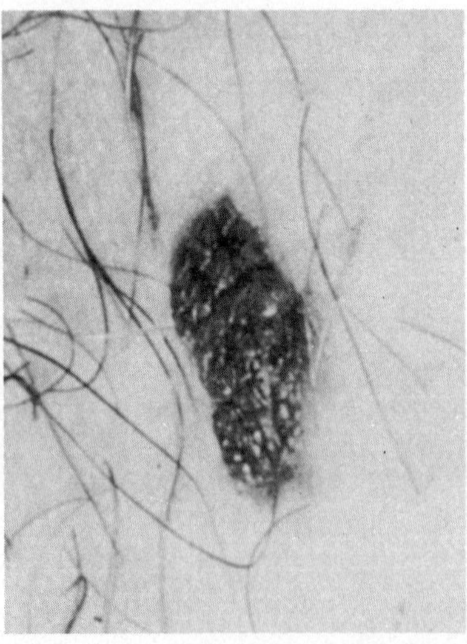

FIGURE 17-5
Compound nevus, usually a slightly elevated pigmented lesion. (From Kaufman RH: Solid tumors. In Gardner HL, Kaufman RH, eds: Benign diseases of the vulva and vagina, 2nd ed. Boston, G.K. Hall, 1981, p. 64. Reproduced with permission.)

Hemangioma

Hemangiomas are rare malformations of blood vessels rather than true neoplasms. Vulvar hemangiomas frequently are discovered first in children. They are usually single, 1 to 2 cm in diameter, flat, and soft, and they range from brown to red or purple. Histologically the multiple channels of hemangiomas are predominantly thin-walled capillaries arranged randomly and separated by thin connective tissue septa. Most hemangiomas are asymptomatic; occasionally they may become ulcerated and bleed.

There are four different types of vulvar hemangiomas. The strawberry or cavernous hemangioma is a congenital defect discovered in young children. It is usually bright red to dark red, is elevated, and rarely increases in size after age 2. Approximately 60% of vulvar hemangiomas discovered during the first year of life spontaneously regress in size. Senile or cherry angiomas are common small lesions that arise on the labia majora of postmenopausal women. They are most often less than 3 mm in diameter, multiple, and red-brown to dark blue. Angiokeratomas are approximately twice the size of cherry angiomas, are purple, and occur in women between the ages of 30 and 50. They are noted for their rapid growth and tendency to bleed during strenuous exercise. Pyogenic granulomas are an overgrowth of inflamed granulation tissue. These lesions grow under the hormonal influence of pregnancy, with similarities to lesions in the oral cavity. Pyogenic granulomas are usually approximately 1 cm in diameter and may be mistaken clinically for malignant melanomas, basal cell carcinomas, vulvar condylomas, or nevi.

The diagnosis is usually established by gross inspection of the vascular lesion. When the differential diagnosis is questionable, excisional biopsy should be performed. A hemangioma that is associated with troublesome bleeding may be destroyed by cryosurgery or use of a laser. Obviously, if the histologic diagnosis is questionable, any bleeding vulvar mass should be treated by excisional biopsy so that the definitive pathologic diagnosis can be established. Lymphangiomas of the vulva do exist but are extremely rare.

Fibroma

Fibromas are the most common benign solid tumors of the vulva. They are more frequent than lipomas, the other common benign tumors of mesenchymal origin. Fibromas occur in all age groups and most commonly originate from the labia majora (Fig. 17-6). They grow

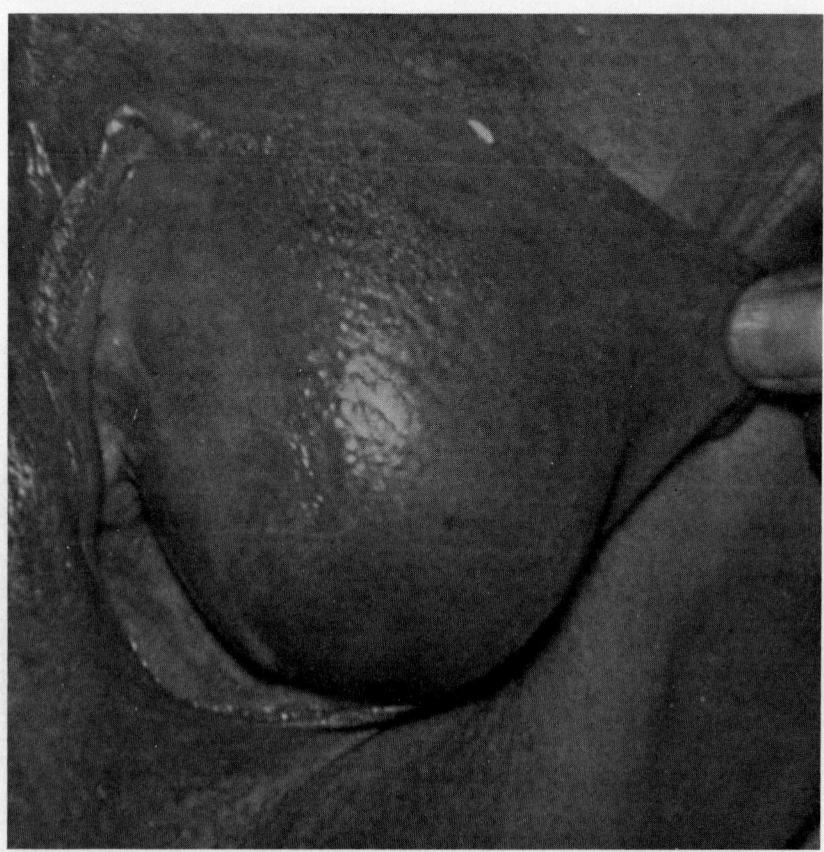

FIGURE 17-6
Fibroma. (From Friedrich EG, ed: Vulvar disease, 2nd ed. Philadelphia, W.B. Saunders Co., 1983, p. 233.)

slowly and vary from a few centimeters to one gigantic vulvar fibroma reported to weigh more than 250 pounds. The smaller fibromas are discovered as subcutaneous nodules. As they increase in size and weight, they become pedunculated. Smaller fibromas are firm; however, larger tumors often become cystic after undergoing myxomatous degeneration.

Fibromas have a smooth surface and a distinct contour. On cut surface the tissue is gray-white. Fat or muscle cells microscopically may be associated with the interlacing fibroblasts. Fibromas have a low-grade potential for becoming malignant. Smaller fibromas are asymptomatic; larger tumors may produce acute pain when they degenerate or chronic pressure symptoms. Treatment is operative removal.

Lipoma

Lipomas are benign, circumscribed tumors of fat cells arising from the subcutaneous tissue of the vulva (Fig. 17-7). Lipomas of the vulva are similar to lipomas of other parts of the body. When discovered they are softer and usually larger than fibromas. The largest vulvar lipoma reported in the literature weighed 44 pounds. Lipomas are the second most frequent benign vulvar mesenchymal tumor. Because of the fat distribution of the vulva, most lipomas are discovered in the labia majora and are superficial in location. They are slow growing, and their malignant potential is low.

When a lipoma is cut, the substance is soft, yellow, and lobulated. Histologically, lipomas are usually more homogeneous than fibromas. Unless extremely large, lipomas do not produce symptoms. Excision is usually performed to establish the diagnosis, although smaller tumors may be followed conservatively.

Hidradenoma

The hidradenoma is a rare, small, benign vulvar tumor that originates from apocrine sweat glands in the inner surface of the labia majora and nearby perineum. For unknown reasons, they are discovered exclusively in Caucasian women between the ages of 30 and 70, most commonly in the fourth decade of life. Hidradenomas may be cystic or solid. In Woodworth's review, 55% were cystic. While 38% originated from the labia majora, 26% arose from the labia minora.

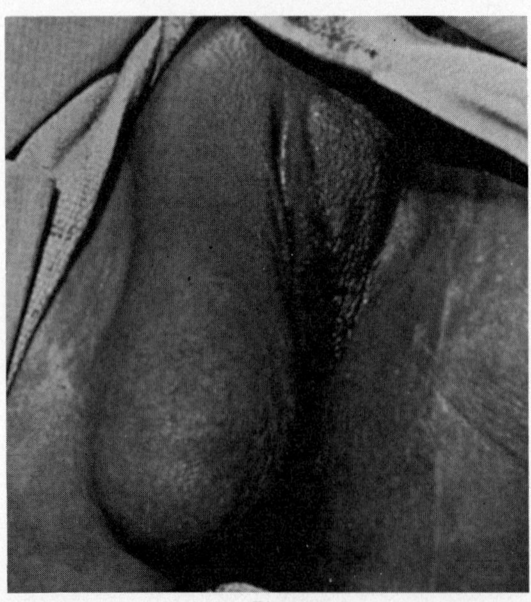

FIGURE 17-7
Lipoma. (From Friedrich EG, ed: Vulvar disease, 2nd ed. Philadelphia, W.B. Saunders Co., 1983, p. 233.)

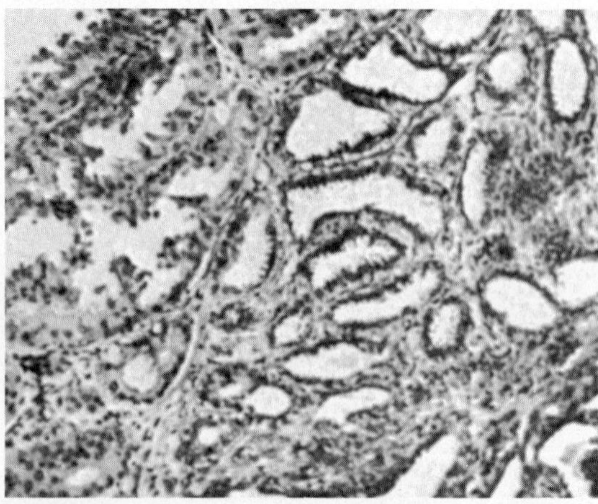

FIGURE 17-8
Hidradenoma. Numerous acini. Distinct apocrine gland–type epithelium is present on left (H&E stain). (From Kaufman RH: Cystic tumors. In Gardner HL, Kaufman RH, eds: Benign diseases of the vulva and vagina, 2nd ed. Boston, G.K. Hall, 1981, p. 101. Reproduced with permission.)

These tumors are well defined and usually sessile, pinkish gray nodules not larger than 1 cm in diameter. In most cases the surface epithelium is white, but occasionally necrosis of a central indented area occurs with a protrusion of reddish brown granulation tissue. These latter lesions may be confused with pyogenic granulomas.

These tumors have well-defined capsules. Histologically because of their hyperplastic, adenomatous pattern, a hidradenoma may be mistaken at first glance for an adenocarcinoma. On close inspection, however, although there is glandular hyperplasia with numerous tubular ducts, there is a paucity of mitotic figures and a lack of significant cellular and nuclear pleomorphism (Fig. 17-8). Unless there is necrosis of the tumor, hidradenomas are asymptomatic. Excisional biopsy is the treatment of choice.

Syringoma

The syringoma is a very rare, benign tumor of the eccrine sweat glands. It appears as small subcutaneous papules that may coalesce to form cords of firm tissue. Identical tumors are often found in the eccrine glands of the eyelids.

Endometriosis

Endometriosis of the vulva is rare. Only 1 in 500 women with endometriosis will present with vulvar lesions. The firm, small nodule or nodules may be cystic or solid and vary from a few millimeters to several centimeters. The subcutaneous lesions are blue, red, or purple, depending on their size, activity, and closeness to the surface of the skin. The gross and microscopic pathologic picture of vulvar endometriosis is similar to endometriosis of the pelvis (Chapter 18).

Endometriosis of the vulva is usually found at the site of an old, healed obstetric laceration, episiotomy site, or an area of operative removal of a Bartholin's duct cyst. The pathophysiology of development of vulvar endometriosis may be secondary to metaplasia, retrograde lymphatic spread, or potential implantation of endometrial tissue during operation. Paull and Tedeschi documented 15 cases of vulvar endometriosis they believed were associated with prophylactic postpartum curettage of the uterus to prevent postpartum bleeding. In their series there was not a single case of vulvar endometriosis in 13,800 deliveries without curettage, but 15 cases of vulvar endometriosis were associated with 2,028 deliveries with prophylactic curettage.

The most common symptoms of endometriosis of the vulva are pain and dyspareunia. The classic history is cyclic discomfort and an enlargement of the mass associated with menstrual periods. Treatment of vulvar endometriosis is by excision or laser vaporization.

Granular Cell Myoblastoma

Granular cell myoblastoma is a rare, slow-growing, solid vulvar tumor. The tumor originates from neural sheath (Schwann) cells and is sometimes called a *schwannoma*. These tumors are found in connective tissues throughout the body, most commonly in the tongue, and occur in any age group. Approximately 7% of solitary granular cell myoblastomas are found in the subcutaneous tissue of the vulva. Twenty percent of multiple myoblastomas are located in the vulva.

These tumors are subcutaneous nodules, usually 1 to 5 cm in diameter. They are benign but characteristically infiltrate the surrounding local tissue. As they grow, they may also cause ulcerations in the skin. The overlying skin often has hyperplastic changes that may look similar to invasive squamous cell carcinoma. Grossly, these tumors are not encapsulated. Histologically, there are irregularly arranged bundles of large, round cells with indistinct borders and pink-staining cytoplasm. Initially the cell of origin was believed to be striated muscle; however, electron microscopic studies have demonstrated that this tumor is from cells of the neural sheath.

The tumor nodules are painless. Treatment involves wide excision to remove the filamentous projections into the surrounding tissue. If the initial excisional biopsy is not wide enough, these benign tumors tend to recur.

von Recklinghausen's Disease

The vulva is sometimes involved with the benign neural sheath tumors of von Recklinghausen's disease (generalized neurofibromatous and café-au-lait spots). The vulvar lesions of this disease are fleshy, brownish red, polypoid tumors. Approximately 18% of women with von Recklinghausen's disease have vulvar involvement. Excision is the treatment of choice for symptomatic tumors.

Other Abnormal Tissue

Other examples of aberrant tissue presenting as vulvar masses include accessory breast tissue and müllerian or wolffian duct remnants.

Hematomas

Hematomas of the vulva are usually secondary to blunt trauma such as a straddle injury from a fall, an automobile accident, or a physical assault. Traumatic injuries producing vulvar hematoma have been reported secondary to a wide range of recreational activities, including bicycle and motorcycle riding, sledding, water skiing, cross-country skiing, riding go-carts, and amusement park rides (Fig. 17-9). Spontaneous hematomas are rare and usually occur from rupture of a varicose vein during pregnancy or the postpartum period.

The management of vulvar hematomas is usually conservative unless the hematoma is rapidly expanding. Compression and application of an ice pack to the area are appropriate therapy. Operative therapy is indicated in an attempt to identify and ligate the damaged vessel only if the hematoma continues to expand.

The majority of hematomas regress with time. However, Reid et al. have emphasized the problems associated with a chronic expanding hematoma. The most familiar clinical example of this problem is the chronic subdural hematoma, but a similar situation may accompany vulvar hematomas. The underlying pathophysiology is the repetitive episodes of bleeding from capillaries in the granulation tissue of the hematoma, which result in a chronic, slowly expanding vulvar mass. Treatment of a chronic expanding hematoma is drainage and debridement.

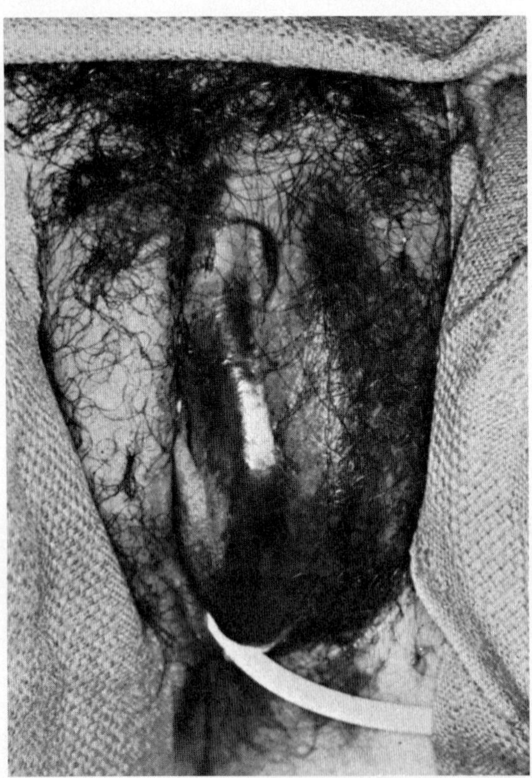

FIGURE 17-9
Vulvar hematoma from a straddle injury that produced urethral obstruction. (From Naumann RO, Droegemueller W: Am J Obstet Gynecol 142:358, 1982.)

DERMATOLOGIC DISEASES

The skin of the vulva is similar to the skin over any surface of the body and is therefore susceptible to any generalized skin disease or involvement by systemic disease. The most common generalized skin diseases involving the vulva include contact dermatitis, neurodermatitis, psoriasis, seborrheic dermatitis, and lichen planus. The diagnosis and treatment of these lesions is often obscured or modified by the environment of the vulva. The moisture and heat of the intertriginous areas may produce irritation, maceration, and a wet weeping surface. The skin of the vulva is susceptible to acute infections produced by streptococcus or staphylococcus, such as folliculitis, furunculitis, impetigo, and a special chronic infection, hidradenitis suppurativa.

The nonspecific symptom complex of vulvar pruritus and burning is presented next as an introduction to the discussion of dermatologic diseases of the vulva.

Pruritus and Vulvodynia

Pruritus is a symptom of intense itching with an associated desire to scratch and rub the affected area. In some women pruritus becomes an almost unrelenting symptom with the development of an "itch-scratch" cycle. The itch-scratch cycle is a complex of itching leading to scratching, producing excoriation and then healing. The healing skin itches, leading to further scratching. *Vulvodynia* is a term recently developed to describe chronic vulvar discomfort, including burning, stinging, and "rawness." Pruritus and vulvodynia are nonspecific symptoms, and their differential diagnosis includes a wide range of vulvar diseases, including skin infections, sexually transmitted diseases, specific dermatosis, vulvar dystrophies, lichen sclerosis, premalignant and malignant disease, contact dermatitis, neurodermatitis, and psychological causes.

The treatment of pruritus and vulvodynia involves establishing a diagnosis, treatment of the offending cause, and improvement of local hygiene. For successful treatment the itch-scratch cycle must be interrupted before the condition becomes chronic, resulting in lichenification of the skin. During the latter process the skin becomes white, thickened, and "leathery." The resulting dry scaly skin frequently cracks, forms fissures, and becomes secondarily infected, thus complicating the treatment. Chapter 30 discusses vulvar dystrophies.

Contact Dermatitis

The vulvar skin, especially the intertriginous areas, is a frequent site of contact dermatitis. Contact dermatitis may be one of two basic pathophysiologic processes: a contact irritant (nonimmunologic) or a truly allergic (immunologic) etiology. The majority of chemicals that produce hypersensitivity of the vulvar skin are cosmetic or therapeutic agents, including vaginal contraceptives, lubricants, sprays, perfumes, douches, fabric dyes, fabric softeners, synthetic fibers, bleaches, soaps, chlorine, dyes in toilet tissues, and local anesthetic creams. Some of the most severe cases of contact dermatitis involve lesions of the vulvar skin secondary to poison ivy or poison oak.

Acute contact dermatitis results in a red, edematous inflamed skin. The skin may become weeping and eczematoid. The most severe skin reactions form vesicles, and any stage may become secondarily infected.

The foundation of treatment of contact dermatitis is to withdraw the offending substance. Sometimes the distribution of the vulvar erythema helps to delineate the irritant. For example, localized erythema often results from vaginal medication, while generalized erythema of the vulva is secondary to an allergen in clothing. It is possible to use a vulvar chemical innocuously for many months or years before the topical vulvar "allergy" develops. Initial treatment of severe lesions is with wet compresses of Burow's solution (diluted 1 to 20) for 30 minutes several times a day. This is followed by drying the vulva with cool air from a hair dryer. The vulvar skin should remain clean and dry. Cotton undergarments that allow the vulvar skin to aerate should be worn, and constrictive, occlusive, or tight-fitting clothing such as pantyhose should be avoided. Vulvar dryness may be facilitated by using a nonmedicated baby powder. Hydrocortisone (0.5% to 1%) and fluorinated corticosteroids (Valisone, 0.1%, or Synalar, 0.01%) as lotions or creams may be rubbed into the skin two to three times a day for a few days to control symptoms. Synthetic systemic corticosteroids (prednisone, 50 mg a day for 7 to 10 days) are sometimes necessary for treatment of poison ivy and poison oak. Antipruritic medications, such as antihistamines, are not of great therapeutic benefit except as soporific agents.

Psoriasis

Psoriasis is a common, generalized skin disease of unknown etiology. Approximately 3% of adult women are affected by this chronic skin disease with an extremely variable and unpredictable course marked by spontaneous remissions and exacerbations. Twenty-five percent of women have a family history of the disease. Common areas of involvement are the scalp and fingernails.

Vulvar psoriasis usually affects intertriginous areas and is manifested by red to red-yellow papules. These papules tend to enlarge, becoming well-circumscribed, dull red plaques. The classic silver scales and bleeding on gentle scraping of the plaque help to establish the diagnosis. In the vulvar region the amount of scales is extremely variable. Under the influence of the moisture and heat of the vulva, vulvar psoriasis may look similar to candidiasis. Initial treatment is a topical fluorinated corticosteroid preparation. If this treatment is not successful, a dermatologist should be consulted.

Seborrheic Dermatitis

Seborrheic dermatitis is a common chronic skin disease of unknown etiology that affects the face, scalp, sternum, and the area behind the ears. Rarely, the mons pubis and vulva area may be involved. Vulvar lesions are erythematous and edematous and are covered by a fine nonadherent scale, which is usually oily. Excessive sweating and emotional tension precipitate attacks. The pruritus associated with seborrheic dermatitis varies from mild to severe. Treatment is similar to contact dermatitis, with hydrocortisone cream being the most effective medication.

Lichen Planus

Lichen planus is a unique, chronic eruption of violaceous papules. These tiny flat papules appear in women over 30 years of age on flexor surfaces, mucous membranes, and vulvar skin. Papules often develop in linear scratch marks. The lesions are intensely pruritic, and the initial onset usually follows a time of intense emotional stress. The etiology of this disease is unknown. Treatment of local lesions is a topical steroid cream. If the patient is intensely symptomatic, oral steroids may be necessary.

Hidradenitis Suppurativa

Hidradenitis suppurativa is a chronic, unrelenting, refractory infection of the skin and subcutaneous tissue. Initially it develops from one or more subcutaneous nodules. It is frequently misdiagnosed and treated unsuccessfully with antibiotics and topical steroids. Gradually a deep-seated chronic infection of apocrine glands develops with occlusion of dilated ducts with inspissated keratin material. The disease progresses to multiple draining abscesses and sinuses. Bhatia et al. recommend

that the diagnosis be confirmed by biopsy. The treatment of choice is early, aggressive, wide operative excision of the infected skin.

Edema

Edema of the vulva may be a symptom of either local or generalized disease. Vulvar edema is often noted before edema in other areas of the female body is noted. The loose connective tissue of the vulva and its dependent position predispose to early development of pitting edema. Systemic causes of vulvar edema include circulatory and renal failure, ascites, and hypoproteinemia. Vulvar edema also may occur after intraperitoneal dextran is given to prevent adhesions following infertility operations. Local causes of vulvar edema include allergy, neurodermatitis, inflammation, trauma, and lymphatic obstruction due to carcinoma or infection.

VAGINA

Urethral Diverticulum

A urethral diverticulum is a common problem, being discovered in approximately 3% of women. The majority of cases are initially diagnosed in reproductive-age females, with the peak incidence in the fourth decade of life. The symptoms of a urethral diverticulum are nonspecific and are identical to the general symptoms of a lower urinary tract infection. To diagnose this elusive condition, one should suspect urethral diverticulum in any woman with chronic or recurrent lower urinary tract symptoms. The urologic aspects of this condition are discussed in Chapter 20.

Urethral diverticula may be congenital or acquired. Few urethral diverticula present in children; therefore it is assumed that most diverticula are not congenital. Huffman made the analogy that anatomically the urethra is similar to a tree with many stunted branches that represent the periurethral ducts and glands. It is assumed that the majority of urethral diverticula result from repetitive or chronic infections of the periurethral glands. The suburethral infection may cause obstruction of the ducts and glands, with subsequent production of cystic enlargement and retention cysts. These cysts may rupture into the urethral lumen and produce a suburethral diverticulum. Occasionally a suburethral diverticulum has associated stone formation in the dilated retention cyst. Urethral diverticula are small, from 3 mm to 3 cm in diameter. The majority of urethral diverticula open into the midportion of the urethra (Table 17-1). Occasionally multiple suburethral diverticula occur in the same woman.

The most common symptoms associated with urethral diverticula are urinary urgency, frequency, and dysuria. Ginsberg and Genadry discovered that 90% of their patients had symptoms of chronic lower urinary tract infection as the presenting complaint. Other authors have stressed the three Ds associated with a diverticula: *dysuria, dyspareunia,* and *dribbling* of the urine. Although for years postvoiding dribbling has been termed a classic symptom of urethral diverticulum, it is reported by fewer than 10% of women with this condition. In Lee's series a palpable, tender mass was felt in 56 of 108 patients. Ginsberg and Genadry found a palpable mass in 46 of 70 women with a urethral diverticulum. It is interesting that in most large series, approximately 20% of the women are asymptomatic. A classic sign of a suburethral diverticulum is the expression of purulent material from the urethra after compressing the suburethral area during a pelvic examination.

The foundation of diagnosing urethral diverticulum is the physician's awareness of the possibility of this defect occurring in women with chronic symptoms of lower urinary tract infection. Subsequently it is important to appreciate that a single diagnostic procedure may not identify the diverticulum. The two most common methods of diagnosing urethral diverticulum are voiding cystourethrography, and cystourethroscopy. Approximately 70% of urethral diverticula will be filled by contrast material on a postvoiding x-ray film with a lateral view. Cystourethroscopy will demonstrate the urethral opening of the urethral diverticulum in approximately 6 of 10 cases. Other diagnostic tests used to identify urethral diverticula include urethral pressure profile recordings and a positive pressure urethrography. The latter test is done with a special double-balloon urethral catheter (Davis catheter) (Fig. 17-10). Ultrasound has been used to diagnose urethral diverticulum but is of limited diagnostic benefit. The differential diagnosis includes Gartner's duct cyst, an ectopic ureter that empties into the urethra, and Skene's glands cysts.

Several different operations can correct urethral diverticula. Operative techniques can be divided into transurethral and transvaginal approaches, with most gynecologists preferring the transvaginal approach as described by Lee. Following operations, approximately 80% of patients obtain complete relief from symptoms. Some diverticula have multiple openings into the urethra. Complete excision of this network of fistulous connections is important. The recurrence rate varies between 10% and 20%, and many failures are due to incomplete surgical resection. The most serious consequences of surgical repair of urethral diverticula are urinary incontinence and urethrovaginal fistula. The incidence of each of these complications is approximately 1% to 2%.

Inclusion Cysts

Inclusion cysts are the most common cystic structures of the vagina. In Deppisch's series of 64 women with cystic masses of the vagina, 34 had inclusion cysts. The cysts are usually discovered in the posterior or lateral walls of the lower third of the vagina. Inclusion cysts vary from 1 mm to 3 cm. Deppisch reported a mean diameter of 1.6 cm. Similar to inclusion cysts of the vulva, inclusion cysts of the vagina are more common in parous women.

TABLE 17-1

Location of the Ostium in 108 Female Patients with Diverticulum of the Urethra

Site	No. of Patients
Distal (external) third of the urethra	11
Middle third of the urethra	55
Proximal (inner) third of the urethra (including vesical neck)	18
Multiple sites	18
Unknown	6

From Lee RA: Diverticulum of the urethra: clinical presentation, diagnosis, and management. Clin Obstet Gynecol 27:491, 1984.

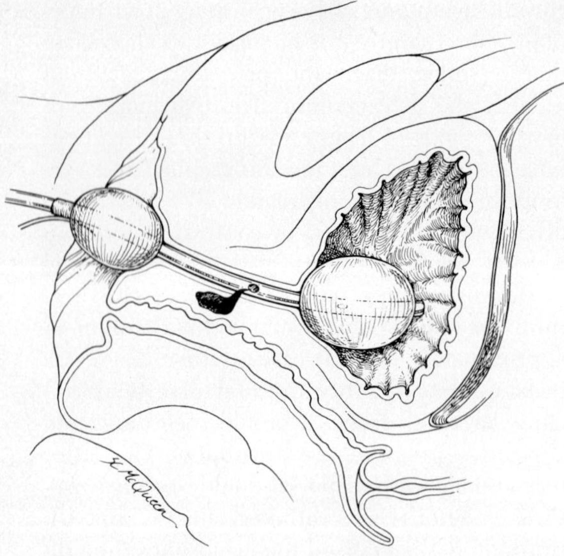

FIGURE 17-10
Double ballooned catheter in use for positive pressure urethrography. (From Mattingly RF, Thompson JD, eds: TeLinde's operative gynecology, 6th ed. Philadelphia, J.B. Lippincott Co., 1985, p. 751.)

Histologically, inclusion cysts are lined by stratified squamous epithelium. These cysts contain a thick, pale yellow substance that is oily and formed by degenerating epithelial cells. Often these cysts are erroneously called sebaceous cysts in the misbelief that the central material is sebaceous. Similar to vulvar inclusion cysts, the etiology is either a small tag of vaginal epithelium buried beneath the surface following a gynecologic or obstetric procedure or a misplaced island of embryonic remnant that was destined to form epithelium.

The majority of inclusion cysts are asymptomatic. If the cyst produces dyspareunia or pain, excisional biopsy is appropriate.

Dysontogenetic Cysts

Dysontogenetic cysts of the vagina are thin-walled, soft cysts of embryonic origin. Though more commonly single, they may be multiple. The cysts vary from 3 to 5 cm in diameter and are usually discovered in the upper one half of the vagina. Sometimes multiple small cysts may present like a string of large, soft beads. A large cyst presenting at the introitus may be mistaken for a cystocele or obstructed aberrant ureter. Approximately 1 in 200 females develop these cysts.

Embryonic cysts of the vagina, especially those on the anterior lateral wall, are usually Gartner's duct cysts. The distal portion of the mesonephric duct runs parallel with the vagina. It is assumed that a segment of this embryonic structure fails to regress, and the obstructed vestigial remnant becomes cystic.

Most of these benign cysts are asymptomatic, sausage-shaped tumors that are discovered only incidentally during pelvic examination. Small asymptomatic Gartner's duct cysts may be followed conservatively. Deppisch, in a series of 25 women undergoing operations for symptomatic dysontogenetic cysts, reported a wide range of symptoms including dyspareunia, vaginal pain, urinary symptoms, and a palpable mass. Sometimes large cysts interfere with the use of tampons.

Operative excision is indicated for chronic mechanical symptoms. Rarely one of these cysts becomes infected, and if operated on during the acute phase, marsupialization of the cyst is preferred. Occasionally, excision of the vaginal cyst is a much more formidable operation than anticipated. The cystic structure may extend up into the broad ligament and anatomically be in proximity to the distal course of the ureter.

Tampon Problems

The vaginal tampon has achieved immense popularity and ubiquitous use by women. It is not surprising that there are rare associated risks with tampon usage: vaginal ulcers, the "forgotten" tampon, and toxic shock syndrome. The latter, related to toxins elaborated by *Staphylococcus aureus*, is discussed in Chapter 21.

Wearing a tampon for a few days has been associated with microscopic epithelial changes. Friedrich, in a study of colposcopic changes related to the tampon, found serial changes of epithelial drying, peeling, layering, and ultimately microulceration. In his study, 15% of women wearing tampons only during the time of normal menstruation developed microulcerations.

Barrett et al. were the first to describe large

macroscopic ulcers of the vaginal fornix in four women who were tampon "abusers." Each of these young women wore vaginal tampons for prolonged lengths of time for persistent vaginal discharge or spotting, changing the individual tampon several times per day. The ulcers had a base of clean granulation tissue with smooth, rolled edges. Jimmerson and Becker found birefractal foreign body fragments in biopsy specimens (fibers from tampons) in the vaginal ulcers of 4 of 10 women. The pathophysiology of the ulcer is believed to be secondary to drying and pressure necrosis induced by the tampon. Obviously, many of these young women use tampons for the identical symptoms that are associated with a vaginal ulcer, that is, spotting and vaginal discharge. Often the intermenstrual spotting is believed to be breakthrough bleeding from oral contraceptives, and the possibility of a vaginal ulcer from chronic tampon usage is overlooked.

Vaginal ulcers are not uncommon with several types of foreign objects, including diaphragms, pessaries, and medicated silicon rings. Management is conservative, as the ulcers heal spontaneously when the foreign object is removed. Any persistent ulcer should be biopsied to rule out carcinoma.

A woman with a "lost" or "forgotten" tampon presents with a classic foul vaginal discharge and occasionally spotting. The tampon is usually found high in the vagina. The odor from a forgotten tampon is overwhelming. The woman should be treated with an antibiotic vaginal cream (Sultrin) for the next 5 to 7 days.

Local Trauma

The most frequent etiology of trauma to the lower genital tract of adult females is coitus. Approximately 80% of vaginal lacerations occur secondary to sexual intercourse. Other causes of vaginal trauma are straddle injuries, penetration injuries by foreign objects, sexual assault, and water skiing accidents. The management of vulvar and vaginal trauma in children is discussed in Chapter 10.

The predisposing factors believed to be related to coital injury include virginity, the postpartum and postmenopausal vaginal epithelium, pregnancy, intercourse after a prolonged period of abstinence, hysterectomy, and inebri-

ation. Smith et al. reviewed 19 injuries from normal coitus; 12 of the women in his series were between the ages of 16 and 25 and 5 were over age 45. The most common injury is a transverse tear of the posterior fornix. Similar linear lacerations often occur in the right or left vaginal fornices. The location of the coital injury is believed to be related to the poor support of the upper vagina, which is supplied only by a thin layer of connective tissue. The most prominent symptom of a coital vaginal laceration is profuse or prolonged vaginal bleeding. Many women experienced sharp pain during intercourse, and 25% noted persistent abdominal pain. The most troublesome but extremely rare complication of vaginal laceration is vaginal evisceration.

Often the history of the coital injury is not obtained, and the patient may even give misleading information. However, coital injury to the vagina should be considered in any woman with profuse or prolonged abnormal vaginal bleeding.

Management of coital lacerations involves prompt suturing under adequate anesthesia. There is no place for conservative management. Secondary injury to the urinary and gastrointestinal tracts should be ruled out.

CERVIX

Endocervical and Cervical Polyps

Endocervical and cervical polyps are the most common benign neoplastic growths of the cervix. In an extensive series Farrar and Nedoss reported an incidence of endocervical polyps in 4% of all gynecologic patients. Endocervical polyps are most common in multiparous women in their forties and fifties (Fig. 17-11). The majority are smooth, soft, reddish purple to cherry red, and fragile. They readily bleed when touched. Cervical polyps may be single or multiple and are a few millimeters to 4 cm in diameter. The stalk of the polyp is of variable length and width (Fig. 17-12). Polyps may arise from either the endocervical canal (endocervical polyp) or ectocervix (cervical polyp). Polyps whose base is in the endocervix usually have a narrow long pedicle and occur during the reproductive years, while polyps that arise from the ectocervix have a

FIGURE 17-11
At the external os a typical cervical polyp with smooth surface and dense vascular network is seen. On the posterior wall of the cervical canal there are some large branched vessels that indicate an old transformation zone. There is no suspicion of malignancy, but the squamocolumnar junction cannot be seen, so the colposcopic findings should be classifed indecisive. (From Kolstad P, Stafl A, eds: Atlas of colposcopy, 2nd ed. Baltimore, University Park Press, 1977, p. 66.)

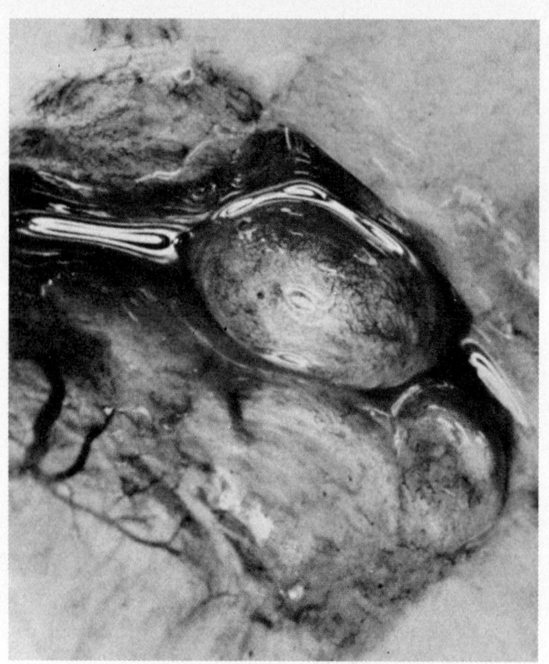

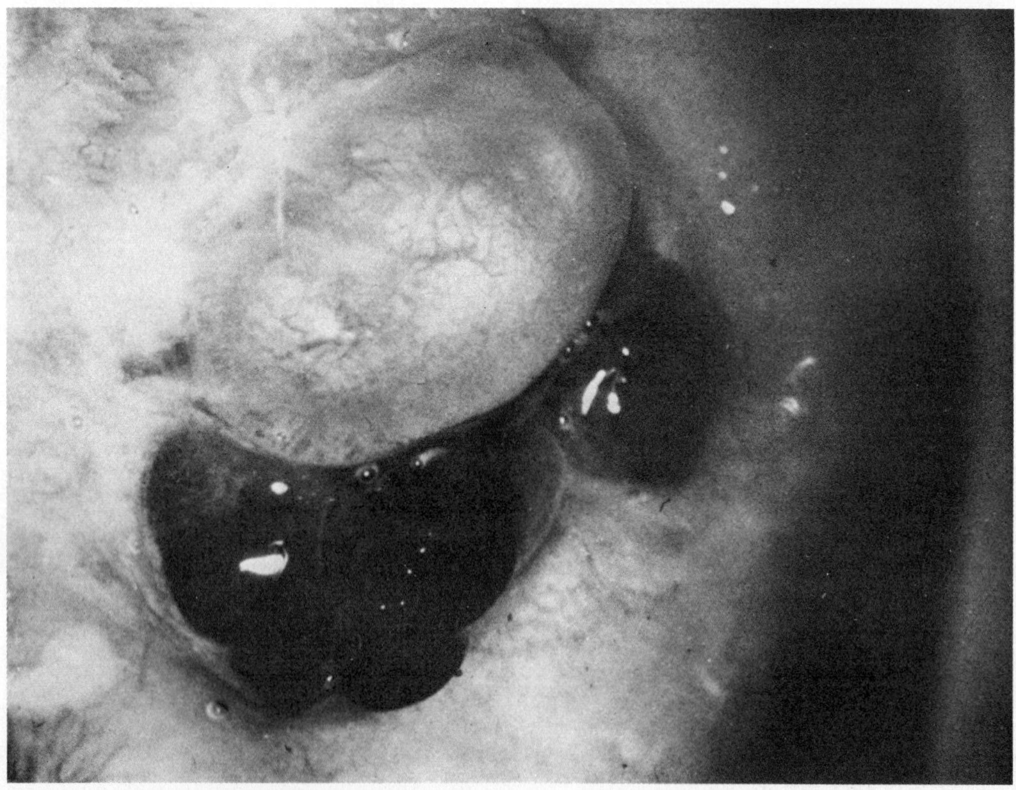

FIGURE 17-12
Endocervical polyp: clinical appearance. (From Gompel C, Silverberg SG, eds: Pathology in gynecology and obstetrics, 2nd ed. Philadelphia, J.B. Lippincott Co., 1977, p. 74.)

short, broad base and usually occur in post-menopausal women.

The general hypothesis of the origin of endocervical polyps is that they are usually secondary to inflammation. Focal hyperplasia and localized proliferation are the response of the cervix to local inflammation. The color of the polyp depends in part on its origin, with most endocervical polyps being cherry red and most cervical polyps grayish white.

The classic symptoms of an endocervical polyp are intermenstrual bleeding, especially following contact such as coitus or an examination. Rarely there may be an associated cervical discharge. A large polyp may dilate the cervix as its dependent portion protrudes into the vagina. Many endocervical polyps are asymptomatic and recognized for the first time during a routine speculum examination. Often the polyp seen on inspection is difficult to palpate because of its soft consistency.

Histologically the surface epithelium of the polyp is columnar or squamous epithelium, depending on the site of origin and the degree of squamous metaplasia (Fig. 17-13). The stalk is composed of an edematous, inflamed, loose, and richly vascular connective tissue. Often there is ulceration of the most dependent portion, which explains the symptom of contact bleeding. Malignant degeneration of an endocervical polyp is extremely rare. Common considerations in the differential diagnosis include endometrial polyps, small prolapsed myomas, and cervical malignancy.

Most endocervical polyps may be managed in the office by grasping the base of the polyp with an appropriately sized clamp. The polyp is avulsed with a twisting motion and sent to the pathology laboratory for microscopic evaluation. If the base is broad or bleeding ensues, the base may be treated with chemical cautery, electrocautery, or cryocautery. If abnormal bleeding continues after the polyp is removed, endometrial sampling should be performed to

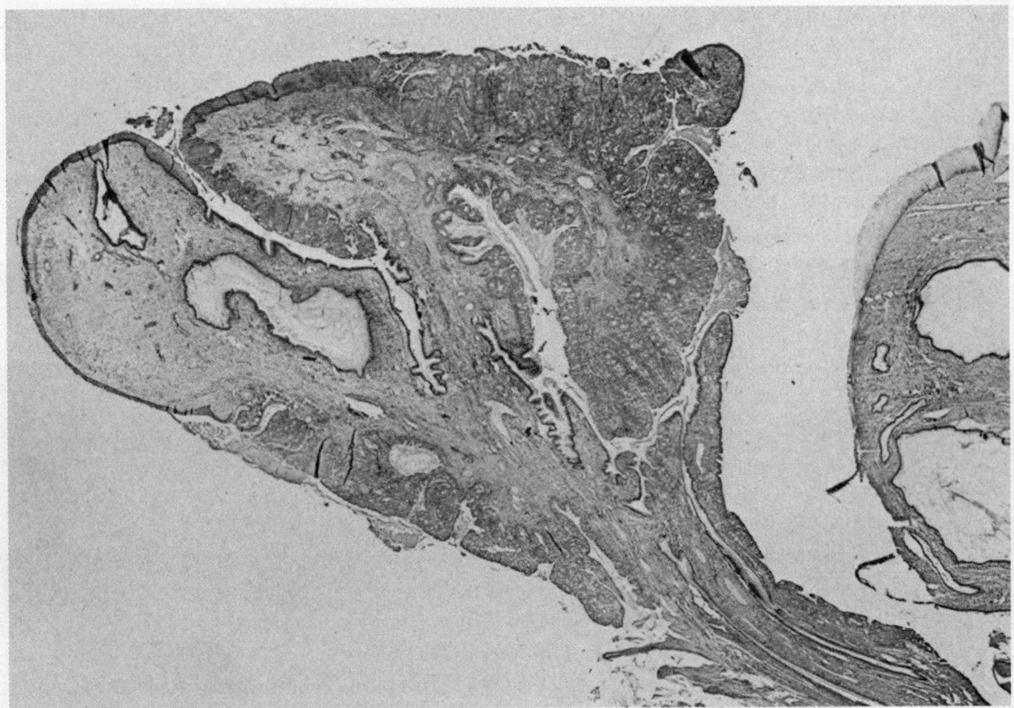

FIGURE 17-13
Endocervical polyp with zones of squamous metaplasia. (From Gompel C, Silverberg SG, eds: Pathology in gynecology and obstetrics, 2nd ed. Philadelphia, J.B. Lippincott Co., 1977, p. 74.)

diagnose an unrelated endometrial hyperplasia or carcinoma that might have produced symptoms identical to those of the polyp.

Nabothian Cysts

Nabothian cysts are retention cysts of endocervical columnar cells occurring where a tunnel or cleft has been covered by squamous metaplasia. These cysts are so common that they are considered a normal feature of the adult cervix. Many women have multiple cysts. Grossly, these cysts may be translucent or opaque whitish blebs. Nabothian cysts vary from microscopic to macroscopic size, with the majority between 3mm and 3 cm in diameter. Rarely, a woman with several large Nabothian cysts may develop gross enlargement of the cervix. These mucous retention cysts are produced by the spontaneous healing process of the cervix. The cervix is in an almost constant process of repair, and squamous cells block the cleft of a gland orifice. The endocervical columnar cells continue to secrete, and thus a mucous retention cyst is formed. Nabothian cysts are asymptomatic, and no treatment is necessary.

Lacerations

Cervical lacerations frequently occur with both normal and abnormal deliveries. Lacerations may occur in nonpregnant women with mechanical dilation of the cervix. Obstetric lacerations vary from minor superficial tears to extensive full-thickness lacerations at 3 and 9 o'clock respectively, which may extend into the broad ligament. In gynecology the atrophic cervix of the postmenopausal woman predisposes to the complication of cervical laceration when the cervix is mechanically dilated for a diagnostic dilation and curettage.

Acute cervical lacerations bleed and should be sutured. Cervical lacerations that are not repaired may give the external os of the cervix a fish-mouthed appearance; however, they are usually asymptomatic. Extensive cervical lacerations may lead to incompetence of the cervix during pregnancy. The use of laminaria tents to slowly soften and dilate the cervix before mechanical instrumentation of the endometrial cavity has reduced the magnitude of ia-

trogenic cervical lacerations. Furthermore the practice of routine inspection of the cervix, stabilized with one or more ring forceps, following every second or third trimester delivery has enabled physicians to discover and repair extensive cervical lacerations.

Cervical Myomas

Cervical myomas are smooth, firm masses that are usually solitary and are similar to myomas of the fundus (Figs. 17-14 and 17-15). Depending on the series, 3% to 8% of myomas are categorized as cervical myomas. In fact, because of the relative paucity of smooth muscle fibers in the cervical stroma the majority of myomas that appear to be cervical actually arise from the isthmus of the uterus.

Most cervical myomas are small and asymptomatic. When symptoms do occur, they are dependent on the direction in which the enlarging myoma expands. Cervical myomas may produce dysuria, urgency, urethral or ureteral obstruction, dyspareunia, or obstruction of the cervix. Occasionally a cervical myoma may become pedunculated and protrude through the external os of the cervix. These prolapsed myomas are often ulcerated and infected. A very large cervical myoma may produce distortion of the cervical canal and upper vagina.

The diagnosis of a cervical myoma is by in-

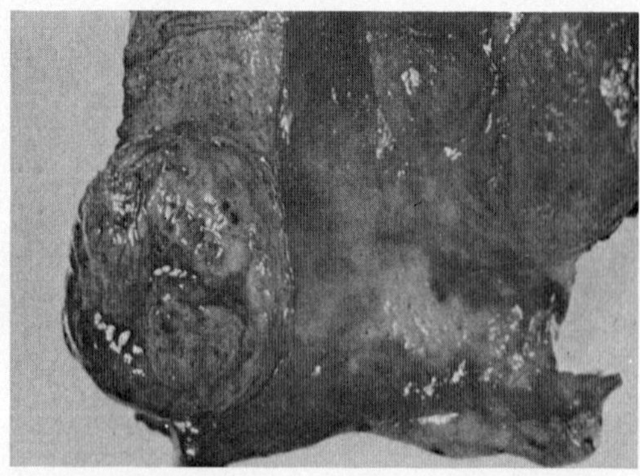

FIGURE 17-14
Leiomyoma, originating in the cervix and dilating the endocervical canal. It is soft, showing degenerative changes. (From Janovski NA, ed: Color atlas of gross gynecologic and obstetric pathology. New York, McGraw-Hill Book Co., 1969, p. 71.)

spection and palpation. Grossly and histologically, cervical myomas are identical to and indistinguishable from myomas of the corpus of the uterus. Management is similar to that of uterine myomas in that asymptomatic, small myomas may be observed for rate of growth. The occurrence and persistence of symptoms from a cervical myoma are an indication for either myomectomy or hysterectomy, depending on the age and future reproductive plans of the patient. Treatment of cervical myomas that grow laterally may become a challenge if myomectomy is the operation of choice, because of both a complex blood supply and involvement with the distal course of the ureter. Prolapsed uterine myomas are discussed later in this chapter.

Cervical Stenosis

Cervical stenosis most often occurs in the region of the internal os. Cervical stenosis may be divided into congenital or acquired types. The causes of acquired cervical stenosis are operative, radiation, infection, neoplasia, or atrophic changes. The most common of the operative procedures that may cause cervical stenosis are cone biopsy and cautery of the cervix, either electrocautery or cryocoagulation.

The symptoms of cervical stenosis depend on

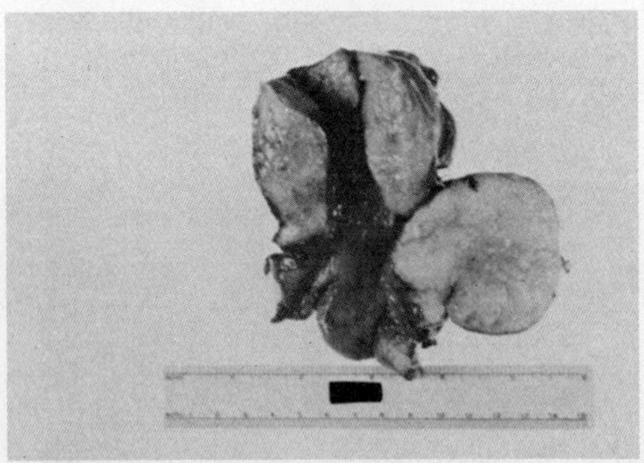

FIGURE 17-15
Leiomyoma of the cervix most likely developing from the lateral endocervix and protruding into the broad ligament. The tumor is whitish, firm, and poorly encapsulated. (From Janovski NA, ed: Color atlas of gross gynecologic and obstetric pathology. New York, McGraw-Hill Book Co., 1969, p. 69.)

whether the patient is premenopausal or postmenopausal and whether the obstruction is complete or partial. Common symptoms in premenopausal women include dysmenorrhea, infertility, abnormal bleeding, and amenorrhea. Postmenopausal women are usually asymptomatic for a long time. Slowly they develop a hematometra (blood), hydrometra (clear fluid), or pyometra (exudate). The collection of fluid inside the uterus may reflux and extend into the fallopian tubes and subsequently the peritoneal cavity. Endometriosis is a commonly associated disease in premenopausal women.

The diagnosis is established by inability to introduce a 1 to 2 mm dilator into the uterine cavity. If the obstruction is complete, a soft, slightly tender, enlarged uterus is appreciated as a midline mass. Management of cervical stenosis is dilation of the cervix with dilators under appropriate anesthesia. If stenosis recurs, monthly laminaria tents may be used. Similarly, office follow-up and sounding of the cervix of women who have had a cone biopsy or cautery of the cervix is necessary to establish patency of the endocervical canal. Postmenopausal women with pyometra usually do not need antibiotics. However, if the cervical stenosis is caused by atrophic changes, a diagnostic curettage of the uterus with biopsies of the endocervical canal to rule out carcinoma of the endometrium should be performed after the acute infection has subsided. After cervical dilation it is often useful to leave a T tube as a stent in the cervical canal for a few days to maintain patency.

UTERUS

Endometrial Polyps

Endometrial polyps are localized overgrowths of endometrial glands and stroma that project beyond the surface of the endometrium. Endometrial polyps are soft and pliable and may be single or multiple. Most polyps arise from the fundus of the uterus. They vary from a few millimeters to several centimeters in diameter, and it is possible for a single large polyp to fill the endometrial cavity. Endometrial polyps may have a broad base (sessile) or be attached by a slender pedicle (pedunculated). In Novak and Woodruff's review of 1100 women with polyps, the growths were discovered in all age groups, with a peak incidence between the ages of 40 and 49. Endometrial polyps are noted in approximately 10% of women when the uterus is examined at autopsy. The etiology of endometrial polyps is unknown. Because polyps are often associated with endometrial hyperplasia, unopposed estrogen may be a partial explanation.

The majority of endometrial polyps are asymptomatic. Those that are symptomatic present with a wide range of abnormal bleeding patterns. No single abnormal bleeding pattern is diagnostic for polyps; however premenstrual and postmenstrual staining and scanty postmenstrual spotting are the most common. Occasionally a pedunculated endometrial polyp with a long pedicle may protrude from the external cervical os.

Polyps are red to brown, succulent, and velvety, and they have a large central vascular core. Histologically an endometrial polyp has three components: endometrial glands, endo-

metrial stroma, and central vascular channels (Figs. 17-16 and 17-17). Epithelium must be identified on three sides, like a peninsula. Approximately two of three polyps consist of immature endometrium that does not respond to cyclic changes in circulating progesterone. This immature endometrium differs from surrounding endometrium and often appears like a "Swiss cheese" cystic hyperplasia during all phases of the menstrual cycle. The other one third of endometrial polyps consists of functional endometrium that will undergo cyclic histologic changes. The tip of a prolapsed polyp often undergoes squamous metaplasia, infection, or ulceration. Often the clinician cannot distinguish whether the abnormal bleeding originates from the polyp or is secondary to the frequently coexisting endometrial hyperplasia.

Malignant transformation in an endometrial polyp has been estimated to be as high as 0.5%. However, a recent epidemiologic, population-based, case control study from Sweden by Petterson et al. estimates that the increased risk of subsequent endometrial carcinoma in

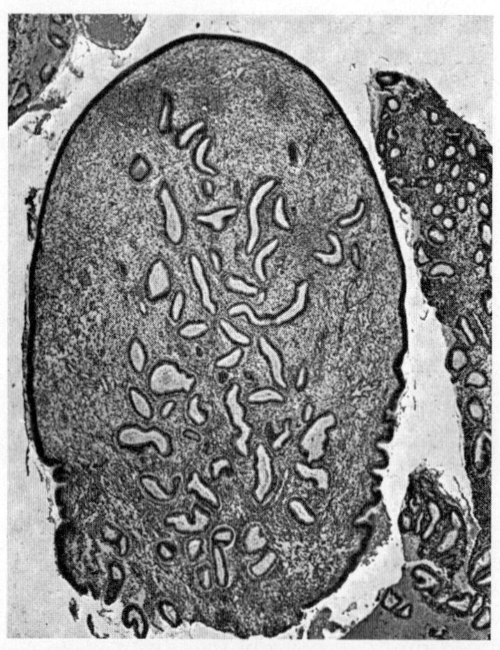

FIGURE 17-16
Typical small endometrial polyp. (From Novak ER, Woodruff JD, eds: Novak's gynecologic and obstetric pathology, 6th ed. Philadelphia, W.B. Saunders Co., 1967, p. 206.)

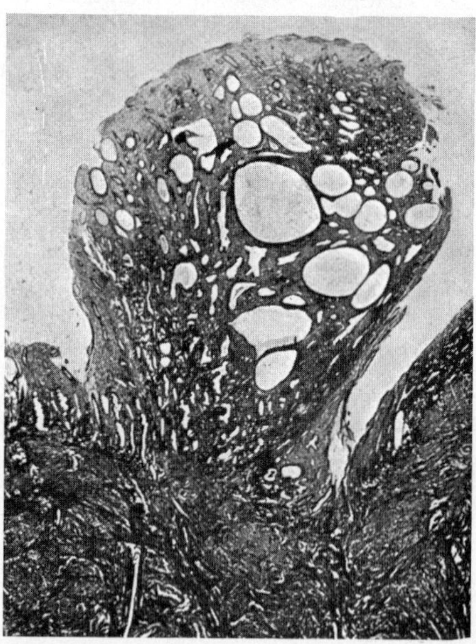

FIGURE 17-17
Endometrial polyp showing hyperplastic, nonfunctioning structure. This is much more common than the functioning type. (From Novak ER, Woodruff JD, eds: Novak's gynecologic and obstetric pathology, 6th ed. Philadelphia, W.B. Saunders Co., 1967, p. 207.)

women with endometrial polyps is only two-fold. This latter study provides a more realistic appraisal of the risk. Malignant change, when found in an endometrial polyp, is usually curable, and the endometrial carcinoma is most often of a low stage and grade.

As most endometrial polyps are asymptomatic, the diagnosis is not usually established until the uterus is opened following hysterectomy for other reasons. Recently endometrial polyps have been discovered by hysteroscopy and hysterosalpingography during the diagnostic work-up of a woman with a refractory case of abnormal uterine bleeding.

The management of endometrial polyps is removal by curettage or via the hysteroscope. Because of the frequent association of endometrial polyps and other endometrial pathology, it is important to examine histologically both the polyp and associated endometrial lining. Polyps, because of their mobility, are often elusive from the curette. Postcurettage hysteroscopic studies have demonstrated that routine use of a long, narrow polyp forceps at the time of curettage at best results in discovery and removal of only approximately one in four endometrial polyps.

Hematometra

A hematometra is a uterus distended with blood and is secondary to partial or complete obstruction of any portion of the lower genital tract. Obstruction of the isthmus of the uterus, cervix, or vagina may be congenital or acquired. The two most common congenital causes of hematometra are an imperforate hymen and a transverse vaginal septum. Among the leading causes of acquired lower tract stenosis are senile atrophy of the endocervical canal, scarring of the isthmus by synechiae, cervical stenosis associated with surgery, radiation therapy, cryocautery or electrocautery, malignant disease of the endocervical canal, and cervical obstruction by tissue following suction curettage.

The symptoms of hematometra depend on the age of the patient, her menstrual history and the rapidity of the accumulation of blood in the uterine cavity, and the possibility of secondary infection producing pyometra. Thus common symptoms of hematometra include primary or secondary amenorrhea and possibly cyclic lower abdominal pain. Occasionally the obstruction is incomplete, and there is associated spotting of dark brown blood. Hematometra in postmenopausal women may be entirely asymptomatic. On pelvic examination a mildly tender, globular uterus is usually palpated.

The diagnosis of hematometra is generally suspected by the history of amenorrhea and cyclic abdominal pain. The diagnosis is usually confirmed by probing the cervix with a narrow metal dilator with release of dark brownish black blood from the endocervical canal. Often the blood retained inside the uterus becomes secondarily infected and has a foul odor.

Management of hematometra is dependent on operative relief of the lower tract obstruction. Treatment of congenital obstruction is discussed in Chapter 9. Appropriate biopsy specimens of the endocervical canal should be obtained to rule out malignancy when the cause of hematometra is not obvious. Hematometra following operations or cryocautery usually resolves with cervical dilation. Hematometra following a first-trimester abortion is treated by repeat suction aspiration of the products of conception that are blocking the internal os.

Leiomyomas

Leiomyomas, also called *myomas*, are benign tumors of muscle cell origin. These tumors are often referred to by their popular names, *fibroids* or *fibromyomas*, but both terms are semantic misnomers if one is referring to the cell of origin. Most leiomyomas contain varying amounts of fibrous tissue, which is believed to be secondary to degeneration of some of the smooth muscle cells.

Leiomyomas are the most frequent pelvic tumors, with the highest incidence occurring during the fifth decade of a woman's life. Although leiomyomas arise throughout the body in any structure containing smooth muscle, in the pelvis the majority are found in the corpus of the uterus. Occasionally, leiomyomas may be found in the fallopian tube or the round ligament, and approximately 5% of uterine myomas originate from the cervix. Myomas may be single but most often are multiple. Myomas

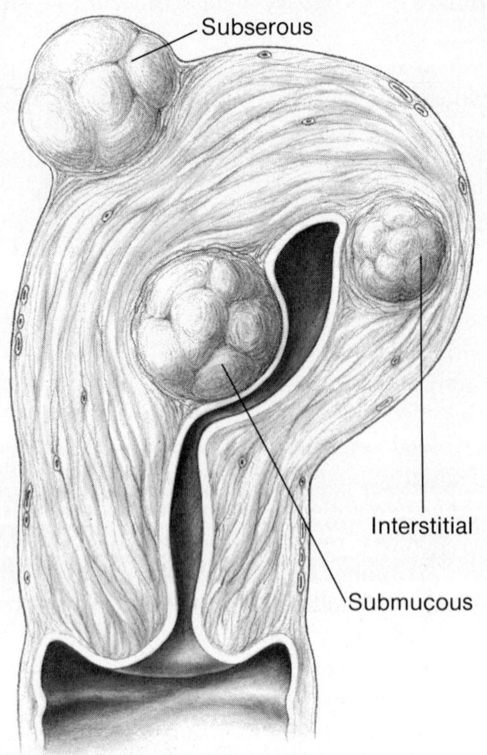

FIGURE 17-18
Drawing of a cut surface of the uterus showing characteristic whorl-like appearance and varying locations of leiomyomas. (From Novak ER, Woodruff JD, eds: Novak's gynecologic and obstetric pathology, 6th ed. Philadelphia, W.B. Saunders Co., 1967, p. 215.)

are discovered in one of four white and one of two black women. They vary greatly in size from microscopic to large, multinodular uterine tumors that may weigh more than 50 pounds and literally fill the patient's abdomen. Myomas are more prone to grow and become symptomatic in nulliparous women. The question as to why some women develop myomas while others do not is unanswered.

All myomas initially develop from the myometrium, beginning as intramural myomas. As they grow, they remain attached to the myometrium with a pedicle of varying width and thickness. Myomas are classed into subgroups by their relative anatomic relationship and position to the layers of the uterus (Fig. 17-18). The three most common types of myomas are intramural (Figs. 17-19 and 17-20), subserous, and submucous, with special nomenclature for broad ligament and parasitic myomas. Continued growth in one direction determines which myomas will be located just below the endometrium, submucosal (Fig. 17-21), while others will be found just beneath the serosa, subserosal. Although only 5% to 10% of myomas become submucosal, they usually are the most troublesome clinically. These submucosal tumors may be associated with abnormal vaginal bleeding or distortion of the uterine cavity that may produce infertility or abortion. Rarely a submucosal myoma enlarges and becomes pedunculated. The uterus will try to expel it, and

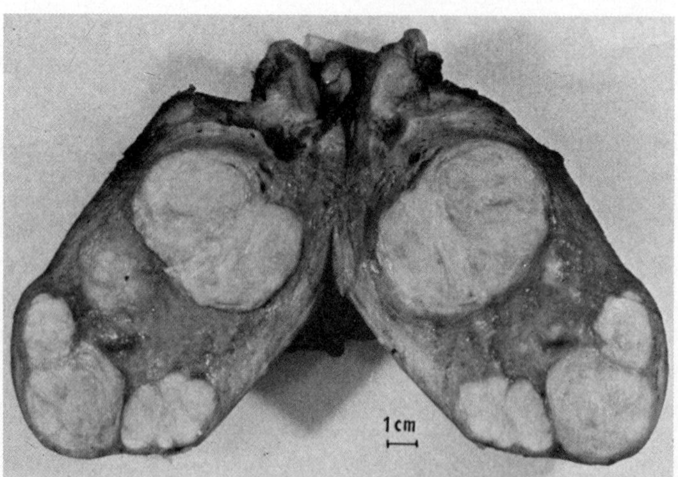

FIGURE 17-19
Intramural leiomyomata. (From Gompel C, Silverberg SG, eds: Pathology in gynecology and obstetrics, 2nd ed. Philadelphia, J.B. Lippincott Co., 1977, p. 186.)

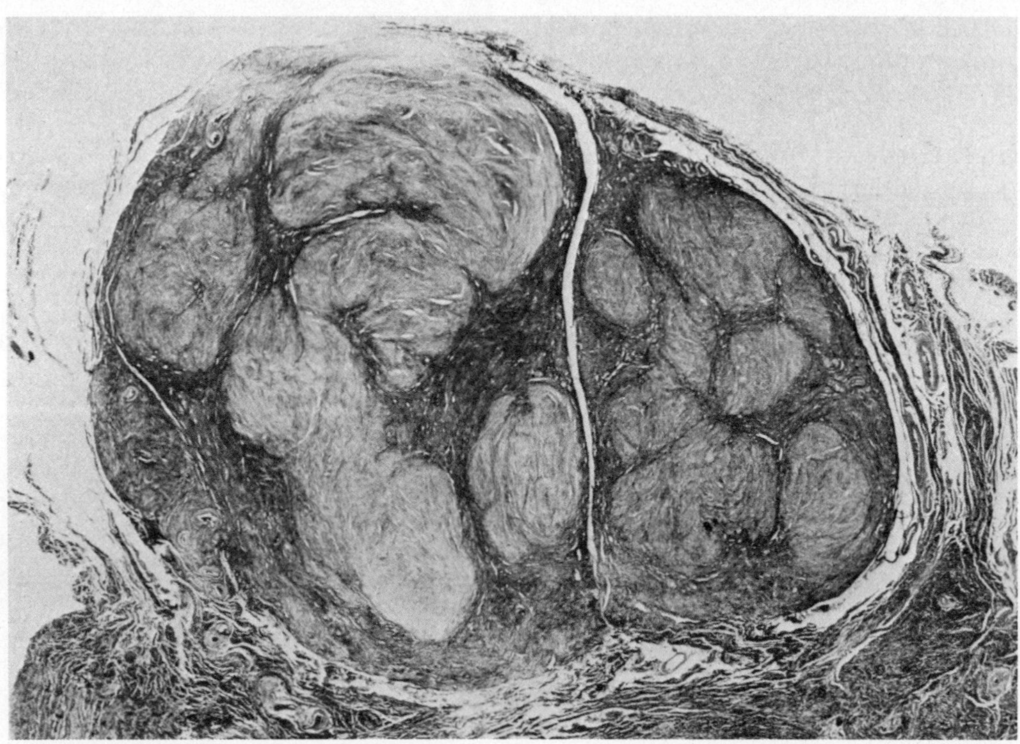

FIGURE 17-20
Intramural leiomyoma. (From Gompel C, Silverberg SG, eds: Pathology in gynecology and obstetrics, 2nd ed. Philadelphia, J.B. Lippincott Co., 1977, p. 187.)

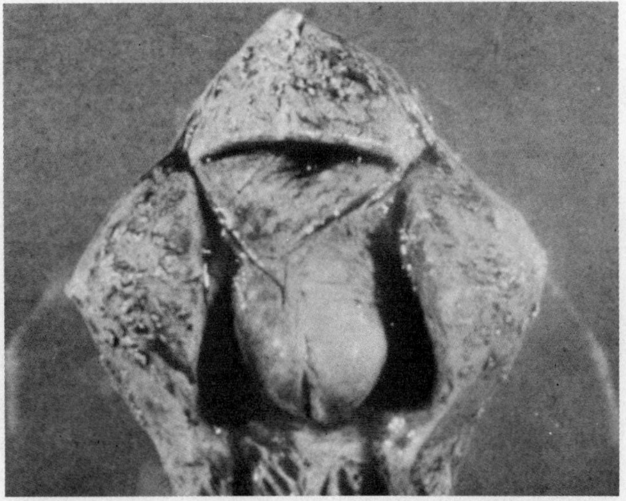

FIGURE 17-21
A large submucosal leiomyoma filling the uterine cavity. (From Demopoulos RI: Benign lesions of the myometrium. In Blaustein A, ed: Pathology of the female genital tract. New York, Springer-Verlag, 1977, p. 301.)

the prolapsed myoma may protrude through the external cervical os. Subserosal myomas give the uterus its knobby contour during pelvic examination.

Further growth of a subserosal myoma may lead to a pedunculated myoma wandering into the peritoneal cavity. This myoma may outgrow its uterine blood supply and obtain a secondary blood supply from another organ, such as the omentum, and become a parasitic myoma. Growth of a myoma in a lateral direction may result in a broad ligament myoma (Fig. 17-22). The clinical significance of broad ligament myomas is that they are difficult to differentiate on pelvic examination from a solid ovarian tumor. Broad ligament myomas often produce a hydroureter as they enlarge.

Small myomas are round, firm, solid tumors. With continued growth the myometrium at the edge of the tumor is compressed and forms a pseudocapsule. Although myomas do not have a true capsule, this pseudocapsule is a valuable surgical plane during a myomectomy.

The etiology of uterine leiomyomas is incompletely understood. It is known that each tumor results from an original single muscle cell. Each uterine myoma is monoclonal in that all cells have identical electrophoretic variance of glucose-6-phosphate dehydrogenase. Pathologists have two different theories as to the cell of origin of this smooth muscle tumor. One hypothesis proposes that the cell of origin is from persistent, small, embryonic cell rests, while the other theory proposes that myomas originate from the smooth muscle of blood vessels.

The stimulus for growth of myomas is similarly unclear. The growth may be partially related to estrogen stimulation. Myomas are rare before menarche, and most myomas diminish in size following menopause or castration, with the reduction of a significant amount of circulating estrogen. Myomas often enlarge during pregnancy and occasionally enlarge secondary to oral contraceptive therapy with relatively high levels of estrogens. Soules and McCarty studied the steroid receptor content of leiomyomas. Estrogen receptors are in higher concentrations in myomas than in the surrounding myometrium. Many women, though, have small myomas that do not grow under the influence of high circulating estrogen levels. Thus the relationship between estrogen and myoma growth is complex. Cramer et al. are studying the growth potential of uterine leiomyomas in vitro and have found heterogeneity in hormonal responsiveness. Other investigators have suggested that growth hormone may also influence the growth of these tumors.

Grossly, a myoma has a lighter color than the normal myometrium. On cut surface the tumor has a glistening, pearl-white appearance, with the smooth muscle arranged in a trabeculated or whorled configuration. Histologically, there is a proliferation of mature smooth muscle

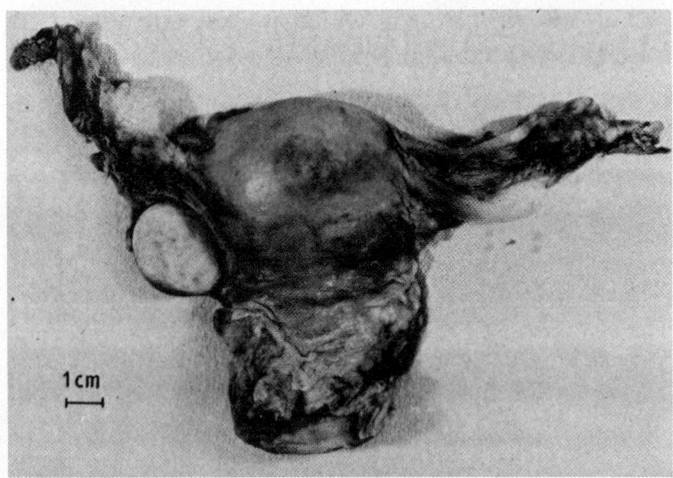

FIGURE 17-22
Leiomyoma of broad ligament. (From Gompel C, Silverberg SG, eds: Pathology in gynecology and obstetrics, 2nd ed. Philadelphia, J.B. Lippincott Co., 1977, p. 187.)

cells. The nonstriated muscle fibers are arranged in interlacing bundles. Between bundles of smooth muscle cells are variable amounts of fibrous connective tissue, especially toward the center of any large tumor (Figs. 17-23 and 17-24). The amount of fibrous tissue is proportional to the extent of atrophy and degeneration that has occurred over time.

The eventual fate of most myomas is determined by their relatively poor vascular supply. This supply is found in one or two major arteries at the base or pedicle of the myoma. The arterial supply of myomas is significantly less than that of a similar sized area of normal myometrium. Thus, with continued growth, degeneration occurs because the tumor outgrows its blood supply. The severity of the discrepancy between the myoma's growth and its blood supply determines the extent of degeneration: hyaline, myxomatous, calcific, cystic, fatty, or red degeneration and necrosis. The mildest form of degeneration of a myoma is hyaline degeneration. Grossly, in this condition the surface of the myoma is homogeneous with loss of the whorled pattern. Histologically with hyaline degeneration, cellular detail is lost as the smooth muscle cells are replaced by fibrous connective tissue.

The most acute form of degeneration is red or carneous infarction. A rapidly growing myoma, most commonly during the second trimester of pregnancy, may acutely outgrow its blood supply. This acute muscular infarction causes severe pain and localized peritoneal irritation. During pregnancy this complication should be treated medically, for attempts at operative removal result in profuse blood loss. If the patient is not pregnant, acute degeneration is not a contraindication to myomectomy. Obviously the more advanced forms of degenerating myomas may become secondarily infected, especially when large necrotic areas exist. The histologic changes of degeneration are found more commonly in larger myomas. However, two thirds of all myomas show some degree of degeneration, with the three most common types being hyaline degeneration (65%), myxomatous degeneration (15%), and calcific degeneration (10%).

The literature emphasizes that the incidence

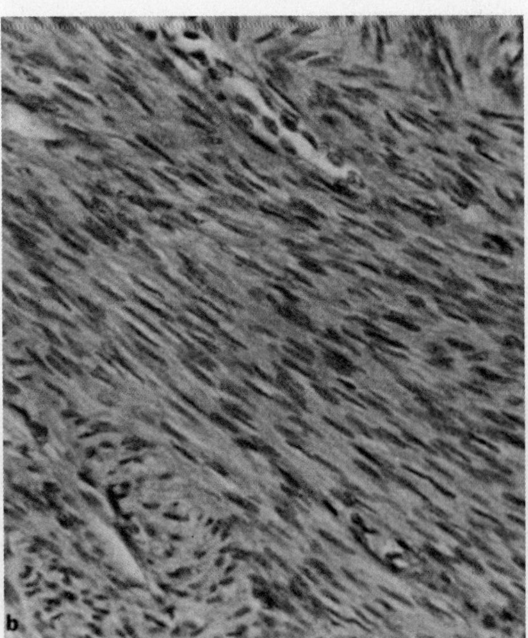

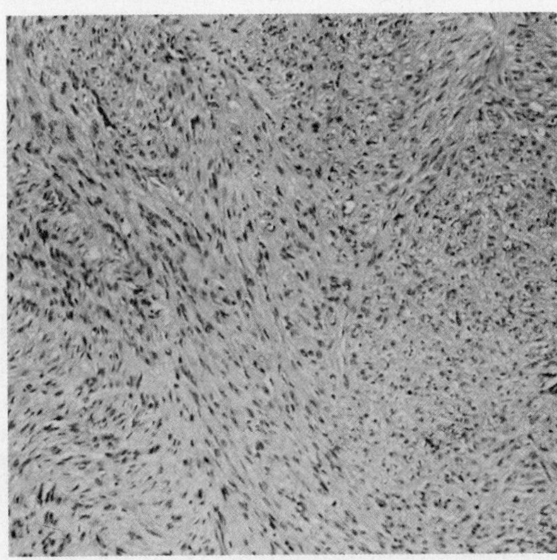

FIGURE 17-23
Leiomyoma: histologic section. (From Gompel C, Silverberg SG, eds: Pathology in gynecology and obstetrics, 2nd ed. Philadelphia, J.B. Lippincott Co., 1977, p. 187.)

FIGURE 17-24
Leiomyoma showing interlacing bundles of smooth muscles with spindle nuclei without degeneration. (From Demopoulos RI: Benign lesions of the myometrium. In Blaustein A, ed: Pathology of the female genital tract. New York, Springer-Verlag, 1977, p. 302.)

of malignant degeneration is estimated to be between 0.3% and 0.7%. However, myomas are so common and leiomyosarcoma is so rare that these figures are overestimates. The term *malignant degeneration* is ambiguous. It is unknown as to whether myomas degenerate into sarcomas or if sarcomas arise spontaneously in myomatous uteri.

The symptoms related to myomas are primarily pressure from an enlarging pelvic mass, pain including dysmenorrhea, abnormal uterine bleeding, infertility, and pregnancy complications, including abortion, premature labor, and dystocia. The severity of symptoms is often directly related to the number, location, and size of the myomas. However, the majority of women with uterine myomas are asymptomatic.

One of three women with myomas experiences pelvic pain. Acquired dysmenorrhea is the most frequent complaint, with a study by Iosif and Akerlund from Sweden documenting an associated increase in myometrial activity. Various forms of vascular compromise, either acute degeneration or torsion of the pedicle, produce severe pelvic pain. Milder pelvic discomfort is described as pelvic heaviness or a dull aching sensation that may be secondary to edematous swelling in the myoma.

An enlarged myoma or myomas often produce pressure symptoms similar to those of an enlarging pregnant uterus. Sometimes a woman will notice that her abdominal girth is increasing without appreciable change in weight. Alternately, an anterior myoma pressing on the bladder may produce urinary frequency and urgency. In general, urinary symptoms are more common than rectal symptoms. Bilateral hydroureter from partial obstruction is a frequent finding with larger masses. Abnormal bleeding is experienced by 30% of women with myomas. The most common symptom is menorrhagia, but intermenstrual spotting and disruption of a normal pattern are other frequent complaints. The exact cause-and-effect relationship between myomas and abnormal bleeding is difficult to determine and is poorly understood. The explanation is straightforward when there are areas of ulceration over submucous myomas. However, ulceration is a clinical rarity. The most popular theory is that myomas result in an abnormal venous pattern with stasis and a change in venous drainage. The

theory that the amount of menorrhagia is directly related to an increase of endometrial surface area has been recently disproven. One of three women with abnormal bleeding and myomas also has endometrial hyperplasia, which may be the cause of the symptom and related to a submucous myoma.

Occasionally myomas are the only identifiable abnormality after a detailed infertility investigation. Myomectomy is indicated in longstanding infertility and recurrent abortion after all other potential factors have been investigated and treated. Successful term pregnancy rates of 40% to 50% have been reported following a myomectomy. The success of an operation is most dependent on the age of the patient, the size of the myomas, and most importantly, the number of compounding factors that affect the couple's fertility.

Growth of a uterine myoma after menopause is a disturbing symptom. This is the classic symptom of a leiomyosarcoma, and thus the patient should have a total abdominal hysterectomy so that the tissue may be examined histologically.

Rarely, a secondary polycythemia is noted in women with uterine myomas. The mechanism is unclear; however, the polycythemia diminishes following removal of the uterus.

The diagnosis of uterine myomas is usually confirmed by palpating an enlarged, firm irregular uterus during pelvic examination. The three conditions that commonly enter into the differential diagnosis include pregnancy, adenomyosis, and an ovarian neoplasm. The discrimination between large ovarian tumors and myomatous uteri may be difficult. Extension of myomas laterally may make palpation of normal ovaries impossible during the pelvic examination. Degeneration of myomas may cause a change of consistency from firm to soft, and some may become cystic. Often, if pregnancy has been excluded, placing a metal sound in the uterine cavity will help to establish the clinical diagnosis. The uterine cavity is generally enlarged and often irregular with myomas, while an ovarian tumor is usually associated with a normal sized uterus. The mobility of the pelvic mass and whether the mass moves independently or as part of the uterus may be helpful diagnostically. Obviously, submucosal myomas may be diagnosed by direct observation during hysteroscopy or indirectly as a filling defect on hysterosalpingography.

Although the majority of uterine myomas may be diagnosed by pelvic examination, difficult cases will benefit from ultrasound examination or a search for concentric calcifications on an abdominal x-ray film. There are several recent reports of computed tomography and magnetic resonant imaging studies of uterine myomas. Until the latter technique can distinguish between benign and malignant myomas, these radiologic imaging techniques will rarely be ordered in routine clinical management of myomas.

The management of a woman with small asymptomatic myomas is judicious observation. When the tumor is first discovered, it is appropriate to perform a pelvic examination at 4- to 6-month intervals to determine the rate of growth. The majority of women will not need an operation, especially those women in the perimenopausal period, where the condition usually improves with diminishing levels of circulating estrogens.

Women with symptomatic leiomyomas should be investigated thoroughly for concurrent problems such as endometrial hyperplasia. If their symptoms do not improve with conservative management, operative therapy should be considered. The choice between a myomectomy and hysterectomy is usually determined by the patient's age, parity, and most importantly, future reproductive plans.

Classic indications for a myomectomy include a rapidly expanding pelvic mass, persistent abnormal bleeding, pain or pressure, previous repetitive abortion, long-standing infertility, or enlargement of an asymptomatic myoma to more than 8 cm in a woman who has not completed childbearing. Contraindications to a myomectomy include pregnancy, advanced adnexal disease, malignancy, and the situation in which enucleation of the myoma would result in a severe reduction of endometrial surface so that the uterus would not be functional. The choice between the two operations is not always an easy one. To quote Richard TeLinde, "All indications and contraindications in medicine are relative, a fact that is especially true when one considers hysterectomy versus myomectomy."

Within 20 years of the myomectomy procedure one in four women subsequently has a hysterectomy performed, the majority for recurrent leiomyomas. With the recent emphasis on endoscopic surgery, women with abnormal bleeding may have their submucous myomas resected via the cervical canal. Neuwirth has been a pioneer in this new technique. In a preliminary study, 17 of 28 women returned to normal menses without difficulty.

The indications for hysterectomy for myomas are similar to indications for myomectomy, with a few additions. Many gynecologists selectively perform a hysterectomy for asymptomatic myomas when the uterus has reached the size of a 12- to 14-week gestation. The hypothesis is that most myomas of this size will eventually produce symptoms. Another previously mentioned indication for hysterectomy is growth of a myoma after the menopause. Prolapse of a myoma through the cervix is occasionally treated by hysterectomy. Sometimes the myoma may be removed vaginally and the base ligated. Finally, the lateral growth of myomas may make it impossible to evaluate the adnexa during pelvic examination.

It is possible to treat leiomyomas medically by reducing the circulating level of estrogen. Medroxyprogesterone (depo-Provera), danazol, and GnRH analogues have undergone preliminary clinical trials. Most series are small and report reduction of tumor size by as much as 50% to 75% in approximately one of two patients given the drugs for usually 4 to 6 months. Myomas often begin to regrow after the therapeutic drug is discontinued; however, this therapy is useful perimenopausally to avoid hysterectomy.

Two associated but rare diseases should be noted: intravenous leiomyomatosis and leiomyomatosis peritonealis disseminata. Intravenous leiomyomatosis is a rare condition in which benign smooth muscle fibers invade and slowly grow into the venous channels of the pelvis. The tumor grows by direct extension and grossly appears like a "spaghetti" tumor. Only 25% of tumors extend beyond the broad ligament, yet case reports exist of tumor growth into the vena cava and right heart.

Leiomyomatosis peritonealis disseminata (LPD) is a benign disease with multiple small nodules over the surface of the pelvis and abdominal peritoneum. Grossly, LPD mimics disseminated carcinoma. However, histologic examination demonstrates benign-appearing myomas. This disorder is usually associated with a recent pregnancy.

OVIDUCT

Leiomyomas

Both benign and malignant tumors of the oviduct are uncommon compared to other gynecologic neoplasms. Although these tumors are underreported, fewer than 100 women with myomas or leiomyomas of the oviduct are described in the literature. Tubal leiomyomas may be single or multiple and usually are discovered in the interstitial portion of the tubes. They usually co-exist with the more common uterine leiomyomas.

Leiomyomas of the tube present as smooth, firm, mobile, usually nontender masses that may be palpated during the bimanual examination. Similar to uterine myomas, they may be subserosal, interstitial, or submucosal. During laparoscopy the myomas appear as a spherical mass that protrudes from beneath the peritoneal surface. They vary from a few millimeters to 15 cm in diameter. Histologically they are identical to uterine leiomyomas.

The majority of the myomas of the oviduct are asymptomatic. Rarely, they may undergo acute degeneration or be associated with unilateral tubal obstruction or torsion. Treatment of a symptomatic tubal leiomyoma is excision.

Another benign tumor of the oviduct is the angiomyoma or adenomatoid tumor. They are small, gray-white, circumscribed nodules, 1 to 2 cm in diameter. These benign tumors are found below the serosa of the fundus of the uterus and the broad ligament. Microscopically they are composed of small tubules lined by a low cuboidal or flat epithelium. Histologic studies have established that the thin-walled channels that comprise these tumors are of mesothelial origin. These tumors do not become malignant; however, they may be mistaken for a low-grade neoplasm when initially viewed during a frozen section evaluation.

Paratubal Cysts

Paratubal cysts are frequently incidental discoveries during gynecologic operations for

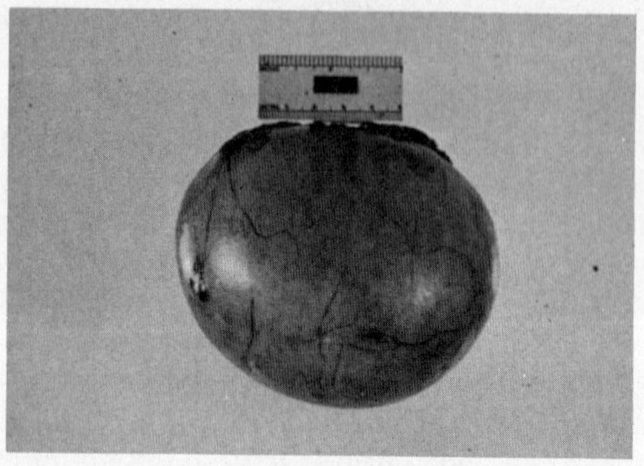

FIGURE 17-25
Parovarian cyst, externally smooth and shiny with a thin, transparent wall. The content of the cyst is a straw-colored, clear fluid. (From Janovski NA, ed: Color atlas of gross gynecologic and obstetric pathology. New York, McGraw-Hill Book Co., 1969, p. 143.)

other abnormalities. They are often multiple and may vary from 0.5 cm to more than 20 cm in diameter (Fig. 17-25). The majority of cysts are asymptomatic and slow growing and are discovered during the third and fourth decade of life. When paratubal cysts are pedunculated and near the fimbrial end of the oviduct, they are called *hydatid cysts of Morgagni* (Fig. 17-26). Cysts near the oviduct may be of mesonephric, mesothelial, or paramesonephric origin. The histogenesis of the majority of paratubal cysts had been believed to be from the mesonephric duct, with the cysts arising from the main duct or accessory tubules. These latter cysts often develop between the leaves of the broad ligament in the mesosalpinx, with the ovary being separate. However, a recent histologic study of 79 paratubal cysts by Samaha and Woodruff has documented that 60 of their series were of tubal origin. Thus the majority of grossly identified "paratubal cysts" are in reality accessory lumina of the fallopian tubes. The remaining 19 cysts in Samaha and Woodruff's series were of mesothelial origin. Paratubal cysts are thin walled and smooth and contain clear fluid. Often there are multiple small cysts. Occasionally there is a papillomatous proliferation on the internal wall of these cysts. When paratubal cysts are symptomatic, they generally produce a dull pain. Often during pelvic examination it is difficult to distin-

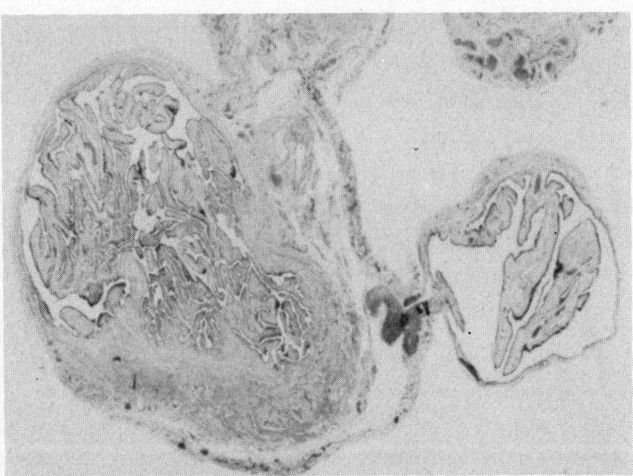

FIGURE 17-26
Normal tube to right with pedunculated hydatid of Morgagni to right (accessory lumen with papillary fronds, really mucosal folds of tube). (From Samaha M, Woodruff JD: Obstet Gynecol 65:692, 1985. Reprinted with permission from The American College of Obstetricians and Gynecologists.)

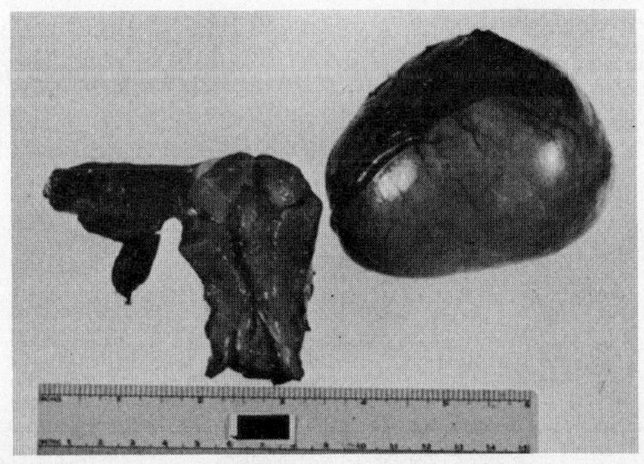

FIGURE 17-27
Parovarian cyst. The cyst occupies the entire mesosalpinx. The oviduct is characteristically stretched over the upper surface of the cyst. It is unilocular. (From Janovski NA, ed: Color atlas of gross gynecologic and obstetric pathology. New York, McGraw-Hill Book Co., 1969, p. 143.)

guish a paratubal cyst from an ovarian mass. At operation the oviduct is often found stretched over a large paratubal cyst (Fig. 17-27). The oviduct should not be removed in these cases, as it will return to normal size after the paratubal cyst is excised.

Paratubal cysts may grow rapidly during pregnancy, and most of the cases of torsion of

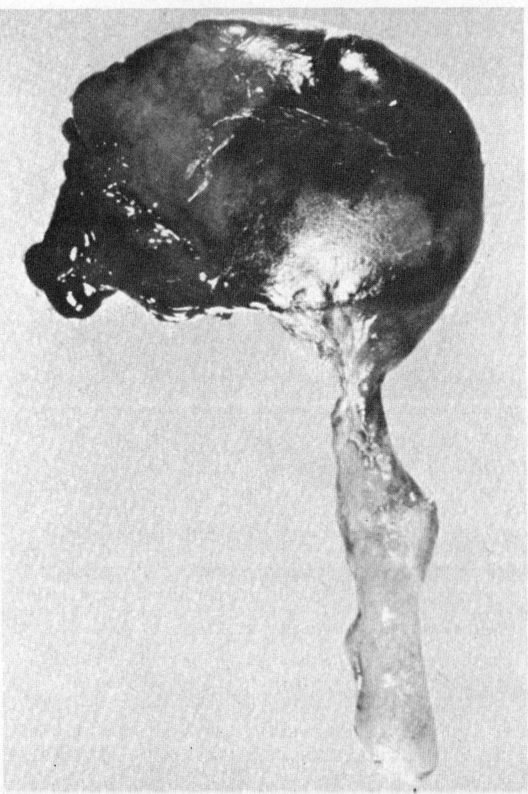

FIGURE 17-28
The right fallopian tube showing hemorrhage, edema, and infarction secondary to torsion. (From Chambers JT, Thiagarajah S, Kitchin JD: Obstet Gynecol 54:488, 1979. Reprinted with permission from The American College of Obstetricians and Gynecologists.)

these cysts have been reported during pregnancy or the puerperium. Treatment is simple excision.

Torsion

Acute torsion of the oviduct is a rare event; however, it has been reported with both normal and pathologic fallopian tubes. Pregnancy predisposes to this problem. Tubal torsion usually accompanies torsion of the ovary, as they have a common vascular pedicle. (See following discussion.) The right tube is involved more frequently than the left (Fig. 17-28). The degree of tubal torsion varies from less than one turn to four complete rotations.

Youssef et al. have subdivided the pathophysiology and etiology of tubal torsion into intrinsic and extrinsic causes. Prominent intrinsic causes include congenital abnormalities such as increased tortuosity due to excessive length of the tube and pathologic processes such as hydrosalpinx, hematosalpinx, tubal neoplasms, and previous operation, especially tubal ligation. Torsion of the fallopian tube after tubal ligation is usually of the distal end. Extrinsic causes of tubal torsion are ovarian and peritubal tumors, adhesions, trauma, and pregnancy.

The most important symptom of tubal torsion is acute lower abdominal and pelvic pain. The onset of this pain may be gradual or sudden, and the pain is usually located in the iliac fossa with radiation to the thigh and flank. The duration of pain is generally less than 48 hours, and it is associated with nausea and vomiting in two thirds of the cases. Unless there is associated torsion of the ovary, a specific mass is usually not palpable on pelvic examination.

The preoperative diagnosis of tubal torsion is made in less than 20% of reported cases. Because of the severity of the pain a wide differential diagnosis of abdominal and pelvic pathology must be considered. The differential diagnosis includes acute appendicitis, ectopic pregnancy, pelvic inflammatory disease, and rupture or torsion of an ovarian cyst.

Exploratory operation determines the extent of hypoxia and the choice of operative techniques. With tubal torsion, usually the tubes are gangrenous and must be excised. The twisted tube is usually filled with a bloody serous fluid. Occasionally, with a minor degree of torsion, it is possible to restore normal circulation to the tube and salvage it. The tube is usually sutured into a secure position to prevent recurrence.

OVARY

Functional Cysts

Follicular Cysts

Follicular cysts are by far the most frequent cystic structures in normal ovaries. The cysts are frequently multiple and may vary from a few millimeters to 8 cm in diameter (Fig. 17-29). The average size of a follicular cyst is 2 cm. These cysts are found most commonly in young, menstruating women. They are not neoplastic and are incapable of autonomous growth. Follicular cysts arise from a temporary pathologic variation of a normal physiologic process. Clinically, they may present with the signs and symptoms of ovarian enlargement and therefore must be differentiated from a true ovarian neoplasm.

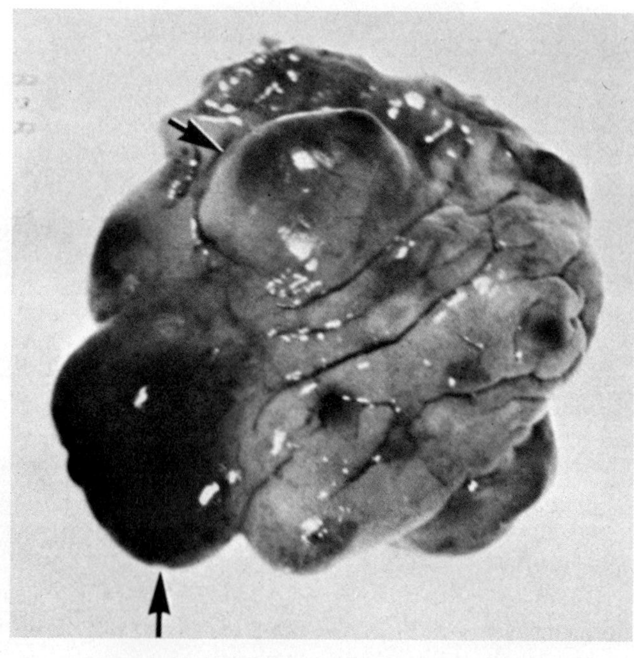

FIGURE 17-29
Multiple small follicular cysts *(arrows)* bulging just beneath the cortex of the ovary. (From Blaustein A: Nonneoplastic cysts of the ovary. In Blaustein A, ed: Pathology of the female genital tract. New York, Springer-Verlag, 1977, p. 395.)

Follicular cysts are translucent and thin walled and are filled with a watery, clear to straw-colored fluid. If a small opening in the capsule of the cyst suddenly develops, the cyst fluid will squirt out under pressure. These cysts are situated in the ovarian cortex, and sometimes they appear as translucent domes on the surface of the ovary. Histologically, the lining of the cyst is usually composed of a closely packed layer of round plump granulosa cells with the spindle-shaped cells of the theca interna deeper in the stroma (Fig. 17-30). In many cysts the lining of granulosa cells is difficult to distinguish, having undergone pressure atrophy. All that remains is a hyalinized connective tissue lining (Fig. 17-31).

The temporary disturbance in follicular function that produces the clinical picture of a follicular cyst is poorly understood. Follicular cysts may result from either the dominant mature follicle's failing to rupture (persistent follicle) or an immature follicle's failing to undergo the normal process of atresia. In the latter circumstance the incompletely developed follicle fails to reabsorb follicular fluid. Some follicular cysts lose their ability to produce estrogen, while in others the granulosa cells remain productive with prolonged secretion of estrogens. Occasionally, follicular cysts are better termed *follicular hematomas,* as blood from the vascular theca zone fills the cavity of the cyst.

The majority of follicular cysts are asymptomatic and are discovered only during a routine pelvic examination. Because of their thin walls, these cysts are often ruptured during examination. The patient experiences a transient tenderness or no pain whatsoever. Only rarely is there significant intraperitoneal bleeding associated with the rupture of a follicular cyst. Occasionally menstrual irregularities and abnormal uterine bleeding may be associated with follicular cysts, which produce prolonged elevated estrogen levels. The syndrome associated with such follicular cysts is of a regular cycle with a prolonged intermenstrual interval, followed by episodes of menorrhagia. Some women with larger follicular cysts notice a vague, dull sensation or a heaviness in the pelvis.

The initial management of a suspected follicular cyst is conservative observation. The majority of follicular cysts disappear spontaneously by either reabsorption of the cyst fluid or silent rupture within 4 to 8 weeks of initial diagnosis. However, a persistent ovarian mass necessitates operative intervention to differentiate a physiologic cyst from a true neoplasm of the ovary. There is no way to make the differentiation on the basis of signs, symptoms, or the initial growth pattern during early development of either process. Spanos suggested prescribing oral contraceptives for young women with adnexal masses for 4 to 6 weeks. This therapy removes any influence that pituitary

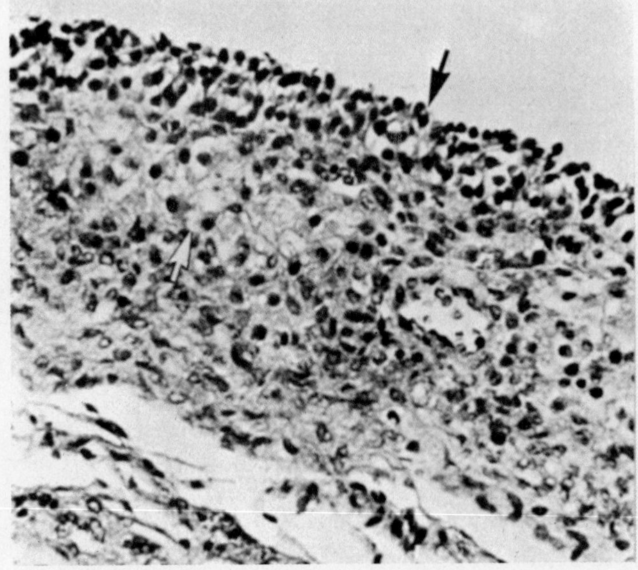

FIGURE 17-30
Lining of a follicular cyst. Granulosa layer *(dark arrow)* is composed of a multicellular layer. Theca interna *(light arrow)* lies immediately beneath the granulosa cells. (From Blaustein A: Nonneoplastic cysts of the ovary. In Blaustein A, ed: Pathology of the female genital tract. New York, Springer-Verlag, 1977, p. 395.)

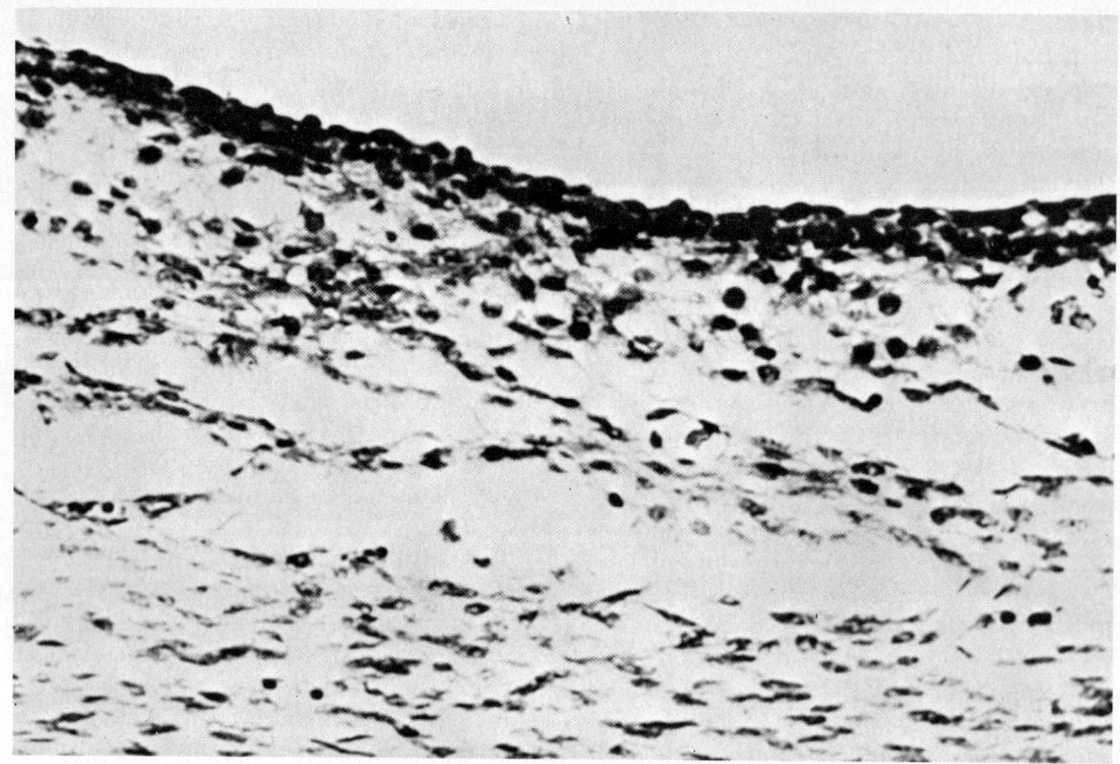

FIGURE 17-31
Lining of a follicular cyst. Compression by the cyst content distorts the granulosa layer. (From Blaustein A: Nonneoplastic cysts of the ovary. In Blaustein A, ed: Pathology of the female genital tract. New York, Springer-Verlag, 1977, p. 395.)

gonadotrophins may have on the persistence of the ovarian cyst. It also allows for several weeks of observation. In Spanos's series, 80% of cystic masses 4 to 6 cm in size disappeared during the time the patient was taking oral contraceptives.

Indications for immediate operation include the presence of any adnexal mass after the menopause or before puberty, a solid adnexal mass at any age, a cystic mass larger than 8 cm, or a cystic mass from 5 to 8 cm that has been observed for longer than 8 weeks in a menstruating woman. Operative management is cystectomy, not oophorectomy.

Corpus Luteum Cysts

Corpus luteum cysts are less common than follicular cysts, but clinically they are more important. This discussion collectively groups corpus luteum cysts and persistently functioning mature corpora lutea (Fig. 17-32). Pathologists

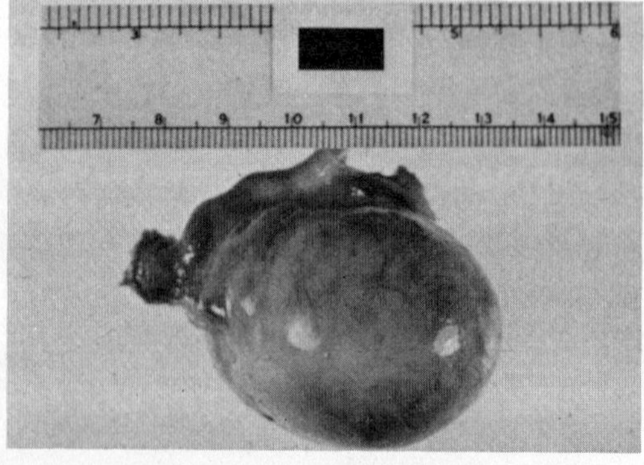

FIGURE 17-32
Corpus luteum cyst, 3 to 4 cm in diameter, externally smooth. (From Janovski NA, ed: Color atlas of gross gynecologic and obstetric pathology. New York, McGraw-Hill Book Co., 1969, p. 155.)

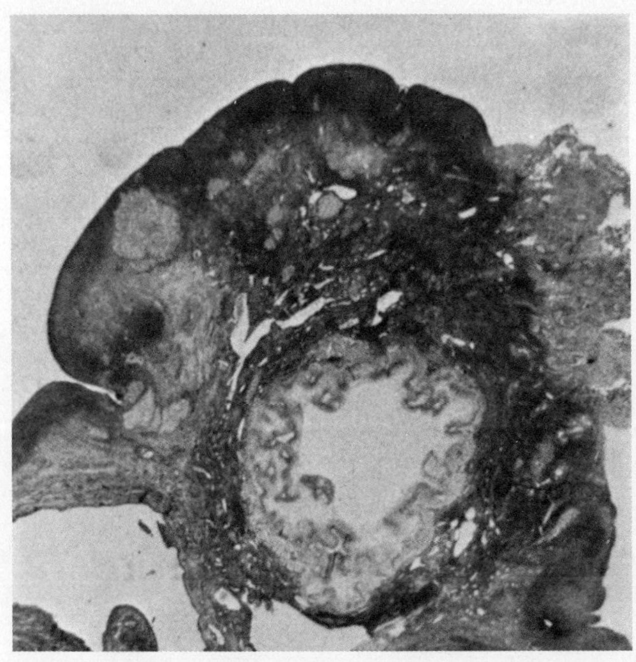

FIGURE 17-33
Corpus albicans cyst. The lining of the cyst is composed of hyalinized connective tissue. (From Blaustein A: Nonneoplastic cysts of the ovary. In Blaustein A, ed: Pathology of the female genital tract. New York, Springer-Verlag, 1977, p. 396.)

are sometimes able to make a distinction between a hemorrhagic cystic corpus luteum and a corpus luteum cyst, but at other times this difference cannot be established. All corpora lutea are cystic with gradual reabsorption of a limited amount of hemorrhage, which may form a cavity. Clinically, corpora lutea are not termed *corpus luteum cysts* unless they are a minimum of 3 cm in diameter. Corpus luteum cysts may be associated with either normal endocrine function or prolonged secretion of progesterone.

Corpora lutea develop from mature graafian follicles. Intrafollicular bleeding does not occur during ovulation. However, 2 to 4 days later, during the stage of vascularization, thin-walled capillaries invade the granulosa cells from the theca interna. Spontaneous but limited bleeding fills the central cavity of the maturing corpus luteum with blood. Subsequently this blood is absorbed, forming a small cystic space. When the hemorrhage is excessive, the cystic space enlarges. If the hemorrhage into the central cavity is brisk, intracystic pressure increases and rupture of the corpus luteum is a possibility. If rupture does not occur, the size of the resulting corpus luteum cyst will vary between 3 and 10 cm. If a cystic central cavity persists, blood is replaced by clear fluid, and

the result is a hormonally inactive corpus albicans cyst (Fig. 17-33). A corpus luteum of pregnancy is normally 3 to 5 cm in diameter with a central cystic structure, occupying at least 50% of the ovarian mass.

Most corpus luteum cysts are small, the average diameter being 4 cm. Grossly, they have a smooth surface and, depending on whether the cyst represents acute or chronic hemorrhage, are purplish red to brown (Fig. 17-34). When a corpus luteum is cut, the lining is yellowish orange, and the center contains an organizing blood clot. Both the granulosa and the theca cells undergo luteinization. In chronic corpus luteum cysts the wall becomes graywhite and the polygonal luteinized cells usually undergo pressure atrophy. Hallatt et al. reviewed 173 ruptured corpora lutea with hemoperitoneum. In their institution the frequency of serious bleeding from a corpus luteum cyst compared to ectopic pregnancy was one in four.

Corpus luteum cysts vary from being asymptomatic masses to those causing catastrophic and massive intraperitoneal bleeding associated with rupture. Many corpus luteum cysts produce dull, unilateral, lower abdominal and pelvic pain. The enlarged ovary is moderately tender on pelvic examination. Depending on the amount of progesterone secretion associ-

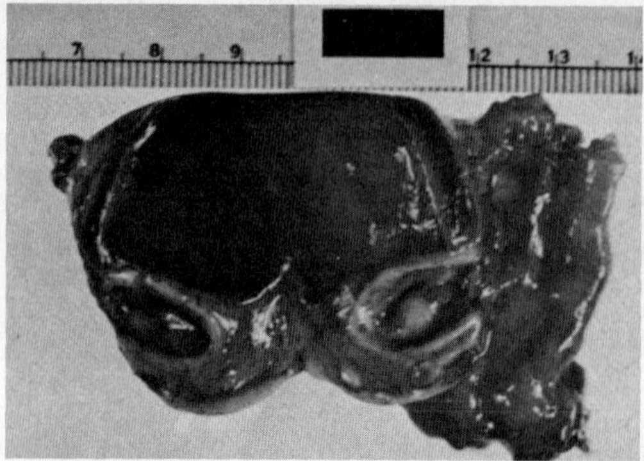

FIGURE 17-34
Corpus luteum cyst with a thickened cyst wall, and definite lutein cell lining recognized by its color. The cyst is filled with hemorrhagic gelatinous material. (From Janovski NA, ed: Color atlas of gross gynecologic and obstetric pathology. New York, McGraw-Hill Book Co., 1969, p. 157.)

ated with cysts, the menstrual bleeding may be normal or delayed several days to weeks with subsequent menorrhagia. Halban in 1915 described a syndrome of a persistently functioning corpus luteum cyst that has clinical features similar to an unruptured ectopic pregnancy. Halban's classic triad was a delay in a normal period followed by spotting, unilateral pelvic pain, and a small, tender adnexal mass.

Corpus luteum cysts may cause intraperitoneal bleeding. The amount of bleeding varies from slight to significant hemorrhage, necessitating blood transfusion. Internal bleeding often follows coitus, exercise, trauma, or a pelvic examination. However, episodes of bleeding usually do not recur, which differs from an ectopic pregnancy. Women undergoing chronic warfarin (Coumadin) therapy are especially prone to develop ovarian hemorrhage from a corpus luteum cyst. Bleeding occurs usually between days 20 to 26 of their cycle, and these women have a 31% chance for subsequent hemorrhage from a recurrent corpus luteum cyst. Oral contraceptives are commonly used to suppress ovulation and avoid recurrent hemorrhage.

Hallatt et al. reported that sudden, severe, lower abdominal pain was a prominent symptom in all patients with hemoperitoneum caused by a ruptured corpus luteum cyst (Table

TABLE 17-2

Symptoms of 173 Women with Ruptured Corpus Luteum

	No.	Percent
Location		
Right ovary	114	66
Left ovary	56	32
Unknown	3	2
Abdominal pain	173	100
Onset with intercourse	29	17
Right ovary	21	72
Left ovary	8	28
Duration		
Less than 24 hours	94	54
1 to 7 days	40	23
Over 7 days	14	8
Unknown	25	15
Nausea or vomiting or diarrhea	60	35

From Hallatt JG, Steele CH, Snyder M: Ruptured corpus luteum with hemoperitoneum: A study of 173 surgical cases. Am J Obstet Gynecol 149:6, 1984.

TABLE 17-3

Menstrual History in 173 Women with Ruptured Corpus Luteum

	No.	No.
Last menstrual period to operation		
Under 14 days		5
14 to 31 days (pregnant = 2)		77
31 to 60 days (pregnant = 15)		56
Over 60 days (pregnant = 10)		18
No menstrual period		14
Hysterectomy	5	
Amenorrhea after oral contraceptives	5	
Secondary amenorrhea	2	
Menarche	1	
Menopause	1	
History of irregular menses		14
Unknown		3

From Hallatt JG, Steele CH, Snyder M: Ruptured corpus luteum with hemoperitoneum: A study of 173 surgical cases. Am J Obstet Gynecol 149:6, 1984.

17-2). One of three women also noted unilateral cramping and lower abdominal pain for 1 to 2 weeks before overt rupture. The right ovary was the source of hemorrhage in 66% of their series. Tang et al. have also reported a right-sided predominance in the incidence of hemorrhage from corpus luteum cysts. They postulated that the difference is related to a higher intraluminal pressure on the right side because of the differences in ovarian vein architecture. Most ruptures occur between days 20 and 26 of the cycle, although in the series of Hallatt et al. 28% of the women had a delay in menses not explained by pregnancy or history (Table 17-3).

The differential diagnosis of a woman with acute pain and suspected ruptured corpus luteum cyst includes ectopic pregnancy, ruptured endometrioma, and adnexal torsion. A sensitive quantitative serum assay for human chorionic gonadotrophin (HCG) may help to differentiate a bleeding corpus luteum from ectopic pregnancy (Chapter 16). Pelvic ultrasound is occasionally useful in establishing a preoperative diagnosis. Culdocentesis is helpful in establishing the rapidity and severity of the hemorrhage. If the hematocrit of the fluid obtained from the posterior cul-de-sac is greater than 15%, exploratory operation is necessary. Cystectomy is the operative treatment of choice, with preservation of the remaining portion of the ovary. However, laparoscopy may be used to establish the differential diagnosis. Unruptured corpus luteum cysts may be followed conservatively.

Theca Lutein Cysts

Theca lutein cysts are by far the least common of the three types of physiologic ovarian cysts (Fig. 17-35). Unlike corpus luteum cysts they are almost always bilateral and asymptomatic. These cysts arise from either prolonged or excessive stimulation of the ovaries by endogenous or exogenous gonadotrophins or increased ovarian sensitivity to gonadotrophins. Approximately 50% of molar pregnancies and 10% of choriocarcinomas have associated bilateral theca lutein cysts (Chapter 29). In these patients the HCG from the trophoblast produces luteinization of the cells in immature, mature, and atretic follicles. The cysts are also discovered in the latter months of pregnancies with conditions that produce a large placenta, such as twins, diabetes, and Rh sensitization. It is not uncommon to iatrogenically produce theca lutein cysts in women receiving drugs to induce ovulation. Theca lutein cysts are occasionally discovered in association with normal pregnancy and in newborn infants sec-

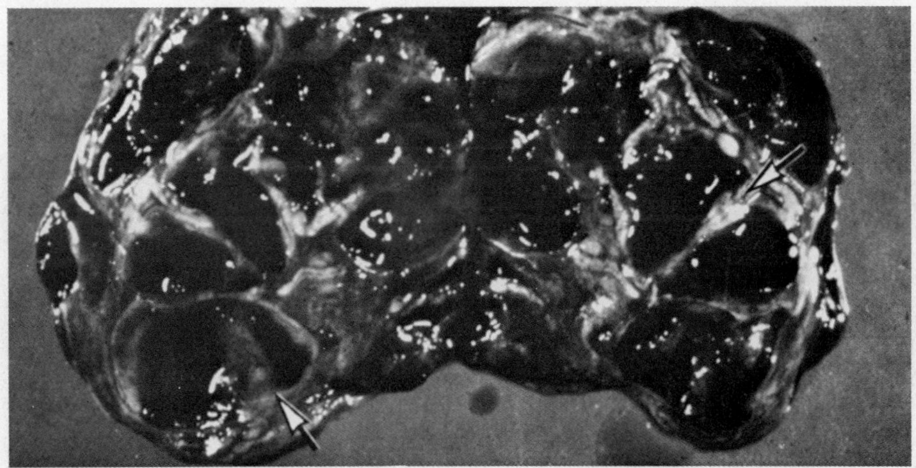

FIGURE 17-35
Theca lutein cyst. Conglomerate of nodular masses *(arrows)*. The cut surface is hemorrhagic. (From Blaustein A: Nonneoplastic cysts of the ovary. In Blaustein A, ed: Pathology of the female genital tract. New York, Springer-Verlag, 1977, p. 397.)

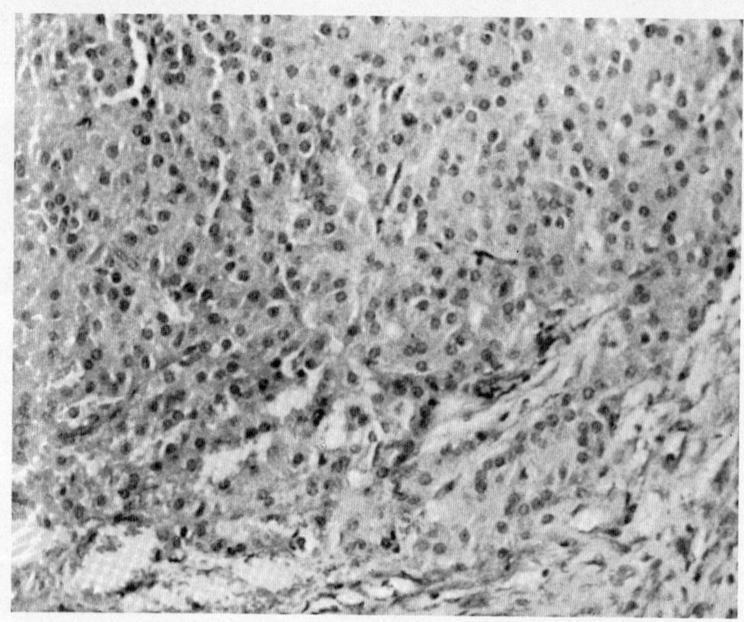

FIGURE 17-36
Luteoma. Solid mass of uniform polygonal "luteinized" cells with spherical nuclei.
H&E; ×220. (From Dische FE, Ritchie JM: J Pathol 100:Plate XXXVI, 1970.)

ondary to transplacental effects of maternal gonadotrophins.

Grossly the total ovarian size may be voluminous, 20 to 30 cm in diameter, with multiple theca lutein cysts. This condition of bilateral ovarian enlargement of gray to bluish tinged cysts is also called *hyperreactio luteinalis*. The bilateral enlargement is secondary to hundreds of thin-walled locules or cysts producing a honeycombed appearance. The small cysts contain a clear to straw-colored fluid. Histologically the lining of the cyst is composed of luteinized theca lutein cells (paralutein cells), believed to originate from ovarian connective tissue. Occasionally there is also luteinization of granulosa cells. These voluminous and congested ovaries are slow growing. Generally only the larger cysts produce vague symptoms, such as a sense of pressure in the pelvis. Ascites and increasing abdominal girth have been reported with hyperstimulation from exogenous gonadotrophins. Rarely, associated adnexal torsion may occur.

The presence of theca lutein cysts is established by palpation and often confirmed by ultrasound examination. Treatment is conservative because these cysts gradually regress. If these cysts are discovered incidentally at cesar-

ean delivery, they should be handled delicately. No attempt should be made to drain or puncture the multiple cysts because of the possibility of hemorrhage. Bleeding is difficult to control in these cases because of the thin walls that comprise the cysts.

A condition related to theca lutein cysts is the luteoma of pregnancy. The condition is rare and not a true neoplasm, but rather a specific, benign, hyperplastic reaction of ovarian theca lutein cells (Fig. 17-36). These nodules do not arise from the corpus luteum of pregnancy. Fifty percent of luteomas are multiple, and approximately 30% of those reported have bilateral nodules. In appearance they are discrete and brown to reddish brown and may be solid or cystic.

The majority of patients with luteomas are asymptomatic, and the nodules are discovered incidentally at cesarean delivery or postpartum tubal ligation. Most reported cases are in multiparous black women. Masculinization of the mother occurs in 30% of cases, and masculinization of the external genitalia of the female fetus may sometimes occur. These tumors regress spontaneously following completion of the pregnancy.

Benign Neoplasms of the Ovary

Benign Cystic Teratoma (Dermoid Cyst, Mature Teratoma)

Benign ovarian teratomas are usually cystic structures that on histologic examination contain elements from all three germ cell layers. The word *teratoma* was first advanced by Virchow and translated literally means monstrous growth. Teratomas of the ovary may be benign or malignant. Though *dermoid* is a misnomer, it is the most common term used to describe the benign cystic tumor, composed of mature cells, whereas the malignant variety is composed of immature cells (immature teratoma). *Dermoid* is a descriptive term in that it emphasizes the preponderance of ectodermal tissue with some mesodermal and rare endodermal derivatives. Malignant teratomas that are immature are usually solid with some cystic areas and histologically contain immature or embryonic-appearing tissue. See Chapter 29 for further discussion of malignant teratomas. Benign teratomas may undergo malignant transformation. This occurs in approximately 1% to 2% of dermoids, usually in women over 40. The malignant component is generally a squamous carcinoma. Nonovarian teratomas may arise in midline structures of the body where the germ cell has resided during embryonic life.

Benign teratomas are among the most common of ovarian neoplasms. Depending on the series, dermoids represent 20% to 25% of all ovarian neoplasms and approximately 33% of all benign tumors, if follicular and corpus luteum cysts are excluded. Dermoids are the most common ovarian neoplasm in prepubertal females and are also common in teenagers. However, more than 50% of benign teratomas are discovered in women between the ages of 25 and 50 years. In the series of Lakkis et al. of 118 patients with dermoids, 86% of the patients were less than 40 years of age, and 3.4% had recurrences (Fig. 17-37). In most large series of benign tumors in postmenopausal women, dermoids account for approximately 20% of the neoplasms.

Dermoids vary from a few millimeters to 25 cm in diameter. However, 80% are less than 10 cm. These tumors may be single or multiple, with as many as nine individual dermoids having been reported in the same ovary. Benign teratomas occur bilaterally 10% to 15% of

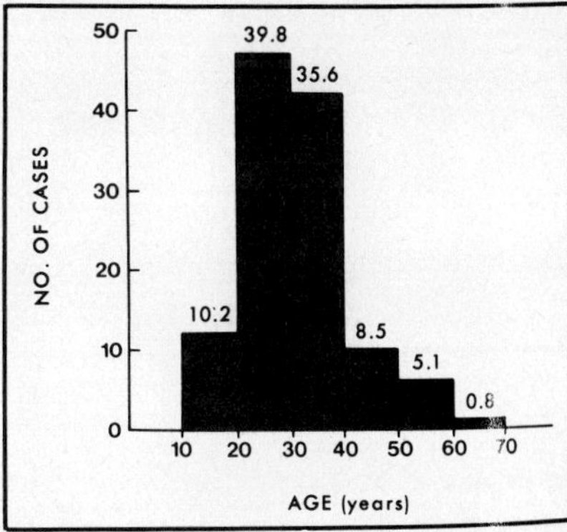

FIGURE 17-37
Age distribution of cystic teratomas. (From Lakkis WG, Martin MC, Gelfand MM: Originally published in Canadian Journal of Surgery 28:444, 1985.)

the time. Often dermoid cysts are pedunculated. These cysts make the ovary heavier than normal, and thus they are usually discovered either in the cul-de-sac or anterior to the broad ligament. Grossly, the cysts are smooth and pearly gray. On palpation these tumors, which have both cystic and solid components, have a doughy consistency.

The cysts are usually unilocular. When they are opened, thick sebaceous fluid, often with tangled masses of hair and firm areas of cartilage and teeth, pours from the cyst (Figs. 17-38 to 17-40). The sebaceous material is a thick fluid at body temperature but solidifies when it cools in room air.

Benign teratomas are believed to arise from a single germ cell after the first meiotic division. Dermoids have a chromosomal makeup of 46XX. Linder et al., in a series of experiments using chromosome banding techniques and electrophoretic variance, discovered that the chromosomes of dermoids were different than the chromosomes of the host. They postulated that dermoids began by parthenogenesis from secondary oocytes. An alternative hypothesis was that the dermoid resulted from fusion of the second polar body with the oocyte. The studies by Linder et al. ruled out the possibility that dermoids arise from somatic cells or from an oogonium before the first stage of meiosis. The first meiotic division occurs at approximately 13 weeks of gestation. Thus dermoids begin in fetal life sometime after this point.

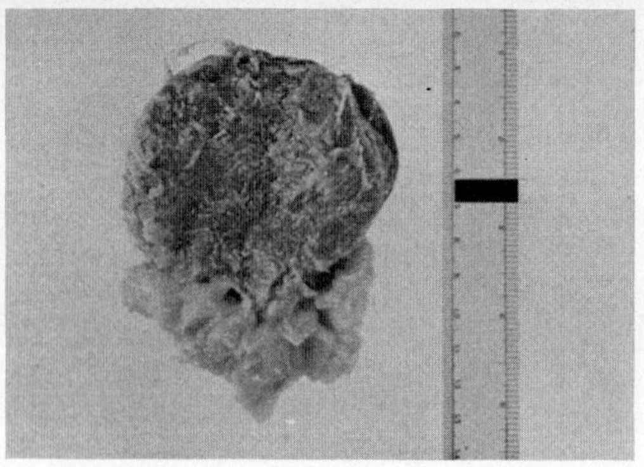

FIGURE 17-38

Benign cystic teratoma of the ovary. In addition to sebaceous material, varying amounts of hair are almost constantly found in the cyst. (From Janovski NA, ed: Color atlas of gross gynecologic and obstetric pathology. New York, McGraw-Hill Book Co., 1969, p. 175.)

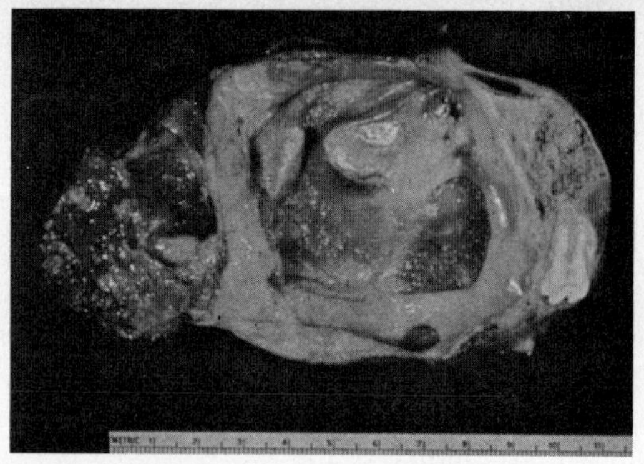

FIGURE 17-39

Benign cystic teratoma of the ovary. There is a rudimentary mandible-like bone and several teeth. The teratoma, although it may contain highly organized structures, is fundamentally nonfetiform. Therefore identifications of caricatures of fetuses (homunculi) and well-developed bones are imaginary. (From Janovski NA, ed: Color atlas of gross gynecologic and obstetric pathology. New York, McGraw-Hill Book Co., 1969, p. 177.)

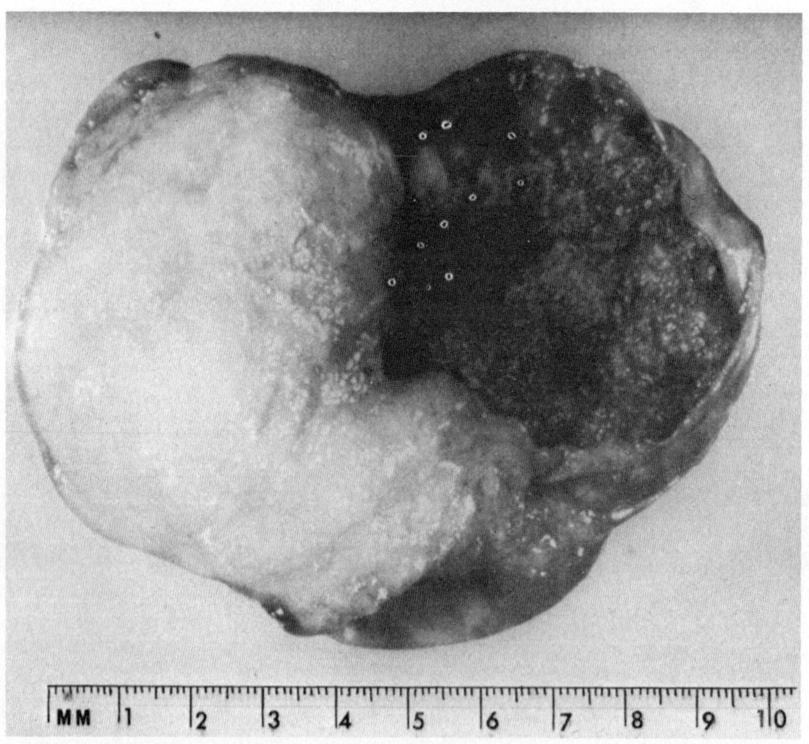

FIGURE 17-40

Cross section through a dermoid cyst of the ovary occupied on the right side by a mass of hair (black area), and on the other by a solid tumor that histologically proved to be epidermoid carcinoma. (From Pantoja E, Rodriguez-Ibanez I, Axtmayer RW, et al: Obstet Gynecol 45:91, 1975. Reprinted with permission from The American College of Obstetricians and Gynecologists.)

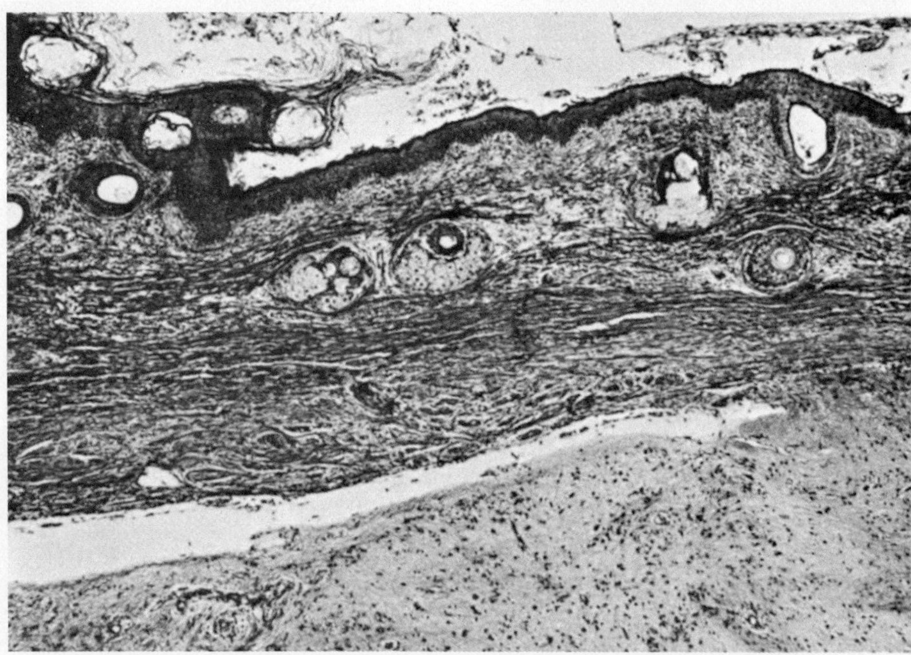

FIGURE 17-41
Mature cystic teratoma. The lining of the cyst is composed of skin with its append-ages. Mature neural tissue is seen beneath the cutaneous structures. (H&E; ×61.) (Reprinted by permission from Talerman A: Germ cell tumors of the ovary. In Blaustein A, ed: Pathology of the female genital tract. New York, Springer-Verlag, 1977, p. 559.)

Histologically, benign teratomas are com-prised of mature cells, usually from all three germ layers (Fig. 17-41). A combination of skin and skin appendages, including sebaceous glands, sweat glands, hair follicles, muscle fi-bers, cartilage, bone, teeth, glial cells, and ep-ithelium of the respiratory and gastrointestinal tracts, may be visualized. Teeth are predomi-nantly premolar and molar forms. The fluid in dermoid cysts is usually sebaceous. Most solid elements arise and are contained in a protru-sion or nipple (mamilla) in the cyst wall termed the *prominence or tubercle of Rokitansky.* The wall of the cyst will often contain granulation tissue, giant cells, and pseudoxanthoma cells.

Approximately 50% of dermoids are asymp-tomatic and are discovered incidentally by pel-vic examination or coincidentally visualized by an abdominal x-ray or ultrasound examination. Specific complications of dermoid cysts include torsion, rupture, infection, hemorrhage, and malignant degeneration. Three medical dis-eases also may be associated with dermoid cysts: thyrotoxicosis, carcinoid syndrome, and autoimmune hemolytic anemia. Torsion of a dermoid is the most frequent complication, oc-curring in 11% of the series by Pantoja et al. of 253 tumors. Because of its weight, the benign teratoma is often pedunculated, which may predispose to torsion. Torsion is more common in younger women.

Rupture or perforation of the contents of a dermoid into the peritoneal cavity or an adja-cent organ is one of the most serious compli-cations. The incidence varies between 0.7% and 4.6%. However, most series report less than 1%. Rupture is more common in preg-nancy. Rupture may occur either catastrophi-cally, which produces an acute abdomen, or by a slow leak of the sebaceous material. The lat-ter is clinically more common, with the seba-ceous material producing a severe chemical granulomatous peritonitis. Waxman and Boyce warn that this possibility should be considered and a frozen section obtained so that the true diagnosis is established. Thus a young woman

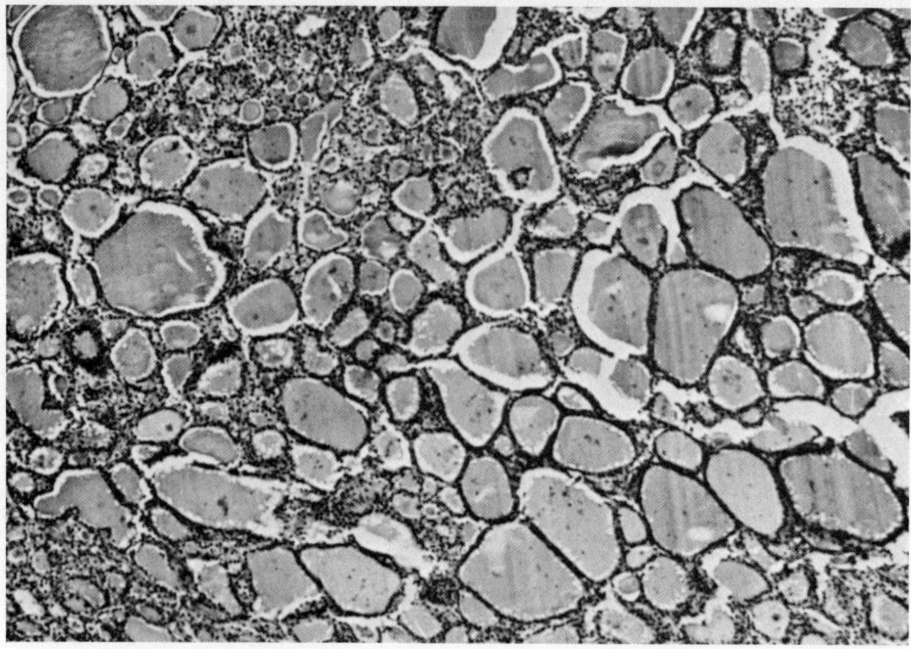

FIGURE 17-42
Struma ovarii. The tumor is composed of normal thyroid tissue. (H&E; ×76.)
(Reprinted by permission from Talerman A: Germ cell tumors of the ovary. In
Blaustein A, ed: Pathology of the female genital tract. New York, Springer-Verlag,
1977, p. 563.)

will not be mistakenly treated for suspected ovarian carcinoma with metastasis, because of the identical gross appearance of a slow-leaking dermoid cyst.

Infection, hemorrhage, and malignant degeneration are all unusual complications of dermoids, occurring in less than 1% of patients.

Adult thyroid tissue is discovered microscopically in approximately 12% of benign teratomas. Struma ovarii is a teratoma in which the thyroid tissue has overgrown other elements and is the predominant tissue (Fig. 17-42). Struma ovarii comprise 2% to 3% of ovarian teratomas. These tumors are usually unilateral and measure less than 10 cm in diameter. Less than 5% of women with struma ovarii develop thyrotoxicosis, which may be secondary to the production of increased thyroid hormone by either the ovarian or the thyroid gland.

Another rare finding with dermoids is the presence of a primary carcinoid tumor from the gastrointestinal or respiratory tract epithelium contained in the dermoid. One of three of these tumors is associated with the typical carcinoid syndrome even without metastatic spread. The autoimmune hemolytic anemia associated with dermoids is the rarest of the three medical complications.

The diagnosis of a dermoid cyst is often established when a semisolid mass is palpated anterior to the broad ligament. Approximately 50% of dermoids have pelvic calcifications on x-ray examination. Often an ovarian teratoma is an incidental finding during radiologic investigation of the genitourinary or gastrointestinal tract. There is an ongoing debate as to whether dermoids have a typical ultrasound picture. Early reports have emphasized an echogenic focus with acoustic shadowing situated within a predominantly cystic mass as classic for dermoid cysts. Laing et al. have found that only one of three dermoids have this "typical picture." In their series of 45 patients with 51 biopsy-proven dermoid cysts, 24% of the dermoid cysts were predominantly solid, 20% were almost entirely cystic, and 24% were not visible (Table 17-4). Treatment of benign cystic teratomas is cystectomy and is discussed in Chapter 29.

TABLE 17-4

Ultrasonographic Appearance of Dermoid Cysts

Appearance	No. of Dermoids	Percent
Cystic	10	20.0
Solid	12	23.5
Cystic and solid	17	33.0
Not visualized	12	23.5
TOTAL	51	100.0

From Laing FC, Van Dalsem VF, Marks WM, et al: Dermoid cysts of the ovary: Their ultrasonographic appearances. Obstet Gynecol 57:103, 1981. Reprinted with permission from The American College of Obstetricians and Gynecologists.

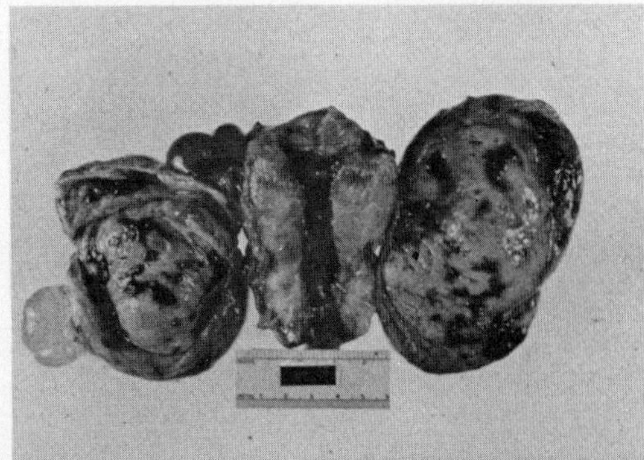

FIGURE 17-43

Endometriosis of the ovaries. The wall of the endometriotic cyst is thickened and fibrotic. The inner surface shows areas of dark brown discoloration. (From Janovski NA, ed: Color atlas of gross gynecologic and obstetric pathology. New York, McGraw-Hill Book Co., 1969, p. 159.)

Endometriomas

Endometriosis of the ovary is often associated with endometriosis in other areas of the pelvic cavity. Approximately two out of three women with endometriosis have ovarian involvement. However, only 5% of these women have enlargement of the ovaries that is detectable by pelvic examination. Because of the frequency of the disease, though, endometriosis is one of the most common causes of enlargement of the ovary. Because most authors do not classify endometriosis as a neoplastic disease, often the diagnosis of endometriosis is not given due consideration in the differential diagnosis of an adnexal mass. Ovarian endometriosis is similar to endometriosis elsewhere and therefore is described in greater detail in Chapter 18.

The size of ovarian endometriomas varies from small, superficial, blue-black implants that are 1 to 5 mm in diameter to large, multiloculated, hemorrhagic cysts that may be 5 to 10 cm in diameter (Fig. 17-43). Rarely, large chocolate cysts of the ovary may reach 15 to 20 cm (Fig. 17-44), and they are frequently bilateral. The surface of an ovary with endometriosis is often irregular, puckered, and scarred.

Although most patients with endometriomas are asymptomatic, the most prominent symptoms of ovarian endometriosis are pelvic pain, dyspareunia, and infertility. Approximately 10% of the operations for endometriosis are for acute symptoms, usually related to a ruptured ovarian endometrioma that was previously asymptomatic. Smaller cysts generally have thinner cyst walls, and thus perforation occurs commonly secondary to cyclic hemorrhage into the cystic cavity.

On pelvic examination the ovaries are usually tender and immobile, secondary to associated inflammation and adhesions. Histologically, endometrial glands, endometrial stroma, and large phagocytic cells containing hemosiderin may be identified (Fig. 17-45). Pressure atrophy may lead to the loss of architecture of the endometrial glands.

The choice between medical and operative management depends on several factors, including the patient's age, future reproductive plans, and severity of symptoms. In general, medical therapy is not successful in treating ovarian endometriosis if the disease has produced ovarian enlargement.

Fibroma

Fibromas are the most common benign, solid neoplasms of the ovary. Their malignant potential is low, less than 1%. These tumors comprise approximately 5% of benign ovarian neoplasms and approximately 20% of all solid tumors of the ovary.

Fibromas vary in size from small nodules to huge pelvic tumors weighing 50 pounds. The

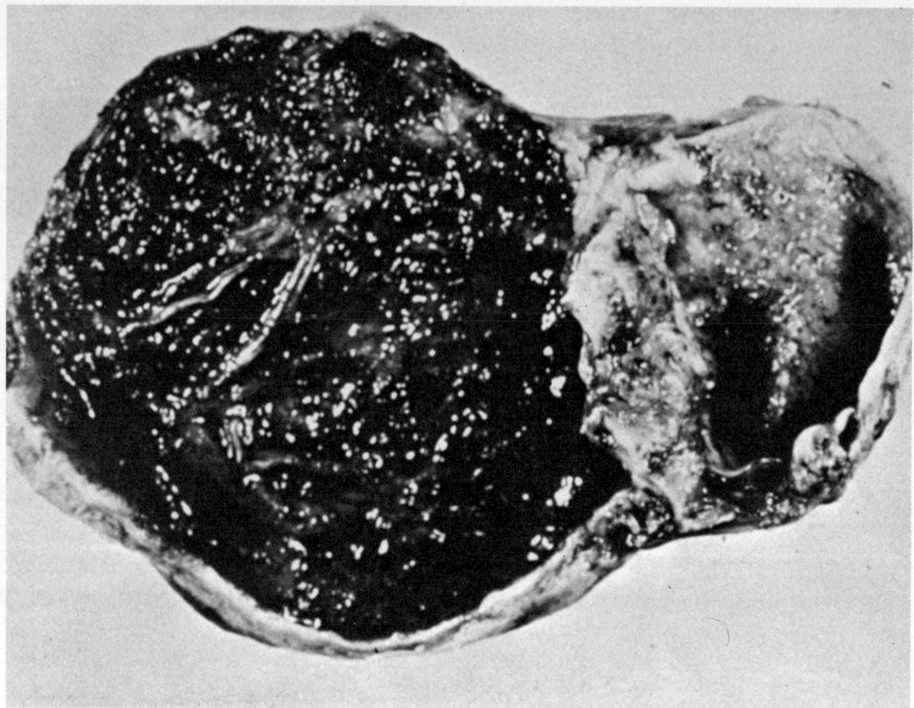

FIGURE 17-44
Opened endometrioma showing a large cyst lined by hemorrhagic tissue. (From Czernobilsky B: Primary epithelial tumors of the ovary. In Blaustein A, ed: Pathology of the female genital tract. New York, Springer-Verlag, 1977, p. 476.)

average diameter of a fibroma is approximately 6 cm; however, larger tumors have reached 30 cm in diameter. In most series, less than 5% of fibromas are greater than 20 cm in diameter. The diameter of a fibroma is important clinically, because the incidence of associated ascites is directly proportional to the size of the tumor. Ninety percent of fibromas are unilateral; however, multiple fibromas are found in the same ovary in 10% to 15% of cases. The average age of a woman with an ovarian fibroma is 48. Thus this tumor often presents in a postmenopausal woman. The tumor arises from the undifferentiated fibrous stroma of the ovary.

The pelvic symptoms that develop with growth of fibromas include pressure and abdominal enlargement, which may be secondary to the size of the tumor and ascites. Smaller tumors are asymptomatic; because these tumors do not elaborate hormones, there is no change in the pattern of menstrual flow. Fibromas may be pedunculated and thus easily palpable during one examination yet difficult to palpate during a subsequent pelvic examination. Meigs' syndrome is the association of an ovarian fibroma, ascites, and hydrothorax. Both the ascites and hydrothorax resolve after removal of the ovarian tumor.

The ascites is caused by transudation of fluid from the ovarian fibroma. Samanth and Black reported that the incidence of ascites was directly related to the size of the fibroma. Fifty percent of patients have ascites if the tumor is greater than 6 cm. Meigs' syndrome occurs in less than 5% of fibromas. The hydrothorax develops secondary to a flow of ascitic fluid into the pleural space via the lymphatics of the diaphragm. Statistically the right pleural space is involved in 75% of reported cases, the left in 10%, and both sides in 15%. The clinical features of Meigs' syndrome are not unique to fibromas, and a similar clinical picture is found with many other ovarian tumors.

Grossly, fibromas are heavy, solid, well encapsulated, and grayish white. The cut surface usually demonstrates a homogeneous white or yellowish white solid tissue with a trabeculated

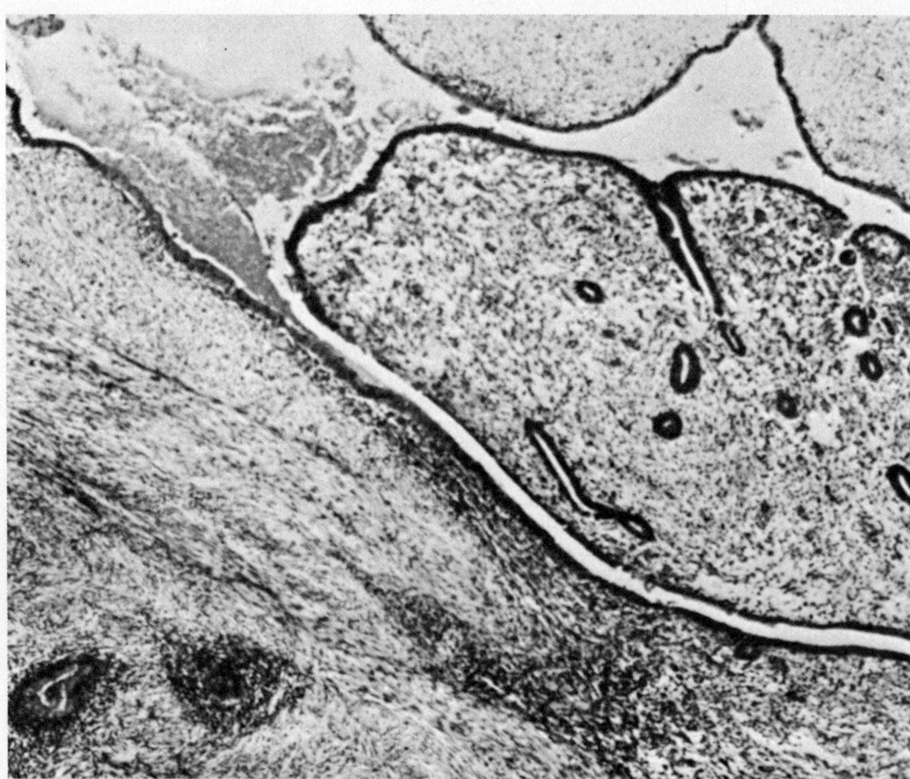

FIGURE 17-45
The wall of an endometrioma lined by endometrial-type epithelium with underlying endometrial stroma. Note the polypoid projections of endometrial tissue projecting into the cyst lumen. (H&E; ×40.) (From Czernobilsky B: Primary epithelial tumors of the ovary. In Blaustein A, ed: Pathology of the female genital tract. New York, Springer-Verlag, 1977, p. 476.)

or whorled appearance similar to that of myomas. The vast majority of fibromas are grossly edematous (Fig. 17-46). Less than 10% of fibromas have calcifications or small areas of hyaline or cystic degeneration. Histologically, fibromas are composed of connective tissue, stromal cells, and varying amounts of collagen interposed between the cells. The connective tissue cells are spindle-shaped, mature fibroblasts. They are arranged in an imperfect pattern. A few smooth muscle fibers may be occasionally identified. It is sometimes difficult to distinguish fibromas from nonneoplastic thecomas. Histologically the pathologist must differentiate fibromas from fibrosarcomas and also look for epithelial elements of an associated Brenner tumor.

The management of fibromas is straightforward; any woman with a solid ovarian neoplasia

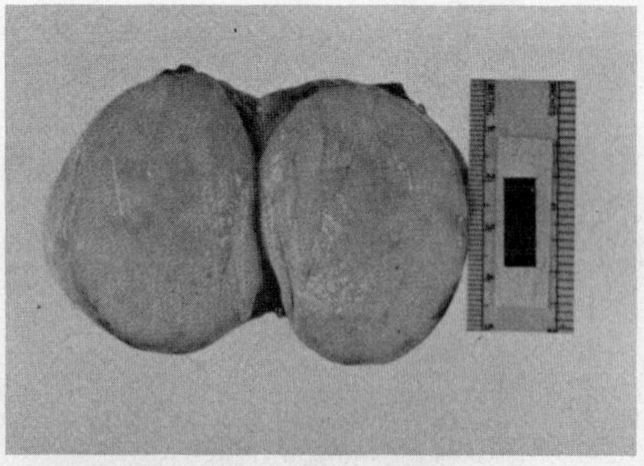

FIGURE 17-46
Fibroma of the ovary. Cut surface shows somewhat edematous, interlacing bundles of connective tissue. (From Janovski NA, ed: Color atlas of gross gynecologic and obstetric pathology. New York, McGraw-Hill Book Co., 1969, p. 163.)

should have an exploratory operation soon after the tumor is discovered. Simple excision of the tumor is all that is necessary. Because these tumors are frequently discovered in postmenopausal women, often a bilateral salpingo-oophorectomy and total abdominal hysterectomy is performed. Most women who preoperatively have a solid ovarian tumor and ascites subsequently are found to have ovarian carcinoma.

Brenner Tumors

Brenner tumors are rare, small, smooth, solid, fibroepithelial ovarian tumors that are generally asymptomatic. The benign proliferative and malignant forms together comprise approximately 2% of ovarian tumors, and they usually occur in women aged 40 to 50 years. Approximately 30% of Brenner tumors are discovered as small, solid tumors in association with serous or mucinous cystadenomas of the ipsilateral ovary. Some are microscopic, with the entire tumor contained in a single low-powered microscopic field, and others may reach a

diameter of 20 cm; the majority are less than 5 cm in diameter. The tumor is usually unilateral, with bilateral Brenner tumors being reported in only 5% to 15% of the women in large series.

The Brenner tumor was first described in 1898. Robert Meyer established that it was a distinct independent neoplasm from granulosa cell tumors in 1932. Since that time there has been a continuing controversy in the gynecologic pathology literature as to the histogenesis of the neoplasm. Most authorities accept the theory that the tumor results from metaplasia of coelomic epithelium into uroepithelium. Others have postulated that the solid nests of epithelial cells of the tumor originate from the rete ovarii, or Walthard rests. Shevchuk et al., in an electron microscopy study, confirmed the histologic and ultrastructural similarity between epithelium in Brenner tumors and transitional epithelium. These authors argue that because of the histogenesis from coelomic inclusion cysts and also the mixture of Müllerian-type epithelium in 30% of Brenner tumors, it

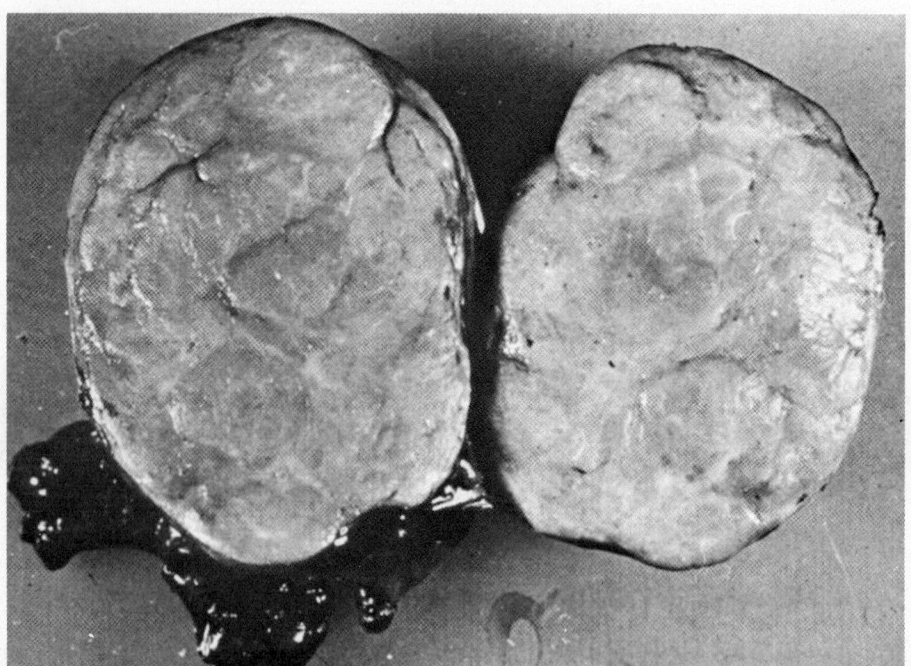

FIGURE 17-47
Cut section of a solid, nodular Brenner tumor. (From Czernobilsky B: Primary epithelial tumors of the ovary. In Blaustein A, ed: Pathology of the female genital tract. New York, Springer-Verlag, 1977, p. 489.)

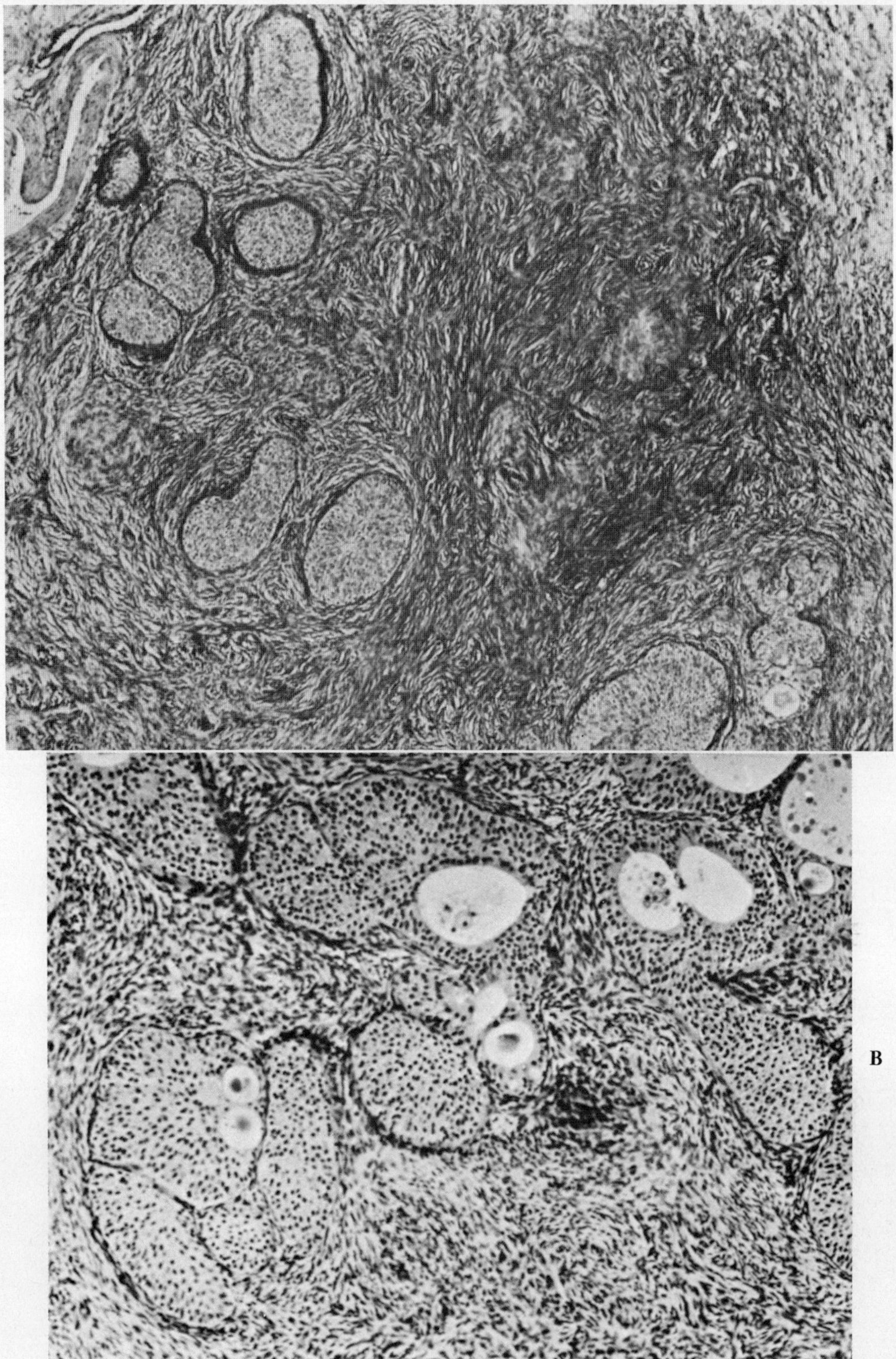

FIGURE 17-48

A, Brenner tumor of the ovary that measured 3 mm in diameter; shows characteristic nests of epithelium in a dense fibrous stroma. The tumor was an incidental microscopic finding (H&E; ×25). **B,** Brenner tumor showing a solid and partly cystic epithelial nest in the dense fibrous stroma. (H&E; ×113.) (**A** from Balasa RW, Adcock LL, Prem KA, et al: Obstet Gynecol 50:121, 1977; **B** from Czernobilsky B: Primary epithelial tumors of the ovary. In Blaustein A, ed: Pathology of the female genital tract. New York, Springer-Verlag, 1977, p. 490.)

might be appropriate to classify Brenner tumors in the epithelial group of ovarian neoplasms.

Approximately 90% of these small neoplasms are discovered incidentally during a gynecologic operation, although large tumors may produce unilateral pelvic discomfort. Postmenopausal bleeding is sometimes associated with Brenner tumors, as endometrial hyperplasia is a coexisting abnormality in 10% to 16% of cases. It is postulated that luteinization of the stroma produces estrogen with resulting hyperplasia.

Grossly, Brenner tumors are smooth, firm, gray-white, solid tumors that grossly resemble fibromas. Upon sectioning, the tumor usually appears gray; however, occasionally there is a yellowish tinge with small cystic spaces (Fig. 17-47). Approximately 1% to 2% of these tumors undergo malignant change (see Chapter 29). Histologically, Brenner tumors have two principal components: solid masses or nests of epithelial cells and a surrounding fibrous stroma. The epithelial cells are uniform and do not appear anaplastic (Fig. 17-48). The histology and ultrastructure of the epithelial cells of a Brenner tumor are similar to transitional epithelium of the urinary bladder. The pale epithelial cells have a "coffee bean"-appearing nucleus, which is also described as a longitudinal groove in the cell's nucleus (Fig. 17-49). Electron microscopy has demonstrated that the longitudinal groove during routine microscopy is produced by prominent indentation of the nuclear membrane. An additional ovarian neoplasm is frequently found associated with Brenner tumors. Balasa et al., in a review of 302 tumors, reported 100 other concurrent neoplasms, with the majority being serous and mucinous cystadenomas or teratomas.

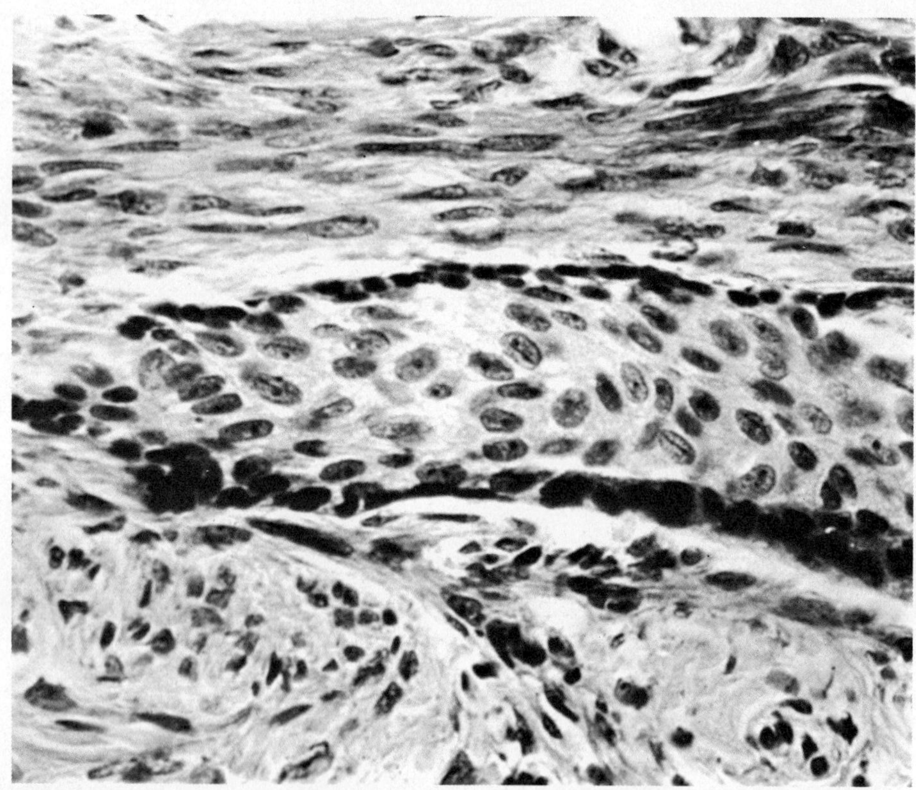

FIGURE 17-49
Detail of epithelial nest of a Brenner tumor demonstrating typical longitudinal grooving or coffee-bean appearance of the nuclei. (H&E; ×400.) (From Czernobilsky B: Primary epithelial tumors of the ovary. In Blaustein A, ed: Pathology of the female genital tract. New York, Springer-Verlag, 1977, p. 490.)

Management of Brenner tumors is operative. As with ovarian fibromas, the patient's age often is the principal factor in deciding the extent of the operation.

Adenofibroma and Cystadenofibroma

Adenofibromas and cystadenofibromas are closely related. Both of these benign firm tumors are rare solid variations of serous cystadenomas. They differ from benign epithelial cystadenomas in that there is a preponderance of connective tissue. The varying degree of fibrous stroma and epithelial elements produces a spectrum of tumors, which have resulted in a confusing nomenclature with terms such as *papilloma*, *fibropapillomas*, and *fibroadenomas*.

Adenofibromas are usually small fibrous tumors that arise from the surface of the ovary. They are bilateral in 20% to 25% of women. They usually occur in postmenopausal women and are 1 to 15 cm in diameter. Grossly, they are gray or white tumors, and it is difficult to distinguish them from fibromas. Papillary adenofibromas, which project from the surface of the ovary, may at first glance appear to be external excrescences of a malignant tumor. Histologically, small precursors of adenofibromas are identified in many normal ovaries. Under the microscope, true cystic gland spaces lined by cuboidal epithelium are characteristic. However, differing from serous cystadenomas, the fibrous connective tissue surrounding the cystic spaces is abundant and is the predominant tissue of the tumor.

Smaller tumors are asymptomatic and are only discovered incidentally during abdominal or pelvic operations. Large tumors may cause pressure symptoms or rarely undergo adnexal torsion.

Because adenofibromas are usually discovered in postmenopausal women, the treatment of choice is bilateral salpingo-oophorectomy and total abdominal hysterectomy. As these tumors are benign and as malignant transformation is rare, simple excision of the tumor and inspection of the contralateral ovary is appropriate in younger women.

Torsion

Torsion of the ovary or both the oviduct and ovary (adnexal torsion) is an unusual but important cause of acute lower abdominal and pelvic pain. Torsion of the ovary may occur separately from torsion of the fallopian tube, but most commonly the two adnexal structures are affected together (Fig. 17-50). In Hibbard's review of 128 cases of adnexal torsion, this syndrome accounted for approximately 3% of gynecologic operative emergencies at the University of Southern California Medical Center.

Adnexal torsion occurs most commonly during the reproductive years, with the average patient being in her mid-twenties. Pregnancy appears to predispose women to adnexal torsion, with approximately one in five women being pregnant when the condition is diagnosed. The most common etiology of adnexal torsion is ovarian enlargement by an 8 to 12 cm benign mass of the ovary. Ovarian tumors are discovered in 50% to 60% of women with adnexal torsion. Torsion of a normal ovary or adnexum is also possible and occurs more frequently in children. Hibbard reports that because of their relative prevalence, dermoids are the tumor most frequently reported in a series of women with adnexal torsion. However, the relative risk of adnexal torsion is higher with paraovarian cysts, solid benign tumors, and serous cysts of the ovary. The right ovary has a greater tendency to twist (3 to 2) than

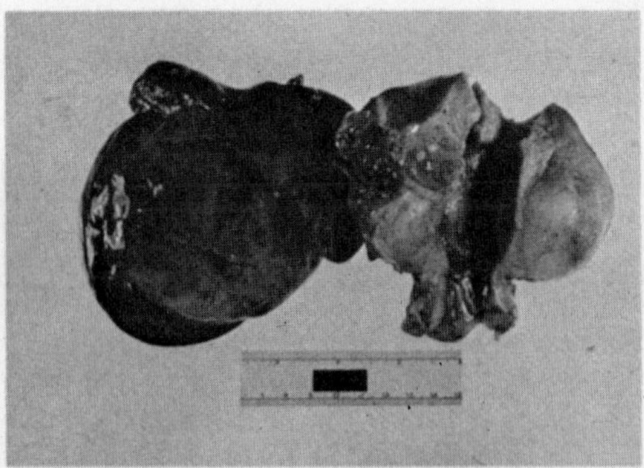

FIGURE 17-50
Torsion of the ovary. The large ovarian cyst is twisted twice around its long axis. The oviduct is included, and both structures are gangrenous. (From Janovski NA, ed: Color atlas of gross gynecologic and obstetric pathology. New York, McGraw-Hill Book Co., 1969, p. 181.)

does the left ovary. Torsion of a malignant ovarian tumor is comparatively rare (2.5% in Hibbard's report).

Patients with adnexal torsion present with acute, severe, unilateral, lower abdominal and pelvic pain. Often the patient relates the onset of the severe pain to an abrupt change of position. Approximately two thirds of patients have associated nausea and vomiting. These associated gastrointestinal symptoms sometimes lead to a preoperative diagnosis of acute appendicitis or small intestinal obstruction. Many patients have noted intermittent previous episodes of similar pain for several days to several weeks. The hypothesis is that previous episodes of pain were secondary to partial torsion, with spontaneous reversal without significant vascular compromise. With progressive torsion, initially venous and lymphatic obstruction occurs. This produces a cyanotic, edematous ovary, which on pelvic examination presents as a unilateral, tender adnexal mass. Further progression of the torsion interrupts the major arterial supply to the ovary, resulting in hypoxia, adnexal necrosis, and a concomitant low-grade fever and leukocystosis. Approximately 10% of women with adnexal torsion have a repetitive episode affecting the contralateral adnexum.

Most patients with adnexal torsion present with symptoms and signs severe enough to demand operative intervention. If the diagnosis is questionable, laparoscopy may be appropriate. The most common gynecologic conditions that may be confused with adnexal torsion are a ruptured corpus luteum or an adnexal abscess.

Because the majority of cases of adnexal torsion occur in young women, a conservative operation is ideal. However, it is often difficult to grossly differentiate between partial torsion and complete torsion. If partial torsion is confirmed, it is acceptable to untwist the pedicle, perform a cystectomy, and stabilize the ovary with sutures so as to prevent recurrence. Conservative operation has the risk of releasing venous thrombi into the general circulation if the degree of torsion is underestimated. Thus, with vascular compromise the proper operation is unilateral salpingo-oophorectomy. The vascular pedicle should be clamped with care so as not to injure the ureter, which may be tented up by the torsion, yet sufficiently distant from the ovary so as to include all areas of vascular thrombosis.

KEY POINTS

- Symptoms of urethral caruncles are variable. Some urethral caruncles are asymptomatic; others cause dysuria, frequency, and urgency. They must be differentiated from urethral carcinoma by biopsy. Treatment of urethral caruncles is topical or oral estrogen therapy.

- The vulva contains 1% of the skin surface of the body, but 5% to 10% of all malignant melanomas in women arise from this region. All vulvar nevi should be excised and examined histologically.

- Symptoms of an early malignant melanoma include *asymmetry, border* irregularity, *color* variegation, and a *diameter* usually greater than 6 mm (ABCD).

- Hidradenomas are asymptomatic vulvar tumors originating from apocrine glands, and are found in white women between 30 and 70 years of age.

- Endometriosis of the vulva is rare, with only 1 in 500 patients with endometriosis having vulvar involvement.

- Treatment of vulvar hematomas is conservative unless they are expanding.

- The most common causes of vulvar contact dermatitis are cosmetic and local therapeutic agents.

- Vulvar psoriasis usually involves intertriginous areas and is manifested by red to red-yellow papules. These lesions enlarge, becoming dull red plaques.

- The treatment of hidradenitis suppurativa is wide operative excision.

- Urethral diverticula occur in approximately 3% of women, and the diagnosis should be suspected in any woman with chronic or recurrent lower urinary tract symptoms.

- Of women with urethral diverticula, 20% are asymptomatic, while tender masses may be palpated in more than half of the patients.

- Prolonged tampon use may be associated with ulcerations of the vagina, discharge, and bleeding.

- Biopsy examination of any persistent vaginal ulcer should be done to rule out carcinoma.

- Endocervical polyps are smooth, soft, red, fragile masses. They are found most commonly in multiparous women in their forties and fifties.

- Malignant transformation of endometrial polyps has been estimated to occur in 0.5% of cases and is most often an endometrial carcinoma of low grade and stage.

- Leiomyomas of the uterus are the most frequent pelvic tumors and occur most commonly in the fifth decade of life.

- Five to ten percent of myomas are submucosal, often presenting with symptoms of abnormal vaginal bleeding and distortion of the uterine cavity that may lead to infertility or abortion.

______________ **KEY POINTS, cont'd** ______________________________

- Broad ligament leiomyomas may produce hydroureters as they enlarge.

- Each individual uterine myoma is monoclonal, arising from a single muscle cell.

- The stimulus for growth of myomas is unclear; however, it is partially related to estrogen levels.

- Acute muscular infarction, as is seen with red degeneration of a myoma, causes severe pain and localized peritoneal irritation.

- The malignant transformation of a fibroid is rare, probably occurring in less than 0.3% of cases.

- The majority of women with uterine myomas are asymptomatic, but one of three will experience pelvic pain, with dysmenorrhea being the most frequent complaint.

- Abnormal bleeding is experienced by 30% of women with myomas, with the most common symptom being menorrhagia, but intermenstrual spotting and disruption of the normal pattern are other frequent complaints.

- The management of women with small, asymptomatic myomas is conservative, and the majority of women will not need operations.

- Women with symptomatic leiomyomas should be investigated thoroughly for concurrent problems, such as endometrial hyperplasia. If their symptoms do not improve with conservative management, operative therapy is indicated.

- Classic indications for myomectomy include rapidly expanding pelvic mass, persistent abnormal bleeding, pain or pressure, previous repetitive abortion, or long-standing infertility.

- Hematometra in postmenopausal women is often asymptomatic.

- The main symptom of torsion of the tube is pain, usually located in the iliac fossa with radiation to the thigh and flank. In two thirds of cases the pain is associated with nausea and vomiting.

- Follicular cysts are the most common cystic structures in normal ovaries.

- Indications for operation on a cyst in the ovary include a mass after the menopause or before puberty, a solid tumor at any age, a cystic mass greater than 8 cm, or a cystic mass 5 to 8 cm in size that has been observed for more than 8 weeks.

- Women taking warfarin (Coumadin) are especially prone to develop hemorrhage from rupture of a corpus luteum cyst.

- The treatment of unruptured corpus luteum cysts is conservative. However, if the cyst persists or intraperitoneal bleeding occurs, necessitating operation, the treatment is cystectomy.

- Benign ovarian teratomas comprise 15% to 25% of all ovarian neoplasms.

- Benign ovarian teratomas vary from a few millimeters to 25 cm, may be single or multiple, and are bilateral 10% to 15% of the time.

- Dermoids are believed to arise during fetal life from a single germ cell. They are 46XX in karyotype.

- Although most dermoids are asymptomatic, torsion and rupture are two important complications.

- Fifty percent of dermoids have calcifications visible on a pelvic x-ray film.

- The most prominent symptoms of ovarian endometriosis are pelvic pain, dyspareunia, and infertility.

- Histologically, ovarian endometriosis usually demonstrates endometrial stroma, large phagocytic cells, and endometrial glands. However, pressure atrophy may lead to loss of architecture of the endometrial glands.

- Fibromas are the most common, benign, solid neoplasms of the ovary. They have a low malignant potential.

—————————— **KEY POINTS, cont'd** ——————————

- Fibromas vary in size from small nodules to huge pelvic tumors weighing as much as 50 pounds. Ninety percent of fibromas are unilateral, and most have an average diameter of 6 cm.

- Fifty percent of patients with an ovarian fibroma will have ascites if the tumor is greater than 6 cm.

- Brenner tumors are smooth, solid, fibroepithelial tumors of the ovary. They usually occur in women between the ages of 40 and 60 years and are predominantly unilateral.

- Adnexal torsion occurs most commonly in the reproductive years, with the average age of patients being mid-twenties, and pregnancy predisposes to adnexal torsion.

- Ovarian tumors are discovered in 50% to 60% of women with adnexal torsion.

BIBLIOGRAPHY

Ahnaimugan S, Asuen MI: Coital laceration of the vagina. Aust NZ J Obstet Gynaecol 20:180, 1980.

Axe S, Parmley T, Woodruff JD, et al: Adenomas in minor vestibular glands. Obstet Gynecol 68:16, 1986.

Babaknia A, Rock JA, Jones HW: Pregnancy success following abdominal myomectomy for infertility. Fertil Steril 30:644, 1978.

Balasa RW, Adcock LL, Prem KA, et al: The Brenner tumor. Obstet Gynecol 50:120, 1977.

Barrett KF, Bledsoe S, Greer BE, et al: Tampon-induced vaginal or cervical ulceration. Am J Obstet Gynecol 127:332, 1977.

Beresford JM, St. George-Hyslop PH: Abscess formation in Gartner's duct cysts associated with ipsilateral renal agenesis. Obstet Gynecol 49:28S, 1977.

Bernardus RE, Van Der Slikke JW, Roex AJM, et al: Torsion of the fallopian tube: some considerations on its etiology. Obstet Gynecol 64:675, 1984.

Bhatia NN, Bergman A, Broen EM: Advanced hidradenitis suppurativa of the vulva. J Reprod Med 29:436, 1984.

Birch HW, Sondag DR: Granular-cell myoblastoma of the vulva. Obstet Gynecol 18:443, 1961.

Blaustein A, ed: Pathology of the female genital tract. New York, Springer-Verlag, 1977.

Buttram VC, Reiter RC: Uterine leiomyomata: etiology, symptomatology, and management. Fertil Steril 36:433, 1981.

Carneiro SJC, Gardner HL, Knox JM: Syringoma: three cases with vulvar involvement. Obstet Gynecol 39:95, 1972.

Chambers JT, Thiagarajah S, Kitchin JD: Torsion of the normal fallopian tube in pregnancy. Obstet Gynecol 54:487, 1979.

Choo YC, Mak KC, Hsu C, et al: Postmenopausal uterine bleeding of nonorganic cause. Obstet Gynecol 66:225, 1985.

Coates JB, Hales JS: Granular cell myoblastoma of the vulva. Obstet Gynecol 41:796, 1973.

Cramer SF, Robertson AL, Ziats NP, et al: Growth potential of human uterine leiomyomas: some in vitro observations and their implications. Obstet Gynecol 66:36, 1985.

Csapo AI, Pulkkinen MO, Ruttner B, et al: The significance of the human corpus in pregnancy maintenance. Am J Obstet Gynecol 112:1061, 1972.

Davis BA: Salivary vulvitis. Obstet Gynecol 37:238, 1971.

Deppisch LM: Cysts of the vagina. Obstet Gynecol 45:623, 1975.

Dick HM, Honore LH: Dental structures in benign ovarian cystic teratomas (dermoid cysts). Oral Surg Oral Med Oral Pathol 60:299, 1985.

Dische FE, Ritche JM: Luteoma of pregnancy. J Pathol 100:77, 1970.

Doss N, Forney P, Vellios F, et al: Covert bilaterality of mature ovarian teratomas. Obstet Gynecol 50:651, 1977.

Dreyer L, Simson IW, Sevenster CBO, et al: Leiomyomatosis peritonealis disseminata. A report of two cases and a review of the literature. Br J Obstet Gynaecol 92:856, 1985.

Dunnihoo DR, Wolff J: Bilateral torsion of the adnexa: a case report and a review of the world literature. Obstet Gynecol 64:55S, 1984.

Evans AT, Symmonds RE, Gaffey TA: Recurrent pelvic intravenous leiomyomatosis. Obstet Gynecol 57:260, 1981.

Farrar HK, Nedoss BR: Benign tumors of the uterine cervix. Am J Obstet Gynecol 81:124, 1961.

Filicori M, Hall DA, Loughlin JS, et al: A conservative approach to the management of uterine leiomyoma: pituitary desensitization by a luteinizing hormone-releasing hormone analogue. Am J Obstet Gynecol 147:726, 1983.

Fogel SR, Slasky BS: Sonography of Nabothian cysts. AJR 138:927, 1982.

Friedel W, Kaiser IH: Vaginal evisceration. Obstet Gynecol 45:315, 1975.

Friedman RJ, Rigel DS, Kopf AW: Early detection of malignant melanoma: the role of physician examination and self-examination of the skin. CA 35:130, 1985.

Friedrich EG: Tampon effects on vaginal health. Clin Obstet Gynecol 24:395, 1981.

Friedrich EG: The vulvar vestibule. J Reprod Med 28:773, 1983.

Friedrich EG: Vulvar disease, 2nd ed. Philadelphia, W.B. Saunders Co., 1983.

Friedrich EG, Wilkinson EJ: Vulvar surgery for neurofibromatosis. Obstet Gynecol 65:135, 1985.

Gardner HL, Kaufman RH: Benign diseases of the vulva and vagina, 2nd ed. Boston, G.K. Hall, 1981.

Ginsburg D, Genadry R: Suburethral diverticulum: classification and therapeutic considerations. Obstet Gynecol 61:685, 1983.

Golditch IM: Endometriosis presenting as an acute abdominal emergency. Obstet Gynecol 26:780, 1965.

Gompel C, Silverberg SG: Pathology in gynecology and obstetrics, 2nd ed. Philadelphia, J.B. Lippincott Co., 1977.

Hague WM, Abdulwahid NA, Jacobs HS, et al: Use of LHRH analogue to obtain reversible castration in a patient with benign metastasizing leiomyoma. Br J Obstet Gynaecol 93:455, 1986.

Hajj SN, Evans MI: Diverticula of the female urethra. Am J Obstet Gynecol 136:335, 1980.

Hakim-Elahi E: Postabortal amenorrhea due to cervical stenosis. Obstet Gynecol 48:723, 1976.

Hallatt JG, Steele CH, Snyder M: Ruptured corpus luteum with hemoperitoneum: A study of 173 surgical cases. Am J Obstet Gynecol 149:5, 1984.

Hamlin DJ, Pettersson H, Fitzsimmons J, et al: MR imaging of uterine leiomyomas and their complications. J Comput Assist Tomogr 9:902, 1985.

Hart WR: Paramesonephric mucinous cysts of the vulva. Am J Obstet Gynecol 107:1079, 1980.

Herndon JH: Itching: the pathophysiology of pruritus. Int J Dermat 14:465, 1975.

Hibbard LT: Adnexal torsion. Am J Obstet Gynecol 152:456, 1985.

Hricak H, Tschalokoff D, Heinrichs L, et al: Uterine leiomyomas: correlation of MR, histopathologic findings, and symptoms. Radiology 158:385, 1986.

Hsu YK, Rosenshein NB, Parmley TH, et al: Leiomyomatosis in pelvic lymph nodes. Obstet Gynecol 57:91S, 1981.

Huddock JJ, Dupayne N, McGeary JA: Traumatic vulvar hematomas. Am J Obstet Gynecol 70:1064, 1955.

Huffman JW: The detailed anatomy of the paraurethral ducts in the adult human female. Am J Obstet Gynecol 55:86, 1948.

Hunter DJS: Management of a massive ovarian cyst. Obstet Gynecol 56:254, 1980.

Imperial R, Helwig EB: Angiokeratoma of the vulva. Obstet Gynecol 29:307, 1967.

Iosif CS, Akerlund M: Fibromyomas and uterine activity. Acta Obstet Gynecol Scand 62:165, 1983.

Israel SL: The clinical similarity of corpus luteum cyst and ectopic pregnancy. Am J Obstet Gynecol 44:22, 1942.

Janovski NA: Color atlas of gross gynecologic and obstetric pathology. New York, McGraw-Hill Book Co., 1969.

Janovski NA: Dysontogenetic cyst of the vulva. Obstet Gynecol 20:227, 1962.

Jimmerson SD, Becker JD: Vaginal ulcers associated with tampon usage. Obstet Gynecol 56:97, 1980.

Jonas HS, Masterson BJ: Giant uterine tumors. Obstet Gynecol 50:2S, 1977.

Junaid TA, Thomas SM: Cysts of the vulva and vagina: a comparative study. Int J Gynaecol Obstet 19:239, 1981.

Klein HZ, Smith RL: Fibromyoma of the uterine tube. Obstet Gynecol 26:515, 1965.

Knox JM: Cutaneous inflammations and infections. Clin Obstet Gynecol 21:991, 1978.

Kolstad P, Stafl A: Atlas of colposcopy, 2nd ed. Baltimore, University Park Press, 1977.

Laing FC, Van Dalsem VF, Marks WM, et al: Dermoid cysts of the ovary: their ultrasonographic appearances. Obstet Gynecol 57:99, 1981.

Lakkis WG, Martin MC, Gelfand MM: Benign cystic teratoma of the ovary: a 6-year review. Can J Surg 28:444, 1985.

Lambert B, De Brux J: Theca lutein cysts of pregnancy without mole or chorioepithelioma. Obstet Gynecol 22:643, 1963.

Lee JKT, Gersell DJ, Balfe DM, et al: The uterus: in vitro MR-anatomic correlation of normal and abnormal specimens. Radiology 157:175, 1985.

Lee RA: Diverticulum of the female urethra: postoperative complications and results. Obstet Gynecol 61:52, 1983.

Lee RA: Diverticulum of the urethra: clinical presentation, diagnosis, and management. Clin Obstet Gynecol 27:490, 1984.

Linder D, McCau BK, Hecht F: Parthenogenic origin of benign ovarian teratomas. N Engl J Med 292:63, 1975.

Lynch PJ: Vulvodynia: a syndrome of unexplained vulvar pain, psychologic disability and sexual dysfunction. J Reprod Med 31:773, 1986.

MacKay B, Bennington JL, Skoglund RW: The adenomatoid tumor: fine structural evidence for a mesothelial origin. Cancer 27:109, 1971.

Maheux R, Guilloteau C, Lemay A, et al: Luteinizing hormone-releasing hormone agonist and uterine leiomyoma: a pilot study. Am J Obstet Gynecol 152:1034, 1985.

Maheux R, Guilloteau C, Lemay A, et al: Regression of leiomyomata uteri following hypoestrogenism induced by repetitive luteinizing hormone-releasing hormone agonist treatment: preliminary report. Fertil Steril 42:644, 1984.

Marshall FC, Uson AC, Melicow MM: Neoplasms and caruncles of the female urethra. Surg Gynecol Obstet 110:723, 1960.

Mathias CGT, Maibach HI: Dermatotoxicology monographs I. Cutaneous irritation: factors influencing the response to irritants. Clin Toxicol 13:333, 1978.

Mattingly RF, Thompson JD, eds: Te Linde's operative gynecology, 6th ed. Philadelphia, J.B. Lippincott Co., 1985.

Mattison DR, Yeh SY: Hemoperitoneum from rupture of a uterine vein overlying a leiomyoma. Am J Obstet Gynecol 136:415, 1980.

McCarthy S, Taylor KJW: Sonography of vaginal masses. AJR 140:1005, 1983.

McKay M: Vulvodynia versus pruritus vulvae. Clin Obstet Gynecol 28:123, 1985.

McLachlan RI, Healy DL, Burger HG: Clinical aspects of LHRH analogues in gynaecology: A review. Br J Obstet Gynaecol 93:431, 1986.

Meigs JV, Armstrong SH, Hamilton HH: A further contribution to the syndrome of fibroma of the ovary with fluid in the abdomen and chest, Meigs' syndrome. Am J Obstet Gynecol 46:19, 1943.

Melody GF: Obstructed cervix. Obstet Gynecol 10:190, 1957.

Mostafa SAM, Bargeron CB, Flower RW, et al: Foreign body granulomas in normal ovaries. Obstet Gynecol 66:701, 1985.

Naumann RO, Droegemueller W: Unusual etiology of vulvar hematomas. Am J Obstet Gynecol 142:357, 1982.

Neuwirth RS: Hysteroscopic management of symptomatic submucous fibroids. Obstet Gynecol 62:509, 1983.

Neuwirth RS: Urethral prolapse—a cause of vaginal bleeding in young girls. Obstet Gynecol 22:290, 1963.

Nichols DH, Julian PJ: Torsion of the adnexa. Clin Obstet Gynecol 28:375, 1985.

Novak ER, Woodruff JD, eds: Novak's gynecologic and obstetric pathology, 6th ed. Philadelphia, W.B. Saunders Co., 1967.

Ong HC, Chan WF: Mucinous cystadenoma, serous cystadenoma and benign cystic teratoma of the ovary. Cancer 41:1538, 1978.

Pantoja E, Rodriguez-Ibanez I, Axtmayer RW, et al: Complications of dermoid tumors of the ovary. Obstet Gynecol 45:89, 1975.

Papadaki L, Beilby JOW: Ovarian cystadenofibroma: a consideration of the role of estrogen in its pathogenesis. Am J Obstet Gynecol 121:501, 1975.

Pauerstein CJ: The fallopian tube: A reappraisal. Philadelphia, Lea & Febiger, 1974.

Paull T, Tedeschi LG: Perineal endometriosis at the site of episiotomy scar. Obstet Gynecol 40:28, 1972.

Persaud V, Arjoon PD: Uterine leiomyoma. Obstet Gynecol 35:432, 1970.

Peters WA, Thiagarajah S, Thornton WN: Ovarian hemorrhage in patients receiving anticoagulant therapy. J Reprod Med 22:82, 1979.

Peters WA, Vaughan ED: Urethral diverticulum in the female. Obstet Gynecol 47:549, 1976.

Peterson WF, Novak ER: Endometrial polyps. Obstet Gynecol 8:40, 1956.

Petterson B, Adami H-O, Lindgren A, et al: Endometrial polyps and hyperplasia as risk factors for endometrial carcinoma. Acta Obstet Gynecol Scand 64:653, 1985.

Piver MS, Williams LJ, Marcuse PM: Influence of luteal cysts on menstrual function. Obstet Gynecol 35:740, 1970.

Radisavljevic SV: The pathogenesis of ovarian inclusion cysts and cystomas. Obstet Gynecol 49:424, 1977.

Ranney B, Frederick I: The occasional need for myomectomy. Obstet Gynecol 53:437, 1979.

Reid JD, Kommareddi S, Lankerani M, et al: Chronic expanding hematomas. JAMA 244:2441, 1980.

Richardson DA, Hajj SN, Herbst AL: Medical treatment of urethral prolapse in children. Obstet Gynecol 59:69, 1982.

Robboy SJ, Ross JS, Prat J, et al: Urogenital sinus origin of mucinous and ciliated cysts of the vulva. Obstet Gynecol 51:347, 1978.

Roberts CL, Marshall HK: Fibromyoma of the fallopian tube. Am J Obstet Gynecol 82:364, 1961.

Rome RM, Fortune DW, Quinn MA, et al: Functioning ovarian tumors in postmenopausal women. Obstet Gynecol 57:705, 1981.

Samaha M, Woodruff JD: Paratubal cysts: frequency, histogenesis, and associated clinical features. Obstet Gynecol 65:691, 1985.

Samanth KK, Black WC: Benign ovarian stromal tumors associated with free peritoneal fluid. Am J Obstet Gynecol 107:538, 1970.

Sauer M, Rodi I, Bustillo M: Unilateral vulvar edema after intraperitoneal Hyskon administration. Fertil Steril 44:546, 1985.

Shevchuk MM, Fenoglio CM, Richart RM: Histogenesis of Brenner tumors, I. Histology and structure. Cancer 46:2607, 1980.

Silvers DN, Halperin AJ: Cutaneous and vulvar melanoma: an update. Clin Obstet Gynecol 21:1117, 1978.

Smith NC, Van Coeverden de Groot HA, Gunston KD: Coital injuries of the vaginal in nonvirginal patients. S Afr Med J 64:746, 1983.

Soules MR, McCarty KS: Leiomyomas: steroid receptor content. Am J Obstet Gynecol 143:6, 1982.

Spanos WJ: Preoperative hormonal therapy of cystic adnexal masses. Am J Obstet Gynecol 116:551, 1973.

Stephenson WM, Laing FC: Sonography of ovarian fibromas. AJR 144:1239, 1985.

Stern JL, Buschema J, Rosenshein NB, et al: Spontaneous rupture of benign cystic teratomas. Obstet Gynecol 57:363, 1981.

Sutherland JA, Wilson EA, Edger DE, et al: Ultrastructure and steroid-binding studies in leiomyomatosis peritonealis disseminata. Am J Obstet Gynecol 136:992, 1980.

Tang LCH, Cho HKM, Chan SYW, et al: Dextropreponderance of corpus luteum rupture. J Reprod Med 30:764, 1985.

Thomas R, Barnhill D, Bibro M, et al: Hidradenitis suppurativa: a case presentation and review of the literature. Obstet Gynecol 66:592, 1985.

Valente PT: Leiomyomatosis peritonealis disseminata. Arch Pathol Lab Med 108:669, 1984.

Valle RF: Hysteroscopic evaluation of patients with abnormal uterine bleeding. Surg Gynecol Obstet 153:521, 1981.

Venter PF, Rohm GF, Slabber CG: Giant neurofibromas of the labia. Obstet Gynecol 57:128, 1981.

Waxman M, Boyce JG: Intraperitoneal rupture of benign cystic ovarian teratoma. Obstet Gynecol 48:9S, 1976.

Weissberg SM, Dodson MG: Recurrent vaginal and cervical ulcers associated with tampon use. JAMA 250:1430, 1983.

Westhoff CL, Beral V: Patterns of ovarian cyst hospital discharge rates in England and Wales, 1962-79. Br Med J 289:1348, 1984.

Williams LJ, Pavlick FJ: Leiomyomatosis peritonealis disseminata. Cancer 45:1726, 1980.

Wolfe SA, Mackles A: Malignant lesions arising from benign endometrial polyps. Obstet Gynecol 20:542, 1962.

Woodworth H, Dockerty MB, Wilson RB, et al: Papillary hidradenoma of the vulva: a clinicopathologic study of 69 cases. Am J Obstet Gynecol 110:501, 1971.

Youssef AF, Fayad MM, Shafeek MA: Torsion of the fallopian tube. Acta Obstet Gynecol Scand 41:291, 1962.

KEY TERMS AND DEFINITIONS

Adenomyoma. An isolated area of endometrial glands and stroma in the uterine musculature that can be identified grossly.

Adenomyosis. The growth of endometrial glands and stroma in the uterine myometrium at a depth of at least 2.5 mm from the basalis layer of the endometrium.

Chocolate Cyst. A cystic area of endometriosis in the ovary.

Coelomic Metaplasia. The potential ability of coelomic epithelium to develop into several different histologic cell types.

Danazol. A synthetic steroid, an attenuated androgen, that is active when taken orally.

Dyschezia. Difficult or painful evacuation of feces from the rectum.

Endometrioma. A small area of endometriosis that can be identified macroscopically.

Endometriosis. The presence and growth of glands and stroma identical to the lining of the uterus in an aberrant location.

Retrograde Menstruation. The flow of menstrual blood, endometrial cells, and debris via the fallopian tubes into the peritoneal cavity.

ENDOMETRIOSIS

Endometriosis is a benign though progressive disease. The wide spectrum of clinical problems that occur with endometriosis has frustrated gynecologists, fascinated pathologists, and burdened patients for years. Though the first histologic description of aberrant endometrial glands and stroma was published in 1860, the classic studies of Sampson in the 1920s were the first to emphasize the clinical and pathologic correlations of endometriosis. Even today, many aspects of the disease remain enigmatic.

By definition, endometriosis is the presence and growth of the glands and stroma of the lining of the uterus in an aberrant or heterotopic location. Adenomyosis is the growth of endometrial glands and stroma in the uterine myometrium at a depth of at least 2.5 mm from the basalis layer of the endometrium. Adenomyosis is sometimes termed *internal endometriosis*.

It is generally believed that the incidence of endometriosis has been increasing over the past 25 years. This "opinion" may be secondary to an enlightened awareness of mild to moderate endometriosis as diagnosed by the increasing use of laparoscopy. Some speculate the "epidemic of endometriosis" is secondary to changes in society that have resulted in delayed childbearing for many women. The age-specific incidence or prevalence of endometriosis is unknown. Any statements concerning the incidence of endometriosis are approximations. Many patients are diagnosed incidentally during laparoscopy or exploratory celiotomy for a variety of other indications. Conservative estimates find endometriosis present in 5% to 15% of laparotomies performed on reproductive-age females. If the women are infertile, the incidence of endometriosis is 30% to 45%.

The etiology of endometriosis is uncertain and may involve retrograde menstruation, vascular dissemination, metaplasia, genetic predisposition, immunologic defects, and hormonal influences. Visualization in the vast majority of endometriosis cases necessitates either laparoscopy or celiotomy. Because few patients have these procedures performed repetitively, the natural history of the disease remains a mystery.

The typical patient with endometriosis is a woman in her mid-thirties who is nulliparous and involuntarily infertile and who has symptoms of secondary dysmenorrhea and pelvic pain. However, in clinical practice the majority of cases are not "classic." Aberrant endometrial tissue grows under the cyclic influence of ovarian hormones; therefore the disease is most commonly found during the reproductive years. Approximately 5% of women with endometriosis are diagnosed following menopause. Postmenopausal endometriosis is usually stimulated by exogenous estrogen. Teenagers with endometriosis should be investigated for obstructive anatomic abnormalities that increase the amount of retrograde menstruation.

Endometriosis is a disease not only of great individual variability but also of contrasting pathophysiologic processes (Table 18-1). It is a benign disease, yet it has the characteristics of a malignancy—locally infiltrative, invasive, and widely disseminating. Although the growth of ectopic endometrium is stimulated by physiologic levels of estrogen and progesterone, both low ("pseudomenopause") and high ("pseudopregnancy") levels of these hormones are usually therapeutic. Another contrast often noted

is the inverse relationship between the extent of pelvic endometriosis and the severity of pelvic pain. Women with extensive endometriosis may be asymptomatic, while other patients with minimal implants may have incapacitating pelvic pain. Finally, there is only speculation as to the underlying pathophysiology that produces infertility in women with endometriosis. Infertility associated with endometriosis is discussed in Chapter 39.

Until the natural history of endometriosis is understood, the clinician will have more questions than answers concerning this benign, progressive, and recurrent disease. These questions are a stimulating challenge to future investigators.

Etiology

There are several theories to explain the histogenesis of endometriosis. However, no single theory adequately explains the protean manifestations of the disease. Most importantly, there is only vague speculation as to why some women develop endometriosis while others do not.

Retrograde Menstruation

The most popular theory is that endometriosis results from retrograde menstruation. Sampson suggested that pelvic endometriosis was secondary to implantation of endometrial cells shed during menstruation. These cells attach to the pelvic peritoneum and under hormonal influence grow as homologous grafts.

A number of experiments in monkeys and clinical observations in humans support this hypothesis. Monkeys developed classic endometriosis when the cervix was sutured to prevent the normal egress of menstrual blood. In these experiments the development of endometriosis was dependent on repetitive "seeding" of the peritoneal cavity. Retrograde menstruation is the rule rather than the exception in all women. This fact has been noted at laparoscopy during the first days of menstrual flow. Recent studies by Blumenkrantz et al. observed bloody dialysate fluid 24 to 48 hours before menstruation in the majority of women being treated with peritoneal dialysis. This bloody peritoneal fluid contained viable endometrial cells.

TABLE 18-1
Endometriosis: A Disease of Clinical Contrasts

Characteristics	Contrasts
Benign disease	Locally invasive
Benign disease	Widespread disseminated foci
Benign disease	Proliferates in pelvic lymph nodes
Minimal disease	Severe pain
Many large endometriomas	Asymptomatic patient
Cyclic hormones cause growth	Continuous hormones reverse the growth pattern

Metaplasia

In contrast to the theory of seeding from retrograde menstruation is the theory of metaplasia from the coelomic epithelium. The müllerian ducts and nearby mesenchymal tissue form the majority of the female reproductive tract. The müllerian duct is derived from the coelomic epithelium during fetal development. The metaplasia hypothesis postulates that the coelomic epithelium retains the ability for multipotential development. It is well known that the surface epithelium of the ovary can differentiate into several different histologic cell types. The decidual reaction of isolated areas of peritoneum during pregnancy is an example of this process.

Metaplasia occurs after an "induction phenomenon" has stimulated the multipotential cell. The induction substance may be a combination of menstrual debris and the influence of estrogen and progesterone. The metaplasia theory helps to explain endometriosis of the umbilicus and deep areas in the rectovaginal septum.

Lymphatic and Vascular Metastasis

The theory of endometrium being transplanted via lymphatic channels and the vascular system helps to explain rare and remote sites of endometriosis such as the spinal column and nose. Endometriosis has been observed in the pelvic lymph nodes of approximately 30% of women with the disease. Hematogenous dissemination of endometrium is the best theory to explain endometriosis of the forearm and thigh, as well as multiple lesions in the lung.

Immunologic Defects

Recent immunologic studies by Dmowski et al. suggest a specific defect in local cell-mediated immunity in women with endometriosis. The investigators were unable to identify a generalized immunologic defect, but their studies documented higher titers of antibodies to endometrial antigens. It is well known that a defect in host response is necessary before antibodies will be developed. The primary defect probably involves a change in function of the peritoneal macrophages so prevalent in the peritoneal fluid of patients with endometriosis. Combining the immunologic etiology with other theories helps partially to explain why some women develop endometriosis while others do not.

Genetic Predisposition

Several studies have documented a familial predisposition to endometriosis with grouping of cases of endometriosis in mothers and their daughters. An investigation by Simpson et al. of the disease demonstrated a sevenfold increase in the incidence of endometriosis in relatives of women with the disease as compared to controls. One out of 10 women with severe endometriosis will have a sister or mother with clinical manifestations of the disease. Women who have a family history of endometriosis are likely to develop the disease earlier in life and have more advanced disease than women whose first-degree relatives are free of the disease. Researchers speculate that the predisposition to develop endometriosis is transmitted via polygenic or multifactorial inheritance patterns. The expression of this genetic tendency may depend on an interaction with environmental factors.

• • •

In summary, most authorities believe that several factors are probably involved in the etiology of endometriosis, including transport of endometrium, a genetic predisposition, and a local immunologic defect. Each factor may contribute to the development of this enigmatic disease (see box below).

Pathology

The majority of endometrial implants are located in the dependent portions of the female

---

ETIOLOGY OF ENDOMETRIOSIS

Retrograde menstruation
Metaplasia
Lymphatic and vascular metastases
Immunologic defect
Genetic predisposition

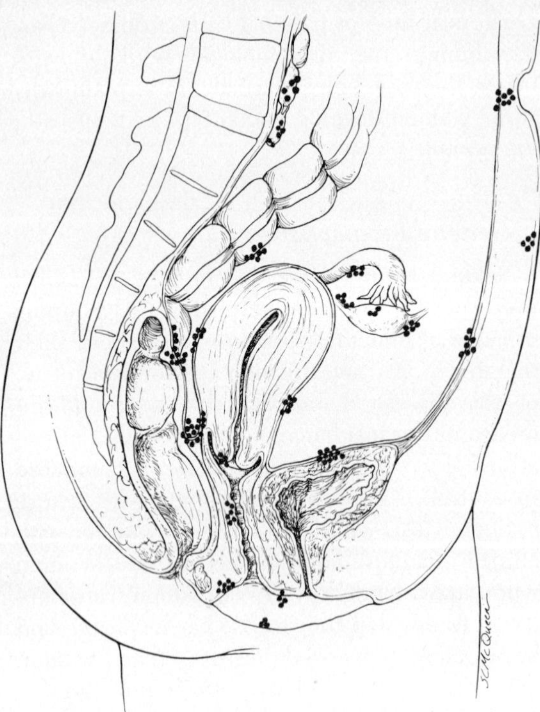

FIGURE 18-1
Common pelvic sites of endometriosis.

pelvis (Fig. 18-1). The ovaries are the most common site, being involved in two of three patients with endometriosis. In most of these patients the involvement is bilateral. The pelvic peritoneum over the uterus, the anterior and posterior cul-de-sac, and the uterosacral, round, and broad ligaments are also frequent sites where endometriosis develops. Pelvic lymph nodes are involved in 30% of cases (Fig. 18-2). The cervix, vagina, and vulva are other possible pelvic locations.

Approximately 10% to 15% of cases involve the rectosigmoid. Depending on the amount of associated scarring, endometriosis of the bowel may be difficult to differentiate grossly from a primary neoplasm of the large intestine.

Rare sites of endometriosis include the umbilicus, areas of previous surgical incisions of the anterior abdominal wall or perineum, bladder, kidney, lung, arms, legs, and even the male urinary tract (Table 18-2).

Gross pathologic changes of endometriosis exhibit wide variability in color, shape, size, and associated inflammatory and fibrotic changes. The gross appearance of the implant

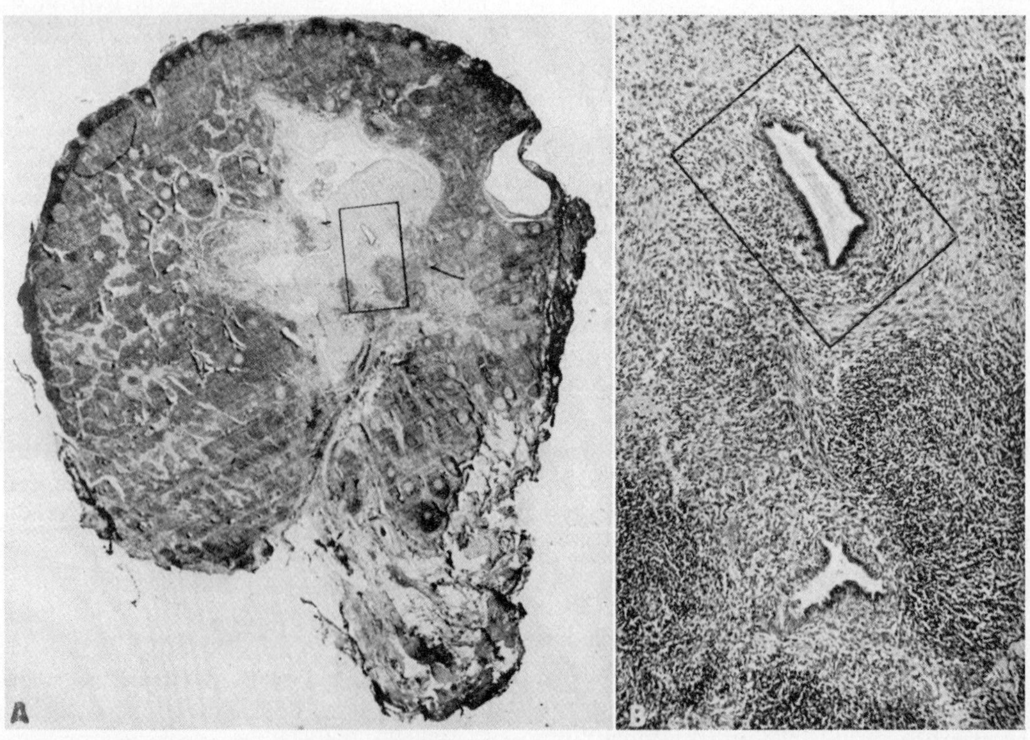

FIGURE 18-2
Endometriosis in right ureteral lymph node. **A,** Low power. **B,** Higher power showing two glands and surrounding stroma. (From Javert CT: Cancer 2:403, 1949.)

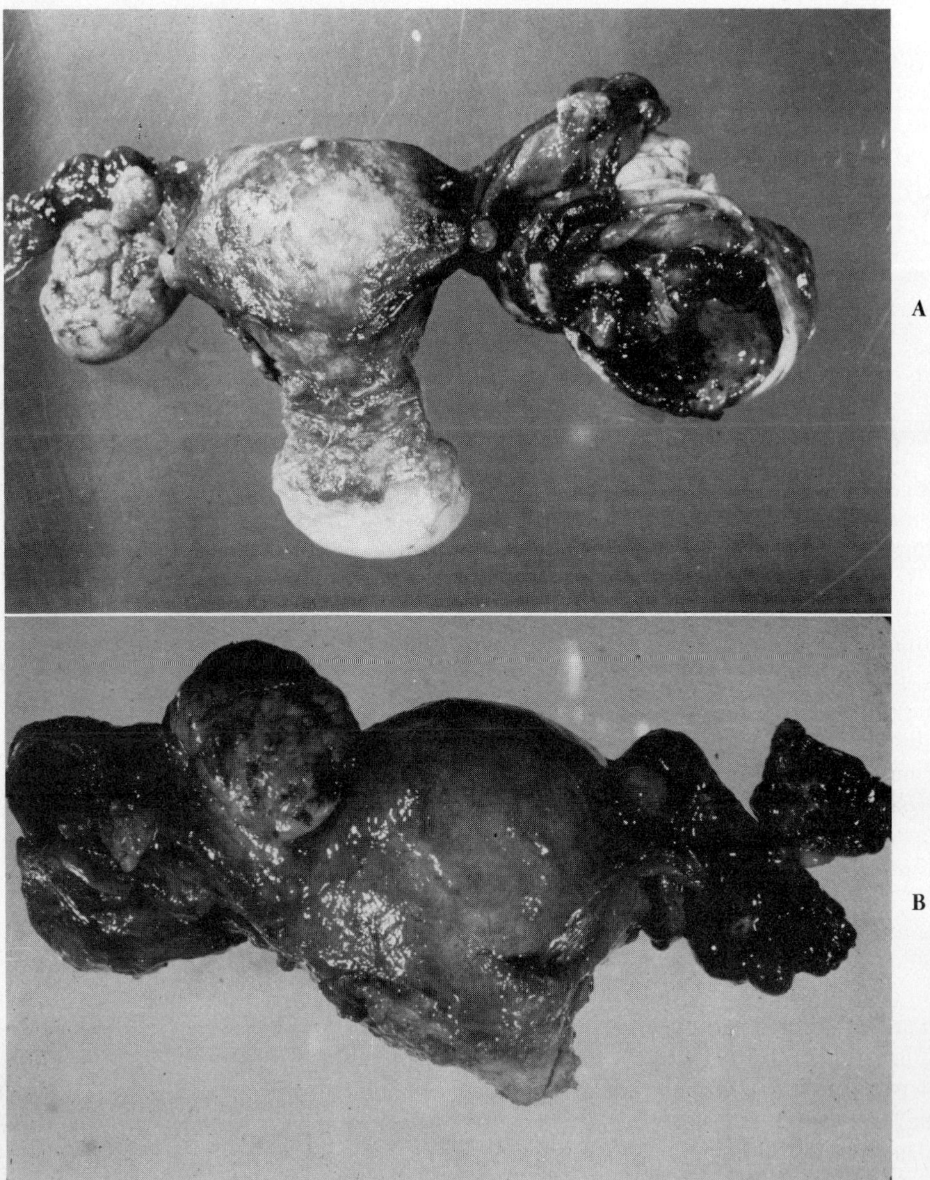

FIGURE 18-3
A, Total hysterectomy specimen from a woman with endometriosis. Right ovary
was partially destroyed by an endometrioma. **B,** Anterior view of same specimen.
Note small endometrial implants on surface of right ovary. (Courtesy Fred Askin,
M.D.)

TABLE 18-2
Anatomic Distribution of Endometriosis

Common Sites	Rare Sites
Ovaries	Umbilicus
Pelvic peritoneum	Episiotomy scar
Ligaments of the uterus	Bladder
Sigmoid colon	Kidney
Appendix	Lungs
Pelvic lymph nodes	Arms
Cervix	Legs
Vagina	Nasal mucosa
Fallopian tubes	Spinal column

depends on the site, activity, and chronicity of the area involved.

New lesions are small, usually blood-filled cysts that are less than 1 cm in diameter. Initially these areas are raised above the surrounding tissues and are either red or bluish black. Colorful adjectives such as "raspberry" or "blueberry" spots describe the gross lesions. With time the areas of endometriosis become larger and assume a light or dark brown color, and they may be described as "powder burn" areas or "chocolate cysts." The older lesions have more intense scarring and are usually puckered or retracted from the surrounding tissue.

The pattern of ovarian endometriosis is also variable (Fig. 18-3). Individual areas vary from 1 mm to large chocolate cysts 8 to 14 cm in diameter. The associated adhesions may be filmy or dense. Larger cysts are usually densely adherent to the surrounding pelvic sidewalls or broad ligament. The pathophysiology of this adhesive process is believed to be repetitive episodes of bloody fluid leaking from the cyst, producing an intense inflammatory response.

The three cardinal histologic features of endometriosis are ectopic endometrial glands, ectopic endometrial stroma, and hemorrhage into the adjacent tissue (Figs. 18-4 and 18-5). Previous hemorrhage can be discovered by identifying large macrophages filled with hemosiderin near the periphery of the lesion. In the majority of cases the aberrant endometrial glands and stroma respond in cyclic fashion to estrogen and progesterone. Depending on the

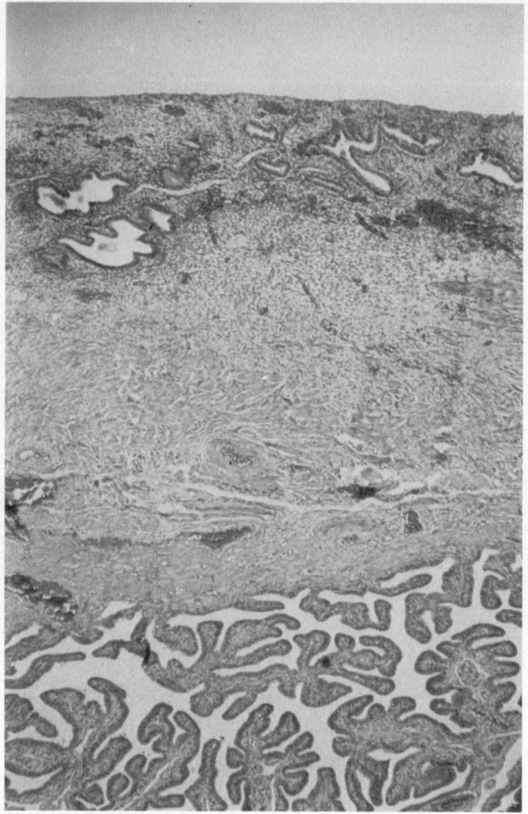

FIGURE 18-4
Endometriosis on fallopian tube. Serosa of tube is being invaded by glands and stroma. (Courtesy Fred Askin, M.D.)

local blood supply, these changes may or may not be in synchrony with the endometrial lining of the uterus. The ectopic endometrial stroma will undergo classic decidual changes similar to pregnancy when exposed to physiologic or pharmacologic levels of progesterone.

In approximately 25% of the cases of endometriosis, viable endometrial glands and stroma cannot be identified. Repetitive episodes of hemorrhage may lead to severe inflammatory changes and result in the glands and stroma undergoing necrobiosis secondary to pressure atrophy or lack of blood supply. In these cases a presumptive diagnosis of endometriosis is made by visualizing the intense inflammatory reaction and the large macrophages filled with blood pigment.

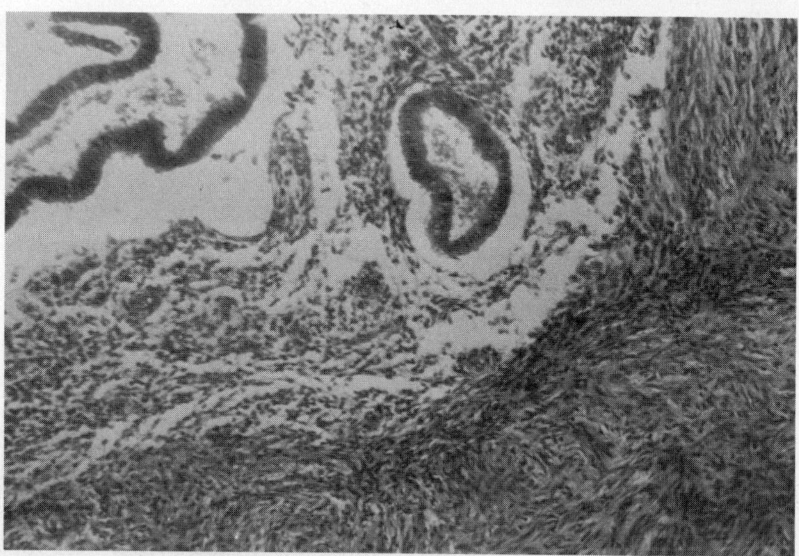

FIGURE 18-5
High-power view of endometrial glands in ovarian stroma. (Courtesy Fred Askin, M.D.)

Clinical Diagnosis

Symptoms

The classic symptoms of endometriosis are cyclic pelvic pain and infertility. The pelvic pain is usually chronic and presents as secondary dysmenorrhea and dyspareunia. However, approximately one third of patients with endometriosis are asymptomatic, with the disease being discovered incidentally during an abdominal operation or visualized at laparoscopy for an unrelated problem.

Clinicians have appreciated the paradox that the extent of pelvic pain is often inversely related to the amount of endometriosis in the female pelvis. Women with large, fixed adnexal masses sometimes have minor symptoms, while other patients with only a few small foci of peritoneal implants may experience moderate to severe chronic pain.

The cyclic pelvic pain is related to the sequential swelling and the extravasation of blood and menstrual debris into the surrounding tissue. The chemical mediator of this intense sterile inflammation and pain is believed to be prostaglandins.

The secondary dysmenorrhea is constant, beginning 24 to 48 hours before menstruation. It varies from a dull ache to severe pelvic pain. It may be unilateral or bilateral and may radiate to the lower back, legs, and groin. Patients often complain of pelvic heaviness or a perception of their internal organs being swollen. Unlike primary dysmenorrhea, the pain may last for several days, including the entire duration of menstrual flow.

The dyspareunia associated with endometriosis is described as pain deep in the pelvis. The etiology of this symptom seems to be immobility of the pelvic organs during coital activity or direct pressure on areas of endometriosis in the uterosacral ligaments or the cul-de-sac of Douglas. Sometimes patients describe areas of point tenderness. The pain, besides being experienced during deep penetration, may continue for several hours following intercourse.

Abnormal bleeding is a symptom noted by 15% to 20% of women with endometriosis. The most frequent complaints are premenstrual spotting and menorrhagia. Usually this abnormal bleeding is not associated with an anovulatory pattern.

Groll recently reported an increased incidence (twofold to threefold) of first trimester abortion in women with untreated endometriosis. The etiology of this association was postulated to be corpus luteum dysfunction or autoimmunity. Medical or surgical therapy for the endometriosis was followed by a decrease in the abortion rate to normal levels.

Less common, yet troublesome, are the symptoms resulting from endometriosis influencing the gastrointestinal and urinary tracts. Cyclic abdominal pain, intermittent constipation, diarrhea, dyschezia, urinary frequency, ysuria, and hematuria are all possible symptoms. Bowel obstruction and hydronephrosis may occur. One rare clinical manifestation of endometriosis is catamenial hemothorax, bloody pleural fluid occurring during menses.

Signs

The most prominent pelvic finding of endometriosis is a fixed retroverted uterus with scarring and tenderness posterior to the uterus. The characteristic nodularity of the uterosacral ligaments and cul-de-sac of Douglas may be palpated on rectovaginal examination. Advanced cases have extensive scarring and narrowing of the posterior vaginal fornix. The ovaries may be enlarged and tender and are often fixed to the broad ligament or lateral pelvic sidewall. The adnexal enlargement is rarely symmetric, as one might expect in other benign pelvic conditions.

Endometriosis is a disease that produces tenderness of the pelvic structures and scarring that restricts movement of the pelvic organs. Occasionally the physician discovers endometriosis in an old surgical incision or a site of a previous amniocentesis. Speculum examination may demonstrate a small area of endometriosis on the cervix or upper vagina.

If a patient presents with secondary dysmenorrhea, deep dyspareunia, and infertility and if on pelvic examination the physician discovers bilateral adnexal tenderness, a fixed posterior uterus, and beading of the uterosacral ligaments, the diagnosis is straightforward. If the diagnosis of endometriosis is in doubt, an experienced clinician will instruct the patient to return for a pelvic examination on the first day of her menstrual flow. This is the time of maximum swelling and tenderness of the areas of endometriosis. The diagnosis can be confirmed in most cases by direct laparoscopic visualiza-

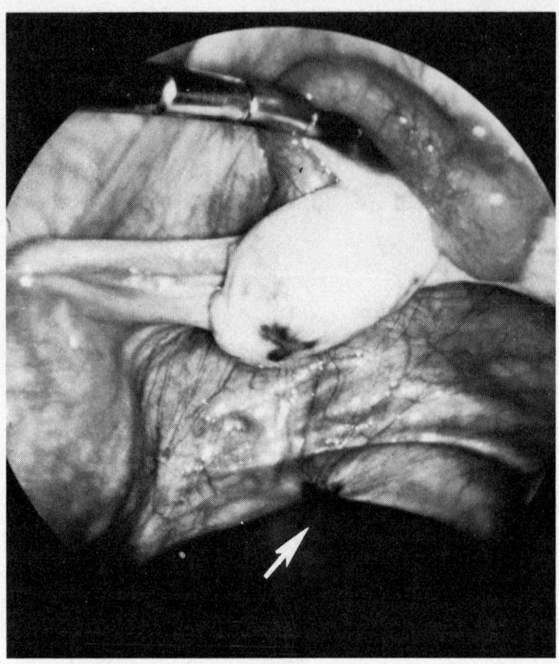

FIGURE 18-6
Laparoscopic view of ovarian and pelvic endometriosis. Tube is being elevated by a probe. Note retracted area of broad ligament around endometriosis *(arrow)*. (Courtesy Jaroslav Hulka, M.D.)

tion of endometriosis with its associated scarring and adhesion formation. In many patients it is discovered for the first time during an infertility investigation. Biopsy of selected implants gives confirmation of the diagnosis. However, biopsy via the laparoscope is not always possible, and sometimes the pathologist may be unable to find glandular elements and endometrial stroma in the biopsy specimens.

When laparoscopy is undertaken to establish the diagnosis of endometriosis, it is important to describe systematically the extent of the pathology (Figs. 18-6 to 18-8). This will help to establish a starting point to measure the results of future therapy. Several systems have been devised to quantitate the extent of the endometriosis. The American Fertility Society classification of endometriosis is useful for patients with infertility (Chapter 39). For patients with pelvic pain the staging system depicted in Table 18-3 is a good model to follow for the success of therapy.

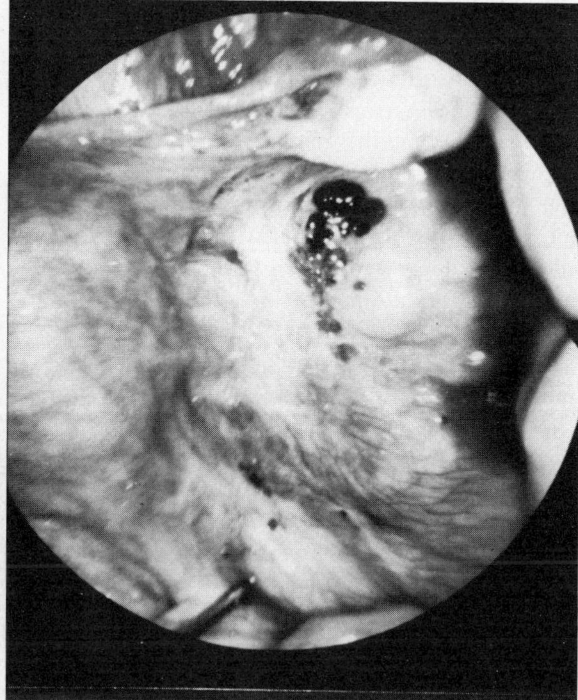

FIGURE 18-7
Laparoscopic view of endometriosis on posterior leaf of broad ligament and cul-de-sac. Note the many adhesions. (Courtesy Jaroslav Hulka, M.D.)

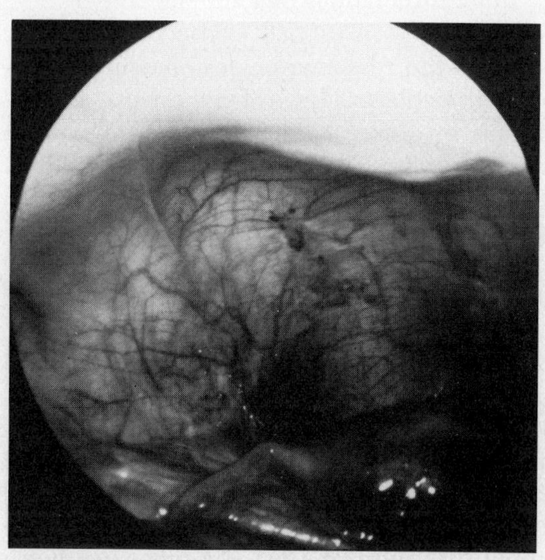

FIGURE 18-8
Laparoscopic view of endometrial implants on sigmoid colon. (Courtesy Jouko Halme, M.D., Ph.D.)

TABLE 18-3
Classification of Endometriosis

Extent of Disease	Findings
Mild	1. Scattered, superficial implants on structures other than uterus, tubes, or ovaries; no scarring 2. Rare, superficial implants on ovaries 3. No significant adhesions
Moderate	1. Involvement of one or both ovaries with multiple implants or small endometriomas (≤ 2 cm) 2. Minimal peritubular or periovarian adhesions 3. Scattered, scarred implants on other structures
Severe	1. Large ovarian endometriomas (≥ 2 cm) 2. Significant tubal or ovarian adhesions 3. Tubal obstruction 4. Obliteration of cul-de-sac, major uterosacral involvement 5. Significant bowel or urinary tract disease

From Puleo JG, Hammond CB: Conservative treatment of endometriosis externa: the effects of danazol therapy. Fertil Steril 40:165, 1983. Reproduced with permission of the publisher, The American Fertility Society.

Although a benign disease, endometriosis exhibits characteristics of both malignancy and sterile inflammation. Therefore the common considerations in the differential diagnosis include chronic pelvic inflammatory disease, ovarian malignancy, degeneration of myomas, adenomyosis, primary dysmenorrhea, and functional bowel disease.

Occasionally a large endometrioma of the ovary may rupture into the peritoneal cavity. This results in an acute surgical abdomen and brings into the differential diagnosis conditions such as ectopic pregnancy, appendicitis, diverticulitis, and a bleeding corpus luteum cyst.

Natural History

Endometriosis is a chronic and progressive disease. The rate of progression of the disease varies widely from one patient to another. Serial pelvic examinations are a poor indicator of progression of the disease. To date, gynecologists do not have a chemical marker or noninvasive test to follow its growth. Therefore the natural history of the disease is largely speculation. In some centers, second-look laparoscopy is routinely performed. These limited studies have given us insight into the success of therapy.

It would be optimal to identify women who are going to develop endometriosis. Clinicians should note the genetic factors in endometriosis and identify family members at risk. The optimal preventive therapy for this progressive disease for a young teenager not desirous of pregnancy until her late twenties is unknown. Clinical options include no treatment, continuous use of oral contraceptives, or cyclic oral contraceptive therapy. Controlled prospective studies are needed to answer the difficult clinical question of the best method to inhibit progression of the disease.

Approximately 10% of teenagers who develop endometriosis have associated congenital outflow obstruction. Therefore teenagers with pelvic pain should be examined for this rare possibility.

Until 20 years ago there was a general belief that pregnancy improved endometriosis. A careful study by McArthur and Ulfelder of external endometriosis, which could be observed throughout the pregnancy, discovered that this generalization was not invariably true. In some cases endometriomas rapidly increase in size during the first few weeks of pregnancy. In general, during the third trimester symptoms are less severe and the size of the external lesions decreases.

Endometriosis is dependent on ovarian hormones to stimulate growth. With a natural menopause there is a gradual relief of symptoms. Following surgical menopause, areas of endometriosis rapidly disappear. However, it is important to note that 5% of symptomatic cases of endometriosis present after the menopause. Many of the cases occurring in women in their late fifties or early sixties are related to the use of exogenous estrogen.

Management

The appropriate treatment for endometriosis varies widely because of the spectrum of clinical symptoms and vast differences in extent of the disease from one patient to another. Therefore the treatment plan must be individualized. Choice of therapy depends on multiple variables, including the patient's age, her future reproductive plans, the location and extent of her disease, her symptoms, and associated pelvic pathology. Most patients should undergo a diagnostic laparoscopy to establish the nature and extent of endometriosis before therapy.

Treatment of endometriosis can be medical, surgical, or a combination of both. The clinical observations that endometriosis regresses after the menopause and that symptoms improve during the latter half of pregnancy have been the basis for hormonal palliation of the disease. The glands and stroma contained in areas of endometriosis and the endometrial glands and stroma of the uterus usually react to hormones in a similar fashion. Most of the sex steroids, alone or in combination, have been tried in clinical studies to suppress the growth of endometriosis. Optimal regression secondary to treatment is observed in small endometriomas that are less than 1 to 2 cm in diameter. Response in larger areas of endometriosis may be minimal with steroid therapy. This poor therapeutic result may be governed by the reduction of blood supply to the mass by surrounding scar tissue.

Surgical therapy is divided into conservative and definitive operations. Conservative surgery involves the resection or destruction of endometrial implants, lysis of adhesions, and attempts to restore normal pelvic anatomy. Definitive surgery involves surgical castration with the removal of both ovaries, the uterus, and all visible ectopic foci of endometriosis.

Medical Therapy

DANAZOL. Since its approval by the Food and Drug Administration in 1975, danazol has been the drug of choice for endometriosis. Danazol also may be prescribed for women with benign cystic mastitis, menorrhagia, and hereditary angioneurotic edema. Danazol is an attenuated androgen that is active when given orally. Chemically it is a synthetic steroid that is the isoxazole derivative of ethisterone (17-alpha-ethinyltestosterone) (Fig. 18-9). The drug is mildly androgenic and anabolic. Many of danazol's side effects are directly related to

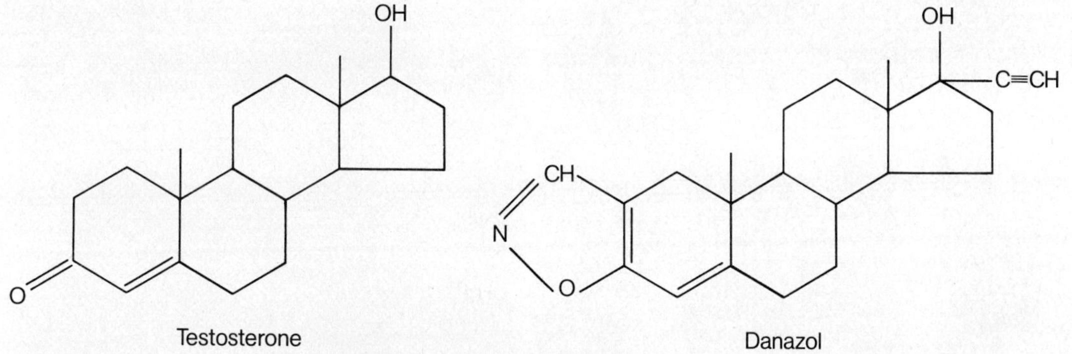

OH

Testosterone

OH

C≡CH

CH

N

O

Danazol

FIGURE 18-9
Chemical structures of danazol and testosterone.

these two properties. Dmowski et al. determined that the androgenic effects of testosterone are approximately 200 times greater than those of danazol.

Danazol was initially prescribed for its "pseudomenopausal effect." The drug significantly decreases follicle-stimulating hormone (FSH) and luteinizing hormone (LH) levels in castrated females. However, in premenopausal women basal levels of gonadotrophins are not influenced. The midcycle surge of FSH and LH is eliminated by a dose of 800 mg a day. The term *pseudomenopause* is a misnomer because during the physiologic menopause gonadotrophins are elevated.

Danazol binds to androgen and progesterone receptors and also binds to sex hormone–binding globulin. The latter effect results in a threefold increase in endogenous free testosterone levels. Danazol directly inhibits several steroidogenic enzymes in both the ovary and the adrenal gland, thus reducing circulating steroid levels. Until the basic mechanisms are further elucidated, the student can remember the misnomer pseudomenopause, which helps to describe the effects at the target organs. For clinicians the effect on the target organ is the desired goal.

The explanations of the exact mechanism of action and underlying pharmacologic properties of danazol are controversial and speculative. Dosages of 800 mg daily produce amenorrhea and inhibition of ovulation within 4 to 6 weeks after the onset of therapy. Danazol definitely produces a hypoestrogenic, hypoprogestational effect on steroid-sensitive end organs. Luciano has found that plasma levels of estro-

gen and progesterone remain in the early follicular range. Danazol induces atrophic changes in the endometrium of the uterus and similar changes in endometrial implants (Fig. 18-10). An endometrial biopsy performed after several weeks of therapy shows endometrial atrophy with few glands and an inactive stroma. It would be difficult to differentiate the biopsy of a young woman taking danazol from the biopsy of a postmenopausal woman.

The standard prescribed dosage of danazol is 400 to 800 mg a day for approximately 6 to 9 months. The half-life of this oral drug is between 4 and 5 hours. Therefore for the 800 mg dosage regimen it is best to recommend one tablet four times a day rather than two tablets in the morning and two at night. The drug is started on the fifth day after the onset of menses. Women should use mechanical contraceptives for the first month, as danazol has produced female pseudohermaphroditism in a developing fetus. If one is certain the patient is not pregnant, danazol is begun on the first day of the menstrual bleeding. By starting the hormone earlier in the cycle the patient will experience less breakthrough bleeding during the first 4 to 6 weeks.

A major drawback of the medication is its expense. A 200 mg tablet costs approximately $1.00 to $1.50, resulting in a total cost of $120 to $180 per month. Because of this factor many investigators have reduced the total daily dosage of the drug. Dmowski et al. and Low et al. compared 600, 400, 200, and even 100 mg of danazol daily. The relief of the symptoms of endometriosis was directly related to the incidence of amenorrhea. The lower dosages of

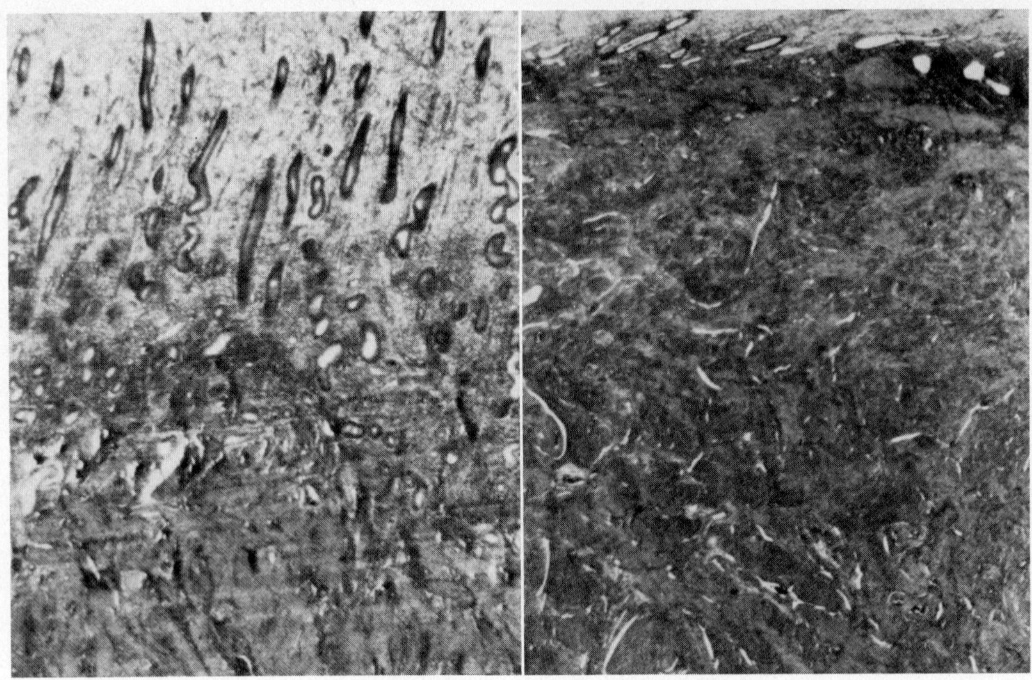

FIGURE 18-10
Left, Untreated endometrium. *Right,* Endometrium after 4 months of treatment with danazol. (From Greenblatt RP, Dmowski WP, Mahesh VB, Scholer HFL: Clinical studies with an antigonadotropin-danazol. Fertil Steril 22:108, 1971. Reproduced with permission of the publisher, The American Fertility Society.)

danazol are not as effective at producing amenorrhea, and the clinical success rates using lower dosages are slightly less with advanced disease than when 400 to 800 mg daily is used. A woman with an atrophic endometrium may occasionally experience breakthrough bleeding.

Side effects of the hormonal pseudomenopause are encountered by 80% of patients taking the drug. Approximately 10% to 20% of women discontinue the drug because of the side effects. Virtually all of the symptoms disappear on cessation of drug therapy. However, there are scattered reports of deepening of the voice that did not resolve after discontinuing the drug. Symptoms that have been related to danazol therapy include menopausal hot flashes, atrophic vaginitis, emotional lability, weight gain averaging 8 to 10 pounds, fluid retention, migraine headaches, dizziness, fatigue, depression, oily skin, facial hair, and deepening of the voice (Table 18-4).

Danazol is metabolized in the liver with cleavage of the isoxazol ring. The biologic effects of danazol are believed to be from the parent compound and not the metabolites. Holt and Keller reported a mild elevation in serum liver enzyme levels in six of seven women treated for endometriosis. Alkaline phosphatase levels were not changed. Clinicians should be alert to these changes, and women who take danazol for longer than 6 months should have serum liver enzyme determinations.

The standard length of treatment with danazol is 6 to 9 months. Approximately three of four patients note significant improvement in their symptoms, and about 90% have objective improvement discovered at second-look laparoscopy. The uncorrected fertility rate following danazol therapy is approximately 40%. Unfortunately, 15% to 30% of patients will have recurrence of symptoms within 2 years following therapy.

Danazol was found superior to continuous oral contraceptives in a comparison study. Noble and Letchworth found greater subjective

TABLE 18-4
Adverse Reactions to Danazol (800 mg/day)

Androgenic Action

Acne	17%
Edema	6%
Weight gain	5%
Hirsutism	6%
Voice changes	3%

Antiestrogenic Action

Flushes and sweats	15%
Uterine spotting	10%
Decrease in breast size	5%
Change in libido	3% to 5%
Atrophic vaginitis	3%

Idiopathic Drug Reactions

GI disturbances	8%
Weakness, dizziness	8%
Muscle cramps	4%
Skin rashes	3%
Headaches	2%
Sleep disturbances	Uncommon

From Luciano AA: A guide to managing endometriosis. Contemp OB/GYN 19:228, 1982. Modified from Greenblatt R, ed: Recent advances in endometriosis: Proceedings of a symposium, Augusta, GA, Mar. 5-6, 1975. Excerpta Medica, 1976, p. 368.

relief of symptoms and more objective regression of endometriosis during second-look laparoscopy in the danazol group. Fewer patients discontinued danazol because of side effects.

ORAL CONTRACEPTIVES. Kistner was the first to popularize the continuous use of high-dosage combination oral contraceptives for endometriosis. In the late 1950s up to 40 mg of norethynodrel with mestranol (Enovid) daily were given to produce amenorrhea and a "pseudopregnancy." Most of the published studies involve the first-generation, high estrogen content oral contraceptives. However, recent reports have established that the present low estrogen combination pills, specifically the ones with a relatively high progestin potency, are equally effective.

The regimen is started by a single daily oral contraceptive tablet beginning on the third day of the patient's period. The pills are taken continuously until breakthrough bleeding occurs, and then the daily dosage is doubled to relieve breakthrough bleeding. After 5 days of a double dose, the majority of patients can return to one to two pills a day, thereby maintaining their amenorrhea on a comparatively low dosage of steroids. As in other hormonal regimens for endometriosis, amenorrhea is the desired endpoint. Most patients are able to maintain the amenorrhea for 6 to 9 months, using at most three to four contraceptive tablets a day. It is important to emphasize to the patient the goal of continuous rather than intermittent oral contraceptive therapy.

The initial histologic response is similar to that of normal pregnancy, with an increase in vascularity and edema in the endometrial implants. This transient growth phase may cause an acute exacerbation of the clinical symptoms. Occasionally, large ovarian endometriomas rupture, resulting in an acute surgical abdomen during the first 6 weeks of oral contraceptive therapy. During prolonged therapy the endometrial glands atrophy and the stroma undergoes a marked decidual reaction. Subsequently in most smaller endometriomas that are less than 1 to 2 cm, there is necrobiosis and absorption.

The many side effects of inducing amenorrhea with oral contraceptives include weight gain, breast tenderness, nausea, chloasma, an increase in appetite, irritability, depression, edema, hypertension, and vaginal discharge. Approximately one of three women discontinue this therapy because of the side effects.

The results of continuous oral contraceptive therapy include a decrease in symptomatology in two thirds of patients following therapy and an uncorrected pregnancy rate of about 30%.

OTHER HORMONAL TREATMENTS. For women who cannot tolerate the high dosage of estrogen in the pseudopregnancy regimen or women who have a contraindication to estrogen therapy, treatment with progestins only has been successful. Medroxyprogesterone (Depo-Provera), if given in a dosage of 100 mg intramuscularly every 2 weeks for four doses and then 200 mg every month for four doses, will produce a prolonged amenorrhea. The medication is acceptable for the older woman who has completed childbearing. The time of resumption of ovulation following discontinuation of injectable medroxyprogesterone is prolonged and extremely variable. Some women will not ovulate for more than a year following their last injection. Therefore this form of therapy should not be prescribed for a young woman who is contemplating pregnancy in the near future. Oral medroxyprogesterone in a dosage of 30 to 40 mg a day is an alternative mode of therapy but is more expensive.

The most persistent side effects while taking medroxyprogesterone are breakthrough spotting or bleeding. If there is no contraindication to estrogen, this symptom can be alleviated by small doses of oral estrogen. Many women find unacceptable the changes in mood, depression, and irritability produced by high-dose progestins.

Clinical results with progestin-only therapy are similar to those with continuous oral contraceptives. Some pathologists postulate that suppression of growth of endometriosis by progestins equals the suppression by oral contraceptives, but there is less necrobiosis and absorption.

For historical interest, it is important to mention two other hormonal regimens, methyltestosterone and stilbestrol. Both therapies enjoyed initial enthusiasm but are rarely prescribed today.

GnRH AGONISTS. The recent isolation and characterization of gonadotrophin releasing hormone (GnRH) has led to the development of two new types of pharmacologic drugs. GnRH analogs that competitively bind with the receptor and have a short biologic half-life are termed *antagonists*. Superagonists have a much longer half-life and induce a downward regulation of LH-RH receptors because of prolonged receptor occupation.

Early clinical studies treating endometriosis involved pharmacologic doses of the superagonists. These drugs dramatically suppressed the pituitary-ovarian axis. Meldrum et al. found that within 2 weeks of initiating daily therapy, not only were levels of FSH and LH suppressed, but serum estrogen levels were in the menopausal range. Endometrial biopsies demonstrated atrophy of both endometrial glands and stroma. These drugs are administered twice daily either by the intranasal or by the subcutaneous route. The greatest advantage of LH-RH agonists is their production of a pseudomenopause or medical castration without the side effects of danazol on other steroid-sensitive organs. Lemay and Quesnel noted in preliminary clinical trials that ovulation resumes within 45 days of discontinuing the drug. Second-look laparoscopy after 6 months of continuous therapy in a small series demonstrated regression of 85% of endometriosis.

Surgical Therapy

The choice between medical treatment to suppress endometriosis and surgical therapy to remove it depends on the patient's age, symptomatology, and reproductive desires. A surgical approach is mandatory in cases involving acute rupture of large endometriomas, ureteral obstruction, compromise in the large bowel's function, or adnexal enlargements that reach a diameter of 8 cm or larger.

The surgical techniques for invasive carcinoma and for endometriosis are similar. The infiltrative nature of both disease processes and the associated scarring from endometriosis result in a loss of cleavage planes and tedious, difficult dissections. Technically it is easier to palpate rather than visualize the extent of the infiltrative process of endometriosis. Special care must be taken so as not to injure the bladder or bowel during excision of areas impinging on these structures.

Laparoscopy is employed frequently for diagnostic reasons and can also be used therapeutically for patients with minimal disease. It is possible to lyse adhesions, obtain tissue for biopsy, remove small implants, and cauterize (using electrocautery) other implants via the laparoscope. Recently the argon laser (photocoagulation) and the Nd-YAG or carbon dioxide laser (vaporization) have been directed toward areas of endometriosis via the laparoscope. The laser is preferable to the electrocautery when endometriosis is adjacent to the ureter, bladder, or bowel because the depth of penetration can be controlled.

Conservative surgery has as its goal the removal of all macroscopic, visible areas of endometriosis with preservation of ovarian function. Conservative operations include resection of all areas of ovarian endometriosis and lysis of adhesions during which the principles of microsurgery and plastic surgery are observed. The goals are careful reperitonealization of the pelvis and an attempt to restore the pelvic anatomy to normal. In selecting a microsurgical approach it is current practice to use a fine suture of Dexon or Vicryl and an anti-inflammatory regimen that may include corticosteroids, intraperitoneal dextran, prostaglandin synthetase inhibitors, and prophylactic antibiotics. At the completion of the operation, most surgeons perform a simple anterior suspension of the uterus by suturing the round ligaments to the anterior rectus fascia. In theory this prevents the adnexa from adhering to raw areas in the posterior cul-de-sac, but the efficacy has not been established.

It is a time-honored tradition to perform a dilation and curettage (D&C) in hopes of decreasing the amount of retrograde menstruation. There are no control studies to document the benefits of either D&C or uterine suspension. If the patient has midline pain, such as dysmenorrhea or dyspareunia, occasionally a presacral neurectomy or resection of the uterosacral ligaments may be performed. Approximately one in four women will have a second operation for a recurrence of their disease.

Somewhere between conservative and definitive surgery for endometriosis there is a place for total abdominal hysterectomy with ovarian preservation. This operation is selected for women who have completed childbearing but are in their late twenties or early thirties. It is interesting that without repetitive episodes of retrograde menstruation the endometriosis remains quiescent in the majority of these patients. In approximately 10% of women the disease is progressive, and they subsequently have a second operation involving oophorectomy.

Definitive surgical treatment is reserved for patients with far-advanced disease and for whom future fertility is not a consideration. Patients with pain that continues after medical and conservative surgery are treated by definitive surgery, which involves castration. Definitive surgery involves total abdominal hysterectomy, bilateral salpingo-oophorectomy, and the removal of all visible endometriosis. If the surgeon believes that it is not possible to surgically remove all the areas of endometriosis, it is best to treat a premenopausal woman with medroxyprogesterone or continuous oral contraceptive therapy for 1 year to relieve menopausal symptoms before beginning cyclic exogenous estrogen therapy.

If a patient has recurrent symptoms following definitive surgery for endometriosis and has not been taking exogenous estrogen, it is possible that she has a remnant of residual ovary, which can be diagnosed by measuring serum gonadotrophin levels. If the FSH and LH levels are not in menopausal range, some viable ovarian tissue remains, usually in the retroperitoneal space.

Most surgeons routinely remove the appendix when performing surgery for endometriosis not related to infertility. Pittaway published a series of more than 100 consecutive patients with endometriosis; 13% had histologic evidence of endometriosis in the appendix. This involvement could be discovered by gross examination in only 60% of patients. Appendectomy is generally contraindicated in infertility surgery because of the remote potential of infection, leakage from the stump, or adhesion formation.

The efficacy of oral contraceptives or danazol immediately before or following surgery for endometriosis is unresolved in clinical practice. Those who advocate hormones before surgery believe that it makes the dissection easier, but most surgeons do not use hormones preoperatively. Oral contraceptives carry the additional hazard of producing a hypercoagulable state during the perioperative period. Oral contraceptives and danazol may help eradicate microscopic endometriosis postoperatively. Obviously, they would not be prescribed for a prolonged period of time if fertility was the primary concern.

Gastrointestinal Tract Endometriosis

One in three women with endometriosis has involvement of the gastrointestinal tract (Fig. 18-11). The severity and extent of involvement of the bowel by ectopic endometrium varies from the incidental finding of a spot on the serosa of the bowel to obstruction of the rectosigmoid. Most cases are insignificant and do not produce clinical symptoms. In the majority of cases, endometriosis of the gastrointestinal tract involves the sigmoid colon and the anterior wall of the rectum. Endometriosis of the appendix is fairly common. The incidence in patients with pelvic endometriosis is reported

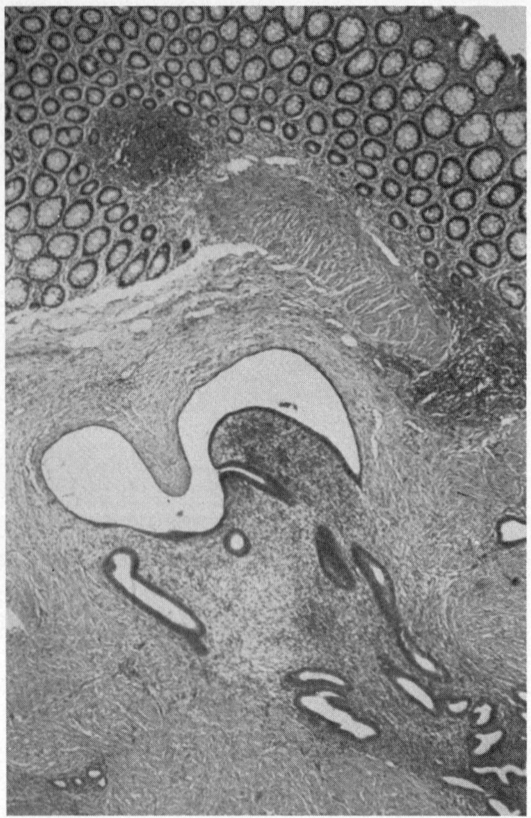

FIGURE 18-11
Endometriosis in bowel wall. (Courtesy Fred Askin, M.D.)

between 1% and 13% (Fig. 18-12). However, endometriosis of the small bowel is rare.

Classic symptoms of endometriosis of the large bowel include cramping, lower abdominal pain, and pain with defecation, especially during the menstrual period. Associated with the abdominal and pelvic pain is a change in bowel function, usually constipation. It is difficult to differentiate the symptoms associated with endometriosis from the constellation of symptoms associated with inflammatory disease of the colon or malignancy. On pathologic examination the aberrant endometrial glands and stroma penetrate the serosa and muscularis of the bowel. It is unusual for endometriosis to involve the submucosa of the bowel. The clinical correlation of this pathologic finding is the statement that women with endometriosis rarely have bleeding from the lumen of the bowel. However, recent series published by Meyers et al., Ruponen and Taina, and Fors-

gren et al. have demonstrated that women with advanced endometriosis of the large bowel experience episodic rectal bleeding, even though the submucosa is not involved by active endometriosis.

Diagnosis of endometriosis invading the rectosigmoid is usually suspected by palpation of a pelvic mass or "rectal shelf" on rectovaginal examination. Sigmoidoscopy demonstrates absence of a mucosal lesion in addition to fixation and immobility of the anterior rectal wall. Meyers et al. boldly state that endometriosis has never been diagnosed by biopsy via colonoscope. A barium enema is an important step in suspected cases, for it helps to establish the differential diagnosis and the degree of obstruction. There is no specific radiologic appearance for endometriosis. However, a filling defect and absence of a mucosal lesion with the presence of extra mucosal involvement are usually demonstrated. The definitive diagnosis and differentiation of endometriosis from carcinoma of the bowel may be delayed until a frozen section is obtained during exploratory surgery.

The treatment of endometriosis of the gastrointestinal tract is dependent on the extent and severity of symptoms. Endocrine therapy is not recommended for advanced cases. The importance of preoperative preparation of the bowel in difficult cases should not be forgotten. Surgical procedures vary from superficial excision of the endometriosis to bowel resection with anastomosis. Superficial excision involves delicate, tedious surgery to ensure that the lumen of the bowel is not entered.

Urinary Tract Endometriosis

Endometriosis in the female pelvis occasionally produces dysfunction in adjacent pelvic organs. Approximately 10% to 20% of women with endometriosis have involvement of the urinary tract by implants of endometriosis and associated retroperitoneal fibrosis. In most cases aberrant endometrial glands and stroma are discovered on the bladder peritoneum and anterior cul-de-sac. The most serious consequence of urinary tract involvement is ureteral obstruction, which occurs in about 1% of women with endometriosis.

Patients with endometriosis involving the urinary tract have nonspecific clinical presen-

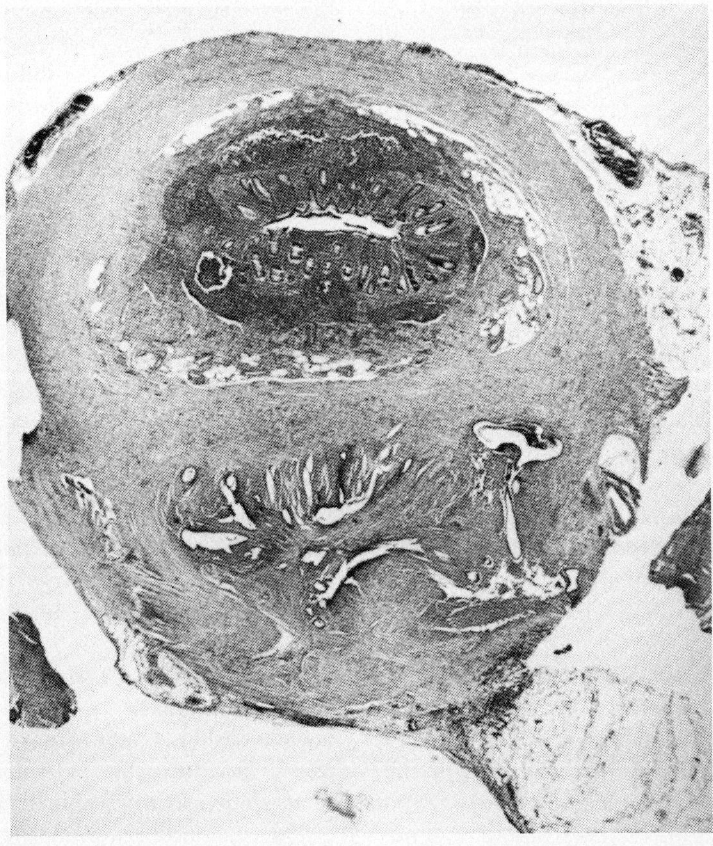

FIGURE 18-12
Cross section of appendix showing lumen of bowel and an island of endometriosis.
(From Dougherty CM: Surgical pathology of gynecologic disease. New York, Harper & Row, Publishers, 1968, p. 636.)

tations. Hematuria and flank pain are experienced by less than 25% of women. One of three women with documented complete ureteral obstruction secondary to endometriosis has no pelvic symptoms whatsoever. The clinical challenge is to diagnose ureteral obstruction at an early stage, before loss of renal function. The obstruction is always in the distal one third of the course of the ureter. The importance of an intravenous pyelogram in all women with retroperitoneal endometriosis cannot be overemphasized.

Treatment of endometriosis of the peritoneum over the bladder can be accomplished by medical or surgical means. Ureteral obstruction may be intrinsic, from active endometriosis, or extrinsic, from long-standing fibrotic reactions to retroperitoneal inflammation. There are few reports of intrinsic endometriosis of the ureter responding to danazol. However, long-term follow-up with serial intravenous pyelograms must be undertaken to ensure that the disease process does not recur.

Surgical therapy is preferred for ureteral obstruction secondary to endometriosis. Because the operations are rare, they must be individualized. However, surgical castration and the relief of urinary obstruction by ureterolysis or by ureteroneocystostomy are the usual alternatives. If ureterolysis is the operation of choice, peristalsis in the involved segment of the ureter should be observed, along with adequate resection of the endometriosis and surrounding inflammation in the retroperitoneal space. Ureteroneocystostomy has the advantage of bypassing the urinary obstruction and making it technically easier to resect the area of endometriosis.

ADENOMYOSIS

Adenomyosis is frequently referred to as *endometriosis interna*. This term is misleading because endometriosis and adenomyosis are discovered in the same patient in less than 20% of women. More importantly, endometriosis and adenomyosis are two clinically different diseases. The only common quality is the presence of ectopic endometrial glands and stroma. Adenomyosis is derived from aberrant glands of the basalis layer of the endometrium. Therefore these glands do not usually undergo the traditional cyclic proliferative and secretory changes that are associated with differing levels of ovarian hormone production.

Adenomyosis is usually diagnosed incidentally by the pathologist examining histologic sections of surgical specimens. The frequency of the histologic diagnosis is directly related to how meticulously the pathologist searches for the disease. If multiple serial sections of the uterus are obtained, the incidence may exceed 60% in women 40 to 50 years of age. Adenomyosis is also a common incidental finding during autopsy. Serial histologic slides confirm the continuity of downward growth of the basalis layer of the endometrium. Thus the histogenesis of adenomyosis is direct extension from the endometrial lining. The pathogenesis of adenomyosis remains unknown. The current theory is that high levels of estrogen stimulate hyperplasia of the basalis layer of the endometrium. For an unknown reason the barrier between the endometrium and myometrium is broken. Initially the stroma and subsequently the glands begin to invade the myometrium along the path of least resistance. In most instances this growth is adjacent to lymphatic and vascular channels.

Pathology

There are two distinctly different pathologic presentations of adenomyosis. Most common is a diffuse involvement of both anterior and posterior walls of the uterus. The individual areas of adenomyosis are not encapsulated. The second presentation is a focal area or adenomyoma. This results in an asymmetric uterus, and this special area of adenomyosis may have a pseudocapsule.

In the more common diffuse type of adenomyosis the uterus is uniformly enlarged, usually two to three times normal size. Sometimes it is difficult to distinguish grossly from uterine leiomyomas. When the myometrium is transected by a knife, the cut surface protrudes convexly and has a spongy appearance. The cut surface of a uterus with adenomyosis is darker than the white surface of a myoma. Sometimes there are discrete areas of adenomyosis that are not densely encapsulated and contain small dark cystic spaces. There is no distinct cleavage plane around focal adenomyomas, as there is with uterine myomas.

Benign endometrial glands and stroma are seen within the myometrium. It is rare for these glands to undergo the same cyclic changes as the normal uterine endometrium. Studies have demonstrated a lack of progesterone receptors in tissue from adenomyosis. There are also fewer estrogen receptors than in normal endometrium. This deficiency of receptors helps to explain the lack of responsiveness of adenomyosis to hormonal therapy.

The standard criterion used in diagnosis of adenomyosis is the finding of endometrial glands and stromas that are more than one low-powered field (2.5 mm) from the basalis layer of the endometrium (Fig. 18-13). The small areas of adenomyosis have the same general appearance as the basalis layers of the endometrium. Histologically the glands exhibit an inactive or proliferative pattern. Occasionally one sees cystic hyperplasia and rarely a secretory pattern. Although the areas do not undergo full menstrual-type changes, bleeding may occur in these ectopic areas as evidenced by both gross and microscopic findings. The reaction of the myometrium to the ectopic endometrium is hyperplasia and hypertrophy of individual muscle fibers (Fig. 18-14). Surrounding most foci of glands and stroma are localized areas of hyperplasia of the smooth muscle of the uterus. It is this change in the myometrium that produces the globular enlargement of the uterus.

Clinical Diagnosis

The majority of women with adenomyosis are asymptomatic or have minor symptoms that do not annoy them enough to seek medical

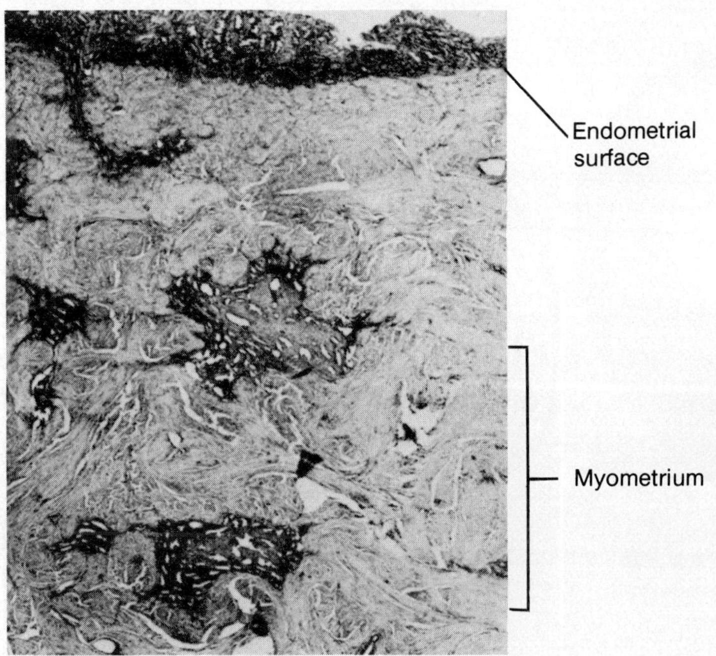

FIGURE 18-13
Adenomyosis. Note islands of endometrial tissue deep within myometrium. (From Janovski NA, Dubrauszky V: Atlas of gynecologic and obstetric diagnostic histopathology. New York, McGraw-Hill Book Co., 1967, p. 217.)

FIGURE 18-14
Adenomyosis. This hysterectomy specimen from a 32-year-old woman has been bisected to demonstrate the hypertrophied myometrium. (From Jeffcoate TNA: Principles of gynaecology, 4th ed. London, Butterworths, 1975, p. 353.)

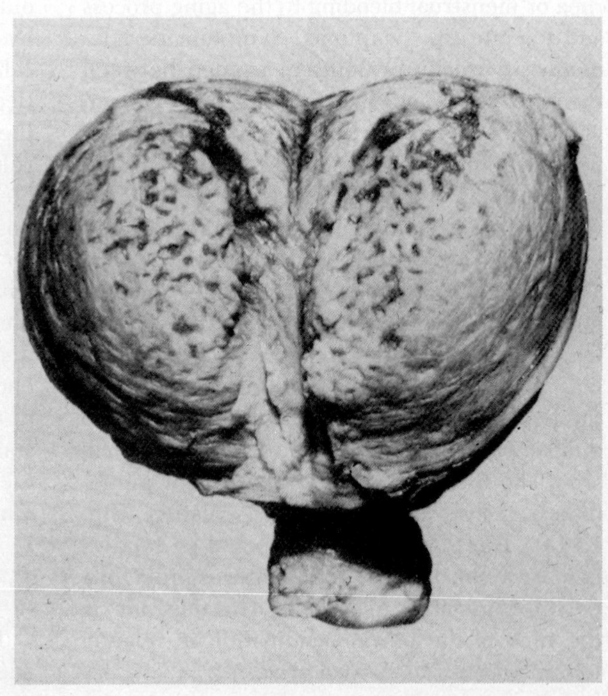

______________ **KEY POINTS, cont'd** ___________________________

- Viable endometrial glands and stroma cannot be identified on pathologic examination in approximately 25% of cases of endometriosis.

- Approximately 10% of teenagers who develop endometriosis have associated congenital outflow obstruction.

- The side effects of danazol are related to its androgenic and anabolic properties as well as to the pseudomenopause produced by the drug.

- Approximately three of four women note significant improvement in symptoms following danazol therapy. One in four will have a recurrence of symptoms within 2 years following completion of medical therapy.

- LH-RH agonists produce a "medical castration" without the side effects of danazol on steroid-sensitive target organs.

- The goals of conservative surgery include removal of macroscopic endometriosis, lysis of adhesions, and restoration of normal anatomy.

- One in three women with endometriosis has involvement of the gastrointestinal tract. Approximately 10% to 20% of women with endometriosis have involvement of the urinary tract.

- Adenomyosis is discovered microscopically in one of three hysterectomy specimens and is frequently asymptomatic.

- Symptomatic adenomyosis primarily occurs in parous women over the age of 35. The classic symptoms are secondary dysmenorrhea and menorrhagia. The most common physical sign is a diffusely enlarged uterus, usually two to three times normal size.

BIBLIOGRAPHY

Andrews WC: Medical versus surgical treatment of endometriosis. Clin Obstet Gynecol 23:917, 1980.

Barbieri RL, Ryan KJ: Danazol: endocrine pharmacology and therapeutic applications. Am J Obstet Gynecol 141:453, 1981.

Bird CC, McElin TW, Manalo-Estrella P: The elusive adenomyosis of the uterus-revisited. Am J Obstet Gynecol 112:583, 1972.

Blumenkrantz MJ, Gallagher N, Bashore RA, et al: Retrograde menstruation in women undergoing chronic peritoneal dialysis. Obstet Gynecol 57:667, 1981.

Buttram VC: Evolution of the revised American Fertility Society classification of endometriosis. Fertil Steril 43:347, 1985.

Buttram VC, Reiter RC, Ward S: Treatment of endometriosis with danazol: Report of a 6-year prospective study. Fertil Steril 43:353, 1985.

Dickey RP, Taylor SN, Curole DN: Serum estradiol and danazol. I. Endometriosis response, side effects, administration interval, concurrent spironolactone and dexamethasone. Fertil Steril 42:709, 1984.

Dmowski WP: Current concepts in the management of endometriosis. Obstet Gynecol Annu 10:279, 1981.

Dmowski WP, Kapetanakis E, Scommegna A: Variable effects of danazol on endometriosis at 4 low-dose levels. Obstet Gynecol 59:408, 1982.

Dmowski WP, Radwanska E: Current concepts on pathology, histogenesis and etiology of endometriosis. Acta Obstet Gynecol Scand Suppl 123:29, 1984.

Dmowski WP, Steele RW, Baker GF: Deficient cellular immunity in endometriosis. Am J Obstet Gynecol 141:377, 1981.

Dougherty CM: Surgical pathology of gynecologic disease. New York, Harper & Row, Publishers, 1968.

Emge LA: The elusive adenomyosis of the uterus. Am J Obstet Gynecol 83:1541, 1962.

Forsgren H, Lindhagen J, Melander S, et al: Colorectal endometriosis. Acta Chir Scand 149:431, 1983.

Greenblatt RP, Dmowski WP, Mahesh VB, et al: Clinical studies with antigonadotropin—danazol. Fertil Steril 22:102, 1971.

Groll M: Endometriosis and spontaneous abortion. Fertil Steril 41:933, 1984.

Holt JP Jr, Keller D: Danazol treatment increases serum enzyme levels. Fertil Steril 41:70, 1984.

Iwasaka T, Okuma Y, Yoshimura T, et al: Endometriosis associated with ascites. Obstet Gynecol 66:72S, 1985.

Janovski NA, Dubrauszky V: Atlas of gynecologic and obstetric diagnostic histopathology. New York, McGraw-Hill Book Co., 1967.

Javert CT: Pathogenesis of endometriosis based on endometrial homeoplasia, direct extension exfoliation and implantation, lymphatic and hematogenous metastasism. Cancer 2:399, 1949.

Jeffcoate TNA: Principles of gynaecology, 4th ed. London, Butterworths, 1975.

Keye WR Jr, Dixon J: Photocoagulation of endometriosis by the argon laser through the laparoscope. Obstet Gynecol 62:383, 1983.

Kistner RW: Infertility with endometriosis. Fertil Steril 13:237, 1962.

Kistner RW: The use of newer progestins in the treatment of endometriosis. Am J Obstet Gynecol 75:264, 1958.

Klein RS, Cattolica EV: Ureteral endometriosis. Urology 13:477, 1979.

Lemay A, Quesnel G: Potential new treatment of endometriosis: reversible inhibition of pituitary-ovarian function by chronic intranasal administration of a luteinizing hormone-releasing hormone (LH-RH) agonist. Fertil Steril 38:376, 1982.

Low RAL, Roberts DGR, Lees DAR: A comparative study of various dosages of danazol in the treatment of endometriosis. Br J Obstet Gynaecol 91:167, 1984.

Luciano AA: A guide to managing endometriosis. Contemp OB/GYN 19:211, 1982.

Malinak LR: Infertility and endometriosis: Operative technique, clinical staging, and prognosis. Clin Obstet Gynecol 23:925, 1980.

McArthur JW, Ulfelder H: The effect of pregnancy upon endometriosis. Obstet Gynecol Surv 20:709, 1965.

Meldrum DR, Pardridge WM, Karow WG, et al: Hormonal effects of danazol and medical oophorectomy in endometriosis. Obstet Gynecol 62:480, 1983.

Meyers WC, Kelvin FM, Jones RS: Diagnosis and surgical treatment of colonic endometriosis. Arch Surg 114:169, 1979.

Moore JG, Hibbard LT, Growdon WA, et al: Urinary tract endometriosis: Enigmas in diagnosis and management. Am J Obstet Gynecol 134:162, 1979.

Noble AD, Letchworth AT: Medical treatment of endometriosis: A comparative trial. Postgrad Med J 55(suppl 5):37, 1979.

Ory SJ: Clinical uses of luteinizing hormone-releasing hormone. Fertil Steril 39:577, 1983.

Pittaway DE: Appendectomy in the surgical treatment of endometriosis. Obstet Gynecol 61:421, 1983.

Pratt JH, Williams TJ: Indications for complete pelvic operations and more radical procedures in the treatment of severe or extensive endometriosis. Clin Obstet Gynecol 23:937, 1980.

Puleo JG, Hammond CB: Conservative treatment of endometriosis externa: The effects of danazol therapy. Fertil Steril 40:164, 1983.

Ranney B: Endometriosis. Obstet Gynecol Annu 7:219, 1978.

Ridley JH: The histogenesis of endometriosis. Obstet Gynecol Surv 23:1, 1968.

Rivlin ME, Krueger RP, Wiser WL: Danazol in the management of ureteral obstruction secondary to endometriosis. Fertil Steril 44:274, 1985.

Rossman F, D'Ablaing III G, Marrs RP: Pregnancy complicated by ruptured endometrioma. Obstet Gynecol 62:519, 1983.

Ruponen S, Taina E: Operative treatment of rectal endometriosis. Acta Obstet Gynecol Scand 57:277, 1978.

Sampson JA: Peritoneal endometriosis due to menstrual dissemination of endometrial tissue into peritoneal cavity. Am J Obstet Gynecol 14:422, 1927.

Sanfilippo JS, Wakim NG, Schikler KN, et al: Endometriosis in association with uterine anomaly. Am J Obstet Gynecol 154:39, 1986.

Schmidt CL: Endometriosis: A reappraisal of pathogenesis and treatment. Fertil Steril 44:157, 1985.

Schriock E, Monroe SE, Henzl M, et al: Treatment of endometriosis with a potent agonist of gonadotropin-releasing hormone (nafarelin). Fertil Steril 44:583, 1985.

Schweppe K-W, Wynn RM: Endocrine dependency of endometriosis: An ultrastructural study. Europ J Obstet Gynecol Reprod Biol 17:193, 1984.

Seibel MM, Berger MJ, Weinstein FG, et al: The effectiveness of danazol on subsequent fertility in minimal endometriosis. Fertil Steril 38:534, 1982.

Simpson JL, Elias S, Malinak LR, et al: Heritable aspects of endometriosis. Am J Obstet Gynecol 137:327, 1980.

Suginami H, Hamada K, Yano K: A case of endometriosis of the lung treated with danazol. Obstet Gynecol 66:68S, 1985.

Vasquez G, Cornillie F, Brosens IA: Peritoneal endometriosis: scanning electron microscopy and histology of minimal pelvic endometriotic lesions. Fertil Steril 42:696, 1984.

Wheeler JM, Malinak LR: Recurrent endometriosis: incidence, management, and prognosis. Am J Obstet Gynecol 146:247, 1983.

Williams TJ, Pratt JH: Endometriosis in 1,000 conservative celiotomies: Incidence and management. Am J Obstet Gynecol 129:245, 1977.

Yen SSC: Clinical applications of gonadotropin-releasing hormone and gonadotropin-releasing hormone analogs. Fertil Steril 39:257, 1983.

Disorders of Abdominal Wall and Pelvic Support

————————— KEY TERMS AND DEFINITIONS —————————

Abdominal Wall Hernia. An outpouching of peritoneum with or without intraabdominal contents through weak areas of the abdominal wall.

Cystocele. Protrusion of the bladder into the vagina, signifying the relaxation of fascial supports of the bladder.

Descensus of Cervix and Uterus (Prolapse, Procidentia). Protrusion of the cervix and uterus into the barrel of the vagina.

 First Degree. Prolapse into the upper vagina.

 Second Degree. Prolapse to or near the introitus.

 Third Degree (Complete). Prolapse through the introitus.

Enterocele. Herniation of the pouch of Douglas (cul-de-sac) between the uterosacral ligaments into the rectovaginal septum; usually contains small bowel.

Femoral Hernia. A hernia that occurs through the femoral triangle. The hernia sac passes beneath the inguinal ligament through Hesselbach's triangle (an area bounded laterally by the inferior epigastric artery, inferiorly by the inguinal ligament, and medially by the lateral margin of the rectus sheath).

Incarcerated Hernia. A hernia whose contents cannot be reduced readily.

Incisional Hernia. A hernia that occurs in a surgical incision.

Inguinal Hernia. A hernia that occurs through the inguinal canal.

Pessary. A prosthesis inserted into the vagina to help support pelvic structures.

Rectocele. Protrusion of the rectum into the vagina, signifying a relaxation of rectal supports.

Reducible Hernia. A hernia whose contents can be reduced from the sac.

Sliding Hernia. A hernia in which the organ protruding makes up a portion of the wall of the hernia sac.

Spigelian Hernia. A rare hernia at a point where the vertical linea semilunaris joins the lateral border of the rectus muscle.

Strangulated Hernia. A hernia whose contents are incarcerated and the blood supply to the content's structures is compromised.

Umbilical Hernia. A hernia protruding through the umbilicus.

Urethrocele. Protrusion of the urethra into the vagina, signifying loss of fascial supports of the urethra.

The structural supports of the abdomen and pelvis are susceptible to a number of stresses. In the female these supports are affected by congenital anatomic weaknesses, the stresses of childbearing, injury, surgical damage, and straining. In addition, a combination of chronic stresses such as lifting heavy objects, straining at stool, or activities that require frequent stretching plus the aging process may make older women more susceptible to such abnormalities. This chapter considers hernias of the abdominal wall and pelvic region as well as conditions that are a result of the loss of pelvic supports.

ABDOMINAL WALL HERNIAS

The abdominal wall is made up of the following structures beginning externally: skin; subcutaneous connective tissue; external oblique, internal oblique, and transversus abdominis muscles with their investing fascia; and parietal peritoneum. The rectus abdominis muscles run longitudinally in the midline from the xiphoid to the pubic symphysis. The investing fasciae of the external oblique, internal oblique, and transversus abdominis muscles completely encase the rectus abdominis muscles cephalic to the semilunar line. Caudally from the semilunar line the muscle is completely behind the aponeurosis of the fasciae of these muscles and lies directly on the peritoneum (Fig. 19-1). Normally the investing fasciae join in the midline after surrounding the rectus abdominis muscles.

In the male the descent of the testes from their original retroperitoneal site to the scrotum necessitates passing through the abdominal wall to the inguinal region. At the level of the transversalis fascia where the descent begins, the internal inguinal ring is formed. The medial margin of this ring is defined by the inferior epigastric artery as it courses from the external iliac artery medially and superiorly into the rectus sheath. The inguinal canal runs from the internal inguinal ring obliquely downward, emerging through the external inguinal ring and opening in the external oblique aponeurosis just above the pubic spine and then continuing into the scrotum. This allows for

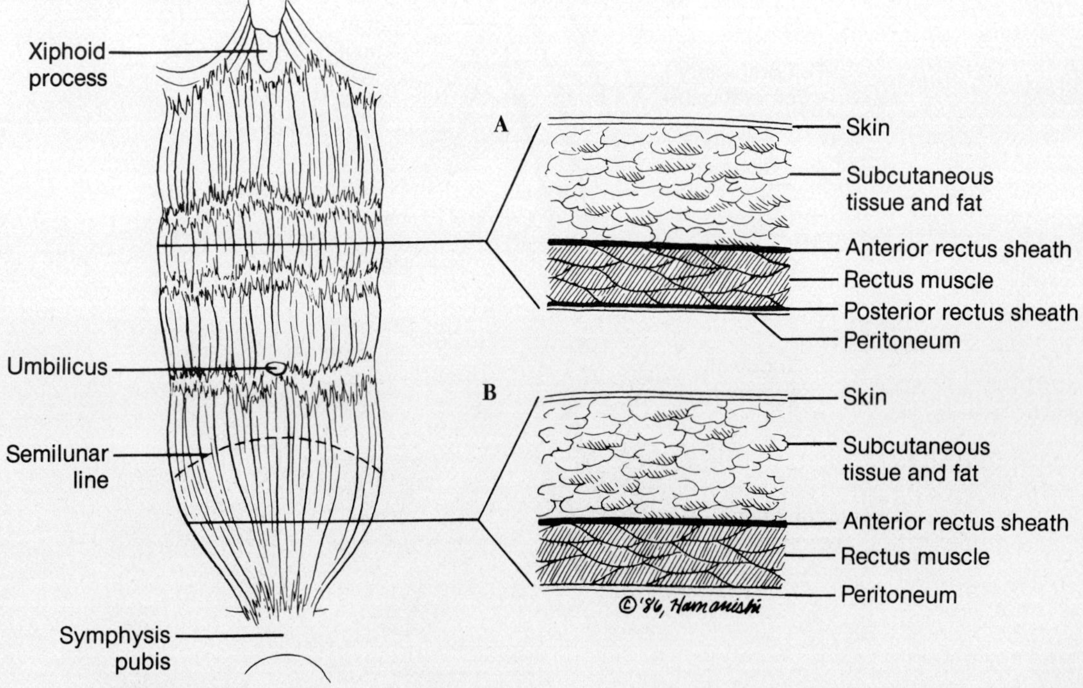

FIGURE 19-1
Graphic representation of layers of the abdominal wall. **A,** Above semilunar line. **B,** Below semilunar line.

passage of the testes and for the presence of part of the spermatic cord.

In the female the round ligament courses in the same direction but ends short of the labia. An inguinal hernia, that is, a bulge of peritoneum through the internal inguinal ring and into the inguinal canal, is less common in the female than in the male and is frequently identified after stretching of the abdominal wall during or following pregnancy. It may be related to a congenital weakness of this area. Occasionally a femoral-type groin hernia may develop. In this case the defect in the transversalis fascia occurs in Hesselbach's triangle, which is an area bounded laterally by the inferior epigastric artery, inferiorly by the inguinal ligament, and medially by the lateral margin of the rectus sheath (Fig. 19-2). The hernia sac passes under the inguinal ligament into the femoral triangle rather than coursing through the inguinal canal. Femoral hernias are more common in females than in males.

The hernia is said to be *reducible* if the con-

tents can be returned to the abdominal cavity. If the contents cannot be reduced, the hernia is said to be incarcerated. An incarcerated hernia may be acute, accompanied by pain, or may be long-standing and asymptomatic. If the blood supply to the incarcerated structure is compromised, the hernia is stated to be *strangulated*. Because the hernia sac is primarily prolapsed peritoneum, the hernia itself is not strangulated but only its contents.

On rare occasions a portion of the wall of the hernia sac is composed of an organ such as the sigmoid colon or the cecum. In these instances the hernia is referred to as a *sliding hernia*.

A ventral hernia occurs in the abdominal wall away from the groin. Examples include umbilical hernias, which are caused by congenital relaxation of the umbilical ring, and incisional hernias, which are herniations through separation of fascial planes following operative incision. Two special ventral hernias include the epigastric hernia, which occurs in a defect of the linea alba above the umbilicus, and the

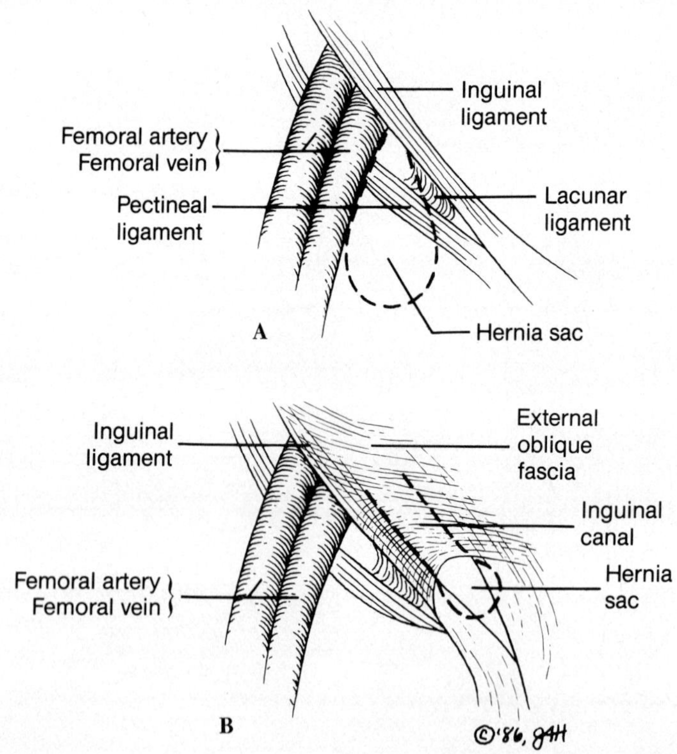

FIGURE 19-2
Graphic representation of right femoral (**A**) and right inguinal (**B**) hernias in the female.

rare spigelian hernia, which is a herniation at a point where the vertical linea semilunaris joins the lateral border of the rectus muscle.

Incisional hernias generally involve the separation of the fascia of the abdominal wall with the hernia sac palpated beneath the skin and subcutaneous tissue. The sac wall is composed of peritoneum.

Because the umbilicus consists of a fusion of skin, fascia, and peritoneum, an umbilical hernia generally occurs because the fascial ring is grossly separated, allowing the hernia sac to protrude. This occurs most frequently in obese women. The hernia sac itself is made up of peritoneum and subcutaneous tissue beneath the skin (Fig. 19-3).

Etiology

Hernias may be the result of a congenital malformation. The umbilical hernia is the best example. Before 10 weeks' gestation the abdominal contents are partially herniated through the umbilicus into the extra embryonic coelomic cavity. However, after 10 weeks the viscera normally return to the abdominal cavity, and the defect in the abdominal wall closes during subsequent fetal growth. Generally at birth only the space occupied by the umbilical cord remains patent. Following the cutting of the cord the area heals so that the skin in the area of the umbilicus fuses above the closed fascial layer. Some infants at birth will show a small umbilical hernia, but in most instances the fascial defect closes during the first 3 years of life. If it does not close, an umbilical hernia will form. In rare cases the abdominal wall closure process is less complete, leading to an omphalocele, which is a hernia sac at the umbilicus covered only by peritoneum and including bowel and other abdominal contents. Omphaloceles are usually seen in infants with other malformations and possibly chromosome anomalies, such as trisomy 13.

Black infants have umbilical hernias more often than do white. Occasionally umbilical hernias occur in adults following the distension of the abdominal cavity with pregnancy or with ascites.

Inguinal hernias are more common in males than in females. Femoral hernias occur primarily in females. Hernias that occur in adults are often associated with trauma or injury. In many instances the hernia bulge develops slowly after years of heavy labor. It is likely that a congenital anatomic defect was always present but became exaggerated over time, leading to the development of a hernia. Zimmerman and Anson felt that such lesions were due to inadequate muscle support at the lower area of the inguinal canal, primarily due to a defect in the internal oblique muscle. Stretching of this area in pregnancy may initiate a hernia, but other factors such as chronic cough due to smoking or chronic respiratory disease may be responsible.

Incisional hernias generally occur because of poor healing of the fascia. This may be secondary to poor nutrition, infection, or necrosis of the fascia secondary to suturing. It may also occur because absorbable suture loses its tensile strength before healing is complete. Stress and strain secondary to chronic cough or retching in the postoperative period may aid the process.

Symptoms and Signs

Bulges in the abdominal wall lead to the discovery of most ventral or groin hernias in women, either by a physician at the time of physical examination or by the patient. These hernias are generally symptom free. Occasionally, excessive straining or trauma will be implicated, and the patient may experience a feeling of tearing of tissue. Frequently the bulges are noted during an increase in intraabdominal pressure such as with pregnancy or ascites. Most hernias are asymptomatic, but in some cases, particularly with larger ones, there may be aching or discomfort. Should intraabdominal

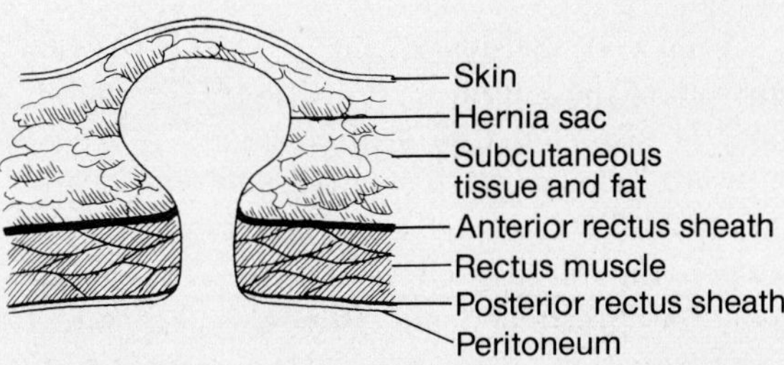

FIGURE 19-3
Graphic representation of umbilical hernia.

organs move into the sac the patient may experience some discomfort. Organs that strangulate within the sac cause acute pain and discomfort. Incarcerated organs may give nonspecific visceral pain, which is most likely due to mesenteric stretching.

In cases where a hernia exists but no contents are within the sac, physical examination reveals a weakening at the site of the hernia. It is often possible to feel the "ring" of the hernia as one palpates the defect through the skin and subcutaneous tissue. The patient's straining will generally accentuate the hernia, making it more palpable and visible. In the case of inguinal and femoral hernias it may be necessary for the patient to be standing for one to palpate the hernia.

When there are intraabdominal contents within the hernia sac, the hernia is more easily palpated. The physician should then decide, based on his or her attempts to gently milk the contents from the sac back through the defect ring, whether the contents are reducible. For hernias that do not reduce easily but in which there is no evidence of vascular compromise it is sometimes useful to apply ice packs to the abdomen in the area of the incarcerated hernia before additional attempts are made to reduce it. In cases of strangulated hernia, evidence for devitalization of an organ, such as fever, leukocytosis, and evidence for an acute abdomen, may be noted.

Management

Nonoperative management of hernias of the ventral wall and groin in women is often feasible. Umbilical hernias in little girls will generally close by age 3 or 4 years and rarely become incarcerated. An incisional hernia, if not too large, can frequently be managed by a corset, which prevents it from becoming incarcerated. Unincarcerated groin hernias are often small and only become uncomfortable with an increase in intraabdominal pressure, such as occurs with pregnancy. Many authors advocate repair, however, because the small neck of these hernias may make incarceration more likely. With pregnancy the opportunity for incarceration is reduced because the increasing size of the uterus pushes bowel contents away from the area of the herniation. Trusses and other supports are generally difficult to fit and are of little value in women.

Larger hernias, hernias that continuously contain intraabdominal contents, hernias that cause continuing discomfort, and those that have been incarcerated should be repaired. Some general principles of operative repair can be stated. The first principle involves the anatomy of the hernia. The hernia almost always consists of a sac of peritoneum with a narrow neck and a fascial defect of some sort. In rare instances, if a peritoneal sac is broad based, it may be possible to simply reduce the sac through the fascial defect without opening it and then to repair the fascial defect. However, if a narrow-necked sac exists, it must be dissected free of the fascial defect, emptied of its contents, and then excised and sutured at the neck (base). The fascial defect is then mobilized completely to remove stress and scarring, and it is closed with permanent suture. In rare cases the fascial defect may be large and the degree of mobilization that is required may be impossible. In such instances, patching with inert material such as Mersilene mesh may be necessary. This is rarely required in women except in the presence of large incisional hernias.

The second principle involves management of the contents of the hernia sac. Usually the hernia sac reduces with ease, but if intraabdominal contents are fixed to the sac wall by adhesions, the sac must be opened and the adhesions carefully separated. Care must be taken not to damage the organs or their blood supply. When these organs are reduced from the sac, the sac may be handled in the usual fashion. When incarceration has occurred, the organs must be inspected for viability before replacement.

Umbilical Hernia

A curved incision is made at the inferior margin of the umbilicus (Fig. 19-4). The umbilicus is dissected free of the sac and reflected upward. The sac is then dissected free of the fascial defect and either reduced or excised, depending on the circumstances. The fascial edges are freshened and either closed by direct approximation anterior to posterior using nonabsorbable sutures or mobilized and closed in a "vest over pants" manner, suturing the ante-

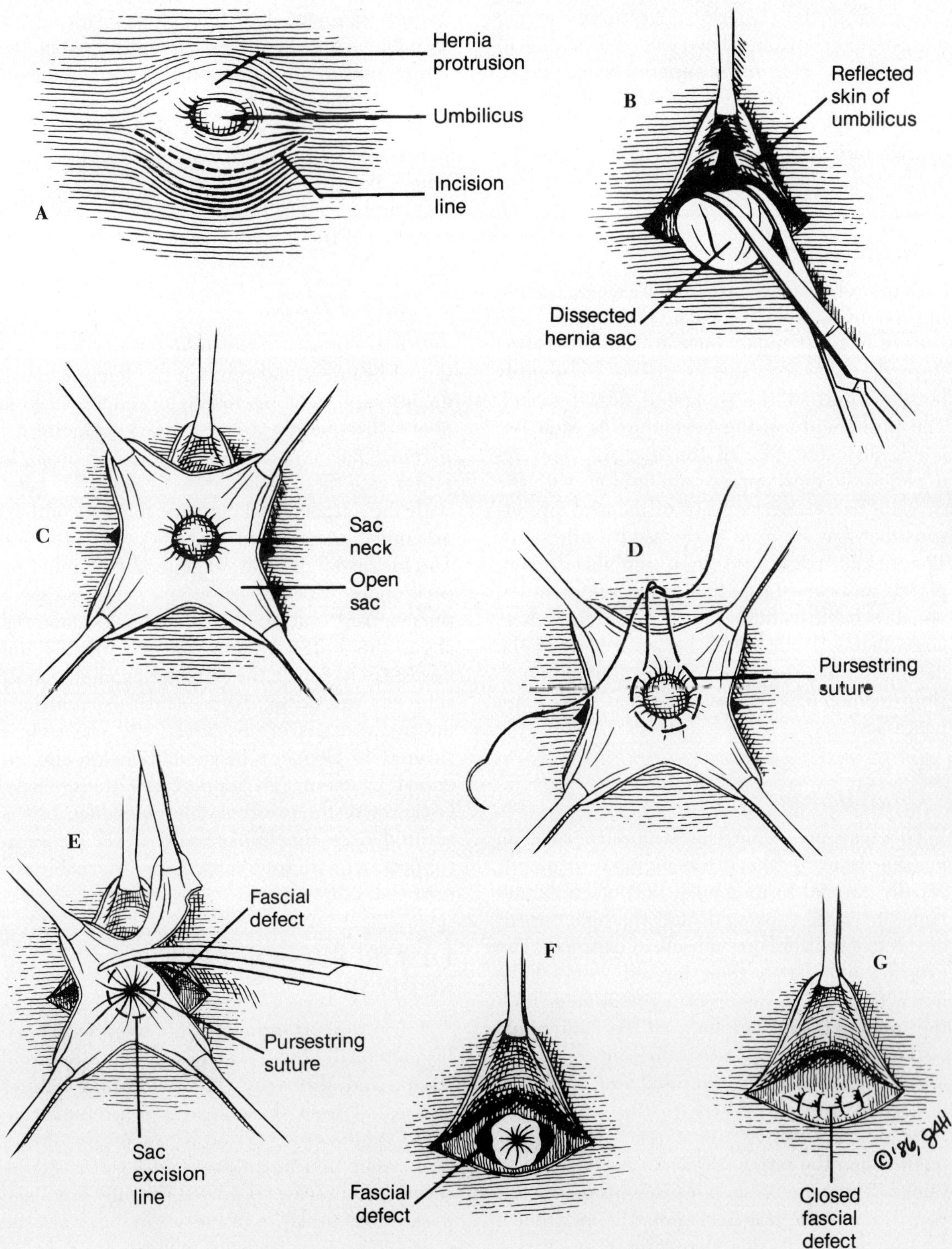

FIGURE 19-4
Repair of umbilical hernia. **A,** Site of incision. **B,** Umbilicus dissected free of sac and reflected upward. **C,** Appearance of sac that is cut open. **D,** Placement of purse-string suture at neck of sac. **E,** Sac dissected free of fascial defect after suture is tied. **F,** Appearance of fascial defect after sac excised. **G,** Fascial defect closed; umbilicus will be tacked to it.

rior edge of the posterior edge in an overlapping fashion. Studies have not shown that either of these closures is superior to the other, and the approach taken generally is the one that best fits the circumstances. The umbilicus is then tacked to the fascial defect and the skin margin approximated.

Incisional Hernia

Repair of an incisional hernia can be accomplished by incising the skin through the old scar or via a parallel incision and dissecting through the subcutaneous tissue to identify both margins of the separated fascial defect. The peritoneum of the hernia sac is then isolated, dissected free of the margins, and reduced in the most appropriate fashion, with the surgeon exercising care not to damage any organs that may be fixed in the sac by adhesions. The fascial edges are then mobilized completely and closed side to side with interrupted nonabsorbable suture. Rarely the defect is so large that a patch has to be sutured over the defect. With care, however, it is generally possible to mobilize the fascia so that this is not necessary.

Groin Hernia

To repair an inguinal or femoral hernia, an incision is made above the inguinal ligament, usually parallel to its medial portion. Subcutaneous tissue is separated, and the aponeurosis of the external oblique muscle is exposed. The external oblique is then incised from above down through the external inguinal ring, with the surgeon taking care to avoid the ilioinguinal nerve, which is frequently adherent to the external ring. The sac is identified and by careful dissection excised down to its emergence through the transversalis fascia. The sac is opened and the intraperitoneal contents are reduced. The surgeon should place his or her finger through the sac neck into the peritoneal cavity and palpate the structures immediately within to be sure that there are no other hernia sacs protruding, particularly into the femoral canal. The sac neck is then ligated and transfixed away from the ring, often to Cooper's ligament. The transversalis fascia is approximated with nonabsorbable suture. The external

oblique aponeurosis is then closed with nonabsorbable suture, and the skin and subcutaneous tissue are closed. Occasionally on opening the external oblique aponeurosis, only a mass of fat is found. In such instances the diagnosis of a hernia was made in error and no sac is present. Often, however, there is both fat and a sac and the surgeon must be careful to determine the contents of the inguinal canal.

Femoral Hernia

When the sac is protruding beneath the inguinal ligament and through the femoral canal, an attempt may be made to reduce it from above. Frequently it is necessary to incise the inguinal ligament to free up the sac neck. In either case the sac should be ligated at its base, with the surgeon making sure that its contents are not damaged and that they are reduced. The sac, as in all cases, is generally handled by excision of excess peritoneum and placing a purse-string suture of absorbable material about the base. Although it is probably not necessary to repair the inguinal ligament, most surgeons will do so. To prevent recurrent hernia in the transversalis fascia, the sac neck is sutured to Cooper's ligament beneath the inguinal ligament. To support the transversalis fascia repair the external oblique aponeurosis is sutured over the transversalis fascia for extra support, all with interrupted nonabsorbable suture material.

DISORDERS OF PELVIC SUPPORT

Pelvic support structures are often weakened by childbirth, other pelvic trauma, stress and strain, and the aging process. Abnormalities that result from these relaxation problems include urethrocele, cystocele, rectocele, enterocele, and uterine prolapse (descensus of the cervix and uterus). If a hysterectomy has been performed, prolapse of the vagina may also be a problem. It is unusual to have only one of these conditions. In most cases the relaxation affects all the support structures of the pelvis. Frequently relaxation of the urethra, the bladder neck, and the bladder (urethrocele, cystocele) is associated with urinary incontinence, which is covered in Chapter 20.

Urethrocele and Cystocele

Attenuation or rupture of the pubovesicle cervical fascia for any reason may allow the descent of the urethra (urethrocele), bladder neck, or bladder (cystocele) into the vaginal canal. Often only a cystocele is present (Fig. 19-5), and generally in these cases the patient is continent. When a urethrocele is present as well, the woman usually suffers from stress incontinence. Urethroceles seem to be more common in women with wide subpubic arches (gynecoid type), which allow the full force of the fetal head against this area during descent in labor. Narrower arches, such as those associated with the android or anthropoid pelvic types, seem to protect this region from the descent of the fetal head.

Symptoms and Signs

Symptoms and signs of urethrocele and cystocele consist of a sensation of fullness or pressure and at times a feeling that organs are falling out, stress incontinence, occasional urgency, and often a feeling of incomplete emptying with voiding. The patient and the physician note a soft bulging mass of the anterior vaginal wall. In some patients this must be replaced manually before the patient can void. Strain or cough accentuates the bulge. The mass may descend to or beyond the introitus. Although urethroceles and cystoceles almost always occur in parous women, they have been noted in nulliparous women who have poor structural supports. This is particularly true in women who have congenital malformations or weaknesses of the endopelvic connective tissue and musculature of the pelvic floor. Most parous women demonstrate some degree of cystocele, and when asymptomatic, they do not require therapy.

Diagnosis

The urethrocele and the cystocele are best demonstrated with a patient in the lithotomy position. A retractor or posterior wall blade of a Graves speculum is used to depress the posterior wall. The patient is then asked to strain, and the degree of the cystocele or urethrocele is noted. The physician should palpate the bladder neck and note whether it is well supported. Generally, if the supports of the bladder neck are adequate, the urethra is adequately supported. If a cystocele and a urethrocele are present, it invariably follows that the bladder neck is not supported. The examination for cystocele and urethrocele is best performed with the bladder at least partially filled (100 to 250 ml).

Urethroceles must be differentiated from inflamed and enlarged Skene's glands and urethral diverticula. Cystoceles must be differentiated from bladder tumors and bladder diverticula, which are both rare but may occur. Urethroceles and cystoceles are generally soft, pliable, and nontender. Although diverticula may be reducible, a sensation of a mass is usually present. Inflamed Skene's glands are generally tender, and it may be possible to express pus from the urethra when they are palpated. Pus may also be expressed in the presence of a diverticulum of the urethra. In such cases gonococcal and chlamydial infections should be considered.

Management

Treatment of urethroceles and cystoceles may be nonoperative or operative. Nonoperative treatment consists of supporting the herniation of the bladder into the vagina using a

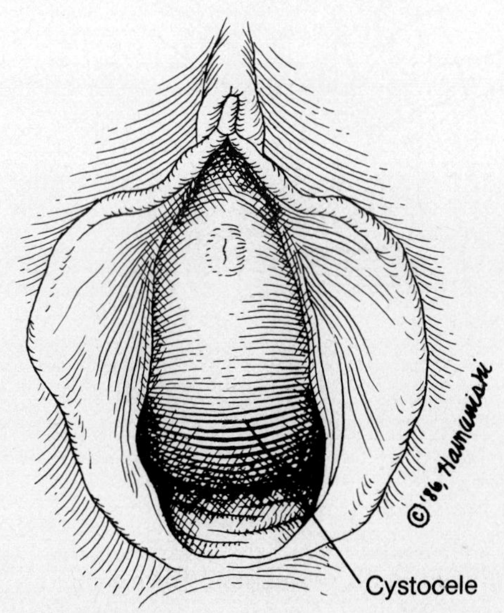

FIGURE 19-5
Cystocele.

pessary of the Smith-Hodge or inflatable type (see Fig. 19-11) or even with the intermittent use of a large tampon. Kegel exercises (see Chapter 20) help to strengthen the pelvic floor musculature and thereby may relieve some of the pressure symptoms produced by the cystocele. In an older woman the use of estrogen systemically or in a vaginal cream may improve both the tone of the pelvic support structures and the vascular supply of these tissues.

A younger woman with a large cystocele should be encouraged to avoid operative repair until she has completed her family. Occasionally the abnormality is so uncomfortable that repair must be performed before childbearing is complete. If this is the case, cesarean delivery should be considered for subsequent pregnancies.

Operative repair of a cystocele is generally performed in conjunction with the repair of a rectocele. It is unusual for anterior supports of the vagina to relax without an accompanying relaxation of the posterior wall. Repair, therefore, usually consists of an anterior and posterior colporrhaphy. If uterine descensus is noted, this must also be treated. Frequently an enterocele accompanies a cystocele and rectocele and where present must be excised. These problems are dealt with later in this chapter.

Anterior wall repair (colporrhaphy) is performed by incising the vaginal epithelium transversally just above the anterior lip of the cervix in the region of the bladder reflection (Fig. 19-6). If the woman has undergone a hysterectomy in the past, the incision may be made approximately 1 to 1.5 cm anterior to the vaginal scar. The vagina is then incised longitudinally from the transverse incision to the level of the bladder neck. If no urethrocele is present, this incision is sufficient. If a urethrocele is present, the incision must be continued under the urethra as well. The longitudinal incision is made by separating the vaginal wall from the underlying tissue progressively, using Metzenbaum scissors. When the longitudinal incision is complete, the cut edge of the vagina is held under tension and the pubocervical fascia that is attached is separated from it by blunt and sharp dissection. This is repeated on each side. At this point the bladder is free of the pubocervical fascia, which is itself free of the vaginal wall. The surgeon then places a suture

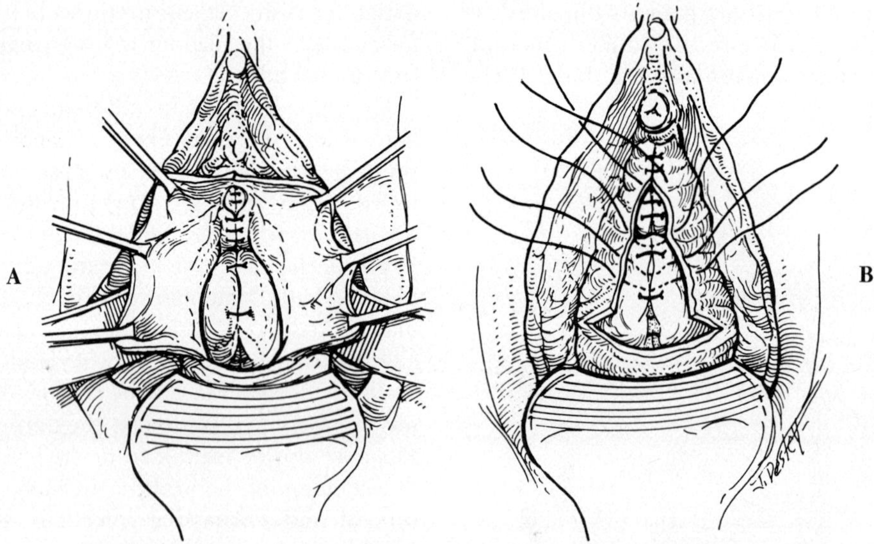

FIGURE 19-6
Cystourethrocele repair. **A,** Appearance of cystourethrocele after plication of bladder neck and repair of cystocele; cut edge of vagina is held apart above repair. **B,** Repair of vagina over cystocele is noted. (Reproduced, with permission, from Symmonds RE: Relaxation of pelvic supports. In Benson, RC, ed: Current obstetric and gynecologic diagnosis and treatment, 5th ed. Copyright 1984 by Lange Medical Publications, Los Altos, Calif.)

over the bladder neck (Kelly stitch), bringing together the pubocervical fasciae on either side. The stitch should be placed in such a fashion that the pubocervical fascia is sutured as far away from the cut edge as possible and parallel to the previous incision. A similar stitch is taken on the opposite side and the suture tied. Zero or 2-0 polyglycol suture is most appropriate for this closure. With the bladder neck well identified and supported, the pubocervical fascia is then closed with progressive similar stitches to completely imbricate the fascia over the bladder. If the urethrocele is present, similar sutures are also placed over the urethra. (In Chapter 20 the replacement of the bladder neck behind the pubic symphysis to correct incontinence is described. The reader may wish to review these steps.) After completing the imbrication of the pubocervical fascia the vaginal edges are trimmed and the vagina closed with a row of interrupted 2-0 polyglycol or catgut sutures.

Postoperatively the bladder should be drained for about 5 days. There are several ways to accomplish this. The first is to leave a No. 16 Foley catheter in place for 5 days, remove the catheter on the fifth day, and allow the patient to try to void. Following voiding of at least 100 to 200 ml the patient should be catheterized for the presence of residual urine. If residual urine is found in a quantity of more than 150 ml on two successive voidings, or if the amount voided is less than 100 ml, the physician should consider replacing the catheter for 24 to 48 hours. If residual urine amounts are less than 150 ml on two consecutive voidings, no further steps are necessary. Occasionally, after an anterior repair, voiding does not occur after 5 days of bladder drainage. At that point the patient may require catheterization for 24 to 48 hours longer, or she may be discharged with a Foley catheter in place for continuous drainage for a week, to be rechecked for voiding and residual urine as an outpatient in 1 week. It is rarely necessary to treat the patient with antibiotics during this period; however, lower urinary tract infections are common and should be treated as they occur. In some patients who have had chronic urinary tract infections, prophylactic antibiotics such as a sulfa preparation or nitrofurantoin (Furadantin) can be administered.

Alternatives to the above regimen include suprapubic catheter drainage or placing an infant feeding tube (No. 5) through the urethra and attaching it with a labial suture. In both methods the drainage tube can be clamped, allowing the patient to void when she can and for residual urine measurements to be taken. The suprapubic technique is simple to use and seems to have a lower incidence of infection than does transurethral catheterization, but patients may complain of extravasation of urine around the site and occasionally of hematoma formation. The surgeon should decide which method is best suited to the needs of his or her institution and develop a system that surgeon and nursing team understand and can follow.

Postoperatively it is important to impress on the patient that heavy lifting, straining, or prolonged periods of standing should be avoided for 3 months. The healing process is slow, and the tissue is generally weak initially. Complete healing should be ensured before the tissue is stressed by normal activities.

Rectocele

Symptoms and Signs

The patient with a rectocele often complains of a heavy or "falling out" feeling in the vagina. She may complain of constipation and occasionally may need to splint the vagina with her fingers to effect a bowel movement. She may also have a feeling of incomplete emptying of the rectum at the time of the bowel movement.

Diagnosis

A rectocele may be identified by retracting the anterior vaginal wall upward and again having the patient strain. The rectum will bulge into the vagina, and this bulge may protrude through the introitus (Fig. 19-7). The physician should then place one finger in the rectum and one in the vagina and palpate the hernia. Often the rectovaginal septum is paper thin and the rectocele can be palpated to its upper margin. If an enterocele is present, it may be possible to differentiate it from the rectocele by having the patient strain. Frequently, however, the diagnosis of a small enterocele is established only at the time of operation.

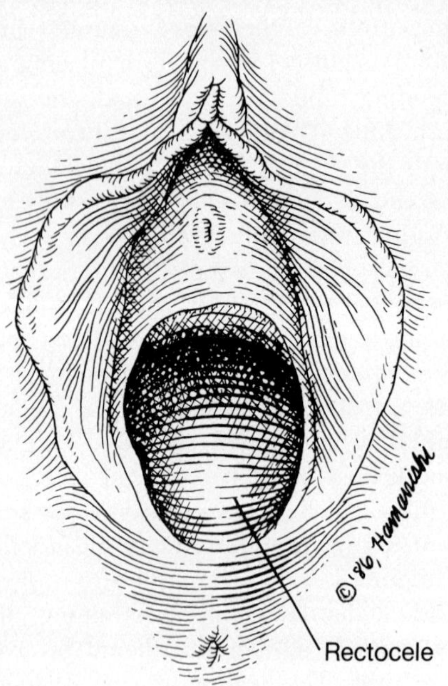

FIGURE 19-7
Rectocele.

Management

Nonoperative management of a rectocele is similar to that mentioned for a cystocele. Pessaries, Kegel exercises, and estrogen may be useful in the appropriate situations.

Operative management of a rectocele (posterior colporrhaphy) is generally performed at the time of an anterior colporrhaphy with or without enterocele repair or operation for descensus. Most women with rectoceles also have gaping vaginas and weakness in their perineal body. Therefore as part of a rectocele repair a perineorrhaphy is performed as well. The surgeon should estimate at the time of starting the posterior repair what degree of perineorrhaphy he or she wishes to perform. The margins of the perineum to be narrowed are generally marked by placing Allis clamps at their extreme at the introital opening (Fig. 19-8). The tissue of the introitus is then incised between these clamps, and the vaginal wall is separated from the underlying tissue and rectum in a progressive manner longitudinally in the midline, beginning at the introital incision and being carried forward to the apex of the vagina above the limit of the rectocele. This is done by progressive separation and incision using the

Metzenbaum scissors in a fashion similar to that reported for cystocele repair.

When the vaginal wall is completely incised, the edges are grasped and placed under tension, and the perirectal connective tissue is separated from the vaginal mucosa by blunt and sharp (if necessary) dissection. This is carried out bilaterally until it is possible for the operator to palpate the perirectal space on each side. The operator then places a finger of his nondominant hand into the rectum using a double-glove technique while an assistant picks up perirectal tissue on either side. The operator then places a 0 nonabsorbable suture (silk or dermalon) into the perirectal tissue on either side. Approximately three or four of these stitches are placed and these are held without tying. The operator should use his or her finger in the rectum to ensure that no suture is placed into the rectum. The perirectal tissue usually includes portions of the levator ani muscles. When the sutures are tied, these tissues are interposed between rectum and vagina, thereby reducing the rectocele. These sutures also serve to tack the vagina to the levator ani area, thereby it is hoped avoiding future vaginal prolapse if a hysterectomy has also been performed. The vaginal edges are then trimmed and the vagina closed with a row of either continuous or interrupted catgut suture.

Attention is then turned to the perineorrhaphy, which is closed in the following fashion. Polyglycol sutures are placed in the lateral margins of the transverse incision, essentially bringing bulbocavernosal muscles together from either side to the midline. The operator should be sure that the bulbocavernosal muscle insertions are included in the sutures by pulling on the suture and noting whether or not the tension identifies the muscle bundles. The remainder of the perineal incision is then closed with a row of 2-0 polyglycol sutures to the deep tissue and the skin of the perineum is closed with either interrupted or continuous subcuticular suture of 3-0 chromic catgut or polyglycol.

Enterocele

Enteroceles frequently occur after an abdominal or vaginal hysterectomy and generally are the result of a weakened support for the

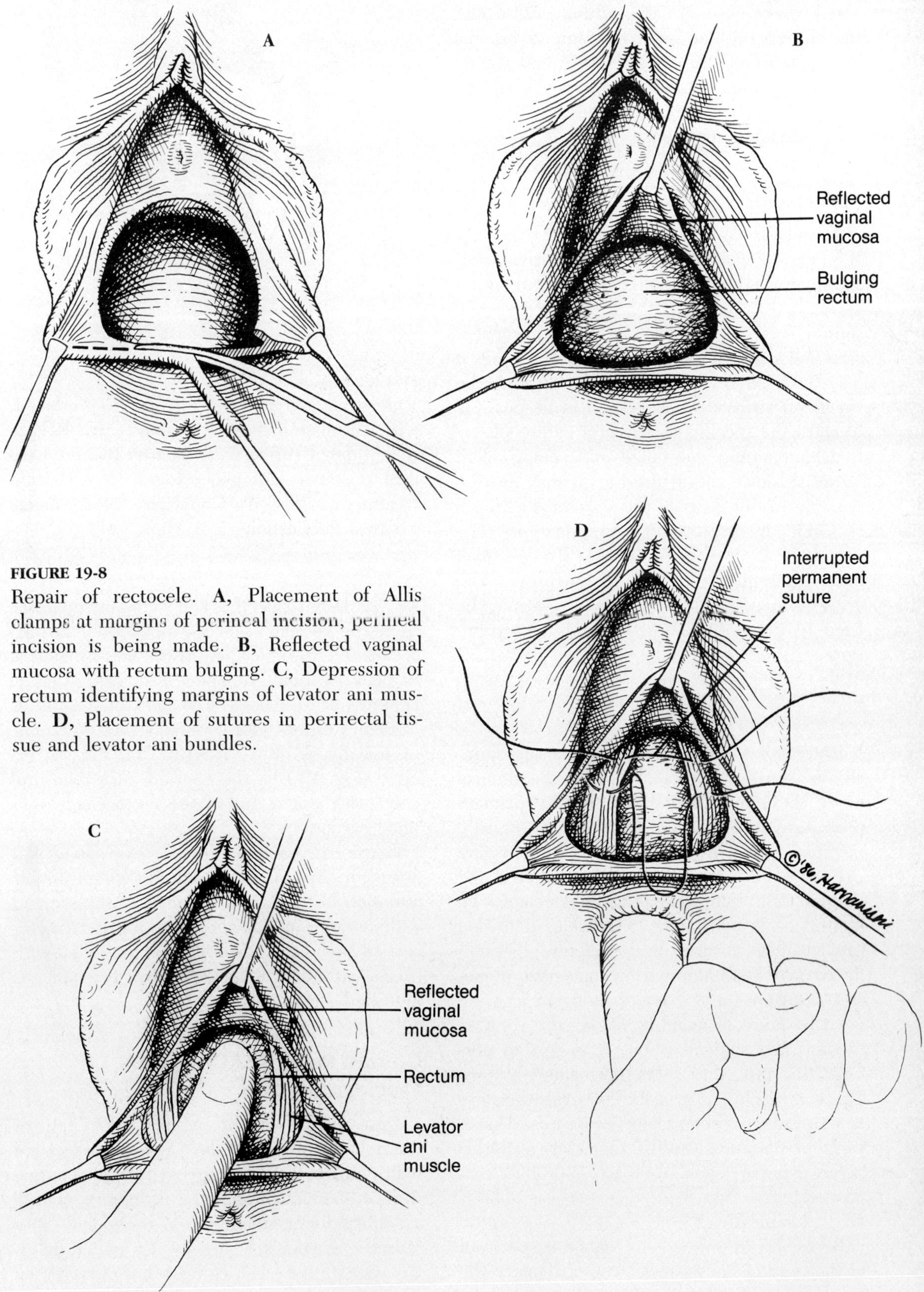

FIGURE 19-8
Repair of rectocele. **A,** Placement of Allis clamps at margins of perineal incision, perineal incision is being made. **B,** Reflected vaginal mucosa with rectum bulging. **C,** Depression of rectum identifying margins of levator ani muscle. **D,** Placement of sutures in perirectal tissue and levator ani bundles.

pouch of Douglas. In preventing enteroceles the uterosacral and cardinal ligaments are the most important support structures and should be incorporated into the vault repair at the time of a hysterectomy, and the ligaments from each side joined together.

Diagnosis

An enterocele is not always easy to diagnose. It is a true hernia of the peritoneal cavity emanating from the pouch of Douglas between the uterosacral ligaments and into the rectovaginal septum (Fig. 19-9). It may be noticed as a separate bulge above the rectocele, and at times it may be large enough to prolapse through the vagina. If such is the case, it may be possible to make the specific diagnosis of enterocele by transilluminating the bulge and seeing small bowel shadows within the sac. It may also be possible to differentiate the enterocele from a rectocele by rectovaginal examination. The contents of an enterocele are always small bowel and may also include omentum. The contents may be easily reducible or may be fixed to the peritoneum of the sac by adhesions.

Management

Enteroceles may be reduced transabdominally as a primary procedure or at the time of other abdominal procedures. In the primary procedure the sac should be reduced upward if possible, and if the uterosacral ligaments are present, these may be brought together in the midline. If the uterosacral ligaments cannot be identified, as with large enteroceles following previously performed hysterectomy, the cul-de-sac may be obliterated by concentric purse-string sutures in the endopelvic fascia. Care must be taken to avoid damaging the ureters, rectum, and sigmoid colon. It is best to perform this procedure with permanent suture. The enterocele has probably occurred because of weakening of pelvic floor structures. Therefore, for optimum results, repair of the lower pelvis using a vaginal approach is probably indicated, even though the enterocele is obliterated abdominally.

Repair of the enterocele can be carried out at the time of the posterior colporrhaphy. The

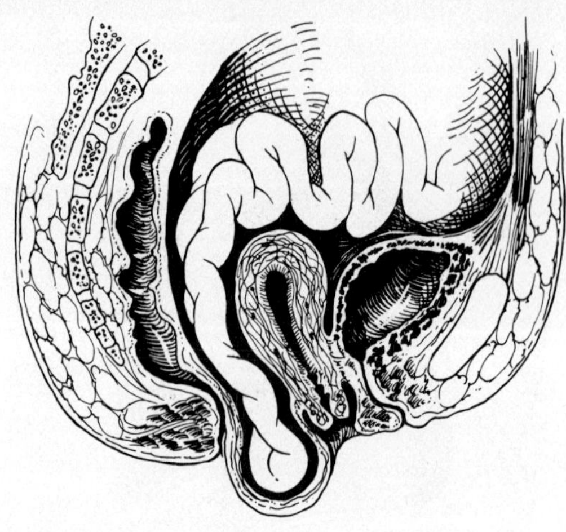

FIGURE 19-9
Enterocele and uterine prolapse. (Reproduced, with permission, from Symmonds RE: Relaxation of pelvic supports. In Benson RC, ed: Current obstetric and gynecologic diagnosis and treatment, 5th ed. Copyright 1984, Lange Medical Publications, Los Altos, Calif.)

sac will be visualized as the vagina is separated from the rectum. The sac must then be dissected free of underlying tissue and isolated at its neck. It should be opened to ensure that all contents are replaced. The neck of the hernia is then sutured with a purse-string 0-chromic or polyglycol suture ligature and the sac excised (Fig. 19-10). The operator may then proceed with the repair of the rectocele as outlined earlier.

Correctly repaired enteroceles usually will not recur. Enteroceles repaired without proper attention to ligation of the neck of the sac and without appropriate rectocele repair may recur. In such cases a subsequent operation with special attention to these surgical principles is indicated.

Uterine Prolapse (Descensus, Procidentia)

Descensus of the uterus and cervix into or through the barrel of the vagina is associated with injuries of the endopelvic fascia, including the cardinal and uterosacral ligaments, as well as injury to or relaxation of the pelvic floor muscles, particularly the levator ani muscles. Occasionally prolapse is the result of increased

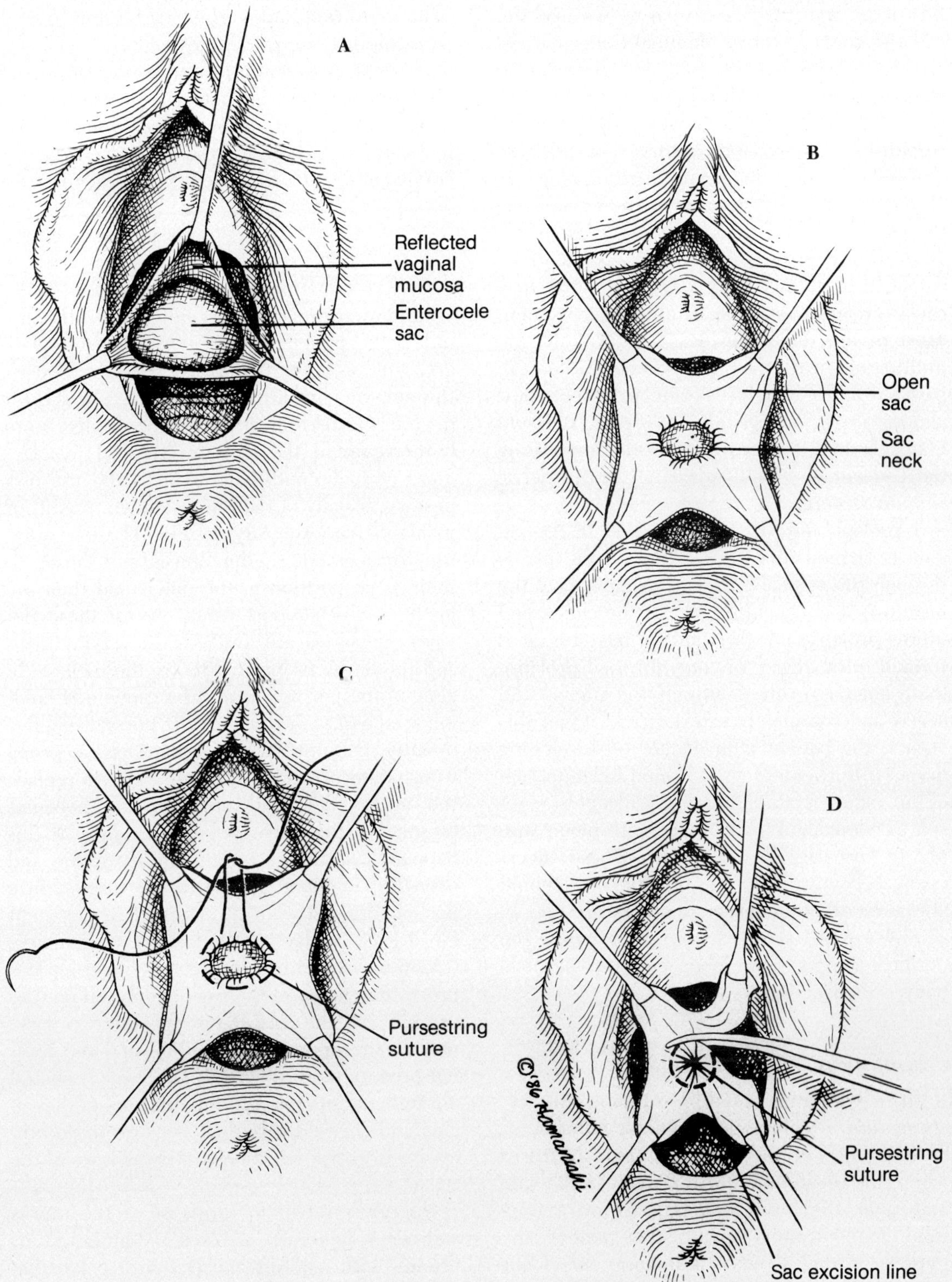

FIGURE 19-10

Repair of enterocele. **A,** Appearance of enterocele sac with vaginal wall reflected. **B,** Appearance of open enterocele sac with sac neck identified. **C,** Placing of pursestring suture at the neck of the enterocele sac. **D,** Excision of enterocele sac.

intraabdominal pressure, such as with ascites or large pelvic or intraabdominal tumors superimposed on poor pelvic supports. In some instances, sacral nerve disorders, especially injuries to S1 to S4, or diabetic neuropathy may be responsible. Associated factors that increase tension on pelvic floor musculature, such as chronic respiratory disease including chronic bronchitis, asthma, and bronchiectasis or severe obesity, may be associated. Congenitally damaged or relaxed pelvic floor supports may cause prolapse in young, nulliparous women. Most of the time, however, the patients are multiparous, with the prolapse being at least in part a result of childbirth trauma. Descensus is almost always associated with rectocele and cystocele and, at times, enterocele, supporting the concept of overall relaxation of the pelvic support structures.

A prolapse into the upper barrel of the vagina is termed *first degree*. If the prolapse is through the vaginal barrel to the region of the introitus, it is *second degree*. If the cervix and uterus prolapse out through the introitus, it is termed *third degree* or *total*. In total prolapse the vagina is everted around the uterus and cervix and completely exteriorized. When this occurs, the patient is in danger of developing dryness, thickening, and chronic inflammation of the vaginal epithelium. Stasis ulcers may result as edema and interference with blood supply to the vaginal wall occur. These ulcers rarely become cancerous, but biopsies should always be taken to ensure that they are not. In almost every case of acquired prolapse, the perineal supports are poor and the perineal body is damaged.

Symptoms and Signs

Major symptoms noted by patients with descensus are a feeling of heaviness, fullness, or "falling out" in the perineal area. In cases where the cervix and uterus are low in the vaginal canal, the cervix may be seen protruding from the introitus, giving the patient the impression that a tumor is bulging out of her vagina. Where total descensus has occurred, the patient is aware that a mass has actually prolapsed out of the introitus. Because prolapse almost always is related to anterior and posterior vaginal wall relaxation, symptoms that were reported earlier for cystocele and rectocele may be present as well.

It is not uncommon for the cervix or vaginal epithelium to become damaged or ulcerated, in which case the patient may report pain or vaginal bleeding. There is often discharge from the cervix and vagina when secondary infection occurs.

Management

Minimum prolapse does not require therapy unless the patient is very uncomfortable. Degrees of prolapse that place the cervix at or through the introitus probably have a greater degree of discomfort and are usually more bothersome to the patient. Medical management of such conditions involves the use of a pessary, usually of the Smith-Hodge, donut, or inflatable variety (Fig. 19-11). These require the replacement of the uterus and cervix to their usual position in the pelvis and then the institution of support using one of these devices. Pessaries are available in varying sizes and should be properly fitted to the patient. In general the perineum must be capable of holding the pessary in place, or the pessary will frequently fall out. If the patient is a young woman and pregnant, it is important to replace the uterus before it enlarges and becomes trapped in the lower pelvis or vagina. If this happens, edema may cause incarceration and even loss of blood supply to the uterus. In a postmenopausal woman, estrogen replacement for at least 30 days in the form of systemic estrogen or vaginal estrogen cream may help improve the vitality of the vaginal epithelium, the cervix, and the vasculature of these organs, making the operative procedure and the healing process more efficient. The patient should not undergo operation until all ulcers of the vagina and cervix are healed, because to do otherwise is to risk infection and breakdown of the repair.

Operative repair for prolapse of the uterus and cervix generally involves a vaginal hysterectomy with anterior and posterior colporrhaphy. The hysterectomy is performed carefully, isolating the uterosacral and cardinal ligaments so that they may be used in the support of the vaginal vault. The uterosacral ligaments should be sutured together so that the cul-de-sac is

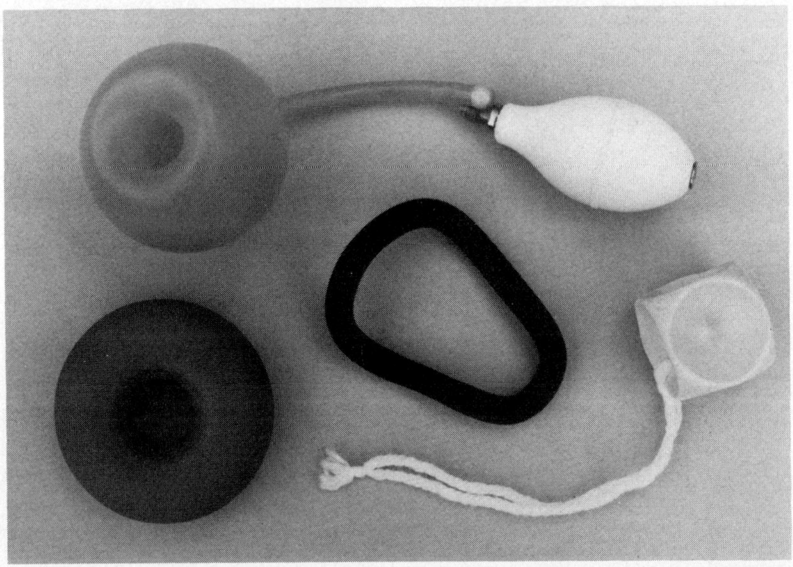

FIGURE 19-11
Examples of pessaries (Smith-Hodge, donut, inflatable types).

shortened or obliterated and the risk of a subsequent enterocele is lessened.

In some cases a vaginal hysterectomy is not advisable. These circumstances would include previous intraabdominal operation for an inflammatory process such as endometriosis or pelvic inflammatory disease. Where such is the case an abdominal hysterectomy may be performed, followed by a vaginal anterior and posterior colporrhaphy. Under these circumstances the cardinal and uterosacral ligaments should be treated as noted earlier.

In some women the cervix is hypertrophied and elongated to the area of the introitus, but the supports of the uterus itself are good. A cystocele and rectocele may be present, and operative repair can consist of a Manchester-Fothergill operation. This operation combines an anterior and posterior colporrhaphy with the amputation of the cervix and the use of the cardinal ligaments to support the anterior vaginal wall and bladder. Although it was suggested for repair in young women who wish to maintain their reproductive abilities, the loss of the cervix may interfere with fertility or lead to incompetence of the internal cervical os. The operation has value in older women who have an elongated cervix and well-supported uterus because it is technically easier and has a shorter

operative time than the vaginal hysterectomy in such cases, and the entering of the peritoneal cavity is avoided.

In older women who are no longer sexually active a simple procedure for reducing prolapse is a partial colpocleisis. The classic procedure was described by Le Fort (Fig. 19-12) and involves the removal of a strip of anterior and posterior vaginal wall, with closure of the margins of the anterior and posterior wall to each other. This procedure may be performed with or without the presence of a uterus and cervix, and when it is completed, a small vaginal canal exists on either side of the septum, which is produced by the suturing of the lateral margins of the excision. The line of dissection of the vaginal wall is carried to the level of the bladder neck anteriorly and to the reflection of bladder onto cervix at the upper margin of the vagina. Posteriorly the dissection is carried from just inside the introitus to a position just posterior to the cervix. If a hysterectomy has been previously performed, the dissection may begin approximately 1 cm on either side of the vaginal scar. When the procedure is completed, the bladder neck is spared from any scarring, and urinary incontinence is generally avoided. Bladder neck plication may be carried out if the patient is incontinent. After healing

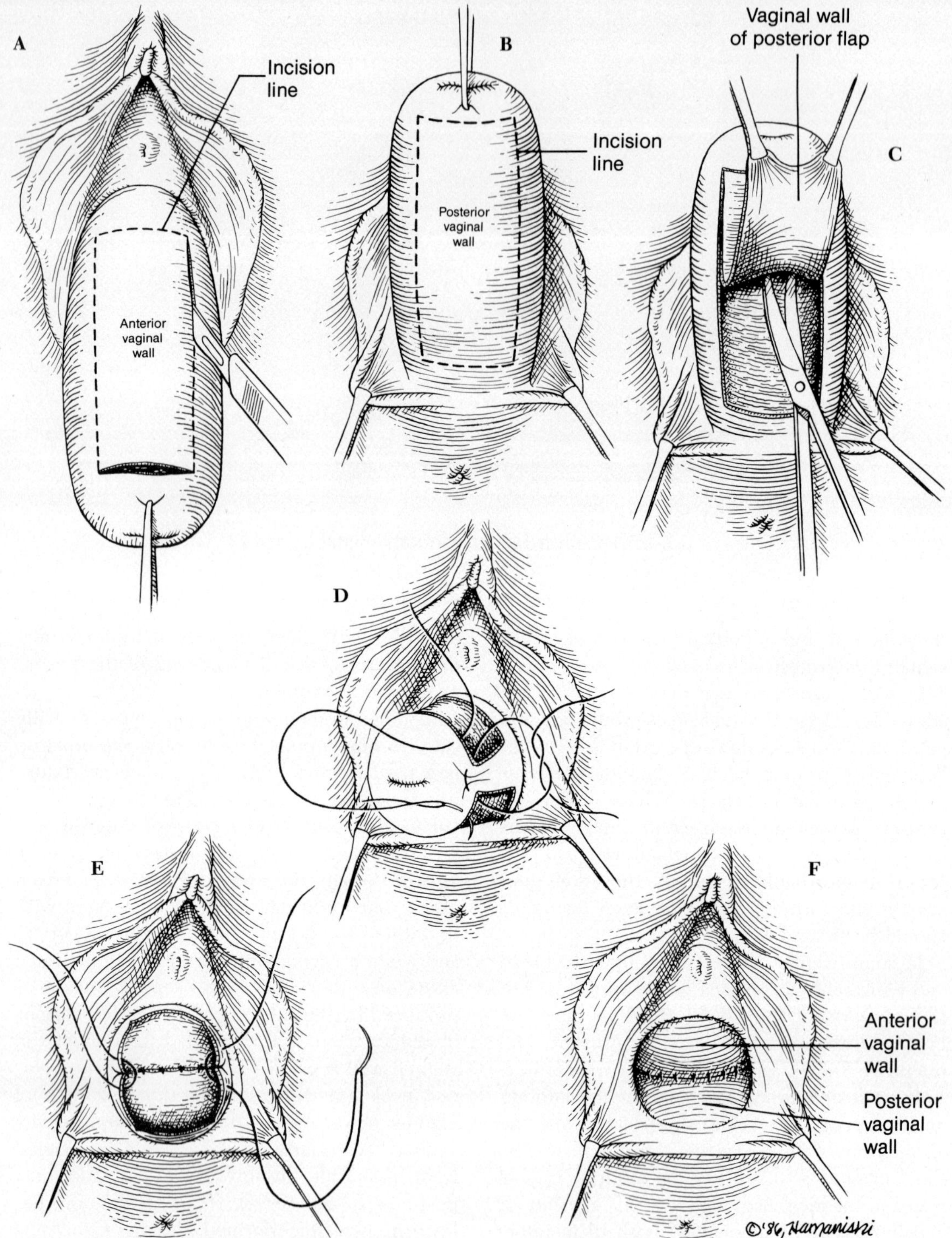

FIGURE 19-12

Le Fort procedure. **A,** Incision of anterior vaginal wall strip. **B,** Incision of posterior wall strip. **C,** Removal of vaginal strip. **D** and **E,** Placement of sutures. **F,** Appearance of vagina after procedure is completed but before perineorrhaphy is performed.

of the plication a small introital area is noted; this has cosmetic benefits in older women. In addition, narrow canals are noted on each lateral vaginal wall. If the cervix and uterus are still present and intrauterine pathology occurs, bleeding along these canals could take place, alerting the physician to a potential problem.

The Goodall-Power modification of the Le Fort operation (Fig. 19-13) allows for the removal of a triangular piece of vaginal wall beginning at the cervical reflection or 1 cm above the vaginal scar at the base of the triangle, with the apex of the triangle just beneath the bladder neck anteriorly and just at the introitus posteriorly. The cut edge of vaginal wall making up the base of the triangle anteriorly is sutured to the similar wall posteriorly, and the vaginal incision is then closed with a row of interrupted sutures beginning beneath the bladder neck and carried side to side to the area of

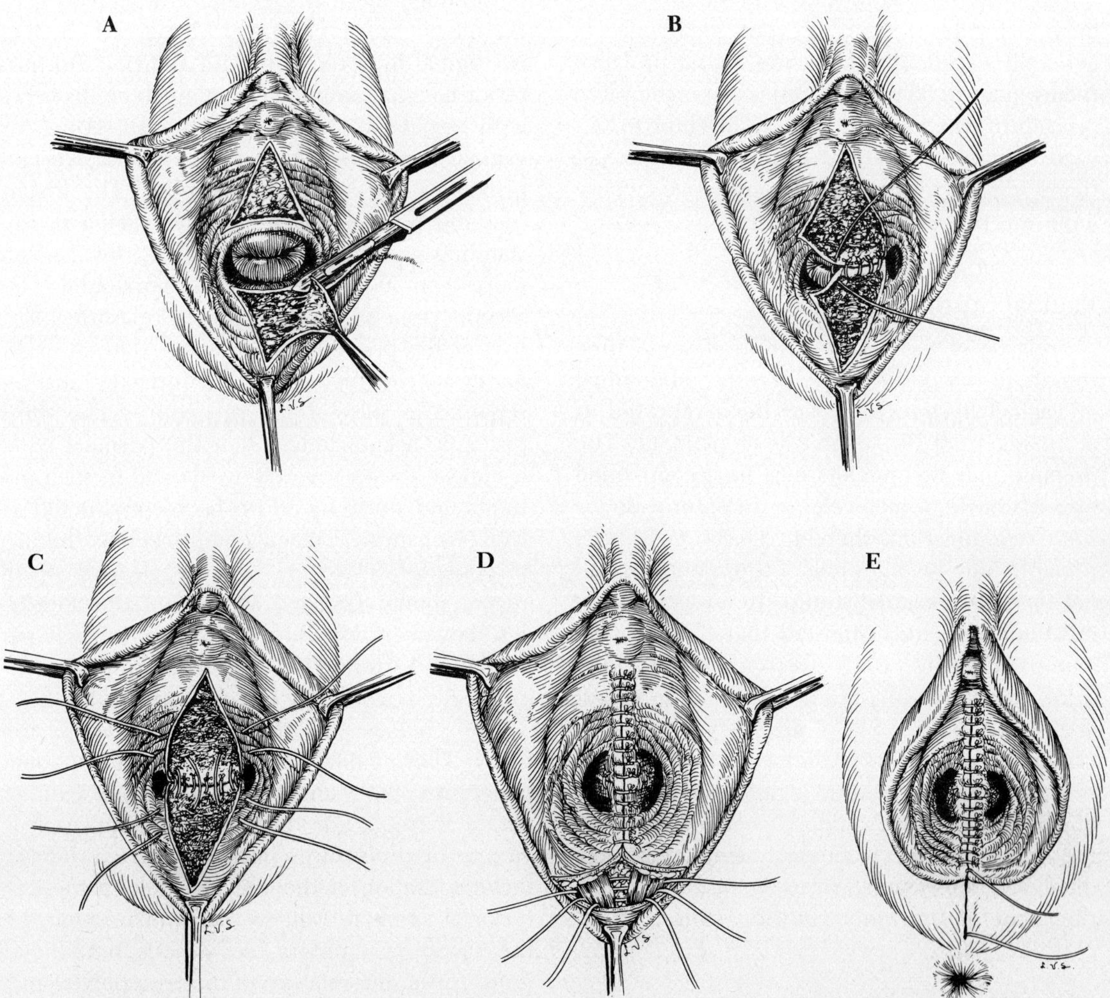

FIGURE 19-13
Goodall-Power modification of Le Fort operation. **A,** Representation of vaginal incision on anterior and posterior wall. **B,** Early placement of sutures. **C,** Later placement of suture. **D,** Vaginal incision completely closed; perineorrhaphy being performed. **E,** Appearance at completion of procedure. (Reprinted, with permission, from Symmonds RE: Relaxation of pelvic supports. In Benson RC, ed: Current obstetric and gynecologic diagnosis and treatment, 5th ed. Copyright 1984, Lange Medical Publications, Los Altos, Calif.)

the introitus. This procedure works well for relatively small prolapses, while the Le Fort is best for larger ones.

When a colpocleisis is performed, if an enterocele is found when the vaginal wall is stripped away, the sac must be identified, its neck ligated, and the peritoneum of the sac excised to prevent recurrence of the enterocele behind the colpocleisis.

In most cases a perineorrhaphy is performed with a colpocleisis to reinforce the introitus.

Prognosis for a colpocleisis procedure to reduce the prolapse and prevent recurrence is generally excellent. Ridley reports no prolapse recurrences in 58 patients unless an incomplete procedure was performed in an attempt to salvage vaginal depth and function. Three patients developed stress incontinence where none was present preoperatively.

Vaginal Stump Prolapse

Prolapse of the vaginal stump at some time remote to the performance of either abdominal or vaginal hysterectomy has been reported as occurring in 0.1% to 18.2% of patients. The prolapse may be total and may be accompanied by a cystocele, a rectocele, or an enterocele, or some combination thereof. Occasionally the prolapse only involves one of those entities and not the entire vaginal stump. In a recent study in Munich, Richter reported that of 97 vaginal stump prolapses, 6.2% were cystocele only, 5.1% rectocele only, 9.3% primarily an enterocele type, and 72.2% of mixed type. Specific classification was not given for 7.2%.

Vaginal stump prolapse is probably the result of continuing pelvic support weakness and failure of the vaginal structures, namely, the cardinal and uterosacral ligaments, to maintain their tone or attachment to the vagina.

Symptoms and Signs

Symptoms and signs of vaginal stump prolapse are similar to those delineated for descensus of the uterus. They include pelvic heaviness, backache, and a mass protruding through the introitus. At times, stress incontinence, urgency, frequency, dribbling, vaginal bleeding or discharge (if there is an ulcer), and, depending on the size of the mass, difficulty with sitting or walking may occur.

Diagnosis

Examination may help determine the contents of the herniation depending on where the vaginal scar is located with respect to the protruding mass and the extent to which the supports of the pelvis are lost. Rectovaginal examination is often helpful in delineating an enterocele from a rectocele.

Management

Although the management of descensus with the uterus present is uniformly agreed on, that is, vaginal hysterectomy with anterior and posterior colporrhaphy, there is much controversy with respect to the choice of the procedure for vaginal stump prolapse. Nevertheless, certain principles and facts are important. The first is that the normal position of the vagina in the standing position is against the rectum and no more than 30 degrees from the horizontal. The second principle is that pelvic relaxation is a part of the problem and dictates that an existing cystocele, rectocele, or enterocele must be repaired as part of the procedure. The third principle acknowledges that the perineal body is almost always severely weakened in such patients and must therefore be reconstructed as well. Nonsurgical management such as the use of pessaries, estrogen, and the clearing up of ulcers should be used as appropriate. Pessaries, however, are rarely retained in such patients, and attempts to treat these patients nonsurgically is generally met with frustration.

The choices of operative procedures are many. These include those that use the abdominal route, the vaginal route, or some combination thereof. For the abdominal approach a variety of procedures have been tried. These include fixation of the vaginal vault to the anterior abdominal wall, to the lumbar spine, to the sacral promontory, to various tendonous lines in the musculature of the true pelvis, and to the sacrospinous ligament. The anterior abdominal wall fixation increases the diameters of the pouch of Douglas and frequently adds to the risk of subsequent enterocele development, often creating a recurrence in short order. Fixation to the lumbar spine or the sacral promontory is often difficult to achieve directly and frequently requires the interposition of a different material. In the past, ox fascia lata, fascial aponeurosis from the patient, or inert materials such as Mersilene have been used. In such procedures it is important to cover the stent with peritoneum, thereby rendering it retroperitoneal to avoid troublesome adhesions and internal hernias at a future date. Following such procedures the pouch of Douglas may still be large enough to allow an enterocele to develop. Fixation to various aspects of the pelvic wall or to the sacrospinous ligament have had encouraging degrees of success, the latter being the most successful. Using the sacrospinous ligament can frequently be accomplished vaginally. Randall and Nichols report excellent success with both abdominal and vaginal approaches. In 18 patients treated with fixation of the vaginal vault to the sacrospinous ligament via the vaginal route, all had successful outcomes.

A variety of vaginal procedures have been designed. The best success, however, occurs in those in which adequate vaginal length is maintained and the vagina is positioned against the rectum nearly parallel to the horizontal. Recently, Thornton reported on 41 women who underwent repair of vaginal stumps, in which the vaginal approach was used with good lasting success. Twenty of these patients required a repair of an enterocele and a posterior repair, which especially detailed the attachment of the posterior wall of the vagina to the perirectal fascia and levator ani muscles. Twenty-one patients underwent a repair of an enterocele with both an anterior and posterior repair because a cystocele was believed to be a major part of their prolapse problem. Long-term follow-ups were effected and the success rate was stated to be excellent.

Richter and Albrich combined the repair of cystocele, rectocele, and enterocele where necessary with a unilateral or bilateral vaginal sacrospinal fixation procedure. They also stressed the importance of suturing the vagina in its physiologic position to the perirectal support tissue. The success in their group of 97 patients was also excellent, in that 61.7% of the patients had what were considered ideal results in long-term follow-up. There was a recurrence of cystocele in 14.8%, rectocele in 8.6%, and enterocele in 3.7%. Stress incontinence was reported in 3.7% of their patients and urgency incontinence in 2.5% with long-term follow-up.

In older women who are no longer sexually active, and particularly in those who have medical reasons to avoid a longer procedure, a Le Fort–type colpocleisis operation may be performed with excellent results.

Vaginal colpocleisis procedures for women who are elderly and are no longer sexually active are appropriate. It is extremely important to identify and repair enteroceles in such women, but this can readily be done as part of the procedure. Perineorrhaphy should always be performed as a part of any procedure to repair a vaginal stump prolapse.

The question of continuing sexual activity after vaginal vault repairs is obviously an important one. With an adequate vaginal operation (with the exception of colpocleisis), intercourse is achievable in most patients who wish to maintain this activity.

KEY POINTS

- Femoral hernias are more common in females than in males, whereas inguinal hernias are more common in males.

- Congenital fascial defects at the umbilicus generally close within the first 3 years of life.

- In the female, large hernias, hernias that continuously contain intraabdominal contents, hernias that cause continuing discomfort, and hernias that have been incarcerated should be operatively repaired.

___________ KEY POINTS, cont'd ___________

- In repairing abdominal wall hernias, fascia should be sutured with nonabsorbable material.

- Urethroceles and cystoceles are more common in women with a gynecoid pelvis than in those with android or anthropoid types.

- Urinary incontinence is usually noted with loss of support of the urethra and bladder neck.

- After cystocele repair, bladder drainage for about 5 days is generally necessary before normal voiding can be anticipated.

- Bladder drainage after cystocele repair may be with a transurethral or suprapubic catheter.

- When an enterocele is present, the sac must be dissected free and ligated at its neck to prevent recurrence.

- Descensus of the uterus and cervix is graded as first degree (prolapse into the upper vagina), second degree (prolapse to or near the introitus), and third degree or complete (prolapse through the introitus).

- Prolapse of the vaginal stump at some time following hysterectomy has been reported in 0.1% to 18.2% of patients.

- Vaginal prolapse after hysterectomy includes a mixture of cystocele, rectocele, and enterocele in 72% of cases.

- Vaginal vault prolapse can be repaired abdominally or vaginally.

- Vaginal vault prolapse repaired using fixation to the sacrospinous ligament will have a success rate approaching 100%.

BIBLIOGRAPHY

Beecham CT: Classification of vaginal relaxation. Am J Obstet Gynecol 136:957, 1980.

Beecham CT, Beecham JB: Correction of prolapsed vagina or enterocele with fascila. Obstet Gynecol 42:542, 1973.

Glassow F: Inguinal and femoral hernia in women. Int Surg 57:34, 1972.

Halverson K, McVay CB: Inguinal and femoral hernioplasty. A 22 year study of author's methods. Arch Surg 101:127, 1970.

Kuhn RJ, Hollyock VE: Observations on the anatomy of the recto-vaginal pouch and septum. Obstet Gynecol 59:445, 1982.

Nichols DH: Transvaginal sacrospinous fixation. Pelvic Surg 1:10, 1981.

Randall CI, Nichols DH: Surgical treatment of vaginal inversion. Obstet Gynecol 38:327, 1971.

Richter K: Massive eversion of the vagina: Pathogenesis, diagnosis and therapy of the "true" prolapse of the vaginal stump. Clin Obstet Gynecol 25:897, 1982.

Richter K, Albrich W: Long-term results following fixation of the vagina on the sacrospinal ligament by the vaginal root (vaginae fixatio sacrospinalis vaginalis). Am J Obstet Gynecol 141:811, 1981.

Ridley JH: Evaluation of the colpocleisis operation: A report of 58 cases. Am J Obstet Gynecol 113:1114, 1972.

Schwartz SI, Shires GT, Spencer FC, Storer EH: Principles of surgery, 4th ed. New York, McGraw-Hill Book Co., 1984.

Seigworth GR: Vaginal vault prolapse with eversion. Obstet Gynecol 54:255, 1979.

Symmonds RE: Relaxation of pelvic supports. In Benson RC, ed. Current obstetric and gynecologic diagnosis and treatment, 5th ed. Los Altos, Calif., Lange Medical Publications, 1984.

Symmonds RE, Williams TJ, Lee RA, Webb MJ: Posthysterectomy, enterocele and vaginal vault prolapse. Am J Obstet Gynecol 140:852, 1981.

Thornton WN Jr, Peters WA: Repair of vaginal prolapse after hysterectomy. Am J Obstet Gynecol 147:140, 1983.

Zacharin RF: Pulsion enterocele: Review of functional anatomy of the pelvic floor. Obstet Gynecol 55:135, 1980.

Zimmerman LM, Anson BJ: The anatomy of surgery of hernia. Baltimore, The Williams & Wilkins Co., 1953.

Gynecologic Urology

————————— KEY TERMS AND DEFINITIONS —————————

Cystometry. Method for measuring pressure-volume relationships of the bladder.

Detrusor Dyssynergia. Involuntary contraction of the bladder during distension with urine or other fluids.

Detrusor Pressure. Component of intravesical pressure created by forces in the bladder wall.

Extra-Urethral Incontinence. The loss of urine through channels other than the urethra.

Flow Rate. Volume of urine expelled via the urethra per unit time expressed in milliliters.

Genuine Stress Incontinence. Condition of immediate involuntary loss of urine when intravesical pressure exceeds the maximum urethral pressure in the absence of detrusor activity.

Incontinence. A condition in which involuntary loss of urine is a social or hygienic problem and one that can be objectively demonstrated.

Intraabdominal Pressure. Pressure surrounding the bladder.

Intravesical Pressure. Pressure within the bladder.

Kegel Exercises. Isometric contractions of the pubococcygeus muscles to improve control of continence.

Osteitis Pubis. An inflammation of the periosteum of the pubic bone, often occurring after suprapubic urethral suspension procedures.

Osteomyelitis Pubis. An infection of the pubic bone, which may occur after pelvic operations.

Overflow Incontinence. Involuntary loss of urine when intravesical pressure exceeds the maximum urethral pressure secondary to an elevation of intravesical pressure associated with bladder distension but in the absence of detrusor activity.

Posterior Urethral Angle (PUV). The angle formed by the posterior aspect of the urethra and the bladder. It is generally less than 120 degrees in continent women.

Reflex Incontinence. The involuntary loss of urine caused by abnormal reflex activity in the spinal cord in the absence of the sensation that is usually associated with the desire to micturate.

Residual Urine. Volume of urine remaining in the bladder immediately following completion of micturition.

Trigone (Bladder). The area of the floor of the urinary bladder that forms a triangle with the urethral opening at the apex and the ureteral openings at the ends of the base.

Trigonitis. Inflammation of the trigone.

Urethral Closure Pressure Profile. Intraluminal pressure along the length of the urethra with the bladder at rest.

Urethral Syndrome. An inflammatory condition of the urethra in which bacterial cultures are found to be negative. In most cases *Chlamydia* can now be cultured.

Urge Incontinence. The involuntary loss of urine associated with a strong desire to void. This may be divided into motor urge incontinence, which is associated with uninhibited detrusor contractions, and sensory urge incontinence, which is not caused by uninhibited detrusor contractions.

The gynecologist is frequently called on for consultation on and treatment of urologic problems in the female patient. Perhaps the most commonly seen of these problems involves infection and inflammation of the lower tract (urethritis, trigonitis, and cystitis). However, as many as 10% of all women suffer from some degree of urinary incontinence. This condition increases in incidence with age, and because the number of older women in our population is growing, it is likely that this problem will grow in magnitude with time.

Continence depends on a number of factors, including the neurologic control of micturition, the anatomic relationships of the urinary tract, and the specific effects of a number of systemic, infectious, and neoplastic conditions. This chapter considers the physiology of micturition and the diagnosis and treatment of pathologic entities that affect the female urologic system, and it offers suggestions on diagnosis and management of urinary incontinence.

PHYSIOLOGY OF MICTURITION

A number of factors are in play to maintain continence. Basically these involve those that maintain a urethral closure mechanism and those that affect detrusor function. In the final analysis it is the balance between urethral closure and detrusor function that determines whether micturition occurs or continence is maintained.

The factors affecting the urethral closure mechanism primarily involve urethral tone and include the basic elasticity of the urethra, the presence of smooth and voluntary (striated) muscle, the vascular component supplying the urethra, and the presence of alpha receptors from the sympathetic nervous system, which when stimulated cause contraction of the urethral sphincter.

Bladder detrusor contractility is stimulated by the activity of the parasympathetic nervous system mediated through the neurotransmitter acetylcholine. This stimulates receptors in the bladder wall, which then activate detrusor contraction. Sympathetic nervous system beta receptors within the bladder cause bladder relaxation when stimulated. Bladder contraction may also be affected by irritation and inflammation of the bladder wall, causing uncoordinated contractions.

The act of voiding is under the control of four basic autonomic and somatic nervous system feedback loops. The first loop (loop I) involves a circuit from the cerebral cortex to the brainstem, which inhibits micturition by modifying sensory stimuli emanating from loop II. Loop II, which originates in the sacral micturition (S2 through S4) center and the detrusor muscle wall itself, represents sensory fibers to the brainstem, where modulation of the stimuli by loop I takes place. If cerebral inhibition is not imposed (loop I), the stimuli are returned to the sacral micturition center as a response to the bladder filling, allowing activation of loop III. Loop III involves sensory flow from the bladder wall to the sacral micturition center with returning motor fibers to the urethral sphincter striated muscle, which allows the voluntary relaxation of the urethral sphincter as the detrusor contracts. Loop IV originates in

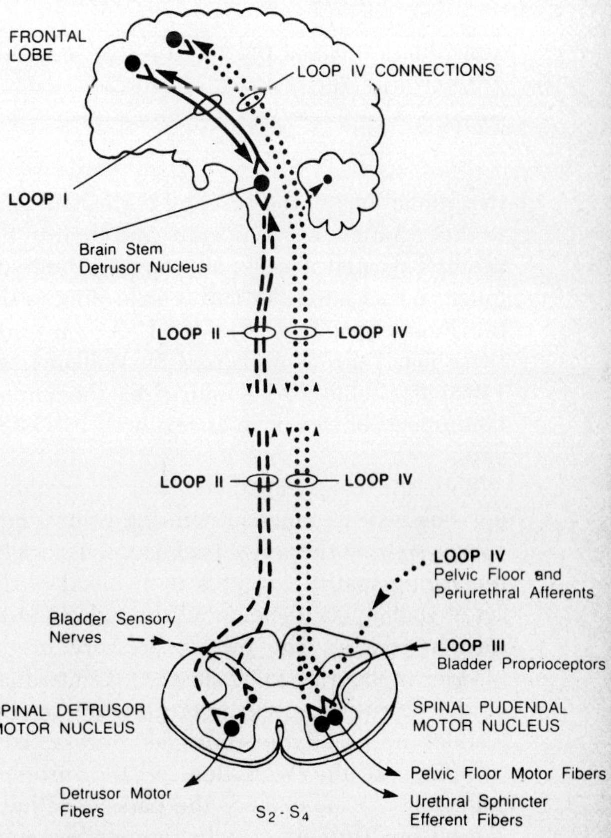

FIGURE 20-1
Central nervous system feedback loops. (From Williams ME, Fitzhugh CP: Ann Intern Med 97:895, 1982.)

TABLE 20-1

Neurologic Control of Micturition: Clinical Considerations on Central Nervous System Reflex Loops

Loop	Origin	Termination	Function	Associated Conditions
I	Frontal lobe	Brainstem	Coordinates volitional control of micturition	Parkinson's disease, brain tumors, trauma, cerebrovascular disease, MS, lower urinary tract disease
II	a. Brainstem b. Bladder wall	Sacral micturition center Brainstem	Detrusor muscle contraction to empty bladder	Spinal cord trauma, MS, spinal cord tumors
III	Sensory afferents of detrusor muscle	Striated muscle of urethral sphincter via pudendal motor nervous and micturition center	Allows relaxation of urethral sphincter in synchrony with detrusor contraction	MS, spinal cord trauma or tumors, diabetic neuropathy, local urinary tract disease
IV	Frontal lobe	Pudendal nucleus	Volitional control of striated external urethral sphincter	Cerebral or spinal trauma or tumor, MS, cerebrovascular disease, lower urinary tract disease

Adapted from Ostergard DR: The neurologic control of micturition and integral voiding reflexes. Obstet Gynecol Surv 34:417, 1979.

the frontal lobe of the cerebral cortex and runs to the sacral micturition center and then to the urethral striated muscle, allowing urethral voluntary muscles to relax and thus leading to the initiation of voiding. Fig. 20-1 demonstrates these four loops as visualized by Williams and Fitzhugh. Table 20-1 summarizes the important aspects of each loop as reviewed by Ostergard.

Both the parasympathetic and sympathetic nervous systems function with the central nervous system in these feedback loops. Basically, the parasympathetic system is involved in the act of voiding via nuclei in S2 through S4 (micturition center). The resting pressure in the bladder is about 20 to 30 cm H_2O. Contraction of the detrusor muscle puts pressure on the bladder neck and the proximal urethra, contributing to the relaxation of the urethral sphincter. As mentioned, the parasympathetic system mediates its activity through the neurotransmitter acetylcholine, directly stimulating receptors in the bladder wall. The sympathetic system, on the other hand, basically acts

to prevent micturition. Via this system norepinephrine is secreted, stimulating both alpha- and beta-adrenergic receptors. The bladder contains primarily beta receptors, stimulation of which causes relaxation of the detrusor muscle. The urethra contains primarily alpha receptors. Stimulation of these alpha receptors causes contraction of the urethral sphincter. Thus the overall effect is to prevent micturition (Fig. 20-2). Because estrogen seems to stimulate alpha receptors and progesterone beta receptors, these hormones play a role in maintaining continence in women in their reproductive years and in women receiving replacement hormone therapy who are postmenopausal.

As the neurogenic control of micturition is so complex and depends on the interaction of so many factors, it is understandable that a host of general systemic diseases, or diseases involving the nervous system, may affect bladder control. These include, but are not limited to, demyelinating diseases, such as multiple sclerosis, diabetes mellitus, vascular diseases, and central

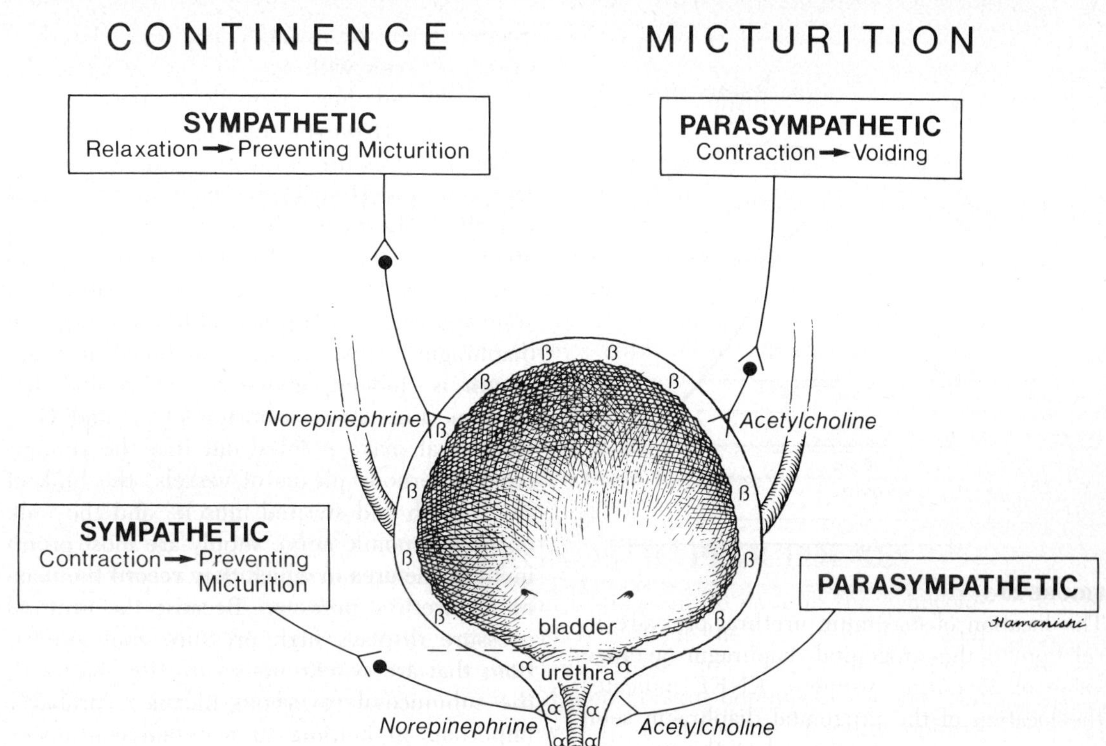

FIGURE 20-2
The innovation of the bladder and urethra. Parasympathetic fibers arising in S2 through S4 have long preganglionic fibers and pelvic ganglia close to the bladder and urethra. These parasympathetic fibers excrete acetylcholine. Sympathetic fibers that have long postganglionic fibers discharge norepinephrine to beta receptors, primarily in the bladder, and alpha receptors, primarily in the urethra. (Redrawn and modified from Raz S: Urol Clin North Am 5:323, 1978.)

nervous system trauma and tumors. In addition, medications that have an effect on the central or autonomic nervous systems may affect bladder control. Compounds with atropinelike effects may interfere with the initiation of micturition, whereas those with cholinergic effects may cause bladder irritability. An appendix to this chapter (pp. 562-566) contains an exhaustive listing developed by Ostergard of agents that affect bladder function.

With the neurologic principles of micturition in mind, it is appropriate to assess other factors that may influence continence. Recently, Asmussen and Ulmsten noted that the bladder and the urethra are essentially a functional unit, with the bladder's subfunction to store urine and the urethra's to allow it to pass. For urine to pass out, the maximum urethral pressure must be lower than the intravesical pressure. Intravesical pressure depends on: (1) the volume of fluid in the bladder, (2) the part of the intraabdominal pressure transmitted to the bladder, and (3) the tension in the bladder wall related to muscular and nervous system activity.

The intraurethral pressure depends on (1) the striatal muscle fibers of the urethral wall, (2) smooth muscle fibers of the urethral wall, (3) the vascular content of the urethral submucosal cavernous plexus, (4) the passive elasticity of the urethral wall, and (5) the part of the intraabdominal pressure transmitted to the urethra.

Anatomically the exact border between the bladder and urethra is difficult to determine. The functional length of the urethra, however,

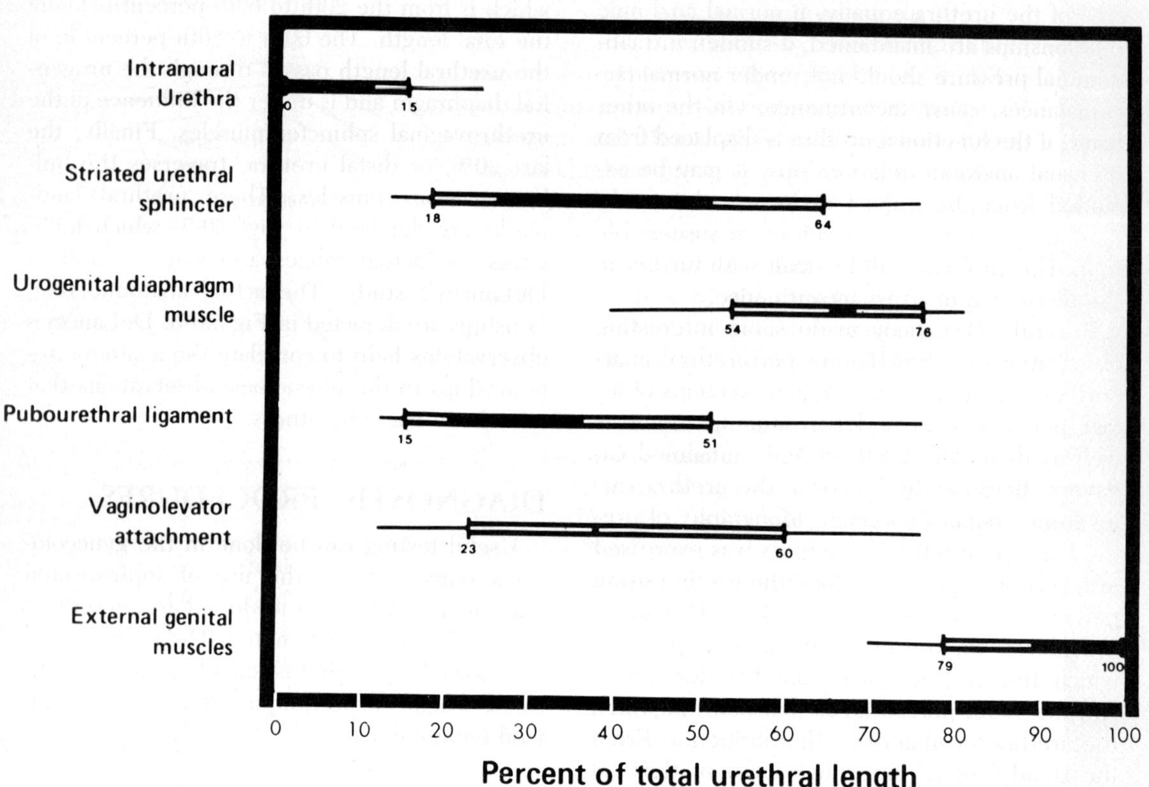

FIGURE 20-5
Average spatial distribution of periurethral structures as well as the range of values found. Urogenital diaphragm muscles are the compressor urethrae and urethrovaginal sphincter. (From DeLancey JO: Obstet Gynecol 68:91, 1986. Reprinted with permission from The American College of Obstetricians and Gynecologists.)

that is infected, trigonitis, or cystitis. Their presence may also suggest an infection in the upper urinary tract such as pyelonephritis. Chronic infection in the lower tract may be associated with urgency, frequency, dysuria, and even incontinence. In such instances the urine analysis and urine culture may be diagnostic.

Test for Residual Urine

This simple procedure can be extremely helpful in the evaluation of a patient with cystocele or overflow incontinence. The patient is asked to void, and a catheter is inserted within 10 to 15 minutes thereafter. The urine remaining in the bladder should be measured and may be sent for analysis and culture. Under normal circumstances the residual should be less than 50 ml after the patient has voided at least 100 to 150 ml. Large residuals suggest overflow incontinence due to inadequate bladder emptying.

Office Cystometrics

Bladder capacity and bladder function may be measured with sophisticated tools, which are discussed later. Nevertheless it is possible to gain a great deal of information about bladder capacity and bladder function with a relatively simple apparatus. If after a catheter is inserted to check for residual urine the catheter is left in place and attached to a graduated Asepto syringe without bulb, it is possible to pour sterile saline into the syringe and measure the amount of saline that first causes the pa-

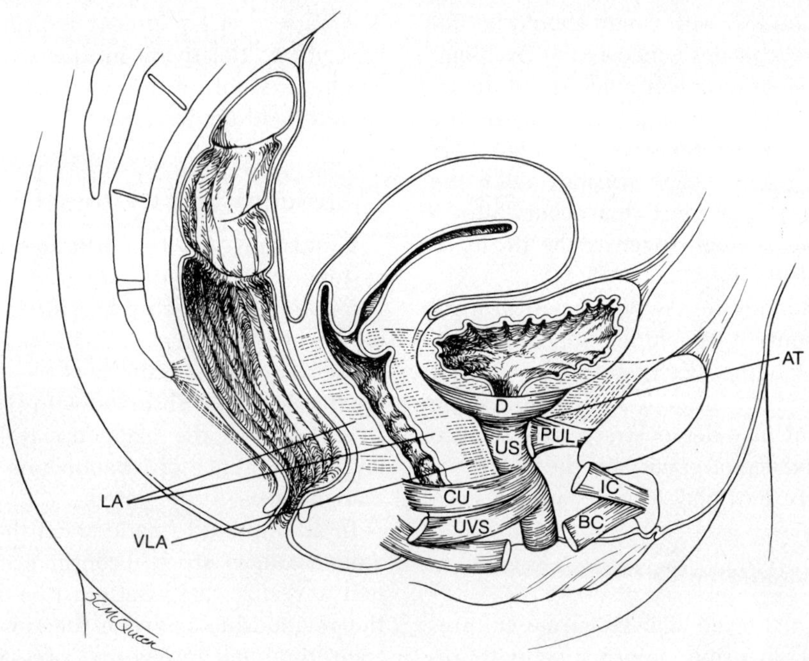

FIGURE 20-6

Interrelationships of approximate location of periurethral structures. Levator ani muscles are shown as light lines running deep to the pelvic viscera. The vaginal levator attachment is shown as a darker area. *VLA,* vaginal levator attachment; *LA,* levator ani muscles; *D,* detrusor muscle; *US,* urethral sphincter; *CU,* compressor urethrae; *UVS,* urethrovaginal sphincter; *AT,* arcus tendineus fasciae pelvis; *PUL,* pubourethral ligament; *IC,* ischiocavernosus muscle; and *BC,* bulbocavernosus muscle. (Redrawn from DeLancey JO: Obstet Gynecol 68:91, 1986. Reproduced with permission from The American College of Obstetricians and Gynecologists.)

tient to have the urge to void. This urge should normally occur after 150 to 200 ml of saline have been infused. However, normal women should be able to continue to maintain continence at that level, with a strong, normally uncontrollable urge to void usually occurring when 400 to 500 ml have been instilled. Thus a normal bladder first transmits an urge to void at 150 to 200 ml, and functional capacity is reached at 400 to 500 ml. Most women can maintain continence with larger volumes, but this is usually accomplished with a great deal of conscious effort.

Stress (Bonney) Test

If a bladder has been previously filled to measure capacity, it should then be emptied to about 250 ml of saline, or if the bladder is empty, 250 ml of saline should be instilled. The catheter is then removed, and the patient is asked to cough while in the recumbent position. If urine spurts from the urethral meatus, stress incontinence may be present. The bladder neck should be gently elevated with the finger or an instrument such as a Kelly clamp, and the patient should be asked to cough once again. Care should be taken not to compress the urethra, thereby mechanically occluding it. If urine no longer spurts from the urethra when the bladder neck is supported, this is suggestive that the bladder neck separation from the pubic symphysis may be responsible for the incontinence, and an appropriate operative repair could be expected to produce continence.

Because urine loss with cough should be immediate if stress incontinence is the problem, it may be possible to detect evidence of detrusor instability by observing the time of the spurt of urine in the Bonney test. Classically the detrusor reacts a few seconds after the stimulus; therefore a spurt that occurs after a delay following a cough suggests the presence of a detrusor instability.

After the Bonney test is performed in a recumbent patient, it should be repeated with the patient standing. Frequently the patient will appear to be continent with stress while lying down but may demonstrate incontinence when the influence of gravity on the pelvic organs is brought into play in the standing position.

. . .

Thus, with the urine analysis, urine culture, tests for residual urine, information with respect to the amount of urine it takes before the first urge to void occurs, information concerning general bladder capacity, and the Bonney test in both the recumbent and the standing positions the physician will have a great deal of information concerning the etiology of the patient's urinary problem. More sophisticated urodynamic evaluations using specific and often costly equipment should be performed by individuals who are trained and experienced in these tests. A short discussion of these procedures and the equipment involved follows.

Urethroscopy

Urethroscopy is excellent for visualizing the urethra and therefore offers information with respect to inflammatory processes within the urethra, urethral diverticula, other anatomic defects, and estrogenic effects and permits some estimation of urethral tone. The use of a gas medium such as carbon dioxide is appropriate for these studies. Although the equipment used for performing gas urethroscopy makes it possible to measure pressures within the urethra and the bladder, caution must be exercised because a rapid instillation of carbon dioxide into the lower urinary tract may stimulate detrusor contraction, which may in itself lead to reflex opening of the vesical neck, thus giving false information about the bladder neck and the urethral sphincter.

A variety of equipment is provided for this procedure. Relatively inexpensive apparatuses can be used for urethroscopy as well as for cystometry and uroflowmetry.

Cystoscopy and Cystometry

Cystoscopy may be performed using a water system or a carbon dioxide gas system. The water system is probably best used for diagnosis of detrusor hyperactivity, because it does not cause the reflex irritability of the detrusor muscle that has been observed with the gas system. In either case the bladder may be visualized and the presence of inflammation or benign or malignant processes noted.

In attempting to understand the basis of anatomic urinary stress incontinence, it is important to realize that what must be determined is the relationship between the simultaneous intraurethral and intravesical pressures (Fig. 20-7). For greatest accuracy these must be measured with the patient in the standing and in the reclining positions at rest and with straining. The ideal means of evaluating a patient for stress incontinence would be to use a multi-

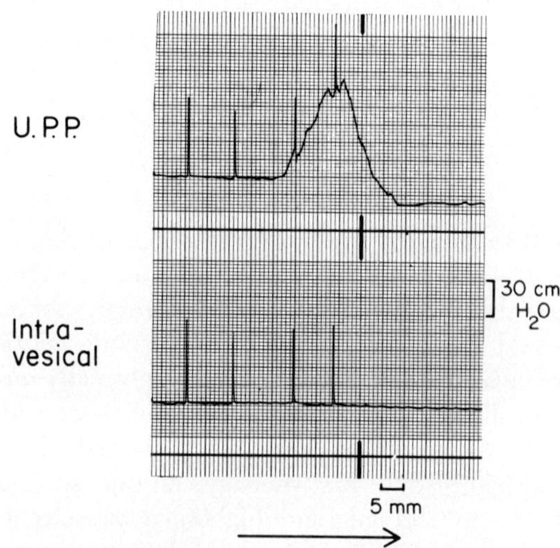

FIGURE 20-7
Simultaneous recordings of urethra and intravesical pressures during coughing. Stress produces a parallel increase of bladder and urethral pressure because the intraabdominal position of the bladder and proximal two thirds of the urethra are displayed. (From Raz S: Urol Clin North Am 5:323, 1978.)

channel recorder that would permit pressure determinations at two points within the urethra (proximal and mid to distal), one within the bladder and one intrabdominally as recorded by an intrarectal sensor or by a sensor within the vagina if the vagina is in a relatively normal position (not prolapsed). Should intraabdominal stress be transmitted equally to the bladder and the urethra and should the intravesical pressure be less than the urethral closing pressure, then one would expect closing pressure to be overcome and stress incontinence to be demonstrated if an intraabdominal pressure increase is transmitted to the bladder but not to the urethra.

Multiple channel devices involves more expensive equipment and require continuous maintenance. It is possible to add a video urodynamic system to the multichannel recorders, making it possible to identify reflux into the ureters under pressure situations. The video system also makes it possible to actually observe the act of micturition and the effect of stress.

INFECTIONS OF THE LOWER URINARY TRACT

Infections of the urethra and bladder are almost always associated with some combination of the following: frequency, urgency, dysuria, pyuria, hematuria, acute or chronic pelvic pain, backache, and at times fever. As many as 20% of all women develop urinary tract infections at some time during their life, and by age 70 as many as 10% of women will have chronic urinary tract infections. At times incontinence is associated with acute and chronic infections. Although *Escherichia coli* is the cause of the majority of the infections, myriad organisms including *Enterobacter, Klebsiella, Pseudomonas, Proteus, Streptococcus faecalis, Morganella, Staphylococcus*, and *Chlamydia* are found. The presence of bacteria in the urine (bacteriuria) does not necessarily prove clinical infection. But the presence of at least 100,000 organisms per milliliter of urine is generally accepted as evidence for a clinical infection. In cases of urethritis and trigonitis the presence of as few as 100 organisms per milliliter may indicate an infection because of the dilution factor of bladder urine. White blood cells are always seen in the urine (pyuria) when urinary

tract infection occurs, and red blood cells may be present in microscopic or macroscopic numbers. Hematuria is frequent in acute infections.

Many explanations have been offered as to why the female urinary tract is vulnerable to infection. These include the fact that the female urethra is short, thereby allowing easier access of bacteria to the bladder; the close proximity of vulva, vagina, and rectum to the opening of the urethra; poor hygiene, including the habit in some women of wiping toward the urethra after a bowel movement; the effects of sexual intercourse on the entrance of bacteria into the urethra and the lower urinary tract; and the effect of loss of estrogen on the reproductive tract of elderly women. To this list it is probably appropriate to add personal immunologic variations that may make one woman more susceptible to certain bacteria than others. Additional circumstances that may be responsible for infections in women include the dilation of the urinary tract in pregnancy, urinary tract obstruction, ureteral reflux, and situations of urinary tract relaxation. Other causes of urinary tract infections in both men and women would be the need for frequent catheterization, instrumentation, the loss of resistance that occurs in general systemic disease, and overdistension of the bladder in neurogenic conditions where stasis becomes a problem.

Urethritis

Patients with urethritis generally have the typical findings of lower urinary tract infection, which include dysuria, frequency, and urgency. They often have a urethra that is tender to palpation. Under certain circumstances it may be possible to express pus from the urethra; this is particularly common in acute infections with the gonococcus or *Chlamydia*. In these situations the infection involves not only the urethra but the periurethral glands as well. Frequently, significant pyuria is noted in a clean-catch urine sample, particularly that taken early in the voiding. The urine should be inspected, since *Trichomonas* infestation is frequently noted in such instances.

Pus expressed from the urethra should be submitted for culture and for smear with Gram's stain. Intracellular diplococci are suggestive of gonorrhea. *Neisseria Gonor-*

rhoeae or *Chlamydia* is usually cultured in such situations. Urine obtained by the clean-catch method should also be cultured.

If no specific organism is identified on smear, a broad-spectrum coverage such as a sulfa preparation or nitrofurantoin (Macrodantin), 50 or 100 mg three times a day, should be prescribed for 10 days. If *Chlamydia* is suspected, tetracycline should be prescribed for at least 10 days. If gonorrhea is diagnosed, a treatment of choice is 4.8 million units of procaine penicillin intramuscularly following 1 g of oral probenecid. It is wise to cover such patients with tetracycline (500 mg four times a day for 7 days) or doxycycline (100 mg twice a day for 7 days) as well because mixed infections are common and also because as many as 20% of cases of gonorrhea are resistant to penicillin.

Urethral Syndrome

The so-called urethral syndrome is characterized by the same symptoms of dysuria, frequency, urgency, and pain that are seen with urethritis, but generally the symptoms are of long standing, and no specific organism can be identified. Classically, urethroscopy has revealed a reddened, chronically inflamed urethra with spasm at the bladder neck. Dilation with progressive urethral dilators has been the treatment of choice. More recently, however, *Chlamydia* and anaerobic organisms have been identified in several such cases. With specific antimicrobial treatment of these organisms symptoms have abated. Therefore the urethral syndrome diagnosis should not be made until all infectious organisms have been ruled out as a cause. When this is done, it is conceivable that the syndrome will disappear.

Cystitis

Cystitis is perhaps the most common of the urinary tract infections. It is diagnosed when a clean voided urine sample or catheterized specimen has a bacteria concentration of 100,000 or more per milliliter of urine and when the patient suffers the symptoms of dysuria, frequency, urgency, and pain. White blood cells are almost always seen in large numbers in the urine, as are bacteria. Red blood cells are frequently present in micro-scopic numbers, but gross hematuria may occur as a result of extravasation of blood across dilated and inflamed capillaries. If the bladder is visualized, it is noted to be uniformly reddened and inflamed. Treatment involves obtaining a culture and beginning the patient on a general antibiotic regimen of sulfa or nitrofurantoin, although a variety of other antibiotics could be used as substitutes for general therapy. These would include tetracycline, ampicillin, cephalosporin, or nalidixic acid (Neg-Gram). When results of the culture are reported, the antibiotic may be changed if the organisms noted are not sensitive to the antibiotic in use. Treatment should be continued for 10 days, and the patient should remain well hydrated and should be encouraged to continue treatment even though symptoms generally disappear within 48 hours. Infections frequently recur and become chronic because they are not adequately eradicated. This may be due to physician error (treating with too low a dose of antibiotic or for too short of a period of time) or patient error (not taking the medication as prescribed). The latter occurrence is generally suspected when the same organism is continuously cultured. Recurrent infections of different organisms should alert the physician to the need for a more complete evaluation of the urinary tract, including intravenous pyelogram (seeking structural abnormalities of the bladder). Occasionally continuous antibiotic therapy at lower doses for more prolonged periods is necessary to ensure that the patient is no longer infected.

Frequent catheterizations or manipulation of the lower urinary tract often cause urinary tract infections. An indwelling catheter left in place for 24 hours leads to bacteriuria in as many as 50% of patients. When left in place for 96 hours an indwelling catheter causes bacteriuria in nearly 100% of patients. Many physicians suggest prophylactic antibiotics in patients who must continue catheter use, but no good evidence supports this thesis. Certainly a patient with an indwelling catheter should be monitored for the possibility of bacteriuria and urinary tract infections, kept well hydrated, and have a urine culture when the catheter is removed. Postoperative and debilitated patients are at greatest risk.

Physicians can counsel their patients about

preventive measures by instructing them on proper hygiene. This consists of cleansing the vulvar region at least daily, wiping the rectum away from the urethra, and encouraging good hygiene with respect to coitus. In women who develop frequent urinary tract infections secondary to coitus, one technique is to encourage voiding immediately after intercourse. This tends to wash out bacteria that have found entrance into the urethra before they can cause an infection. Elderly, sexually active women may be benefited by either external or systemic estrogen therapy.

Urethral Diverticulum

Etiology

Urethral diverticula occur in perhaps as many as 3% to 4% of all women sometime during their lifetime. Age distribution in published reports ranges from 19 to 76 years, but the majority of diverticula seem to occur between the ages of 30 and 50. Andersen has suggested that the disease occurs more frequently in blacks, with a ratio perhaps as high as 6 to 1.

A variety of etiologies has been suggested, including congenital, acute and chronic inflammatory, and traumatic. The congenital theory stems from the fact that cases have been reported in children and neonates. Evidence for acute and chronic infection stems from the fact that several observers have noted infection and obstruction of periurethral glands, which result in the formation of retention cysts that when repeatedly infected may rupture into the lumen of the urethra, giving rise to the diverticulum. Several authors have suggested that the gonococcus is the cause of this, but *E. coli* and other organisms have been found in such processes. Urethral trauma from multiple catheterizations or via childbirth has also been suggested as an etiologic factor. However, many women with diverticula have neither been catheterized nor have they given birth. The infectious etiology is probably the most common.

Signs and Symptoms

The usual symptoms and signs of a patient with diverticulitis include urgency, frequency, dysuria, and dyspareunia. Frequently a history of recurrent urinary tract infection, dribbling, and incontinence is noted. Occasionally hematuria occurs. In a recent series reported from the Mayo Clinic, Lee noted that a palpable, tender suburethral mass was present in 51 of 85 patients (60%) and that protrusion of the diverticulum from the vaginal introitus occurred in four patients. Occasionally patients have urinary stones within the diverticula.

Diagnosis

Diagnosis is generally suspected by physical examination and confirmed by cystourethroscopy or voiding cystourethrogram. At times it may be necessary to use a double-catheter balloon technique that essentially closes the urethra at each end and forces contrast medium into the diverticulum under pressure during cystogram.

Management

A variety of procedures has been suggested for the management of urethral diverticula. Lapides has suggested a technique for transurethral marsupialization that involves the resection of the roof of the diverticulum, using transurethral electrocautery. Essentially this technique enlarges the orifice of the diverticulum by incising its roof. Spence and Duckett reported a marsupialization technique in which the diverticulum was opened and sutured to the vaginal epithelial surface. Generally this leads to a fistula and requires secondary closure, making this technique useful in only rare circumstances.

A classic operative approach uses urethroscopy to identify the location of the diverticulum. It is important at this point to note the presence of multiple diverticula. In Lee's report from the Mayo Clinic the diverticulum was noted coming from the distal third of the urethra in only 10 of the 85 patients, whereas 38 patients demonstrated an origin from the middle third, and 13 from the proximal third including the bladder neck. Lee noted multiple diverticula in 18 of his 85 patients.

After the diverticulum is identified and evaluated, an incision is made in the anterior vaginal wall and the diverticulum is dissected free of the pubocervical fascia. The diverticulum's attachment to the urethra is noted; it is excised by sharp dissection, and the urethral wall is closed with a row of interrupted 4-0 catgut sutures. The closure line is generally in the longitudinal axis. Occasionally, however, a transverse closure is necessary because of the nature of the attachment. The pubocervical fascia is then reinforced with a row of 3-0 polyglycol reabsorbable interrupted sutures. Hemostasis is scrupulously secured with electrocautery, and the vaginal incision is closed with polyglycol sutures (Fig. 20-8).

Most diverticula emanate from the ventral wall of the urethra. Occasionally, however, the diverticulum is noted to be arising from the lateral wall of the urethra or even from the anterior wall. In such cases the dissection must be

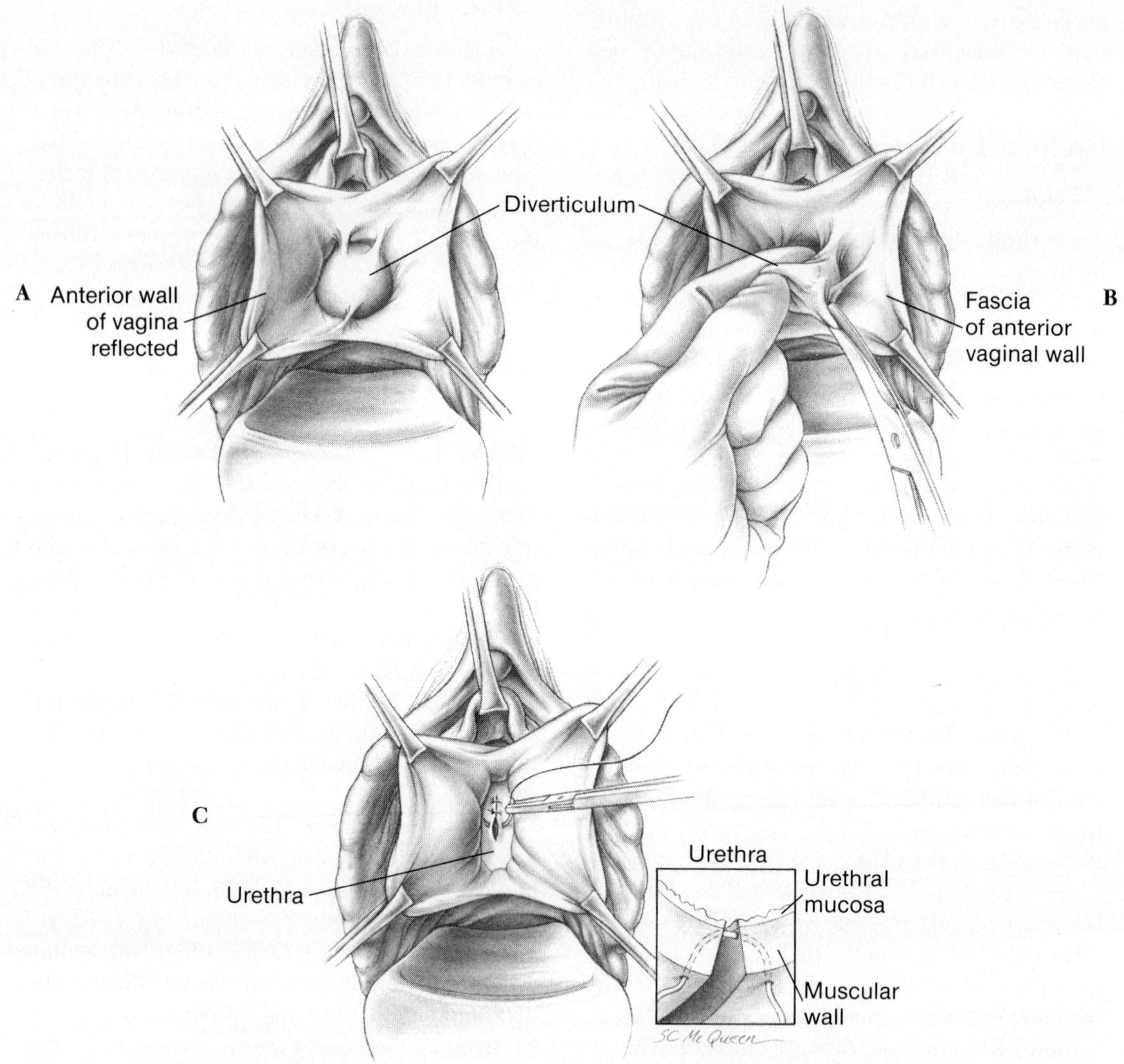

FIGURE 20-8
Resection of urethral diverticulum. **A,** Diverticulum exposed with vaginal lining and endopelvic fascia retracted. **B,** Fingers hold diverticulum on traction, which aids in dissection and identification of ostium. **C,** After complete resection of diverticulum, urethra is closed with fine uninterrupted extramucosal sutures. (Redrawn from Lee RA: Obstet Gynecol 61:52, 1983. Reprinted with permission from The American College of Obstetricians and Gynecologists.)

carefully carried to the base of the diverticulum and the procedure carried out as stated. In cases of diverticula arising from the dorsal wall of the urethra, it is appropriate to simply excise the diverticulum at its neck and allow the tissue of the urethra to retract. In all cases a No. 16 or 18 Foley catheter is left in place for 6 or 7 days.

Several nuances have been offered to make dissection and subsequent repair easier. One of these is placing a ureteral catheter into the diverticulum and allowing it to coil up so that the diverticulum is more easily observable during dissection. Other surgeons have attempted to dilate the neck of the diverticulum before beginning the excision and occasionally have even tried to pack foreign substances such as gauze through the neck to make the dissection easier.

Complications

Major complications of this procedure include urethrovaginal fistula formation, recurrence of the diverticulum, and stricture of the urethra.

In a study from the Mayo Clinic, MacKinnon et al. reported on 140 patients treated operatively, seven of whom (5%) developed urethrovaginal fistulas. In Lee's report of a later study from the Mayo Clinic only one patient developed a fistula. In another series, Spraitz and Welch, reporting on 94 patients repaired, found four with urethrovaginal fistulas.

Recurrence of diverticula is reported in about 5% to 10% of patients in various series. If the diverticulum recurs within the first few months after operation, it may represent a second diverticulum that was overlooked or an inappropriate repair of the diagnosed diverticulum. If the recurrence occurs after 1 year it is probably a new lesion.

Stricture of the urethra has rarely been reported in any of the operative series. It is a theoretic possibility.

Other complications involve stress incontinence, which may be related to the dissection of the bladder neck away from its usual location, and the development of the urethral syndrome, probably caused by continuing inflammation and irritation. These conditions generally respond to appropriate specific therapy.

Urolithiasis

Urinary tract stones may occur in patients of either sex and at any age. They may be related to metabolic abnormalities such as gout or errors of calcium metabolism, but most often they relate to chronic infection and stasis of urine. Risk factors for calculi in women include pregnancy, during which time the urinary tract becomes dilated and stasis is more common; large cystoceles; and obstruction of outflow secondary to anatomic variations or external pressure from other organs. A variety of management techniques is available, but the major consideration should be correction of the basic problem.

GENUINE STRESS INCONTINENCE

Genuine stress incontinence occurs when increased intraabdominal pressure is not transmitted equally to the bladder and the functional urethra. If intraabdominal pressure plus bladder pressure is sufficient to overcome urethral closing pressure, incontinence will occur. The real problem is the fact that the bladder neck, the base of the bladder, and the proximal urethra are no longer adequately supported. This may be due to a separation of the supports that hold the upper vagina and urethra to the pubic symphysis, to a relaxation of pelvic fascia and musculature secondary to childbearing or the aging process, or to some sort of trauma. Because the proximal two thirds of the urethra normally is an intraabdominal structure, an increased intraabdominal pressure would normally be exerted against it as well as the bladder. However, with a change in the anatomic relationships of this portion of the urethra, its intraabdominal position may be lost, thereby making it the brunt of such pressure rather than allowing it this degree of protection.

Over the years urethral length has been implicated as a related factor in stress incontinence. Lapides et al. measured urethral length using calibrated intraurethral catheters before and after operative correction of stress incontinence and found the urethra was shorter in cases of incontinence. However, during their procedure, downward traction was exerted to give the most meaningful measurement. Because the bladder neck in such women frequently funnels, accuracy of the measurements by Lapides et al. has been considered suspect. Other studies by multiple investigators using bead-chain urethrocystography have failed to show any change in urethral length before or after standard repair procedures. Thus it would seem that except for the most unusual circumstances, anatomic urethral length is not a major factor in stress incontinence.

The importance of a posterior urethrovesical angle in maintaining continence was first discussed by Jeffcoate and Roberts using urethrocystographic techniques in both continent and incontinent women. They concluded that a normal posterior urethrovesical angle (PUV) of less than 120 degrees was an important aspect of the continence mechanism, because such an angle was characteristically greater than 120 degrees in patients suffering from stress incontinence. This point has been verified by several authors since then. It has been noted that the relationship of the bladder neck and urethra to the pubic symphysis is not the major anatomic feature of the etiology of stress incontinence, because many patients with bladder descent but with a normal PUV angle were continent, whereas some incontinent women had bladders and urethras appropriately positioned to the pubic symphysis but had lost their PUV. Normal continent women demonstrate a bladder base nearly parallel to the horizontal in a standing position and have a sharply defined PUV angle of 90 to 100 degrees. When such bladders are visualized by cystourethrography it is noted that the angle is maintained even with cough, and funneling does not occur. Most women with stress incontinence usually demonstrate near complete loss of the PUV angle and funneling and posterior descent of the vesical neck.

In the past Green and others have attempted to separate the severity of stress incontinence by the amount of loss of PUV angle. They defined type I loss as showing complete or almost complete loss of PUV angle but with the angle of inclination to the vertical of the urethral axis as being normal (10 to 30 degrees) or at least 45 degrees in the lateral standing-straining configuration, as measured by urethrocystogram. They define a type II defect as representing loss of the PUV angle with an abnormal angle

of inclination to the vertical of the urethral axis generally being between 45 and 90 degrees. In 1971 the concept of a Q-tip test was introduced to differentiate these two types of defects. This test involved placing a Q-tip into the urethra and observing the angle the urethra made with the horizontal in the relaxed and voiding positions. Recently Montz and Stanton reevaluated the Q-tip test and discovered that 32% of patients with a positive Q-tip test had either pure detrusor instability or pure sensory urgency after a complete urologic workup. Further, 29% of the patients who had a negative Q-tip test were finally diagnosed as pure genuine stress incontinence. Although these authors noted that the Q-tip test was more likely to be positive in younger patients with a cystourethrocele who had undergone minimal bladder neck repair, they believed that the Q-tip test was not sensitive enough to differentiate stress incontinence from other forms of incontinence and recommended that more sensitive and specific urodynamic investigations be carried out in incontinent women. This is now a widely accepted concept.

A second test developed to help identify abnormalities of the bladder neck was the bead-chain cystourethrogram. This involved placing a sterile bead chain through the urethra into the bladder and x-raying the patient during the resting stage and during voiding. Recently, however, Fantl et al. demonstrated that 83 cystourethrograms interpreted by three radiologists using five specific radiologic landmarks failed to identify any agreement in interpretation, with a variation in interpretation being from 19.3% to 54.2%. Further, Fantl's group could find no statistically significant difference in the distribution of radiographic characteristics between patients with stress incontinence and detrusor instability.

It is well accepted today that the degree of loss of PUV angle is not as critical as the position of the bladder neck within the abdominal cavity, and Green's classification is no longer used in most centers.

A frequent area of confusion in diagnosis is caused by the presence of a cystocele. A cystocele is a herniation of the bladder into the vagina and is visualized with the patient in the lithotomy position as a bulge of the anterior vaginal wall. Most patients with cystoceles, however, have well-supported bladder necks and are continent. At times the anatomic defect involves the urethra and the bladder neck as well, forming a cystourethrocele. In such cases in addition to the presence of the cystocele the bladder neck is displaced also. Whereas the patient with a cystocele rarely has stress incontinence, the patient with the cystourethrocele frequently has stress incontinence.

Management

Before considering the operative approaches to the treatment of stress incontinence, it is reasonable to discuss other means of management. The first of these is directed toward the strengthening of the levator ani and pubococcygeal muscles. This can be effected by isometric exercises as described by Kegel. Although a number of modifications of these exercises exist, one useful application is to teach the patient to contract these muscles for the count of 10, 5 to 10 times, and to repeat this series several times a day. Interestingly, Kegal in 1956 suggested that the patient contract her pubococcygeal muscles 5 times on waking, 5 times on rising, and 5 times every half hour throughout the day. The patient can be instructed on how to contract these muscles by being told to attempt to stop the urinary stream while she is voiding. After she learns which muscles to contract, she may perform the exercises at any time without any relationship to voiding. These exercises improve the muscular supports of the bladder neck, and in some cases this may be enough to overcome the anatomic weakness that led to the stress incontinence.

In postmenopausal women, estrogen therapy may increase the vasculature and the tone of the bladder neck, thereby increasing urethral closing pressure and again overcoming the effects that have led to mild degrees of stress incontinence. Estrogen also has a positive effect on pelvic supports in many women, and the combination of estrogen and Kegel exercises may occasionally be all that some women require to overcome their stress incontinence.

Other drugs and combinations of drugs have been studied to determine whether nonoperative therapy could aid stress incontinent women. In a study of 30 stress incontinent women using clinical and urodynamic assessment, Kiesswetter et al. compared continence profiles after treatment with an alpha-adrenergic stimulant, midodrine; a cholinesterase inhibitor, distigmine bromide; a tricyclic antidepressant, imipramine; or an estriol, triodurin. In each case the patients were treated for 4 weeks and reevaluated. Finally, a suspensory sling operation was performed. After a successful sling operation the profile for continence as outlined by the authors increased 45% as compared to an increase of 9% for midodrine, 8.9% for imipramine, and 7.9% for the combination of estriol and distigmine bromide. The urethral pressures showed an increase of mean value of 8.1% after operation, 8.3% after midodrine, 7.9% after imipramine, 3.5% after estriol, and 3.5% after distigmine bromide. The authors believed that subjectively estriol plus midodrine and estriol plus imipramine were favored by the patients over single-drug therapy, but little difference was noted in urodynamic assessment to show the advantage of one drug or combination over another. Although imipramine is a tricyclic antidepressant, it has alpha-adrenergic enhancement characteristics. Table 20-3 is a summary by Corlett of classes of other agents that may affect urinary function or therapy.

Before the 1950s the operative approach to treat stress incontinence primarily involved vaginal procedures, which included plication of the bladder neck (Kelly procedure) with anterior colporrhaphy to reduce a cystocele. However, after Green attempted to grade the degree of PUV angle loss in such patients, it was demonstrated by Bailey and others that the success rate using the vaginal approach varied according to the etiology. Patients showing an almost complete loss of PUV angle had a 90% success rate when followed for 5 to 10 years following a bladder neck plication and anterior colporrhaphy, but only 50% of patients with lesser PUV angle loss remained continent over that period. However, after the introduction of suprapubic urethrovesical suspension operations the 5-year cure rate for these latter patients surpassed 90% in most series. It thus seemed important to determine the type of anatomic defect the patient had and to design appropriate operative management.

For the patient with a definite relaxation of the anterior vaginal wall and a bladder neck

TABLE 20-3
Drugs With Possible Effects on the Lower Urinary Tract

Class	Possible Side Effects	Drug and Usual Indication	Action
Antihypertensives	Incontinence	Reserpine—hypertension Methyldopa—hypertension	Pharmacologic sympathectomy by depleting catecholamines
Dopaminergic agonists	Bladder neck obstruction	Bromocriptine—galactorrhea Levodopa—Parkinson's disease	Increased urethral resistance and decreased detrusor contractions
Cholinergic agonists	Decreased bladder capacity and increased intravesical pressure	Digitalis—cardiotropic	Increased bladder wall tension
Neuroleptics	Incontinence	Major tranquilizers: prochlorperazine, promethazine, trifluoperazine, chlorpromazine, haloperidol	Dopamine receptor blockade, with internal sphincter relaxation
β-Adrenergic agents	Urinary retention	Isoxsuprine—vasodilator Terbutaline—bronchodilator Ritodrine—tocolytic agent	Inhibited bladder muscle contractility
Xanthines	Incontinence	Caffeine	Decreased urethral closure pressure

From Corlett RC: Gynecologic urology. I. Urinary incontinence. Female Patient 10:20, 1985.

that is displaced into the lower pelvis, an anterior colporrhaphy with bladder neck plication is appropriate. This is frequently performed in conjunction with a vaginal hysterectomy if there is evidence for uterine prolapse and a posterior colporrhaphy, because such patients frequently have relaxation of the support structures of both anterior and posterior vaginal walls. The decision of whether to perform a vaginal hysterectomy and posterior wall repair depends on the circumstances of the patient and does not modify the success rate of the anterior colporrhaphy and bladder neck plication with respect to stress incontinence.

The anterior colporrhaphy is carried out by incising the vaginal mucosa in the midline and separating the pubocervical fascia from the vaginal mucosa by blunt and sharp dissection. The dissection is carried to the area of the bladder neck, and the first plication suture is placed on either side of the bladder neck using a 2-0 polyglycol suture. The slowly absorbable suture is ideal for this type of repair. Bladder plication is then continued from the area of the bladder neck to reduce an existing cystocele (Fig. 20-9). In a patient with a displaced bladder neck and a cystourethrocele it is often useful to place sutures in paravaginal tissue lateral to the bladder neck and fix this area to the pubic symphysis during the vaginal procedure. The vaginal tissue parallel to the bladder neck is identified and sutured with a polyglycol suture that is placed into the pubic symphysis. One suture on either side frequently suffices; the procedure requires a certain amount of dexterity, but the operator can quickly achieve this with practice.

Modifications of this procedure have been described. Special needles have been developed by Pereyra that can be used to guide sutures from the paravaginal tissue through the space of Retzius. Nonabsorbable material is

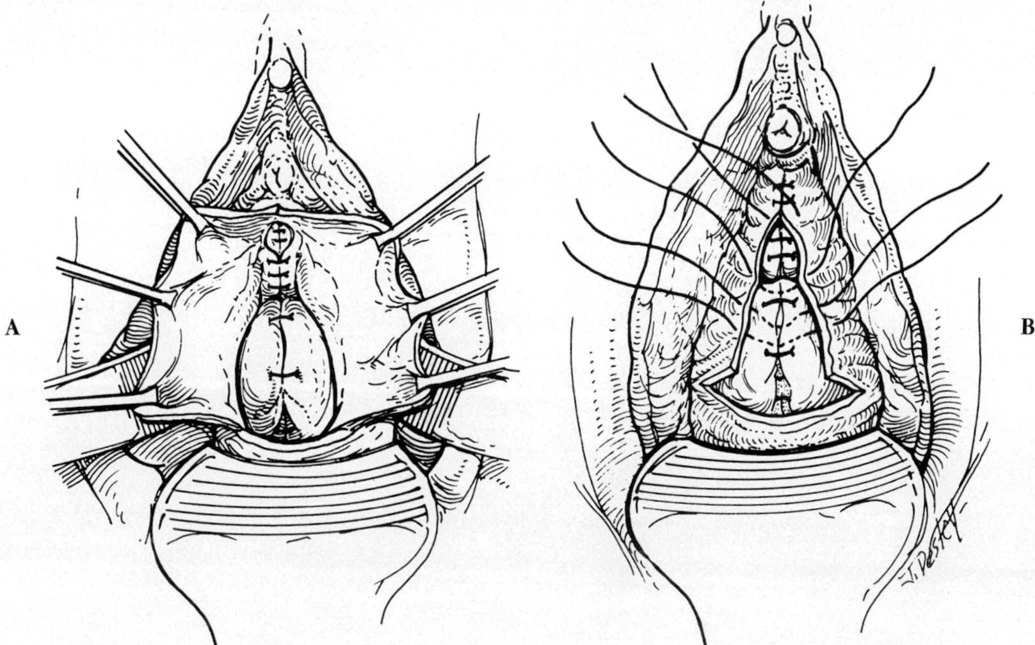

FIGURE 20-9
Cystourethrocele repair. **A,** Appearance of cystourethrocele after plication of bladder neck and repair of cystocele; cut edge of vagina is held apart above repair. **B,** Repair of vagina over cystocele is noted. (From Symmonds RE: Relaxation of pelvic supports. In Benson, RC, ed: Current obstetric and gynecologic diagnosis and treatment, 5th ed. Los Altos, Calif., Lange Medical Publications, 1984.)

used, and the suture is tied over the rectus fascia just above the bladder neck. This is carried out through a small suprapubic incision. It is appropriate to follow the steps of this procedure under direct urethrocystoscopy to avoid injuring the bladder neck during the needle placement. Stamey's modification of the Pereyra procedure uses a small tube of Dacron material to buttress the suture, thereby keeping it from pulling through. Stamey reports about 3% of the patients in his series required a removal of the suprapubic suture because of pain or infection.

Appropriate therapy for patients with bladder neck displacement, without significant anterior vaginal wall relaxation but with incontinence, in most instances is by a suprapubic approach. The Marshall-Marchetti-Krantz suprapubic urethrovesical suspension operation was first reported in 1949 and has been the mainstay of most surgeons attempting to ac-

complish alleviation of stress incontinence in such patients. The procedure may be done by itself or in conjunction with other abdominal procedures such as an abdominal hysterectomy. The space of Retzius is entered, the bladder neck is identified generally with a 30 cc bulb Foley catheter in the bladder, and the paravaginal tissue adjacent to the bladder neck is identified and sutured to the pubic symphysis using two or three interrupted sutures on either side of the bladder neck. Again, 2-0 polyglycol suture is ideal for this procedure but many operators prefer catgut and even nonabsorbable suture. The operator must be careful not to place undue stress on the bladder neck. Stress can generally be assessed by placing one hand in the vagina and palpating the tension on the bladder neck at the time the sutures are tied (Fig. 20-10). The space of Retzius is then drained for 48 hours with a small Penrose drain and the patient is followed for 5 days with con-

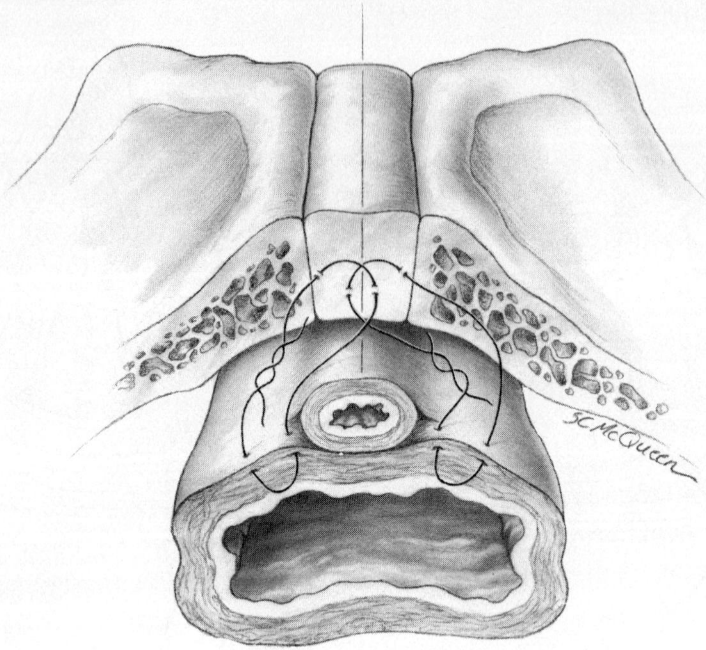

FIGURE 20-10

Demonstration of the relative position of a pair of sutures adjacent to the urethra securely placed into the pubic symphysis. (Redrawn from Buchsbaum HJ, Schmidt JD, eds: Gynecologic and obstetric urology. Reprinted with permission from W.B. Saunders Co., Philadelphia, 1982.)

tinuous catheter drainage. In most cases after the removal of the catheter the patient will void. Occasionally, voiding is delayed and the patient may need to be discharged with an indwelling catheter in the bladder to be checked 1 week hence. It is usual to check a patient for residual urine after she voids; residuals of less than 100 cc, after the patient voids at least 100 to 200 ml, are considered acceptable. Larger residuals should signal continuing catheterization for 48 to 72 hours.

A rare (1% to 2%) but painful complication of the Marshall-Marchetti-Krantz procedure is osteitis pubis. This condition is an inflammatory reaction in the periosteum of the pubic bone more often associated with permanent suture material. This complication following suprapubic cystotomy was first reported in 1923 by Legueu and Rochet. The following year Beer described six patients with pubic symphysis periostitis after suprapubic procedures. It is important to differentiate this condition from true osteomyelitis. The latter condition, seen occasionally after radical pelvic operations

and other pelvic procedures, involves infection of the bone and is often associated with positive blood cultures. Hoyme et al. recently reviewed this subject with respect to radical gynecologic operations. Treatment of osteomyelitis often involves prolonged antibiotic therapy and surgical debridement. Treatment of osteitis pubis includes antibiotics and analgesics and may require the removal of permanent sutures.

In 1961, Burch advocated a modification of the suprapubic bladder neck suspension by suspending the vaginal wall to Cooper's ligament. The original description uses 2-0 chromic catgut suture, but polyglycol sutures are probably more appropriate now. Postoperative care similiar to that described for the Marshall-Marchetti-Krantz operation is appropriate. At times patients have difficulty voiding for prolonged periods, and the occasional patient may report that she needs to rise off the commode to a semistanding position to void.

Both the Marshall-Marchetti-Krantz and Burch procedures have their advocates. When properly performed each procedure cures patients with stress incontinence in 90% to 95% of cases. Frequently failures can be resolved by performing the same procedure again, indicating that the problem was technical performance of the procedure rather than a failure of the type of procedure.

In situations where the Marshall-Marchetti-Krantz or Burch operations fail and the operator does not wish to attempt a similar suspension, a fascial sling procedure may be considered. This procedure, which mobilizes the bladder neck completely using a vaginal and abdominal approach, allows for the imposition of a strip of anterior rectus fascia still attached surrounding the bladder neck and then reattached to the anterior rectus fascia on the opposite side. This creates a pulley effect, and with intraabdominal stress, contraction of the abdominal wall muscles allows for a "pulling up" effect on the bladder neck. This procedure is generally effective in creating continence. The surgeon must exercise care in determining the tension to be applied on the bladder neck when the fascia is fixed. Making the sling too tight may interfere with voiding and may actually damage the bladder neck; making it too loose will abrogate its effectiveness. Generally with a No. 16 or 18 Foley catheter in the urethra it should be possible for the surgeon to judge the tension so that the sling fits comfortably against the urethra without compressing it. Concomitant cystoscopy may also be used.

Although an anterior rectus sheath fascial sling procedure is probably as effective as a Marshall-Marchetti-Krantz or Burch procedure, it involves a greater degree of dissection as well as entry into the vagina with the potential risk of ascending infection. It is a more complicated procedure than necessary in most cases.

Other types of sling procedures have been advocated over the years, including using inert materials such as Mersilene and polypropylene (Marlex) and a variety of human and nonhuman fascial strips. These slings have been fashioned to encircle the urethra and to be put in place by vaginal, abdominal, or combined procedures. In many cases the inert material or nonhuman fascial strips have been rejected or in the case of the latter reabsorbed. Risk of morbidity, especially by infection, has been considerable. The anterior rectus sheath sling operation is the most successful and safest, but it should be used only after a Marshall-Marchetti-Krantz or Burch procedure failure.

Urodynamic Studies After Retropubic Urethropexy for Stress Incontinence

In a study of 29 women with stress incontinence investigated urodynamically before and after Marshall-Marchetti-Krantz operation by Beisland et al. no major changes in the urethral pressure profile could be demonstrated. The authors did note a good correlation between clinical results and the changes in transmission of increased abdominal pressure to the urethra. The operative procedure did not seem to increase the urethral pressure. Those patients with low maximal urethral pressure preoperatively continued to have insufficient urethral sphincter function after the operation. Indeed the operation in some cases may have caused injury to the sphincter because of too extensive dissection around the urethra. The authors pointed out that patients with a low urethral closure pressure but with good transmission to the urethra of pressure are not suitable candidates for urethropexy. Insufficiency of the urethral sphincter in postmenopausal women is usually associated with atrophy of the mucosa of the urethra and the epithelium of the vagina as well as decreased blood supply in the periurethral tissue. The authors suggested such patients should be treated with a combination of alpha-receptor stimulating drugs and estrogen and not by operation.

In a study of 25 women after Burch colposuspension in which 88% had objective evidence of cure, an increase in voiding difficulty and urodynamic evidence of outflow obstruction was seen 6 months after the procedure. Beisland et al. also noted that the Burch procedure, like the Marshall-Marchetti-Krantz operation, does not induce any significant change in resting urethral profile; they believed the changes noted were most likely a mechanical obstruction of the bladder neck.

DETRUSOR DYSSYNERGIA

Walter and Olesen studied 303 patients complaining of urinary incontinence and discovered that 43% had stress incontinence, 21% urge incontinence, and 36% had both urge and stress incontinence. Most patients with urge incontinence suffer from detrusor dyssynergia. This condition is generally chronic and is associated with an urgency-frequency type of problem often accompanied by painless urine loss. Generally a large volume of urine is lost; leakage may occur in any position and often with a change in position. Stress secondary to running, walking, coughing, sneezing, or laughing may trigger this type of incontinence, but it is generally delayed until several seconds after the stress has occurred. Stress incontinence frequently disappears during the night but urge incontinence continues often with nocturia. Patients are often unable to stop their stream during the act of voiding, whereas women with stress incontinence can accomplish this.

Detrusor dyssynergia is the result of sudden, spontaneous detrusor muscle activity and has previously been termed *detrusor instability* or *detrusor irritability*. Some 50% to 80% of patients have an underlying functional or psychosomatic component. Patients, however, may suffer from generalized diseases affecting the bladder or its innervation.

The loss of urine is probably triggered by sudden, uninhibited stimulation of receptors in the bladder wall. These may be hyperreactive for emotional reasons or may be a result of chronic irritation. The problem may also be caused by the breakdown of normal neurologic and inhibitory reflexes. Frequently such patients demonstrate symptoms of chronic anxiety.

Diagnosis

Electronic urethrocystometry as well as fluid cystometrographic techniques allow the detection of spontaneous involuntary pressure changes within the bladder, which are noted as the bladder fills. These techniques are also useful in detecting patients with true stress incontinence who have an urgency incontinence (detrusor dyssynergic) component to their incontinence. It is important that in such cases both problems be treated, or it is not likely that incontinence will be cured.

Management

Operative procedures to treat urgency incontinence are useless. In fact, they can be expected to have no influence on the problem at all. In those patients who have stress incontinence and detrusor dyssynergia an operation may have a place in the specific therapy. However, if the major part of the problem seems to be detrusor dyssynergia, this should be treated first, as an operative procedure may frequently not be necessary. Likewise, patients who have undergone an operation for stress urinary incontinence and continue to be incontinent should be evaluated for detrusor dyssynergia. Bates et al. demonstrated that a high percentage of such failures will be found on urethrocystometric studies to have detrusor dyssynergia.

Because the majority of patients with detrusor dyssynergia have psychosomatic problems, retraining or bladder drills may be of use. This should take the form of bladder retraining, which involves a programmed progressive lengthening of the period between voiding with or without the addition of biofeedback techniques. In a recent study Millard and Oldenburg demonstrated improvement in 74% of women with detrusor dyssynergia using such techniques. Cystometric studies performed on these patients revealed a reversion to stable bladder function.

Postmenopausal women may benefit from estrogen therapy; estrogen not only improves the vasculature of the bladder neck and the mucosa of the urethra and trigone but also has an alpha-adrenergic stimulating capacity that may help overall urinary control.

Anticholinergic drugs or beta-adrenergic stimulation that will relax the detrusor muscle may be useful. The following may be tried: propantheline (Pro-Banthine) at doses of 15 to 30 mg 4 times a day, oxybutynin chloride (Ditropan) 5 mg every 8 to 12 hours, flavoxate (Urispas) 200 mg every 6 hours, imipramine (Tofranil) 50 mg every 8 hours, or ephedrine sulfate 25 mg every 6 hours. At times these medications in conjunction with bladder retraining have greater efficacy than either alone.

TRUE INCONTINENCE

True incontinence is a loss of urine without abnormal bladder function. This is generally caused by fistulas or by other damage to the urinary tract. Such damage may occur congenitally or secondary to trauma.

OVERFLOW INCONTINENCE

This condition occurs when a bladder is overdistended because of its inability to empty. The problem may be caused by a neurologic disorder that interferes with normal bladder reflexes or by partial obstruction of the urethra.

Typically the patient complains of voiding small amounts and still having the feeling that there is urine in the bladder. In addition, the patient frequently loses small amounts of urine without any control. This condition is commonly seen in patients with multiple sclerosis, diabetic neuropathy, and trauma or tumors of the central nervous system. A complete general medical and urologic workup is necessary to clarify the patient's condition. Therapy directed at the primary cause may be beneficial. Often the patient must be trained in techniques of intermittent self-catheterization.

KEY POINTS

- At least 10% of all women suffer from some degree of urinary incontinence during their lifetime.

- Continence is determined by the balance between those forces that maintain urethral closure and those that affect detrusor function.

- Parasympathetic nervous system activity via the neurotransmitter acetylcholine stimulates receptors in the bladder wall to activate detrusor contraction.

- Anticholinergic agents decrease detrusor activity.

- Sympathetic nervous system receptors in the bladder are mostly beta receptors and when stimulated cause relaxation.

- Sympathetic nervous system receptors in the urethra are basically alpha receptors. Stimulation causes contraction.

- The highest pressure zone in the urethra is about midpoint in the functional urethra, which is roughly 0.5 cm proximal to the urogenital diaphragm.

- Resting pressure within the bladder is between 20 and 30 cm H_2O.

- A normal bladder transmits a voiding urge at 150 to 200 ml volume, and functional capacity is generally 400 to 500 ml.

—————————— **KEY POINTS, cont'd** ——————————

- About 20% of all women will develop urinary infections at some time in their life, and by age 70 as many as 10% of women will have chronic urinary tract infections.

- Bacterial counts of 100,000 or greater per milliliter of urine are usually indicative of a urinary tract infection. *Escherichia coli* is the most common organism seen.

- Bacterial counts of 100 per milliliter may be seen in patients with urethritis.

- Some 3% to 4% of all women will suffer from urethral diverticula, with the majority of cases occurring between the ages of 30 and 50. Most urethral diverticula originate in the middle third of the urethra, but diverticula may occur from any area of the urethra and may be multiple.

- Urethral syndrome should not be diagnosed until all infectious organisms have been ruled out.

- Some 75% to 80% of women with urinary incontinence suffer from stress incontinence.

- The cure rate for Marshall-Marchetti-Krantz and Burch procedures is 90% to 95%.

- Osteitis pubis occurs in 1% to 2% of suprapubic suspension operations.

- About 20% of women with urinary incontinence suffer from detrusor dyssynergia.

- Some 50% to 80% of patients with detrusor dyssynergia have an underlying functional or psychosomatic component.

- Operative procedures are of no value in treating detrusor dyssynergia unless there is a stress incontinence component as well.

- An indwelling catheter for more than 24 hours leads to urinary tract infection in about 50% of cases and in nearly 100% after 96 hours.

BIBLIOGRAPHY

Andersen MTF: The incidence of diverticula in the female urethra. J Urol 98:96, 1967.

Arnold EP, Webster JR, Loose H, et al: Urodynamics of female incontinence: factors influencing the results of surgery. Am J Obstet Gynecol 117:805, 1973.

Asmussen M, Ulmsten U: A new technique for measurement of the urethra pressure profile. Acta Obstet Gynecol Scand 55:167, 1976.

Asmussen M, Ulmsten U: On the physiology of continence and pathophysiology of stress incontinence in the female. Controversies in gynecology and obstetrics, vol. 10. S. Karger, Basel, 1983.

Asmussen M, Ulmsten U: Simultaneous urethrocystometry with a new technique. Scand J Urol Nephrol 10:7, 1976.

Bailey KV: A clinical investigation into uterine prolapse with stress incontinence. Treatment by modified Manchester colporrhaphy. J Obstet Gynaecol Br Comm Part I, 61:291, 1954; Part II, 63:663, 1956; Part III, 70:947, 1963.

Barnett RM: The modern Kelly plication. Obstet Gynecol 34:667, 1969.

Bates CP, Bradley W, Glen E, et al: First report of the standardization of terminology of lower urinary tract function. J Urol 48:39, 1976.

Bates P, Bradley WE, Glen E, et al.: The standardization of terminology of lower urinary tract function. J Urol 121:551, 1979.

Bates CP, Loose H, Stanton SLR: The objective study of incontinence after repair operations. Surg Gynecol Obstet 136:17, 1973.

Beck RP, Maughan GB: Simultaneous intaurethral and intravesical pressure studies in normal women and those with stress incontinence. Am J Obstet Gynecol 89:746, 1964.

Beer E: Periostitis of the symphysis and descending rami of the pubes following suprapubic operations. Int J Med 37:224, 1924.

Beisland HO, Fossberg E, Sander S: Urodynamic studies before and after retropubic urethropexy for stress incontinence in females. Surg Gynecol Obstet 155:333, 1982.

Bhatia NN, Ostergard DR: Urodynamics in women with stress urinary incontinence. Obstet Gynecol 60:552, 1982.

Buchsbaum HJ, Schmidt JD, eds: Gynecologic and obstetric urology. Philadelphia, W.B. Saunders Co., 1982.

Burch JC: Cooper's ligament urethrovesical suspension for stress incontinence. Am J Obstet Gynecol 100:764, 1968.

Corlett RC: Gynecologic urology. I. Urinary incontinence. Female Patient 10:20, 1985.

DeLancey JO: Correlative study of periurethral anatomy. Obstet Gynecol 68:91, 1986.

Enhorning G: Simultaneous recording of intravesical and intraurethral pressure. Acta Chir Scand Suppl 276:1, 1971.

Fantl JA, Beachley MC, Bosch HA, et al: Bead-chain cystourethrogram: An evaluation. Obstet Gynecol 58:237, 1981.

Fernie GR, Jewett MAS, Halsall P, et al: Urodynamic characterization of incontinence in the elderly by bladder volume. J Urol 129:772, 1983.

Fossberg E, Veisland HO, Lundgren RA: Stress incontinence in females: Treatment with phenylpropanolamine. A urodynamic and pharmacological evaluation. Urol Int 38:293, 1983.

Frewen WK: Urgency incontinence. J Obstet Gynaecol Br Comm 79:77, 1972.

Gossling JA, Dixon JS, Critchley, et al: Comparative studies of the human external sphincter and periurethral levator ani muscles. Br J Urol 53:35, 1981.

Green TH Jr: Development of a plan for diagnosis and treatment of urinary stress incontinence. Am J Obstet Gynecol 83:632, 1962.

Green TH Jr: The problem of urinary stress incontinence in the female: An appraisal of its current status. Obstet Gynecol Surv 23:603, 1968.

Green TH Jr: Urinary stress incontinence differential diagnosis pathophysiology and management. Am J Obstet Gynecol 122:368, 1975.

Hajj SN. Female urinary incontinence: A dynamic evaluation. J Reprod Med 23:33, 1979.

Henriksson L, Ulmsten U: Urodynamic evaluation of the effects of abdominal urethrocystopexy and vaginal sling urethroplasty in women with stress incontinence. Am J Obstet Gynecol 131:77, 1978.

Hilton P, Stanton SL: A clinical and urodynamic assessment of the Burch colposuspension for genuine stress incontinence. Br J Obstet Gynaecol 90:934, 1983.

Hilton P, Stanton SL: Urethral pressure measurements by microtransducer: The results of symptom free women and in those with genuine stress incontinence. Br J Obstet Gynaecol 90:919, 1983.

Hilton P, Stanton SL: Use of intravaginal oestrogen cream in genuine stress incontinence. Br J Obstet Gynaecol 90:940, 1983.

Hodgkinson CP: Relationships of the female urethra and bladder in urinary stress incontinence. Am J Obstet Gynecol 65:506, 1953.

Hodgkinson CP, Cobert N: Direct urethrocystommetry. Am J Obstet Gynecol 79:648, 1960.

Hodgkinson CP, Ayers MA, Drukker BH: Dyssynergic detrusor dysfunction in the apparently normal female. Am J Obstet Gynecol 87:717, 1963.

Hodgkinson CP, Drukker BH, Hershey GJG: Stress urinary incontinence in the female. VIII. Etiology significance of the short urethra. Am J Obstet Gynecol 86:16, 1963.

Hoyme UB, Tamimi HK, Eschenbach DA, et al: Osteomyelitis pubis after radical gynecologic operations. Obstet Gynecol 63:47S, 1984.

Jeffcoate TNA, Roberts H: Observations of stress incontinence of urine. Am J Obstet Gynecol 64:721, 1952.

Kegel AH: Stress incontinence of urine in women: Physiologic treatment. J Int Coll Surg 25:487, 1956.

Kiesswetter H, Hennrich F, Englisch M: Clinical and urodynamic assessment of pharmacologic therapy of stress incontinence. Urol Int 38:58, 1983.

Kujansuu E: The effect of pelvic floor exercises on urethral function in female stress incontinence and urodynamic study. Ann Chir Gynaecol 72:28, 1983.

Lapides J: Transurethral treatment of urethral diverticula in women. Trans Am Assoc Genitourin Surg 70:135, 1978.

Lapides J, Ajemian EP, Stewart BH, et al: Physiopathology of stress incontinence. Surg Gynecol Obstet 111:224, 1960.

Lee RA: Diverticulum of the female urethra: Postoperative complications and results. Obstet Gynecol 61:52, 1983.

Legueu and Rochet: Les cellulites perivesicales et pelviennes. J Urol Med Chir 15:1, 1923.

Low JA: Clinical characteristics of patients with demonstrable urinary incontinence. Am J Obstet Gynecol 88:322, 1964.

MacKinnon M, Pratt JH, Pool TL: Diverticulum of the female urethra. Surg Clin North Am 39:953, 1959.

Marchetti AA, Marshall VF, Shultis LD: Simple vesicourethral suspension for stress incontinence of urine. Am J Obstet Gynecol 74:57, 1957.

Millard RJ, Oldenburg BF: The symptomatic urodynamic and psychodynamic results of bladder reeducation programs. J Urol 130:715, 1983.

Mohr JA, Rogers J Jr, Brown TN, et al: Stress urinary incontinence. The simple and practical approach to diagnosis and treatment. J Am Geriatr Soc 31:476, 1983.

Montz FJ, Stanton SL: Q-tip test in female urinary incontinence. Obstet Gynecol 67:258, 1986.

Muellner SR, Fleischner FG: Normal and abnormal micturition study of the bladder behavior by means of fluoroscopy. J Urol 61:233, 1949.

Nichols DH: A Mersilene mesh gauze hammock for severe urinary stress incontinence. Obstet Gynecol 41:88, 1973.

Ostergard DR: The effect of drugs on the lower urinary tract. Obstet Gynecol Surv 34:424, 1979.

Ostergard DR: The neurologic control of micturition and integral voiding reflexes. Obstet Gynecol Surv 34:417, 1979.

Pereyra AJ: A simplified surgical procedure for the correction of stress incontinence in women. West J Surg 67:223, 1959.

Pereyra AJ, Lebherz TB: Combined urethrovesical suspension and vaginal urethroplasty for correction of stress incontinence. Obstet Gynecol 30:537, 1967.

Rudd T: Urethral pressure profile in continent women from childhood to old age. Acta Obstet Gynecol Scand 59:331, 1979.

Sjoberg B, Nyman CR: Hydrodynamics of micturition in stress incontinent women. Comparisons of pressure and flow at different micturition volumes in stress incontinent and continent women. Scand J Urol Nephrol 16:1, 1982.

Spence HM, Duckett JW, Jr: Diverticulum of the female urethra. Clinical aspects and presentation of a simple operative technique for cure. J Urol 104:432, 1970.

Spraitz AF, Jr, Welch JS: Diverticulum of the female urethra. Am J Obstet Gynecol 91:1013, 1965.

Stamey TA: Endoscopic suspension of the vesical neck for urinary incontinence in females: Report of 203 consecutive cases. Ann Surg 192:465, 1980.

Te Linde RW: Urethral sling operation. Clin Obstet Gynecol 6:206, 1963.

Walter S, Olesen KP: Urinary incontinence in genital prolapse in the female: Clinical urodynamic and radiologic examinations. Br J Obstet Gynaecol 89:393, 1982.

Westby M, Asmussen M, Ulmsten U: Localization of maximum intraurethral pressure related to urogenital diaphragm in the female subject as studied by simultaneous urethrocystommetry and voiding urethrocystography. Am J Obstet Gynecol 144:408, 1982.

Williams ME, Fitzhugh CP: Urinary incontinence in the elderly. Ann Intern Med 97:895, 1982.

APPENDIX

Drugs That Affect Bladder Functions

Generic Name	Trade Name	Generic Name	Trade Name
DRUGS AFFECTING SYMPATHETIC NERVOUS SYSTEM		Isopropylmethoxamine	—
Alpha-adrenergic blockers		Ko692	—
		LB-46	Prinololol
Azapetine	Ilidar	M 1999	Sotalol
Dihydroergotoxine	Hydergine	Oxprenolol	—
Ergot alkaloids	—	Practolol	Eraldin
Phenothiazines	(Various; see below: Drugs Affecting Autonomic Nervous System— Causing Retention)	**General adrenergic stimulators**	
		Adrenalone	Kephrine
		Aminorex*	—
		—	Aranthol
Phentolamine	Regitine	Benzphetamine	Didrex
Piperoxan	Benodaine	Chlorphentermine	Pre-Sate
Tolazoline	Priscoline	Clortemine	Voranil
		Cyclopantamine	Clopane
Beta-adrenergic blockers		Deoxyepinephrine	Epinine
		Dextroamphetamine	Dexedrine
Alprenolol	—	Diethylpropion	Tenuate, Tepanil
Butidrine	—	Epinephrine	—
Butoxamine	—	Ethylnorepinephrine	Bronkephrine
Dichloroisoproterenol	Alderlin, Nethalide, Pronethalol	Fenfluramine	Pondimin
		Hydroxyamphetamine	Paredrine

*Not available in the United States.

Drugs That Affect Bladder Functions, cont'd

Generic Name	Trade Name	Generic Name	Trade Name
H1032*	—	**Beta-adrenergic stimulators**	
Isometheptene	Octin	Albuterol	Proventil, Ventolin
Levamphetamine	Ad-Nil, Amodril, Cydril, Maigret	Bamethan*	—
		Chlorprenaline	—
Mazindol	Sanorex	Dioxethedrine	—
Methamphetamine	Dexoxyn	Etafedrine	—
Mephentermine	Wyamine	Ethylnorepinephrine	Butanefrine, Bronkephrine
Methylaminoheptane	Oenethyl		
Methylhexamine	Forthane	Hydroxyephedrine	—
Naphazoline	Privine	Isoethamine	—
Oxymetazoline	Afrin	Isoproterenol	Aludrine, Isuprel, Norisodrine
Phedrazine*	—		
Phendimetrazine	Dietrol, Plegine	Methoxyphenamine	Orthoxine
Phenmetrazine	Preludin	Nylidrin	Arlidin
Phentermine	Ionamin, Wilpo	Protokylol	Caytine
Pholedrine	Paredrinal	Salbutanal	—
Propylhexedrine	Benzedrex	Soterenol	—
Pseudoephedrine	Sudafed, Ro-Fedrin	Terbutaline	Bricamyl
Racephedrine	—	**Adrenergic neuron blockers**	
Synephrine*	—		
Tenaphtoxaline*	—	Alseroxylon	Rautensin, Rauwiloid
Tetrahydrozoline	Tyzine		
Tramazoline	—	Bethanidine	Esbatal
Tuaminoheptane	Tuamine	Bretylium	Darenthin
Tymazoline*	Pernazene	Debrisoquin	Declinax
Xylometazoline	Otrivin	Deserpidine	Harmonyl
		Guanadrel	—
Alpha adrenergic stimulators		Guanethidine	Ismelin
Amidephrine	—	Guanoclor	Vatensol
Cyclopentamine	Clopane	Guanoxan	Envacar
Dopamine	Intropin	Hydralazine	Apresoline
Etafedrine	—	Methyldopa	Aldomet
Ethylphenylephrine	Effortil	Methyldopate	Aldomet Ester
Hydroxyamphetamine	Paredrine	Nialamide	—
Metaraminol	Aramine	Pargyline	Eutonyl
Methamphetamine	Desoxyn, Efroxine, Methedrine, Norodin, Synodroy	Rauwolfia	Hyperloid, Raudixin, Rauja, Raulfin, Rautina, Rauval, Venibar
Methoxamine	Vasoxyl		
Methylhexaneamine	Forthane	Rescinnamine	Cinatabs, Moderil
Nordefrin	Cobefrin	Reserpine	Lemiserp, Rau-Sed, Resercen, Reserpoid, Rolserp, Sandril, Serpasil, Sertina, Vio-Serpine
Norepinephrine	Levarterenol		
Novadral	—		
Phenylephrine	Neosynephrine, Isophrin, Synasal, Alcon-Efrin Biomydrin, Isohalent Improved		
		Syrosingopine	Singoserp
		Tranylcypromine	—
Phenylpropylmethylamine	Vonedrine	Veratrum alkaloids	Unitensin, Veralba, Veriloid, Vertairs
Propylhexedrine	Benzedrex		
Tyramine	—		

Drugs That Affect Bladder Functions, cont'd

Generic Name	Trade Name	Generic Name	Trade Name
DRUGS AFFECTING PARASYMPATHETIC NERVOUS SYSTEM		Pipenzolate	Piptal
		Piperidolate	Dactil
Stimulators		Poldine	Nacton
		Scopolamine	—
Ambenonium	Mytelase	Thihexinol	Sorboquel
Carbachol	Carcholin, Isopto Carbachol	Thiphenamil	Trocinate
		Tincture of belladonna	—
Echothiophate	Phospholine	Tricyclamol	Elorine
Demecarium	Humorsol	Tridihexethyl	Pathilon
Edrophonium	Tensilon	Tropicamide	Mydriacyl
Isoflurophate	Floropryl	Valethamate	Murel
Methacholine	Mecholyl		
Pilocarpine	Pilocar	**DRUGS AFFECTING SYMPATHETIC AND PARASYMPATHETIC NERVOUS SYSTEM— GANGLIONIC BLOCKERS**	
Pralidoxime	Protopam		
Pyridostigmine	Mestinon		
Inhibitors		Azamethonium	Pendiomid
		Chlorisondamine	Ecolid
Adiphenine	Trasentine	Hexamethonium	—
Alverine	Prafenil, Spacolin	Mecamylamine	Inversine
Anisotropine	Valpin	Methaphan	Arfonad
Atropine	—	Pentolinium	Ansolysen
Belladonna extract	—	Sparteine	Spartocin, Tocosamine
Carbofluorene	Pavatrine		
Clidinium	Librax, Quarzan	Trimethidinium	Ostensin
Cyclopentolate	Cyclogyl		
Diphemanil	Prantal	**DRUGS AFFECTING AUTONOMIC NERVOUS SYSTEM**	
Ethaverine	Ethaquin, Laverin, Neopavrin		
		Causing retention	
Eucatropine	Euphthalmine	Acetophenazine	Tindal
Glycopyrrolate	Robinul	Amitriptyline	Elavil
Hexocyclium	Tral	Amphotericin B	Fungizone
Homatropine hydrobromide	—	Benztropine	Cogentin
Homatropine methylbromide	Homapin, Malcotran, Mesopin, Novatrin	Biperiden	Akineton
		Bromodiphenhydramine	Ambodryl
		Brompheniramine	Dimetane
Hyoscyamine sulfate	Levsin	Butaperazine	Repoise
Isometheptene	Isometene, Octin	Carbinoxamine	Clistin
Mepenzolate	Cantil	Carphenazine	Proketazine
Methixene	Trest	Chlorpheniramine	Chlor-Trimeton, Histaspan, Teldrin
Methscopolamine bromide	Pamine		
		Chlorphenoxamine	Systral, Phenoxene
Methylatropine nitrate (atropine methylnitrate)	Metropine	Chlorpromazine	Thorazine
		Chlorprothixene	Taractan
Oxyphenonium	Antrenyl	Cycrimine	Pagitane
Papaverine	Cerespan, Pap-Kaps, Pavabid, Pavacap, Pavacen, Pavarine, Pavatest, Paveril, Vasal, Vasospan	Deanol	Deaner
		Desipramine	Norpramin, Pertofrane
		Dexbrompheniramine	Disomer
		Dexchlorpheniramine	Polaramine
		Dimethindene	Forhistal, Triten
Pentapiperium	Quilene	Diphenhydramine	Benadryl
Penthienate	Monodral	Diphenylpyraline	Diafen, Hispril

Drugs That Affect Bladder Functions, cont'd

Generic Name	Trade Name	Generic Name	Trade Name
Doxepin	Adapin, Sinequan	Thioridazine	Mellaril
Doxylamine	Decapryn	Thiothixene	Navane
Droperidol	Inapsine	Tranylcypromine	Parnate
Ethopropazine	Parsidol	Trifluoperazine	Stelazine
Fluphenazine	Prolixin, Permitil	Triflupromazine	Vesprin
Haloperidol	Haldol	Trihexyphenidyl	Artane, Pipanol, Tremin
Imipramine	Tofranil, Presamine		
Isocarboxazid	Marplan	Trimeprazine	Temaril
Mepazine	—	Tripelennamine	Pyribenzamine
Mesoridazine	Serentil	Triprolidine	Actidil
Metaxalone	Skelaxin		
Methapyrilene	Histadyl		

Causing miscellaneous urologic symptoms

Generic Name	Trade Name
Frequency	
Dantrolene	Dantrium Triavil (mixture)
Iron Sorbitex	Jectofer Etrafon (mixture)
Incontinence	
Estrogens	—
Hydroxystilbamidine	—
Urgency	
Disodium Edetate	Endrate
Frequency, retention, and incontinence	
Levodopa	Bendopa, Dopar, Larodopa, Levo-dopa
Levopropoxyphene	Novrad

Generic Name	Trade Name
Methdilazine	Tacaryl
Methylphenidate	Ritalin
Methysergide	Sansert
Molindone	Moban
Nortriptyline	Aventyl
Orphenadrine	Norflex
Perphenazine	Trilafon
Phenelzine	Nardil
Phenindamine	Thephorin
Piperacetazine	Quide
Pipradrol	Meratran
Prochlorperazine	Compazine
Procyclidine	Kemadrin
Promazine	Sparine
Promethazine	Phenergan
Protriptyline	Vivactil
Pyrilamine	—
Rotoxamine	Turiston
Thiopropazate	Dartal

From Ostergard, DR: The effect of drugs on the lower urinary tract. Obstet Gynecol Surv 34:424, 1979.

Combined Preparation Drugs

Drugs affecting sympathetic nervous system

Actifed-C Expectorant
Acutuss
Acutuss Expectorant
  with Codeine
Aerolone Compound
Amesec
Amodrine
Asbron
Ayrcap
AyrLiquid
Bihisdin
Brondilate
Bronkometer
Bronkosol
Bronkotabs
Calcidrine Syrup
Cerose Expectorant
Chlor-Trimeton Expec-
  torant with Codeine
Citra
Colrex Compound
Copavin
Copavin Compound
Coricidin Nasal Mist
Co-Xan
Dainite
Dainite-K1
Deltasmyl
Duo-Medihaler
Duovent
Dylephrine

Ephed-Organidin
Ephedrine and Chlor-
  cyclizine
Ephedrine and Nem-
  butal
Ephedrine and Seconal
  Sodium
Ephoxamine
Glynazan/EP
Hyadrine
Hydryllin with Ra-
  cephedrine Hy-
  drochloride
Iso-Tabs
Isuprel Compound
Lufyllin-EP
Marax
Neo-Vadrin
Norisodrine with
  Calcium Iodide
Novalene
NTZ
Numa
Orthoxine and
  Aminophylline
Pyracort
Quadrinal
Tedral
Tedral-25
Tedral Anti-H
Thalfed
Triaminicin

Drugs inhibiting sympathetic nervous system

Aldoclor
Aldoril
Butiserpazide
Diupres
Diutensen
Enduronyl
Esimil
Eutron
Exna-R
Hydromox-R
Hydropres
Maxitate with Rauwol-
  fia
Metatensin
Naquival

Nyomin
Oreticyl
Protalba-R
Rautrax
Rawiloid + Veri-
  loid
Regroton
Renese-R
Salutensin
Sandril with Py-
  ronil
Serpasil-Esidrix
Singoserp-Esidrix

Drugs inhibiting parasympathetic nervous system

Belbarb
Belladenal
Bellergal
Butibel
Cantil with Phenobar-
  bital
Chardonna
Combid
Daricon-PB
Donnatal
Donphen
Enarax
Histalet
Hybephen
Kinesed
Kolantyl

Levsin with Phe-
  nobarbital
Milpath
Nolamine
Pamine
Pathibamate
Pathilon with Phe-
  nobarbital
Phenobarbitol and
  Belladonna
Probanthine with
  Dartal
Probanthine with
  Phenobarbitol
Robinul-PH
Sidonna
Trasentine-pheno-
  barbitol
Valpin-PB

From Ostergard DR: The effect of drugs on the lower urinary tract. Obstet Gynecol Surv 34:424, 1979.

Infections of the Lower Genital Tract

KEY TERMS AND DEFINITIONS

Acyclovir. An antiviral agent, a purine nucleoside analogue used in the treatment of herpes. This agent comes in oral, topical, and intravenous preparations.

Calymmatobacterium granulomatis. The gram-negative, nonmotile rod that causes granuloma inguinale.

Clue Cells. Epithelial cells with clusters of bacteria adherent to their external surfaces, obscuring their normal, fine border. They have a granular or stippled appearance and are associated with bacterial vaginosis.

Condyloma Acuminatum. A sexually transmitted viral disease of the vulva, vagina, and cervix caused by the human papillomavirus.

Condyloma Latum. The large, raised, flattened, grayish white lesions of secondary syphilis, most often found on the vulva.

Dark-Field Microscopy. A technique used to identify the spirochetes of syphilis, *Treponema pallidum.*

Donovan Bodies. The pathognomonic clusters of dark-staining bacteria (bipolar in appearance) found in the cytoplasm of large mononuclear cells in patients with granuloma inguinale.

Forme Fruste. A mild form of a disease.

Groove Sign. A depression between groups of inflamed nodes producing a double genitocrural fold in patients with lymphogranuloma venereum.

Gumma. An infectious granuloma characteristic of late or tertiary syphilis.

HTLV-III. The human T cell lymphocytotropic virus type III thought to be responsible for acquired immune deficiency syndrome (AIDS), now commonly referred to as HIV or human immunodeficiency virus.

Mucopurulent Cervicitis. The counterpart to urethritis in men, diagnosed by gross visualization of yellow mucopurulent material or the presence of 10 or more polymorphonucleocytes per high-powered field on Gram stain of the endocervix.

Nit. The egg of the crab louse.

Podophyllin. A topical resin mixed with benzoin and alcohol used to treat the lesions of condyloma acuminatum.

Sexually Transmitted Disease (STD). A term used to describe an infection acquired primarily through sexual contact; venereal disease.

Toxin I (One). The toxin involved in producing the signs and symptoms of toxic shock syndrome. It is a small protein with a molecular weight of 22,000. Its primary effects are the production of increased vascular permeability and profuse leaking of fluid from the intravascular space to the extravascular space.

Whiff Test. A test used clinically. The smell of vaginal discharge after the addition of 10% potassium hydroxide. A positive sample associated with either bacterial vaginosis or *Trichomonas* infections will give off a fishy or aminelike smell.

Western Blot Test. A technique to a identify antibodies to a protein of a specific molecular weight. This test is more specific than the ELISA test for AIDS.

Word Catheter. A short catheter with an inflatable Foley balloon used to help develop a fistulous tract from a Bartholin's duct to the vestibule.

The discussion of infectious diseases of the female genital tract is divided into two chapters. Infections involving the vulva, vagina, and cervix are discussed in this chapter, and infections involving the uterus, oviducts, and ovaries are discussed in Chapter 22. This separation has been made only to be similar to other chapters of the book and for clarity of presentation. The female genital tract has anatomic and physiologic continuity. Thus infectious agents that colonize and involve one organ often infect adjacent organs. To understand the pathophysiology and natural history of infectious diseases of the genital tract, one must always keep this continuity in mind.

This chapter will focus on infections of the lower genital tract. The symptoms caused by infections in this area produce the most common conditions seen by gynecologists. Therefore, the focus of this chapter is on clinical presentation and differential diagnosis of vulvitis, vaginitis, and cervicitis. For more detailed discussions of microbiology and pharmacology, the reader is directed to the bibliography.

Toxic shock syndrome, acquired immune deficiency syndrome (AIDS), and syphilis are discussed in this chapter. Although the most devastating pathologic processes from these diseases occur in sites other than the genital tract, they obtain entry into the body most often through the vagina.

Many of the infections discussed in this chapter may be acquired through sexual contact and are termed sexually transmitted diseases (STDs). These often coexist—for example, herpes and condyloma or infections of *Chlamydia trachomatis* and *Neisseria gonorrhoeae.* When one disease is suspected, appropriate diagnostic methods must be used to detect other infections. This principle cannot be overemphasized.

INFECTIONS OF THE VULVA

The skin of the vulva is composed of a stratified squamous epithelium containing hair follicles and sebaceous, sweat, and apocrine glands. The subcutaneous tissue of the vulva also contains specialized structures such as the Bartholin glands. Similar to skin elsewhere on the body, the vulvar area is subject to both primary and secondary infections. The three most prevalent primary viral infections of the vulva are herpes genitalis, condyloma acuminatum, and molluscum contagiosum. However, symptoms from secondary infections of the vulva caused by organisms that produce vulvovaginitis are among the most common of all gynecologic conditions. To understand the differential diagnosis of vulvar infections, one must consider that vulvar skin is also sensitive to hormonal, metabolic, and allergic influences.

Vulvar itching or burning of acute onset and short duration suggests infection. Approximately 10% of outpatient visits to gynecologists are for vulvar pruritus. The signs of erythema, edema, and superficial skin ulcers of the vulva also suggest infection. Skin fissures and excoriation may be signs of primary infection or may be caused by the patient's scratching as a result of irritation from a vaginal discharge.

Acute Urethral Syndrome

Dysuria, urinary frequency, and urinary urgency are the classic symptoms of infections of the lower urinary tract. It is estimated that 10% to 20% of adult women experience these symptoms each year. Women are prone to ascending infections because of the shortness of the female urethra and the fact that the distal one third of the urethra is constantly colonized by bacteria from the vulvar vestibule.

A woman with urinary frequency and dysuria who does not have significant bacterial growth in the urine (less than 10^2 organisms per milliliter) has acute urethral syndrome. Another name for this condition is dysuria–sterile pyuria syndrome. The diagnosis of acute urethral syndrome is made by exclusion of other diseases, primarily cystitis and vulvovaginitis. Cystitis is characterized by identical symptoms except for the presence of more than 100 uropathogens per milliliter of urine. Vulvovaginitis also produces a similar symptom complex and must be excluded from the diagnosis during the physical examination.

The most common cause of acute urethral syndrome is ascending infection from the introitus and distal urethra. The most frequent pathogens involved in premenopausal women are *Escherichia coli, Staphylococcus saprophyticus, C. trachomatis,* and *N. gonorrhoeae.* Postmenopausal women often experience similar symptoms related to estrogen deficiency without significant bacterial colonization of the bladder.

The diagnosis of acute urethral syndrome is established primarily by excluding the possibility that the symptom complex is secondary to cervicitis, vulvovaginitis, or cystitis. The patient's perception of the anatomic site of the dysuria may be helpful. Vulvovaginitis tends to produce "external" dysuria in contrast to a deeper, "internal" dysuria associated with cystitis. There are two basic diagnostic steps in the workup of a woman with dysuria and urinary frequency. Initially, pelvic examination is performed to discover whether the patient has an associated vaginal or cervical infection. Second, a clean-catch, midstream urine specimen is obtained. The urine should be examined for both white cells and bacteria. A urine culture is obtained if bacteria are present and the patient has been treated for similar symptoms in the past. To obtain accurate estimates of the number of bacteria per milliliter, it is important to culture the urine within 2 hours or refrigerate the specimen until it is sent to the laboratory. The "gold standard" of more than 10^5 uropathogens per milliliter had been the criterion used to make the diagnosis of significant bacteriuria. However, recently bacterial concentrations of as few as 10^2 per milliliter are accepted as bacteriologic confirmation of cystitis. In large series, 50% of women with dysuria and frequency did not have significant bacteriuria. Women, especially in the age group of 15 to 25, with pyuria and a sterile urine culture often have urethral infection by *Chlamydia* or gonorrhea. In general, women with urethral syndrome secondary to *Chlamydia* have more chronic symptoms with a gradual onset and less urgency than women with acute bacterial cystitis.

The initial treatment of choice for women with bacteriuria or acute cystitis is identical: single-dose regimens of trimethoprim-sulfamethoxazole (three tablets of double strength, 480 mg of trimethoprim and 2400 mg of sulfamethoxazole) or amoxicillin (3 g). The advantages of single-dose therapy are simplicity, better patient compliance, lower cost, and reduction of side effects such as diarrhea and vaginitis. Contraindications to single-dose therapy include chronic infections, systemic mani-

festations of infection, renal disease, anatomic abnormalities of the urinary tract, and diabetes mellitus. If bacteriuria is not present, the patient should be treated with tetracycline (500 mg every 6 hours) for 7 days to treat a presumptive diagnosis of *Chlamydia* infection. Failure to respond necessitates quantitative cultures of the urine for bacteria and culture of the endocervix for *Chlamydia* and gonorrhea organisms. It is important to stress that uncomplicated lower urinary tract infection is not a threat to renal function in an ambulatory adult woman.

Chronic urethral syndrome has many causes, including estrogen deficiency, trauma (especially during intercourse), chronic infection (most commonly with genital *Mycoplasma*), anatomic obstruction, allergy, and neurologic and psychogenic conditions. Chronic urethral syndrome is discussed in detail in Chapter 20.

Infections of Bartholin's glands

Bartholin's glands normally are two rounded, pea-sized glands deep in the perineum. They are located at the entrance of the vagina at 5 and 7 o'clock. A normal Bartholin's gland cannot be palpated. Approximately 2% of adult women develop enlargements of one or both glands, of which there are three common causes. The most common cause is cystic dilation of Bartholin's duct. Symptomatic enlargement of Bartholin's glands may be secondary to adenitis or abscess formation (Fig. 21-1). Mechanical obstruction of the duct usually precedes overt infection. The most serious sequela of infection is a polymicrobial necrotizing subcutaneous infection, especially in diabetics. In women over the age of 40, enlargement may be caused by the rare adenocarcinoma of Bartholin's glands.

The etiology of a Bartholin's duct cyst is obstruction of the duct secondary to nonspecific inflammation or trauma. Twenty years ago bilateral enlargement of Bartholin's glands was believed to be a pathognomonic sign of gonococcal infection. This is no longer true. Unilateral or bilateral Bartholin's gland infection in the majority of cases is not caused by a sexually transmitted disease. Lee et al. obtained bacterial cultures of fluid from Bartholin's duct cysts and abscesses. More than 80% of cultures from

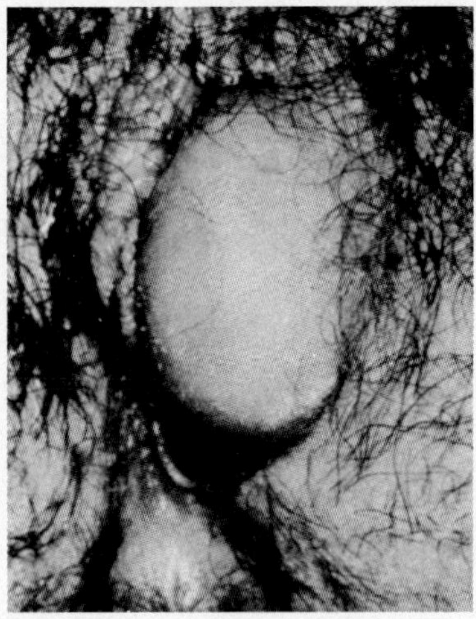

FIGURE 21-1
Bartholin's abscess. Mass is tender and fluctuant and is situated on lower lateral aspect of labium minus at 5 o'clock. (From Kaufman RH: Cystic tumors. In Gardner HL, Kaufman RH, eds: Benign diseases of the vulva and vagina, 2nd ed. Chicago, Year Book Medical Publishers, 1981, p. 120.)

cysts were sterile, as were one in three cultures from Bartholin's abscesses. Positive cultures from Bartholin's gland abscesses are often polymicrobial and contain a wide range of bacteria similar to the natural flora of the vagina.

The differential diagnosis of Bartholin's gland cysts includes mesonephric cysts of the vagina and epithelial inclusion cysts. Mesonephric cysts are generally more cephalad in the vagina, and epithelial inclusion cysts are more superficial. Rarely, a lipoma, fibroma, hernia, or hydrocele may be confused with a Bartholin's duct cyst. Bartholin's duct cysts are found in the labia majora, whereas Bartholin's glands are at the base of the labia minora.

Most women with Bartholin's duct cysts are asymptomatic. The cysts may vary from 1 to 8 cm in diameter, and they are usually unilateral, tense, and nonpainful. An abscess of a Bartholin gland tends to develop rapidly over 2 to 4 days. Symptoms include acute vulvar pain, dyspareunia, and pain during walking. Local symptoms of acute pain and tenderness are secondary to rapid enlargement, hemorrhage, or secondary infection. The signs are those of a classic abscess: erythema, acute tenderness,

edema, and occasionally cellulitis of the surrounding subcutaneous tissue. Without therapy, most abscesses tend to rupture spontaneously by the third or fourth day.

The treatment of infections or enlargement of Bartholin's glands depends on their symptomatology. Asymptomatic cysts in women under the age of 40 do not need treatment. The therapy for acute adenitis without abscess formation is broad-spectrum antibiotics and frequent hot sitz baths.

The treatment of choice for a symptomatic cyst or abscess is the development of a fistulous tract from the dilated duct to the vestibule. Simple incision and drainage of a Bartholin's gland abscess are complicated by a tendency for the abscess to recur. The classic surgical treatment is to develop a fistulous tract to "marsupialize" the duct. After an elliptical wedge of tissue has been removed, the remaining edges of the duct or abscess are everted and sutured to the surrounding skin with interrupted sutures. This forms an epithelialized pouch that provides drainage for the gland. An alternate surgical approach is to insert a Word catheter (a short catheter with an inflatable Foley balloon) through a stab incision into the duct or abscess and leave it in place for 4 to 6 weeks (Fig. 21-2). During this period a tract of epithelium will form. Davis has recently described a procedure using a carbon dioxide laser to produce a neostoma in a Bartholin's duct cyst. All of the above-mentioned operations may be performed with local anesthesia. Antibiotics are not necessary unless there is an associated cellulitis surrounding the Bartholin's gland abscess.

Excision of a Bartholin duct and gland is indicated for persistent deep infection, multiple recurrences of abscesses, or enlargement of the gland in women over the age of 40. Excision for gland enlargement in women over 40 is performed to diagnose adenocarcinoma of Bartholin's gland. Because of the richness of the vascular supply to the region, including the vestibular bulbs directly below Bartholin's gland, excision is a more formidable task than one would expect. It is best to have either regional block or general anesthesia for excision. Bartholin's gland secretions are not important for providing lubrication during sexual intercourse. Mucinous secretions from Bartholin's

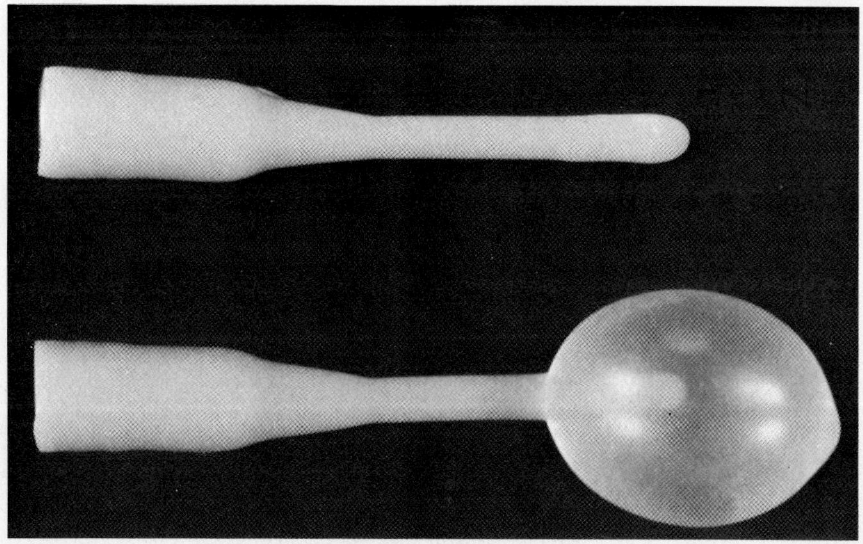

FIGURE 21-2

Word catheters before and after inflation. They are used to develop a fistula from Bartholin's cyst or abscess to vestibule. (From Friedrich EG: Vulvar disease, 2nd ed. Philadelphia, W.B. Saunders Co., 1983, p. 71.)

glands do provide moisture for the epithelium of the vestibule but are not important for vaginal lubrication.

Pediculosis Pubis and Scabies

The skin of the vulva is a frequent site of infestation by animal parasites, the two most common being the crab louse and the itch mite. Ideally, early diagnosis and treatment are of the utmost importance to control parasitic infection. However, because many women experience embarrassment, guilt, and anxiety over the potential diagnosis of this infection, delay in diagnosis often interferes with ideal treatment.

Pediculosis pubis is an infestation by the crab louse, *Phthirus pubis*. The crab louse is also called the pubic louse and is a different species than the body or head louse. The louse is transmitted usually by close contact, although it may be acquired from towels or bedding. *P. pubis* is generally confined to the hairy areas of the vulva. It may occasionally be found in other areas such as the eyelids. The major nourishment of the louse is human blood.

There are three stages in the louse's life cycle: egg (nit), nymph, and adult. The entire life cycle is spent on the host. Eggs are deposited at the base of hair follicles. The adult parasite is approximately 1 mm long and dark gray when its alimentary tract is not filled with blood (Fig. 21-3). Of clinical importance for diagnosis is the fact that the louse moves slowly.

Scabies is a parasitic infection of the itch mite, *Sarcoptes scabiei*. Similar to the crab louse, it is transmitted by close contact. Unlike louse infestation, scabies is an infection that is widespread over the body without a predilection for hairy areas. The adult female itch mite digs a burrow just beneath the skin. She lays eggs in this home during her life span of approximately 1 month. The adult itch mite is usually less than 0.5 mm long. Unlike the crab louse, an itch mite travels rapidly over skin and may move up to 2.5 cm in 1 minute.

The predominant clinical symptom of louse infestation is constant itching in the pubic area, which is secondary to allergic sensitization. Examination of the vulvar area without magnification demonstrates eggs and adult lice (Fig. 21-4). The tiny rough spots visualized with the naked eye are the alimentary tracts of lice filled with human blood. The vulvar skin may become secondarily irritated or infected by constant scratching. For definitive diagnosis one

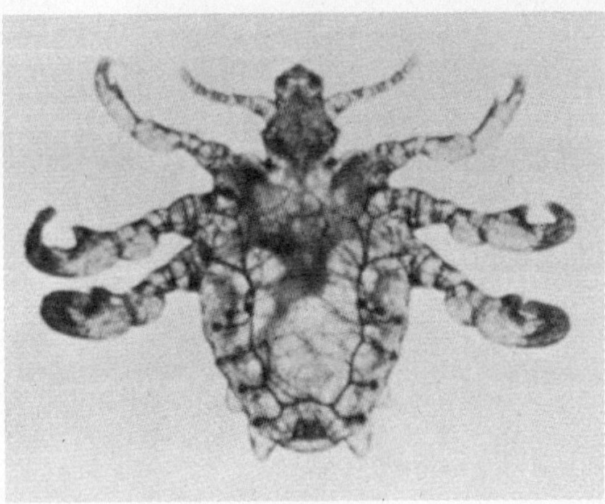

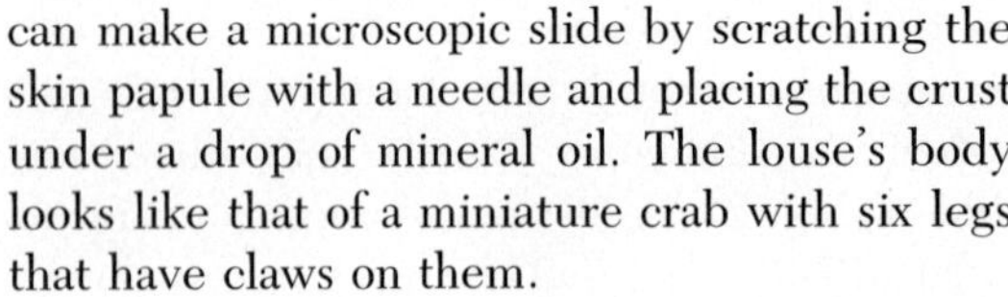

FIGURE 21-3
Pubic louse, *Phthirus pubis*, after blood meal. (From Billstein S: Human lice. In Holmes KK, Mårdh PA, Sparling PF, et al, eds: Sexually transmitted diseases. New York, McGraw-Hill Book Co., 1984, p. 514.)

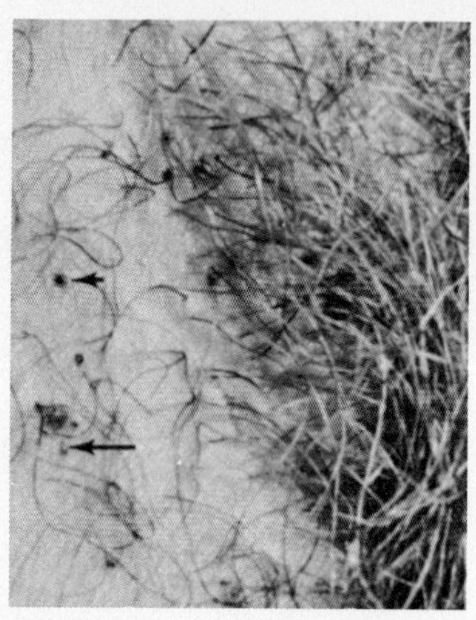

FIGURE 21-4
Crab lice and nits of pediculosis pubis *(arrows)*. (From Gardner HL: Miscellaneous conditions. In Gardner HL, Kaufman RH, eds: Benign diseases of the vulva and vagina, 2nd ed. Chicago, Year Book Medical Publishers, 1981, p. 509.)

can make a microscopic slide by scratching the skin papule with a needle and placing the crust under a drop of mineral oil. The louse's body looks like that of a miniature crab with six legs that have claws on them.

The predominant clinical symptom of scabies is severe but intermittent itching. Generally, more intense pruritus occurs at night when the skin is warmer and the mites are more active. Scabies may present as papules, vesicles, or burrows. Any area of the skin may be infected, with the hands, wrists, breasts, vulva, and buttocks being most commonly involved. A handheld magnifying lens is helpful for examining suspicious areas. Microscopic slides may be made by use of mineral oil and a scratch technique (Fig. 21-5). Mites lack lateral claw legs but have two anterior triangular hairy buds.

The treatment of pediculosis pubis and scabies involves an agent that kills both the adult parasite and eggs. Lindane, which is a 1% gamma-benzene hexachloride preparation (Kwell), is available as a cream, lotion, and shampoo. The infected individual should take a shower and then apply Kwell to the infested areas of the body for 12 hours on 2 successive days. Lindane must remain in direct contact for at least 1 hour to kill eggs. For scabies, approximately 30 ml of lotion covers the entire skin surface of an adult patient. Patients with scabies have intense pruritus that may persist for several days following effective therapy. An antihistamine will help to alleviate this symptom. The treatment of other family members should be prescribed to avoid reinfection. Obviously, clothes, bedding, and the home environment must be disinfected.

Molluscum Contagiosum

Molluscum contagiosum in adults is an asymptomatic viral disease of the vulvar skin. In contrast, molluscum contagiosum in children may present over the entire body. This benign skin disease is caused by the poxvirus. Poxvirus does not grow on mucous membranes and is spread by close contact. Unlike most sexually transmitted diseases, poxvirus is only mildly contagious. The incubation period is several weeks, and many of the skin lesions result from autoinoculation.

The small nodules or domed papules of molluscum contagiosum are usually 1 to 5 mm in diameter (Fig. 21-6). A descriptive name for

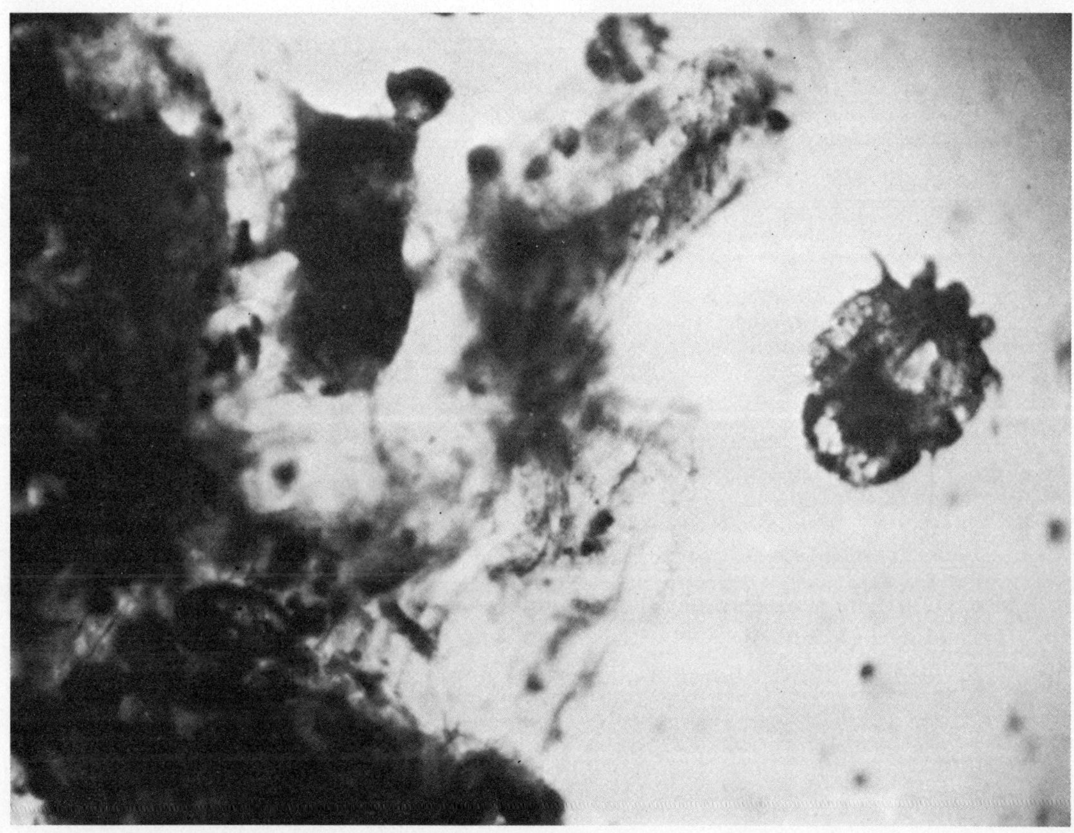

FIGURE 21-5
Skin scrapings of unexcoriated papules fortuitously disclose adults, larva, eggs, and fecal pellets, any of which would be diagnostic of scabies. (From Orkin M, Howard IM: Scabies. In Holmes KK, Mårdh PA, Sparling PF, et al, eds: Sexually transmitted diseases. New York, McGraw-Hill Book Co., 1984, p. 521.)

the small nodule is the "water wart." Close inspection reveals that many of the more mature nodules have an umbilicated center. Characteristically, an infected woman will have 1 to 20 solitary lesions randomly distributed over the vulvar skin. A crop of new nodules will persist from several months to years. If the diagnosis cannot be made by simple inspection, the white, waxy material from inside the nodule should be expressed on a microscopic slide. The finding of intracytoplasmic molluscum bodies with Wright's or Giemsa stain confirms the diagnosis (Fig. 21-7).

Treatment of individual papules is initiated with injection of a local anesthetic with a small subdermal wheel of 1% lidocaine (Xylocaine). The caseous material is then evacuated and the nodule excised with a sharp dermal curet. The base of the papule is subsequently chemically treated with either ferric subsulfate (Monsel's solution) or 85% trichloroacetic acid. As an alternative the base of the papule may be treated with cryosurgery, electrocautery, or laser therapy.

Condyloma Acuminatum

Condyloma acuminatum is a sexually transmitted viral disease of the vulva, vagina, and cervix caused by the human papillomavirus (HPV). Synonyms for vulvar condylomata acuminata include genital, venereal, or anogenital warts. In the past few years this disease has reached epidemic levels. It is estimated that in

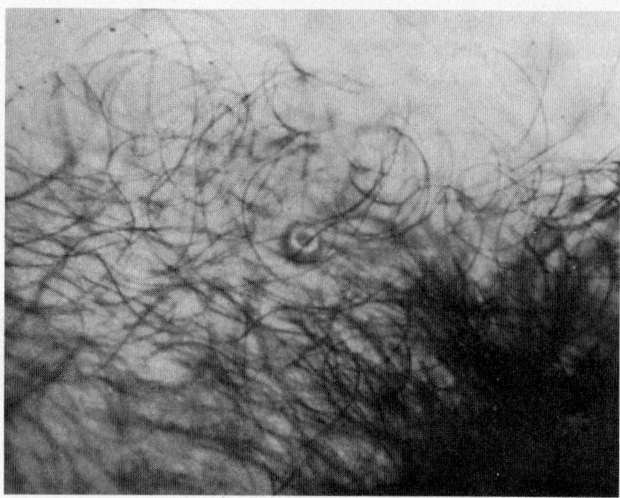

FIGURE 21-6
Papule of molluscum contagiosum with umbilicated center. (From Brown ST: Molluscum contagiosum. In Holmes KK, Mårdh PA, Sparling PF, et al, eds: Sexually transmitted diseases. New York, McGraw-Hill Book Co., 1984, p. 510.)

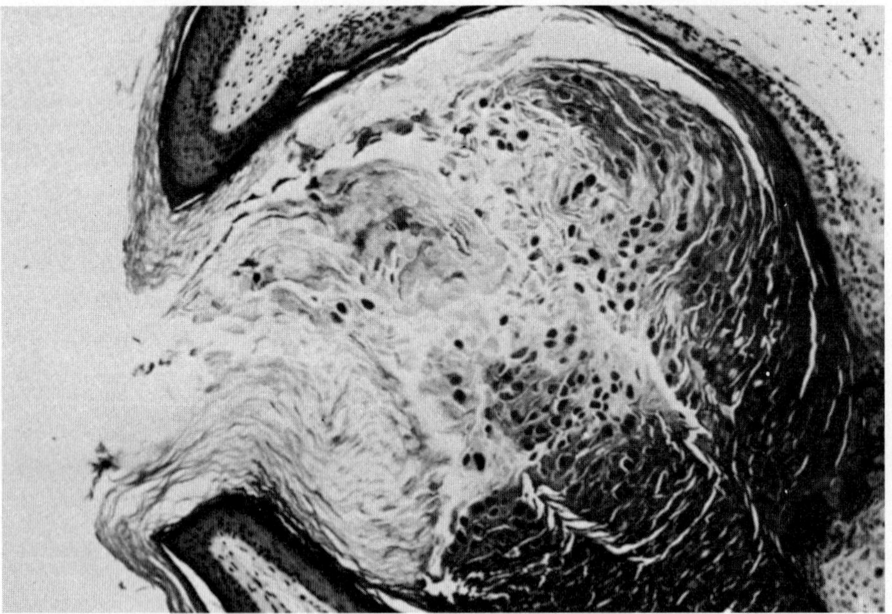

FIGURE 21-7
Papule of molluscum contagiosum with plug of acanthotic and hyperkeratolytic epidermis containing numerous intracytoplasmic inclusions opening to the surface through an apical hole. (H&E stain; ×75.) (From Brown ST: Molluscum contagiosum. In Holmes KK, Mårdh PA, Sparling PF, et al, eds: Sexually transmitted diseases. New York, McGraw-Hill Book Co., 1984, p. 510.)

the past 15 years the number of infected individuals has increased approximately 500%. The increasing incidence and the awareness of the relationship between HPV infection and early cervical intraepithelial neoplasia have been the stimuli for expanding research efforts into this complex group of viruses.

Recent advances in molecular biology have identified more than 45 subtypes of HPV, which differ from one another in their amino acid sequences. Many different subtypes of HPV have been involved in genital infection. HPV 6, 11, 16, and 18 are the most frequently identified. HPV types 16 and 18 may be asso-

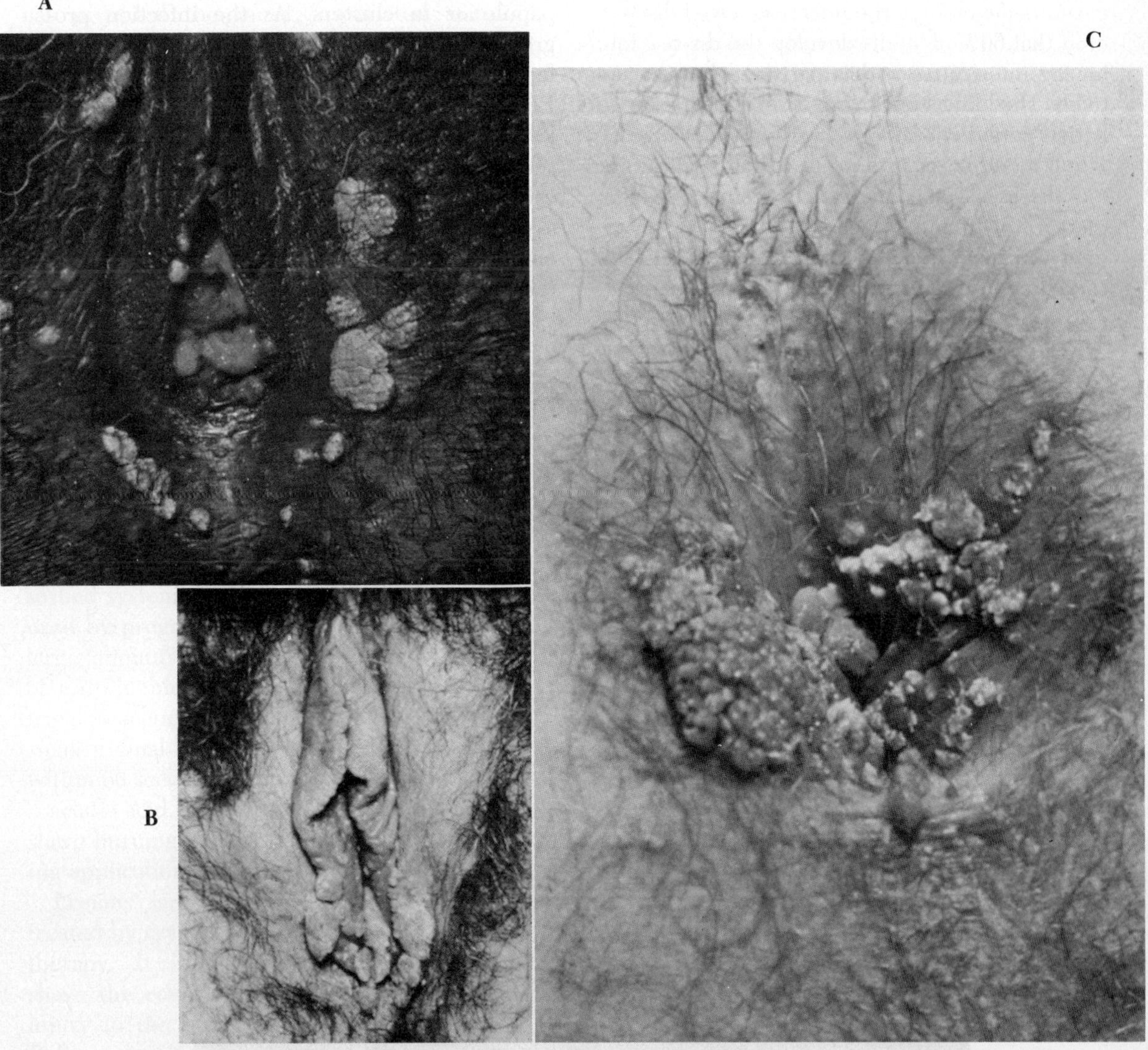

FIGURE 21-8
A, Condylomata acuminata. **B,** Multiple, discrete, papillary lesions of condylomata acuminata. **C,** Anal condylomata acuminata. (**A** from Friedrich EG: Vulvar disease, 2nd ed. Philadelphia, W.B. Saunders Co., 1983. **B** from Kaufman RH: Viral infections. In Gardner HL, Kaufman RH, eds: Benign diseases of the vulva and vagina, 2nd ed. Chicago, Year Book Medical Publishers, 1981. **C** from Oriel JD: Genital warts. In Holmes KK, Mårdh PA, Sparling PF, et al, eds: Sexually transmitted diseases. New York, McGraw-Hill Book Co., 1984.)

TABLE 21-1
Characteristics of Sexually Transmitted Genital Ulcers

	Syphilis	Chancroid	Herpes	Lymphogranuloma Venereum	Granuloma Inguinale
Primary lesion	Papule	Erythematous papule or pustule	Vesicle*	Papule, pustule, or vesicle	Papule
Number of lesions	Usually one; occasionally multiple	Usually one to three, may be multiple	Multiple,* may coalesce	Usually one	Single or multiple
Border	Sharply demarcated	Erythematous and undermined*	Erythematous	Variable	Rolled and elevated*
Depth	Superficial	Excavated*	Superficial	Superficial	Elevated
Base	Red and smooth	Yellow to gray	Red and smooth	Variable	Red and rough*
Secretion	Serous	Purulent and hemorrhagic	Serous	Variable	Rare, may be hemorrhagic
Induration	Firm*	Rare, soft	None	None	Firm*
Pain	Rare*	Often*	Common	Variable	Rare
Lymph nodes	Nontender, firm	Tender, may suppurate	Tender, firm	Tender, may suppurate	Pseudoadenopathy

From Kraus SJ: Genital ulcer adenopathy syndrome. In Holmes KK, Mårdh PA, Sparling PF, et al, eds: Sexually transmitted diseases. New York, McGraw-Hill Book Co., 1984, p. 708.
*Useful in differential diagnosis.

predict the time of the next recurrence. Luby and Klinge and Bierman have excellent reviews of the psychologic fears and anxieties created by herpes and the perception of its being "an incurable disease."

There are two distinct types of herpes simplex virus—type I (HSV-I) and type II (HSV-II). As a broad generalization, HSV-I tends to infect epithelium above the waist, and HSV-II tends to cause ulceration below the waist. However, depending on the series, HSV-I may cause pelvic infections between 13% and 40% of the time. From a molecular biologic standpoint the classification of HSV-I and HSV-II is an oversimplification. Multiple strains of each virus have been discovered. From a clinical standpoint the only important difference is that the frequency of recurrence is 4 times greater following a primary infection with HSV-II in comparison to HSV-I.

The primary infection by herpes is both a local and a systemic disease (Fig. 21-10). The incubation period is between 3 and 7 days, with an average of 6 days. Often the patient experiences paresthesias of the vulvar skin before vesicle formation. Usually there are multiple vesicles that become shallow, superficial ulcers over a large area of the vulva. There is often simultaneous involvement of the vagina and cervix (Fig. 21-11). Patients experience multiple crops of ulcers for 2 to 6 weeks. Often the ulcers coalesce; however, the ulcers heal spontaneously without scarring. Viral shedding may occur for 2 to 3 weeks after vulvar lesions appear. Positive cultures for herpesvirus may be obtained from the cervix in 75% of women and from the urine in 50% of women with primary infections. The vast majority of women have severe vulvar pain, tenderness, and inguinal adenopathy.

Systemic symptoms, including general malaise and fever, are experienced by 70% of women during the primary infection. Rarely there is central nervous system infection, with the reported mortality from herpes encephalitis being approximately 50%. Primary infections of the urethra and bladder may result in acute urinary retention, necessitating catheterization. The symptoms of vulvar pain, pruritus, and discharge peak between days 7 and 11 of the primary infection. The average woman experiences severe symptoms for approximately 14 days. The severity of symptoms necessitates hospitalization for approximately 10% of women. Occasionally a primary pelvic infection is subclinical.

Recurrent genital herpes is a local disease, and the symptoms are much less severe. In 50% of women the first recurrence occurs within 6 months of the initial infection. There is a general clinical opinion that recurrences are frequently related to the onset of a menstrual period or emotional stress. To generalize, most clinical manifestations of recurrent infection are half as severe as those of primary infections. That is, vulvar involvement is usually unilateral, recurrent attacks last an average of 7 days, and viral shedding occurs for approximately 5 days. The ability to successfully culture herpesvirus from the cervix during that period varies from 20% to 60%, depending on the study cited. Recurrent herpetic ulcers are small—1 to 5 mm in diameter (Fig. 21-12). A common feature of recurrence is a prodromal phase of sacroneuralgia, vulvar burning, tenderness, and pruritus for 5 to 10 days before vesicle formation.

The herpesvirus resides in a latent phase in the dorsal root ganglia of S-2, S-3, and S-4. Corey has reviewed the two current hypotheses regarding the etiology of recurrent attacks. The "ganglion trigger theory" proposes a constant viral replication in the privileged immune site of the dorsal root ganglia. Unknown stimuli, possibly hormonal, trigger the release of virus, which travels in a retrograde fashion via the peripheral nerves to the female genital organs. The alternate "skin trigger theory" proposes a regular production and retrograde flow of virus from the nerve ganglion down the sensory axon. Normally, local immunity inactivates the virus and recurrence results from a local immunologic defect.

The clinical diagnosis of genital herpes usually can be made by simple clinical inspection. Women come to the physician when they de-

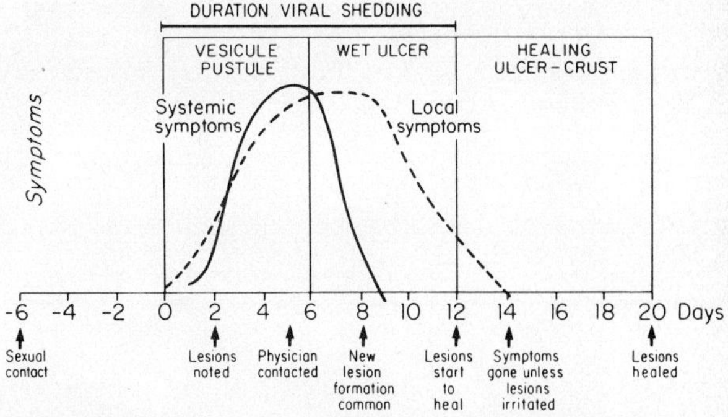

FIGURE 21-10
Schematic graph of clinical course of primary genital herpes. (From Corey L: Genital herpes. In Holmes KK, Mårdh PA, Sparling PF, et al, eds: Sexually transmitted diseases. New York, McGraw-Hill Book Co., 1984, p. 453.)

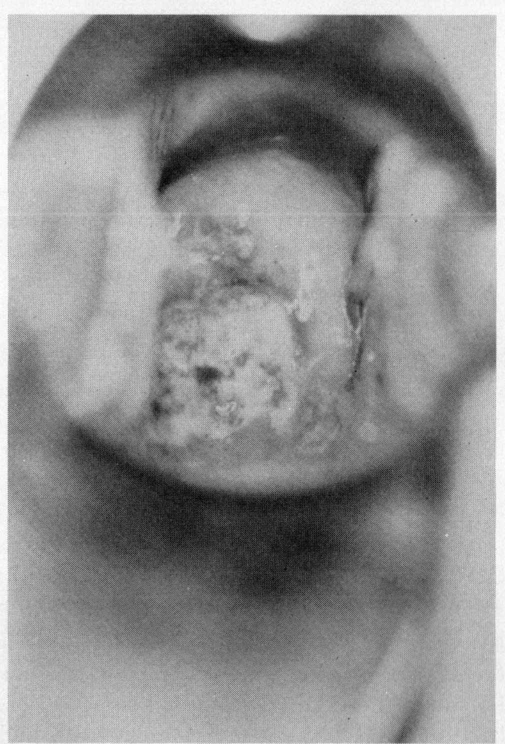

FIGURE 21-11
Primary herpes involving cervix. Necrotic, exophytic mass is seen on posterior lip. This was clinically thought to be invasive carcinoma. Herpes simplex virus culture was positive. Lesion spontaneously disappeared. (Reproduced with permission from Kaufman, RH: Viral infections, in Gardner, HL and Kaufman, RH (eds.): Benign Diseases of the Vulva and Vagina, 2nd edition. Copyright © 1981 by Year Book Medical Publishers, Inc., Chicago.)

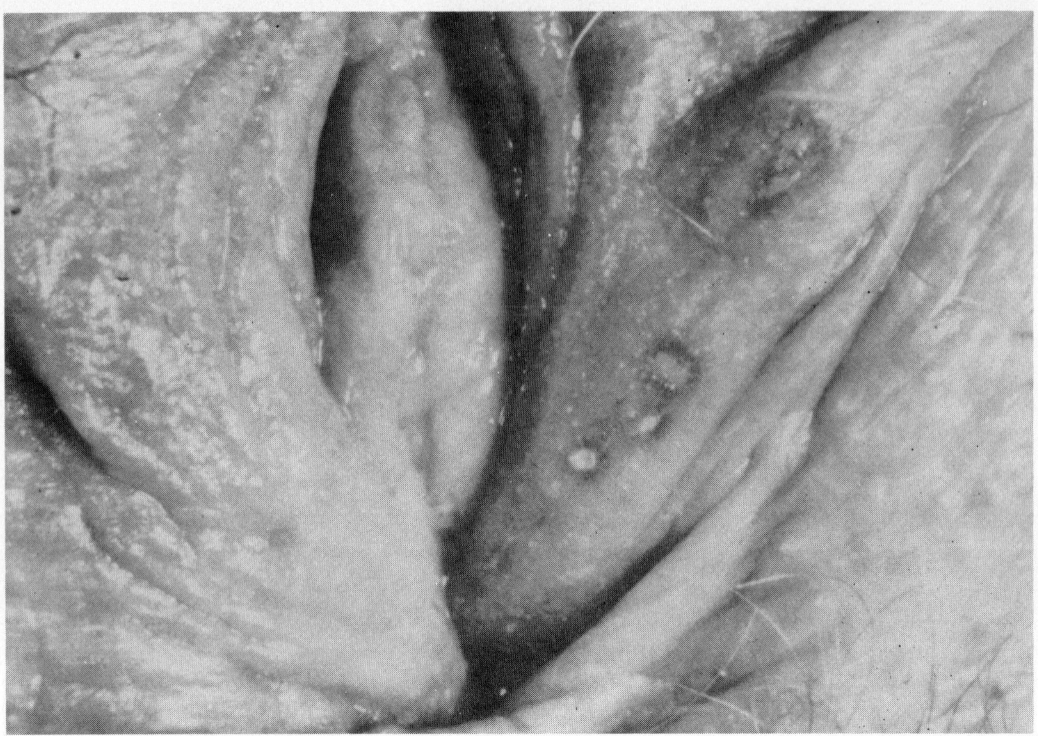

FIGURE 21-12
Recurrent herpes genitalis. Superficial ulcers are noted following rupture of vesi-
cles. (Reproduced with permission from Kaufman, RH: Viral infections, in Gardner,
HL and Kaufman, RH (eds): Benign Diseases of the Vulva and Vagina, 2nd edition.
Copyright © 1981 by Year Book Medical Publishers, Inc., Chicago.)

velop symptoms from vulvar ulcers. Herpetic
ulcers are painful when touched with a cotton-
tipped applicator, whereas the ulcers of syphilis are painless. Of the laboratory tests, viral
cultures of the lesions are the most accurate in
confirming the diagnosis. Most herpesvirus cultures will become positive within 2 to 4 days of
inoculation. Rapid immunologic tests (10% to
30% false negatives) or cytologic studies (30%
false negatives) are significantly less reliable
than viral cultures. Serologic tests are only
helpful in determining whether a patient has
been infected in the past with herpesvirus. Obviously, cultures for other sexually transmitted
diseases should be obtained, as they may co-
exist with herpes.

Approximately 10% of women with primary
infection have symptoms severe enough to require hospitalization. Common indications for
hospitalization include severe headache, central nervous system involvement, extreme
pain, difficulty in walking, and severe pain on
urination or acute urinary retention.

The treatment of choice for either severe primary genital herpes or herpes genitalis in an
immunosuppressed woman is intravenous acyclovir (5 mg/kg every 8 hours). The drug is
given as an infusion over approximately 1 hour.
Acyclovir is an antiviral agent that is a purine
nucleoside analogue. The drug is available in
oral, topical, and intravenous preparations. The
pharmacology of intravenous acyclovir is similar to that of aminoglycocides, although they do
not share similar structures. Care must be
taken that the patient has normal renal function. Side effects of intravenous acyclovir include local phlebitis and a transient increase in
serum creatinine levels in 15% of cases.

If the patient does not require hospitalization, first episodes of genital herpes infections
may be treated with oral acyclovir. Large, collaborative, double-blind studies published by
Nilsen, Mertz, and Bryson and their co-workers documented that oral acyclovir 200 mg 5
times daily for 5 days was extremely efficacious
in primary episodes of genital herpes. Acyclo-

vir significantly reduced the median duration of viral shedding, time to crusting and healing of lesions, and the duration of both constitutional symptoms and local pain as compared with times for control subjects. The clinical course of the disease was shortened approximately 1 week. Treating the patient with oral acyclovir for 5 to 10 days during the primary infection did not influence viral latency—that is, either the frequency of or time to first recurrence.

Topical acyclovir in a 5% ointment is sometimes prescribed for primary episodes. The ointment is applied to blisters every 3 to 4 hours for 7 days. Topical acyclovir does decrease the duration of viral shedding by 60% and the duration of pain and healing by approximately 2 days. Because of the possibility of spreading the infection with topical medication, the oral drug is preferred.

The major fears of women with recurrent genital herpes are the rate of recurrence and possible transmission of the disease to their sexual partners. Women should be instructed to abstain from sexual intercourse from the time of prodromal symptoms or the time that lesions appear until the time that all lesions have completely reepithelialized. Active viral shedding may occur from the time of the prodromal period and does occur in women with ulcers even though the ulcers have crusted over.

Patients with frequent episodes of recurrent genital herpes may be successfully treated with prophylactic oral acyclovir. Douglas et al. studied 91 women given 200 mg acyclovir tablets (two to five tablets daily) for 4 months and 47 placebo recipients. The median time to first clinical recurrence was 120 days in the acyclovir group versus 18 days in women receiving the placebo. After acyclovir had been discontinued, the recurrence rate returned to the same frequency as the pretreatment rate.

There are several areas of concern in the use of oral acyclovir to suppress recurrent disease. Resistant strains of herpesvirus have been identified from women treated with suppressive acyclovir. Acyclovir is a drug with minimum toxicity if given for a few months, but the long-term safety of the drug, especially as it relates to the patient's immune system, is unknown. Also, acyclovir does not alter the rate of asymptomatic shedding of the virus. There-fore, the drug probably does not influence the transmission of the disease to sexual partners.

A vaccine would be the logical approach for optimum prevention of herpes. There have been extensive attempts to develop a safe vaccine. To date researchers have not been successful. It is important that the vaccine be free of viral DNA because of the potential oncogenicity of the viral genetic material. However, there is promise that a successful vaccine against surface glycoproteins will be developed in the future.

Granuloma Inguinale

Granuloma inguinale, also known as donovanosis, is a chronic, ulcerative, bacterial infection of the skin and subcutaneous tissue of the vulva. Rarely, the vagina and cervix are involved in advanced, untreated cases. Granuloma inguinale is common in tropical climates such as New Guinea and the Caribbean islands, but fewer than 100 cases are reported each year in the United States.

This chronic disease is caused by a gram-negative, nonmotile, encapsulated rod—*Calymmatobacterium granulomatis*. This bacterium shares common antigens with *Klebsiella*. It cannot be cultured on standard media, and serologic tests are nonspecific. This disease can be spread both as a sexually transmitted disease and through close nonsexual contact. However, it is not highly contagious, and chronic exposure is usually necessary to contract the disease. The incubation period is extremely variable—from 1 to 12 weeks.

The initial growth of granuloma inguinale is an asymptomatic nodule. The skin over the nodule ulcerates, and the characteristic lesion is a beefy-red ulcer with fresh granulation tissue. Adjacent areas of ulceration grow and coalesce and, if not treated, will eventually destroy the normal vulvar architecture. The ulcers are painless unless secondarily infected. Adenopathy is not a prominent feature unless there is a superimposed infection.

The diagnosis is established by identifying Donovan bodies in smears and specimens taken from the ulcers (Fig. 21-13). Both the deep aspects of the ulcer crater and the fresh edge of an expanding lesion should be sampled. The pathognomonic Donovan bodies are

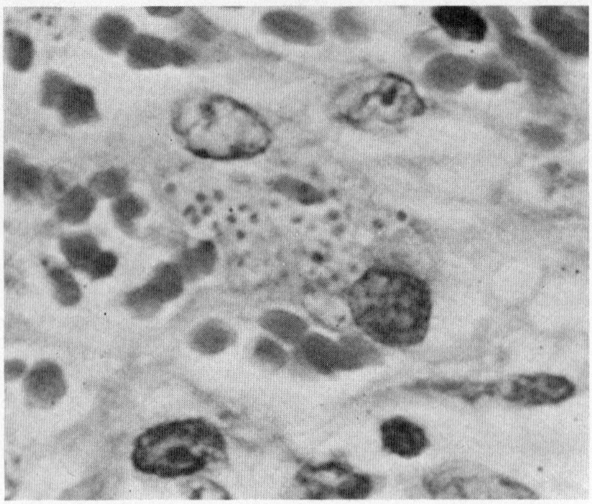

FIGURE 21-13
Donovanosis. Biopsy specimen shows intracytoplasmic Donovan bodies. (H&E stain.) (From Hart G: Donovanosis. In Holmes KK, Mårdh PA, Sparling PF, et al, eds: Sexually transmitted diseases. New York, McGraw-Hill Book Co., 1984, p. 394.)

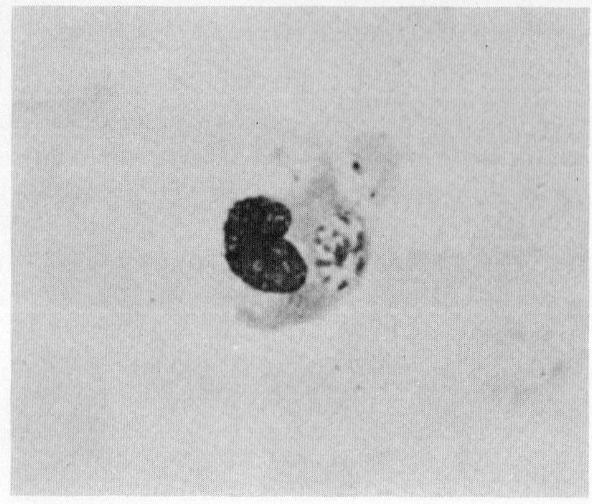

FIGURE 21-14
Donovanosis. Crust preparation from biopsy specimen shows single cell with many intracytoplasmic Donovan bodies (Giemsa stain.) (From Hart G: Donovanosis. In Holmes KK, Mårdh PA, Sparling PF, et al, eds: Sexually transmitted diseases. New York, McGraw-Hill Book Co., 1984, p. 394.)

clusters of dark-staining bacteria with a bipolar (safety pin) appearance found in the cytoplasm of large mononuclear cells (Fig. 21-14). Special silver stains highlight the Donovan bodies. However, even a brief period of previous antibiotic therapy may result in an absence of Donovan bodies in women who have granuloma inguinale. The differential diagnosis includes lymphogranuloma venereum, vulvar carcinoma, syphilis, and other granulomatous diseases.

Granuloma inguinale may be managed by a wide range of oral broad-spectrum antibiotics. Tetracycline is the most popular choice and should be prescribed for a minimum of 2 to 3 weeks (500 mg orally every 6 hours). It is best to continue antibiotics until a complete clinical response is noted with healing of the ulcerative lesions. Alternate antibiotic therapy such as an aminoglycoside has been used in refractory cases. Rarely, medical therapy fails and surgical excision is required.

Lymphogranuloma Venereum

Lymphogranuloma venereum (LGV) is a chronic infection of lymphatic tissue produced by *Chlamydia trachomatis*. It is found most commonly in the tropics. Cases occur infrequently in the United States, with fewer than 500 new cases being reported each year. The majority of cases are reported to occur in men. The vulva is the most frequent site of infection in women, but the urethra, rectum, and cervix may also be involved. Subclinical infection is common. Studies have demonstrated positive complement fixation tests in more than 50% of prostitutes without demonstrable disease. This sexually transmitted disease is produced by serotypes L_1, L_2, and L_3 of *C. trachomatis*. These serotypes are similar to the serotypes that produce trachoma. The incubation period is between 4 and 21 days.

There are three distinct phases of vulvar and perirectal LGV. The primary infection is a shallow, painless ulcer of the vestibule or labia. Occasionally this ulcer is near the urethra or rectum. The ulcer heals rapidly without therapy. The patient usually consults a physician during the secondary phase of the disease, which begins 1 to 4 weeks after the primary infection. The secondary phase is marked by painful adenopathy in the inguinal and perirectal areas. Two thirds of women have unilateral

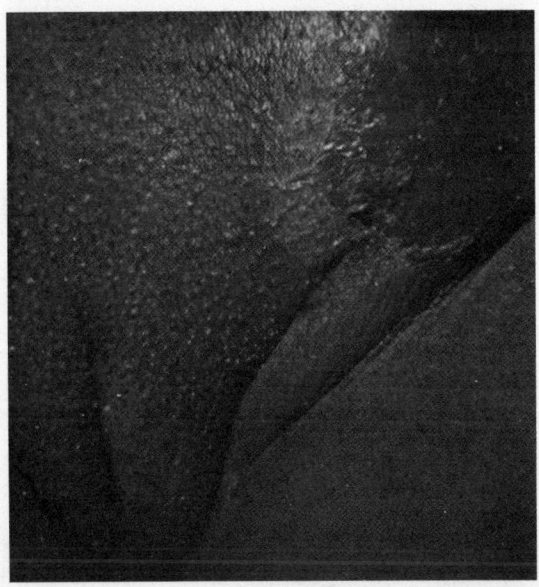

FIGURE 21-15
Lymphogranuloma venereum bubo with "groove" sign. (From Friedrich EG: Vulvar disease, 2nd ed. Philadelphia, W.B. Saunders Co., 1983, p. 229.)

adenopathy, and half have systemic symptoms, including general malaise and fever. When the disease is not treated, the infected nodes become increasingly tender, enlarged, matted together, and adherent to overlying skin, forming bubos. A classic clinical sign of LGV is the double genitocrural fold or "groove sign" (Fig. 21-15), a depression between groups of inflamed nodes. Within 7 to 15 days the bubo will rupture spontaneously and form multiple draining sinuses and fistulas. These are classic of the tertiary phase of the infection. Extensive tissue destruction of the external genitalia and anorectal region may occur during the tertiary phase. This tissue destruction and secondary extensive scarring and fibrosis may result in elephantiasis, multiple fistulas, and stricture formation of the anal canal and rectum.

Diagnosis is established by culture of pus or aspirate from a tender lymph node. With the recent development of monoclonal antibodies for *Chlamydia*, the diagnosis may be confirmed with this technique. The complement fixation antibody titer is the most frequently used serum method for diagnosis. Antibody titers greater than 1:64 are indicative of active infec-

tion. The Frei skin test has been abandoned because of its low sensitivity. The differential diagnosis of LGV includes syphilis, chancroid, granuloma inguinale, vulvar carcinoma, genital herpes, and Hodgkin's disease.

Oral tetracycline or erythromycin (500 mg every 6 hours) for 3 to 6 weeks is the preferred treatment. Fluctuant nodes may be aspirated with a large-bore needle, but incision and drainage are contraindicated. The late sequelae of the destructive tertiary phase of LGV often require extensive surgical reconstruction. It is important to administer antibiotics during the perioperative period.

Chancroid

Chancroid is a sexually transmitted, acute, ulcerative disease of the vulva. The soft chancre of chancroid is always painful and tender. In comparison, the hard chancre of syphilis is usually asymptomatic. Chancroid is a common disease in the third world, but fewer than 1500 new cases are discovered in the United States each year. Symptomatic disease is more common in males than females.

Chancroid is caused by *Haemophilus ducreyi*, a highly contagious, small, gram-negative rod. *H. ducreyi* is a nonmotile, facultative anaerobe. This bacterium on Gram stain exhibits a classic appearance of streptobacillary chains, or what has been described as an extracellular "school of fish." The incubation period is short—usually 3 to 6 days. Tissue trauma and excoriation of the skin must precede initial infection because *H. ducreyi* is unable to penetrate and invade normal skin.

Women with chancroid who consult a physician have solitary or multiple ulcers, most commonly of the vulvar vestibule and rarely of the vagina or cervix. The initial lesion is a small papule. Within 48 to 72 hours the papule evolves into a pustule and subsequently ulcerates. Multiple papules and ulcers may be in different phases of maturation secondary to autoinoculation. The painful ulcers are shallow with a characteristic ragged edge. The ulcers have a dirty, gray, necrotic exudate, and there is an absence of induration at the base (the soft chancre). Approximately 50% of women develop acutely tender inguinal adenopathy, usually within the first 2 weeks of an untreated infection. In most cases the inguinal adenopathy is unilateral, on the same side of the vulva as the preponderance of infection.

The diagnosis is made by Gram stain and culture of purulent material or by aspiration of tender lymph nodes. *H. ducreyi* may be difficult to grow in culture, depending on the experience of the bacteriology laboratory. Tissue biopsy helps to differentiate the other common vulvar diseases, including granuloma inguinale, syphilis, and genital herpes.

For years tetracycline was the standard treatment for chancroid. Recently Hammond et al. reported bacterial resistance to tetracycline. Therefore, trimethoprim 160 mg and sulfamethoxazole 800 mg (orally every 12 hours for 10 days) or erythromycin 500 mg (orally every 6 hours for 10 days) are the drugs of choice. Many other antibiotics, including second and third generation cephalosporins, are active against *H. ducreyi*.

Syphilis

Syphilis is a chronic disease produced by the spirochete *Treponema pallidum*. The initial infection primarily involves mucus membranes. Syphilis remains one of the important sexually transmitted diseases in the United States. Epidemiologists speculate that only one out of four new cases of syphilis is reported. Thus there will be approximately 280,000 new cases of primary and secondary syphilis in the United States this year. Even with mandatory screening, congenital syphilis also continues to be a public health problem. Careful follow-up has documented that mothers experiencing the tragedy of stillbirth or neonatal death from syphilis usually have not received prenatal care. Syphilis should be included in the differential diagnosis of all genital ulcers and cutaneous rashes of unknown etiology.

Sir William Osler emphasized that syphilis was the great imitator of clinical medicine. He taught that if a physician had mastered all the systemic manifestations of syphilis, he would understand clinical medicine. The present discussion will deal with the gynecologic manifestations of the disease.

T. pallidum is an anaerobic, elongated, tightly wound spirochete. Because of its extreme thinness, it is difficult to detect by light

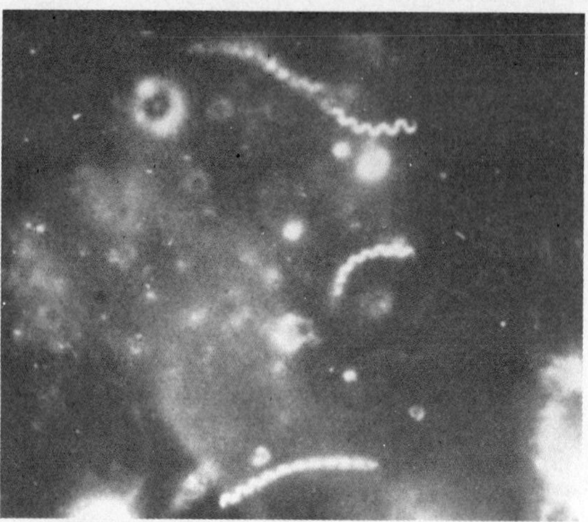

FIGURE 21-16
Dark-field microscopic appearance of *T. pallidum*. (From Larsen SA, McGrew BE, Hunter EF, et al: Syphilis serology and dark field microscopy. In Holmes KK, Mårdh PA, Sparling PF, et al, eds: Sexually transmitted diseases. New York, McGraw-Hill Book Co., 1984, p. 884.)

microscopy. Therefore, spirochetes are diagnosed by use of a specially adapted technique—dark-field microscopy (Fig. 21-16). These organisms have the ability to penetrate either skin or mucous membranes. The incubation period is between 10 and 90 days, with the average being 3 weeks. They replicate every 30 to 36 hours, which accounts for the comparatively long incubation period.

Syphilis is a moderately contagious disease. Approximately 10% of patients contract the disease from a single sexual encounter with an infected partner. Similar studies have documented that 30% of individuals become infected following a 1-month exposure to a sexual partner with primary or secondary syphilis. Patients are contagious during primary, secondary, and probably the first year of latent syphilis.

Serologic tests have been the foundation of screening programs to detect early syphilis, and there are two types of serologic tests—the nonspecific, nontreponemal and the specific, antitreponemal antibody tests. The nonspecific tests such as the VDRL (Veneral Disease Research Laboratory) slide test and the RPR

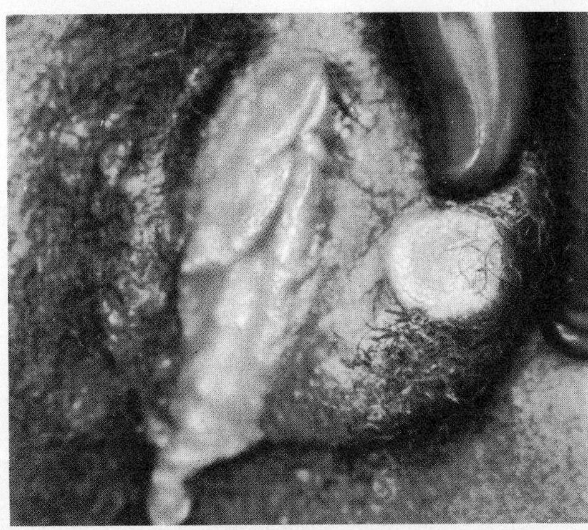

FIGURE 21-17
Hard chancre of primary syphilis. (From Kissane JM: Bacterial diseases. In Kissane JM, Anderson WAD, eds: Anderson's pathology. St. Louis, The C.V. Mosby Co., 1985, vol. 1, plate 1, A.)

(rapid plasma reagin) card test are inexpensive and easy to perform. These tests evaluate the patient's serum for the presence of reagin antibodies as they react with an antigen from beef heart. Approximately 1% of patients have technical or biologic false positive results with the nonspecific tests. Many conditions produce biologic false positive results, including a recent febrile illness, pregnancy, immunization, chronic active hepatitis, malaria, sarcoidosis, intravenous drug use, and autoimmune diseases such as lupus erythematosus or rheumatoid arthritis. Biologic false positive serum tests usually are of extremely low titers ($< 1:8$).

If a nonspecific test result is positive, the significance of this result must be confirmed by a specific antitreponemal test. Specific tests are more sensitive; however, occasionally they may also produce false positive results. Most false positive results occur among women with lupus erythematosus. The standard for specific tests had been the TPI (*Treponema* immobilization test). It has largely been replaced by the FTA-ABS (fluorescent-labeled *Treponema* antibody absorption), the MHA-TP (microhemagglutination assay for antibodies to *T. pallidum*), and the HATTS (hemagglutination treponemal test for syphilis).

Clinically, syphilis is divided into primary, secondary, and tertiary stages. The classic finding of primary syphilis is a hard chancre (Fig. 21-17). The chancre is a painless ulcer, with an indurated base that develops at the site of entry of the spirochete. The chancre is often solitary and painless and is usually found on the vulva, vagina, or cervix. However, a recent increase in extragenital primary lesions has been reported, including lesions of the mouth, anal canal, and nipple of the breast. A primary chancre develops approximately 3 weeks after sexual contact with an infected partner. The ulcer heals spontaneously within 2 to 6 weeks. Confirmation that the ulcer is primary or secondary syphilis depends on identification of *T. pallidum* by dark-field microscopy from wet smears of the ulcer. Special preparations must be made to obtain suitable smears. It is important to clean and abrade the ulcer with gauze before obtaining the serum for the slides. Nontender regional adenopathy develops during the first week of clinical disease.

Serologic tests for syphilis generally become positive 4 to 6 weeks after exposure—thus 1 to 2 weeks after development of the chancre. At the time of positive dark-field identification of *T. pallidum* from a primary chancre, approximately 70% of women will have a positive serologic test. If the serologic test result remains negative for 3 months, it is unlikely that the ulcer was syphilis.

Secondary syphilis is the result of hematogenous dissemination of the spirochetes and thus is a systemic disease. Secondary syphilis develops between 6 weeks and 6 months (with an average of 9 weeks) after the primary chancre. During an attack of secondary syphilis, which if untreated will last 2 to 6 weeks, there is a multitude of systemic symptoms depending on the major organs involved. The classic rash of secondary syphilis is red macules and papules over the palms of the hands and the soles of the feet (Fig. 21-18). Vulvar lesions include mucous patches and condyloma latum associated with painless lymphadenopathy. The vulvar lesions of condyloma latum are large, raised, flattened, grayish-white areas (Fig. 21-19). On wet surfaces of the vulva, soft papules that often coalesce form ulcers. These ulcers are larger than herpetic ulcers and are not tender unless secondarily infected.

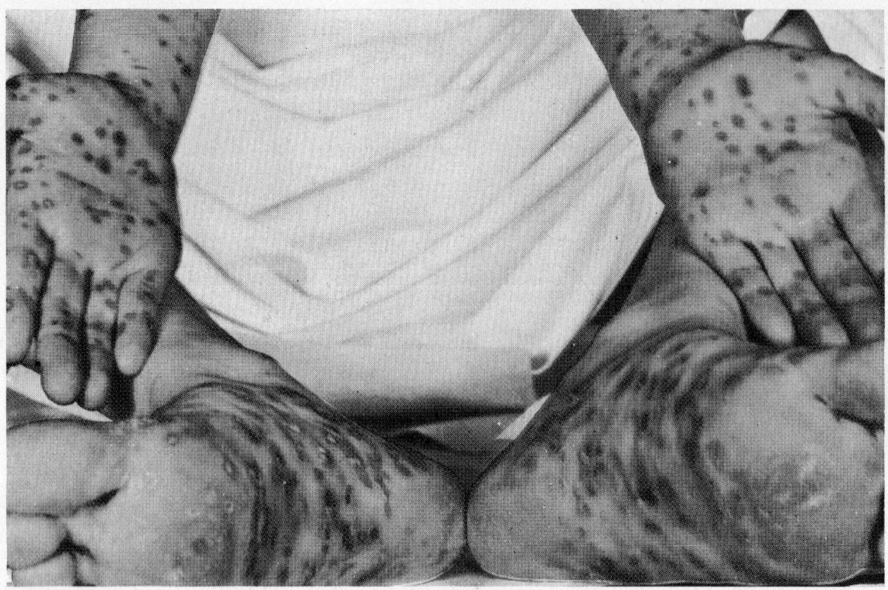

FIGURE 21-18
Rash of secondary syphilis: Red maculopapular lesions that involve palms and soles. (From Kissane JM: Bacterial diseases. In Kissane JM, Anderson WAD, eds: Anderson's pathology. St. Louis, The C.V. Mosby Co., 1985, vol. 1, plate 1, *B*.)

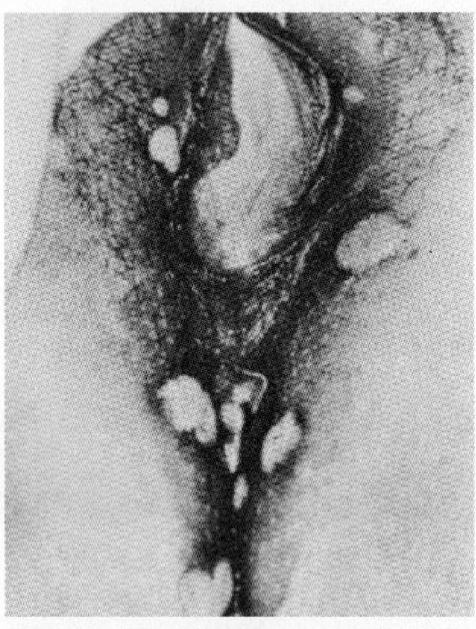

FIGURE 21-19
Multiple lesions of condylomata lata on vulva and perineum. Dark-field microscopic findings were positive. (From Gardner HL: Venereal diseases. In Gardner HL, Kaufman RH, eds: Benign diseases of the vulva and vagina, 2nd ed. Chicago, Year Book Medical Publishers, 1981, p. 463.)

The latent stage of syphilis follows the secondary stage and varies in duration from 2 to 20 years. During the first 3 to 4 years of the latent phase an individual may experience relapses of secondary syphilis.

The tertiary phase of syphilis is devastating in its potentially destructive effects on the central nervous, cardiovascular, and musculoskeletal systems. The manifestations of late syphilis include optic atrophy, tabes dorsalis, generalized paresis, aortic aneurysm, and gummas of the skin and bones. A gumma is similar to a cold abscess with a necrotic center and the obliteration of small vessels by endarteritis.

Penicillin is the drug of choice for syphilis. *T. pallidum* is exquisitely sensitive to penicillin. However, because of the slow replication time of the spirochete, blood levels must be maintained for 7 to 14 days. The Centers for Disease Control recommend 2.4 million U of benzathine penicillin G in a single session for early syphilis (primary and secondary syphilis and the first year of latent syphilis). Patients who are allergic to penicillin should receive oral tetracycline 500 mg every 6 hours for 15

eraliz
impo
TSS e
the d
Cent
demi
prese
grade
sion.
  Th
are th
the sl
burn.
will b
relate
there
the fa

TABL
Labor
Syndr

Coagu
  yloc
  vagi
Imma
  poly
  cell
Total
  <65
Total
  <5.
Serum
  <3.
Serum
  <7.
Serum
  anc
Serum
  >1.
Serum
  ≤1
Proth

From
manife
1981. (
*Resul
with t
patient
time (l

TABLE 21-2
Treatment of Syphilis

Stage of Disease	Drugs of Choice	Alternative Drugs	Comments
Primary, secondary or early latent	Benzathine penicillin G, 2.4 million units intramuscularly as single dose—one half the total dose into two separate sites, *or* aqueous procaine penicillin G, 600,000 units intramuscularly daily for 8 days	Tetracycline, 500 mg orally four times daily for 15 days, *or* erythromycin, 500 mg orally four times daily for 15 days	The alternative drugs should be prescribed for patients who are allergic to penicillin; it should be noted that the treatment of gonococcal infections with procaine penicillin will treat incubating syphilis but not primary disease
Late latent or latent of undetermined duration	Benzathine penicillin G, 2.4 million units intramuscularly weekly for 3 weeks	Tetracycline, 500 mg orally four times daily for 30 days, *or* erythromycin, 500 mg orally four times daily for 30 days	
During pregnancy	Benzathine penicillin G, 2.4 million units intramuscularly weekly for 3 weeks	Erythromycin, 750 mg orally four times a day for 20 days	Although tetracycline cannot be used in pregnancy, for patients who are allergic to both penicillin and erythromycin, doxycycline, 200 mg every 12 hours for 15 days, has prevented congenital syphilis in infants

From Charles D: Syphilis. Clin Obstet Gynecol 26:133, 1983.

days. Standard treatment protocols for syphilis are detailed in Table 21-2. All women with early syphilis should have repeat, quantitative, nontreponemal serum antibody tests every 3 months for the first year following therapy. With successful treatment the VDRL titer will become nonreactive or at most be reactive with a lower titer within 1 year. There is a 1% to 2% chance that the patient will not exhibit a fourfold titer decline, and these cases are considered therapeutic failures. These women should be treated once again. Patients with syphilis lasting longer than 1 year should have quantitative VDRL titers for 2 years following therapy, because their titers will decline more slowly. A specific test for syphilis, such as the FTA-ABS, remains reactive indefinitely.

Vulvar Irritation Caused by Vaginitis

Anatomic distribution of symptoms occasionally creates a semantic misinterpretation of the clinical reality. This is true for vulvar disease. The first symptom of vaginal infection is often vulvar pruritus, and the first sign of vaginal infection may be secondary erythema and edema of the vulvar skin. Often, self-medication for a vaginal infection may produce irritation of the vulva. Women whose chief complaint is vaginal itching or burning have symptoms because of irritation of the vestibule and adjacent vulvar epithelium. The sensory nerve endings are more numerous in the vulvar skin than in the vagina. The presence of excessive vaginal fluid is not appreciated until the fluid flows from the vagina onto the vulva.

involvement of individual organ systems. Not all patients develop a temperature of greater than 38.9° C and hypotension. Thus clinicians and patients should be aware of the "forme fruste" manifestations of the syndrome.

It is possible to significantly decrease the incidence of TSS by a change in use of catamenial products. Women should be encouraged to change tampons every 4 to 6 hours. The intermittent use of external pads is also good preventive medicine. Women will usually accept the recommendation to wear external pads during sleep. The incidence of TSS has decreased dramatically with the removal of super-absorbing tampons from the market.

Acquired Immune Deficiency Syndrome

Acquired immune deficiency syndrome (AIDS) has been defined as a disease of severe defects in cell-mediated immunity occurring in previously healthy people without a known cause for their immunologic deficiencies. AIDS is believed to be caused by a unique retrovirus. Associated with AIDS are unusual neoplasias such as Kaposi's sarcoma and opportunistic infections, the most common of which is *Pneumocystis carinii* pneumonia. The disease was first described in June 1981 when a small cluster of patients with an unexplained defect in cellular immunity developed *P. carinii* pneumonia. In the next 5 and a half years, approximately 28,000 cases were reported in the United States. The disease has reached epidemic proportions in the United States, causing widespread fear, anxiety, and even hysteria in the general public. The Centers for Disease Control estimated that by the end of 1986, between 1 and 2 million Americans became infected with the human T-cell leukemia (lymphocytotropic) virus type III (HTLV-III) or HIV (human immunodeficiency virus), the etiologic agent for AIDS.

Several features of the infection with HIV make AIDS a difficult clinical challenge. The virus may be transmitted from an individual several years before that person's development of symptoms. There is a recognized latency of 2 months to more than 5 years between transmission of the virus and appearance of clinical symptoms. After the infection is transmitted, most hosts, even persons who have no symptoms, have active virus in their blood. The present hypothesis is that 10% to 20% of infected individuals develop symptomatic disease each year. Thus 80% to 90% of individuals with the virus are asymptomatic carriers. However, 80% to 90% of individuals who develop the full-blown syndrome die within 2 years of diagnosis of the disease.

In the United States the high-risk populations for AIDS include homosexual men, intravenous drug users, and hemophiliacs. Originally, immigrants of Haitian descent were believed to be at high risk, but they were removed from this category. The prevalence of infection in the general population in late 1986 was 9 per 100,000. The mean age at diagnosis is 35 years, and in the United States men are affected more commonly than women. The prevalence rate of HIV varies among high-risk groups, with homosexual men clustered in large urban centers affected at a rate of 80%. Transmission of the virus occurs by both horizontal and vertical routes. There are three primary methods of contracting the virus: intimate sexual contact, use of contaminated needles or blood products especially in hemophiliacs, and perinatal transmission from mother to child. Presently, approximately 70% of people contracting the disease do so through sexual contact. Multiple reports of heterosexual transmission of the virus denote that the demographic groups at risk are expanding. In a study of hospital personnel by Hirsch et al. of 85 individuals with nosocomial exposure to AIDS, including needle stick accidents, no subjects have developed antibodies to HIV.

The wide spectrum of immunologic abnormalities in patients with AIDS includes lymphopenia, a decreased number of T helper cells, a decreased number of T-lymphocytes, hypergammaglobulinemia, and also an inverted T_4/T_8 ratio. Seligmann et al. have outlined (see box on p. 591) the many variations in immunologic abnormalities that have been associated with AIDS. In the most severe cases there is a persistent quantitative and functional depression of the T_4 lymphocytes associated with hyperactivity of the B cells.

AIDS is most likely caused by HIV, which has been isolated from 85% of symptomatic individuals with AIDS. Because of the variable

IMMUNOLOGIC ABNORMALITIES IN AIDS

I. Abnormalities that characterize the syndrome
  1. Lymphopenia
  2. Selective T cell deficiency based on a quantitative reduction with the antigenic subset designated by T_4 or Leu_3 monoclonal antibodies
  3. Decreased or absent delayed cutaneous hypersensitivity to both recall and new antigens
  4. Elevated serum immunoglobulins, predominantly IgG and IgA in adults and including IgM in children
  5. Increased spontaneous immunoglobulin secretion by individual B lymphocytes

II. Consistently observed abnormalities
  1. Decreased in vitro lymphocyte proliferative responses
    a. Mitogens
    b. Antigens
    c. Alloantigens, autoantigens
  2. Decreased cytotoxic responses
    a. Natural killer cells
    b. Cell-mediated cytotoxicity (T cell)
  3. Decreased ability to mount a de novo antibody response to a new antigen
  4. Altered monocyte function
  5. Elevated serum levels of immune complexes

III. Other reported abnormalities
  1. Increased levels of acid-labile alpha-interferon
  2. Antilymphocyte antibodies
  3. Suppressor factors
  4. Increased levels of beta-2 microglobulin and alpha-1 thymosin; decreased serum thymulin levels

From Seligmann M, Chess L, Fahey HL, et al: AIDS—an immunologic reevaluation. N Engl J Med 311:1287, 1984. Reprinted by permission of The New England Journal of Medicine.

length of time between transmission of the virus and appearance of clinical symptoms, it has been postulated that certain host characteristics may be cofactors that lower resistance to the virus. Again, it is important to note that the viremia is present for years in both symptomatic and asymptomatic individuals.

Presently there are three different clinical patterns associated with active clinical AIDS: lymphadenopathy, Kaposi's sarcoma, and multiple opportunistic infections. Patients with the lymphadenopathy pattern have a syndrome of persistent generalized lymphadenopathy, general malaise, nausea and vomiting, and often a fever of undetermined origin. This mildest form of AIDS may persist for years, with approximately 10% of persons subsequently developing either Kaposi's sarcoma or one or more of the severe opportunistic infections. Kaposi's sarcoma before the AIDS epidemic was an extremely rare neoplasia of connective tissue and blood vessels. However, it is the most common cancer found in AIDS victims. It is usually a slowly growing carcinoma involving purple or reddish nodules or plaques on the skin and epithelium of the gastrointestinal tract. Kaposi's sarcoma associated with AIDS may involve lymph nodes and occasionally has a rapid downhill course. Most individuals with Kaposi's sarcoma subsequently die of opportunistic infections.

Patients with AIDS are subject to opportunistic infections similar to immunosuppressed patients taking corticosteroids or chemotherapy for cancer. The most common opportunistic infection is *P. carinii* pneumonia. The clinical course of this pneumonia varies from an intermittent, slowly progressive disease to a fulminating infection with death in a few days. Two out of three patients survive the initial episode of *P. carinii* pneumonia. However, it has a recurrence rate of at least 20%. Other common opportunistic infections in AIDS patients are listed here, including disseminated viral infections, fungal infections, parasitic infections, and disseminated bacterial infections*:

- Bacteria
  Mycobacterium tuberculosis
  Mycobacterium avium-intracellulare
  Mycobacterium fortuitum
  Salmonella sp.
  Legionella pneumophila
- Fungi
  Cryptococcus carinii

*From Curran JW, Gold J, Jaffe HW: The acquired immunodeficiency syndrome (AIDS). In Holmes KK, Mårdh PA, Sparling PF, et al, eds: Sexually transmitted diseases. New York, McGraw-Hill Book Co., 1984.

Candida sp.
Aspergillus sp.
Histoplasma capsulatum
Coccidioides immitis
- Parasites
Pneumocystis carinii
Toxoplasma gondii
Cryptosporidium sp.
Isospora belli
Strongyloides stercoralis
- Viruses
Cytomegalovirus
Herpes simplex virus
- Varicella-zoster virus
- JC virus (progressive multifocal leukoencephalopathy)

Symptomatic infections with the following organisms have not been reported yet but are to be anticipated: bacteria—*Listeria monocytogenes, Nocardia asteroides;* viruses—Epstein-Barr virus, adenovirus.

A "forme fruste" or prodromal illness to full-blown AIDS has been noted, AIDS related complex (ARC). This nonspecific illness in seropositive individuals may produce a generalized lymphadenopathy, wasting with weight loss, diarrhea, and malabsorption. Recent interest has also focused on the central nervous system manifestations of AIDS. Multiple neurologic problems, including severe dementia and chronic central nervous system degeneration, have been identified. HIV has a high affinity for nervous tissue, with the majority of AIDS victims having CNS lesions at autopsy.

To protect recipients of blood transfusions, donors are currently screened for antibodies to HIV. The screening test is an enzyme-linked immunosorbent assay (ELISA). This serologic screening, though, is not a test for AIDS. There are biologic false positive and false negative results related to nonspecific test factors and infections by viruses with similar antigens. The sensitivity of the ELISA test is approximately 95%, and the specificity 99.7%. Thus in a population group with a low disease prevalence for AIDS, of 100 positive ELISA tests, 99 will be false positive and one will be truly positive. False positive results are more common in multiparous women and women taking oral contraceptives. A more specific assay, the Western blot technique, is used to investigate individuals with persistently positive ELISA

tests. The Western blot technique identifies antibodies to proteins of a specific molecular weight; it is, therefore, more specific than the ELISA test.

There is no standard treatment for the immunologic defects associated with AIDS. The hope for the future is that a successful vaccine will be developed, although the current outlook is not promising. Currently in progress are several experimental trials of drugs that interfere with replication of the AIDS virus. However, even if these clinical trials are successful, most experts believe these antiviral drugs will have to be combined with immunomodulators to have an impact on patients with the full-blown disease. The greatest impact on the spread of the disease will be made in the near future through prevention. It is hoped that changes in sexual practice and the use of condoms will decrease the incidence of this fatal disease.

VAGINITIS

Vaginal discharge resulting from primary infections of the vagina is one of the most common gynecologic symptoms. A gynecologist in private practice will see on the average two to four patients per day with vaginal infections. There are three common infections of the vagina—one produced by a fungus (candidiasis), another by a protozoon *(Trichomonas)*, and the third a synergistic bacterial infection (bacterial vaginosis). Relative prevalence differs depending on the population being studied. However, in a group of middle-class women in the reproductive range, bacterial vaginosis represents approximately 50% of cases, whereas candidiasis and *Trichomonas* infection each constitute approximately 25% of cases. Vaginal discharge resulting from viral infections such as herpes was discussed earlier in the chapter. Vaginitis in prepubertal and postmenopausal women is discussed in chapters dedicated to gynecologic problems in those age groups (Chapter 10 and 40).

The vaginal environment has been described as both a dynamic and a delicate ecosystem. The normal vaginal pH is 3.8 to 4.2. The maintenance of an optimum pH balance involves a complex interplay of hormonal, microbiologic, and other unknown factors. In reproductive age women, estrogen stimulates the glycogen content of vaginal epithelial cells. The glycogen is metabolized to lactic acid and other short-chain organic acids, principally by the lactobacilli but also by other vaginal bacteria and enzymes. This interplay maintains the acidic environment of the vagina at a pH of approximately 4.0, which in turn limits the growth of potentially pathogenic bacteria and protozoa. One of the most helpful diagnostic aids in the differential diagnosis of vaginitis is to measure vaginal acidity with pH indicator paper. A vaginal pH of greater than 5.0 indicates bacterial vaginosis or *Trichomonas* infection or possibly an atrophic vaginal discharge. A vaginal pH of less than 4.5 represents either a physiologic discharge or a fungal infection. Cervical mucus, vaginal fluids produced during sexual excitement, and semen are all of a neutral or basic pH and may temporarily change the normal acidity. Semen has been found to buffer vaginal acidity for 6 to 8 hours following intercourse. Douching has little effect on vaginal pH.

Normal physiologic vaginal discharge consists of cervical and vaginal epithelium, normal bacterial flora, water, electrolytes, and other chemicals. The quantitative concentration of bacterial organisms is 10^8 to 10^9 colonies per milliliter of vaginal fluid. Döderlein in 1894 was the first to study the bacterial flora. Recently Larsen and Galask as well as Bartlett and Polk have published extensive reviews of both qualitative and quantitative studies of normal bacterial flora of the vagina. In the latter study, the investigators serially sampled several women throughout the same cycle. Bartlett and Polk discovered that the concentration of anaerobic and aerobic bacteria varied considerably during the menstrual cycle. Qualitatively the number of bacterial species varied from 17 to 29. Anaerobic bacteria were quantitatively the most prevalent—5 times more common than aerobic bacteria.

Lactobacillus, an aerobic gram-positive rod, is found in 62% to 88% of asymptomatic women. Other common aerobic bacteria are diphtheroids, streptococci, *Staphylococcus epidermidis*, and *Gardnerella vaginalis*. The most common gram-negative bacillus is *E. coli*. Anaerobic bacteria have been detected in approximately 80% of women, the most prevalent being *Peptococcus, Peptostreptococcus,* and

TABLE 21-4
Bacterial Vaginal Flora among Asymptomatic Women without Vaginitis

Organism	Range of Recovery (%)
Facultative Organisms	
Gram-positive rods	
Lactobacilli	50-75
Diphtheroids	40
Gram-positive cocci	
Staphylococcus epidermidis	40-55
Staphylococcus aureus	0-5
Beta-hemolytic streptococci	20
Group D streptococci	35-55
Gram-negative organisms	
Escherichia coli	10-30
Klebsiella sp.	10
Other organisms	2-10
Anaerobic Organisms	
Peptococcus sp.	5-65
Peptostreptococcus spp.	25-35
Bacteroides spp.	20-40
Bacteroides fragilis	5-15
Fusobacterium sp.	5-25
Clostridium sp.	5-20
Eubacterium sp.	5-35
Veillonella sp.	10-30

From Eschenbach DA: Vaginal infection. Clin Obstet Gynecol 26:187, 1983.

Bacteroides species (Table 21-4). *Candida* species and mycoplasmas are also common inhabitants of asymptomatic women.

The ultimate diagnosis of the etiology of vaginitis depends on examination of the vaginal secretions under the microscope and measurement of vaginal pH. Nevertheless it is helpful to generalize about the classic characteristics of normal secretions and the three common vaginal infections (Table 21-5).

Normal vaginal secretions are white, floccular or curdy, and odorless. Godley has recently quantified normal vaginal secretions. Although the amount varies with the day of the menstrual cycle, asymptomatic women averaged 1.6 g every 8 hours. If the vaginal discharge is white and curdy, fungal infections are more likely. Gray-white discharges that are thin and usually profuse indicate a differential diagnosis

TABLE 21-5

Appearance of Vaginal Discharge

	Normal	Bacterial Vaginosis	Trichomoniasis	Candidiasis
Discharge present at introitus	No	Yes	Yes	No
Color	White	Gray	Yellow-gray	White
Viscosity	High	Low	Low	High
Consistency	Floccular	Homogeneous	Homogeneous	Floccular
Presence in vagina	Dependent portion	Adherent to vaginal walls	Adherent to vaginal walls	Adherent to vaginal walls

From Eschenbach DA: Vaginal infection. Clin Obstet Gynecol 26:186, 1983.

of *Trichomonas* or bacterial vaginosis. Vaginal discharges that have a foul odor are usually caused by either *Trichomonas* or bacterial vaginosis.

Bacterial Vaginosis (Nonspecific Vaginitis)

Bacterial vaginosis, referred to as nonspecific vaginitis by many, is the most frequent infectious vaginitis. The majority of experts consider it to be a sexually transmitted disease. The incubation period is 5 to 10 days following exposure.

Concepts of the etiology of this disease have changed over the past few years. An associated semantic debate concerning the best descriptive name for the type of vaginitis caused by one or more bacteria has accompanied the changing concepts. Twenty years ago the offending organism was called *Haemophilus* or *Corynebacterium vaginale*. Subsequently a specific species was named after Herman Gardner and called *Gardnerella vaginalis*. The latter is classified as a gram-negative, small bacillus. In practice the organism is a coccobacillus that is gram variable (sometimes gram positive, sometimes gram negative), depending on the age of the cultures. As more sophisticated culture techniques have been developed, it is apparent that *G. vaginalis* may be recovered from the vaginas of 30% to 40% of asymptomatic women.

Holmes and Eschenbach and their colleagues from Seattle proposed that nonspecific vaginitis was a symbiotic infection of anaerobic bacteria and *Gardnerella*, both organisms contributing to produce the clinical symptoms. They discovered that the prevalence and concentration of *Gardnerella* organisms were increased from 10^4 bacteria per milliliter in asymptomatic women to 10^7 bacteria per milliliter in symptomatic women. Concentrations of anaerobic bacteria increased tenfold in symptomatic women. The name of the infection was therefore changed from nonspecific vaginitis to bacterial vaginosis. To further complicate the picture, several groups have recently reported the association of vaginal vibrios in approximately 50% of symptomatic women. These small, curved anaerobic rods are from the *Mobiluncus* group, and their exact role in the production of vaginal infection is unclear.

Women with bacterial vaginosis have the most uniform spectrum of symptoms of all the types of infectious vaginitis (Table 21-6). The most frequent symptom is an unpleasant vaginal odor, which patients describe as "musty," or "fishy." The odor is often sensed following intercourse, when the alkaline semen results in a release of aromatic amines.

The vaginal discharge associated with bacterial vaginosis is thin and gray-white. Speculum examination reveals that the discharge is mildly adherent to the vaginal walls in contrast to a physiologic discharge, which is discovered in the most dependent areas of the vagina. The vaginal discharge is frothy in approximately 10% of women, and it is rare to have associated vulvar irritation.

The diagnosis of bacterial vaginosis is confirmed by a saline wet smear. The classic find-

TABLE 21-6
Major Categories of Vaginitis

	C. albicans	*C. glabrata*	*Gardnerella*	*Trichomonas*
Symptom	Itch	Burn	Odor	Discharge
Mucosal erythema*	+ + +	+	None	Variable
pH	4-5	4-5	5-6	6-7
Wet smear	Budding filaments	Spores only	Clue cells	Many white blood cell protozoa

From Friedrich EG: Vaginitis. Am J Obstet Gynecol 152:248, 1985.
*Degree of severity: +, mild; + + +, severe.

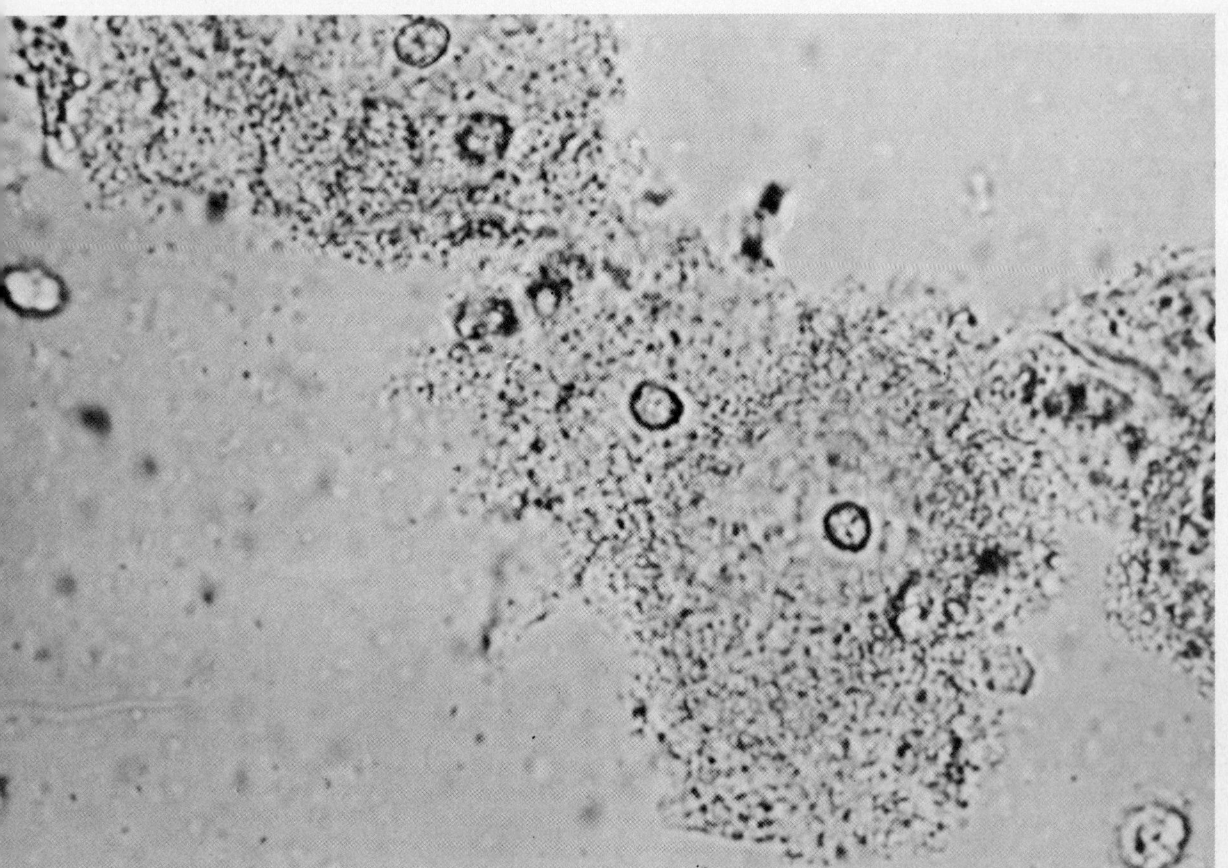

FIGURE 21-20
Vaginal epithelial cells from woman with bacterial vaginosis. These are typical clue cells, being heavily covered by coccobacilli, with loss of distinct cell margins. (×400.) (From Holmes KK: Lower genital tract infections in women: Cystitis/urethritis, vulvovaginitis, and cervicitis. In Holmes KK, Mårdh PA, Sparling PF, et al, eds: Sexually transmitted diseases. New York, McGraw-Hill Book Co., 1984, p. 565.)

ings on wet smear are clumps of bacteria and "clue cells," which are vaginal epithelial cells with clusters of bacteria adherent to their external surfaces (Fig. 21-20). The bacteria give the clue cell a granular or stippled appearance by obscuring their cellular borders. The percentage of clue cells may vary widely, ranging from 2% to 50% of infected women. The wet smear also demonstrates a comparative lack of inflammatory cells and lactobacilli. If inflammatory cells are visualized on wet smear, there is usually associated cervical infection or *Trichomonas vaginalis* infection. In experimental studies where vaginal biopsies have been performed in women with bacterial vaginosis, there is no histologic evidence of vaginal inflammation.

The vaginal pH associated with bacterial vaginosis is 5.0 to 6.0. When 10% potassium hydroxide is placed on the vaginal speculum or a glass slide containing vaginal secretions, an aromatic amine will be vaporized. A positive "whiff test" may be obtained with either bacterial vaginosis or *Trichomonas* infection. It is usually more prominent with bacterial infections because of the amount of anaerobic metabolism. The common aromatic amines are cadaverine and putrescine, both of which result from anaerobic metabolism. In all likelihood, bacterial vaginosis is a sexually transmitted disease. The *Gardnerella* organism may be recovered from approximately 90% of male partners. Women with multiple sexual partners are in a high-risk group for the disease. It has been postulated that the associated increased prevalence and concentration of anaerobic bacteria in the vagina may also predispose certain women to upper tract pelvic infection.

The treatment of choice for bacterial vaginosis is metronidazole (Protostat, Flagyl) 500 mg twice daily for 7 days. Metronidazole has excellent activity against anaerobic bacteria, and its hydroxy metabolite is active against *G. vaginalis*. Pfeifer et al. found clinical cures in 80 of 81 women treated with metronidazole but mediocre reponses to ampicillin, tetracycline, or sulfa cream. More important, facultative *Lactobacillus* organisms return after treatment with metronidazole but not with ampicillin. Most investigators report a cure rate of approximately two out of three women with a 1-week course of ampicillin 500 mg every 6 hours.

Blackwell et al. have recently contrasted treatment of 7 days of metronidazole with a regimen of 2 g of metronidazole divided over 12 hours. They described a 95% cure rate with 7 days versus a 75% cure rate with single-day therapy. Purdon et al. found similar results with 67% of women treated with single-day therapy and 86% of patients cured receiving the 7-day course. The alternate treatment to metronidazole is cephradine 500 mg every 6 hours for 7 days.

Bump et al. have added to the therapeutic dilemma by a study of prevalence and persistence of *G. vaginalis* in asymptomatic women over a 6-month period. They believe that the *Gardnerella* bacterium is indigenous flora and is often transient. They advise not treating a patient unless she exhibits classic symptoms.

Concurrent treatment of the male partner is most controversial. The literature is divided on this subject. We favor treating the male partner if there is recurrent vaginitis or any suspicion of associated upper genital tract infection.

Trichomonas Vaginal Infection

Trichomonas vaginalis is a protozoon that inhabits the vagina and lower urinary tract, especially Skene's ducts in the female. The relative importance of *Trichomonas* as a cause of vaginitis has decreased since the introduction of metronidazole 25 years ago. It is estimated that there are between 2.5 and 3 million cases of vaginitis secondary to *Trichomonas* infection in the United States each year. *Trichomonas* is the etiologic factor for approximately one in four episodes of infectious vaginitis. Many women who harbor *Trichomonas* in their vaginal secretions are free of symptoms. McLellan et al. discovered that only one out of two women with positive vaginal cultures had symptoms of a vaginal discharge. In the same study only one out of six women complained of vulvar pruritus. Positive wet smears or cultures for *Trichomonas* are reported in 5% to 15% of asymptomatic gynecology patients, with a much higher percentage being found in women attending a sexually transmitted disease clinic. Trichomoniasis is definitely a sexually transmitted disease, with the protozoa being isolated from 67% to 100% of the sexual partners of an individual with a positive culture. *Trichomonas* is a hardy organism and will survive for up to 24 hours on a wet towel and up to 6 hours on a surface. However, experimental studies have established that successful vaginal infection depends on the deposition of an inoculum of several thousand organisms. Thus it is unlikely that infection may be related to exposure from infected towels or swimming pools.

Trichomonas vaginitis is caused by the anaerobic, flagellated protozoon, *T. vaginalis* (Fig. 21-21). There are other species of *Trichomonas* that reside in the oral pharynx and rectum. These species are site specific and do not produce disease in the vagina. *T. vaginalis* resides in the paraurethral glands of both the male and female. Before systemic medication,

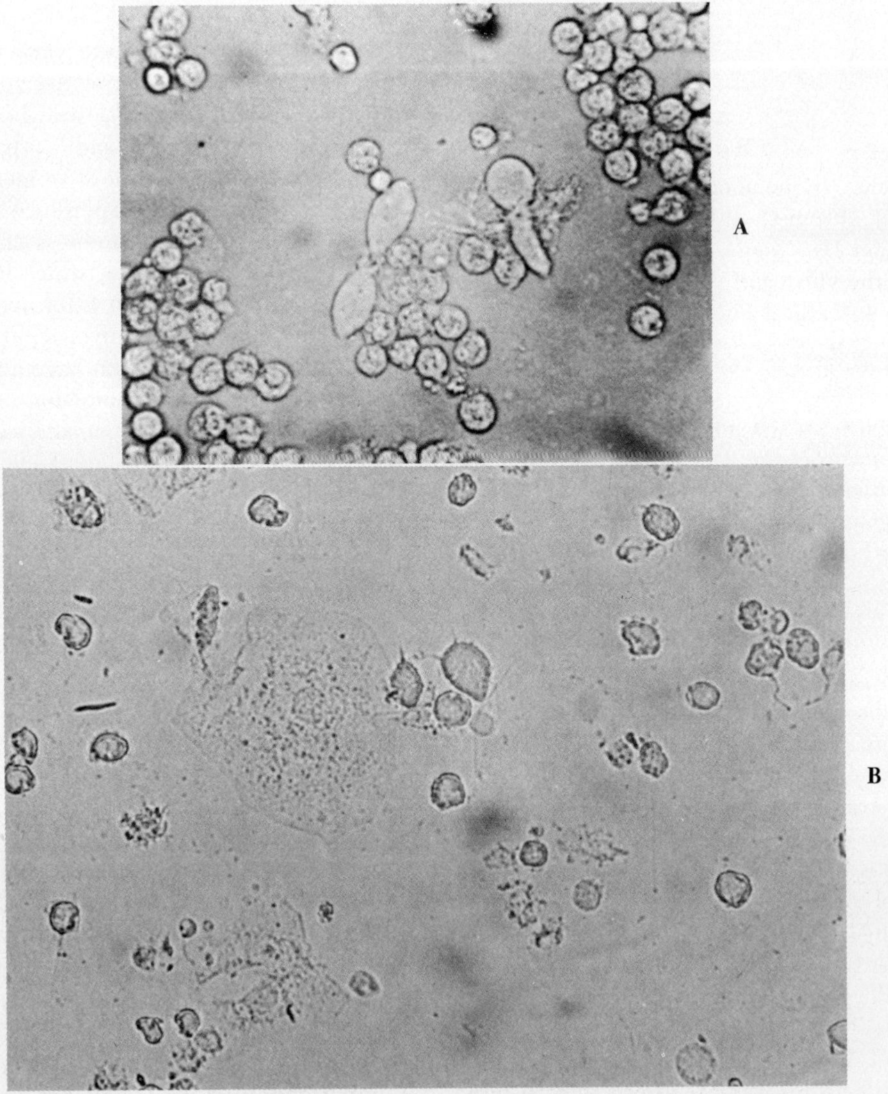

FIGURE 21-21
A and **B,** Trichomonads in wet mount prepared with physiologic saline. (**A** from Gardner HL: Trichomoniasis. In Gardner HL, Kaufman RH, eds: Benign diseases of the vulva and vagina, 2nd ed. Chicago, Year Book Medical Publishers, 1981, p. 260. **B** from Friedrich EG: Vulvar disease, 2nd ed. Philadelphia, W.B. Saunders Co., 1983, p. 23.)

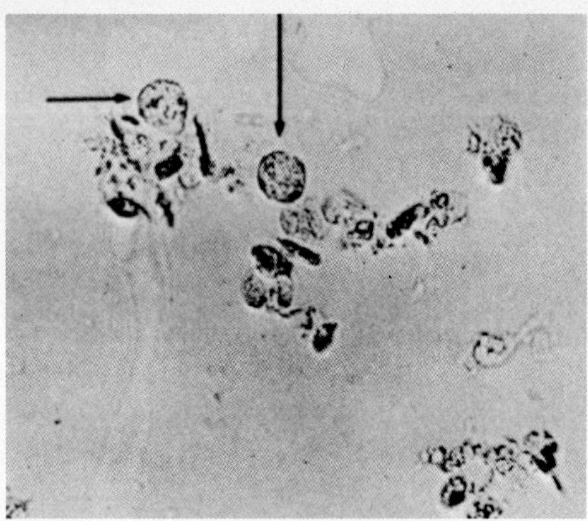

FIGURE 21-22
"Balled-up" trichomonads *(arrow)* in urinary sediment. (From Gardner HL: Trichomoniasis. In Gardner HL, Kaufman RH, eds: Benign diseases of the vulva and vagina, 2nd ed. Chicago, Year Book Medical Publishers, 1981, p. 260.)

reinfection occurred not only from an infected partner but from the patient's own urethra and Skene's ducts.

T. vaginalis is a unicellular protozoon that is normally fusiform in shape. It is slightly larger than a white blood cell. Three to five flagella extend from one end of the organism. The flagella provide the active movement of the protozoon with the direction of motion usually toward the end with the flagella. The *Trichomonas* organism assumes a spherical shape in an acidic environment (Fig. 21-22). Motion is then restricted to waves of the undulating membrane of the protozoon.

Vaginitis from *Trichomonas* is a disease primarily of women in the reproductive years. The normal highly acidic vaginal environment is resistant to *Trichomonas* infection. When lactobacilli predominate in the vaginal fluid, a woman will not develop symptoms. However, menstrual blood or other vaginal pathogens that transform the vaginal pH to a more basic level favor the growth of *Trichomonas* organisms.

Trichomonas produces a wide variety of patterns of vaginal infection. Women may or may not have symptoms and signs of acute or chronic infection. The primary symptom of *Tri-*

chomonas vaginal infection is profuse vaginal discharge. Patients often complain that the copious discharge makes them feel "wet." The discharge may be white, gray, yellow, or green. The classic discharge of *Trichomonas* infection has been termed "frothy" (with bubbles) and often has an unpleasant odor. However, a frothy discharge is only noted in 10% to 25% of women with proven *Trichomonas* infection. This discharge is not diagnostic, because it may be seen also with nonspecific bacterial vaginal infections.

Associated with the acute vaginal discharge are erythema and edema of the vulva and vagina. The classic sign of a strawberry appearance of the upper vagina and cervix is rare and is noted in less than 10% of women. Approximately 25% of women experience vulvar pruritus. Vulvar skin involvement is limited to the vestibule and labia minora, which helps to distinguish it from the more extensive vulvar involvement of monilial vulvovaginitis. Women with chronic infection often have a malodorous discharge as their only complaint.

The diagnosis of *Trichomonas* vaginal infection is confirmed by examination of vaginal fluid mixed with physiologic saline under the microscope (Fig. 21-21). To optimally visualize *Trichomonas* organisms, it is best to use high power and dampen the condenser to produce the greatest contrast. If the wet smear is fresh and warm, the organisms will exhibit forward motion. If the slide is cold, if the organisms are surrounded by white blood cells, or if the saline is too hypertonic, the *Trichomonas* organisms will assume an ovoid configuration and exhibit minimal motion. The wet smear usually contains a large number of inflammatory cells and many vaginal epithelial cells. The only other vaginitis with an abundance of white blood cells is atrophic vaginitis. The epithelial cells are normal in appearance and have distinct edges. It is postulated that *Trichomonas* excretes a cytotoxic substance that lyses intracellular bridges. This may explain the large number of normal epithelial cells on wet smear seen with severe infection.

The accuracy of diagnosis by wet smear equals or exceeds that made by culture. Therefore, a culture for *Trichomonas* is rarely indicated. Attempts to diagnose *T. vaginalis* infection by Papanicolaou (pap) smear results in an error rate of at least 50%. There is a large number of both false positive and false negative reports. A complementary laboratory test to the wet smear is the measurement of pH of the vaginal fluid with colorimetric paper. The vaginal pH associated with *T. vaginalis* is between 5.0 and 7.0.

Metronidazole (Flagyl, Protostat) is the treatment of choice for *T. vaginalis* infection. Metronidazole is marketed in the United States as 250 and 500 mg tablets and an intravenous preparation for severe anaerobic infections. The drug is completely absorbed orally and has a half-life of 8 hours. Phenobarbital decreases the serum concentration approximately 50% by activating liver enzymes. There are two standard treatment regimens, which yield equal results of an approximately 90% cure rate. Single-day therapy is 1 g of metronidazole in the morning and another 1 g at night. Alternate therapy is 250 mg every 8 hours for 7 days. Single-day therapy is preferable, because it is less expensive and has fewer side effects and greater patient compliance. The major side effects of metronidazole therapy include nausea, vomiting, a metallic taste, and secondary yeast infections. Nausea is the most frequent complication and is experienced by 5% of women. Patients should be warned that metronidazole inhibits ethanol metabolism. Therefore, they may experience a disulfiram-like reaction if the two drugs are used concurrently. Metronidazole is contraindicated in the first trimester of pregnancy because of possible mutagenesis. Several reports have noted an association between chronic high-dose metronidazole treatment and pulmonary cancers in mice. However, studies of humans have not confirmed any relationship between metronidazole therapy and oncogenesis.

One of the continuing debates regarding therapy is treatment of the asymptomatic male partner. Gardner and Dukes documented a 2.5-fold greater reinfection rate when the sexual partner was not treated. Some physicians elect to treat the male partner only when the vaginitis is recurrent. We believe that *Trichomonas* infection should be treated in a similar fashion to any sexually transmitted disease. Thus it is our practice to treat male sexual partners with 2 g of metronidazole (single-day therapy).

Women who have recurrence have in most cases either been reinfected or complied poorly with therapy. Recently a few resistant strains of *Trichomonas* have been documented. These resistant cases usually respond to daily doses of 1 to 2 g of metronidazole for 7 days.

If a woman is allergic to metronidazole, topical clotrimazole, an imidazole derivative, is the appropriate drug. Friedrich has advocated douching with hypertonic (20%) saline solution to reduce the vaginal inoculum.

Candida Vaginitis

Candida vaginitis is produced by a ubiquitous, airborne, gram-positive fungus. The vast majority of cases are caused by *Candida albicans*, with a rare vaginal infection produced by *C. glabrata* or *C. tropicalis*. *Candida* species are part of the normal flora of approximately 25% of women, being a commensal saprophytic organism on the mucosal surface of the vagina. Its prevalence in the rectum is three to four times greater and in the mouth two times greater than in the vagina. When the ecosystem of the vagina is disturbed, *C. albicans* becomes an opportunistic pathogen. Lactobacilli inhibit the growth of fungi in the vagina. However, when the relative concentration of lactobacilli declines, rapid overgrowth of *Candida* species occurs.

Vulvovaginal candidiasis has a variety of names, such as "moniliasis." This term is semantically incorrect, because the name is reserved for plant pathogens. Candidiasis is also often referred to as a yeast infection because of its similarity to true yeast cells.

Candida vaginitis has several features unlike those of protozoal or bacterial vaginitis. *Candida* is rarely found in a mixed infection, with *Trichomonas* or bacterial vaginosis. *Candida* vulvovaginitis is not associated with other sexually transmitted diseases and is not seen more frequently in STD clinics. Unlike other vaginal infections, there is no direct relationship between the number of organisms and the patient's signs and symptoms. Some women with a small amount of yeast may have extensive symptoms. It has been postulated that such patients may be hypersensitive to the fungus. Also, candidiasis is not considered a sexually transmitted disease. However, 10% of male

type discharge is often visualized with adherent clumps and plaques (thrush patches) attached to the walls of the vagina. The pH of the vagina associated with this infection is below 4.5.

The diagnosis is established by obtaining a wet smear of vaginal secretion and mixing this with 10% to 20% potassium hydroxide (Fig. 21-24). The alkali rapidly lyse both red blood cells and inflammatory cells. It is important to always use a coverslip, because potassium hydroxide will destroy the glass lens of the microscope. Active disease is associated with filamentous forms rather than spores. However, it may be necessary to search the slide and scan many different microscopic fields to identify hyphae or pseudohyphae. The average concentration of organisms is 10^3 to 10^4 per milliliter, but as stated previously, there is no direct relationship between the concentration of organism and the severity of the signs and symptoms. The microscopic diagnosis of fungal infection has a sensitivity of approximately 65%. A negative smear does not exclude *Candida* vulvovaginitis. The diagnosis can be established by culture with either Nickerson or Sabouraud medium. These cultures will become positive in 24 to 72 hours and are a simple office procedure, because they can be grown at room temperature.

The treatment of choice for *Candida* vaginitis is the topical application of one of the synthetic imidazoles—miconazole (Monistat), clotrimazole (Lotrimin, Mycelex), or butoconazole (Femstat). These compounds are marketed in an array of carrier vehicles, primarily as suppositories or creams. They exert their action by changing the permeability of the surface membrane of the fungus. The most recent therapeutic advance has been found in several comparative studies that have documented equal effectiveness between the traditional 7-day therapy and the newer 3-day therapy. The 3-day course is less expensive and provides improved patient compliance. Symptom cure rates are greater than 90%; however, approximately 20% of women will have positive cultures when followed for 4 to 6 weeks after therapy.

Before the introduction of synthetic imidazoles, polyenes, primarily nystatin (Mycostatin), were the standard therapy. Nystatin was prescribed for 10 to 14 days and resulted in clinical cure rates of approximately 80%. Povidone-iodine douche has been used for years, but when used alone it is only 60% effective.

One of the most perplexing problems in clinical gynecology is recurrent vaginal infection caused by *C. albicans*. Often it is difficult to distinguish a relapse from a reinfection. It is important to first confirm that the woman's symptoms are not the result of drug sensitivity. A screening test for diabetes should be performed. The vaginal discharge should be cultured and the identity of the fungus species determined. Horowitz et al. have demonstrated a twofold rate of recurrence with *C. tropicalis*, because this organism is not as susceptible to the imidazoles as *C. albicans*. Similarly, *C. glabrata* infections are often resistant to imidazoles. The latter fungus produces a clinical syndrome of vulvar burning with little to no vaginal discharge. Both *C. tropicalis* and *C. glabrata* should be treated with topical gentian violet.

Sobel and Eschenbach have each reported clinical trials for recurrent or persistent vulvovaginal candidiasis using ketoconazole (400 mg daily), an oral preparation. Both studies reported greater than 50% recurrence rates after the drug was discontinued. Liver toxicity is a worrisome side effect of ketoconazole; thus it is unlikely that it will be prescribed for long periods for vaginal infection. Treatment of the male partner and elimination of *Candida* species from the gastrointestinal tract have not been beneficial in alleviating the problem.

Potential therapy for recurrent disease includes gentian violet, boric acid, povidone-iodine douching, and dietary changes. Painting the vagina with 1% gentian violet is messy, and patients must be warned to wear a minipad so that their clothes will not be stained. The vagina should not be treated with gentian violet at intervals of less than 3 to 4 days, for the patient may develop a chemical "burn." Van Slyke et al. recommended that 600 mg boric acid in gelatin capsules be placed high in the vagina twice a day. Douching with povidone-iodine is sometimes helpful as adjunctive therapy to other methods. There are anecdotal reports of successful therapy with instructions to restrict sugar in the diet. Also, prophylactic treatment either immediately before or following menses or at the first sign of recurrence is often beneficial.

CERVICITIS

With the current epidemic of sexually transmitted diseases, cervical infections have drawn increasing interest from both clinicians and epidemiologists. The cervix may be a reservoir for *Neisseria gonorrhoeae, Chlamydia trachomatis,* and *Mycoplasma* species. Often the patient is asymptomatic, even though the cervix is colonized with either gonorrheal or chlamydial organisms. The cervix acts as a barrier between the bacterial flora of the vagina and the bacteriologically sterile endometrial cavity and oviducts. Viral infections of the cervix such as herpes simplex and human papillomavirus are frequently associated with the development of cervical intraepithelial neoplasia. Whether this relationship is induction or promotion of neoplasia remains a matter of debate.

The semantics of cervical infections have recently been dramatically revised. Colposcopy has demonstrated that the redness that was believed to be inflammation is often the capillary bed below an area of ectopic columnar epithelia (ectopy). Cervicitis used to be diagnosed erroneously when the clinician was viewing an area of metaplasia or erosion. Therefore descriptive clinical terms such as acute cervicitis, chronic cervicitis, and follicular and hypertrophic cervicitis have been abandoned. In a similar fashion the histologic diagnosis of chronic cervicitis is so prevalent that it should be considered the norm for parous women of reproductive age.

The pathophysiologic relationship between cervical mucus and both lower and upper genital tract infections is beginning to be elucidated. Mucus is much more than a simple physical barrier; it exerts a definite bacteriostatic effect. Mucus may also act as a competitive inhibitor with bacteria for receptors on the endocervical epithelial cells. Cervical mucus also contains antibodies and inflammatory cells that are active against various sexually transmitted organisms. The present debate concerning the effect of oral contraceptives on the prevalence of serious upper tract pelvic infection may yield insight into the pathophysiology of cervical infection. Women taking oral contra-

ceptives have a twofold to threefold increase in incidence of positive endocervical cultures for *C. trachomatis.* There are several hypotheses to explain this association. It may relate to differences in sexual activity. Alternatively, the cervical ectopy produced by oral contraceptives may preferentially facilitate adherence of *Chlamydia* organisms (Fig. 21-25). Cultures of *Chlamydia* may be more productive from smears of columnar cells. The higher prevalence may simply reflect a higher isolation rate.

The cervix may become infected by a wide variety of viral, protozoal, and fungal organisms. All of the sexually transmitted diseases may produce ulcerative lesions of the cervix. However, the principal infections of the cervix are caused by *N. gonorrhoeae, C. trachomatis,* genital herpes, and human papillomavirus. This section will focus on mucopurulent cervicitis and techniques to diagnose common cervical infections. The clinical diagnosis of mucopurulent cervicitis may be easily established. It is hoped that by diagnosing and treating mucopurulent cervicitis the prevalence of upper genital tract pelvic infection will be curtailed.

Mucopurulent Cervicitis

Brunham et al. have recently described objective criteria to diagnose endocervical infections. They have suggested the term *mucopurulent cervicitis* for the clinical diagnosis of active cervical infection. Mucopurulent cervicitis is directly analogous to, and the female counterpart of, urethritis in men. Two simple, definitive, objective criteria have been developed to establish this diagnosis—gross visualization of yellow mucopurulent material on a white swab and the presence of 10 or more polymorphonuclear leukocytes per microscopic field (magnification $\times 1000$) on gram-stained smears obtained from the endocervix. In their original study the Seattle group discovered that 40% of patients with sexually transmitted diseases had mucopurulent cervicitis (24% diagnosed by grossly visualized purulent material and 16% without mucopus but positive Gram stains of cervical mucus).

The prevalence of mucopurulent cervicitis depends on the population being studied. Approximately 30% to 40% of women attending clinics for sexually transmitted diseases and 8%

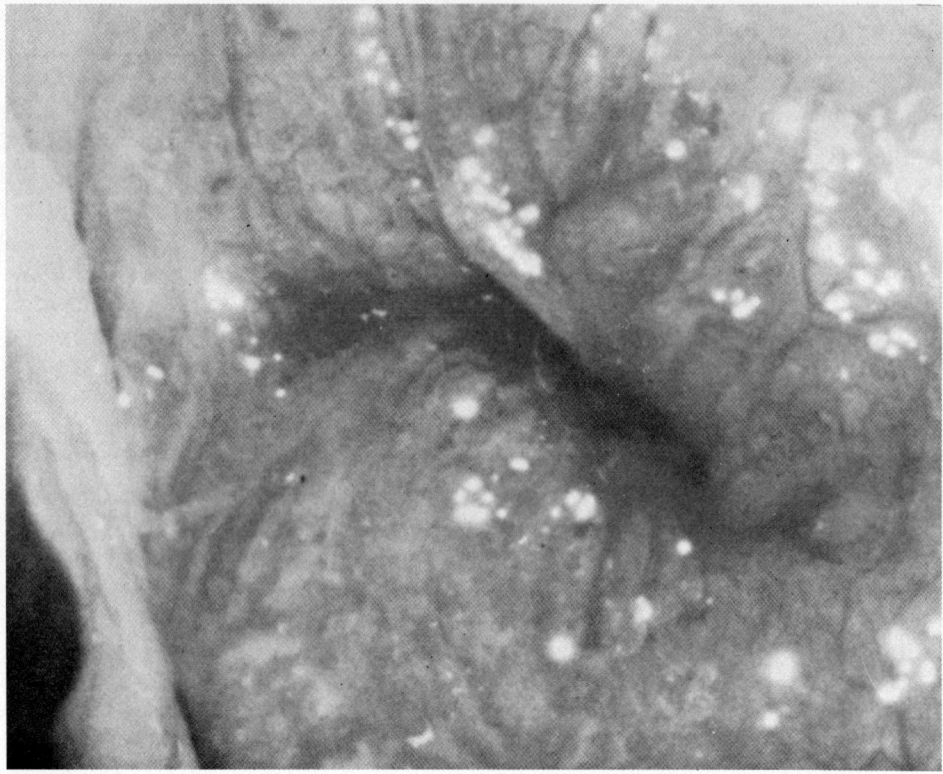

FIGURE 21-25
Colpophotograph of cervix infected with *Chlamydia trachomatis*, showing proliferation and dilation of subepithelial capillaries in zone of ectopy. (From Holmes KK: Lower genital tract infections in women: Cystitis/urethritis, vulvovaginitis, and cervicitis. In Holmes KK, Mårdh PA, Sparling PF, et al, eds: Sexually transmitted diseases. New York, McGraw-Hill Book Co., 1984, p. 579.)

to 10% of women in university student health clinics have the condition. The majority of women with this disease are asymptomatic. Symptoms that suggest cervical infection include vaginal discharge, deep dyspareunia, and postcoital bleeding.

C. trachomatis is the cause of cervical infection in most women with mucopurulent cervicitis (Fig. 21-26). In the initial study in Seattle, *Chlamydia* organisms were isolated from specimens of 20 of 40 women with mucopurulent cervicitis but only 2 of 60 without mucopurulent cervicitis. Subsequent studies have documented that up to two thirds of women with mucopurulent cervicitis have a positive endocervical chlamydial culture. Mucopurulent cervicitis is present in approximately 12% of women in whom no cervical pathogen can be

identified. The presence of active herpes infection was correlated with ulceration of the exocervix but not mucopus. *N. gonorrhoeae* was frequently isolated in this study, but its presence was not statistically significantly associated with either mucopus or 10 or more inflammatory cells per high-powered field. The mean number of inflammatory cells with positive gonorrheal cultures was 1.9 per high-powered field.

Special care must be taken in obtaining the cervical smears to establish a diagnosis of mucopurulent cervicitis. Initially a large cotton swab is used to absorb the vaginal secretions from the upper vagina and wipe away the mucus from the exocervix. Next a small white swab is inserted into the endocervical canal. It is inspected grossly for the presence of yellow

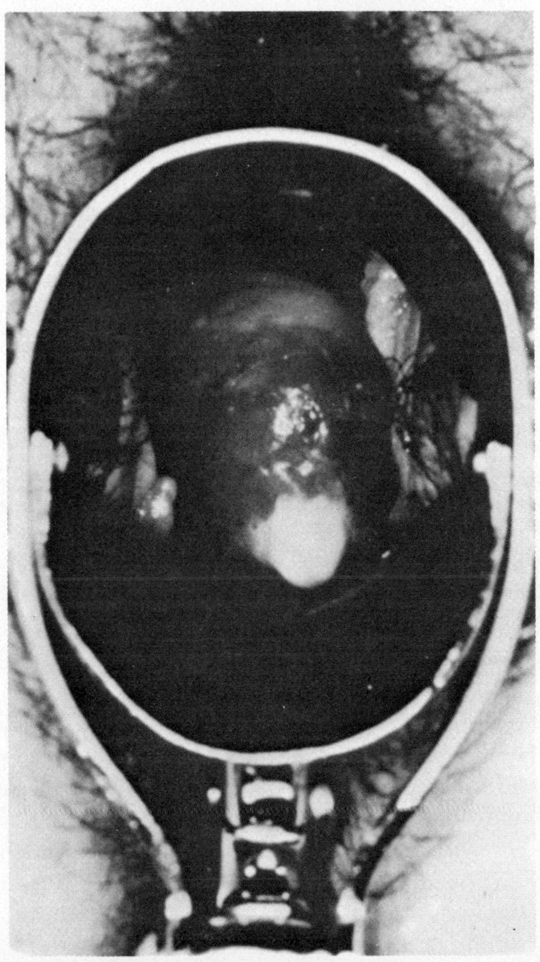

FIGURE 21-26
Mucopurulent cervicitis caused by *C. trachomatis*. (From Holmes KK: Lower genital tract infections in women: Cystitis/urethritis, vulvovaginitis and cervicitis. In Holmes KK, Mårdh PA, Sparling PF, et al, eds: Sexually transmitted diseases. New York, McGraw-Hill Book Co., 1984, p. 577.)

purulent material, gross pus from the endocervix being similar to the purulent urethral discharge in a male. Subsequently, the swab is rolled on a glass slide, and the slide is dried and gram stained. The slide is scanned to identify strands of cervical mucus containing areas of inflammatory cells. If 10 or more polymorphonuclear leukocytes are seen at a magnification of 1000, a positive diagnosis has been made. A culture for gonorrheal organisms should also be obtained, as the two organisms will be found simultaneously in approximately one third of cervical infections. Menstruation or the presence of vaginal squamous cells destroys the validity of the slide. Pandya and Cohen have discovered that endocervical leukocytes are a normal physiologic response to the deposition of sperm in the cervical canal. Therefore, if sperm are present, leukocyte presence indicates only a physiologic response of the cervix and not a pathologic reaction.

The treatment of choice for mucopurulent cervicitis is oral tetracycline 500 mg every 6 hours for at least 7 days. Doxycycline, 100 mg twice a day for 1 week, is an alternate oral therapy with better patient compliance. If a patient is allergic to tetracycline, erythromycin, 500 mg every 6 hours for 7 days, is acceptable. Another alternative is trimethoprim 160 mg plus sulfamethoxazole 800 mg twice a day for 10 days. The male partner should receive identical therapy.

The genital mycoplasmas, *Mycoplasma hominis* and *Ureaplasma urealyticum*, are frequently isolated from both the vagina and endocervix. Colonization rates as high as 75% have been reported. The exact role of genital mycoplasmas in producing either bacterial vaginosis or active cervical infection is unclear. Paavonen et al. reported that genital mycoplasmas do not produce mucopurulent cervicitis.

Detection of Pathogenic Cervical Bacteria

Neisseria gonorrhoeae

The diagnosis of cervical infection from *N. gonorrhoeae* is made by culture of the endocervical mucus. Gram staining of the endocervical mucus is diagnostic for only 50% of women with positive cultures for *N. gonorrhoeae* because other bacteria may appear similar on Gram stain. Thus culture of endocervical mucus directly on modified Thayer-Martin or similar medium is the diagnostic standard. A cotton swab should be rotated deep in the endocervical canal for 15 to 20 seconds. A single endocervical culture will detect approximately 85% of cervical infections. If a separate rectal swab specimen is cultured, the accuracy of diagnosing gonorrhea increases to 93%. Additional cultures of the pharynx, urethra, and ducts of accessory sex glands may be obtained depending on the patient's symptoms and sexual habits. Although transport media are available, it is important for the culture to reach the laboratory within 24 hours or there will be a loss of sensitivity. Growth of *N. gonorrhoeae* in culture is best at 37° C and in an environment between 2% and 10% carbon dioxide.

It is important to test positive cultures for sensitivity to penicillin. Penicillinase-producing strains of *N. gonorrhoeae* cause approximately 2% of gonorrheal infections in the United States. However, these strains are common in Africa and Asia. ELISA procedures such as the Gonozyme test for antigens do not depend on the viability of the organisms. Martin et al. reported that Gonozyme had a sensitivity of 95% and a specificity of 99%. Others have reported a lower sensitivity rate in females. Disadvantages of this test are that multiple steps are involved, which take over 1 hour, and that results must be interpreted by a spectrophotometer.

The treatment for gonococcal urethritis and cervicitis as recommended by the Centers for Disease Control is oral amoxicillin (3 g) or ampicillin (3.5 g) or intramuscular aqueous procaine penicillin (4.8 million units) or ceftriaxone (250 mg). Amoxicillin, ampicillin, and penicillin (but not ceftriaxone) are accompanied by oral probenecid (1 g). In addition to this regimen the CDC recommends also treating with oral tetracycline hydrochloride 500 mg four times daily for 7 days or oral doxycycline 100 mg twice daily for 7 days, because 45% of patients with gonorrhea have coexisting chlamydial infection. Follow-up cultures should be obtained 4 to 7 days after completion of treatment. Culture specimens should be obtained from the rectum of all women who have been treated for gonorrhea, regardless of whether rectal gonorrhea was documented before therapy.

Chlamydia trachomatis

The standard technique used to identify *C. trachomatis* infection is isolation of this intra-

cellular organism in tissue culture. A dacron, rayon, or calcium alginate swab is placed in the endocervical canal. It is rotated for 15 to 20 seconds to gently abrade the columnar epithelium. The swab is placed in an antibiotic containing transport medium and stored at 4° C. It is important to perform the definitive culture within 24 hours. Freezing and thawing of the transport medium decrease the eventual yield of positive cultures. Cultures are incubated on McCoy cell monolayers. Subsequently, in approximately 48 to 72 hours the monolayers are stained and examined microscopically for inclusions. The exact sensitivity of culture techniques is not known. Most experts estimate the sensitivity to be approximately 75%, depending primarily on the adequacy of sampling infected epithelial cells.

Recently, rapid, simple, and sensitive methods to detect chlamydial antigens have been introduced. One test uses fluorescein-conjugated monocolonal antibodies to detect elementary bodies of *C. trachomatis*. This slide test may be performed on endocervical smears and takes less than 30 minutes to complete. Tam et al. and Stamm et al. have published large series comparing this monocolonal antibody test with traditional tissue culture methods. For women the rapid slide test (MicroTrak, Syva) has a sensitivity of 85% to 93% and a specificity of 99%. False positive and false negative results were discovered in slide specimens containing a limited number of organisms. This slide test is approximately one third as expensive as cell culture techniques. There is only one major drawback to the direct test. There is a subjective assessment in reading the immunofluorescence, which necessitates several hours of training by laboratory personnel. The ELISA takes about 3 to 4 hours, requires a spectrophotometer, and has a sensitivity of 67% to 90% and a specificity of 92% to 97%. It is approximately half the cost of the direct fluorescent antibody test. Attempts have been made to diagnose chlamydial cervical infection from routine pap smears. However, at best this is an insensitive, nonspecific method to judge acute cervical inflammation.

KEY POINTS

- The three most prevalent primary viral infections of the skin of the vulva are genital herpes, condyloma acuminatum, and molluscum contagiosum.

- From 10% to 20% of adult women experience the symptoms of dysuria, frequency, and urgency each year. About 50% of women with these symptoms do not have significant bacteriuria.

- The most frequent pathogens causing acute urethral syndrome are *Escherichia coli*, *Staphylococcus saprophyticus*, *Chlamydia trachomatis*, and *Neisseria gonorrhoeae*.

- Women with pyuria and a "sterile" urine culture often have infection with chlamydial or gonorrheal organisms.

- Approximately 2% of adult women develop enlargement of both Bartholin's glands.

- The treatment of choice for a symptomatic cyst or abscess is the development of a fistulous tract from the dilated Bartholin's duct to the vestibule.

- Excision of Bartholin's duct and gland is indicated for persistent deep infection, multiple recurrences of abscesses, or enlargement of the gland in a woman over the age of 40.

- Pediculosis pubis, an infestation by the crab louse *Phthirus pubis*, is characterized by constant itching, predominantly vulvar involvement, and the finding of eggs and lice by visual inspection. It is treated by topical application of lindane (Kwell).

- Scabies, an infection by the itch mite *Sarcoptes scabiei*, is characterized by intermittent pruritus, most commonly in the hands, wrists, breasts, vulva, and buttocks. It is diagnosed by a scraping of the papules, vesicles, or burrows in which the mites live and inspection under the microscope. It is treated by topical application of lindane (Kwell).

- Condyloma acuminatum is a sexually transmitted disease spread by skin-to-skin contact. Autoinoculation also occurs. It is a highly contagious disease, with 25% to 65% of sexual partners developing the infection.

_______________ **KEY POINTS, cont'd** _______________

- There are approximately 280,000 new cases of syphilis, both primary and secondary, in the United States per year. Syphilis should be included in the differential diagnosis of all genital ulcers. Antibiotic treatment protocols depend on the stage of the disease.

- Dark-field microscopy rather than normal light microscopy is used for detection of syphilis because of the extreme thinness of the spirochete *Treponema pallidum*.

- Nonspecific tests for syphilis, the VDRL and RPR, have a 1% false positive rate. Therefore, specific tests such as the FTA-ABS, HATTS, and MHA-TP must be employed when a positive nonspecific test result is encountered.

- After successful treatment of syphilis the VDRL titer will become nonreactive or, at most, reactive with at least a fourfold titer decline within 1 year. The FTA-ABS may remain reactive indefinitely.

- Herpes is highly contagious, with 75% of sexual partners contracting the disease. One out of 200 American women are estimated to be asymptomatic shedders of herpesvirus from their reproductive tracts.

- Herpes genital infections are caused by both type I and type II virus. HSV-I is found in 13% to 40% of cases.

- The incubation period of primary herpes is 3 to 7 days, with an average of 6 days, and ulcers last for 2 to 6 weeks in multiple crops. Systemic symptoms for primary herpes are experienced by 70% of women. Secondary or recurrent genital herpes will occur in 50% of women by 6 months after the initial infection and last for approximately 7 days.

- Granuloma inguinale may be managed by a wide range of oral broad-spectrum antibiotics. Tetracycline is the most popular choice and should be prescribed for a minimum of 2 to 3 weeks.

- The treatment for lymphogranuloma venereum is oral tetracycline or erythromycin 500 mg every 6 hours for 3 to 6 weeks.

- The treatment of chancroid is oral trimethoprim 160 mg and sulfamethaxole 800 mg every 12 hours for 10 days or oral erythromycin 500 mg every 6 hours for 10 days.

- The risk of recurrence of toxic shock syndrome (TSS) without antibiotic therapy is approximately 33%.

- Studies of the vagina of normal menstruating females have documented 5% to 17% colonization with *Staphylococcus aureus* with 5% at midcycle and 10% to 17% during the menses.

- The initial rash of TSS over the first 48 hours is similar in appearance to an intense sunburn. Over the next several days it evolves into a macular rash with fine, flaky desquamation over the face and trunk and sloughing of the entire skin thickness over the palms and soles.

- Women with TSS should be treated with beta-lactamase resistant antistaphylococcal antibiotics for 10 to 14 days.

- Individuals with acquired immune deficiency syndrome (AIDS) may shed HTLV-III (HIV) and have active viremias throughout the asymptomatic phase of their disease, which may last for several years.

- There are three primary methods of contracting the HTLV-III virus: intimate sexual contact, use of contaminated needles or blood products especially in hemophiliacs, and perinatal transmission from mother to child.

- The present hypothesis of AIDS is that each year 10% to 20% of infected individuals develop symptomatic disease. Thus 80% to 90% of individuals with the virus are asymptomatic carriers. However, 80% to 90% of individuals who develop the full-blown syndrome die within 2 years of diagnosis of the disease.

- In middle-class women in the reproductive age range, bacterial vaginosis represents approximately 50% of vaginitis, while candidiasis and *Trichomonas* infection represent approximately 25% each.

- The normal vaginal environment is a dynamic and delicate ecosystem, with a pH of 3.8 to 4.2.

_______________ **KEY POINTS, cont'd** _______________

- A vaginal pH of greater than 5.0 indicates bacterial vaginosis or *Trichomonas* infection, whereas a vaginal pH of less than 4.5 is either a physiologic discharge or fungal in etiology.

- *Trichomonas* is a hardy organism and will survive for up to 24 hours on a wet towel and up to 6 hours on a wet surface. However, since a large inoculum is needed for infection, it is unlikely that infection is related to exposure from infected towels or swimming pools. *Trichomonas* vaginitis is treated with oral metronidazole (Flagyl).

- The most frequent symptom of bacterial vaginosis is an unpleasant vaginal odor described by patients as musty or fishy. Bacterial vaginosis is treated by oral metronidazole (Flagyl) 500 mg twice daily for 7 days.

- *Candida albicans* causes the majority of fungal vaginitis. It is found on most mucosal and skin surfaces and is the normal flora of approximately 25% of women, but it becomes an opportunistic pathogen when the normal ecosystem of the vagina is disturbed. *Candida* vaginitis is treated by means of topical application of one of the synthetic imidazoles.

- A negative wet smear of the vagina does not exclude *Candida* vulvovaginitis. The diagnosis can be established by culture with either Nickerson or Sabouraud medium.

- Symptoms that suggest cervical infection include vaginal discharge, deep dyspareunia, and postcoital bleeding. *Chlamydia trachomatis* is the major etiologic agent in women with mucopurulent cervicitis.

- Sperm-induced leukocyte presence in the endocervical mucus is a physiologic response.

- Culture is the standard technique for diagnosis of *Neisseria gonorrhoeae* because Gram stain smears are positive for only 50% of women with positive cultures. Sensitivity should also be evaluated, because approximately 2% of gonorrheal infections in the United States are resistant to penicillin.

- The standard technique used to identify *Chlamydia trachomatis* infection is isolation of this intracellular organism in tissue culture. The cultures are incubated on McCoy cell monolayers.

BIBLIOGRAPHY

Abramowicz M, ed: Treatment of sexually transmitted diseases. Med Lett 28:23, 1986.

Abrams AJ: Lymphogranuloma venereum. JAMA 205:199, 1968.

Bartlett JG, Polk R: Bacterial flora of the vagina: Quantitative study. Rev Infect Dis 6:S67, 1984.

Beard CM, Noller KL, O'Fallon M, et al: Lack of evidence for cancer due to use of metronidazole. N Engl J Med 301:519, 1979.

Becker TM, Blount JH, Guinan ME: Genital herpes infections in private practice in the United States, 1966 to 1981. JAMA 253:1601, 1985.

Bellina JH: The use of the carbon dioxide laser in the management of condylomata acuminatum with eight-year follow-up. Am J Obstet Gynecol 147:375, 1983.

Bierman SM: Recurrent genital herpes simplex infection: A trivial disorder. Arch Dermatol 121:513, 1985.

Blackwell AL, Phillips I, Fox AR, et al: Anaerobic vaginosis (non-specific vaginitis): Clinical, microbiological, and therapeutic findings. Lancet 2:1379, 1983.

Bolan RK, Sands M, Schachter J, et al: Lymphogranuloma venereum and acute ulcerative proctitis. Am J Med 72:703, 1982.

Bongard F, Landers DV, Lewis F: Differential diagnosis of appendicitis and pelvic inflammatory disease. Am J Surg 150:90, 1985.

Britigan BE, Cohen MS, Sparling PF: Gonococcal infection: A model of molecular pathogenesis. N Engl J Med 312:1683, 1985.

Brown D, Kaufman RH, Gardner HL: *Gardnerella vaginalis* vaginitis. J Reprod Med 29:300, 1984.

Brown ST, Nalley JF, Kraus SJ: Molluscum contagiosum. Sex Transm Dis 8:227, 1981.

Brunham RC, Paavonen J, Stevens CE, et al: Mucopurulent cervicitis—the ignored counterpart in women of urethritis in men. N Engl J Med 311:1, 1984.

Bryson YJ, Dillon M, Lovett M, et al: Treatment of first episodes of genital herpes simplex virus infection with oral acyclovir: A randomized double-blind controlled trial in normal subjects. N Engl J Med 308:916, 1983.

Bump RC, Copeland WE: Urethral isolation of the genital mycoplasmas and *Chlamydia trachomatis* in women with chronic urologic complaints. Am J Obstet Gynecol 152:38, 1985.

Bump RC, Zuspan FP, Buesching WJ, et al: The prevalence, six-month persistence and predictive values of laboratory indicators of bacterial vaginosis (nonspecific vaginitis) in asymptomatic women. Am J Obstet Gynecol 150:917, 1984.

Campbell-Brown M, McFadyen IR: Bacteriuria in pregnancy treated with a single dose of cephalexin. Br J Obstet Gynaecol 90:1054, 1983.

Carlson JR, Bryant ML, Hinrichs SH, et al: AIDS serology testing in low- and high-risk groups. JAMA 253:3405, 1985.

Carpenter JL, Back A, Gehle D, et al: Treatment of chancroid with erythromycin. Sex Transm Dis 8:192, 1981.

Centers for Disease Control: Sexually transmitted disease treatment guidelines 1985. MMWR 35(suppl 4):1, 1985.

Chapel TA: The signs and symptoms of secondary syphilis. Sex Transm Dis 7:161, 1980.

Chapel TA: The variability of syphilitic chancres. Sex Transm Dis 5:68, 1978.

Charles D: Syphilis. Clin Obstet Gynecol 26:125, 1983.

Chesney PJ, Davis JP, Purdy WK, et al: Clinical manifestations of toxic shock syndrome. JAMA 246:741, 1981.

Corey L, Adams HG, Brown ZA, et al: Genital herpes simplex virus infections: Clinical manifestations, course, and complications. Ann Intern Med 98:958, 1983.

Dan BB: Prevention and treatment of toxic shock syndrome: A retrospective look. JAMA 252:3411, 1984.

Davis GD: Management of Bartholin duct cysts with the carbon dioxide laser. Obstet Gynecol 65:279, 1985.

Dodson RF, Fritz GS, Hubler WR, et al: Donovanosis: A morphologic study. J Invest Dermatol 62:611, 1974.

Douglas CP: Lymphogranuloma venereum and granuloma inguinale of the vulva. J Obstet Gynaecol Br Cmmwlth 69:871, 1962.

Douglas JM, Critchlow C, Benedetti J, et al: A double-blind study of oral acyclovir for suppression of recurrences of genital herpes simplex virus infection. N Engl J Med 310:1551, 1984.

Droegemueller W, Adamson DG, Brown D, et al: Three-day treatment with butoconazole nitrate for vulvovaginal candidiasis. Obstet Gynecol 64:530, 1984.

Elion GB: Mechanism of action and selectivity of acyclovir. Am J Med 73:7, 1982.

Eschenbach DA: Vaginal infection. Clin Obstet Gynecol 26:186, 1983.

Eschenbach DA, Hummel D, Gravett MG: Recurrent and persistent vulvovaginal candidiasis: Treatment with ketoconazole. Obstet Gynecol 66:248, 1985.

Ferenczy A: Laser therapy of genital condylomata acuminata. Obstet Gynecol 63:703, 1984.

Fish EN, Tobin SM, Cooter NBE, et al: Update on the relation of herpesvirus hominis type II to carcinoma of the cervix. Obstet Gynecol 59:220, 1982.

Fitzpatrick JE, Tyler H, Gramstad ND: Treatment of chancroid: comparison of sulfamethoxazole trimethoprim with recommended therapies. JAMA 246:1804, 1981.

Fiumara NJ: Treatment of primary and secondary syphilis. JAMA 243:2500, 1980.

Friedrich EG: Vaginitis. Am J Obstet Gynecol 152:247, 1985.

Friedrich EG: Vulvar disease, 2nd ed. Philadelphia, W.B. Saunders Co., 1983.

Gaisin A, Heaton CL: Chancroid: Alias the soft chancre. Int J Dermatol 14:188, 1975.

Gardner HL: *Haemophilus vaginalis* vaginitis after twenty-five years. Am J Obstet Gynecol 137:385, 1980.

Gardner HL, Dukes CD: Clinical and laboratory effects of metronidazole. Am J Obstet Gynecol 89:990, 1964.

Gardner HL, Kaufman RH, eds: Benign diseases of the vulva and vagina, 2nd ed. Chicago, Year Book Medical Publishers, 1981, p. 120.

Godley MJ: Quantitation of vaginal discharge in healthy volunteers. Br J Obstet Gynaecol 92:739, 1985.

Goedert JJ, Biggar RJ, Weiss SH, et al: Three-year incidence of AIDS in five cohorts of HTLV-III-infected risk group members. Science 231:992, 1986.

Goldman P: Metronidazole. N Engl J Med 303:1212, 1980.

Hahn GA: Carbon dioxide laser surgery in treatment of condyloma. Am J Obstet Gynecol 141:1000, 1981.

Hammond GW, Lian CJ, Wilt JC, et al: Antimicrobial susceptibility of *Haemophilus ducreyi*. Antimicrob Agents Chemother 13:608, 1978.

Hammond GW, Slutchuk M, Scatliff J, et al: Epidemiological, clinical, laboratory and therapeutic features of an urban outbreak of chancroid in North America. Rev Infect Dis 2:867, 1980.

Helgerson SD, Mallery BL, Foster LR: Toxic shock syndrome in Oregon. JAMA 252:3402, 1984.

Hirsch MS, Wormser GP, Schooley RT, et al: Risk of nosocomial infection with human T-cell lymphotropic virus III (HTLV-III). N Engl J Med 312:1, 1985.

Holmes KK, Mårdh PA, Sparling PF, et al: Sexually transmitted diseases. New York, McGraw-Hill Book Co., 1984, p. 389.

Horowitz BJ, Edelstein SW, Lippman L: *Candida tropicalis* vulvovaginitis. Obstet Gynecol 66:229, 1985.

Jaffe HW: The laboratory diagnosis of syphilis. Ann Intern Med 83:846, 1975.

Johannisson G, Lowhagen GB, Lycke E: Genital *Chlamydia trachomatis* infection in women. Obstet Gynecol 56:671, 1980.

Kampmeier RH: Herpes genitalis: A clinical puzzle for two centuries. Sex Transm Dis 11:41, 1984.

Kaufman RH, Faro S: Herpes genitalis: Clinical features and treatment. Clin Obstet Gynecol 28:152, 1985.

Kissane JM, Anderson WAD: Anderson's pathology. St. Louis, The C.V. Mosby Co., 1985.

Kit S, Trkula D, Qavi H, et al: Sequential genital infections by herpes simplex viruses types 1 and 2: Restriction nuclease analyses of viruses from recurrent infections. Sex Transm Dis 10:67, 1983.

Kiviat NB, Paavonen JA, Brockway J, et al: Cytologic manifestations of cervical and vaginal infections. JAMA 253:989, 1985.

Lal S, Nicholas C: Epidemiological and clinical features in 165 cases of granuloma inguinale. Br J Vener Dis 46:461, 1970.

Larsen B, Galask RP: Vaginal microbial flora: Composition and influences of host physiology. Ann Intern Med 96:926, 1982.

Lee YH, Rankin JS, Alpert S, et al: Microbiological investigation of Bartholin's gland abscesses and cysts. Am J Obstet Gynecol 129:150, 1977.

Luby ED, Klinge V: Genital herpes: A pervasive psychosocial disorder. Arch Dermatol 121:494, 1985.

Lutzner MA: The human papillomaviruses: A review. Arch Dermatol 119:631, 1983.

Martin R, Wentworth BB, Coopes S, et al: Comparison of Transgrow and Gonozyme for the detection of *Neisseria gonorrhoeae* in mailed specimens. J Clin Microbiol 19:893, 1984.

McLellan R, Spence MR, Brockman M, et al: The clinical diagnosis of trichomoniasis. Obstet Gynecol 60:30, 1982.

Merkus JMWM, Bisschop MPJM, Stolte LAM: The proper nature of vaginal candidosis and the problem of recurrence. Obstet Gynecol Surv 40:493, 1985.

Mertz GJ, Critchlow CW, Benedetti J, et al: Double-blind placebo-controlled trial of oral acyclovir in first-episode genital herpes simplex virus infection. JAMA 252:1147, 1984.

Mindel A, Faherty A, Hindel D, et al: Prophylactic oral acyclovir in recurrent genital herpes. Lancet 2:57, 1984.

Moller BR, Jorgensen AS, From E, et al: *Chlamydia*, mycoplasmas, ureaplasmas, and yeasts in the lower genital tract of females. Acta Obstet Gynecol Scand 64:145, 1985.

Monif GRG: Infectious diseases in obstetrics and gynecology, 2nd ed. Philadelphia, Harper & Row, Publishers, 1982.

Montes LF, Wilborn WH: Fungus-host relationship in candidiasis. Arch Dermatol 121:119, 1985.

Morton RS: Metronidazole in the single-dose treatment of trichomoniasis in men and women. Br J Vener Dis 48:525, 1972.

Navia BA, Jordan BD, Price RW: The AIDS dementia complex. I. Clinical features. Ann Neurol 19:517, 1986.

Nilsen AE, Aasen T, Halsos AM, et al: Efficacy of oral acyclovir in the treatment of initial and recurrent genital herpes. Lancet 2:571, 1982.

Norris SJ: In vitro cultivation of *Treponema pallidum:* Independent confirmation. Infect Immun 36:437, 1982.

Oriel JD: Natural history of genital warts. Br J Vener Dis 47:1, 1971.

Oriel JD, Partridge BM, Denny MJ, et al: Genital yeast infections. Br Med J 4:761, 1972.

Orkin M, Epstein E, Maibach HI: Treatment of today's scabies and pediculosis. JAMA 236:1136, 1976.

Osborne NG, Grubin L, Pratson L: Vaginitis in sexually active women: Relationship to nine sexually transmitted organisms. Am J Obstet Gynecol 142:962, 1982.

Paavonen J, Miettinen A, Stevens CE, et al: *Mycoplasma hominis* in cervicitis and endometritis. Sex Transm Dis 10:276, 1983.

Pandya IJ, Cohen J: The leukocytic reaction of the human cervix to spermatozoa. Fertil Steril 43:417, 1985.

Peterman TA, Curran JW: Sexual transmission of human immunodeficiency virus. JAMA 256:2222, 1986.

Pfeifer TA, Forsyth PS, Durfee MA, et al: Nonspecific vaginitis: Role of *Haemophilus vaginalis* and treatment with metronidazole. N Engl J Med 298:1429, 1978.

Purdon A, Hanna JH, Morse PL, et al: An evaluation of single-dose metronidazole treatment of *Gardnerella vaginalis*. Obstet Gynecol 64:271, 1984.

Quinn TC, Goodell SE, Mkrtichian E, et al: *Chlamydia trachomatis* proctitis. N Engl J Med 305:195, 1981.

Redfield RR, Markham PD, Salahuddin SZ, et al: Frequent transmission of HTLV-III among spouses of patients with AIDS-related complex and AIDS. JAMA 253:1571, 1985.

Reeves WC, Corey L, Adams HG, et al: Risk of recurrence after first episodes of genital herpes. N Engl J Med 305:315, 1981.

Reichman RC, Badger GJ, Mertz GJ, et al: Treatment of recurrent genital herpes simplex infections with oral acyclovir: A controlled trial. JAMA 251:2103, 1984.

Resnick L, Veren K, Salahuddin SZ, et al: Stability and inactivation of HTLV-III/LAV under clinical and laboratory environments. JAMA 255:1887, 1986.

Schlievert PM, Blomster DA, Kelly JA: Toxic shock syndrome *Staphylococcus aureus:* Effect of tampons on toxic shock syndrome toxin 1 production. Obstet Gynecol 64:666, 1984.

Schupbach J, Haller O, Vogt M, et al: Antibodies to HTLV-III in Swiss patients with AIDS and pre-AIDS and in groups at risk for AIDS. N Engl J Med 312:265, 1985.

Scotti RJ, Ostergard DR: The urethral syndrome. Clin Obstet Gynecol 27:515, 1984.

Seligmann M, Chess L, Fahey HL, et al: AIDS—an immunologic reevaluation. N Engl J Med 311:1286, 1984.

Shacter B: Treatment of scabies and pediculosis with lindane preparations: An evaluation. J Am Acad Dermatol 5:517, 1981.

Shafer MA, Chew KL, Kromhout LK, et al: Chlamydial endocervical infections and cytologic findings in sexually active female adolescents. Am J Obstet Gynecol 151:765, 1985.

Sheenan G, Harding GKM, Ronald AR: Advances in the treatment of urinary tract infection. Am J Med 76:141, 1984.

Sobel JD: Management of recurrent vulvovaginal candidiasis with intermittent ketoconazole prophylaxis. Obstet Gynecol 65:435, 1985.

Sprott MS, Ingham HS, Pattman RS, et al: Characteristics of motile curved rods in vaginal secretions. J Med Microbiol 16:175, 1983.

Stamm WE, Guinan ME, Johnson C, et al: Effect of treatment regimens for *Neisseria gonorrhoeae* on simultaneous infection with *Chlamydia trachomatis*. N Engl J Med 310:545, 1984.

Stamm WE, Harrison HR, Alexander ER, et al: Diagnosis

of *Chlamydia trachomatis* infections by direct immunofluorescence staining of genital secretions. Ann Intern Med 101:638, 1984.

Straus SE, Takiff HE, Seidlin M, et al: Suppression of frequently recurring genital herpes: a placebo-controlled double-blind trial of oral acyclovir. N Engl J Med 310:1545, 1984.

Sweet RL, Gibbs RS: Infectious diseases of the female genital tract. Baltimore, The Williams & Wilkins Co., 1985.

Tam MR, Stamm WE, Handsfield H, et al: Culture-independent diagnosis of *Chlamydia trachomatis* using monoclonal antibodies. N Engl J Med 310:1146, 1984.

Taylor E, Barlow D, Blackwell AL, et al: *Gardnerella vaginalis*, anaerobes, and vaginal discharge. Lancet 1:1376, 1982.

Todd JK, Ressman M, Caston SA, et al: Corticosteroid therapy for patients with toxic shock syndrome. JAMA 252:3399, 1984.

Tofte RW, Williams DN: Toxic shock syndrome: Evidence of a broad clinical spectrum. JAMA 246:2163, 1981.

Van Slyke KK, Michel VP, Rein MF: Treatment of vulvovaginal candidiasis with boric acid powder. Am J Obstet Gynecol 141:145, 1981.

Vesterinen E, Meyer B, Cantell K, et al: Topical treatment of flat vaginal condyloma with human leukocyte interferon. Obstet Gynecol 63:535, 1984.

Vontver LA, Eschenbach DA: The role of *Gardnerella vaginalis* in nonspecific vaginitis. Clin Obstet Gynecol 24:439, 1981.

Wager GP: Toxic shock syndrome: A review. Am J Obstet Gynecol 146:93, 1983.

Washington AE, Gove S, Schachter J, et al: Oral contraceptives, *Chlamydia trachomatis* infection, and pelvic inflammatory disease. JAMA 253:2246, 1985.

Weber DJ, Redfield RR, Lemon SM: Acquired immunodeficiency syndrome: epidemiology and significance for the obstetrician and gynecologist. Am J Obstet Gynecol 155:235, 1986.

Weiss A, Hollander H, Stobo J: Acquired immunodeficiency syndrome: epidemiology, virology and immunology. Annu Rev Med 36:545, 1985.

Wilkin JK: Molluscum contagiosum venereum in a women's outpatient clinic: A venereally transmitted disease. Am J Obstet Gynecol 128:531, 1977.

Word B: Office treatment of cyst and abscess of Bartholin's gland duct. South Med J 61:514, 1968.

Upper Genital Tract Infections

———————— KEY TERMS AND DEFINITIONS ————————

Canaliculus. A small, canallike opening forming a channel for ascension of bacteria from the lower to the upper genital tract.

Commensal Bacteria. An organism that may exist in the genital tract without actually causing disease.

Fitz-Hugh–Curtis Syndrome. A syndrome of perihepatic inflammation that develops in 5% to 10% of women with acute pelvic inflammatory disease, originating from transperitoneal or vascular dissemination of either *Neisseria gonorrhoeae* or *Chlamydia trachomatis.*

"Iatrogenic" Pelvic Inflammatory Disease. An upper genital tract infection secondary to a penetration of the cervical mucus barrier caused by an operative procedure.

Nonoxynol-9. A chemical detergent used in spermicidal preparations that is also bactericidal and viricidal.

Penicillinase-Producing Gonorrhea. Strains of *N. gonorrhoeae* that become resistant to penicillin by acquiring a resistance factor plasmid that enables the gonococcus to produce an enzyme that destroys penicillin.

Hydrosalpinx. A collection of watery, sterile fluid in the fallopian tube, an end stage of a pyosalpinx.

Pelvic Inflammatory Disease. A nonspecific term, used in gynecology, that most commonly refers to inflammation caused by infection in the upper genital tract; often used synonymously with the term *acute salpingitis.*

Tuboovarian Complex. A collection of pus within an anatomic space created by adherence of adjacent organs, involving the oviducts, ovaries, and occasionally the intestines.

This chapter considers upper genital tract infections. The primary focus is on acute pelvic inflammatory disease, which is the ultimate devastation of sexually transmitted diseases. Although this discussion considers the epidemiology, diagnosis, and treatment of acute pelvic inflammatory disease, the hope of the future is the prevention of the sexually transmitted diseases. The direct and indirect monetary costs of pelvic inflammatory disease are estimated to be in the billions of dollars in the United States each year. The sequelae of ectopic pregnancies, chronic pain, and infertility cannot be measured. This chapter will also consider uncommon causes of upper genital tract infection such as tuberculosis and actinomycosis. For more detail of the infections with *Neisseria gonorrhoeae* and *Chlamydia trachomatis*, the reader is referred to Chapter 21.

ENDOMETRITIS

Nonpuerperal endometritis is an obscure chronic infection of the lining of the uterus. The obstetric counterpart of an acute endometritis that develops following a delivery or an abortion is well known. Since acute pelvic inflammatory disease is an ascending infection along the mucosa of the reproductive tract, endometritis must be an intermediate state of ascending infection from the endocervical canal. Regretfully, the temporal development of endometritis has not been studied extensively in women with either mucopurulent cervicitis or acute pelvic inflammatory disease. Many of the pertinent clinical questions such as the time it takes for an ascending infection to colonize various areas of the upper genital tract are unknown.

Chronic endometritis is often undiagnosed unless there is a high degree of suspicion by both the clinician and the pathologist. Paavonen et al. have found that 72% of women with laparoscopically proven acute pelvic inflammatory disease had associated histologic evidence of endometritis. Similar studies have found that 40% of women with mucopurulent cervicitis and 58% of women with positive endocervical cultures for either *C. trachomatis* or *N. gonorrhoeae* have concomitant endometritis.

The pathophysiology of endometritis is straightforward. A cervical infection leads to canalicular spread of organisms from the endocervix to the endometrium and subsequently to the endosalpinx. Microorganisms that have been commonly associated with chronic endometritis include *C. trachomatis*, *N. gonorrhoeae*, *Streptococcus agalactiae*, cytomegalovirus, and herpes simplex virus. Paavonen et al. have found a correlation between serum antibody levels of *Mycoplasma hominis* and *C. trachomatis* and the prevalence of endometritis.

Many women with chronic endometritis are asymptomatic. Conversely, when endometritis coexists with acute pelvic inflammatory disease it is difficult to differentiate whether inflammation of the oviducts or the endometrium is producing the pelvic symptoms. The classic symptom of chronic endometritis is intermenstrual vaginal bleeding. Some women experience postcoital bleeding or menorrhagia. Other women complain of a dull, constant lower abdominal pain. Chronic endometritis is a rare cause of infertility.

The diagnosis of chronic endometritis is established by endometrial biopsy and culture. It is possible to have a positive endometrial culture and at the same time a negative endocervical culture. The histologic findings of chronic endometritis are an inflammatory reaction of monocytes and plasma cells in the endometrial stroma (five plasma cells per high-power field). In severe cases, diffuse inflammatory infiltrates of lymphocytes and plasma cells are seen throughout the endometrial stroma. This may be associated with lymphoid follicles and stromal necrosis. No correlation has been found between the presence of polymorphonuclear leukocytes and chronic endometritis.

The treatment of chronic endometritis is oral tetracycline 2 g per day or Vibramycin 100 mg twice daily for 10 days. Many women have clinically persistent endometritis following treatment of acute pelvic inflammatory disease if they are not given either a tetracycline or erythromycin as part of their primary therapy.

PELVIC INFLAMMATORY DISEASE

Pelvic inflammatory disease is a gynecologic condition that lacks a precise definition. The term is used most commonly to refer to inflammation caused by an infection in the upper genital tract. Thus it may include infection of any or all of the following anatomic locations: the endometrium (endometritis), the oviducts (salpingitis), the ovary (oophoritis), the uterine wall (myometritis), the uterine serosa and broad ligaments (parametritis), and infection of the pelvic peritoneum. Many authors prefer the term *salpingitis*, because infection of the oviducts is the most characteristic and common component of pelvic inflammatory disease. Importantly, most long-term sequelae of pelvic inflammatory disease result from destruction of the tubal architecture by acute infection. In most clinical situations the terms acute *salpingitis* and *pelvic inflammatory disease* are used synonymously to describe an acute infection. *Chronic pelvic inflammatory disease* is a term that has largely been abandoned because the long-term sequelae of acute infection such as adhesions and hydrosalpinx are bacteriologically sterile. With the exception of infection with extremely rare organisms such as tuberculosis or actinomycosis, pelvic infections are not chronic.

The present and growing epidemic of sexually transmitted diseases and corresponding pelvic inflammatory disease is a major public health concern. Washington et al. estimate that

TABLE 22-2
Studies of Patients with Isolation of *N. gonorrhoeae,* Anaerobes, and Aerobes from Culdocentesis Aspirates of Women with Acute PID*

		Culdocentesis		
No. of Patients	Endocervical *N. gonorrhoeae*	*N. gonorrhoeae* only	*N. gonorrhoeae* plus Anaerobes and Aerobes	Anaerobes and Aerobes Only
104	56 (54)	12 (22)	18 (32)	26 (46)
30	24 (80)	5 (21)	5 (21)	14 (58)
54	21 (39)	6 (28)	1 (5)	5 (24)
17	16 (94)	5 (31)	5 (31)	6 (38)
26	13 (50)	4 (31)	4 (31)	4 (31)
20	13 (65)	—	1 (5)	18 (95)

From Sweet RL: Pelvic inflammatory disease. Sex Transm Dis 13:193, 1986.
*Results expressed as number (percentage) with indicated isolate.

TABLE 22-3
Comparison of *C. trachomatis* and *N. gonorrhoeae* Cervical Isolation and *N. gonorrhoeae* Tubal Isolation among Women with Acute PID

First Author of Study	No. of Patients	Cervical Infection		Tubal/ Peritoneal Infection*
		C. trachomatis	*N. gonorrhoeae*	*N. gonorrhoeae*
Henry-Suchet	17	(38%)	0/4	1/4 (25%)
Møller	166	(22%)	9 (5%)	
Mårdh	60	(38%)	4 (7%)	
Gjønnaess	65	(46%)	5 (8%)	0/65
Mårdh	63	(36%)	11 (17%)	1/14 (7%)
Adler	78	(5%)	14 (18%)	
Ripa	206	(33%)	39 (19%)	
Osser	209	(47%)	41 (20%)	
Paavonen	106	(25%)	27 (25%)	
Paavonen	101	(32%)	25 (25%)	
Paavonen	228	(30%)	60 (26%)	
Eilard	22	(27%)	7 (32%)	1/22 (5%)
Bowie	43	(51%)	15 (35%)	
Eschenbach	204	(20%)	90 (44%)	7/54 (13%)
Sweet	39	(5%)	18 (46%)	8/35 (23%)
Cunningham	104		56 (54%)	30/104 (29%)
Thompson	30	(10%)	24 (80%)	10/30 (33%)
TOTAL	1741	400/1365 (29%)	445/1728 (26%)	58/328 (18%)

From Eschenbach DA: Acute pelvic inflammatory disease, vol. 1. In Gynecology and obstetrics. Philadelphia, Harper & Row, Publishers, 1985, p. 8.
*Isolation of *N. gonorrhoeae* from the peritoneum of the total number of women studied.

at the time of acute pelvic inflammatory disease will have the same organism cultured from the fallopian tubes. If *N. gonorrhoeae* is the only organism cultured from the tubes, a patient will usually respond rapidly to treatment.

The virulence of the strain or colony type of *N. gonorrhoeae* helps to predict the incidence of upper genital tract infection. Transparent colonies of *N. gonorrhoeae* on culture medium attach more readily to epithelial cells and thus produce tubal infection more frequently than opaque-appearing colonies. Immunologic studies have demonstrated that an antibody against the outer membrane protein of the gonococcus develops in approximately 70% of women following severe pelvic infection. The lack of significant antibody titers may help explain why teenagers are more likely to develop upper genital tract disease than women in their late twenties.

There is an extremely wide variation in the recovery rates of *N. gonorrhoeae*, depending on the geographic location of the study (Table 22-3). The highest recovery rates occur in young, urban, black females in the United States.

The gonococcus produces an intense inflammatory reaction in the tubes, which causes the tubal lumen to swell with necrotic debris and purulent material. This cellular destruction is much more extensive than the reaction associated with a chlamydial infection.

Penicillinase-producing *N. gonorrhoeae* organisms were first identified 10 years ago. These strains of gonorrhea become resistant to penicillin by acquiring a resistance factor plasmid that enables the gonococcus to produce an enzyme that destroys penicillin. In 1983 another form of resistance to penicillin, chromosomally mediated, was first reported.

C. trachomatis is an intracellular, sexually transmitted bacterial pathogen. This organism

TABLE 22-4
C. trachomatis Infection Among Women with PID

First Author of Study	No. Patients	*C. trachomatis* Present in Cervix	Present in Tubes/Peritoneum	Antibody Titer IgM or Fourfold IgGΔ
Adler	78	4 (5%)		24/78 (31%)*
Sweet	39	2 (5%)	0/35	5/22 (23%)
Thompson	30	3 (10%)	3/30 (10%)	
Eschenbach	100	20 (20%)	1/54 (2%)	15/74 (20%)
Møller	166	37 (22%)		34 (20%)
Paavonen	106	27 (25%)		19/72 (26%)
Eilard	22	6 (27%)	2 (9%)	
Paavonen	228	69 (30%)		32/167 (19%)
Paavonen	101	32 (32%)		18 (18%)
Mårdh	63	19/53 (36%)	6/20 (30%)	
Ripa	156	52 (33%)		37/80 (46%)
Henry-Suchet	16	6 (38%)	4/17 (24%)	
Mårdh	60	23 (38%)		22/60 (37%)
Gjønnaess	65	26/56 (46%)	5/31 (16%)†	24/60 (40%)
Osser	111	52 (47%)		37/72 (51%)
Bowie	43	22 (51%)		
Skaug	34	19 (56%)		16 (47%)
TOTAL	1418	419/1399 (30%)	21/209 (10%)	281/986 (28%)

From Eschenbach DA: Acute pelvic inflammatory disease, vol. 1. In Gynecology and obstetrics. Philadelphia, Harper & Row, Publishers, 1985, p. 9.
Δ, Antibody change.
*Criteria of antibody response not given.
†Additional women had *C. trachomatis* organisms in the peritoneum but not in the cervix.

is the leading cause of acute pelvic inflammatory disease in Sweden. However, there is a widespread difference in isolation rates depending on the series and the geographic location (Table 22-4). One of the primary reasons that chlamydial organisms were not recovered in early studies in the United States was the reluctance to perform a biopsy of the fallopian tubes to obtain culture material. *Chlamydia* has recently become more prevalent than gonorrhea. From 20% to 40% of sexually active women have antibodies against *C. trachomatis*. From 10% to 30% of women with acute pelvic inflammatory disease who do not have cultures positive for *Chlamydia* have evidence of acute chlamydial infection by serial antibody titer testing.

C. trachomatis infection of either the lower or upper genital tract is seen most frequently in young women who are sexually active. Clinically, *Chlamydia* produces a mild form of salpingitis with an insidious onset. Whereas gonorrhea remains in the fallopian tubes for at most a few days in untreated patients, *Chlamydia* may remain in the fallopian tubes for months following initial colonization of the upper genital tract. In experimental studies the salpingitis produced by *Chlamydia* is confined to the tubal mucosa. Chlamydiae probably produce a disruption of the tubal mucosa by an immunopathologic mechanism rather than by a direct cytotoxicity, as is the case with *N. gonorrhoeae*.

The role of genital mycoplasmas in the etiology of acute pelvic inflammatory disease is unclear. Cervical cultures positive for both *Mycoplasma hominis* and *Ureaplasma urealyticum* may be obtained from the majority of young, sexually active women. The rate of isolation of genital mycoplasmas from the cervix is approximately 75% and similar in populations of women who are sexually active both with and without pelvic inflammatory disease.

Direct tubal cultures demonstrated *M. hominis* in 4% to 17% and *U. urealyticum* in 2% to 20% of women with acute pelvic inflammatory disease (Table 22-5). However, serologic studies in women with acute pelvic inflammatory disease have demonstrated that approximately one in four women develops a significant rise in antibody titers to these organisms. Experimental inoculation of the cervix of the Grivet monkey demonstrated that the route of spread of mycoplasmas is via the parametria rather

TABLE 22-5

Evidence of Genital *Mycoplasma* Infection among Women with Acute Salpingitis

Isolate/First Author of Study	Cervical Isolation (%)	Tubal Isolation (%)	Antibody Change (%)
M. hominis			
Sweet	73	4	
Eschenbach	72	4	20
Mårdh and Weström	62	8	
Thompson	60	17	
Møller	55		30
Mårdh			12
U. urealyticum			
Eschenbach	81	2	18
Mårdh and Weström	56	4	
Sweet	54	15	
Thompson	33	20	
Henry-Suchet	24	17	
Sweet		9	

From Eschenbach DA: Acute pelvic inflammatory disease, vol. 1. In Gynecology and obstetrics. Philadelphia, Harper & Row, Publishers, 1985, p. 11.

than the mucosa. Thus the primary upper genital tract infection is in the parametria and the tissue surrounding the tubes, not in the tubal lumen. This fact may help to explain the low success rate of direct tubal cultures. Histologically, *Mycoplasma* does not appear to produce damage to the tubal mucosa. In summary, in vitro and in vivo studies suggest that *Mycoplasma* may be a commensal bacterium rather than a pathogen in the oviducts.

The endogenous aerobic and anaerobic flora of the vagina frequently ascend to colonize and infect the upper reproductive tract. Direct cultures of purulent material from the tubal lumen or posterior cul-de-sac have demonstrated a wide range of organisms (Table 22-6). The most common aerobic organisms are nonhemolytic *Streptococcus, Escherichia coli*, group B *Streptococcus*, and coagulase-negative *Staphylococcus*. Anaerobic organisms tend to predominate over aerobes, and the most common anaerobic organisms are *Bacteroides* species, *Peptostreptococcus*, and *Peptococcus*. Anaerobic organisms are almost ubiquitous in pelvic abscesses associated with acute pelvic inflammatory disease. Presently there is a controversy as to which species of *Bacteroides* is the predomi-

nant agent in acute disease. Some investigators have discovered primarily *Bacteroides fragilis*, whereas others believe *Bacteroides bivius* is the most important anaerobe. With recent emphasis on the predominant anaerobic flora associated with bacterial vaginosis, there has been speculation that this condition predisposes women to acute pelvic inflammatory disease. This hypothesis is plausible and epidemiologically interesting but is difficult to prove.

Risk Factors

Risk factors are important considerations in both the clinical management and prevention of upper genital tract infections. The woman who is classically at highest risk is the menstruating teenager who has multiple sexual partners, does not use contraception, and lives in an area with a high prevalence of sexually transmitted disease. There is a strong correlation between the incidence of sexually transmitted disease and acute pelvic inflammatory disease in any given population. The age distribution of uncomplicated sexually transmitted disease is usually the same as that for acute pelvic inflammatory disease.

In epidemiologic studies, age at first intercourse, marital status, coital frequency, and number of sexual partners are all gross indicators of the frequency of exposure to sexually transmitted diseases. Having multiple sexual partners increases the chance of acquiring acute pelvic inflammatory disease approximately fivefold, and women who are not sexually active rarely acquire upper genital tract infection. The frequency of intercourse with a monogamous partner is not a risk factor. Women with a monogamous partner who has had a vasectomy appear to have a lower incidence of the disease.

The incidence of acute pelvic inflammatory disease decreases with advancing age (Fig. 22-1). Acute pelvic inflammatory disease is a condition of young females, with 75% of cases occurring in women less than 25 years of age. The risk that a sexually active adolescent female will develop acute pelvic inflammatory disease is 1 in 8. This risk factor decreases to 1 in 80 for women over the age of 25. Obviously the sexual habits of teenagers, including contact with multiple partners and lack of contra-

TABLE 22-6
Nongonococcal, Nonchlamydial Bacteria Recovered from the Upper Genital Tract of 74 Patients with Acute Salpingitis at San Francisco General Hospital

Species	No. of Isolates
Bacteroides species	48
Bacteroides bivius	35
Peptococcus asaccharolyticus	38
Peptococcus prevotii	16
Peptostreptococcus anaerobius	24
Veillonella parvula	19
Gardnerella vaginalis	30
Escherichia coli	18
Nonhemolytic streptococci	16
Group B streptococci	16
Coagulase-negative staphylococci	22

From Sweet RL: Pelvic inflammatory disease. Sex Transm Dis 13:194, 1986.

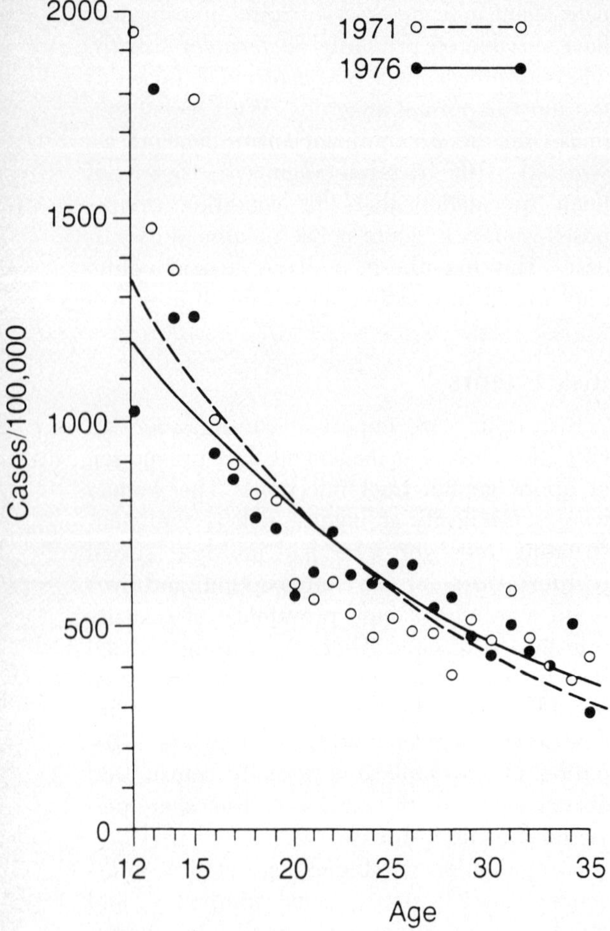

FIGURE 22-1

Estimated incidences of hospitalized pelvic inflammatory disease in sexually active females aged 12 to 35 years (United States, 1971 and 1976). (From Bell TA, Holmes KK: Sex Transm Dis 11:293, 1984.)

ception, predispose them to sexually transmitted diseases and, correspondingly, acute pelvic inflammatory disease. However, relative youth in itself increases the incidence of acute pelvic inflammatory disease. For unknown reasons young women with colonization of the cervix by *Chlamydia* have a higher incidence of upper genital tract infection than older women do. An unproven hypothesis to explain the increased infection rate in teenagers includes the comparative lack of antibody protection and the wider area of cervical columnar epithelium, which allows colonization by *C. trachomatis* and *N. gonorrhoeae*.

Stone et al. have tabulated (Table 22-7) both proven and hypothetical methods of preventing sexually transmitted disease and acute pelvic inflammatory disease. Both clinical and laboratory studies have documented that the use of contraceptives changes the relative risk of developing acute pelvic inflammatory disease. Weström has developed an arbitrary risk rating scale in which the risk of developing acute pelvic inflammatory disease in sexually active women not using contraception is assigned a score of 1. The corresponding risk among women wearing an IUD is 2 to 4, among women using oral contraceptives 0.3, and among women using a barrier method of contraception 0.4.

Barrier methods—condoms, diaphragms, and spermicidal preparations—are effective both as mechanical obstructive devices and as chemical barriers. Nonoxynol 9, the material ubiquitous in spermicidal preparations, is both bactericidal and viricidal. Laboratory tests have demonstrated that Nonoxynol 9 kills *N. gonorrhoeae*, genital *Mycoplasma* species, *Trichomonas vaginalis*, *Treponema pallidum*, herpes simplex virus, and human immunodeficiency virus (HIV). The porosity of latex in condoms is more than 1000 times smaller than viral particles. Thus routine condom use prevents deposition and transmission of infected organisms from the semen to the endocervix.

Oral contraceptive use has two preventive effects: a lower incidence of acute pelvic inflammatory disease and a milder form of upper genital tract infection when it does occur. The decrease in incidence of upper genital tract infection is believed to be secondary to thicker cervical mucus produced by the progestin component of oral contraceptives, which inhibits sperm and bacterial penetration. The decrease in duration of menstrual flow accompanying oral contraceptive use theoretically creates a shorter interval for bacterial colonization of the upper tract. Wolner-Hanssen et al. correlated laparoscopic findings of women with acute pelvic inflammatory disease and contraceptive use in a case-controlled study. Not only was there less pelvic inflammatory disease in the oral contraceptive group but also the spread of inflammation to the fallopian tubes seemed to be inhibited in oral contraceptive users (Table 22-8). Washington et al. have urged caution in the

TABLE 22-7
Methods of Preventing STDs, Mechanisms of Action, and Efficacy

Method	Mechanism	Efficacy in Prevention of STDs
Behavioral		
Monogamy Reducing number of partners Avoiding certain sexual practices Inspecting and questioning partners	Decreases likelihood of exposure to infected persons Decreases likelihood of contact with infectious agents	Not well studied; theoretical efficacy
Barriers		
Condom	Protects partner from direct contact with semen, urethral discharge, or penile lesion Protects wearer from direct contact with partner's mucosal secretions	Effective in vitro barrier to chlamydiae, CMV, HSV, and HIV Appears to decrease risk of acquiring urethral/cervical GC, PID, cervical cancer, and male urethral *Ureaplasma* colonization Effect on risk of acquiring NGU not established
Spermicide	Chemically inactivates infectious agents	Nonvaginal use has not been studied Inactivates gonococci, syphilis spirochetes, trichomonads, HSV, ureaplasmas, and HIV in vitro Appears to decrease risk of acquiring cervical GC, PID, and cervical cancer; chlamydiae studies in progress
Diaphragm/spermicide	Mechanical barrier covers cervix Used with spermicides	Diaphragm alone has not been studied Appears to decrease risk of acquiring cervical GC and PID
Vaccines	Induce antibody response that renders host immune to disease	Commercially available hepatitis B vaccine is safe and effective Results of clinical trials of gonococcal and herpes simplex vaccines not encouraging Gonococcal, HIV, and HSV vaccines research in progress
Oral Antibiotics Penicillin Sulfathiazole Tetracycline analogues	Kill infectious agent on or shortly after exposure before infection is established	No studies among women or civilian men Appears to decrease risk of acquiring GC and hard and soft chancre, but use not recommended
Local Postcoital urination Postcoital washing	Flushes infectious agents out of urethra and washes infectious agents off genital skin and mucous membranes	Poorly studied
Postcoital antiseptic douching	Inactivates and washes infectious agents out of vagina	Poorly studied

From Stone KM, Grimes DA, Magder LS: Primary prevention of sexually transmitted diseases. JAMA 255:1764, 1986. Copyright 1986, American Medical Association.
CMV, Cytomegalovirus; *HSV*, herpes simplex virus; *HIV*, human immunodeficiency virus; *GC*, gonorrhea; *PID*, pelvic inflammatory disease; *NGU*, nongonococcal urethritis.

TABLE 22-8

Comparison of Laparoscopic Findings with Type of Contraceptive Use in 738 Women with Signs and Symptoms Suggestive of Acute Salpingitis

Laparoscopic Findings	Contraceptive Method*		
	Oral Contraceptive (%)	Intrauterine Device (%)	Reference† (%)
Salpingitis	171 (59.8)	183 (80.6)	190 (84.4)
Nonsalpingitis	115 (40.2)	44 (19.4)	35 (15.6)

From Wolner-Hanssen P, Svensson L, Mårdh PA, et al: Laparoscopic findings and contraceptive use in women with signs and symptoms suggestive of acute salpingitis. Obstet Gynecol 66:234, 1985. Reprinted with permission from the American College of Obstetricians and Gynecologists.

*Relative risk of oral contraceptive use versus reference = 0.27 (X_1^2 = 36.9, $P < .0001$); relative risk of IUD use versus reference = 0.77 (95% confidence interval .47 to 1.26, X_1^2 = 1.1, $P = .28$); and relative risk of oral contraceptive versus IUD use = 0.36 (95% confidence interval .24 to .54, X_1^2 = 25.7, $P < .0001$).

†Reference = barrier methods or no contraception.

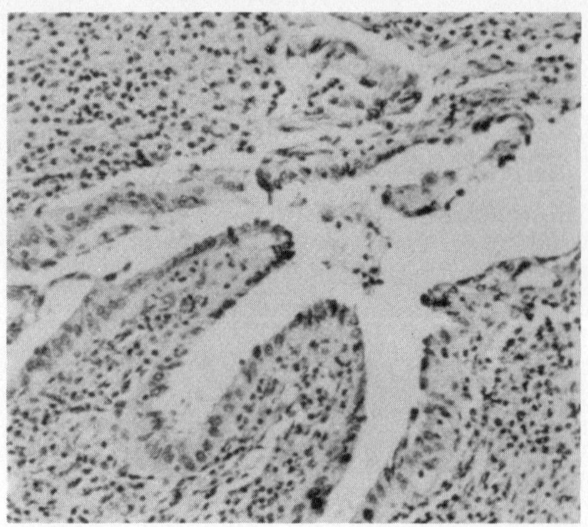

FIGURE 22-2
Tubal mucous membrane of proximal stump with lamina propria extensively infiltrated by numerous acute and chronic inflammatory cells in woman with a previous tubal ligation. (From Phillips AJ, D'Ablainge G: Obstet Gynecol 67: 56S, 1986. Reprinted with permission from The American College of Obstetricians and Gynecologists.)

conclusion that oral contraceptives protect against all forms of acute pelvic inflammatory disease. A twofold to threefold increase in the prevalence of endocervical infection by *C. trachomatis* has been demonstrated in multiple epidemiologic studies of women using oral contraceptives. Whether the colonization of the endocervix results in more upper genital tract disease is presently being studied.

Multiple case-controlled studies have shown an increased risk of acute pelvic inflammatory disease in women who wear an IUD. There has been just criticism of some of the early epidemiologic studies for their selection of control groups and the bias of including women with Dalkon Shields in their statistics. Nevertheless, the risk of acute pelvic inflammatory disease in women who wear an IUD is two to three times greater during the first three months after an IUD is inserted than in women who do not use contraceptives.

Acute salpingitis occurring in a woman with a previous tubal ligation is rare. Phillips and D'Ablaing reported the incidence of acute pelvic inflammatory disease developing in the proximal stump of previously ligated fallopian tubes as 1 in 450 women hospitalized for acute salpingitis (Fig. 22-2).

Epidemiologic studies have documented that previous acute pelvic inflammatory disease is a definite risk factor for future attacks of the disease. Approximately 25% of women with acute pelvic inflammatory disease subsequently develop acute tubal infection. Ten years ago this reinfection was believed to be "chronic infection" or exacerbations of a "latent" tubal process. Direct cultures have proven that the disease is another primary infection. This increased risk may be related to the sexual habits of the woman involved or to an untreated male partner. Studies have documented that greater than 80% of male contacts are not treated. Approximately 50% of men with sexually transmitted diseases are free of symptoms, and thus they do not seek treatment. Also, the microscopic tubal damage produced by the initial upper genital tract infection may facilitate repeat infection.

"Iatrogenic" acute pelvic inflammatory disease that follows transcervical penetration of the cervical mucus barrier with instrumentation of the uterus is a risk factor. Approxi-

TABLE 22-9
Laparoscopic Findings in Patients with False Positive Clinical Diagnosis of Acute PID but with Pelvic Disorders Other than PID

Laparoscopic Finding	No.
Acute appendicitis	24
Endometriosis	16
Corpus luteum bleeding	12
Ectopic pregnancy	11
Pelvic adhesions only	7
Benign ovarian tumor	7
Chronic salpingitis	6
Miscellaneous	15
TOTAL	98

From Jacobson LJ: Differential diagnosis of acute pelvic inflammatory disease. Am J Obstet Gynecol 138:1007, 1980.

TABLE 22-10
Laparoscopy/Laparotomy Diagnoses in Patients with False Negative Clinical Diagnosis of Acute PID by Laparoscopy

Clinical Diagnosis	Visual Diagnosis: Acute PID (No.)
Ovarian tumor	20
Acute appendicitis	18
Ectopic pregnancy	16
Chronic salpingitis	10
Acute peritonitis	6
Endometriosis	5
Uterine myoma	5
Uncharacteristic pelvic pain	5
Miscellaneous	6
TOTAL	91

From Jacobson LJ: Differential diagnosis of acute pelvic inflammatory disease. Am J Obstet Gynecol 138:1007, 1980.

mately 1 million first trimester abortions are performed each year in the United States. The incidence of upper genital tract infection associated with this procedure is approximately 1 in 200 cases. Thus 5000 cases of acute upper tract infection will result each year from pregnancy terminations. Recent practice has emphasized the use of prophylactic antibiotics in high-risk cases to attempt to decrease the incidence of iatrogenic acute pelvic inflammatory disease.

Symptoms and Signs

Patients with acute pelvic inflammatory disease present with a wide range of nonspecific clinical symptoms. This great variation in clinical presentation is exemplified by the extremes of asymptomatic women versus women with diffuse peritonitis and a life-threatening illness. Since the diagnosis is usually based on clinical criteria, there is both a high false positive rate and a high false negative rate. The differential diagnosis of acute pelvic inflammatory disease includes lower genital tract pelvic infection, ectopic pregnancy, torsion or rupture of an adnexal mass, acute appendicitis, and endometriosis.

Laparoscopic studies of women with a clinical diagnosis of acute pelvic inflammatory disease have established the inadequacy of diagnosis by the usual criteria of history and physical and laboratory examination. In these studies approximately 20% to 25% of women had no identifiable intraabdominal or pelvic disease. Another 10% to 15% of patients were found to have other pathologic conditions such as ectopic pregnancy, acute appendicitis, or torsion of the adnexa. In one of these studies Jacobson reported a series of 814 women in whom laparoscopy was done because of clinically suspected acute pelvic inflammatory disease. The clinical diagnosis was confirmed at laparoscopy in 532 women (65%). This study also documented the laparoscopic findings in 98 women with a false positive clinical diagnosis of acute pelvic inflammatory disease and 91 cases of false negative clinical diagnosis of acute pelvic inflammatory disease (Tables 22-9 and 22-10). Another interesting finding of laparoscopic studies is the lack of correlation between the number and intensity of symptoms and the severity of tubal inflammation. Women with *C. trachomatis* infections may exhibit minor symptoms but have a severe inflammatory process visualized by laparoscopic examination. Criteria for establishing the severity of acute pelvic inflammatory disease by laparoscopic examination are listed in Table 22-11.

Historically, the diagnosis of acute pelvic inflammatory disease was not established unless the patient had the triad of fever, elevated erythrocyte sedimentation rate, and adnexal tenderness or a mass. Only 17% of laparoscop-

TABLE 22-11
Severity of Disease by Laparoscopic
Examination

Severity	Findings
Mild	Erythema, edema, no spontaneous purulent exudate*; tubes freely movable
Moderate	Gross purulent material evident; erythema and edema more marked; tubes may not be freely movable, and fimbria stoma may not be patent
Severe	Pyosalpinx or inflammatory complex Abscess†

From Hager WD, Eschenbach DA, Spence MR, et al: Criteria for diagnosis and grading of salpingitis. Obstet Gynecol 61:114, 1983. Reprinted with permission from The American College of Obstetricians and Gynecologists.
*The tubes may require manipulation to produce purulent exudate.
†The size of any pelvic abscess should be measured.

TABLE 22-12
Salpingitis: Clinical Criteria for Diagnosis

Criteria	
Abdominal direct tenderness, with or without rebound tenderness	All 3 necessary for diagnosis
Tenderness with motion of cervix and uterus	
Adnexal tenderness	
	plus
Gram stain of endocervix—positive for gram-negative, intracellular diplococci	
Temperature (>38° C)	
Leukocytosis (>10,000)	1 or more necessary for diagnosis
Purulent material (white blood cells present) from peritoneal cavity by culdocentesis or laparoscopy	
Pelvic abscess or inflammatory complex on bimanual examination or on sonography	

From Hager WD, Eschenbach DA, Spence MR, et al: Criteria for diagnosis and grading of salpingitis. Obstet Gynecol 61:114, 1983. Reprinted with permission from The American College of Obstetricians and Gynecologists.

ically identified cases have this classic triad. Jacobson described the reverse logic that has been applied to the syndrome of acute pelvic inflammatory disease. He points out that the disorder had been made to fit the criteria established for it and not vice versa, as is usually the clinical practice. Thus reliance on stringent clinical criteria for establishing the diagnosis of the disease would result in the majority of cases being overlooked and not treated. Obviously, more frequent and liberal use of diagnostic laparoscopy is an important advance in the management of the disease. Laparoscopy allows precise diagnosis and also the opportunity to collect culture material from the site of the infection. However, in practice the majority of women with acute pelvic inflammatory disease do not undergo laparoscopy because of the expense of this invasive technique.

Hager and Eschenbach have established clinical criteria for acute pelvic inflammatory disease that they hope will standardize the diagnosis from one institution to another (Table 22-12). These uniform criteria have recently been adopted by the Obstetrical and Gynecologic Infectious Disease Society. If the criteria are too narrow, women with mild disease will be excluded. If the criteria are too broad, the

number of falsely diagnosed cases abruptly increases. Hadgu and Weström have recently published a multivariate logistic regression analysis of symptoms, signs, and laboratory findings of women laparoscopically diagnosed as having their first episode of acute pelvic inflammatory disease. This mathematic model correctly predicted 87% of cases and had an overall correct classification rate of 76%. The frequencies of various symptoms, signs, and laboratory data from this series of 414 women are depicted in Tables 22-13 and 22-14.

Pain in the lower abdomen and pelvis is by far the most frequent symptom of acute pelvic inflammatory disease. In all large series, more than 90% of women present with diffuse bilateral lower abdominal pain. This pain is usually described as constant and dull. On occasion the pain may become cramping, and it is accentuated by motion or sexual activity. Generally the pain is of short duration, usually less than 7 days. If the pain has been present for longer than 3 weeks, it is unlikely that the patient has acute pelvic inflammatory disease. Approxi-

TABLE 22-13

Frequency of Various Symptoms as Reported by Patients in Acute PID and Visually Normal Groups (first-time PID patients)

| | Laparoscopic Diagnosis | | | | |
| | Acute PID (No. = 414) | | Normal (No. = 138) | | |
Symptom	No.	%	No.	%	P Value
Lower abdominal pain	411	99.3	135	98.6	NS
Vaginal discharge	287	69.3	85	61.6	NS
Temperature ≥38° C	142	34.4	34	24.6	0.05
Irregular bleeding	165	40.0	54	39.1	NS
Urinary symptoms	82	19.8	29	21.8	NS
Vomiting	43	10.4	13	9.4	NS
Proctitis symptoms	30	7.3	4	2.9	NS
Other	33	8.0	8	5.8	NS

From Hadgu A, Weström L, Brooks CA, et al: Predicting acute pelvic inflammatory disease: A multivariate analysis. Am J Obstet Gynecol 155:956, 1986.

TABLE 22-14

Frequency of Various Objective Findings at Admission in Acute PID and Visually Normal Groups

| | Laparoscopic Diagnosis | | | | |
| | Acute PID (No. = 414) | | Normal (No. = 138) | | |
Clinical Findings at Admission	No.	%	No.	%	P Value
Bimanual examination					
Marked tenderness	395	95.4	128	92.8	NS
Palpable mass or swelling	198	47.8	36	26.1	0.001
Erythrocyte sedimentation rate >15 mm/h	336	81.2	78	56.5	0.001
Abnormal vaginal discharge	337	81.4	80	58.0	0.001
Fever (38° C)	146	35.3	21	15.2	0.001

From Hadgu A, Weström L, Brooks CA, et al: Predicting acute pelvic inflammatory disease: A multivariate analysis. Am J Obstet Gynecol 155:956, 1986.

mately 75% of patients with acute pelvic inflammatory disease have an associated endocervical infection and coexistent purulent vaginal discharge. Abnormal vaginal bleeding, especially spotting or menorrhagia, is noted in about 40% of patients. The latter symptom often leads to a suspected diagnosis of ectopic pregnancy. Nausea and vomiting are comparably late symptoms in the course of the disease.

When one compares the frequency of individual symptoms and signs between women with laparoscopically proven acute pelvic inflammatory disease and those without the disease, there is no significant difference with the exception of fever (Fig. 22-3). Acute pelvic inflammatory disease often occurs with minimum symptoms. Approximately 50% of women who are infertile as a result of tubal obstruction do not remember ever having symptoms of acute pelvic infection.

The symptoms of acute pelvic infection secondary to *N. gonorrhoeae* are of rapid onset,

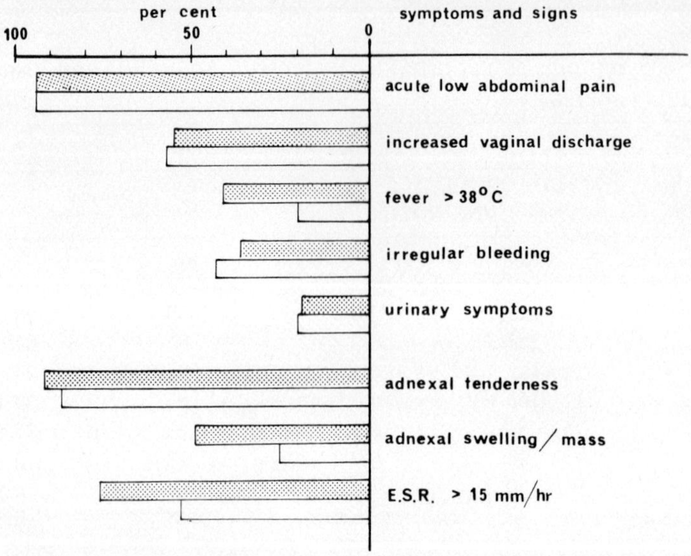

FIGURE 22-3

Comparison of frequency of symptoms, signs, and laboratory findings between patients with acute pelvic inflammatory disease (PID) *(dotted bars)* and suspected PID without pelvic pathology *(open bars)* by laparoscopic examination. (From Jacobson LJ: Am J Obstet Gynecol 138:1008, 1980.)

and the pelvic pain usually begins a few days after the onset of a menstrual period. Acute pelvic infection caused by *C. trachomatis* has an indolent course with slow onset, less pain, and less fever.

Five to ten percent of women with acute pelvic inflammatory disease develop symptoms of perihepatic inflammation—the Fitz-Hugh–Curtis syndrome. The condition is often mistakenly diagnosed as either pneumonia or acute cholecystitis. Persistent symptoms and signs include right upper quadrant pain, pleuritic pain, and tenderness in the right upper quadrant when the liver is palpated. Fitz-Hugh–Curtis syndrome develops from transperitoneal or vascular dissemination of either the gonococcus or *Chlamydia* organism to produce the perihepatic inflammation.

Women with laparoscopically confirmed acute pelvic inflammatory disease are often afebrile. Only one out of three women with acute pelvic inflammatory disease presents with a temperature greater than 38° C. Lower abdominal and pelvic tenderness during examination is the hallmark of acute pelvic inflammatory disease. Most women have tenderness to direct palpation in the lower abdomen and sometimes may have rebound tenderness. Bilateral tenderness of the parametria and adnexa is usually discovered during pelvic examination. This tenderness is especially noted with movement of the uterus or cervix during the pelvic examination. An ill-defined adnexal fullness is frequently noted. This may represent edema, inflammatory adhesions to either the small or large intestine, or an adnexal complex or abscess. The incidence of true adnexal abscess is approximately 10% in women with acute pelvic inflammatory disease.

Diagnosis

Direct visualization via the laparoscope is the most accurate method of diagnosis of acute pelvic inflammatory disease. Laparoscopy is also indispensable in the clinical research of the disease. Nevertheless the diagnosis of the majority of episodes of acute pelvic inflammatory disease is made on the basis of clinical history and physical examination. Laboratory tests may be obtained, but their results lack sufficient sensitivity and specificity to make them an important factor in establishing the diagnosis. For example, the criteria of the infectious disease society (see Table 22-12) assign a minor role to positive laboratory data. Since clinical symptoms and signs are nonspecific for the disease, when the diagnosis is based on clinical criteria there is a high percentage of both false positive and false negative rates. Because of the long-term sequelae of the disease, clinicians readily accept that they are treating many women who actually do not have pelvic infection in order not to omit treating women with early or mild disease.

Leukocytosis is not a reliable indicator of acute pelvic inflammatory disease, nor does it correlate with the need for hospitalization or the severity of tubal inflammation. Less than 50% of women with acute pelvic inflammatory disease have a white blood cell count of greater than 10,000 cells per milliliter. For years, erythrocyte sedimentation rate was a standard laboratory test for women with acute pelvic inflammatory disease. This laboratory test is nonspecific. The sedimentation rate is elevated, greater than 15 mm per hour, in approximately 75% of women with laparoscopically confirmed acute pelvic infection. However, 53% of women with pelvic pain and visually normal pelvic organs have an elevated erythrocyte sedimentation rate. Similarly, the sedimentation rate is a crude indicator of severity of disease and is no longer used to guide therapy.

Women with acute pelvic inflammatory disease should have a sensitive test for human chorionic gonadotrophin to help in the differential diagnosis of ectopic pregnancy. About 3 to 4 of every 100 women who are admitted to a hospital with a diagnosis of acute pelvic infection have an ectopic pregnancy. The diagnosis is often made by aspirating nonclotting bloody fluid by culdocentesis or by diagnostic laparoscopy.

Because most cases of upper genital tract infection are associated with and preceded by lower genital tract infection, it is important to examine the endocervical mucus for inflammatory cells, perform a Gram stain, and culture for both *N. gonorrhoeae* and *C. trachomatis*. A positive gram-stained smear of the endocervical mucus is nonspecific, and a negative smear does not rule out upper tract infection. However, Scandinavian studies have found that acute pelvic inflammatory disease is rare without a concomitant increase in inflammatory

cells in the vagina and the cervix. Because acute pelvic inflammatory disease is usually secondary to a sexually transmitted disease, it is ideal to examine, culture, and smear urethral secretions from the male partner. Often this step is not performed for a variety of nonmedical reasons.

European investigators have measured plasma protein levels, "acute phase reactants" including C-reactive protein, and antichymotrypsin to help in the diagnosis of acute pelvic inflammatory disease. These tests are only slightly more sensitive than the sedimentation rate. Other investigators have found that measuring specific genital isoamylases in peritoneal fluid is the best nonculture laboratory test for the disease. These isoamylases may be electrophoretically separated from pancreatic and salivary isoamylases. These enzymes are decreased or absent in peritoneal fluid in cases of acute pelvic inflammatory disease. The major disadvantage of this diagnostic technique is that the test requires several hours to complete.

Ultrasonography is of limited value for patients with mild or moderate pelvic inflammatory disease. Thus sonography should not be routinely ordered for women with acute disease. However, ultrasonography is helpful in distinguishing an adnexal abscess. Sonography is also a noninvasive diagnostic aid for patients who are so tender during pelvic examination that the physician cannot determine the presence or absence of a pelvic mass.

Culdocentesis sometimes helps in the diagnosis of acute pelvic inflammatory disease when purulent peritoneal fluid is aspirated. With acute pelvic inflammatory disease, the white blood count of peritoneal fluid is greater than 30,000 cells per milliliter. The white blood count of women without peritoneal inflammation is less than 1000 cells per milliliter. In some cases endometrial biopsy may be helpful in confirming the diagnosis of coexisting endometritis.

Laparoscopy, as already noted, is the gold standard in the diagnosis of acute pelvic inflammatory disease. Direct visualization of the pelvic organs is the most accurate method of diagnosis. The appearance of the pelvic organs may vary from red, indurated, edematous oviducts, to pockets of purulent material, to a large pyosalpinx or tuboovarian abscess. In recent years there has been increasing use of the laparoscope in women with acute pelvic pain. Laparoscopy is definitely indicated for patients who are not responding to therapy, both to confirm the diagnosis and to obtain cultures of purulent material.

Management

The two most important goals of the medical therapy of acute pelvic inflammatory disease are the resolution of symptoms and the preservation of tubal function. Antibiotic therapy should be started as soon as cultures have been obtained and the diagnosis is suspected; only early diagnosis and early treatment will help reduce the number of women who suffer from the long-term sequelae of the disease. In the management of acute pelvic inflammatory disease, one should not forget the treatment of the male partner and education for the prevention of the disease, including the use of proper contraceptives, which help to reduce the rate of upper genital tract infection.

The choice of antibiotic therapy for an infectious disease is usually based on culture and sensitivity of bacteria obtained directly from the site of the infection. This approach may be accomplished via laparoscopy. However, in most cases this is not financially feasible. Thus selection of antibiotic protocols is largely empirical. In addition to financial factors, laparoscopy is not without its risks. If every woman with acute salpingitis were to undergo laparoscopy, there would be 14 deaths directly associated with this diagnostic technique in the United States each year.

Empirical antibiotic protocols should cover a wide range of bacteria including *N. gonorrhoeae*, *C. trachomatis*, anaerobic rods and cocci, gram-negative aerobic rods, gram-positive aerobes, and *Mycoplasma* species (Table 22-15). Selection of one antibiotic protocol over another will often depend on the clinical history (see Table 22-16). For example, acute pelvic inflammatory disease following an operative procedure is usually caused by endogenous flora of the vagina.

Grimes analyzed more than 25 million prescriptions written between 1966 and 1983 in the United States for treatment of acute pelvic infections. He discovered that most women were treated as outpatients and received only a single antibiotic. Less than one third of women

TABLE 22-15

Microorganisms Isolated from the Fallopian Tubes of Patients with Pelvic Inflammatory Disease

Type of Agent	Organism
Sexually transmitted disease	*Chlamydia trachomatis*
	Neisseria gonorrhoeae
	Mycoplasma hominis
Endogenous agent	*Streptococcus* species
Aerobic or facultative	*Staphylococcus* species
	Haemophilus species
	Escherichia coli
Anaerobic	*Bacteroides* species
	Peptococcus species
	Peptostreptococcus species
	Clostridium species
	Actinomyces species

From Weström L: Introductory address: Treatment of pelvic inflammatory disease in view of etiology and risk factors. Sex Transm Dis 11:439, 1984.

TABLE 22-16

Probability of PID Being Associated or Not Associated with STD

	Risk of Indicated Type of PID	
Factor	Probably STD Associated	Probably Not STD Associated
Age < 25 years	+ + +	+
Age > 30 years	+	+ + +
Mild disease	+ + +	—
Severe disease	+	+ + +
Abscess formation	+	+ + +
Numerous sexual partners	+ + +	+
Symptoms in partners	+ + +	—
Use of IUD	+	+ + +
Earlier PID episode	+ +	+ + +
Good general condition	+ + +	+
Poor general condition	+	+ + +

From Weström L: Introductory address: Treatment of pelvic inflammatory disease in view of etiology and risk factors. Sex Transm Dis 11:439, 1984.
+ + +, most likely; + +, likely; +, less likely.

received tetracycline to treat possible chlamydial infection. It is hoped that these statistics will rapidly change as the polymicrobial etiology of acute pelvic inflammatory disease receives greater appreciation.

In the United States, for economic reasons, most women with acute pelvic inflammatory disease are not hospitalized. In Scandinavia, with a different health care system, the vast majority of women are treated as inpatients. Studies have documented a 10% to 20% treatment failure rate (persistence of symptoms and signs) for women receiving oral antibiotics as outpatients. Inpatient failure rates with intravenous antibiotics are approximately 5% to 10%.

Presently in the United States approximately three out of every four women with acute pelvic infection are being treated as outpatients for their disease. The Centers for Disease Control (CDC) has recommended one of five antibiotics for outpatient therapy (cefoxitin, amoxicillin, ampicillin, aqueous procaine penicillin G, and ceftriaxone) (see box below). Three of these antibiotics are administered parenterally, and two are given by mouth. The CDC recommends that all patients also receive doxycycline (100 mg by mouth twice per day for 10 to 14 days). Treatment by one drug alone without tetracycline does not cover the possibility that both *N. gonorrhoeae* and *C. trachomatis* are present. The failure rate of outpatient oral therapy may be related to noncompliance, reinfection, or inadequate antibiotic coverage for penicillinase-producing or chromosomally mediated resistant *N. gonorrhoeae* or facultative or anaerobic organisms involved in upper genital tract infection that are resistant to the drug prescribed. If penicillinase-producing *N. gonorrhoeae* or chromosomally mediated resistant organisms are recovered on culture, then the appropriate treatment is spectinomycin (2 g intramuscularly).

It is important to reexamine women within 48 to 72 hours of initiating outpatient therapy to evaluate the response of the disease to oral antibiotics. The patient should be hospitalized when the therapeutic response is not optimal. If the disease is responding well, approximately 2 weeks after therapy another specimen should be cultured to test for clinical cure.

Both rectal and pharyngeal gonorrheal infections are more difficult to cure than endocervical infections. Handsfield reports that pharyngeal gonorrhea is the most difficult to cure, with a cure rate of 50% to 70%. He advises using ceftriaxone in a single dose of 125 to 250 mg for infections of either gastrointestinal anatomic site.

Ideally, every woman with acute pelvic inflammatory disease would be hospitalized for the first few days of antibiotic treatment. Because this therapy is not practical financially, it is important to develop a list of criteria or indications for hospitalization (see box on p. 632). If possible, young nulliparous women should be hospitalized with their first episode of acute pelvic inflammatory disease. This would ensure maximum levels of antibiotics in the hope of preventing microscopic tubal damage. A strong indicator for hospitalization is an adnexal mass. Outpatient therapy does not provide high enough levels of appropriate antibiotics to successfully penetrate an abscess cavity. The association of a viable pregnancy and pelvic inflammatory disease, without a foreign body being inserted into the uterus, is a rare event. However, the second trimester uterus is a fertile ground for severe pelvic infection, since the in-

---

**CENTERS FOR DISEASE CONTROL–
RECOMMENDED REGIMENS FOR
OUTPATIENT THERAPY OF ACUTE PID**

Cefoxitin 2 g intramuscularly *or* amoxicillin 3 g by mouth *or* ampicillin 3.5 g by mouth *or* aqueous procaine penicillin G 4.8 million units intramuscularly at two sites *or* ceftriaxone 250 mg intramuscularly. Each of these regimens except ceftriaxone is accompanied by probenecid 1 g by mouth.

FOLLOWED BY

Doxycycline 100 mg by mouth twice daily for 10 to 14 days. Tetracycline hydrochloride 500 mg 4 times daily may be substituted for doxycycline but is less active against certain anaerobes and requires more frequent administration; these are potentially important drawbacks in the treatment of pelvic inflammatory disease.

From Centers for Disease Control: STD Treatment Guidelines 1985. MMWR 34(4S):20, 1985.

INDICATIONS FOR HOSPITALIZING PATIENTS WITH PELVIC INFLAMMATORY DISEASE

Nulliparity
Presence of tuboovarian complex or abscess
Pregnancy
Uncertain diagnosis
Gastrointestinal symptoms
Peritonitis in upper quadrants
Presence of an intrauterine device
History of operative or diagnostic procedures
Inadequate response to outpatient therapy

fection does not become localized. A patient may develop widespread signs and symptoms of sepsis before the subtle inflammatory changes in the pelvis are recognized.

Women for whom the definitive diagnosis of acute pelvic inflammatory disease is questionable are best admitted to the hospital. Any large series of 100 consecutive suspected cases of pelvic inflammatory disease will include three or four patients with ectopic pregnancy and three or four patients with acute appendicitis. Both the wide clinical spectrum of pelvic inflammatory disease and the difficulty of establishing a correct diagnosis without direct visualization of the pelvic organs are uncertainties that are best clarified in the hospital. The foundation of outpatient therapy of acute pelvic inflammatory disease is broad-spectrum oral antibiotics. If the patient presents with gastrointestinal symptoms, such as nausea and vomiting, there is a good chance that she will not be able to tolerate her medications. Acute peritonitis in the right upper quadrant, especially liver tenderness without hepatomegaly, is another indication for hospital admission.

Acute pelvic inflammatory disease associated with the presence of an IUD is usually more advanced at the time of diagnosis than infection without a foreign body. Both patient and physician delays in diagnosis are not unusual. Often women misinterpret the early signs and symptoms of an infection as being related to the IUD. Pelvic infections with an IUD in place and pelvic infections following operative or diagnostic procedures often are due to an-

aerobic bacteria. Thus it is best to hospitalize these patients and use intravenous antibiotics. The IUD should be removed and cultured as soon as appropriate levels of intravenous antibiotics have been obtained. Finally, if a therapeutic response or compliance with oral medications has not been optimal, the patient should be admitted for intravenous antibiotic therapy.

In October 1985 the CDC published their most recent guidelines for impatient treatment of acute pelvic inflammatory disease. Their recommendations have been widely accepted with only minor modifications. Their protocols stress two concepts: the polymicrobial etiology of acute pelvic infection and an increasing importance of *C. trachomatis.* Thus each protocol includes at least two antibiotics (see box on p. 633). With both intravenous protocols the CDC recommends a minimum of 4 days of therapy and continuation of the intravenous antibiotics at least 48 hours after the patient's fever abates. We follow these guidelines when the patient has a mass; however, for patients without a mass we switch to oral antibiotics when the symptoms have diminished and the patient has been afebrile for 24 hours.

Regimen A (see box) is a combination of intravenous doxycycline and intravenous cefoxitin. It is excellent for community-acquired infection because it treats both gonorrhea and chlamydial infection. Doxycycline and cefoxitin provide excellent coverage for *N. gonorrhoeae, C. trachomatis,* and also penicillinase-producing *N. gonorrhoeae.* Cefoxitin is an excellent antibiotic against *Peptococcus, Peptostreptococcus,* and *E. coli.* The disadvantage of this combination is that the two drugs are less than ideal for a pelvic abscess or for anaerobic infections.

Doxycycline should be included in the regimen of follow-up oral therapy. Sweet observed 17 women with pelvic inflammatory disease who initially had endometrial cultures positive for *Chlamydia.* Clinically, 16 out of 17 women responded to treatment with cephalosporins alone. However, posttreatment endometrial cultures remained positive for *Chlamydia* in 12 of 13 women. Therefore, without tetracycline or erythromycin a patient may appear free of symptoms but may still be harboring *Chlamydia.*

CENTERS FOR DISEASE CONTROL–RECOMMENDED REGIMENS FOR INPATIENT THERAPY FOR ACUTE PID

Regimen A

Doxycycline 100 mg intravenously twice daily *plus* cefoxitin 2 g intravenously 4 times daily. Continue intravenous drugs for at least 4 days and at least 48 hours after the patient's condition improves. Then continue doxycycline 100 mg by mouth twice per day to complete 10 to 14 days total therapy.

Regimen B

Clindamycin 600 mg intravenously 4 times daily *plus* gentamicin 2 mg/kg intravenously followed by 1.5 mg/kg 3 times daily in patients with normal renal function. Continue intravenous drugs for at least 4 days and at least 48 hours after the patient's condition improves. Then continue clindamycin 450 mg by mouth 4 times daily to complete 10 to 14 days total therapy.

From Centers for Disease Control: STD Treatment Guidelines 1985. MMWR 34(4S):1, 1985.

Regimen B is a combination of clindamycin and an aminoglycoside (gentamicin). Regimen B has the advantage of providing excellent coverage for anaerobic infections and facultative gram-negative rods. Therefore it is preferred for patients with an abscess, IUD-related infections, and pelvic infections following a diagnostic or operative procedure. Since the CDC recommendation was published there has been a practical change, and most centers are now giving clindamycin 900 mg every 8 hours. The serum levels are identical and it is more economical to give the drug every 8 hours. The disadvantage of this combination is a lack of optimum activity against *C. trachomatis* and *N. gonorrhoeae*. Studies have demonstrated that high intravenous levels of clindamycin, such as 900 mg every 8 hours, provide some activity against *Chlamydia*. To overcome this theoretical disadvantage we have discharged patients from the hospital on a treatment regimen of oral doxycycline as well as clindamycin. It is important with aminoglycoside therapy to obtain peak and trough serum levels. Peak levels should be approximately 8 µg/ml and trough

levels less than 2 µg/ml. Peak and trough levels should be obtained after 24 hours of intravenous therapy and approximately every 4 days thereafter. The incidence of aminoglycoside toxicity is 2% to 3%, and approximately 25% of women require an adjustment in their intravenous dosage.

In summary, neither regimen A nor regimen B is uniformly effective for all patients. To date there are not sufficient clinical data to suggest superiority of one regimen over another, either with respect to initial response or subsequent fertility. One must individualize using the clinical history, which will generally indicate the types of microorganisms causing the disease.

Operative treatment of acute pelvic inflammatory disease has decreased markedly in the past 10 years. Operations are restricted to life-threatening infections, ruptured tuboovarian abscesses, drainage of a pelvic abscess that is pointing into the cul-de-sac, persistent masses in some older women for whom future childbearing is not a consideration, and removal of a persistent symptomatic mass. Because of the techniques of in vitro fertilization, every effort is made to perform conservative surgery and preserve ovarian and uterine function in women who have not completed their families. Unilateral removal of a tuboovarian complex or an abscess is a frequent conservative operation for acute pelvic inflammatory disease. Similarly, drainage of a cul-de-sac abscess via culpotomy incision results in preservation of the reproductive organs. Recently there have been reports of small series of percutaneous aspiration or drainage of pelvic abscesses under ultrasonic guidance. This technique has been advocated in only a few centers and should be considered investigational.

Rigorously defined, an abscess is a collection of pus within a newly created space. In contrast, a tuboovarian complex is a collection of pus within an anatomic space created by adherence of adjacent organs. Clinically, they are treated in similar fashions. Landers and Sweet have published a large series of 232 women with tuboovarian abscesses or complexes initially treated conservatively with antibiotics (Tables 22-17 and 22-18).

Unilateral tuboovarian abscesses were discovered in 164 (71%) of the women. Seven women (3%) suffered acute rupture of their

TABLE 22-17
Epidemiologic Correlates of Tuboovarian Abscesses (TOAs) Diagnosed Clinically and Those of TOAs Confirmed Surgically

Patient Category (No. of Patients)	No. of Patients (%) with Indicated Epidemiologic Correlate			
	Nulliparous	Prior History of Gonorrhea	Prior History of Salpingitis	IUD Usage
TOA clinically diagnosed only (160)	90 (56)	48 (30)	52 (32.5)	53 (33)
TOA surgically confirmed (72)	30 (42)	23 (32)	24 (33)	23 (32)
TOA not excised (20)	9 (45)	6 (30)	6 (30)	4 (20)
TOA excised (52)	21 (40)	17 (33)	18 (35)	19 (36)
Total (232)	120 (52)	71 (31)	76 (33)	76 (33)

From Landers DV, Sweet RL: Tubo-ovarian abscess: Contemporary approach to management. Rev Infect Dis 5:878, 1983.

tuboovarian abscesses. There was no statistical difference between the incidence of unilateral tuboovarian abscess in women with IUDs and those without IUDs. Landers and Sweet described a 20% rate of early treatment failure after 48 to 72 hours of antibiotic therapy as a result of persistent pain or enlargement of the tuboovarian abscess or complex. In addition, 31% required an operation several weeks to

months following their acute infections. A fact that was brought to light from this study was that even though women had prior tuboovarian abscesses, 14% subsequently experienced an intrauterine pregnancy.

Abscesses caused by acute pelvic inflammatory disease contain a mixture of anaerobes and facultative or aerobic organisms (Fig. 22-4). The environment of an abscess cavity results in a low level of oxygen tension. Therefore anaerobic organisms predominate and have been cultured from 60% to 100% of reported cases. Landers and Sweet noted that in 68% of their cases the abscess decreased in size if the anti-

TABLE 22-18
Presenting Symptoms and Findings among 232 Patients with Tuboovarian Abscess

Symptom/Finding	No. of Patients in Indicated Group (%) with Presenting Symptom or Finding	
	Medically Treated (No. = 175)	Surgically Treated (No. = 57)
Acute pain	158 (90)	48 (84)
Chronic pain	29 (17)	14 (25)
Fever/chills	86 (49)	31 (53)
Vaginal discharge	53 (30)	11 (19)
Abnormal uterine bleeding	37 (21)	11 (19)
Nausea	44 (25)	17 (30)
Vomiting	23 (13)	13 (23)
Temperature >100° F	102 (58)	37 (65)
White blood cell count >10,000/mm^3	114 (72)	44 (77)

From Landers DV, Sweet RL: Tubo-ovarian abscess: Contemporary approach to management. Rev Infect Dis 5:879, 1983.

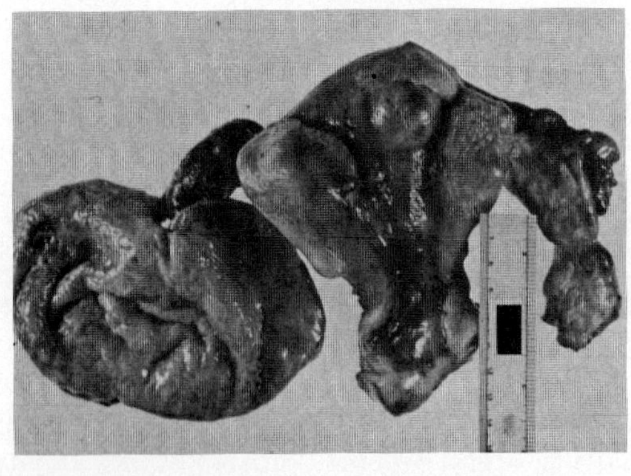

FIGURE 22-4
Pyosalpinx. Right tube is markedly enlarged and contains 50 ml of creamy pus. Tubal wall is thickened. (From Janovski NA, ed: Color atlas of gross gynecologic and obstetric pathology. New York, McGraw-Hill Book Co., 1969, p. 131.)

biotic protocol contained clindamycin versus a decrease in mass size in only 37% of cases when clindamycin was not included in the antibiotic therapy. Basic investigations have discovered that clindamycin penetrates the human neutrophil, and it is possible that this property facilitates the level of clindamycin within the abscess. Clindamycin is also stable in the abscess environment, which is not true of many other antibiotics. Thus a combination of clindamycin and an aminoglycoside is considered the gold standard for treatment of tuboovarian abscess. This combination does not treat the enterococcus, and ampicillin should be added if there is suspicion that this organism is involved. Metronidazole is an effective alternative to clindamycin for anaerobic infections.

Sequelae

Before antibiotic therapy the mortality associated with acute pelvic inflammatory disease was 1%. Grimes has estimated that there is presently one death every other day in the United States directly related to pelvic inflammatory disease. Most of these deaths result from rupture of tuboovarian abscesses. The mortality today is 5% to 10% for ruptured tuboovarian abscesses even with modern medical and operative therapy. Each year approximately 40 women die of ectopic pregnancy in the United States, and at least 50% of these ectopic implantations are secondary to the tubal damage produced by acute salpingitis.

Recurrent acute pelvic inflammatory disease is experienced by approximately 25% of women. Younger women become reinfected twice as often as older women. A great challenge to health care providers is to educate women with pelvic inflammatory disease to reduce their chances of a second episode of infection. Preventive medicine should include treatment and education of the male partner, selection of contraceptives that will reduce the chance of upper genital tract infections, and liberal prescriptions for treatment of lower genital tract disease for these women.

The number of ectopic pregnancies has doubled over the past 10 years. This increased rate is directly parallel and proportional to the increase in sexually transmitted diseases and

TABLE 22-19

Ratios of Ectopic to Intrauterine Pregnancies (EP/IU ratio) in women 15 to 39 Years of Age (Lund, 1960-1977)

Years	No. of Intrauterine Pregnancies	No. of Ectopic Pregnancies	EP/IU Ratio
1960-1964	6143	35	1:177
1965-1969	7730	51	1:133
1970-1974	9977	70	1:144
1975-1977	6293	71	1:90

From Weström L: Incidence, prevalence, and trends of acute pelvic inflammatory disease and its consequences in industrialized countries. Am J Obstet Gynecol 138:888, 1980.

acute pelvic inflammatory diseases (Table 22-19). Pathologic studies estimate that approximately 50% of ectopic pregnancies occur in oviducts damaged by previous salpingitis (Fig. 22-5). The microscopic tubal damage either retards transport of or entraps fertilized ovum, thereby producing implantation in the tube rather than the endometrial cavity. Weström, in a prospective long-term follow-up of women with acute salpingitis in Sweden, discovered a rate of 1 ectopic pregnancy to every 24 intrauterine pregnancies for women treated for acute pelvic infection in the 1960s. In a later study the rate increased to 1 ectopic pregnancy to 16 intrauterine pregnancies for women treated in the 1970s. The ratio of ectopic pregnancies to intrauterine pregnancies was 1 to 147 in a controlled group of women who had not experienced tubal infection.

The chance that a women will develop chronic pelvic pain following acute salpingitis is four times greater than the risk for control subjects. Approximately 20% of women with acute pelvic infections subsequently develop chronic pelvic pain, versus approximately 5% in a control group without pelvic infection. Among women with chronic pelvic pain, approximately two out of three are involuntarily infertile, and a similar percentage have deep dyspareunia. Chronic pelvic pain may be caused by a hydrosalpinx, a collection of sterile, watery fluid in the fallopian tube. A hydrosalpinx is the end-stage development of a pyosalpinx. Chronic pain often develops in a woman even

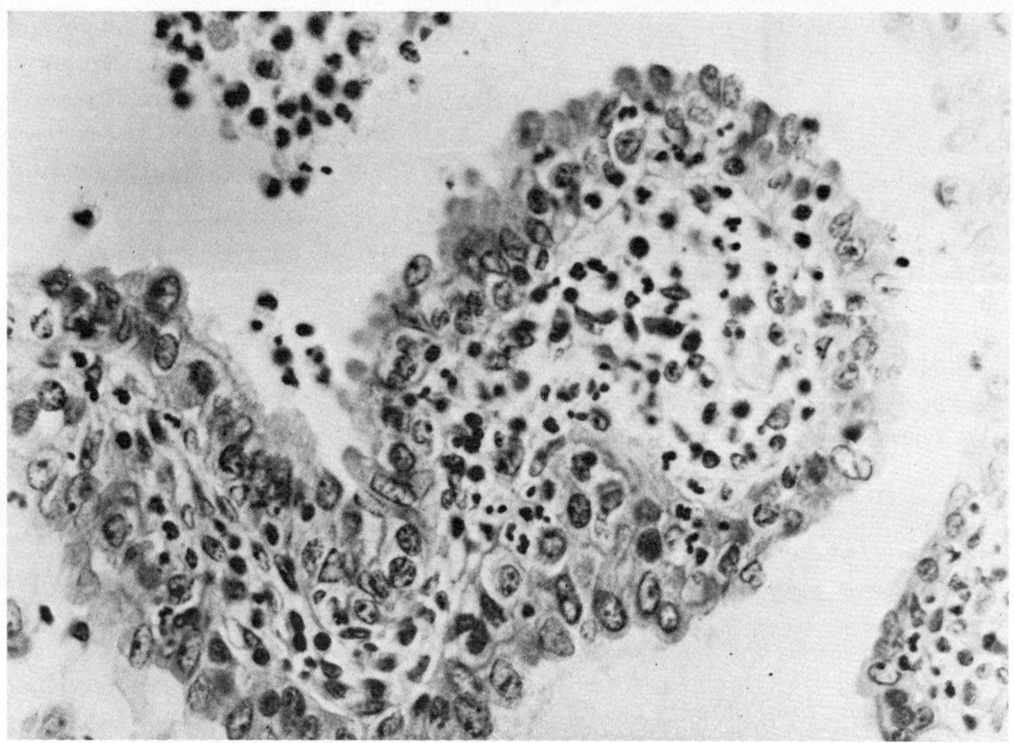

FIGURE 22-5
Microscopic appearance of salpingitis. (From Gompel C, Silverberg SG, eds: Pathology in gynecology and obstetrics, 2nd ed. Philadelphia, J.B. Lippincott Co., 1977, p. 253.)

though she may have had a normal pelvic examination when examined 4 to 8 weeks following her acute infection. The pain may be related to adhesions surrounding the ovary. The hypothesis has been advanced that the chronic dull pain is secondary to menstrual cycle–related changes in the volume of the ovary, which produce tension in the surrounding adhesions. Some women with chronic pelvic pain benefit from long-term progestin or danazol therapy. All women with chronic pelvic pain believed to be caused by acute pelvic inflammatory disease should undergo laparoscopy to establish the diagnosis and rule out other diseases such as endometriosis. Recently emphasis has focused on conservative surgery for this sequela via either laparoscopy or celiotomy.

Acute pelvic infection is one of the major causes of female infertility. Epidemiologic studies estimate that between 4% and 13% of women either are infertile or have an operative procedure secondary to acute pelvic inflammatory disease. In one survey of women not using contraception, 15% of the women considered themselves sterile as a result of salpingitis. Before antibiotic therapy, 50% to 75% of women who had experienced upper genital tract infections were sterile.

The sequelae of infections vary from a patent oviduct, to peritubular and periovarian adhesions that may hinder ovum pickup, to complete tubal obstruction. Tubal obstructions that are secondary to infection are commonly found at the fimbrial end or the cornual region of the oviduct.

Weström has presented long-term follow-up statistics for women with pelvic inflammatory disease in Sweden (Table 22-20). He discovered that the infertility rate was significantly lower in the younger group than in the older age group following a single episode of infection (Table 22-21). Women with mild episodes of acute pelvic inflammatory disease were

TABLE 22-20
Reproductive Events After One or More Tubal Infections in 1000 Women 15 to 34 Years of Age (Lund, 1960-1974) Followed to First Pregnancy or, if Not Pregnant, for 8 Years

	No./1000 Women
Pregnant	
Intrauterine	624
Ectopic	41
Not pregnant	
Voluntarily	171
Involuntarily	
Tubal occlusion	126
Other causes	38

From Weström L: Incidence, prevalence, and trends of acute pelvic inflammatory disease and its consequences in industrialized countries. Am J Obstet Gynecol 138:888, 1980.

TABLE 22-21
Percent Infertility Because of Tubal Occlusion After Mild, Moderately Severe, and Severe Infections in Women with One Episode of Salpingitis and Exposure to Chance of Pregnancy

Inflammatory Changes	% Infertility Postsalpingitis in Age Group		
	15-24 Years	25-34 Years	Total
Mild	5.8	7.8	6.1
Moderately severe	10.8	22.0	13.4
Severe	27.3	40.0	30.0

From Weström L: Incidence, prevalence, and trends of acute pelvic inflammatory disease and its consequences in industrialized countries. Am J Obstet Gynecol 138:888, 1980.

seven times less likely to suffer tubal obstruction than women with severe disease. The infertility rate increased directly with the number of episodes of acute pelvic infection. The latter is not surprising, because the prevalence of most long-term sequelae is directly proportional to the number of episodes of acute pelvic inflammatory disease.

ACTINOMYCES INFECTION

Actinomyces is a rare cause of upper genital tract infection. *Actinomyces israelii* is the most common species found and is a gram-positive anaerobe, which is difficult to culture. To successfully culture this organism, an anaerobic environment must be maintained for 2 to 3 weeks.

A. israelii is discovered either by histologic examination or culture from women with tuboovarian abscesses. There are many large series of tuboovarian abscesses without a single case of *A. israelii* described. Most cases described have been in women wearing an IUD. Usually *A. israelii* is part of a polymicrobial infection, and whether its role is primary or secondary in the infectious process is unknown.

Recently there has been a controversy as to the significance of discovering actinomycetes on a Papanicolaou smear of women wearing an IUD. Burkman et al. reported that women with a positive smear had a 3.5-fold risk of hospitalization for acute pelvic inflammatory disease. Also, these investigators found that when women developed acute infections, there was a higher tendency to develop tuboovarian abscesses. Other investigations have disagreed with this hypothesis. Conflicting studies have found that approximately 3% of women with or without an IUD have actinomycetes on a Papanicolaou smear.

Although some investigators suggest that actinomycetes produce a chronic endometritis with an associated foul-smelling discharge, the diagnosis of *Actinomyces* infection is usually not made until a tuboovarian abscess is examined by the pathologist. Then the classic "sulfur granules" are observed histologically.

Although much has been written about chronic draining sinuses with *Actinomyces* infection, this complication is unusual in gynecology. However, when this organism is present, the patient should receive oral penicillin for 12 weeks following an operative procedure.

TUBERCULOSIS

Tuberculosis of the upper genital tract, primarily chronic salpingitis and chronic endometritis, is a rare disease in the United States.

Most gynecologists will practice a lifetime and not encounter a single case. However, it is a frequent cause of chronic pelvic inflammatory disease and infertility in other parts of the world. Thus it should be suspected in immigrants, especially those from Asia, the Middle East, and Latin America.

Pelvic tuberculosis may be produced by either *Mycobacterium tuberculosis* or *Mycobacterium bovis*. The primary site of infection for tuberculosis is usually the lung. Within 1 to 2 years of the pulmonary infection the bacteria spread hematogenously and the infection becomes located in the oviduct. Subsequently the bacilli usually spread to the endometrium and occasionally to the ovaries. However, the oviducts are the primary and predominant site of pelvic tuberculosis. In Third World countries without pasteurization of milk, bovine tuberculosis produces primary infections in the human gastrointestinal tract. Subsequent lymphatic or hematogenous dissemination results in pelvic tuberculosis.

The predominant presentations of this chronic infection are infertility and abnormal uterine bleeding. Mild to moderate chronic abdominal and pelvic pain occur in 35% of women with the disease. Advanced cases are often accompanied by ascites. Some women may be asymptomatic. The findings at pelvic examination are normal in approximately 50% of cases. The remaining patients have mild adnexal tenderness and bilateral adnexal masses, with an inability to manipulate the adnexa because of scarring and fixation.

Tuberculous salpingitis should be suspected when a patient is not responding to conventional antibiotic therapy for acute bacterial pelvic inflammatory disease. Results of a tuberculin skin test will be positive. However, approximately one in three women do not have evidence of pulmonary tuberculosis on chest x-

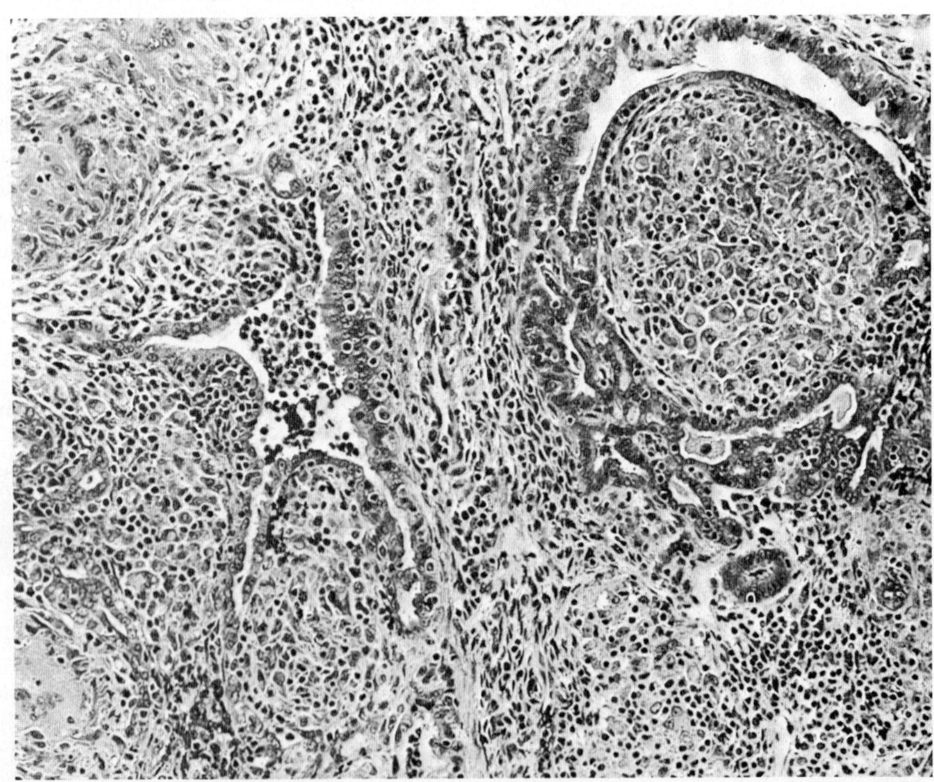

FIGURE 22-6
Tuberculous salpingitis: Langhans' giant cell granuloma. (From Gompel C, Silverberg SG, eds: Pathology in gynecology and obstetrics, 2nd ed. Philadelphia, J.B. Lippincott Co., 1977, p. 258.)

ray films. The diagnosis may be established by performing an endometrial biopsy late in the secretory phase of the cycle. A portion of the endometrial biopsy should be sent for culture and animal inoculation, while the remaining portion should be examined histologically. The findings of classic giant cells, granulomas, and caseous necrosis confirm the diagnosis (Fig. 22-6). Approximately two out of three women with tuberculous salpingitis will have concomitant tuberculous endometritis. Pelvic tuberculosis may not be diagnosed until laparotomy or celiotomy when the characteristic changes may be visualized. The distal ends of the oviduct remain everted, producing a "tobacco pouch" appearance. When the diagnosis has been established, the patient should have a chest x-ray examination, intravenous pyleogram, serial gastric washings, and urine cultures for tuberculosis. Approximately 10% of women with pelvic tuberculosis have concomitant urinary tract tuberculosis.

Treatment of pelvic tuberculosis is medical, with a combination of two antibiotics for 24 months. Occasionally a woman becomes pregnant following medical therapy. Combination therapy is used to decrease the rate of drug-resistant organisms. Present antibiotic therapy includes isoniazid (INH) (300 mg per day) and ethambutol (Myambutol) (1200 mg per day). Operative therapy is reserved for women with persistent pelvic masses, women with resistant organisms, women over 40 years of age, and women whose endometrial cultures remain positive.

KEY POINTS

- The diagnosis of chronic endometritis is established by the finding of plasma cells on endometrial biopsy.

- Acute pelvic inflammatory disease is usually caused by a polymicrobial infection of organisms ascending from the vagina and cervix, traveling along the mucosa of the endometrium to infect the mucosa of the oviduct. The primary bacterial organisms cultured from tubal fluid and mucosa include *Neisseria gonorrhoeae, Chlamydia trachomatis,* endogenous aerobic and anaerobic bacteria, and genital *Mycoplasma* species.

- Approximately one in four women with acute pelvic inflammatory disease experience further medical sequelae.

- Approximately 15% of women with cervical infection by gonorrhea subsequently develop pelvic inflammatory disease. The virulence of the strain of *N. gonorrhoeae* helps to predict the incidence of upper genital tract infection.

- *C. trachomatis* is rapidly becoming the most prevalent organism causing pelvic inflammatory disease. The salpingitis it produces is insidious in onset.

———————— KEY POINTS, cont'd ————————

- There is a strong correlation between the incidence of sexually transmitted disease within a population and the incidence of acute pelvic inflammatory disease.

- Acute pelvic inflammatory disease is a condition of young menstruating women, with 75% of cases occurring in women less than 25 years of age. The risk for a sexually active adolescent female is 1 in 8. This decreases to 1 in 80 for women over the age of 25.

- Oral contraceptive use provides a twofold preventive effect in inhibiting the development of pelvic inflammatory disease. One mechanism may be the thickening of cervical mucus caused by the progestin component of the oral contraceptives. The other may be the decrease in the duration of menstrual flow, which creates a shorter interval for bacterial colonization of the upper genital tract.

- Because acute pelvic inflammatory disease has a wide range of nonspecific clinical symptoms, there is both a high false positive rate and a high false negative rate when the diagnosis is based on clinical findings and laboratory results.

- Approximately 20% to 25% of women have no identifiable intraabdominal or pelvic disease by laparoscopy when diagnosed as having acute pelvic inflammatory disease on the basis of history or physical or laboratory examination.

- Pain in the lower abdomen and pelvis is the most frequent symptom of acute pelvic inflammatory disease, and in all large series more than 90% of women with the diagnosis have some type of abdominal pain.

- Seventy-five percent of patients with acute pelvic inflammatory disease have an associated endocervical infection and coexistent purulent vaginal discharge.

- Nausea and vomiting are comparatively late symptoms in the course of acute pelvic inflammatory disease.

- From 5% to 10% of women with acute pelvic inflammatory disease develop perihepatic inflammation, Fitz-Hugh–Curtis syndrome.

- Approximately one third of women with acute pelvic inflammatory disease present with a temperature of greater than 38° C.

- The incidence of true adnexal abscess is approximately 10% in women with acute pelvic inflammatory disease.

- Less than 50% of women with acute pelvic inflammatory disease have a white blood cell count of greater than 10,000 cells per milliliter.

- Laparoscopy is the optimum method to accurately establish the diagnosis of acute pelvic inflammatory disease.

- Women who are being treated as outpatients for acute pelvic inflammatory disease should be reexamined within 48 to 72 hours of initiation of therapy to evaluate the response of the disease to oral antibiotics.

- Surgical treatment for acute pelvic inflammatory disease is restricted to life-threatening infections, ruptured tuboovarian abscesses, drainage of a pelvic abscess that is pointing into the cul-de-sac, persistent masses in some older women for whom future childbearing is not a consideration, and removal of a persistent symptomatic mass. Unilateral removal of a tuboovarian complex or abscess is a frequent conservative operation for acute pelvic inflammatory disease for women desiring future childbearing.

- Recurrent acute pelvic inflammatory disease is experienced by approximately 25% of women. The chance that a woman will develop chronic pelvic pain following acute pelvic inflammatory disease is four times greater than the risk for control subjects.

- Pelvic tuberculosis may be produced by either *Mycobacterium tuberculosis* or *Mycobacterium bovis*. The primary site of infection is usually the lung.

- The predominant presentations of tuberculous salpingitis are infertility and abnormal uterine bleeding.

BIBLIOGRAPHY

Bell TA, Holmes KK: Age-specific risks of syphilis, gonorrhea, and hospitalized pelvic inflammatory disease in sexually experienced U.S. women. Sex Transm Dis 11:291, 1984.

Burkman R, Schlesselman S, McCaffrey L, et al: The relationship of genital tract actinomycetes and the development of pelvic inflammatory disease. Am J Obstet Gynecol 143:585, 1982.

Burnakis TG, Hildebrandt NB: Pelvic inflammatory disease: A review with emphasis on antimicrobial therapy. Rev Infect Dis 8:86, 1986.

Centers for Disease Control: STD Treatment Guidelines 1985. MMWR 34(4S):1, 1985.

Conway D, Caul EO, Hull MGR, et al: Chlamydial serology in fertile and infertile women. Lancet 1:191, 1984.

Darling MRN, Golan A, Rubin A: Colpotomy drainage of pelvic abscesses. Acta Obstet Gynecol Scand 62:257, 1983.

Dodson MG, Faro S: The polymicrobial etiology of acute pelvic inflammatory disease and treatment regimens. Rev Infect Dis 7:S696, 1985.

Eschenbach DA: Epidemiology and diagnosis of acute pelvic inflammatory disease. Obstet Gynecol 55:142S, 1980.

Eschenbach DA: New concepts of obstetric and gynecologic infection. Arch Intern Med 142:2039, 1982.

Eschenbach DA: Acute pelvic inflammatory disease, vol. 1. In Gynecology and obstetrics. Philadelphia, Harper & Row, Publishers, 1985.

Gompel C, Silverberg SG, eds: Pathology in gynecology and obstetrics, 2nd ed. Philadelphia, J.B. Lippincott Co., 1977.

Grimes DA: Deaths due to sexually transmitted diseases. JAMA 255:1727, 1986.

Grimes DA, Blount JH, Patrick J, et al: Antibiotic treatment of pelvic inflammatory disease. JAMA 256:3233, 1986.

Hadgu A, Weström L, Brooks CA, et al: Predicting acute pelvic inflammatory disease: A multivariate analysis. Am J Obstet Gynecol 155:954, 1986.

Hager WD: Follow-up of patients with tubo-ovarian abscess(es) in association with salpingitis. Obstet Gynecol 61:680, 1983.

Hager WD, Eschenbach DA, Spence MR, et al: Criteria for diagnosis and grading of salpingitis. Obstet Gynecol 61:113, 1983.

Handsfield HH: Problems in the treatment of bacterial sexually transmitted diseases. Sex Transm Dis 13:179, 1986.

Jacobson L: Differential diagnosis of acute pelvic inflammatory disease. Am J Obstet Gynecol 138:1006, 1980.

Janovski NA, ed: Color atlas of gross gynecologic and obstetric pathology. New York, McGraw-Hill Book Co., 1969.

Landers DV, Sweet RL: Tubo-ovarian abscess: Contemporary approach to management. Rev Infect Dis 5:876, 1983.

Paavonen J, Aine R, Teisala K, et al: Chlamydial endometritis. J Clin Pathol 38:726, 1985.

Paavonen J, Kiviat N, Brunham RC, et al: Prevalence and manifestations of endometritis among women with cervicitis. Am J Obstet Gynecol 152:280, 1985.

Paavonen J, Miettinen A, Stevens CE, et al: Mycoplasma hominis in cervicitis and endometritis. Sex Transm Dis 10:276, 1983.

Phillips AJ, D'Ablaing G: Acute salpingitis subsequent to tubal ligation. Obstet Gynecol 67:55S, 1986.

Pine L, Curtis EM, Brown JM: Actinomyces and the intrauterine contraceptive device: Aspects of the fluorescent antibody stain. Am J Obstet Gynecol 152:287, 1985.

Rice RJ, Biddle JW, JeanLouis YA, et al: Chromosomally mediated resistance in Neisseria gonorrhoeae in the United States: Results of surveillance and reporting, 1983-1984. J Infect Dis 153:340, 1986.

Ristuccia AM, Cunha BA, eds: Antimicrobial therapy. New York, Raven Press, 1984.

Schaefer G: Female genital tuberculosis. Clin Obstet Gynecol 19:223, 1976.

Siegenthaler WE, Bonetti A, Luthy R: Aminogylcoside antibiotics in infectious diseases. Am J Med 80(suppl. 6B):2, 1986.

Stone KM, Grimes DA, Magder LS: Primary prevention of sexually transmitted diseases. JAMA 255:1763, 1986.

Sweet RL: Pelvic inflammatory disease. Sex Transm Dis 13:192, 1986.

Sweet RL, Blankfort-Doyle M, Robbie MO, et al: The occurrence of chlamydial and gonococcal salpingitis during the menstrual cycle. JAMA 255:2062, 1986.

Sweet RL, Schachter J, Robbie MO: Failure of β-lactam antibiotics to eradicate Chlamydia trachomatis in the endometrium despite apparent clinical cure of acute salpingitis. JAMA 250:2641, 1983.

Sweet RL, Yonekura ML, Hill G, et al: Appropriate use of antibiotics in serious obstetric and gynecologic infections. Am J Obstet Gynecol 146:719, 1983.

Toth A, O'Leary WM, Ledger W: Evidence for microbial transfer by spermatozoa. Obstet Gynecol 59:556, 1982.

Washington AE, Arno PS, Brooks MA: The economic cost of pelvic inflammatory disease. JAMA 255:1735, 1986.

Washington AE, Gove S, Schachter J, et al: Oral contraceptives, Chlamydia trachomatis infection, and pelvic inflammatory disease. JAMA 253:2246, 1985.

Weström L: Incidence, prevalence, and trends of acute pelvic inflammatory disease and its consequences in industrialized countries. Am J Obstet Gynecol 138:880, 1980.

Weström L: Introductory address: Treatment of pelvic inflammatory disease in view of etiology and risk factors. Sex Transm Dis 11:437, 1984.

Winkler B, Reumann W, Mitao M, et al: Chlamydial endometritis. Am J Surg Pathol 8:771, 1984.

Wolner-Hanssen P, Svensson L, Mårdh P-A, et al: Laparoscopic findings and contraceptive use in women with signs and symptoms suggestive of acute salpingitis. Obstet Gynecol 66:233, 1985.

Preoperative Management

KEY TERMS AND DEFINITIONS

Antisialagogue. An agent that decreases the production and amount of saliva.

Effective Period. The first 3 hours of decreased tissue resistance following a surgical insult. Prophylactic antibiotics must be at the site of damaged tissue during this interval.

Informed Consent. An agreement by the patient that she understands the following: the nature and extent of the disease process, the nature and extent of the contemplated operation, the anticipated benefits and results of the surgery including a conservative estimate of successful outcome, the risks and potential complications of the operative procedure, and alternative methods of therapy.

Minidose Heparin. A low dose (5000 units) of heparin given 2 hours preoperatively and usually every 8 to 12 hours postoperatively, subcutaneously, as a prophylactic agent to decrease the incidence of venous thrombosis.

Nosocomial Infection. An infection acquired in a hospital.

Prophylactic Antibiotics. The administration of antibiotics to patients without evidence of infection to prevent postoperative morbidity related to infection.

Preoperative evaluation is a challenge to the gynecologist, for it involves both the art and the science of clinical medicine. Optimum preparation involves two personality traits: compulsive attention to detailed planning and a deep empathy for the patient. Preoperative planning can be divided into three basic aspects: obtaining preoperative information, reducing the patient's anxieties and fears, and obtaining informed consent. Francis D. Moore states that the first aphorism of preoperative preparation is to avoid "surprises." This dictum should be applied to protect both the patient and the physician.

The gynecologist, as leader of the surgical team, has an obligation to prepare the patient, her family, and the hospital personnel, including nurses, anesthesiologists, and the operating room team, for what to anticipate surrounding the surgical procedure. The majority of gynecologic operations are elective and thus allow sufficient time to prepare. However, even in emergency situations, preoperative preparation should be as detailed as possible because short cuts during an emergency can result in further compromise to the patient.

For the patient, there are no small, insignificant or minor operations. Almost any operation is a major event in her life. Associated with an elective operation are the anxiety and apprehension of hospitalization coupled with the ambivalence of deciding whether to have the operation. To help her decide, it is important for the physician to outline the natural history of the gynecologic disease so that the patient is able to understand the benefits of surgery. Most women have questions concerning the return of normal body functions; these questions must be discussed.

There are not many events that assault human dignity as much as admission to a hospital for an elective operation. The woman is usually stripped of her clothing, bombarded with questions, given multiple enemas, and shaved of pubic hair. It is important for the physician to protect the patient's privacy and human dignity during the preoperative period. The gynecologist must appreciate that the preoperative period is one of great psychological stress for the patient. The time of the anticipated surgical procedure is a catalyst for emotional responses ranging from vulnerability and helplessness to the grief produced by anticipated loss of a reproductive organ. The physician-patient relationship is far more than the legally described contractual one. An important aspect of the relationship that builds confidence is the physician's encouragement of the patient to be a partner in the mutual goal of a return to normal function. The understanding and trust built between the patient and physician during the preoperative period will help the patient cope with the stress of the postoperative period.

One of the most important aspects of the preoperative preparation is a discussion with the physician before the procedure. Ideally the physician, the patient, and her family meet without other members of the hospital staff. During this time, it is important for the physician to answer all the patient's questions as well as those of her family and not skip details. It is acceptable to answer a question with the statement, "I don't know." Patients admire the honesty this expresses. The gynecologist must remember that just as he or she studies the patient for both verbal and nonverbal information, so does the patient watch the gynecologist. Gentleness and patience are essential for the gynecologist to display at this time. Sincere interest may be reinforced by eye-to-eye contact and a gentle touch of the hands.

A thorough and detailed history and physical examination, considering the entire patient, not just the pelvis, detects approximately 90% of the facts pertinent to the surgical procedure. Preoperative laboratory screening tests discover fewer than 10% of significant surgical risk factors. It is an established surgical axiom that operative morbidity and mortality are directly proportional to preexisting conditions. Thus it is important to evaluate the influence of gynecologic disease on other organ systems. For ex-

ample, is a pelvic mass producing obstruction of the ureters?

This chapter outlines the preoperative preparations for gynecologic operations for benign disease. Emphasis is placed on obtaining a standard history, performing a physical examination, and on educating the patient and family (including obtaining informed consent). Special considerations of women with concurrent common medical disease are also included. Two recurrent themes are stressed in the chapter: avoiding surprises during each step in the preoperative period and alleviating the patient's fears and anxiety. This chapter is not intended to be an exhaustive discussion of all medical and surgical conditions that may have some impact on preoperative planning. Rather, the focus is on common preoperative problems faced in benign gynecologic surgery.

PREOPERATIVE HISTORY

A detailed history not only obtains information but also helps to relieve the patient's fears and anxieties. If the history is obtained in an unhurried manner, the process is reassuring to the patient. The patient should perceive the gynecologist as a gentle and reassuring clinician rather than a detective trying to rapidly solve a crime. The extent and depth of the general history are modified to a minor degree by the age and general health of the woman and the operation contemplated. However, even minor operations may have major complications. Therefore it is best to be overprepared. The possibility of degenerative multiple organ disease necessitates a detailed review before any surgical procedure in geriatric patients. Even for an emergency operation a detailed history is important.

For elective operations the preoperative history is taken on two separate occasions. The interview occurs initially in the physician's office several days or weeks before the operation and is repeated the day before the procedure is done. The interval is valuable, for it gives the patient an opportunity to reconsider her decision. Similarly, the physician uses the time to collect necessary information, such as records of previous surgical procedures. In reviewing the history the second time, often the patient recalls important information that she omitted during the initial history. For example, she may have recently talked to a sister who has a history of excessive bleeding during an operation.

There are two purposes in obtaining an optimum history from the patient. The first is to put the patient at ease; the second is to cover a formalized and extremely thorough set of questions. The two processes demand time and gentle consideration of the patient's anxiety. It is best to let the patient ramble at first. Subsequently the physician may direct the questions to a standard format. Obviously the format must be covered in a systematic manner so that essential areas are not omitted.

Although this chapter does not review all the components of a complete history (see Chapter 5), it is advantageous to group questions under the specific organ systems: pulmonary, cardiovascular, renal, hepatic, metabolic, endocrine, hematologic, and immunologic. Several specific questions should be included to fill any holes and to crosscheck on the review of symptoms. These questions cover problems with surgery, anesthesia, or bleeding in the patient or her family. An example is, "Are there personal or family histories of bleeding problems?"

The next general category is drug allergy and current medications. Questions must be constructed so as to include both prescribed and over-the-counter medications. Many women do not consider aspirin or oral contraceptives as medication; therefore specific questions regarding these substances are needed. General questions regarding smoking, exercise tolerance, and recent upper respiratory infections are often grouped together.

The woman's contraceptive history, including any recent change, must be known. Over the years there has been no greater embarrassment in the operating room than the realization that a recent contraceptive practice has been abandoned and the patient is pregnant.

PHYSICAL EXAMINATION

The preoperative physical examination should answer three basic questions: Has the primary gynecologic disease process changed since the initial diagnosis? What is the impact of the primary gynecologic disease on other organ systems? What deficiencies in other organ systems may affect the proposed surgery and

hospitalization? A pelvic examination performed the night before surgery may demonstrate that a myoma has undergone acute degeneration or an ovarian cyst may have ruptured and "disappeared." Pelvic masses that are adherent to the large intestine suggest the necessity of mechanical cleansing of the bowel before surgery. A patient with cardiac murmurs from rheumatic heart disease needs antibiotic prophylaxis against subacute bacterial endocarditis.

The most important feature of the preoperative physical examination is that it should be performed in a thorough and compulsive manner. The gynecologist should use the same routine sequence each time to help focus attention on the evaluation of each organ system.

The physical examination is best performed in the privacy of a room with a single bed or examining table. Then the patient need not worry about being embarrassed by hospital personnel or visitors entering the hospital room during the physical examination. To diminish the patient's anxiety, the physical examination should not be performed in silence. Conversation with the patient may involve further history taking or questions and answers about the proposed operation. Gentle palpation is important. A gentle touch helps to build the trust and confidence that are the foundation of the physician-patient relationship.

Two important axioms should be stressed. First, in emergency situations it is imperative to perform a complete physical examination. This examination should include an evaluation of the patient's blood pressure and pulse in both the recumbent and sitting positions; orthostatic hypotension and tachycardia are crude indexes of a decrease in circulating intravascular volume. Second, it is important to perform a pelvic examination the afternoon or night before the operation and again in the operating room immediately before the surgical incision. Pelvic masses sometimes "disappear" when the bladder and gastrointestinal tracts are empty. These measures help avoid surprises.

STANDARD LABORATORY PROCEDURES

The general purpose of preoperative laboratory procedures is to identify conditions that will alter or aid in perioperative management. Specifically, screening tests are used to find unsuspected, asymptomatic diseases that may affect, alter, or postpone the anticipated surgical procedure. Preoperative laboratory tests also help to establish the extent of known disease that may influence the scheduling of elective surgery. Some special laboratory procedures are used to determine the effects of pelvic disease on other organ systems. Special laboratory tests such as intravenous pyelograms or barium enemas are discussed later.

Presently there is an extensive debate over which preoperative laboratory procedures should be standard. Attention has been drawn to the cost-benefit ratio of preoperative screening. Although the cost of each individual test is usually low, the aggregate costs are substantial. The cost argument is often overcome by the individual gynecologist's concern to practice defensive medicine in the present medicolegal climate. Many preoperative laboratory tests are ordered simply by convention, for years being standard orders in an individual's or hospital's practice.

Kaplan et al. have retrospectively studied the usefulness of preoperative laboratory procedures. They estimate that 60% of the routinely ordered tests such as differential cell count, platelet count, and 12-factor automated multiple analyses would not have been performed if tests had been ordered only for an indication discovered by history or physical examination. Most importantly, only 0.22% of these tests demonstrated an abnormality that might influence perioperative management. These authors predict that rigid cost-benefit analysis will soon affect physicians' habits of routine preoperative testing. The final conclusion in their assessment of 2,000 patients undergoing elective operations was that in the absence of specific indications, routine preoperative laboratory tests do not significantly contribute to patient care and could be eliminated.

Two of the most important considerations in the choice of preoperative tests are the age of the patient and the extent of the surgical procedure. Ideally, preoperative laboratory procedures should be determined in each patient based on the findings of both a complete history and a physical examination. Most impor-

tantly, abnormal results from any laboratory test should result in some change in perioperative management. Regretfully, unexpected abnormalities in many standard preoperative laboratory tests are frequently overlooked or ignored.

Preoperative complete blood count and urinalysis are required by nearly all hospitals. By far the most important of these tests for gynecologists is the test for anemia. A woman should not be admitted for elective gynecologic surgery with a low hematocrit level that will necessitate transfusion during the perioperative period, unless a delay in surgery is contraindicated or medical therapy to improve the hematocrit level has been unsuccessful. The results of the urinalysis, white blood cell count, and differential count rarely alter management. A blood sample should be sent to the blood bank for typing and screening for unusual antibodies before major gynecologic surgery, to replace the expensive routine typing and crossmatch. However, it is important that the blood bank have the capability of providing crossmatched blood within a reasonable period of time if serious intraoperative bleeding does occur. Routine clotting studies are not cost-effective unless indicated by history and physical examination.

It is beneficial to order the following three blood screening tests in women over 40 years of age or in women who have positive family histories or questionable past histories of hepatic or renal disease: blood urea nitrogen (BUN) or creatinine, blood sugar, and serum transaminase. A preoperative creatinine or BUN is especially important if the patient is going to be treated with antibiotics excreted by the kidneys. A test for human chorionic gonadotrophin may be appropriate, depending on contraceptive and sexual history. Menstrual history is at best an imperfect indication of early pregnancy. Serum electrolytes are ordered in women taking diuretics or giving a history of conditions that affect water or electrolyte balance.

The tradition of ordering chest x-ray films on all patients has been seriously questioned. Roizen performed a detailed cost analysis of routine chest x-ray films and determined the practice was not cost effective unless the patient was over the age of 60. Rucker et al., in a similar study, concluded that a history and physical examination are sufficient to screen patients, and chest x-ray films need only be ordered for patients with positive findings. In the latter study of 368 patients without risk factors, only one had a positive chest x-ray finding, and that finding did not alter the surgical procedure.

A baseline preoperative electrocardiogram has been found to be cost effective in asymptomatic women only after the age of 40. It sometimes detects a recent asymptomatic myocardial infarction or serious cardiac arrhythmias. The results of several screening tests should be reviewed in the office visit just before hospitalization. These include a Papanicolaou smear on all patients and mammography, depending on the patient's age and risk factors. Testing the stool for occult blood in women over 40 detects bleeding from a colon cancer in approximately 2 of 1000 asymptomatic women.

PATIENT-FAMILY EDUCATION AND INFORMED CONSENT

One of the primary responsibilities of the gynecologic surgeon is to educate the patient and her family about the anticipated hospitalization and surgical procedure. Giving this information is both an ethical and legal responsibility. More importantly, in most circumstances the patient and her family want to know about the operation. Similar to the history and physical examination, educational discussions should take place on at least two occasions, both in the outpatient and inpatient environments.

Educating the patient is a great step in relieving anxiety. If the patient is aware of the sequence of events following admission, the stress of this time becomes more tolerable. It is difficult to overeducate the patient on details of the hospitalization, the operating room, and recovery room routines. Psychological preparation of the family is equally important, and arrangements should be made for a meeting with family members immediately following the operation. An informed family is one of the surgeon's greatest assistants. An uninformed family will often harrass the entire health care delivery team.

Few concepts bring more anxiety, concern, and fear to the physician than the doctrine of informed consent. In the present medicolegal climate, the absence of informed consent is cited as a major problem in many lawsuits. Some critics have pointed out that true informed consent would involve sending the patient to medical school and then through several hours of intensive discussion.

It is important to differentiate the concepts of consent and informed consent. Consent involves a simple yes-or-no decision, while informed consent is an educational process. If a gynecologist were to operate without consent, he or she would be vulnerable to charges of assault and battery. The right of an adult woman to have final authority to consent to an operation has over 200 years of legal precedent. The preoperative consent form that is standard in most hospitals simply documents that consent, hopefully informed consent, has been obtained.

To obtain informed consent the surgeon must explain to the patient in understandable terms the following: the nature and extent of the disease process; the nature and extent of the contemplated operation; the anticipated benefits and results of the surgery, including a conservative estimate of successful outcome; the risks and potential complications of the operative procedure; and alternative methods of therapy. The gynecologist should also discuss with the patient what the operation will not accomplish. Many patients expect surgery to magically cure a large constellation of symptoms. After being educated and considering the information, the patient acquires an understanding of the risks and benefits of the proposed surgery and may make a "fully informed" decision and give informed consent for the operation to be performed.

The possibility of unanticipated pathologic conditions should be discussed with the patient and permission obtained on the written consent form for the most extensive operative procedure that may be necessary. Patients readily accept the necessity of freedom of judgment by the gynecologist during the operation as to the extent of the surgical procedure needed, depending on what is discovered during surgery. For example, written permission to remove both fallopian tubes and ovaries along with the uterus should be obtained in the event that extensive adnexal disease is an unanticipated finding.

One of the greatest dilemmas in the doctrine of informed consent is the extent and depth of discussions concerning potential complications of an operation. Attorneys who specialize in defending gynecologists in medical malpractice litigation strongly advise discussing all major complications, including death from surgery and rare serious complications such as urinary tract fistulas following hysterectomy. Wingo et al. from the Centers for Disease Control recently reviewed the overall mortality associated with hysterectomy in the United States. This study, which gathered data from approximately 40% of the gynecologic operations performed each year, documented an overall mortality of 12 per 10,000 hysterectomy procedures. The death rate per 10,000 operations was higher in women who were pregnant (29 per 10,000) and women with cancer (38 per 10,000), whereas if the surgery were performed for benign gynecologic disease there were 6 deaths per 10,000 operations. To protect the gynecologist the final discussion of the informed consent process should be witnessed by a family member and another member of the health delivery team. Highlights of this discussion should be documented by a paragraph written by the gynecologist in the progress notes of the chart.

ADMISSION AND PREOPERATIVE ORDERS

The admission and preoperative orders should communicate the gynecologist's preoperative preparation for his or her patient. To avoid omissions, it is important to develop a systematic method of writing preoperative orders. A simple outline is depicted in the box above. The orders should be individualized depending on the history and physical examination obtained as an outpatient, the patient's age, and the extent of the proposed surgical procedure. Unusual or infrequent orders should be written in specific detail to avoid confusion by nursing and other hospital personnel.

The first two or three lines of the order sheet should include the reasons for admission, the proposed operation, and a list of the patient's diseases. Further orders are subdivided into four broad categories: general measures, medication, laboratory tests, and preventive therapies.

SAMPLE ADMISSION AND PREOPERATIVE ORDERS

A. General measures
 1. Activity
 2. Diet
 3. Vital signs
 4. N.P.O. after midnight
B. Medications
 1. Pain
 2. Sleep
 3. Prophylactic antibiotics
 4. Special (for medical illness)
C. Laboratory tests
 1. Routine
 2. Special
 3. Blood for typing and screening
 4. Pregnancy test
D. Preventive therapies
 1. Elastic stockings
 2. Enemas until clear

General measures include orders for activity, diet, and vital signs. The patient should have nothing by mouth (NPO) for at least 6 hours before elective surgery. If the patient's operation is not scheduled until the middle of the afternoon, it is acceptable for the patient to have an early liquid breakfast.

The second category of orders is for medications. The three common subgroups of medications are for pain, sleep, and antibiotics. When prophylactic antibiotics are ordered, the time of injection should ensure that significant blood and tissue levels will be present at the time of bacterial contamination during the surgical procedure. An additional subgroup is special medications for specific medical illness. It is presumed that the anesthesiologist will write orders for preoperative medication to alleviate anxiety and reduce tracheobronchial secretions.

The third major group of orders involve preoperative laboratory tests. This group includes standard laboratory tests, specifically indicated laboratory tests or procedures such as an intravenous pyelogram, or blood samples for typing and screening for unusual antibodies.

The fourth and last group of orders involves preventive therapies. Thrombophlebitis remains a major complication of gynecologic surgery. Patients often are advised to wear elastic stockings up to the knee to help overcome venous stasis. Prophylactic subcutaneous heparin is indicated in women at high risk for thromboembolic disease. Because the lower intestinal tract should be empty before an operation, it is appropriate to order enemas to cleanse the lower intestine. One of the time-honored traditions in gynecologic surgery has been douching the evening before the operation. The medical value of this habit is unproven. Amstey and Jones found no advantage to washing the vagina with an iodine solution. The vagina recolonizes with similar quantiative bacterial counts within 30 to 60 minutes. Another unnecessary order involves having the patient empty her bladder before going to the operating room, because catheterization should be performed before the pelvic examination on the operating room table. If removal of hair is necessary for the operation, it should be clipped immediately before the operation.

CONSULTATION WITH THE ANESTHESIOLOGIST

The preoperative interaction between the patient and the anesthesiologist is most important. For the patient, both the reassurance of meeting the anesthesiologist and their exchange of information greatly alleviate anxiety. For the anesthesiologist, it is an opportunity to obtain necessary medical information, evaluate the patient, determine the risk of the perioperative period, and write preoperative medication orders. This meeting has traditionally occurred the afternoon or evening before surgery. However, with emphasis on cost containment and greater use of outpatient facilities, and with admission to the hospital the morning of the operation, this meeting frequently occurs on an outpatient basis several days before surgery.

Anesthesiologists classify surgical procedures according to the patient's risk of mortality. Dripps, in 1961, first published guidelines to determine the risk of death related to major operative procedures. This Physical Status Scale (Table 23-1) has been adopted by the American Society of Anesthesiologists. An emergency operation doubles the mortality risks for classes 1, 2, and 3, produces a slightly increased risk in class 4, and does not change the risk in class 5. Hirsch is of the opinion that

TABLE 23-1
Dripps-American Society of Anesthesiologists Classification

Class	Description
1	A normal healthy patient
2	A patient with mild-to-moderate systemic disease
3	A patient with severe systemic disease with limited activity but not incapacitated
4	A patient with incapacitating, constantly life-threatening systemic disease
5	A moribund patient not expected to survive 24 hours with or without operation

Adapted from New classification of physical status. Anesthesiology 24:111, 1963.
From Jewell ER, Persson AV: Preoperative evaluation of the high-risk patient. Surg Clin North Am 65:4, 1985.

5% to 10% of the total perioperative mortality rate is directly related to anesthetic problems. The majority of deaths due to anesthesia are ascribable to human error.

A problem frequently encountered by both gynecologists and anesthesiologists is whether to continue or interrupt medications that the patient is taking. If the drug is prescribed for a medical illness it is best to continue the drug through the perioperative period. It is acceptable to have the patient take oral medications the morning of surgery. The 30 to 60 ml of water needed to swallow the oral medication is negligible compared to gastric fluid volumes. Roizen has listed several drugs as special exceptions to routine administration before the operation, for they interfere or interact with either anesthesia or surgery. This list includes monoamine oxidase inhibitors, nicotinic acid, insulin, corticosteroids, and anticoagulants.

Three special gynecologic situations should be considered by the anesthesiologist in his or her choice of general or conduction anesthesia. Spinal anesthesia should be avoided during rectovaginal fistula repairs so that the surgeon may judge the "tightness" of the external sphincter in consideration of performing a relaxing sphincterotomy incision. It has also been our clinical impression that the incidence of spinal headache may be increased in operations performed in the extreme lithotomy position.

TABLE 23-2
Drugs and Doses Used for Preoperative Medication

Classification	Drug	Typical Adult Dose (mg)	Route of Administration
Barbiturates	Secobarbital	50-150	Oral, IM
	Pentobarbital	50-150	Oral, IM
Narcotics	Morphine	5-15	IM
	Meperidine	50-100	IM
Tranquilizers and	Diazepam	5-10	Oral
sedative-hypnotics	Droperidol	2.5-5	IM
	Hydroxyzine*	50-150	IM
	Promethazine*	25-50	IM
Anticholinergics	Atropine	0.3-0.6	IM
	Scopolamine	0.3-0.5	IM
	Glycopyrrolate	0.2-0.3	IM
Histamine H_2-receptor antagonist	Cimetidine	300	Oral, IM, IV

From Stoelting RK: Psychological preparation and preoperative medication. In Miller RD, ed: Anesthesia, 2nd ed. New York, Churchill Livingstone, 1986. Reprinted by permission.
*May also be classified as antihistamine.

Finally, the choice of conduction anesthesia for surgery on an adnexal mass must take into account the possibility of upper abdominal exploration and biopsy if the adnexal mass is malignant.

The general types of drugs used for premedication include barbiturates, narcotics, tranquilizers, sedatives, hypnotics, anticholinergics, antihistamines, and H_2-receptor antagonists (Table 23-2). Sedation is easy to accomplish; however, relief of anxiety does not invariably accompany sedation. Narcotics and sedatives are contraindicated in patients with chronic respiratory or liver disease.

Stoelting has outlined ideal preoperative medications for the majority of patients (see box p. 651). He recommended flurazepam orally the evening before surgery followed by diazepam and cimetidine orally 1 to 2 hours before induction of anesthesia. For an antisialagogue effect, atropine or scopolamine is given intramuscularly immediately before the patient is transported to the operating room. This alleviates the dry-mouth feeling produced by anticholinergics given 1 or 2 hours before surgery. If the central nervous system effects of atropine and scopolamine are worrisome, glycopyrrolate is the drug of choice. The latter drug has the advantage of producing minimal cardiovascular and visual side effects.

PROPHYLACTIC ANTIBIOTICS

When a significant risk of postoperative infection exists, the use of prophylactic antibiotics in gynecologic surgical procedures has become standard practice. Rigidly defined, prophylactic antibiotic use involves the administration of antibiotics to women without evidence of pelvic infection to prevent postoperative morbidity related to infection. The major use of prophylactic antibiotics is in operations such as vaginal hysterectomy, following which there is a high incidence of postoperative pelvic cellulitis. The goal of antibiotic therapy is to prevent infection by the endogenous flora of the lower female reproductive tract. Prophylactic antibiotics are given occasionally when the incidence of postoperative infection is low, but the results of the surgical procedure would be severely compromised if an infection did occur, such as with reconstructive operations on the fallopian tubes. Presently, approximately 40% of all antibiotics used in hospitals are ordered

RECOMMENDED APPROACH TO PREOPERATIVE MEDICATION

1. Patient interview by anesthesiologist the day before an elective operation
2. Flurazepam orally the evening before the operation to prevent insomnia
3. Diazepam orally 1 to 2 hours before induction of anesthesia

     Substitute morphine intramuscularly if analgesia is desired

     Scopolamine intramuscularly at the same time as diazepam or morphine if reliable sedation and amnesia are desired—otherwise recommendation number 5
4. Cimetidine orally 1 to 2 hours before induction of anesthesia
5. Glycopyrrolate intramuscularly when patient is sent to the operating room

From Stoelting RK: Psychological preparation and preoperative medication. In Miller RD, ed: Anesthesia, 2nd ed. New York, Churchill Livingstone, 1986. Reprinted by permission.

as prophylaxis. The use of prophylactic antibiotics in gynecologic surgery has been the subject of much debate. As in any discussion of preventive medicine, one has to evaluate the benefits, risks, and costs. In general, the use of prophylactic antibiotics result in fewer operative site infections (abdominal wound and pelvic infections), reduced febrile morbidity, and shorter hospital stays. The major risk of allergic or toxic reactions is small, especially with a short course of prophylactic antibiotics. The increased cost of the antibiotics is balanced by a lower total cost from a shorter hospitalization. Certainly the economic costs of prolonged hospitalization for even a minor postoperative infection are substantial.

The foundation of our understanding of prophylactic antibiotics is the classic study of John Burke published in 1961. He stressed the fact that maximum antibacterial activity in subcutaneous wounds results from a combination of host resistance and antibiotics. His experimental studies proved that the antibiotic must be present in damaged tissue at the time of contamination with bacteria or very shortly thereafter. Burke termed the first 3 hours of decreased tissue resistance following a surgical insult as the *effective period*. He found that there was no protective effect in preventing the development of subcutaneous wound infections if the antibiotics were given later than 3 hours following bacterial contamination. Subsequent studies have documented two other important facts concerning prophylactic antibiotics in gynecology. First, the goal of prophylactic antibiotics is to reduce the total number of bacteria present in the operative incision. It is not necessary to kill all of the bacteria. Second, for prophylaxis to be successful, adequate tissue levels of antibiotics need to be maintained only for the duration of the operation. The normal endogenous vaginal flora has 1×10^8 bacteria per milliliter of vaginal secretions, consisting of a wide spectrum of both aerobic and anaerobic organisms. Thus, theoretically, the choice of a single antibiotic for prophylaxis in gynecology is a most difficult one. Ideally the drug chosen as a prophylactic antibiotic should be nontoxic, inexpensive, and effective against most organisms encountered in the endogenous flora.

There is abundant literature supporting the use of prophylactic antibiotics in gynecology. At least 48 studies summarize the data from more than 3000 women who received prophylactic antibiotics for vaginal hysterectomy. The results of these studies show that the incidence of febrile morbidity was reduced from 40% to 15% and the incidence of pelvic infection from 25% to 5%. The results of 30 studies of 2165 women having abdominal hysterectomies are not as decisive. Some studies demonstrated no significant improvement, whereas positive studies demonstrated less dramatic declines in febrile morbidity, pelvic infection, and wound infection. The average reduction in febrile morbidity was 12%, and the average reduction in operation site infection was 5%. In many studies it is difficult to determine whether the investigators equated postoperative fever with postoperative infection.

No center or expert has demonstrated the antibiotic of choice for prophylaxis in gynecology. It is most difficult to compare one prophylactic antibiotic with another. Not only are there differences in methodology between studies but also differences in terminology between definitions of febrile morbidity and documented pelvic infections. There do not seem to be significant differences no matter which modern single broad-spectrum antibiotic (ampicillin, tetracyclines, cephalosporins) is used. Presently, first- or second-generation cephalosporins are the most popular choice for prophylactic antibiotics in gynecology (for example, a single dose of first-generation, cefazolin [Kefzol] 1 to 2 g intramuscularly or intravenously 30 minutes before the operation, or a second-generation, cefoxitin [Mefoxin] 1 to 2 g intramuscularly or intravenously 30 minutes before the operation).

There is universal agreement that the third-generation cephalosporins should be reserved as alternatives to aminoglycosides for life-threatening infections. With the wide spectrum of bacteria involved in the constantly changing ecologic system of the vagina, a single antibiotic does not have the spectrum to be bacteriocidal or bacteriostatic against all the bacteria present. The important feature sought in a prophylactic antibiotic is an ability to reduce the total number of bacteria present in the bacterial innoculum; it does not have to affect all organisms. A reduction in overall number allows the woman's natural defense mechanisms to eradicate the remaining bacteria.

Shapiro et al. performed a cost-benefit analysis of prophylactic antibiotics for both abdominal and vaginal hysterectomy. They estimated the excessive cost per patient with infection or febrile morbidity was $1,777 for vaginal hysterectomies and $716 for abdominal hysterectomies. They performed a randomized, placebo-controlled clinical trial of 515 patients, giving three injections of a cephalosporin for prophylaxis. The computer program estimated the cost savings of prophylactic antibiotics as $492 per patient with vaginal hysterectomy and $102 per patient for abdominal hysterectomy. These calculations included the cost of the prophylactic antibiotics (Table 23-3).

Recent emphasis has focused on an extremely short duration of therapy for prophylactic antibiotics. Comparative studies have documented that single-dose therapy is as effective as 24 hours of antibiotics. This short duration of administration also reduces cost and complications. The incidence of serious complications such as drug allergy and resistant bacteria is directly related to the length of administration of the antibiotic. With prophylactic antibiotics the major concern is the potential threat of increasing bacterial resistance. This results in two problems: more nosocomial infections with resistant organisms, and alterations of the normal vaginal flora. If infection does develop following prophylactic antibiotics, one must obtain cultures and select antibiotic coverage different from the antibiotic used for prophylaxis.

TABLE 23-3

Derivation of Excess Costs for In-Hospital Infectious Morbidity After Vaginal or Abdominal Hysterectomy

Cost Variable	With Morbidity	Without Morbidity	Difference	Excess Cost, $
Vaginal hysterectomy				
Hospital stay, days*	9.16	7.35	1.81	507
Bacterial cultures, No.	3.04	2.04	1.00	30
Antimicrobials, $	1,276	36	1,240	<u>1,240</u>
TOTAL, $	. . .	. . .	. . .	1,777
Abdominal hysterectomy				
Hospital stay, days*	8.78	7.99	.79	221
Bacterial cultures, No.	2.47	1.26	1.21	36
Antimicrobials, $	580	121	459	<u>459</u>
TOTAL, $	. . .	. . .	. . .	716

From Shapiro M, Schoenbaum SC, Tager IB, et al: Benefit-cost analysis of antimicrobial prophylaxis in abdominal and vaginal hysterectomy. JAMA 249:1291, 1983. Copyright 1983, American Medical Association.
*Geometric mean.

Many significant factors affect the risk of postoperative infection. The length of the operation, whether the woman is premenopausal or postmenopausal, obesity, indigency, the use of prophylactic antibiotics, and the operative approach are the most important of these factors and correlate directly with the incidence of operative site infection. Most studies have not documented that prophylactic antibiotics decrease the incidence of serious pelvic infections such as pelvic abscess. Some studies have questioned the benefits of prophylactic antibiotics in operative procedures that last more than 3½ hours.

In summary, prophylactic antibiotics are the standard of care for vaginal or abdominal hysterectomies and gynecologic operations that carry a substantial risk of postoperative infection. The most popular choice is a first- or second-generation cephalosporin such as cefazolin or cefoxitin. Whatever broad-spectrum antibiotic is selected, the gynecologist must know the pharmacokinetics of the drug. The half-life of the antibiotic is important in selecting the proper timing and route of preoperative administration and the possible necessity of an intraoperative dose for longer operations. The amount of antibiotic bound to plasma proteins is important, for it determines the concentration of free antibiotic in the tissues (Table 23-4). The antibiotic selected should be active against the majority of endogenous flora of the vagina. The drug should be present at the time of surgical insult, and it should be used for fewer than 24 hours.

THROMBOEMBOLIC DISEASE

Thrombophlebitis of either the pelvic or the leg veins is a frequent complication of gynecologic surgery (Table 23-5). Many aspects of pelvic surgery predispose to thrombophlebitis, including venous stasis, surgical injury to the walls of large veins, and often associated anaerobic infection. Because of the significant morbidity and mortality associated with a postoperative pulmonary embolus, every effort should be made to reduce the incidence of thrombophlebitis. Although the initial venous injury most often occurs at the time of the operation, approximately 15% of symptomatic emboli do not occur until the first week following discharge from the hospital.

During the perioperative period the patient should be evaluated for factors that place her at increased risk for thromboembolic disease. Such factors include a history of previous thrombophlebitis or embolus, family history of hypercoagulability, malignant disease, previous radiation therapy, morbid obesity, venous disease, active pelvic infection, use of oral contraceptives up to the time of the operation, and

TABLE 23-4
Pharmacologic Properties of Cephalosporins

	Peak Serum Concentration (µg/ml)			
	Intravenous*	Intramuscular†	Half-Life (min)	Protein Binding (%)
Parenteral (1 g dose)				
Cephalothin	15	20	40	70
Cephapirin	15	20	40	45
Cephradine	15	15	20	10
Cefazolin	80	60	100	80
Cefamandole	55	25	40	80
Cefoxitin	30	20	40	70
Cefotaxime	50	20	60	40
Moxalactam	90	25	120	50

From Thompson RL, Wright AJ: Cephalosporin antibiotics. Mayo Clin Proc 58:82, 1983.
*At 30 minutes after rapid infusion.
†At 30 minutes after intramuscular injection.

TABLE 23-5
Incidence of Venous Thrombosis After Gynecologic Operations with I-Fibrinogen Scanning

Reference	No. of Patients	Type of Operation	Incidence of Leg-Vein Thrombosis
Adolf et al.	75	Major	29
Ballard et al.	55	Major benign disease	29
Clayton et al.	231	Major	16
Endl and Auinger	43	Major	37
Walsh et al.	100	Vaginal hysterectomy	7
	117	Abdominal hysterectomy	13
	23	Wertheim's operation	25
	22	Other malignant disease	45

From Bonnar J: Venous thromboembolism and gynecologic surgery. Clin Obstet Gynecol 28:433, 1985.

TABLE 23-6
Assessment of Risk of Venous Thromboembolism in Gynecologic Patients

Thromboembolic Complications	Low Risk (Under 40 years; operative procedures less than 30 minutes; no immobilization)	Moderate Risk (Over 40 years; estrogen therapy; operative procedures more than 30 minutes; varicose veins; obesity; postoperative infection)	High Risk (Previous thromboembolism; abdominal or pelvic operation for malignant disease; immobilization)
Calf-vein thrombosis	<3%	10%-30%	30%-60%
Proximal-vein thrombosis	<1%	2%-8%	6%-12%
Pulmonary embolism	<0.01%	0.1%-0.7%	1%-2%

From Bonnar J: Venous thromboembolism and gynecologic surgery. Clin Obstet Gynecol 28:435, 1985.

length of preoperative hospitalization (Table 23-6). Lengthy surgical procedures, especially associated with profuse bleeding, are also significant risk factors.

Various means are used to prevent thromboembolic disease. The first prophylactic measure to reduce the incidence of embolic disease is to discontinue oral contraceptives 4 weeks before *major* elective operations. Oral contraceptives decrease the concentration of the body's major coagulation inhibitor, antithrombin III. Oral contraceptives also modify the effect of plasminogen activator, which activates the fibrinolytic defense system. Several clotting factors are elevated by oral contraceptive use, but the significance of this elevation in thrombogenesis has not been established. There is no evidence of increased venous thrombosis with estrogen doses used for menopausal replacement therapy. Thus, replacement estrogen does not have to be discontinued. Other empirical prophylactic measures include elastic stockings, early ambulation, leg exercises in bed, and elevating the foot of the bed. Support hose should be only knee-high so as to avoid venous stasis at the knee. The appearance of the support hose probably serves more of a teaching function to remind patients and nursing personnel of the importance of ambulation and exercise to prevent venous stasis.

The key decision for the prophylaxis of thromboembolic diseases is whether to order prophylactic mini-heparin, intraoperative dextran, or pneumatic inflated sleeve devices (see

Chapter 24). It is our practice to order mini-heparin for the patient at substantially high risk. Subcutaneous heparin (dose of 5000 units) with 0.5 mg of dihydroergotamine mesylate (Embolex) is given 2 hours before the operation and every 8 to 12 hours thereafter throughout the hospital stay. Critics of prophylactic heparin argue that it may reduce the incidence of venous thrombosis in the calf, but has little or no effect in preventing embolic phenomena from pelvic veins. Another problem is that some women are fully anticoagulated by the mini-heparin dose of 5000 units every 8 to 12 hours and thus may experience excessive bleeding during or following the operative procedure.

GASTROINTESTINAL TRACT

Gastrointestinal symptoms are rare in women being evaluated for elective operations for benign gynecologic conditions. However, if the patient has such symptoms, the gynecologist should consider preoperative endoscopy and radiologic studies of the gastrointestinal tract. The impact of nausea, vomiting, or diarrhea on serum electrolytes and on the nutritional status of the patient also needs to be evaluated.

In this era of cost containment a barium enema and sigmoidoscopy need not be routinely performed on all patients with adnexal masses. These tests do help to establish the differential diagnosis between diverticulitis, carcinoma of the colon, and endometriosis. Therefore a barium enema and endoscopy are indicated if there is a left-sided adnexal mass in a woman over the age of 40, a positive stool guaiac test, or bowel symptoms. Again, the evaluation of each patient must be individualized in an attempt to determine if a primary gynecologic process is pressing on the bowel or directly invading the large intestine.

The preoperative nutritional state of the patient must be assessed. Many women with pelvic cancer need hyperalimentation before an elective operation. The two most common complications of parenteral nutrition are sepsis and metabolic abnormalities.

Proper mechanical cleansing of the gastrointestinal tract is important before every elective gynecologic operation. The patient should not have eaten for 6 hours before surgery. Clear liquids are emptied from the stomach within minutes; however, fatty foods greatly delay gastric emptying. Obviously, incomplete preparation of the upper gastrointestinal tract increases the risk of aspiration, which is a serious complication of anesthesia and operations.

Preoperative enemas to mechanically cleanse the large bowel are one of the simplest of preoperative orders. When properly performed, the cleansing enemas hasten the return of normal bowel function postoperatively and help to reduce the incidence of fecal impaction during the immediate postoperative period. An empty large bowel also facilitates the accuracy of the pelvic examination under anesthesia. It is important that enemas are given early on the evening before the operation so that most gas and all fluid and stool are properly expelled from the distal colon. If an enema is given the morning of the operation and subsequently not totally evacuated, the patient is likely to expel the contents during the operation.

If there is a suspicion that the operation will necessitate entry into the lumen of the large intestine, both mechanical cleansing and antibiotics to reduce the bacterial count of the colon should be ordered. Colon and rectal surgeons have debated for years about the best methods to accomplish this. Traditionally, mechanical preparation has been accomplished by 3 days of liquid diet, cathartics, and enemas. Recently, many gynecologists have modified their mechanical preparation to a single day of an oral gut lavage solution (Golytely and bisacodyl) (Table 23-7). Golytely is ingested at a rate of 1.5 L per hour until diarrheal effluent is clear. Beck et al. have contrasted the standard 3-day bowel preparation with Golytely the day before surgery. Quantitative stool cultures obtained before, following preparation of the bowel, and intraoperatively were similar. The Golytely preparation was preferred by patients. The patients experienced less weight loss, and superior mechanical cleansing of the colon was discovered at their operations.

In summary, the advantages of oral gut lavage are that it is rapid and safe with negligible water and sodium absorption or intestinal secretion. The alternative choices concerning antibiotic coverage have focused on whether to reduce the high bacterial count inside the

TABLE 23-7
Golytely Formulation

Components	Concentration
Polyethylene glycol 4000 (PEG)	59.1 g L
Sodium sulfate (Na_2SO_4)	40 mmol/L
Potassium chloride (KCl)	10 mmol/L
Sodium chloride (NaCl)	25 mmol/L
Sodium bicarbonate ($NaHCO_3$)	20 mmol/L
Distilled water*	
Parabens†	
Final osmolarity	280-300 mosm/L

From Beck DE, Harford FJ, DiPalma JA: Comparison of cleansing methods in preparation for colonic surgery. Dis Colon Rectum 28:492, 1985.
*Distilled to a final volume of 1000 ml.
†Methylparabens 0.2 g; prophylparabens 0.1 g.

TABLE 23-8
Mechanical and Antibiotic Preparation of Intestine

Day Before the Operation	Day of the Operation
Golytely orally 1.5 L/h until effluent is clear	Cefoxitin 2 g IV or IM 30 min before the operation
Neomycin 1 g and erythromycin base 1 g orally at 2, 4, and 10 PM	

bowel lumen (neomycin 1 g and erythromycin base 1 g each given 3 or 4 times the day before the operation) or to use parenteral prophylactic antibiotics as to obtain high tissue levels before possible contamination by colon bacteria. We believe both types of antibiotic prophylaxis are important and both should be utilized (Table 23-8).

URINARY TRACT

The lower urinary tract is in close anatomic proximity to the pelvic organs. Both benign and malignant gynecologic diseases frequently produce anatomic distortion, partial obstruction, hydroureter, or hydronephrosis. Preoperative evaluation may include both radiologic and blood chemistry studies. A decade ago many gynecologists ordered a routine preoperative intravenous pyelogram (IVP) before all major gynecologic operations in an attempt to identify anatomic or functional abnormalities of the lower urinary tract. Recently, indications for a preoperative IVP have become more restricted in women without pelvic malignancy or large pelvic masses such as leiomyomata.

An IVP helps to diagnose congenital abnormalities of the urinary tract. Congenital urinary anomalies are rare but are more common in women with congenital anomalies of the reproductive tract. If only a single kidney is visualized by an IVP, it is important to determine if the other kidney is congenitally absent or nonfunctioning. The presence of a pelvic kidney is important information in the differential diagnosis of a large fixed adnexal mass. The presence of a double ureter is another anomaly discovered by preoperative radiologic studies.

A preoperative IVP also helps to confirm the patency of the lower urinary tract. It is important to establish whether the enlargement, inflammation, or displacement of the gynecologic organs has produced distortion, obstruction, and possibly associated chronic infection in the corresponding area of the urinary tract. Common indications for the preoperative IVP with benign gynecologic disease include cervical myomas, lateral projection of uterine myomas, adnexal masses that are fixed and adherent, complete uterine prolapse, and large pelvic masses that produce urinary symptoms. However, a preoperative IVP will not give the gynecologist information that will necessarily reduce the incidence of operative injury to the ureters. During the operation the ureters must be identified along their entire course. The exact incidence of ureteral injury associated with benign surgery is unknown, for many injuries do not produce symptoms. However, Symmonds and others have estimated that ureteral injury occurs in 0.5% to 2.5% of all gynecologic operations.

One serious problem with IVPs is an allergic reaction to the radiologic contrast medium. Approximately 5% to 8% of women have an allergic reaction during an IVP, with 1% to 2% of these reactions being life-threatening. The fatality rate with IVPs is estimated to be approximately 1 in 100,000 procedures.

Insufficient renal function is a major risk factor in elective operations because of the patient's decreased ability to excrete drugs. Women with insufficient renal function do poorly if they develop perioperative infections. Patients with azotemia have a threefold greater risk of adverse drug reactions than women with normal renal function. However, renal insufficiency is very infrequent in an asymptomatic woman under age 40, especially compared to the incidence of unsuspected respiratory disease. The frequency of abnormal serum BUN or creatinine levels is directly dependent on the patient's age. If all patients are screened regardless of whether the history is positive or negative for renal disease, the incidence of abnormal values is 2.5% in women under age 40, 5% in women ages 40 to 59, and 7.5% in women over the age of 60. Baseline and interval tests of renal function in women who are going to be treated with aminoglycosides are necessary and valuable studies.

More than 28,000 Americans have received renal transplant operations. Thus the gynecologist may encounter such a woman in his or her practice. These women need sufficient supplemental amounts of parenteral corticosteroids (hydrocortisone, 300 mg total over 24 hours) during the perioperative period to protect against acute adrenal insufficiency.

RESPIRATORY SYSTEM

The goals of the preoperative assessment of the respiratory system are to identify women at risk for developing postoperative pulmonary complications and to prescribe appropriate preoperative therapy to reduce these risks. Similar to the evaluation of other organ systems, the history and physical examination are the most important parts of the pulmonary evaluation. Pulmonary function tests of lung volumes and flow rates are indicated to evaluate women with history or physical findings suggestive of restrictive or obstructive pulmonary disease.

Preoperative assessment must determine if the patient has the pulmonary reserve to overcome the normal postoperative decrease in pulmonary function. Women who have mildly compromised preoperative pulmonary function are especially susceptible to develop postoperative atelectasis, which occurs following approximately 10% of gynecologic operations. Women with severely diminished pulmonary reserve sometimes develop fulminating postoperative respiratory failure. Predisposing factors that increase the incidence of atelectasis include obesity, smoking, pulmonary disease, and advanced age. Increased pain, the supine position, abdominal distension, and sedation also contribute to decreased lung volumes and reduced dynamic measurements of pulmonary function for the postoperative patient.

Important questions in the history relate to smoking, recent upper respiratory infection, cough, amount of sputum production, degree of dyspnea, wheezing, and most importantly exercise tolerance. In women with known respiratory disease, a complete medication history should be obtained, including antibiotics, bronchodilators, mucolytic agents, and corticosteroids. If either oral or inhalation corticosteroids have been taken during the past 6 to 9 months, the patient needs parenteral hydrocortisone to cover adrenal insufficiency during the perioperative period. The history should also include questions about exposure to industrial air pollution.

Obesity is a significant independent risk factor for postoperative complications. A weight of greater than 30% over ideal body weight increases pulmonary complications twofold by reducing the functional residual capacity by approximately 15%. If the woman is currently a smoker, the risk of postoperative pulmonary complications increases approximately sixfold. The basic defense mechanisms of the lungs, such as the ciliary action of the epithelial cells that line the respiratory tract, are significantly impaired by smoking. Even young women with "normal lungs" who smoke one-half pack of cigarettes a day are at an increased risk. Ideally, patients should abstain from smoking for 2 to 4 weeks preoperatively. However, even a few days of abstinence from nicotine decreases excessive sputum production. Smoking is most detrimental in women with chronic bronchitis or chronic obstructive pulmonary disease.

There should be at least a 10-day interval between an upper respiratory infection and the date of an elective operation. If the patient has productive sputum, the amount of sputum should be estimated, purulent sputum cultured, and appropriate antibiotics given.

During the physical examination, special attention should be given to findings of tachypnea, wheezing, rales, and prolonged expiration. Direct observation of exercise tolerance, such as climbing a flight of stairs, is helpful in evaluating the extent of pulmonary reserve. This is a crude index of pulmonary function. Patients with any positive findings on history or physical examination should have a chest x-ray examination and in selected cases arterial blood gases and pulmonary function tests. Lockwood has estimated the extent of respiratory disease and the probability of pulmonary complications from the results of pulmonary function tests. If arterial blood gases are measured, the oxygen tension should exceed 65 mm Hg, and the carbon dioxide tension should be less than 45 mm Hg.

Pulmonary function tests help both to assess the pulmonary reserve and to identify the extent to which the dysfunction is reversible. Pulmonary function tests that measure lung volumes and flow rates help to distinguish restrictive defects or a decrease in the amount of lung tissue from obstructive defects in which there is a reduction and prolongation of airflow during expiration. The two most common pulmonary function tests used for screening are vital capacity and forced expiratory volume in 1 second. A woman with a vital capacity volume of less than 50% of the predicted normal for her age and body size should have more extensive testing for significant lung disease. Similarly, the forced expiratory volume in 1 second should be greater than 75% of the predicted normal volume.

Twenty-five million Americans have asthma. Thus this condition is frequently encountered during the preoperative evaluation. Asthma increases the incidence of perioperative respiratory problems approximately fourfold. Preoperative preparation of patients with asthma or other chronic obstructive pulmonary disease includes cessation of smoking; instruction in incentive spirometry, bronchodilators, and postural drainage; adequate hydration; and antibiotics for purulent sputum for several days before the anticipated surgery. Improvements in pulmonary function by intensive treatment several days before an operation should be documented by serial pulmonary function tests. Gilmour has emphasized that the major factors in postoperative respiratory morbidity are underlying pulmonary disease and the associated decrease in functional respiratory capacity normally produced by the events surrounding an operation.

DIABETES MELLITUS

Diabetes mellitus is encountered more frequently in women undergoing gynecologic surgery than any other disease of the endocrine system. Elective operations should be scheduled for the diabetic patient only if she is in nutritional balance and under good diabetic control. The stress of an operation and of anesthesia often produces changes in glucose tolerance and insulin resistance. There is a threefold increase in morbidity and a doubling of mortality if an operation is performed in diabetic patients in poor control.

During the perioperative period the additional release of catecholamines, cortisol, and glucagon may produce hyperglycemia. The combined effects of these three hormones tend to elevate the blood sugar levels by 20 to 40 mg/100 ml. The principal postoperative complications in diabetic patients are increased operative site infections and wound disruptions. The increase in infection rate is believed to be secondary to a decrease in both cellular and humoral responses to bacteria. The increased incidence of wound disruptions is due to a decreased tensile strength during healing.

Preoperative evaluation requires meticulous attention to the details of the patient's disease during the history and physical examination. Important questions center around the severity of the diabetes, types of medications, and recent diabetic control, including blood and urine glucose levels. Specific inquiries should be made about the complications of chronic diabetes, especially those affecting the cardiovascular and renal systems. During the physical examination attention should be directed toward the diagnosis of peripheral neuropathy. Diabetic neuropathy may be the explanation of persistent pain during the perioperative period. Autonomic neuropathy may cause postoperative gastrointestinal or genitourinary dysfunction. Autonomic dysfunction also predisposes the diabetic patient to cardiac arrest. Preoperative blood studies should include complete electrolyte, renal, and liver profiles. An electrocardiogram and chest film should be obtained regardless of the woman's age. Diabetic patients have an unusual predisposition to develop acute renal failure following intravenous injection of iodine dyes used in radiology. Thus, noninvasive imaging tests should be used when they will give appropriately useful information.

The medical sequelae of diabetes mellitus, such as renal and cardiac insufficiency, peripheral neuropathy, and peripheral vascular disease, are related to both the severity and chronicity of the disease. The patient's history will help to differentiate mild insulin-dependent diabetes from severe insulin-dependent diabetes. When diabetes is treated with oral agents, consideration should be directed to preoperative dosage. Long-acting sulfonylureas have long half-lives and should be discontinued 3 days before surgery to avoid hyperosmolar coma. Short-acting sulfonylureas should be discontinued 24 hours before operation. During major elective surgery mildly diabetic patients are usually treated with small doses of regular insulin.

There are three current rationales of perioperative management of insulin-dependent diabetes. The general goals of all regimens are to avoid ketosis, hyperglycemia, and hypoglycemia. The first regimen uses no insulin and no glucose. This method is appropriate only for diabetic women under excellent control whose proposed surgery will have a short operative time, with limited disruption of gastrointestinal function. The second regimen is the administration of one third to one half of a woman's usual insulin dosage given subcutaneously the morning of surgery. An intravenous infusion of 5% dextrose and water at 125 ml/h is begun 1 hour before surgery. The availability of rapid bedside measurements of blood sugar allows the adjustment of blood sugar levels by supplemental intravenous regular insulin. The third regimen is one of rigid glucose control. The goal of the rigid protocol is to maintain the blood glucose level between 100 and 200 mg/ 100 ml throughout the perioperative period. Patients are admitted 48 to 72 hours before surgery and placed on a continuous intravenous infusion of regular insulin. Levels of blood glucose are obtained at frequent intervals and insulin adjusted until a steady state is obtained. Thereafter the blood glucose level is measured at least every 4 hours.

CARDIOVASCULAR DISEASE

The vast majority of women with heart disease, who have compensated cardiac function, tolerate surgery well. The presence of congestive failure is the single most predictive factor of cardiovascular complications during the perioperative period. If a patient with cardiac disease is not in failure and does not have severe coronary artery disease, she will do as well as a woman without heart disease. Elective surgery should be scheduled only when a patient is not in cardiac failure and her blood pressure is under proper control. Physiologically, surgery and anesthesia decrease cardiac output by reducing cardiac function and decreasing effective intravascular volume. The stress of surgery results in increased production of catecholamines, cortisol, and antidiuretic hormone. Anesthetic agents depress myocardial function and have varying effects on the autonomic nervous system and peripheral vascular tone. Surgery and anesthesia are an additional burden to a cardiovascular system without adequate reserve.

The severity of cardiac disease may be assessed in the history by questions regarding exercise tolerance, dyspnea, chest pain, and orthopnea. On physical examination the presence of an abnormal heart rate or rhythm, cardiac size, murmurs, and signs of cardiac failure should be noted. A large, appropriately sized blood pressure cuff should be obtained for obese women. Routine ECGs obtained on postmenopausal women may diagnose asymptomatic myocardial infarctions or serious arrhythmias, which will necessitate postponing elective surgery. When women with severe heart disease have major surgery, optimum control of fluid balance and filling pressures are determined by arterial lines and Swan-Ganz catheters.

In 1977 Goldman et al. published a classic study predicting perioperative cardiac risk. Their study involved 1001 patients over the age of 40. By multivariable analysis, they identified nine factors related to life-threatening cardiac complications (Table 23-9). Using Goldman's

TABLE 23-9
Cardiac Risk Factors for Patients Going to Surgery

Criteria	Finding	Points
History	Age over 70	5
	Myocardial infarction in previous 6 months	10*
Physical examination	Third heart sound or jugular venous distension	11*
	Significant aortic stenosis	3
Electrocardiogram	*Any* rhythm other than normal sinus	7
	Premature atrial contractions on last preoperative ECG	7*
	More than 5 premature contractions per minute on *any* previous ECG	7
General status	Po_2 less than 60 mm Hg, Pco_2 greater than 50 mm Hg K^+ less than 3.0 mEq/L, HCO_3 less than 20 mEq/L BUN greater than 50 mg/dl, creatinine greater than 3.0 mg/dl	
	Abnormal SGOT or signs of chronic liver disease	3*
Operation	Emergency surgery	4*
	Intraperitoneal, thoracic, or major vascular procedure	3
		53

Adapted from Goldman et al (1977). From Salem DN, Homans D, McNally JW, et al: Cardiology. In Molitch ME, ed: *Management of medical problems in surgical patients.* Philadelphia, F.A. Davis Co., 1982, p. 75.
*Risk factors that may be altered by preoperative intervention or delay in surgery.

criteria, patients can be rated via a numerical score (Table 23-10) as to the risk of cardiac death or significant cardiac morbidity.

HYPERTENSIVE DISEASE. Women with controlled essential hypertension in the absence of cardiac or renal complications are not at an increased risk for major problems with elective surgery. However, women with poorly controlled hypertension and a diastolic pressure greater than 110 mm Hg should have more intense medical management of their hypertension before elective surgery. During the induction of anesthesia there is a potential abrupt rise of blood pressure of 20 to 50 mm Hg. This transient hypertension is experienced during intubation in 6% of normotensive patients and 17% of women with hypertension. Rapid hemodynamic fluctuations are directly related to morbidity in hypertensive women. Major differences between preoperative and intraoperative blood pressures correlate directly with episodes of myocardial ischemia.

Antihypertensive medication should be continued throughout the perioperative period. The only exception is monoamine oxidase in-

hibitors, which should be discontinued for at least 2 weeks before surgery. Discontinuing some antihypertensive agents is potentially harmful. For example, if beta-blockers are withdrawn, patients may develop a hypersensitivity to adrenergic stimulation and an exacerbation of ischemic heart disease. Similarly, patients taking clonidine develop abrupt hypertensive rebound if the drug is withdrawn. Diuretic therapy need not be discontinued before surgery. Potential hazards of diuretics include a relative hypovolemia and hypokalemia. Although diuretics often produce hypokalemia, and associated arrhythmias are a major concern in women with organic heart disease, they are rarely seen in women without significant heart disease.

CORONARY ARTERY DISEASE. Medically significant coronary artery disease is a problem of older women. It is most unusual for a premenopausal woman to have ischemic heart disease unless she has diabetes, hyperlipidemia, severe hypertension, or a strong family history of coronary disease. Nevertheless, women over the age of 50 often have elective gynecologic

TABLE 23-10
Cardiac Risk Classes for Patients Going to Surgery

Risk Class	Point Score	No or Minor Complications (percentage)	Life-threatening Complications* (percentage)	Cardiac Death (percentage)
I	0-5	99	0.7	0.2
II	6-12	93	5	2
III	13-25	86	11	2
IV	>26	22	22	56

Adapted from Goldman et al (1978). From Salem DN, Homans D, McNally JW, et al: Cardiology. In Molitch ME, ed: Management of medical problems in surgical patients. Philadelphia, F.A. Davis Co., 1982, p. 76.
*Myocardial infarction, ventricular tachycardia, pulmonary edema.

surgery. Thus considerations of angina and previous myocardial infarctions are essential in planning elective surgery.

Unstable angina of less than 3 months' duration is a strong contraindication to an elective operation. Conversely, women with stable angina without a previous history of myocardial infarction do not have an increased risk of infarction during operations. When a woman has had a myocardial infarction, it is important to delay an elective operation for at least 6 months. The excessive mortality associated with a noncardiac operative procedure within 3 months of an acute myocardial infarct is 27% to 37%. Following a 6-month interval the chance of a reinfarction is 4% to 6% with elective operations.

The induction of anesthesia is an especially vulnerable period of time for myocardial ischemia. Myocardial ischemia occurs when the heart has to increase its rate and respond to an increase in systemic blood pressure. Recurrent myocardial infarctions are infrequently accompanied by chest pains, and one third occur on the third or fourth postoperative day. Thus women with coronary artery disease should be closely monitored both hemodynamically and electrocardiographically for at least 4 days postoperatively.

The potential dangers of operations in a woman with multiple premature ventricular contractions are only significant if the premature ventricular contractions are associated with a decrease in left ventricular function.

VALVULAR HEART DISEASE. The major perioperative consideration in women with valvular heart disease is the use of prophylactic antibiotics to reduce the incidence of subacute bacterial endocarditis developing from a bacteremia associated with the surgical procedure. Even without antibiotic coverage this is a rare complication. However, because of the substantial morbidity and mortality associated with bacterial endocarditis, antibiotic prophylaxis is the standard of care.

Women with heart disease who should receive antibiotic coverage include women with congenital or acquired valvular heart disease, high-pressure congenital cardiac shunts, operatively repaired congenital defects or heart valves, and previous episodes of endocarditis. The incidence of rheumatic fever has declined recently, and mitral valve prolapse is presently the leading indication for endocarditis prophylaxis. Mitral valve prolapse is a common finding, being diagnosed in 6% to 8% of women having gynecologic surgery. We believe that it is necessary to give antibiotic prophylaxis only to those women with mitral valve prolapse associated with mitral insufficiency. The risk of bacterial endocarditis is low if the extent of mitral valve prolapse is an isolated systolic click. An appropriate antibiotic coverage for gynecologic surgery is ampicillin (2 g intramuscularly or intravenously) and gentamicin (1.5 mg/kg intramuscularly) approximately 1 hour before the operation. Depending on the time of expected bacteremia, often the same dosage of both drugs is repeated 8 hours later. If the woman is allergic to ampicillin, vancomycin (1 g given slowly intravenously) may be substituted.

THE MORNING OF THE OPERATION

Preoperative Note

A brief preoperative note helps to serve as a final summary of preoperative preparation. This abbreviated checklist should summarize important findings in the preoperative history, physical examination, and laboratory screening tests. This note is designed to assure the gynecologist that no step has been forgotten and to summarize in a few words pertinent details for other individuals who subsequently attend the patient.

Shaving

Many centers have abandoned the ancient ritual of shaving the abdomen and vulvar areas the day before surgery. Shaving is not necessary unless dense hair presents a mechanical problem in preoperative washing of the skin. Multiple studies have documented a twofold to threefold increase in infection rate directly related to perioperative shaving. Cruse and Foord studied approximately 63,000 operations over a 10-year period and found a 0.9% incidence of infection when patients were not shaved as opposed to 2.5% when they were shaved. Razors produce macroscopic and microscopic nicks and cuts that allow a protective environment for colonization by skin bacteria. Depilatory agents often produce intense burning if used on the perineum. In general, gynecologists should abandon the humiliating and crude procedure of preoperative shaving. If the hair is mechanically in the way, it should be clipped just before the operation.

Reassurance

Many women are extremely anxious on the morning of their operation. The physical presence of "her" gynecologist when she enters the operating room provides great reassurance. The kindess of touching the patient's hand or standing by her side as the induction of anesthesia begins is never forgotten.

Pelvic Examination

After the patient is asleep or the conduction anesthesia has taken effect, the gynecologic surgeon has two important responsibilities: performing the preoperative pelvic examination and supervising the positioning of the patient. A pelvic examination following catheterization and just before surgical incision should be standard practice, regardless of the type or extent of the proposed gynecologic operation. The relaxation of the abdominal wall produced by anesthesia and the advantage of an empty bladder and lower intestinal tract affords the surgeon the optimum environment for performing a pelvic examination. The findings may change the choice of incision or operative approach. For example, a scheduled laparoscopic procedure for chronic pelvic pain may be changed to an exploratory celiotomy if previously unrecognized adnexal pathology is palpated. Following the pelvic examination it is sometimes beneficial to measure the depth and direction of the uterine cavity with a metal sound. This procedure helps to distinguish the uterus from adnexal pathology. Before draping the patient, the gynecologist should make sure that the patient is properly positioned on the operating room table. This is especially true to obtain good exposure in the lithotomy position. Pressure points should be avoided to protect against neuromuscular injury.

_________________ **KEY POINTS** _________________

- The goals of preoperative planning are to obtain appropriate information, reduce the patient's anxieties and fears, and obtain informed consent.

- Eye-to-eye contact and gentle touching of the hands are appropriate and effective ways to express the physician's sincere interest in caring for the patient.

- A detailed history and physical examination will detect approximately 90% of the information pertinent to the surgical procedure.

- Surgical morbidity and mortality are directly proportional to the amount of a patient's preexisting medical disease.

- It is important in taking the history to ask specifically about oral contraceptives as well as nonprescription medicine such as aspirin, for they are often not considered "medicines" by the patient.

- The most important feature of the preoperative physical examination is that it be performed in a thorough and compulsive manner.

- The choice of which preoperative tests to perform should be based on the age of the patient and the extent of the surgical procedure, as well as details from the history and physical examination.

- Routine clotting studies are not cost effective unless indicated by history or physical examination.

- Blood urea nitrogen and creatinine measurements should be ordered preoperatively if there is a history suggestive of renal disease or the woman is over age 40.

- Routine chest x-ray films are not cost effective unless the patient is over the age of 60 or has findings in the history or physical examination suggestive of respiratory disease.

- A baseline preoperative electrocardiogram is appropriate and cost effective in women over the age of 40.

_______________ **KEY POINTS, cont'd** _______________

- An operation without consent makes the gynecologist vulnerable to charges of assault and battery except in an emergency.

- Highlights of the discussion regarding informed consent should be documented by a paragraph written by the gynecologist in the progress notes of the chart.

- Perioperative shaving of the patient is inappropriate because studies have documented a twofold to threefold increase in infection rate related to shaving. If the hair will interfere with the operation, it should be clipped immediately before the operation.

- Douching the evening before surgery is not an effective way of cleaning the vagina and is not necessary. Emptying the bladder before going to the operating room is also unnecessary because catheterization should be performed before surgery.

- Oral contraceptives should be discontinued 4 weeks before major elective surgery. Postmenopausal replacement estrogens need not be discontinued.

- The factors that make a woman at high risk for thromboembolic disease include a previous history of thromboembolic disease, a family history of hypercoagulability, malignant disease, previous radiation therapy, obesity, venous disease, active pelvic infection, and lengthy preoperative hospitalization.

- Patients at high risk for thromboembolic disease should be considered as candidates for prophylactic heparin in a dose of 5000 units of subcutaneous heparin combined with 0.5 mg of dihydroergotamine mesylate 2 hours before operation and every 8 to 12 hours afterward for 5 to 7 days or until the patient is fully ambulatory.

- Antibiotic prophylaxis works by reducing the number of bacteria present, not by killing all bacteria. To be effective, the antibiotic must be present at the time of tissue injury or shortly thereafter.

- Oral medications that a patient may be taking for a specific condition or illness may be taken the morning before surgery with 30 to 60 ml of water.

- Barium enema and endoscopy need not be performed routinely on all patients with adnexal masses. These tests are indicated in women over 40 with left-sided masses, women with positive stool guaiac tests, or women with bowel symptoms.

- If there is a possibility that the pelvic pathology may necessitate entry in the lumen of the large intestine, both mechanical cleansing of the bowel and antibiotics to reduce the bacterial count should be ordered before surgery.

- Allergic reactions to the radiologic contrast medium occur during intravenous pyelograms in approximately 5% to 8% of women.

- Factors that increase the incidence of atelectasis include obesity, smoking, pulmonary disease, and advanced age.

- A weight of greater than 30% over ideal body weight increases pulmonary complications twofold, primarily by reducing the functional residual capacity by up to 15%.

- If a woman is currently a smoker, her risk of postoperative pulmonary complications increases approximately sixfold.

- If an operation is elective, there should be at least a 10-day interval between resolution of an upper respiratory infection and the date of the operation.

- If preoperative arterial blood gases are measured, the oxygen tension should exceed 65 mm Hg, and the carbon dioxide tension should be less than 45 mm Hg.

- Asthma increases the incidence of perioperative respiratory problems approximately fourfold.

- There is a threefold increase in morbidity and a doubling of the mortality if surgery is performed on diabetic patients who are in poor glucose control.

- The preoperative workup of a diabetic patient should include electrolyte levels, renal panel, liver profiles, an electrocardiogram, and a chest film, regardless of the woman's age.

—————————— KEY POINTS, cont'd ——————————

- The presence of congestive failure is the single most predictive factor of cardio-vascular complications during the perioperative period.

- The excessive mortality associated with noncardiac surgery within 3 months of an acute myocardial infarction is 27% to 37%.

- The recommended protocol for bacterial endocarditis prophylaxis is ampicillin, 2 g intramuscularly or intravenously, and gentamicin, 1.5 mg/kg intramuscularly or intravenously, 1 hour before the operation.

BIBLIOGRAPHY

Amstey MS, Jones AP: Preparation of the vagina for surgery. JAMA 245:839, 1981.

Astedt B: Does estrogen replacement therapy predispose to thrombosis? Acta Obstet Gynecol Scand Suppl 130:71, 1985.

Beck DE, Harford FJ, DiPalma JA: Comparison of cleansing methods in preparation for colonic surgery. Dis Colon Rectum 28:491, 1985.

Bird BJ, Chrisp DB, Scrimgeour G: Extensive pre-operative shaving: A costly exercise. NZ Med J 97:727, 1984.

Bonnar J: Venous thromboembolism and gynecologic surgery. Clin Obstet Gynecol 28:432, 1985.

Burke JF: The effective period of preventive antibiotic action in experimental incisions and dermal lesions. Surgery 50:161, 1961.

Cartwright PS, Pittaway DE, Jones HW, et al: The use of prophylactic antibiotics in obstetrics and gynecology: A review. Obstet Gynecol Surv 39:537, 1984.

Cruse PJ, Foord R: A 10 year prospective study of 62,939 wounds. Surg Clin North Am 60:27, 1980.

Dudrick SJ, Baue AE, Eiseman B, et al, eds: Manual of preoperative and postoperative care, 3rd ed. Philadelphia, W.B. Saunders Co., 1983.

Gilmour IJ: Perioperative respiratory care. Urol Clin North Am 10:65, 1983.

Goldman DR, Brown FH, Levy WK, et al, eds: Medical care of the surgical patient. Philadelphia, J.B. Lippincott Co., 1982.

Goldman L, Caldera DL, Nussbaum SR, et al: Multifactorial index of cardiac risk in noncardiac surgical procedures. N Engl J Med 297:845, 1977.

Goldman L, Caldera DL, Southwick FS, et al: Cardiac risk factors and complications in non-cardiac surgery. Medicine 57:357, 1978.

Guillebaud J: Surgery and the pill. Br Med J 291:498, 1985.

Hirsch HA: Prophylactic antibiotics in obstetrics and gynecology. Am J Med 78(suppl 6B):170, 1985.

Hirsh RA: An approach to assessing perioperative risk. In Goldman DR, Brown FH, Levy WK, et al, eds: Medical care of the surgical patient. Philadelphia, J.B. Lippincott Co., 1982.

Hubbell FA, Greenfield S, Tyler JL, et al: The impact of routine admission chest x-ray films on patient care. N Engl J Med 312:209, 1985.

Jewell ER, Persson AV: Preoperative evaluation of the high-risk patient. Surg Clin North Am 65:3, 1985.

Kaplan EB, Sheiner LB, Boeckmann AJ, et al: The usefulness of preoperative laboratory screening. JAMA 253:3576, 1985.

Lockwood P: Lung function test results and the risk of post-thoracotomy complications. Respiration 30:529, 1973.

Lockwood P: The principles of predicting the risk of post-thoracotomy function-related complications in bronchial carcinoma. Respiration 30:329, 1973.

Mader JT, Cierny G: The principles of the use of preventive antibiotics. Clin Orthop 190:75, 1984.

Panton ONM, Atkinson KG, Crichton EP, et al: Mechanical preparation of the large bowel for elective surgery. Am J Surg 149:615, 1985.

Pennock JL: Perioperative management of drug therapy. Surg Clin North Am 63:1049, 1983.

Roizen MF: Preoperative evaluation of patients with diseases that require special preoperative evaluation and intraoperative management. In Miller RD, ed: Anesthesia, vol. 1. New York, Churchill Livingston, 1981.

Roizen MF: Routine preoperative evaluation. In Miller RD, ed: Anesthesia, vol. 1. New York, Churchill Livingston, 1981.

Rucker L, Frey EB, Staten MA: Usefulness of screening chest roentgenograms in preoperative patients. JAMA 250:3209, 1983.

Salem DN, Homans D, McNally JW, et al: Cardiology. In Molitch ME, ed: Management of medical problems in surgical patients. Philadelphia, F.A. Davis Co., 1982.

Shapiro M, Munoz A, Tager IB, et al: Risk factors for infection at the operative site after abdominal or vaginal hysterectomy. N Engl J Med 307:1661, 1982.

Shapiro M, Schoenbaum SC, Tager IB, et al: Benefit-cost analysis of antimicrobial prophylaxis in abdominal and vaginal hysterectomy. JAMA 249:1290, 1983.

Stoelting RK: Psychological preparation and preoperative medication. In Miller RD, ed: Anesthesia, 2nd ed. New York, Churchill Livingstone, 1986.

Symmonds RE: Ureteral injuries associated with gynecologic surgery: Prevention and management. Clin Obstet Gynecol 19:632, 1976.

Thompson RL, Wright AJ: Cephalosporin antibiotics. Mayo Clin Proc 58:79, 1983.

Wingo PA, Huezo CM, Rubin GL, et al: The mortality risk associated with hysterectomy. Am J Obstet Gynecol 152:803, 1985.

Postoperative Complications

KEY TERMS AND DEFINITIONS

Adynamic (Paralytic) Ileus. A temporary loss of intestinal peristalsis that leads to a functional intestinal obstruction.

Atelectasis. Imperfect expansion of the lung.

Cuff Cellulitis. One of many terms used for the cellulitis caused by an infection from endogenous bacteria in the serosanguineous fluid that collects in the retroperitoneal space at the vaginal apex.

Dihydroergotamine. A venotonic drug exerting a selective constrictive effect on capacitance blood vessels with only minimum constrictive effects on resistance vessels.

Homan's Sign. Discomfort behind the knee on forced dorsiflexion of the foot; a sign of thrombosis in the calf.

Impedance Plethysmography. A noninvasive screening method using changes in blood volume as measured by changes in electrical resistance for the detection of deep vein thrombophlebitis.

Latzko's Operation. A technique for repair of a fistula at the vaginal apex that includes partial colpocleisis with denudation of the vaginal mucosa surrounding the fistula and subsequent multilayer closure without entering the bladder.

Lymphocyst. A local collection of lymphatic fluid.

Necrotizing Fasciitis. A virulent, rapidly progressing soft tissue infection that is sometimes fatal.

Phlebography (Venography). Radiography of the venous system, the most accurate current method of detecting deep vein thrombophlebitis.

Shock. A condition in which circulatory insufficiency prevents adequate vascular perfusion of vital organs.

Therapeutic Window. The range of effective blood concentration of a medication before undesired side effects occur.

Thrombophlebitis. The process of venous thrombosis formation, secondary coagulation of blood, and fibrin formation in the presence of venous stasis.

Ventilation-Perfusion Scan (V-Q Scan). A safe imaging technique that is the first step in establishing or excluding the diagnosis of pulmonary embolus.

Wound Dehiscence. Disruption of any layers of the surgical incision caused by a failure of normal healing with intact peritoneum.

Wound Evisceration. Complete breakdown of the healing process through all levels of the incision, with omentum or bowel presenting through the incision.

Postoperative complications may occur even after minor operations. The period of hospitalization following an operation is as important in ensuring a successful outcome as the preoperative preparation and the operation itself. The goal of postoperative care is to restore the woman to normal physiologic and psychological health. Some problems are inherently nonpreventable, and therefore early recognition and treatment are necessary. If minor complications are overlooked, they may evolve into major problems for both the patient and her physician.

During the first 24 hours following an operation, the cardiovascular, renal, and respiratory systems should be closely monitored. If the patient is in good health and has had a gynecologic operation for a benign disease, she may be returned to her preoperative location after being monitored for 1 to 3 hours in the recovery room. The expert monitoring and skilled assistance of an intensive care unit are preferable for patients with coexisting illness or extensive operations for malignancy.

An outline of general guidelines for postoperative orders for a woman following an abdominal or vaginal hysterectomy is included in the box below. Flexibility and individual considerations should take precedence over standard orders, but the guidelines can help the physician develop his or her own preferences.

Two major considerations in the postoperative course are pyrexia and blood loss. The causes of fever encompass the majority of postoperative complications. All gynecologic organs are endowed with a rich blood supply. Thus hemorrhage and hematoma formation are also frequent postoperative complications.

POSTOPERATIVE FEVER

The exact definition of postoperative febrile morbidity varies greatly among authors. Although a normal temperature is usually below 37° C, most definitions use a temperature greater than 38° C as the febrile indicator of morbidity. It is not unusual for gynecologic patients to have a mild temperature elevation during the first 72 hours of the postoperative period, especially during the late afternoon or evening. Approximately 25% of women following abdominal hysterectomy and 35% after vaginal hysterectomy exhibit febrile morbidity. Agents that produce fever are either endogenous or exogenous pyrogens.

The physician's primary goal in examining the postoperatively febrile patient is to determine whether the fever is caused by an infection. Some conditions necessitate active intervention, whereas others are self-limiting. Approximately 20% of postoperative fevers are directly related to infection, and 80% are related to noninfectious causes. Thus it is imperative not to empirically treat a postoperatively febrile patient with broad-spectrum antibiotics; in addition, it is usually unnecessary to give antipyretics to lower the temperature of an adult. As Duff has emphasized in a recent review, fever is a phylogenic host response to infection in fish, lizards, and in higher mammals including humans. Fever may be a beneficial response to the host.

Fever is a common postoperative finding, especially a mild temperature elevation during the first 48 to 72 hours following an operation. The cause of a postoperative fever may be simple and common, such as atelectasis or dehydration, or unusual, such as malignant hyper-

---

SAMPLE POSTOPERATIVE ORDERS

1. Admit to recovery room; to ward when stable
2. Diagnosis: abdominal hysterectomy for myomas
3. Condition: stable
4. Vital signs: q15min ×4, q30min ×2, q1h ×4, q4h
5. I & O (intake and output)
6. No known allergies
7. Turn, cough, and deep breathe in bed q2h
8. Dangle feet this evening
9. Ambulate in halls ×4 on postop. day 1
10. IV solutions: 5% dextrose and 0.45% sodium chloride 125 ml/h
11. NPO (nothing by mouth)
12. Medications: 100 mg meperidine (Demerol) and 50 mg promethazine (Phenergan) IM q3h, prn, pain
13. Catheter to gravity drainage
14. Hematocrit on postop. days 1 and 3

thermia or thyroid storm. The temporal relationship of the *onset* of a patient's febrile response to common postoperative complications is depicted in Table 24-1.

Workup for Fever

The initial workup for a postoperatively febrile patient should emphasize the most common problems. Medical students memorize the five Ws in the differential diagnosis: wind (atelectasis), water (urinary tract infection), wound (infection or hematoma), walk (superficial or deep vein phlebitis), and wonder drugs (drug-induced fever).

The proper workup of a postoperative fever, similar to that of any problem in gynecology, involves the three classic steps of history, physical examination, and laboratory evaluations. A chart review and history from the patient may highlight preoperative problems that might cause fever, intraoperative complications such as aspiration of gastric or oral contents, placement of foreign bodies such as drains, recent infusion of blood products or drugs, and known allergies. The physical examination emphasizes examination of the lungs for atelectasis or pneumonia, the wound and operative site for infection or hematoma formation, the costovertebral angles for tenderness, which might suggest pyelonephritis, and veins in the arms for superficial phlebitis and deep veins in the legs for deep vein phlebitis.

The findings of the history and physical examination and considerations of cost containment all influence the extent of laboratory tests ordered. The three most commonly ordered laboratory tests are complete blood count, chest roentgenograph, and urinalysis. Other common tests include a sputum and urine Gram smear and culture and serial blood cultures. Refractory patients may need tests of liver function or special imaging studies such as an intravenous pyelogram, computerized axial tomography, or magnetic resonance imaging to detect problems such as compromised ureters, abscesses, or foreign bodies.

Each major complication will be discussed in detail later in the chapter. However, several specific generalizations concerning the type and characteristics of fever patterns should be emphasized. Atelectasis is the cause of more than 90% of fevers occurring in the first 48 hours after operation. Patients who develop fever as a result of foreign bodies such as plastic intravenous lines or Foley catheters are afe-

TABLE 24-1
Time of Usual Onset of Fever for Various Postoperative Complications

Causes	1	2	3	4	5	6	1 Week or More
Atelectasis	├—	—	—→				
Pneumonia			├—	—	—	—	—→
Wound infection							
Streptococcal							
or	├—	—	—→				
Clostridial							
Other bacterial				├—	—	—	—→
Ovarian abscess							├—→
Cuff cellulitis				├—	—	—→	
Phlebitis							
Superficial			├—	—	—→		
Deep			├—	—	—	—	—→
Urinary tract infection			├—	—	—	—	—→
Ureteral or bladder injury							├—→

brile for several days, then have an abrupt temperature spike. In contrast, wound or pelvic infections (which are usually clinically diagnosed from the fourth to seventh postoperative days), in retrospect, are associated with a low-grade fever that begins early in the postoperative period. An empiric trial of intravenous heparin for 72 hours is often a diagnostic and therapeutic trial for pelvic thrombophlebitis in refractory cases of postoperative fever of unknown origin.

A patient with a drug-induced fever both feels better and does not look as ill as her temperature course indicates. The presence of eosinophilia suggests a drug-induced fever. However, it is often a diagnosis of exclusion. Presumptive evidence of a drug-induced fever is established when the fever disappears after discontinuation of the drug. The diagnosis can only be confirmed by challenging the patient with the medication again after the fever has subsided. Clinically, this latter technique is not pragmatic.

Superficial thrombophlebitis often produces an enigmatic fever. Thus it is important to empirically change any intravenous lines that have been in place for longer than 48 hours. Febrile transfusion reactions generally are caused by leukocyte or platelet antibodies. As long as a major blood type incompatibility is not found, treatment may be conservative.

The basic fever workup should be repeated at intervals until the diagnosis is established. The patient should be reexamined and selective laboratory tests reordered. Rare causes of postoperative fever include malignant neoplasms, pelvic thrombophlebitis, halothane hepatitis, thyroid storm, and malignant hyperthermia.

MANAGEMENT OF A FALLING HEMATOCRIT

Postoperative bleeding is one of the most feared postoperative complications because it not only prolongs hospital stay but also in rare cases may lead to the patient's death. Significant bleeding in the first 24 hours often necessitates reoperation. This complication is discussed along with the management of shock and pelvic hematomas later in the chapter.

Vital signs should be ordered at frequent intervals during the first 24 hours to detect hypovolemia secondary to postoperative bleeding. However, following an operation, sizable amounts of unrecognized intraperitoneal or retroperitoneal bleeding sometimes are present without the patient's having subjective symptoms or appreciable changes in her vital signs or urine output. Thus a hematocrit is necessary at two times during the postoperative course. We prefer a hematocrit at 24 and 72 hours following the operative procedure. A hematocrit drawn 24 hours following an operation may not give a true reflection of postoperative blood loss. The normal physiologic response to the stress of the operation and tissue destruction is a release of increased levels of aldosterone and antidiuretic hormone. The higher levels of aldosterone produces an increase in both sodium and water retention, while increased levels of antidiuretic hormone promote free water retention. Depending on the type and amount of postoperative intravenous fluids, the hematocrit on the first postoperative day may be misleading and reflect fluid changes rather than postoperative hemorrhage. The hematocrit from the third postoperative day is a more valid measurement of postoperative change. Hematocrits should be obtained in a standard fashion so as to eliminate sampling errors. For example, hematocrit samples drawn from central lines or during blood gas determinations often give false values because of the heparin or saline flush solutions.

After the effects of the operative blood loss are subtracted from the preoperative hematocrit, each further reduction in hematocrit of 3 to 5 points reflects a postoperative hemorrhage of approximately 500 ml. The safe level of postoperative anemia is a controversial issue. Certainly it is not identical to the level needed before an operation. Most young, healthy women without complicating medical illness will tolerate hematocrits of 24% to 25% without needing transfusion. These patients should be observed for orthostatic changes in their vital signs. Obviously the site of the hidden hematoma should be discovered by abdominal and bimanual examination (see discussions on the diagnosis and management of wound and pelvic hematomas).

RESPIRATORY COMPLICATIONS

Atelectasis

The term *atelectasis* is derived from two Greek words that mean "imperfect expansion." Atelectasis is a common complication, developing in approximately 10% of women following pelvic operation, and is the most common cause of postoperative fever. Ninety percent of all postoperative respiratory complications are related to atelectasis. The immediate postoperative period is characterized by a decrease in functional residual capacity and lung compliance (Fig. 24-1). Thus the work of breathing is increased. Microatelectasis is most common where small airways less than 1 mm in diameter become blocked by secretions. When small airways remain closed, the gas distal to the obstruction is absorbed, resulting in atelectasis. These changes occur during the first 72 hours following an operation. When atelectasis becomes progressive and involves a large area of lung tissue, there is an associated decrease in oxygen saturation and a decrease in arterial PO_2. This is associated with a normal to low arterial PCO_2.

Wellman has listed both nonpulmonary and pulmonary factors that favor premature airway closure and development of atelectasis (see box on p. 672). The supine position decreases the functional residual capacity approximately 20% as compared with the erect position. Obesity, smoking, age greater than 60 years, prolonged operative time, and coexisting medical conditions such as cardiac disease and pulmonary infection all predispose patients to atelectasis.

In normal breathing there are periodic, involuntary, deep inspirations that help to expand all areas of the lung. Pain, the supine position, and abdominal distension all contribute to a pattern of monotonous shallow breathing without spontaneous deep sighs in the postoperative period. A further decrease in functional residual capacity, a decrease in surfactant, and a depression of mucociliary transport all contribute to ventilation-perfusion readjustments and reduced ventilation-perfusion ratios. The end results are gas trapping, atelectasis, and vascular shunting. In the majority of individuals microatelectasis is patchy and localized to small areas. However, the severity of atelectasis may vary from a small area to a complete lung.

The endotracheal tube may contribute to the development of atelectasis. Even correctly placed endotracheal tubes have been associated with destruction of cilia in the respiratory tract epithelium. Women with nasogastric tubes have a higher incidence of atelectasis more commonly related to a decrease in deep

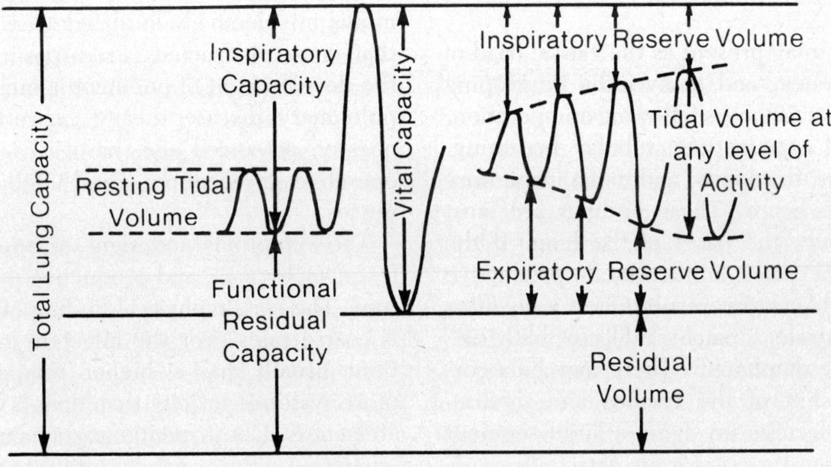

FIGURE 24-1
Graphic illustration of lung volumes and capacities. (From Wellman JJ: Respiratory care in the surgical patient. In Lubin MF, Walker HD, Smith RB, eds: Medical management of the surgical patient. Boston, Butterworths, 1982, p. 285. Used with permission.)

and the systolic blood pressure drops below 80 mm Hg. Again, because of adaptive cardiovascular changes, it takes a rapid loss of approximately one third of the blood volume to produce significant hypotension.

After an operation both intraperitoneal and retroperitoneal bleeding often occur without significant local symptoms. Extraperitoneal bleeding may present as bleeding from the vaginal vault if the vaginal cuff was left open. There may be mild flank or back tenderness with rebound on abdominal palpation. However, abdominal distension, muscle rigidity, and shoulder pain are late signs of intraperitoneal hemorrhage. The diagnosis of significant postoperative bleeding may be confirmed by serial changes in hematocrits or by paracentesis. Bimanual examination with the patient under anesthesia will help in the diagnosis of silent retroperitoneal bleeding immediately before reoperation. An intravenous pyelogram will sometimes demonstrate obliteration of the psoas shadow and deviation of the ureter by a large retroperitoneal hematoma.

The goals of management of a woman who has developed postoperative shock are to replace and restore the effective circulating blood volume and establish normal cellular perfusion and oxygenation. The first priority is to provide adequate ventilation; poor respiratory gas exchange is the most frequent cause of death in these patients. The second, almost simultaneous, priority is rapid fluid replacement with adequate amounts of blood and crystalloid solution (normal saline or lactated Ringer's solution). The three-to-one rule suggests a ratio of 3 ml of crystalloid solution for every 1 ml of blood loss. Table 24-2 lists types of blood components used for replacement therapy. To monitor the rapid replacement of large volumes of intravenous fluid, a Swan-Ganz catheter is usually inserted to determine pulmonary artery pressure, pulmonary wedge pressure, central venous pressure, and cardiac output. These values allow adjustments in the rate of vascular volume replacement. A Foley catheter facilitates measurement of hourly urine outputs.

TABLE 24-2
Available Blood Components

Component	Content	Vol. (ml)	Indications	Risk	Comments
Whole blood	All components	500	Massive acute blood loss	Hepatitis, volume overload	Consider component therapy
Packed cells	Red cells	200	Blood replacement	Hepatitis, allosensitization	Increases hematocrit 3%-5%
Frozen plasma	Clotting factors	200	DIC, factor and immunoglobulin deficiency	Hepatitis	Increase fibrinogen 10 mg/dl per unit infused
Platelet concentrate	Platelets	50	Hereditary and acquired thrombocytopenia	Rh isoimmunization	Increase platelet count 7500/μl per unit infused
Cryoprecipitate	I, V, VIII, XIII	40	DIC, von Willebrand's hemophilia A	Hepatitis	Increase fibrinogen 10 mg/dl per unit infused
Factor concentrates	VIII, IX	20	Hemophilia A, IX deficiency	Hepatitis	1 unit equals factor activity in 1 ml pooled plasma

From American College of Obstetricians and Gynecologists: Blood component therapy. (ACOG Tech Bull 78:1). Washington DC, ACOG, 1984.

Returning a patient to the operating room to control hemorrhage is often a difficult decision. However, this decision should not be postponed, and the patient should have an exploratory operation as soon as possible following volume replacement. During this operation excellent anesthesia, a full selection of surgical instruments, and the value of good assistance cannot be overemphasized. Proper exposure is paramount for the success of this operation. Initially the old clots are removed, and further bleeding is reduced by direct pressure over the pelvic vessels. A systematic search is conducted in an effort to identify the individual vessels that are bleeding. Often the offending artery or vein cannot be identified, or friability of the tissues results in further bleeding.

Bilateral ligation of the hypogastric arteries is an effective operation to control persistent postoperative pelvic hemorrhage. This procedure results in a reduction of pulse pressure, which allows a stable clot to form at the site where the pelvic vessels are injured. Classically, two ligatures are placed and tied around each hypogastric artery (Fig. 24-2). The major potential complication of this procedure is injury to the hypogastric vein. If there is generalized oozing, then thrombocytopenia, disseminated intravascular coagulation, or factor VIII deficiency should be suspected. If these conditions are excluded, venous oozing from small vessels in the pelvis may be controlled by local application of microfibrillar collagen (Avitene).

Many centers use angiographic embolization in place of hypogastric artery ligation. To permit visualization of a bleeding vessel, a flow of 1 ml/per minute is required. Rosenthal et al. have described treatment of recurrent postoperative hemorrhage or hemorrhage late in the postoperative course (7 to 14 days) with angiographic arterial embolization using small particles of a gelatin sponge or a minicoil.

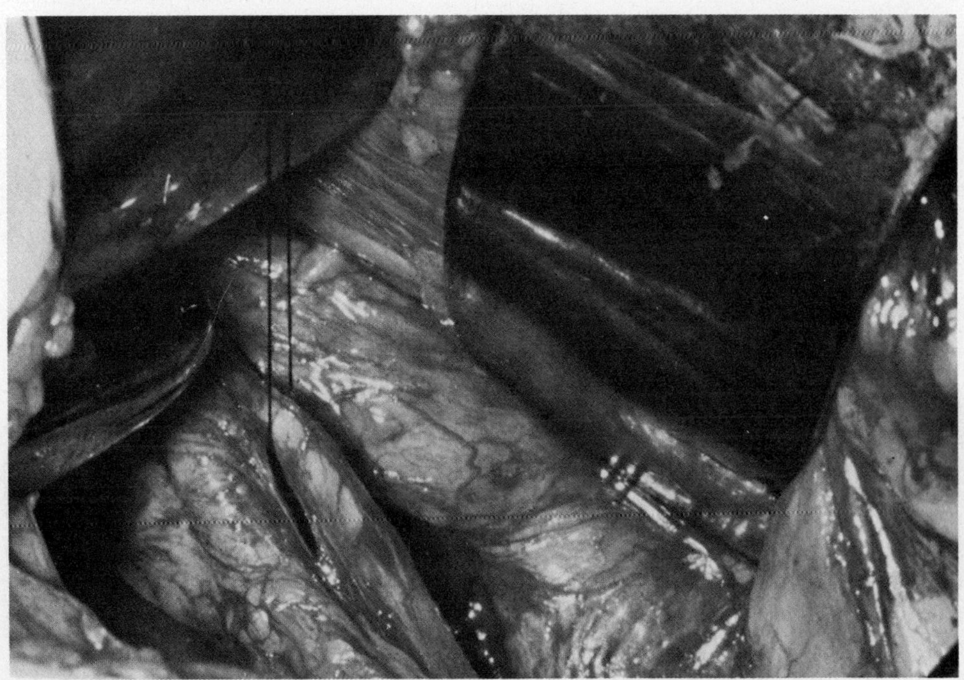

FIGURE 24-2
Ligation of internal iliac artery. Double loop is being directed toward bifurcation of common iliac artery. (From Breen JL, Gregori CA, Kindzierski JA: Hemorrhage in gynecologic surgery. In Schaefer G, Graber EA, eds: Complications in obstetric and gynecologic surgery. Hagerstown, Md, Harper & Row, Publishers, 1981, p. 439.)

Hematomas

This section will describe the management of wounds or pelvic hematomas that develop slowly and are diagnosed after the first postoperative day. These hematomas result from intermittent or slow, continuous venous bleeding and are self-limited. Eventually the pressure of the expanding hematoma will exceed the venous pressure, and a stable clot will form. The extent of the hematoma is determined by the potential size of the compartment into which the bleeding occurs. Retroperitoneal or broad ligament hematomas may contain several units of blood.

The diagnosis of a wound or pelvic hematoma is usually suspected on the morning of the third postoperative day when the laboratory reports an unexpectedly low hematocrit. The patient may have mild to moderate tenderness over the affected area. By the fifth postoperative day the hematoma liquefies and is easier to outline during bimanual examination. The differential diagnosis between an uninfected hematoma and a hematoma that has become secondarily infected is difficult before its incision and drainage. Both clinical situations produce tenderness and fever secondary to the inflammation surrounding the hematoma. The diagnosis of the majority of retroperitoneal hematomas may be made by physical examination. Most important is a careful rectovaginal examination. Rarely, radiologic imaging studies are indicated when the hematoma cannot be palpated.

Hematomas less than 5 cm in diameter may be treated conservatively. Larger hematomas should be drained via an extraperitoneal approach as soon as they liquefy. If not treated by incision and drainage, most hematomas will become secondarily infected even when the patient is treated with parenteral antibiotics. Effective drainage of most pelvic and broad ligament hematomas usually can be accomplished vaginally. Whenever a surgeon punctures a hematoma with a syringe and needle to confirm the diagnosis, incision and drainage should be performed soon afterward, since introduction of the needle from the vagina to the hematoma results in inoculation of the hematoma with vaginal flora.

Thrombophlebitis and Pulmonary Embolus
Superficial Thrombophlebitis

Superficial thrombophlebitis is one of the most frequent postoperative complications and is most commonly associated with intravenous catheters. Women with established superficial varicosities in the lower extremities are especially susceptible because of localized stasis or pressure during the operative procedure and inactivity during the first 24 hours after operation. Patients with superficial thrombophlebitis

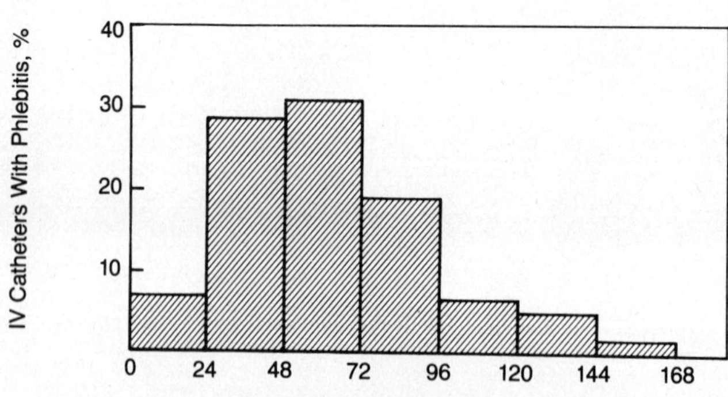

FIGURE 24-3

Hours after insertion that phlebitis was diagnosed. Time of diagnosis of phlebitis from time of intravenous catheter insertion. (From Hershey CO, Tomford JW, McLaren CE, et al: Arch Intern Med 144:1374, 1984. Copyright 1984, American Medical Association.)

of the legs may also have concomitant deep venous disease. Thus the finding of superficial thrombophlebitis does not eliminate the necessity to consider deep venous thrombosis as well.

Detailed basic investigations have identified fibrin sheaths surrounding intravenous catheters in 60% to 100% of patients studied. The exact fate of the several inches of clot and fibrin sheath after the removal of the intravenous catheter is uncertain. Venography studies have found that these clots and fibrin sheaths do not break up on catheter removal but initially remain in situ. The most serious complication of intravenous catheter use is infection of the thrombus, producing suppurative phlebitis or catheter sepsis. The infection may occur via the bloodstream or via bacteria from the skin reaching the thrombus along the catheter line.

The natural history of intravenous catheter–associated phlebitis has been documented by Hershey et al. The classic symptoms of phlebitis are those of inflammation of the subcutaneous tissue along the course of a vein or over the area of merging varicosities. The patient develops a painful, tender, erythematous induration (nodule or core). In the majority of severe cases there is associated fever. However, milder forms may not involve fever. In studying 202 episodes of superficial phlebitis, Hershey et al. discovered that the disease develops relatively rapidly, giving few symptoms or signs that allow removal of the catheter to prevent the disease (Figs. 24-3 and 24-4). After the process has begun, the inflammation does not consistently terminate with removal of the catheter. In their study more than 40% of cases occurred 24 hours or more after withdrawal of the intravenous line. Nevertheless the duration of phlebitis is prolonged if the catheter is not immediately removed when the diagnosis of superficial phlebitis is made. Hershey et al. recommended that all intravenous catheters should be removed and replaced at 48-hour intervals regardless of whether signs or symptoms of superficial phlebitis are present. In addition, the use of an intravenous team decreased the incidence of catheter-associated phlebitis from 32% to 15% in their series. Strict aseptic techniques should be used during catheter insertion. Catheters inserted into the hand or forearm, through which antibiotics are infused, should be changed at least every 36 hours.

The clinical management of mild superficial thrombophlebitis includes rest, elevation, and local heat. Moderate to severe superficial thrombophlebitis may be treated with a nonsteroidal antiinflammatory agent such as ibuprofen (Motrin, 600 mg every 8 hours). The rare case of proximal progression of the inflammatory process should be treated with therapeutic doses of intravenous heparin and antibiotics.

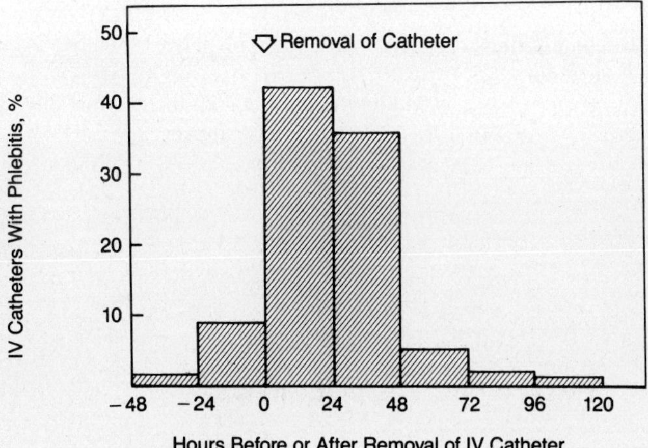

FIGURE 24-4
Distribution of intravenous catheter–induced phlebitis relative to interval between diagnosis of phlebitis and removal of catheter. (From Hershey CO, Tomford JW, McLaren CE, et al: Arch Intern Med 144:1374, 1984. Copyright 1984, American Medical Association.)

Deep Vein Thrombophlebitis

Thrombophlebitis is a common intraoperative and postoperative complication. It is the process of venous thrombosis formation occurring in any deep vein, secondary to coagulation of blood, and fibrin formation in the presence of venous stasis. Generally, thromboembolic complications occur early in the postoperative course—50% within the first 24 hours and 75% within 72 hours. Approximately 15% occur after the seventh postoperative day. Thus the potential threat is present even after the woman is discharged from the hospital.

Venous thrombosis and pulmonary embolus are the direct causes of approximately 40% of deaths in gynecologic cases. The incidence of fatal pulmonary emboli following gynecologic operations is between 0.1% and 0.8%. Because patients often die within a few hours of the appearance of initial symptoms, emphasis must be placed on prevention rather than treatment of this complication. Pulmonary embolus is not the only major consequence of deep venous thrombophlebitis. Many women develop chronic venous insufficiency or "postphlebitic syndrome" as a major sequela following thrombophlebitis. The resulting damage to valves of the deep veins produces shunting of blood to superficial veins, chronic edema, pain on exercise, and skin ulceration.

The reported incidence of deep vein thrombosis with gynecologic operations varies from 7% to 45%, with an average of approximately 15%. Fatal pulmonary emboli occur in approximately 1% of these cases. Walsh et al. found the incidence of deep venous thrombosis to be 7% following vaginal hysterectomy, 13% following abdominal hysterectomy for benign disease, 25% following Wertheim hysterectomy, and 45% following extensive gynecologic cancer operations. The incidence of thrombophlebitis is directly dependent on risk factors such as the type and duration of operation, the age of patient, obesity, immobility, malignancy, sepsis, severe diabetes, and conditions that produce venous stasis such as ascites and heart failure (Table 24-3). Older and obese women have an increased incidence of thrombophlebi-

TABLE 24-3
Risk Categories of Thromboembolism in Gynecologic Operations

Risk Category	Low Risk	Medium Risk	High Risk
Age	40 years	40 years	50 years
Contributing factors			
Operation	Uncomplicated or minor	Major abdominal or pelvic	Major, extensive malignant disease
Weight		Moderately obese—75 to 90 kg or > 20% above ideal weight	Morbidly obese— >115 kg or >30% above ideal weight Previous venous thrombosis Varicose veins Cardiac disease Diabetes (insulin dependent)
Calf vein thrombosis	2%	10%-35%	30%-60%
Iliofemoral vein thrombosis	0.4%	2%-8%	5%-10%
Fatal pulmonary emboli	0.2%	0.1%-0.5%	1%
Recommended prophylaxis	Early ambulation	Low-dose heparin or intermittent pneumatic compression	Low-dose heparin or intermittent pneumatic compression

From Mattingly RF, Thompson JD, eds: Te Linde's operative gynecology, 6th ed. Philadelphia, J.B. Lippincott Co., 1985, p. 106.

tis because of dilation of their deep venous system.

The process of thrombosis most often begins in the deep veins of the calf. It is estimated that 75% of pulmonary emboli originate from a thrombus that began in the leg veins. If one leg is involved, the other leg has thrombophlebitis in approximately 33% of women. Usually the thrombophlebitis remains localized and the clot lyses spontaneously, and the patient is free of symptoms. In approximately 1 in 20 cases the process extends centrally to the veins of the upper leg and pelvis. Involvement of the femoral vein often results in swelling caused by obstruction of this large vein. Pulmonary emboli from calf veins alone are rare, with only 4% to 10% of pulmonary emboli originating from this area. In contrast there is a 50% risk of a pulmonary embolus if thrombophlebitis of the femoral vein is not treated.

In 1854 Virchow described the three key predisposing or precipitating factors in the production of thrombi: an increase in coagulation factors, damage to the vessel wall, and venous stasis. Subsequent studies have documented that all three events occur with gynecologic operations. Blood flow in the iliac vein decreases by approximately 55% during an operation. After an operation a patient normally undergoes several changes that produce hypercoagulability, including an increase in factors VIII, IX, and X; increased number of platelets; increase in platelet aggregation and adherence; increase in fibrinogen; and an increase in thromboplastin-like substance from tissue necrosis.

Kakkar has described the cascade of events leading to the development of thrombophlebitis. The initial event in the cascade was stasis. Stasis leads to localized anoxia with subsequent generation of thrombi at the anoxic site. This produces changes in the lining of the vessel with exposure of the basement membrane and platelet adhesion and local coagulation. Kakkar further postulated that the interaction of this process with activators of fibrinolysis and inhibitors of coagulation determines and regulates whether fibrin is deposited and a venous thrombus develops. Thus the most important event in thrombophlebitis is the generation of thrombi in the presence of venous stasis. A thrombus may generate in an area of stasis, or it may generate wherever a vessel wall is damaged during the operative procedure with resultant exposure of the subendothelial collagen to which platelets will adhere.

The site of initial formation of the thrombus is most often near the base of a valve cusp in the calf of the leg (Fig. 24-5). The thrombus propagates and grows by repetitive layers of platelet aggregation and deposition of fibrin from fibrinogen. The most recently formed portion of the propagating thrombi are free-floating (not attached to the vein) and are most likely to become pulmonary emboli. The body attempts to repair the area of thrombosis through an invasion of fibroblasts from the vein wall to encompass the base of the thrombus. Eventually the thrombus is attached to the vein wall, the area is reepithelialized, organization occurs, and symptoms resolve.

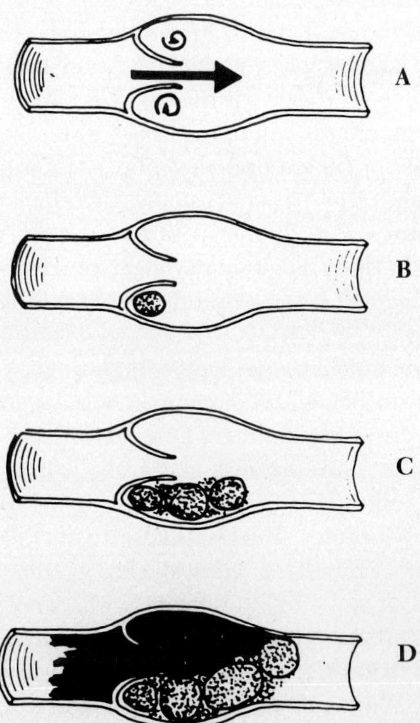

FIGURE 24-5
Stages in development of thrombus in valve pocket of deep veins of leg. **A,** Stasis in valve pocket results in thrombin generation. **B,** Platelet aggregation and fibrin formation. **C,** Propagation of platelet-fibrin nidus. **D,** Blockage of venous flow with resultant retrograde extension. (From Bloom AL, Thomas DP, eds: Haemostases and thrombosis. Churchill Livingstone, Edinburgh, 1981, p. 684.)

The signs and symptoms of deep vein thrombophlebitis depend directly on the severity and extent of the process. Many localized cases of deep vein thrombophlebitis in the calf are asymptomatic and are only recognized by screening procedures such as scanning for thrombus formation using fibrinogen labeled with iodine 125. However, even extensive areas of deep vein thrombophlebitis may be asymptomatic, and the first sign may be the development of a pulmonary embolus.

Studies using fibrinogen ^{125}I to screen the legs have documented that approximately one out of two patients who develop deep vein thrombophlebitis following gynecologic operation is totally free of symptoms. Among women who develop signs and symptoms, approximately 68% have induration of the calf muscles, 52% have minimum edema, 25% have calf tenderness, and 11% develop a difference of more than 1 cm in diameter of the leg. Homans' sign is present in 10%, and differential pain over the calf with a blood pressure cuff is present in approximately 40%. The clinical diagnosis of iliofemoral thrombosis is much easier, and the patient usually develops severe symptoms due to obstruction of venous return. Usually there is an acute onset of severe pain, swelling, and a sensation that the leg will "burst."

The clinician must have a high degree of suspicion to begin the diagnostic workup for deep vein thrombophlebitis. One disturbing fact is that the more symptomatic the disease, the more adherent the thrombus. Thus patients with symptoms are less likely to develop pulmonary emboli. A clinical clue is the persistence of a low-grade fever with unexplained tachycardia. The tachycardia is often more rapid than one would expect with a low-grade fever. Physical examination of the legs produces false positive findings in approximately 50% of cases. Thus if the signs and symptoms are suspicious, the diagnosis should be confirmed by one of the imaging techniques currently available to detect deep vein thrombophlebitis.

Venography (phlebography) is the gold standard—the most accurate current method—for detecting deep vein thrombophlebitis (Fig. 24-6). The diagnostic accuracy of venography is estimated to be 95% for peripheral disease and 90% for iliofemoral thrombophlebitis. The major drawback is that this imaging procedure is quite painful when there is extravasation of the contrast material into the tissue.

Scanning the leg with fibrinogen ^{125}I is the best method to screen women for occult thrombi. Initially, the patient is given an oral dose of potassium iodide to block the thyroid gland. The test is performed by repetitive scanning of the leg for radioactivity for several days following the single intravenous injection of 100 μCi of fibrinogen [125]I. The test result is positive when the area of thrombophlebitis incorporates the radioactive fibrinogen into the propagating thrombus. This test correlates 85% to 95% with venography. The test is not diagnostic above the midthigh because of the amount of radiation emanating from the femoral artery and urinary bladder.

Doppler ultrasound is a noninvasive screening test for deep vein thrombophlebitis that depends on changes in venous blood flow for a positive diagnosis. The accuracy of Doppler ultrasound varies widely in the literature, between 46% and 96%. This technique is associated with high false positive and high false negative rates. Doppler ultrasound accuracy is limited in small vessels in the calf but is more accurate in the thigh.

Impedance plethysmography is another noninvasive screening method to detect deep venous thrombosis. A pneumatic cuff is applied around the thigh, and changes in blood volume are measured by changes in electrical resistance (impedance). Obviously, impedance is reduced with venous thrombi. This method has at least a 15% false negative rate and a 20% false positive rate. As with Doppler studies the accuracy of this method to detect thrombi of small vessels is limited.

The objectives of clinical management of deep vein thrombophlebitis associated with gynecologic operations are preventive medicine, early detection, and early therapy. In reality all antithrombotic therapy, whether with heparin or warfarin sodium (Coumadin), is prophylactic since the therapeutic agent interrupts progression of the disease (thrombus formation) but does not actively resolve the disease process.

The NIH Consensus Conference recently published recommended guidelines for preven-

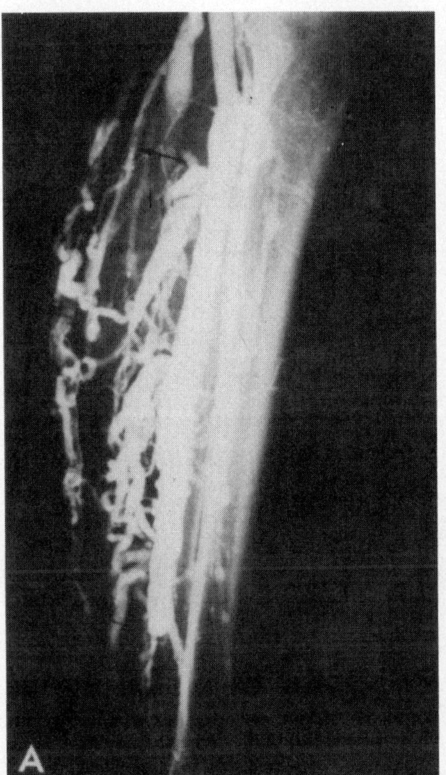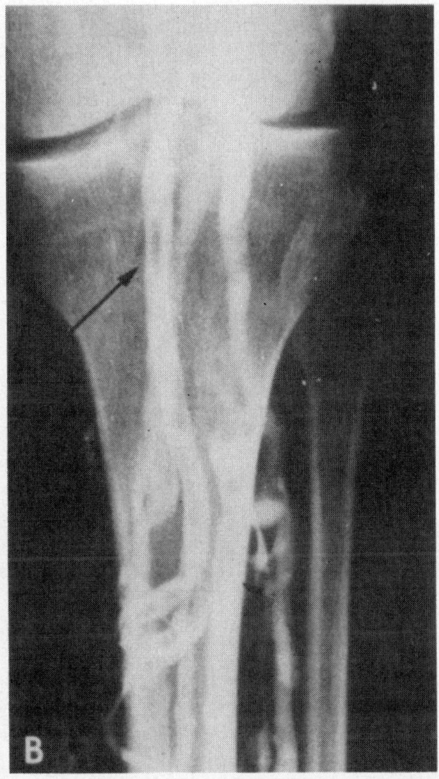

FIGURE 24-6
A, Phlebogram showing small thrombi in veins of calf, which are usually of no clinical significance. **B,** Thrombi in deep vein of calf showing extension into popliteal vein. (From Bonnar J: Clin Obstet Gynecol 28:439, 1985.)

tion of venous thrombosis and pulmonary embolism in gynecology. For the low-risk patient under 40 years of age with an operative procedure of less than 30 minutes' duration, early ambulation and graduated compression stockings are "sufficient prophylaxis." Women at moderate to high risk undergoing gynecologic operations for benign conditions can be managed with low-dose heparin, dextran, external pneumatic compression, or a combination of these with comparable results (Table 24-4). The Consensus Conference stated that data are not conclusive to determine the optimum management of high-risk patients with malignant disease.

Low-dose heparin (5000 IU given prophylactically 2 hours before operation and every 8 to 12 hours subcutaneously thereafter) reduces substantially the frequency and morbidity of deep venous thrombophlebitis (see Chapter 23). Two studies of patients with benign gyne-

cologic conditions have documented a reduction in the incidence of deep venous thrombosis: one from 23% to 6% and the other from 29% to 4%. Wound hematomas were reported in 7% of cases in one series; however, they occur much less frequently if low-dose heparin is given every 12 hours. Low-dose heparin prolongs the activated partial thromboplastin time more than 1.5 times control values in 10% to 15% of women. Furthermore, 6% experience an associated thrombocytopenia with low-dose heparin. Recently a multicentered investigation of prophylaxis of postoperative thrombosis in 880 patients has suggested that a combination of 0.5 mg of dihydroergotamine mesylate plus 5000 IU of heparin (Embolex) every 12 hours is more effective than either drug given alone (Table 24-5). Dihydroergotamine is a venotonic drug that exerts a selective constrictive effect on capacitance blood vessels (veins and venoles) with only minimum effects on re-

TABLE 24-4
Antithrombotic Agents and Procedures in Venous Thromboembolism

Agent	Mechanism of Action	Onset of Action	Application	Route of Administration	Contraindication
Heparin 25,000-35,000 units per day	Prevents extension of active, established venous thromboembolism by inhibiting thrombin activity via the cofactor (ATIII)	Immediate	Treatment of established pulmonary embolism and deep venous thrombosis	IV or subcutaneous	Severe active bleeding documented; hypersensitivity; heparin-induced thrombocytopenia and thrombosis
Heparin 10,000-15,000 units per day	Prevents formation of venous thrombi by inhibiting factor Xa activity via the cofactor (ATIII)	Immediate	Prevention of venous thromboembolic disease in selected postoperative patients	Subcutaneous	Established venous thromboembolic disease documented; hypersensitivity; heparin-induced thrombocytopenia and thrombosis
Warfarin	Inhibits proper synthesis of vitamin K–dependent coagulation factors (II, VII, IX, X)	4-5 days	Long-term treatment of established disease; prevention of disease	Oral	Severe active bleeding; pregnancy
Dextran	Inhibits platelet function and fibrin polymerization	Immediate	Prevention of venous thromboembolic disease in selected high-risk patients	IV	Established venous thromboembolism; congestive heart failure; dextran hypersensitivity
Aspirin	Inhibits platelet function by suppressing prostaglandin synthesis	Hours	Possible prevention in selected high-risk orthopedic patients	Oral	Established venous thromboembolism; sensitivity to aspirin (e.g., triad asthma)
External pneumatic leg compression	Prevents venous stasis, activates fibrinolytic system	Immediate	Prevention in high-risk patients	Local application	Established venous thromboembolism; severe peripheral arterial disease with compromised tissue viability, skin ulcers

From Hyers TM, Hull RD, Web JG: Antithrombotic therapy for venous thromboembolic disease. Chest 89:26S, 1986.
ATIII, Antithrombin III.

TABLE 24-5

Comparison of Deep Vein Thrombosis (DVT) Incidence Rates for All Patients

Treatment Group	No. of Patients	Frequency (%)		Pairwise Comparisons Exact *P* Level by Group*			
		With DVT	Without DVT	2	3	4	5
Dihydroergotamine mesylate, 0.5 mg, and heparin sodium, 5000 IU	181	17 (9.4)	164 (90.6)	0.0241	0.0241	0.0174	0.0011
Dihydroergotamine mesylate, 0.5 mg, and heparin sodium 2500 IU	190	32 (16.8)	158 (83.2)	—	1.0000	0.3575	0.0908
Heparin sodium, 5000 IU	190	32 (16.8)	158 (83.2)	—	—	0.6209	0.0908
Dihydroergotamine mesylate, 0.5 mg	93	18 (19.4)	75 (80.6)	—	—	—	0.2566
Placebo	90	22 (24.4)	68 (75.6)	—	—	—	—

From Multicenter Trial Committee: Dihydroergotamine-heparin prophylaxis of postoperative deep vein thrombosis. JAMA 251:2963, 1984. Copyright 1984, American Medical Association.
*One-tailed tests used when comparing a combination to a component or to a lower dose or when making comparisons to a placebo. All other tests are two tailed.

sistance vessels (arteries and arterioles). Thus its prophylactic effect is via correction of venous stasis and increase of venous return from the lower extremities. In this large series the placebo group had an incidence of deep vein thrombophlebitis of 24.4%, whereas the group given dihydroergotamine alone had an incidence of 19.4%, the group given heparin alone 16.8%, and the group given a combination of heparin and dihydroergotamine 9.4%. Dihydroergotamine is contraindicated for patients with sepsis, hypertension, or atherosclerotic vascular disease.

An alternative to low-dose heparin for prevention of deep venous thrombosis is the intravenous infusion of dextran, either 40,000 or 70,000 molecular weight. Protocols for the use of dextran differ. However, usually 500 ml is infused during the operation, with 500 ml given during the first 6 hours after the operation and another 500 ml on the first postoperative day. Dextran is expensive, and anaphylaxis occurs in approximately 1 in 3500 patients. Dextran's method of action is not understood. It may decrease platelet adhesion, or it may decrease blood viscosity.

Several studies have documented that external pneumatic intraoperative and postoperative compression of the legs by pneumatic inflated sleeve devices decreases the incidence of deep venous thrombosis to approximately one third of the incidence in control patients. These mechanical devices not only increase venous return from the legs but also are believed to increase endogenous fibrinolysis. The cost for external pneumatic compression is approximately the same as the cost for low-dose heparin, and either is approximately 50% of the cost for prophylactic dextran.

For the future there is the promise that new, low-molecular-weight heparins or heparinoids will be available with similar antithrombin effects but fewer hemorrhagic complications.

Heparin is the drug of choice for the initial treatment of deep venous thrombosis or pulmonary embolism once the diagnosis is confirmed. An initial loading dose of 5000 IU is given intravenously, followed by continuous infusion of 1000 to 1500 IU per hour. The dosage of continuous intravenous heparin should be adjusted to prolong the Lee-White clotting time to 2 to 3 times control values, or alternatively, to prolong an activated partial thromboplastin time to 1.5 to 2 times control values. Continuous heparin infusion is preferred over periodic bolus injections because there are fewer hemorrhagic complications. The half-life of heparin on the average is 1 to 2 hours after

is more frequent and lasts longer after an operation that involves the urethra or bladder neck. The etiology of postoperative voiding problems is complex. The differential diagnosis includes anxiety, mechanical interference, obstruction by swelling and edema, neurologic imbalance, and tranquilizer associated detrusor hypotonia.

The patient's initial attempts at voiding should be made *in privacy* to minimize performance anxiety and should be made in a sitting position. It is best not to remove the Foley catheter until the patient is ambulatory. Most women have difficulty in completely emptying their bladders either on a bedpan or in a semirecumbent position during the first 24 hours following abdominal hysterectomy. Catheter drainage keeps the bladder at rest and avoids acute bladder distension with resulting detrusor dysfunction and possibly retrograde reflux of urine. Most problems with voiding resolve without medication and with time. If mechanical obstruction is not suspected to be a major factor, intermittent straight catheterization is indicated. This will result in a lower incidence of urinary tract infection and a more rapid return to normal function than periodic replacement and removal of a Foley catheter for the evaluation of residual urine volume.

Rarely, medications may be given to patients who experience prolonged periods of inability to void. Reflex urethral spasm is common after plastic surgery to repair an enterocele or rectocele. Urethral spasm may be diminished by an alpha-adrenergic receptor blocking agent, phenoxybenzamine (Dibenzyline), in a dosage of 10 mg every 8 hours. However, hypotension is commonly associated with use of this drug. Bladder hypotonia may occur as a result of overdistension, prolonged inactivity, or use of medications such as beta blockers. Bladder hypotonia may be treated with bethanechol (Urecholine) in a dosage of 25 to 50 mg every 8 hours. Urecholine effectively produces detrusor contractions. We do not prescribe this medication for patients who have had operations on the bladder neck until postoperative edema has begun to regress (usually 5 days).

Infection

The most commonly acquired infection in the hospital and the most frequent cause of gram-negative bacteremia in hospitalized patients is catheter-associated urinary tract infection. Patients without catheters, however, may develop overdistension and bladder atony as a result of pain. Overdistension produces a temporary paralysis of the detrusor activity that may take several days to resolve. The atonic bladder is also prone to urinary tract infection. Thus after a gynecologic operation the patient is susceptible to urinary tract infection either with or without a Foley catheter in place.

The normal uroepithelium inhibits adherence of surface bacteria to the walls of the urethra and bladder. A Foley catheter disrupts this property, and surface bacteria are able to colonize the lower urinary tract. The incidence of a positive culture increases dramatically with

TABLE 24-8

Occurrence of Antecedent Urethral or Rectal Bacterial Colonization in Patients with Catheter-Associated Urinary Tract Infections

	Women		Men	
	Urethral Colonization	Rectal Colonization	Urethral Colonization	Rectal Colonization
Gram-positive cocci	4/5	5/5	3/12	2/12
Gram-negative rods	6/9	7/9	1/4	3/4
Candida	2/4	2/4	1/1	0/1
All microorganisms	12/18	14/18	5/17	5/17

From Daifuku R, Stamm WE: Association of rectal and urethral colonization with urinary tract infection in patients with indwelling catheters. JAMA 252:2029, 1984. Copyright 1984, American Medical Association.

time. After a Foley catheter has been in place for 36 hours, approximately 20% of women have bacterial colonization, and after 72 hours more than 75% have positive cultures. The incidence of infection is directly related to the length of time the catheter is in place. Daifuku and Stamm performed a series of cultures which documented that rectal or urethral colonization precedes lower urinary tract infection by 24 to 48 hours (Table 24-8). The incidence of a positive urine culture after a single in-and-out catheterization is approximately 4%.

Sterile technique used during insertion, strict aseptic catheter care, and maintenance of a closed drainage system are all important steps to reduce the incidence of infection through reduced colonization. Studies have documented a lower risk of infection with a suprapubic, transabdominal urinary catheter. The latter technique also decreases patient discomfort and permits earlier spontaneous voidings. Systemic prophylactic antibiotics exert a short-term effect, decreasing the initial incidence of infection. However, the negative effect of prophylactic antibiotics is an increased emergence of antibiotic-resistant bacteria. Therefore, prophylactic antibiotics are not used to "cover a catheter" except in immunocompromised patients. With catheterization for longer than 3 weeks, all patients have bacterial colonization regardless of the use of prophylactic antibiotics.

The symptoms of urinary tract infection usually develop 24 to 48 hours after the Foley catheter is removed. Patients with lower urinary tract infections usually do not have fever but experience urinary frequency and mild dysuria that are difficult to distinguish from normal postoperative discomfort. Women with upper urinary tract infections usually have a high fever, chills, and flank pain. If urinary tract symptoms persist after appropriate antibiotic therapy, one should obtain an intravenous pyelogram to evaluate the possibility of obstruction in the urinary tract. Obstruction of the ureter without associated infection may be asymptomatic or produce only mild flank tenderness. No appreciable change will be noted in urinary output with an isolated unilateral ureteral obstruction.

The diagnosis of urinary tract infection is established by urinalysis and urine culture. Stark and Maki have emphasized that a bacterial concentration of 10^2 organisms per milliliter is significant. In their studies more than 95% of patients with 10^2 colony forming units per milliliter subsequently developed the standard criterion of infection, which is 100,000 colonies per millilter.

To reduce the incidence of urinary tract infection, the Foley catheter should be used judiciously. When possible use of a suprapubic catheter or intermittent in-and-out catheterization is preferable to continuous drainage with a Foley catheter. If a Foley catheter is used, retrograde flow of urine from the bag to the bladder during ambulation should be avoided. Preventive measures such as aseptic care of the catheter and a closed, sterile drainage system are also important. Modern practice is not to treat catheter-associated urinary tract infections unless the patient is febrile. Prophylactic antibiotics are not used unless the patient is immunosuppressed, for they often result in a urinary tract infection with a *Proteus* or *Pseudomonas* species rather than the more common *Escherichia coli*.

Urinary Fistula

Vesicovaginal and ureterovaginal fistulas are infrequent yet troublesome complications of operations for benign gynecologic conditions. In recent series, gynecologic operations have been found to be the cause of approximately 75% of urinary tract fistulas. Surprisingly, it is not the difficult cancer operation but rather the simple total abdominal hysterectomy for benign disease such as myomas or abnormal bleeding that is the most frequent cause of this complication. Fistulas following gynecologic operations are secondary to abdominal hysterectomy in 75% of cases and vaginal operations in the remaining 25%.

The classic clinical symptom of a urinary tract fistula is the painless and almost continuous loss of urine, usually from the vagina. On occasion the uncontrolled loss of urine is not continuous but may be related to change in position or posture. When urine loss is intermittent and related to position one should suspect a ureterovaginal rather than vesicovaginal fistula. Urinary incontinence may be present within a few hours of the operative procedure. This symptom is secondary to a direct surgical injury to the bladder or ureter that was not appreciated during the operative procedure. The majority of fistulas present 8 to 12 days and occasionally as late as 25 to 30 days following an operation. In these cases, avascular necrosis of the tissue resulting from occlusion of the blood supply from clamping or figure-of-eight sutures has resulted in sloughing of the urogenital tissues. On pelvic examination there is often a small reddened area of granulation tissue at the site of the fistula.

The differential diagnosis of a ureterovaginal fistula includes spontaneous loss of peritoneal fluid or serosanguineous fluid from the retroperitoneal space. A small fistula may be localized by placing a tampon in the vagina and instilling a dilute solution of methylene blue dye into the urinary bladder. This will also help differentiate between a vesicovaginal fistula and a ureterovaginal fistula. If the blue coloring is discovered on the tampon, then a defect in the bladder should be suspected. If the tampon is not colored, 1 to 2 ml of indigo carmine should be injected intravenously. The subsequent finding of blue coloring on the tampon is presumptive evidence of a ureterovaginal fistula. An intravenous pyelogram should be obtained in either case to detect obstruction of the ureter and diagnose compound (ureter and vesical) fistulas.

As with most other postoperative complications, preventive medicine is paramount. Optimum operative technique should emphasize the standard axioms in the prevention of urinary tract injury: the patient should have an empty bladder, and the physician should obtain adequate exposure of the site. Sharp dissection should be made along tissue planes with proper traction and countertraction. When operating near the bladder or ureter, bleeding vessels should be ligated individually rather than with random clamping of tissue. Opening of the dome of the bladder and palpation with the index finger and thumb may help to identify the proper surgical plane in the most difficult cases where anatomic landmarks are obscure. The urinary system, especially the bladder, is very "forgiving" if given a short period of rest to recover. If trauma to the bladder is suspected, continuous catheter drainage for 3 to 5 days often results in spontaneous healing of multiple defects.

When leakage from the urinary tract is first discovered, the bladder should be drained with a large-bore Foley catheter. Ureteral injuries should be treated with retrograde ureteral catheters. Approximately 20% of bladder injuries and 30% of ureteral injuries heal spontaneously without further operations. In these cases, splinting of the urinary tract facilitates healing of the defect before epithelization of the aberrant tract occurs, which would result in a true fistula. Spontaneous healing usually occurs within the first 4 weeks. With a ureteral fistula, follow-up intravenous pyelograms should be ordered at 3, 6, and 12 months to detect delayed ureteral strictures.

Operative repair should usually be delayed 2 to 6 months after the initial injury to obtain optimum results. The workup of a patient before operative repair of a vesicovaginal fistula includes intravenous pyelography, cystoscopy, and biopsy of the margins of the fistula if carcinoma is suspected. Cystoscopy is mandatory and should be performed for two reasons: to establish that edema and inflammation have subsided surrounding the fistulous tract and to establish the relationship of the fistulous tract to the trigone of the bladder, especially the ureteral orifices. Occasionally repair of a fistula within 1 cm of the ureteral orifice compromises the ureter, and the ureter must be reimplanted into the bladder.

Operative repair of a vesicovaginal fistula is usually accomplished via a multilayered closure performed by the vaginal route. The principles for a successful operation include adequate exposure, dissection and mobilization of each tissue layer, excision of the fistulous tract, closure of each layer without tension on the suture line, and excellent hemostasis with closure of the dead space. Reliable bladder drainage is provided to avoid tension on the suture line for approximately 10 days. Latzko's operation is the simplest means of repairing a fistula at the vaginal apex. This technique of partial colpoclesis involves denudation of the vaginal mucosa surrounding the fistula and subsequent multilayer closure without entering the bladder. The primary disadvantage of the procedure is postoperative shortening of the vagina.

Ureterovaginal fistulas that do not heal spontaneously are usually repaired 2 to 3 months following the original operation. There are several choices as to the operative technique. However, most cases of persistent ureterovaginal fistulas, involving the lower third of the ureter, are repaired by reimplanting the ureter into the bladder.

GASTROINTESTINAL COMPLICATIONS

Ileus

Minor disturbances in gastrointestinal function are a normal consequence of anesthesia. The patient usually experiences nausea for approximately 12 hours, passes flatus sometime during the first 3 postoperative days, and has a spontaneous bowel movement by the third or fourth postoperative day.

Ileus is an intestinal dysfunction that causes a functional intestinal obstruction. Adynamic (paralytic) ileus is a normal event defined as an ileus of minor to moderate degree. It may be expected to follow any intraperitoneal or pelvic operation. The incidence and duration of adynamic ileus are less following vaginal hysterectomy than with abdominal hysterectomy. If adynamic ileus persists for longer than 3 days, a diagnosis of mechanical bowel obstruction should be strongly considered.

Adynamic ileus is believed to result from a lack of coordinated motor activity of the small intestine, which results in disorganized, propulsive activity. Electrical activity is present, but the basic defect is continuous activity of the intrinsic inhibitor neurons in the wall of the small intestine. Usually the process is generalized, but occasionally it may be localized, involving only an isolated loop of small intestine.

Major factors that result in intensification of adynamic ileus are peritoneal contamination by purulent material or blood, extensive handling of the small intestine, and inadequate replacement of fluids or electrolytes, specifically potassium. Early feeding of the postoperative patient may intensify adynamic ileus and certainly will not improve the condition. Other factors predisposing to the development of ileus include obesity, age of the patient, preoperative immobility, and the removal of large pelvic-abdominal masses.

The classic symptoms of ileus include absence of flatus, abdominal distension, and obstipation. These symptoms are often associated with nausea and vomiting. Bowel sounds may be hyperactive or absent. This condition may be associated with abdominal tenderness, and the abdomen is usually tympanic to percussion. Nausea and vomiting persisting longer than 24 hours after operation constitute cause for concern. The difference between small bowel obstruction and adynamic ileus is a subtle one, for adynamic ileus is normally associated with partial obstruction of the small intestine.

Diagnostic films of the abdomen (supine, erect, and lateral) help to establish the correct diagnosis (Table 24-9). In a woman with adynamic ileus, the intestinal gas is scattered throughout the gastrointestinal tract, including the small intestine and colon. Air-fluid levels, if present, tend to be at the same level.

Watkins and Robertson have suggested that

TABLE 24-9

Differential Radiographic Findings in Ileus and Mechanical Obstruction

Adynamic Ileus	Mechanical Obstruction
Small and large bowel are distended in proportion to each other	In small-bowel obstruction there is dilated small bowel proximal to site of obstruction; in colonic obstruction the colon is distended and small-bowel distension is present with incompetent ileocecal valve
Air-fluid levels in small bowel are infrequent; when present, they are at the same levels	Air-fluid levels are common and at different levels in the bowel
Quantitative difference in small-bowel distension	Greater small-bowel distension than with ileus
Small-bowel distension in central part of abdomen with colon in periphery	Small-bowel distension present in central part of abdomen; no peripheral large-bowel distension

From Buchsbaum HJ, Mazer J: The gastrointestinal tract. In Buchsbaum HJ, Walton LA, eds: Strategies in gynecologic surgery. New York, Springer-Verlag, 1986, p. 100.

the oral administration of radiocontrast material may be both a therapeutic and diagnostic test. After preliminary abdominal films were obtained, 120 mg of 66% diatrizoate meglumine, 10% diatrizoate sodium (Gastrografin) was administrated orally or via nasogastric tube. The osmolality of the radiocontrast material is approximately six times greater than that of normal saline. Thus a large amount of fluid enters the small bowel and acts as a direct stimulant of peristalsis. They noted that passage of liquid stool occurred within a few hours in patients with adynamic ileus (Table 24-10). This material, unlike barium, is nontoxic if it accidentally contaminates the peritoneal cavity during an operation for bowel obstruction.

Adynamic ileus is a self-limiting condition that responds to gastrointestinal rest and time. During the period of watchful expectancy, adequate fluid and electrolyte replacement is necessary. If adequate bowel sounds are present, a rectal tube, Fleet's enema, or rectal suppository may facilitate the initial passage of flatus. Some advocate the routine postoperative administration of a wetting agent such as simethicone (Mylicon) to reduce surface tension of intestinal mucus and liberate entrapped gas. Opinions are mixed as to whether such an agent reduces the incidence or intensity of adynamic ileus.

Severe cases of ileus should be treated with intravenous fluids and gastrointestinal and nasogastric suctioning. Nasogastric suction prevents progression of the intestinal distension. During periods when nasogastric suctioning is used, special attention should be given to correct replacement of fluid and electrolytes (Tables 24-11 and 24-12). The use of drugs that stimulate peristalsis is usually ineffective.

Intestinal Obstruction

Adhesions are the most common cause of intestinal obstruction postoperatively. Less common causes are hernias, mesenteric defects, intussusception, volvulus, and neoplasm. Large raw areas of the pelvis facilitate the attachment of small intestine following pelvic operations. Fortunately the fibrous adhesions that form during the first 2 to 3 weeks after an operation are soft and filmy. Thus intestinal strangulation during the postoperative period is extremely rare. Dense adhesions may develop several months after an operation. In their review of bowel obstruction, Ratcliff et al. point out that gynecologic operations are the most common cause of small-bowel obstruction in women. As mentioned previously, the differential diagnosis between bowel obstruction and ileus is a difficult one (Table 24-13).

The acute symptoms of intestinal obstruction present most commonly between the fifth and seventh postoperative day. Women with bowel obstruction appear to have more toxicity and more acute distress than women with ileus. The abdominal pain is intermittent, colicky, and sharp in nature. Bowel sounds are loud, high pitched, and metallic. Occasionally they may be heard without a stethoscope. Nasogastric drainage is more profuse than in patients with severe adynamic ileus. A patient with a small-bowel obstruction may have a bowel movement, eliminating fecal material that already existed in the colon.

TABLE 24-10
Study of 47 Cases of Adynamic Ileus Treated with Ingestion of Contrast Material

	Average	Range
Interim from operation to time of study	4.2 days	2-14 days
Approximate duration of ileus	35 h	12-96 h
Transit time from ingestion to large bowel	3 h 20 min	25 min-6 h
Transit time from ingestion to first stool	6 h 20 min	1-18 h
Duration of hospitalization after study	3.8 days	1-8 days
Obstetric-gynecologic patients	2.8 days	1-7 days

From Watkins DT, Robertson CL: Water-soluble radiocontrast material in the treatment of postoperative ileus. Am J Obstet Gynecol 152:451, 1985.

Abdominal x-ray films demonstrate a step-ladder appearance—multiple air-fluid levels throughout the small intestine with an absence of gas in the colon and rectum. Pneumoperitoneum from an exploratory celiotomy usually persists for 7 to 10 days. Thus free air under the diaphragm is not diagnostic of perforation of a hollow viscus in a postoperative patient.

Obstruction of the colon may be diagnosed by retrograde infusion of contrast material or by flexible endoscopy.

The foundation of early treatment of postoperative intestinal obstruction is decompression of the small intestine. On some occasions, such as with a ruptured tuboovarian abscess, a nasogastric tube should be used in the immediate

TABLE 24-11

Average Daily Volume and Electrolyte Concentrations of Gastrointestinal Secretions

	Volume (ml/day)	Electrolyte Concentrations (mEq/L)		
		Na^+	K^+	C^-
Saliva	1000-1500	10-40	10-20	6-30
Gastric juice	2000-2500	60-120	10-20	10-30
Hepatic bile	600-800	130-155	2-12	80-100
Pancreatic juice	700-1000	150-155	5-10	30-50
Duodenal secretions	300-800	90-140	2-10	70-120
Jejunal and ileal secretions	2000-3000	125-140	5-10	100-130
Colonic mucosal secretions	200-500	140-148	5-10	60-90
TOTAL	8000-10,000			

From Buchsbaum HJ, Mazer J: The gastrointesinal tract. In Buchsbaum HJ, Walton LA, eds: Strategies in gynecologic surgery. New York, Springer-Verlag, 1986, p. 103.

TABLE 24-12

Composition of Intravenous Solutions

Solutions	Glucose (g/L)	Na	Cl	HCO_3	K	Ca	Mg	HPO_4	NH_4
				(mEq/L)					
Extracellular fluid	1000	140	102	27	4.2	5	3	0.3	
5% Dextrose and water	50								
10% Dextrose and water	100								
0.9% Sodium chloride (normal saline)		154	154						
0.45% Sodium chloride (half-normal saline)		77	77						
0.21% Sodium chloride (¼ normal saline)		34	34						
3% Sodium chloride (hypertonic saline)		513	513						
Lactated Ringer's solution		130	109	28*	4	2.7			
0.9% Ammonium chloride			168						168

From Miller TA, Duke JH: Fluid and electrolyte management. In Dudrick SJ, Baue AE, Eiseman B, et al, eds: Manual of preoperative and postoperative care, 3rd ed. Philadelphia, W.B. Saunders Co, 1983, p. 47.
*Present in solution as lactate but is metabolized to bicarbonate.

TABLE 24-13
Differential Diagnosis Between Postoperative Ileus and Postoperative Obstruction

Clinical Features	Postoperative Ileus	Postoperative Obstruction
Abdominal pain	Discomfort from distension but not cramping pains	Cramping, progressively severe
Relationship to previous operation	Usually within 48-72 hours of operation	Usually delayed; may be 5-7 days for remote onset
Nausea and vomiting	Present	Present
Distension	Present	Present
Bowel sounds	Absent or hypoactive	Borborygmi with peristaltic rushes and high-pitched tinkles
Fever	Only if related to associated peritonitis	Rarely present unless bowel becomes gangrenous
Abdominal x-ray film	Distended loops of small and large bowels; gas usually present in colon	Single or multiple loops of distended bowel, usually small bowel with air-fluid levels
Treatment	Conservative with nasogastric suction, enemas, cholinergic stimulation	Partial: conservative with nasogastric decompression; or Complete: surgical

From Mattingly RF, Thompson JD, eds: Te Linde's operative gynecology, 6th ed. Philadelphia, J.B. Lippincott Co., 1985, p. 102.

postoperative period for its prophylactic value. Decompression may be accomplished by means of a nasogastric tube or, preferably, a long tube (Miller-Abbott or Cantor tube). Serial monitoring of white blood cell counts with differentials should be performed. Repeat abdominal x-ray examinations at regular intervals are used to assess the degree of intestinal distension. Expectant management is successful in many patients. In the series by Wolfson et al., less than 40% of 112 patients with small-bowel obstruction due to adhesions required operation. Conservative therapy was most successful in those patients in whom the long intestinal drainage tube was successfully advanced from the stomach into the small intestine.

The major cause of morbidity and death with bowel obstruction is delay in diagnosis with resultant strangulation and secondary sepsis. Women who develop strangulation experience a dramatic increase in the intensity of abdominal pain, and it becomes continuous. Generally, strangulation of the small bowel is associated with localized peritoneal irritation, increase in temperature, and marked leukocytosis.

Rectovaginal Fistula

Rectovaginal fistulas and fecal incontinence secondary to complete perineal tears are most commonly obstetric complications and are only rarely associated with gynecologic operations. In general, rectovaginal fistulas following hysterectomy or repair of an enterocele are usually located in the upper third of the vagina, while those secondary to a posterior colporrhaphy are in the lower third of the vagina. Other causes of rectovaginal fistula are carcinoma, radiation therapy, perirectal abscess, inflammatory bowel disease, lymphogranuloma venereum, and trauma.

Fistulous tracts between the rectum and vagina usually present 7 to 14 days after an operation. The first warning may be the rectal passage of several blood clots indicating that a hematoma has ruptured into the rectum. Distressing symptoms include involuntary passage of gas and, depending on the size of the opening, the passage of fecal material from the vagina. Associated with these two classic symptoms are chronic, foul-smelling vaginal discharge and subsequent dyspareunia. Aside from the physical symptoms of the anatomic defect, these fistulas cause severe emotional distress because they affect almost every aspect of the patient's daily life.

The diagnosis is not difficult to establish, and only very small openings present a diagnostic problem. What appears to be granulation tissue in the posterior aspect of the vagina is the dark red rectal mucosa, which stands out in contrast to the lighter vaginal mucosa. Usually the defect may be successfully defined with a small, malleable metal probe. If this is not successful, a Foley catheter should be placed in the rectum. Methylene blue dye or milk may then be instilled into the rectum with a tampon in the vagina as is done for the diagnosis of a vesicovaginal fistula.

For initial treatment the patient should be obstipated with a low-residue diet and diphenoxylate hydrochloride (Lomotil). Approximately one in four anatomic defects heals spontaneously before epithelialization of the tract. Hyperalimentation may be helpful in the closure of some fistulas by allowing the patient to abstain from oral intake.

Timing of the operative repair is important. Repairs should not be undertaken before 8 to 12 weeks after the injury. The gynecologist should inspect the area surrounding the fistula to make sure that the tissues are free of edema, induration, and infection. Preoperative evaluation includes visualization of the entire vagina and sigmoidoscopy of the rectal mucosa for attempts to discover more than one opening. A barium enema or flexible endoscopy is important if there is any suspicion of coexistence of Crohn's disease.

The operative technique employed depends on the size and location of the fistula. Standard operative principles include removal of the entire fistulous tract and closure of tissue layers without tension on the suture line. In the repair of large rectovaginal fistulas in the lower part of the vagina, it is usually easier to convert the rectovaginal fistula into a fourth-degree laceration. Diverting colostomy should be used for all radiation-induced fistulas, the majority of fistulas associated with inflammatory bowel disease, and some large postoperative fistulas at the apex of the vagina. Postoperative care is minimal in that the patient may be discharged from the hospital after the first bowel movement. The stool should be kept soft with low-residue diets and stool softeners for the first 2 weeks after the operation.

WOUND COMPLICATIONS

Infection

Most major wound infections prolong a hospital stay approximately 6 to 8 days. In his extensive review of 23,649 operations, Cruse and Foord determined that the incidence of abdominal wound infection varied depending on risk factors; however, for abdominal hysterectomy the incidence was approximately 5%.

The pathophysiology of wound infection depends on an interaction of two factors: the number and virulence of bacterial contamination and the resistance of the patient. Inoculation of bacteria into the wound occurs in the operating room during the operative procedure. There is a wide spectrum of common, endogenous bacteria that produce wound infections, including most gram-positive cocci and both aerobic and anaerobic rods. Small numbers of bacteria are present in all surgical wounds; however, bacterial growth is facilitated by decreased tissue oxygen and excessive amounts of necrotic tissue.

Both local and systemic factors contribute to the level of host resistance and thus to the incidence of wound infections. Local factors are more significant and include the presence of hematomas, necrotic tissue, foreign bodies, dead space, use of cautery, and decreased local tissue perfusion. Systemic factors include obesity, diabetes, liver disease, malnutrition, immunosuppression, defects in the reticuloendothelial system, age, and the duration of preoperative hospitalization. Pitkin discovered that the incidence of postoperative wound infection is increased eightfold when the woman's preoperative weight exceeds 200 pounds. Corticosteroid therapy may deplete systemic protein and suppress the inflammatory phase of the healing process. However, after the first 5 days of wound healing, corticosteroid therapy has no effect on an uninfected wound.

The first symptom of most wound infections appears between the fifth and the tenth postoperative day. Wound infection may occur as late as several months following surgery, but more than 90% of cases present within the first

2 weeks of the postoperative period. The first sign is usually fever, followed by tachycardia and varying degrees of increased tenderness or pain. As the infection progresses, many wounds develop areas that are either fluctuant or firm, and some develop crepitus. The incision is swollen, erythematous, edematous, and tender. Later in the course of the infection there may be associated spontaneous purulent drainage from the wound.

Fever during the first 24 to 48 hours is usually secondary to atelectasis. However, two rare types of wound infections are so virulent that they produce toxicity within the first 48 hours: those produced by *Clostridium* species and acute beta-hemolytic streptococcal infection. Clinically, wound infections secondary to beta-hemolytic streptococci appear swollen and red and have an odorless discharge. In contrast, infections secondary to *Clostridium* are boggy and edematous, and the discharge has a sweet odor.

Initial management consists of opening and drainage of the wound. On removal of the skin sutures or skin clips the wound opens easily. Gram stain and both aerobic and anaerobic cultures of the wound should be obtained at this point. These initial cultures are most valuable if the patient does not respond to initial management. In such cases the differential diagnosis would be between infections involving deeper tissue planes and infection for which host resistance has failed even after drainage of the wound.

Once a wound infection has been opened and drained, care is directed toward initial packing of the wound with gauze to effect debridement and periodic irrigation. Rarely are antibiotics needed, unless there is a surrounding cellulitis. Most women with a wound infection will become afebrile within 72 hours after the wound has been opened and debrided.

Prevention is the foundation of any approach to the management of wound infections. Prevention involves consideration of both local and systemic factors, which if unattended, predispose to infection. Prophylactic antibiotics, especially in high-risk cases, definitely decrease the incidence of wound infection. If the wound is grossly contaminated, then delayed primary closure on the third or fourth postoperative day is appropriate. In a small series, Brown et al. reported that the latter technique reduced the incidence of wound infection from 23% in a control group to 2% in the group having delayed closure.

A virulent, rapidly progressing form of soft tissue wound infection is necrotizing fasciitis. This extremely rare but potentially fatal condition necessitates wide debridement of all necrotic tissue, high levels of systemic antibiotics, and sometimes hyperbaric oxygen. Stamenkovic and Lew have suggested the use of frozen section biopsy to help establish the early diagnosis of this condition.

Dehiscence and Evisceration

Dehiscence is a failure of normal healing and literally means disruption of any of the layers of a surgical incision. Clinically, dehiscence usually means that the incision of the skin, subcutaneous tissue, and fascia has separated, but not the peritoneum, usually during the first 2 postoperative weeks. Evisceration is a complete breakdown of the healing process through all levels of the abdominal incision with omentum or bowel presenting through the incision. The incidence of wound dehiscence is approximately 1 in 200 gynecologic operations. The major short-term result of wound dehiscence is the prolongation of hospital stay. Over the long term, dehiscence predisposes to incisional hernias. Wound infection is present in approximately 50% of women with wound disruption. As with wound infections, preventive management is the most important therapeutic consideration. The incidence of dehiscence has decreased with the introduction of synthetic absorbable sutures, such as Dexon and Vicryl (Table 24-14). They are superior to catgut in their more predictable absorption, reduction of tissue reaction, and greater tensile strength (Table 24-15).

Poole has reviewed the literature concerning prevention of disruption of fascial closure. The consensus of authorities is that local factors are much more important in the pathophysiology of wound disruption than systemic factors, although both should be considered in preventive management. Important mechanical factors predisposing to disruption are conditions that increase the tension on the incision line, such as abdominal distension and chronic lung

TABLE 24-14
Classification of Suture Material

Type	Generic Name	Raw Material	Trade Names
Absorbable			
Natural collagen	Plain catgut	Submucosa of sheep intestine	—
	Chromic catgut	+ Buffered chromicizing	—
Synthetics	Polyglycolic acid	Homopolymer of glycolide	Dexon, Dexon-S, Dexon-Plus
		+ Poloxamer 188 coating	
	Polyglactin 910	Copolymer lactic and glycolic acid	Vicryl
		+ Calcium stearate coating	Coated Vicryl
	Polydioxanone	Monofilament	PDS
Nonabsorbable			
Natural fiber	Surgical cotton	Twisted natural cotton	—
	Surgical silk	Braided protein, natural spun by silk worm	—
Synthetics	Nylon	Polyamide polymer	—
		Monofilament	Dermalon, Ethilon
		Multifilament	Neurolon
		Multifilament-silicone treated	Surgilon
	Polypropylene	Polymer of polypropylene	—
		Monofilament	Surgilene, Prolene, NovaFil
	Polybutester		
	Polyethylene	Thermoplastic synthetic resin	Dermalene
	Polyester	Polyethylene terephthalate-multifilament	
		Braided-plain	Dacron, Mersilene
		Braided-silicone treated	Ti-Cron
		Braided-polybutilate coated	Ethibond
		Braided-PFTE* (Teflon) coated	Polydek, Ethiflex
		Braided-heavy PFTE (Teflon) impregnated	Tevdek
Metal	Stainless steel wire	Ferrous alloy	—
		Twisted multistrand	Flexon
		Monofilament strand	—
	Silver wire	Silver wire	—

From Sanz L, Smith S: Mechanisms of wound healing, suture material, and wound closure. In Buchsbaum HJ, Walton LA, eds: Strategies in gynecologic surgery. New York, Springer-Verlag, 1986, p. 62.
*Polytetrafluoroethylene.

TABLE 24-15
Qualities of Absorbable Sutures

Type	Knot Security	Tensile Strength	Wound Security
Gut	+	+ +	5-7 days (50%)
Chromic	+ +	+ +	10-14 days (50%)
Dexon*	+ + + +	+ + + +	25 days (50%)
Vicryl†	+ + +	+ + + +	30 days (50%)

From Sanz L, Smith S: Mechanisms of wound healing, suture material, and wound closure. In Buchsbaum HJ, Walton LA, eds: Strategies in gynecologic surgery. New York, Springer-Verlag, 1986, p. 63.
*Polyglycolic acid.
†Polyglactin 910.

disease. Other factors are obesity, the patient's age, malignant disease, prior radiation therapy, and whether the incision is made through an area of a previous incision. Malt has shown that whether an incision is horizontal or vertical has little effect on the incidence of wound disruption. The pathophysiology of fascial dehiscence involves exaggerated collagen lysis in the wound. Clinically the sutures "tear through the fascia" rather than dissolving or becoming "untied."

The classic symptom and sign of an impending wound disruption is the spontaneous passage of serosanguineous fluid from the abdominal incision. Most often this occurs between the fifth and eighth postoperative days. Patients with uninfected wounds generally have been asymptomatic.

Imperative for prevention of wound dehiscence is proper closure of the incision in a woman at high risk for anything less than optimum healing. Although there are many regional preferences for the choice of suture and method of closure, the most popular technique is the Smead-Jones closure with permanent suture (Fig. 24-7). Closure with the Smead-Jones technique results in a dehiscence rate of approximately 1 in 1000 operations. With this technique it is important to place individual sutures at least 1 to 1.5 cm away from the adjacent sutures and include at least 2 cm of fascia on either side of the incision. The alternate technique is a mass closure using a monifilament permanent suture material such as nylon

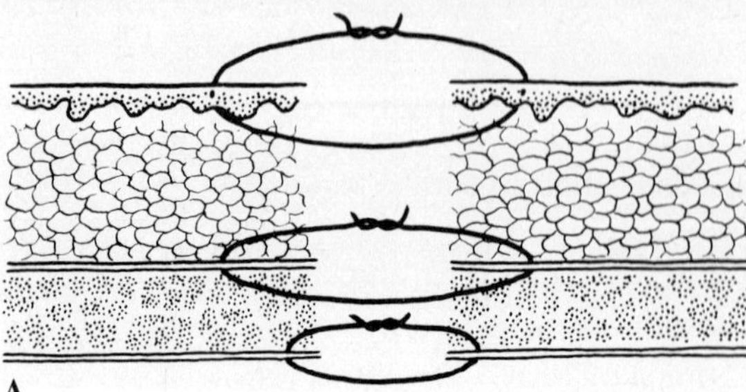

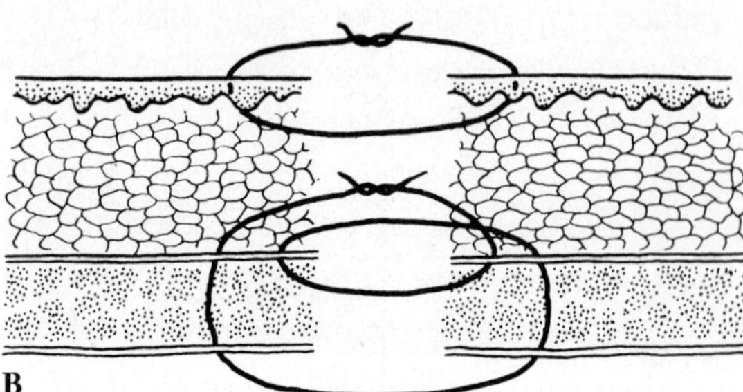

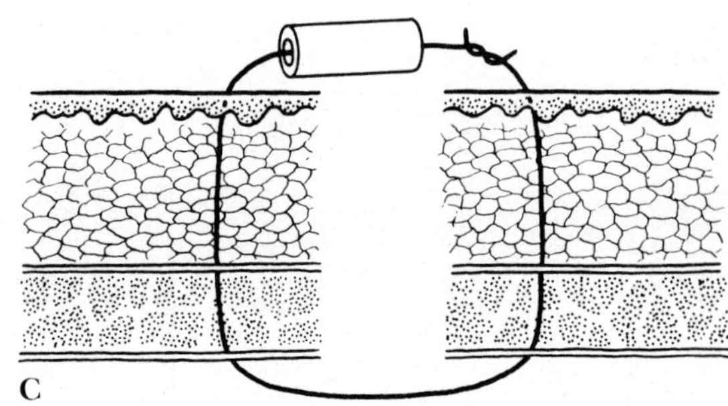

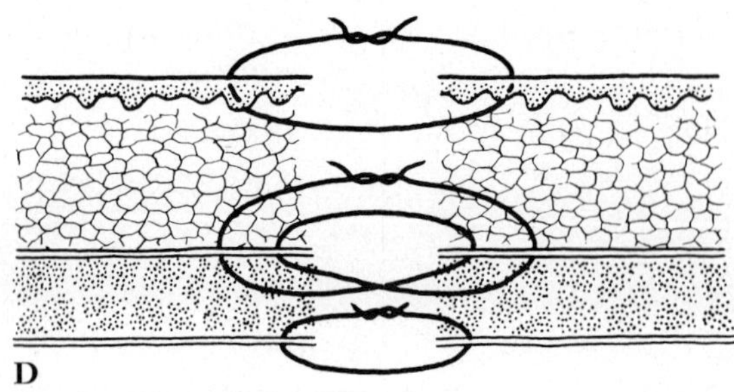

FIGURE 24-7
Types of abdominal incision closures. **A,** Layered. **B,** Smead-Jones. **C,** Through-and-through. **D,** Far-near. (From Braun TE: Wound dehiscence. In Schaefer G, Graber EA, eds: Complications in obstetric and gynecological surgery. Hagerstown, Md, Harper & Row, Publishers, 1981, p. 159.)

or polypropylene (Proline). Delayed primary wound closure 3 to 5 days after the operation should be considered if the wound was contaminated during the procedure, such as with rupture of a tuboovarian abscess. Delayed closure should also be considered for any patient already at high risk for wound complications, such as the malnourished patient, the diabetic patient, or the woman who is immunosuppressed.

The treatment of wound disruption depends on the size and the depth of the defect. Similar to the management of wound infections, digital examination of the defect is important so that the full extent of the problem will be recognized. With larger defects the wound edges must be debrided and the wound closed with the Smead-Jones or mass closure technique.

OPERATIVE SITE COMPLICATIONS

Pelvic Cellulitis and Abscess

Infections of the contiguous retroperitoneal space immediately above the vaginal apex are common complications following abdominal or vaginal hysterectomy. These soft tissue infections range in severity from localized, minor cellulitis to large pelvic abscesses and have many names from "cuff cellulitis" to "infected hematoma." Nevertheless they are similar to soft tissue infections in other parts of the body and are either a cellulitis or an abscess. These infections prolong hospital stay and increase the cost of patient care. The bacterial spectrum that produces these infections includes aerobic and anaerobic bacteria from both exogenous and endogenous sources. Most postoperative pelvic infections are polymicrobial, usually from endogenous vaginal flora, and approximately 60% to 80% involve anaerobic organisms.

The pathophysiology of development of retroperitoneal infection is straightforward. The normal hysterectomy site produces an average of 40 ml of serosanguineous fluid each day during the first 72 postoperative hours. The endogenous flora of the upper vagina colonize and multiply in this retroperitoneal serosanguineous fluid or in pelvic hematomas after the operation.

The major symptoms of an operative site infection are fever and lower quadrant abdominal and pelvic pain. The fever usually becomes prominent between the third and fifth postoperative days. As the infection becomes more severe, the fever becomes spiking in character, the pain intensifies, and the patient develops moderate leukocytosis.

The diagnosis of cuff cellulitis is confirmed by pelvic examination. Pelvic tenderness and induration are prominent during the bimanual examination. Cuff cellulitis sometimes responds to drainage, by opening of the vaginal cuff. Appropriate cultures of the site are difficult with cellulitis because of surface contamination. Both persistent cellulitis, or one encompassing a large area, and abscess necessitate parenteral antibiotic therapy. Because of their polymicrobial etiology the infections are usually treated with an aminoglycocide (gentamicin 2 mg/kg intravenously followed by 1.5 mg/kg intravenously every 8 hours in patients with normal renal function) and an antibiotic specific for anaerobic infection (clindamycin 900 mg intravenously every 8 hours). It is important with an aminoglycoside to obtain peak and trough levels. They should be obtained 30 minutes after intravenous injection or 1 hour after intramuscular injection and 30 minutes before the next dose of the drug. Peak levels should be approximately 8 μg/ml of gentamicin and trough levels less than 2 μg/ml. The prevalance of aminoglycoside toxicity is 2% to 3%, and approximately 25% of women will require an adjustment in intravenous dosage. It is important to obtain peak and trough levels after 24 hours of antibiotic therapy and approximately every 3 to 4 days thereafter.

Although many pelvic abscesses drain spontaneously, patients should have serial pelvic examinations to determine the necessity of or most appropriate time to effect operative drainage. Appropriate cultures should be obtained from the center of an abscess cavity when the abscess is operatively incised. If a patient does not become afebrile within 48 hours of proper drainage of a retroperitoneal abscess, a concomitant complication of pelvic thrombophlebitis should be suspected. The appropriate management is a 72-hour trial of intravenous heparin therapy.

Granulation Tissue

Granulation tissue at the apex of the vaginal vault is a frequent complication following abdominal hysterectomy. Small areas of friable, red granulation tissue are seen at the 6-week postoperative pelvic examination in more than 50% of women. Granulation tissue is more common following abdominal than vaginal hysterectomy and is more frequently found when the vaginal cuff is left open rather than closed.

Excessive granulation tissue is the result of an exaggerated healing response of the vascular-rich pelvic tissues. One of the causes is believed to be inversion of the vaginal epithelium between the margins of the edges of the incision at the apex of the vaginal vault.

Most patients are asymptomatic, but some women experience a slight bloody discharge after intercourse. The rare patient may have mild pelvic discomfort. On speculum examination the granulation tissue appears as a polypoid projection hanging from the vaginal suture line. The differential diagnosis includes a prolapsed fallopian tube and recurrent carcinoma in a patient with a pelvic malignancy. The polypoid mass is easily avulsed from the vaginal apex. The remaining areas of granulation tissue should be treated with a chemical cautery (silver nitrate or Monsel's solution) or by cryocautery or electrocautery.

Prolapsed Fallopian Tube

Prolapse of the distal end of the fallopian tube is a rare complication of abdominal or vaginal hysterectomy. It is usually discovered during a routine visit during the first few months following the operation.

Many women with this complication are free of symptoms, but others experience a watery discharge, postcoital spotting, or moderate lower abdominal and pelvic pain. Differing from granulation tissue, the fallopian tube is not friable and is firmly attached. The fallopian tube may be removed during an outpatient procedure using conduction anesthesia. Most clinicians opt for a vaginal approach with ligation of the fallopian tube as high as possible. The stump of the tube is buried retroperitoneally and the vaginal epithelium closed. An alternate treatment is coagulation of the segment of fallopian tube protruding through the vaginal

apex with cryocautery. Often the vaginal wall reepithelializes over the area, thereby excluding the tube from any connection with the vaginal cavity.

MISCELLANEOUS COMPLICATIONS

Lymphocyst

A lymphocyst is a local collection of lymphatic fluid within the pelvis resulting from retrograde drainage of lymph. It is a rare complication, found most frequently after pelvic node dissections. In the past this complication occurred in approximately 20% of patients having undergone radical operations. However, with meticulous attention to ligation of distal lymphatic channels and routine postoperative suction drainage of the retroperitoneal space, this complication is now reported in only 1% to 3% of such cases. Conditions that predispose the patient to formation of a lymphocyst are previous radiation and anticoagulation.

Lymphocysts usually present during the first 4 postoperative weeks. The cyst begins anterior and medial to the iliac vessels. As it expands, it may produce obstruction of the ureter or pressure symptoms on the bladder. Small lymphocysts, less than 4 cm in diameter, are usually asymptomatic and regress spontaneously. Larger cysts necessitate treatment either by intermittent aspiration followed by pressure dressings or insertion of an indwelling catheter under ultrasound guidance. Simple incision and drainage is usually unsuccessful as the condition recurs. Choo et al. have advised peritoneal marsupialization for lymphocysts that do not respond to traditional operative management.

Ovarian Abscess

Ovarian abscess is a rare but serious postoperative complication. If the diagnosis is not established, this condition is potentially fatal because of intraperitoneal rupture of the abscess. Ovarian abscesses arise from bacterial colonization of the ovarian cortex. This may occur either via disruption of the ovarian capsule by the presence of a corpus luteum or via an operative disruption such as cystectomy performed during vaginal hysterectomy.

The disease may follow either a slow, indolent course or a rapidly progressive one. Some patients with this complication present during the first postoperative week with a high fever and severe pain, which is continuous until rupture occurs. Others become afebrile following the operation but return sometime during the first few months with a persistent low-grade fever and mild pain. Willson and Black in a classic work describing 28 patients with ovarian abscess noted that the predominant symptom was abdominal pain associated with persistent tachycardia and high fever.

Initial treatment is medical therapy with intravenous antibiotics; however, most patients do not respond to medical therapy, and operative removal of the adnexa becomes a necessity. This rare problem should be considered in any woman having a gynecologic operation in which the integrity of the ovarian capsule is disrupted either physiologically or operatively.

Femoral Neuropathy

The femoral nerve is the largest branch of the lumbar plexus and arises from the primary rami of L2, L3, and L4. It provides motor function to several leg muscles, including the quadriceps, and sensory fibers that innervate the anterior and medial surfaces of the thigh and leg. The vascular supply to the femoral nerve may be compromised during an abdominal or vaginal hysterectomy. Rosenblum et al. have described the pathophysiology of this complication as being secondary to continuous pressure, usually by a self-retaining retractor producing ischemic necrosis of the nerve. The vascular circulation of the nerve itself is compromised by diminished blood flow in the vaso nervosa. The most common site of nerve compression is 4 to 6 cm above the inguinal ligament where the nerve pierces the psoas muscle. Factors that contribute to the development of this complication are thinness, long retractor blades, prolonged operative time, and diabetes mellitus. A similar problem may develop following vaginal operations in thin women with exaggerated hip flexion or abduction in the lithotomy position.

Patients with this complication may experience numbness, paresthesias, and difficulty with their gait. These symptoms are causes of great anxiety to the patient. Because of the inability to lift the leg, climbing stairs is a particular problem. The muscle and sensory function recovers spontaneously over several weeks to several months. To prevent this complication, it is important to palpate the lateral pelvic wall and femoral artery after placement of a self-retaining retractor. In a thin patient, placing folded towels between the skin surface and the self-retaining retractor helps to prevent this complication by decreasing the depth of penetration of the lateral retractor blades.

ESTROGEN REPLACEMENT

Bilateral salpingo-oophorectomy is often performed on young women for conditions such as pelvic inflammatory disease. National surveys have documented that bilateral castration concomitant with hysterectomy is performed in approximately 25% of premenopausal women undergoing this operation. The possible consequences of estrogen deprivation include vasomotor symptoms, urogenital tissue atrophy (atrophic vaginitis, dyspareunia, and urethral syndrome), and osteoporosis. For premenopausal women an additional risk of castration is the development of atherosclerotic heart disease at an earlier age than for a woman with normal ovarian function. The pathophysiology of premature coronary vascular disease is complex and multifactorial, but the change in the ratio of high-density lipoproteins (HDLs) to low-density lipoproteins (LDLs) is a critical factor.

Estrogen replacement is indicated in the vast majority of premenopausal women having bilateral oophorectomy. The increase in hypercoagulability produced by the doses of estrogen used for postmenopausal symptoms is negligible. Nevertheless, because of the hypercoagulability and injury to the intima of vessels associated with the operative procedure, high dose estrogen therapy should not be started immediately after the procedure. A dosage of 0.625 mg of conjugated estrogens daily is sufficient to protect from bone demineralization and osteoporosis. A higher dose may be required to alleviate hot flushes (see Chapter 40). All patients should continue estrogen therapy until age 50. The decision for further therapy after age 50 must be made on an individual basis.

PSYCHOLOGICAL COMPLICATIONS

Pain Relief

The proper management of pain during the postoperative period is a primary goal of all surgeons. Most women experience moderate to severe pain during the first 36 to 48 hours following a gynecologic operation. However, pain and suffering are personal, internal events, the extent and presence of which may only be measured by direct communication with the patient.

For many patients who undergo gynecologic operations, dosages of analgesics are prescribed that are less than adequate to relieve pain, and many nurses further reduce the amount of medication. White has presented a schematic diagram of the pain cycle and the potential delays in pain relief with traditional "prn" analgesic regimens (Fig. 24-8). Many studies have confirmed that regular interval preventive pain relief is superior to conventional "on demand" analgesic medication during the first 36 to 48 hours following the operation. Relative potencies of common analgesic medications are listed in Table 24-16. However, there is great variability in absorption. In addition, the therapeutic window (the range of effective blood concentration before undesired side effects occur) is narrow. When 100 mg of meperidine hydrochloride (Demerol) is given every 4 hours intramuscularly, the concentration of the drug in the blood exceeds the minimum level necessary to produce adequate pain relief only 35% of the 4-hour period (Table 24-17).

In White's study, peak concentrations varied as much as fivefold among the 10 different individuals, and the time to reach peak blood level varied as much as sevenfold. Thus patient-controlled analgesic systems will probably be the preferred method of pain relief during the immediate postoperative period in the future.

After the first 48 hours, pain relief may be successfully controlled with prostaglandin synthetase inhibitors. Morrison et al. reported in a study of 161 women that 50 mg of flurbiprofen (Ansaid) was as effective as 10 mg of intramuscular morphine for postoperative gynecologic pain. This oral medication was as effective in pain intensity scores, duration of pain relief, and clinical appreciation of pain by the patients.

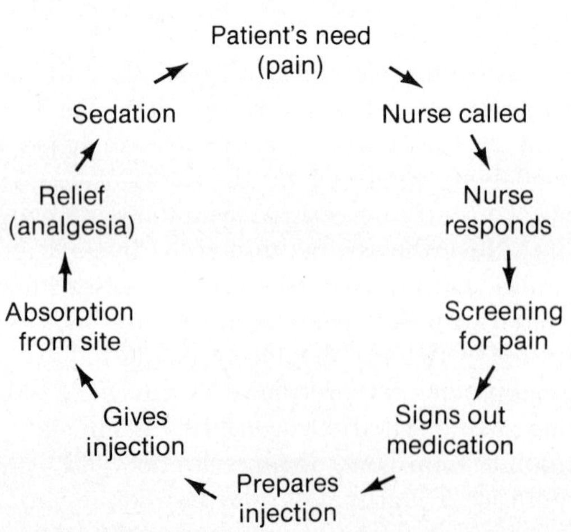

FIGURE 24-8
Pain cycle. (From White PF: Postgrad Med 80:8, 1986.)

TABLE 24-16
Relative* Potencies of Analgesics (mg/mg)

	Intramuscular	Oral
Alphaprodine	45	—
Buprenorphine	2.5-5	0.4 (sublingual)
Butorphanol	2-3	—
Codeine	130	200
Fentanyl	0.125	—
Heroin	4	—
Hydromorphone	1.5	7.5
Levorphanol	2	4
Meperidine	75	300
Methadone	10	20
Morphine	10	30-60
Nalbuphine	10	—
Oxycodone	10	30
Pentazocine	60	180
Propoxyphene	240	300
Sufentanil	0.0125	—

From Gorman ES, Warfield CA: The use of opioids in the management of pain. Hosp Prac 21:48B, 1986.
*To 10 mg morphine, intramuscular.

TABLE 24-17

Blood Meperidine Concentrations After Intramuscular Administration of 100 mg
Every 4 Hours in 10 Patients

	Peak Level (μg/ml)	Time to Peak Level (min)	Minimum Analgesic Concentration* (μg/ml)	Time Level Exceeded Minimum Analgesic Concentration* (min)
Initial Postoperative Injections				
Mean	0.51	57	0.43	42
Range	0.24-0.82	18-108	0.26-0.85	0-240
SD	0.14	27	0.14	57
Second Postoperative Day				
Mean	0.77	39	0.49	150
Range	0.51-1.21	18-108	0.28-0.66	54-240
SD	0.23	24	0.10	72

From White PF: Pain management (special report). Postgrad Med 80:9, 1986.
*Minimum analgesic concentration refers to the minimum level required to provide adequate pain relief.

Psychosexual Problems and Depression

Any operation on the female reproductive organs stimulates questions and conflicts concerning body image, feminine identity, sexuality, and possibly future childbearing. The period following a gynecologic operation is one of transition and is a unique psychological challenge to the patient. The reader should review Chapter 7 to emphasize the problems of loss and grief and the four stages of depression: impact, retreat, acknowledgment, and reconstitution. After gynecologic operations every patient needs support to overcome this challenge, and it is important to emphasize that it may take many months to complete the process.

KEY POINTS

- Postoperative febrile morbidity is related to infection in approximately 20% of cases and noninfectious causes in 80% of cases.

- Atelectasis is the cause of more than 90% of cases of postoperative fever presenting in the first 48 hours.

- The normal physiologic response to the stress of an operation and tissue destruction is release of increased levels of antidiuretic hormone and aldosterone, producing both sodium and water retention.

- Because of the shifts in water balance the postoperative hematocrit at 72 hours is a more accurate measurement of operative and postoperative blood loss than a hematocrit at 24 hours.

______________ **KEY POINTS, cont'd** ______________

- After subtracting the effects of the operative blood loss from the preoperative hematocrit, a further reduction in hematocrit of 3 to 5 points reflects a postoperative hemorrhage of approximately 500 ml.

- Factors that predispose patients to atelectasis include supine position, obesity, smoking, age greater than 60 years, prolonged operative time, and coexisting medical conditions such as cardiac disease or pulmonary infection.

- The clinical presentation of fever, tachypnea, and tachycardia within 72 hours of an operation is pathognomonic for atelectasis.

- Postoperative pneumonia is commonly associated with atelectasis with predisposing factors including chronic pulmonary disease, heavy cigarette smoking, obesity, older age, nasogastric tubes, long procedures, and debilitating illnesses.

- The differential diagnosis of hemorrhagic shock in the postoperative patient includes pneumothorax, pulmonary embolus, massive pulmonary aspiration, myocardial infarction, and acute gastric dilation.

- In the healthy reproductive age female, because of normal adaptive changes, it takes a rapid loss of approximately one third of the blood volume to produce significant hypotension.

- The goals of management of shock are to replace and restore effective circulating blood volume and to establish normal cellular perfusion and oxygenation.

- The extent of wound or pelvic hematomas is determined by the potential size of the compartment into which the bleeding occurs. Retroperitoneal or broad ligament hematomas may contain several units of blood.

- Generally, thromboembolic complications occur early in the postoperative course, with 75% occurring within the first 72 hours. Approximately 15% occur after the seventh postoperative day.

- The incidence of fatal pulmonary emboli following gynecologic operations is between 0.1% and 0.8%.

- Operative repair of a urinary tract fistula should be delayed 2 to 6 months after the initial injury to obtain optimum results. Preoperative workup of such an injury includes intravenous pyelography, cystoscopy, and biopsy of the margins if carcinoma is suspected.

- Superficial thrombophlebitis is a frequent problem both in the lower extremities and along intravenous catheter sites. The finding of superficial thrombophlebitis does not rule out concomitant inflammation in the deep veins.

- The clinical management of mild superficial thrombophlebitis includes rest, elevation, and local heat. Moderate to severe superficial thrombophlebitis may be treated with nonsteroidal antiinflammatory agents.

- The incidence of thrombophlebitis is directly dependent on the risk factors of type and duration of operation, age of the patient, obesity, immobility, malignancy, sepsis, diabetes, and conditions producing venous stasis.

- Thrombophlebitis most often begins in the deep veins of the calf. Approximately 75% of pulmonary emboli originate from a thrombus that begins in the leg veins and extends to the femoral veins.

- If thrombophlebitis affects one leg, the other leg is involved in approximately 33% of women.

- The three precipitating factors that produce thrombi as described by Virchow are an increase in coagulability, damage to the vessel wall, and venous stasis.

- Venography is the gold standard for detecting deep vein thrombophlebitis.

- Recently published guidelines from the NIH Consensus suggest that low-risk patients under 40 years of age who undergo an operation of less than 30 minutes' duration need early ambulation and compression stocking for prophylaxis for deep vein thrombophlebitis. Women at moderate to high risk should be treated with low-dose heparin, dextran, or external pneumatic compression for prophylaxis.

- Low-dose heparin (5000 IU given 2 hours before and every 8 to 12 hours after operation) reduces the incidence of deep vein thrombophlebitis.

________________ **KEY POINTS, cont'd** ________________

- External pneumatic compression of the legs by pneumatic inflated sleeve devices is as effective as low-dose heparin in the prevention of deep vein thrombophlebitis. It is approximately equal in cost.

- Heparin is the drug of choice for the initial treatment of thrombosis or pulmonary embolus once the diagnosis is confirmed. An IV bolus of 5000 IU is given initially, after which an infusion of 1000 to 1500 IU per hour is appropriate.

- Patients with pulmonary emboli have a mortality rate of 30% in untreated cases versus 8% in treated cases.

- Signs and symptoms of pulmonary emboli are nonspecific; however, a national study found the most common to include chest pain, dyspnea, apprehension, tachypnea, rales, and an increase in the second heart sound over the pulmonic area.

- Ventilation-perfusion scans are the first line in imaging techniques to rule out the diagnosis of pulmonary embolus. However, pulmonary angiography is the most definitive test in establishing the diagnosis. Five percent of patients experience complications from pulmonary angiography.

- The etiology of postoperative voiding problems includes anxiety, mechanical interference, obstruction by swelling and edema, neurologic imbalance, and tranquilizer-associated detrusor hypotonia.

- The most commonly acquired infection in the hospital and most frequent cause of gram-negative bacteremia in hospitalized patients is catheter-associated urinary tract infection.

- The incidence of positive urine culture after a single in-and-out catheterization is 4%. When a Foley catheter has been in place for 36 hours, approximately 20% of women have bacterial colonization. After 72 hours of catheterization, 75% of patients will have positive cultures.

- Prophylactic antibiotics should not be used with a Foley catheter to cover for the possibility of urinary tract infection unless the patient is immunocompromised.

- Fistulas following gynecologic operations are secondary to abdominal hysterectomy in 75% and to vaginal procedures in the remaining 25%.

- Although symptoms of urinary incontinence may present within a few hours of the operative procedure, the majority of fistulas usually present 8 to 12 days after operation, occasionally as late as 25 to 30 days after operation.

- If there is a suspicion that trauma to the bladder has occurred during an operative procedure, continuous catheter drainage for 3 to 5 days will often result in spontaneous healing of multiple defects.

- Approximately 20% of bladder injuries and 30% of ureteral injuries heal spontaneously without further operation if adequate drainage is obtained.

- Major factors that result in intensification of adynamic ileus include peritoneal contamination by purulent material or blood, extensive handling of the small intestine, and inadequate replacement of fluids and electrolytes.

- Predisposing factors to the development of ileus include obesity, age of the patient, preoperative immobility, and removal of large pelvic and abdominal masses.

- Previous gynecologic operations are the most common cause of bowel obstruction in women.

- Pneumoperitoneum from an exploratory celiotomy usually persists for 7 to 10 days; thus after operation, free air under the diaphragm is not diagnostic of perforation of a viscus.

- The foundation of early treatment of postoperative intestinal obstruction is decompression of the small intestine, accomplished by nasogastric tube or, preferably, a long tube.

- The etiology of rectovaginal fistula includes gynecologic operations, carcinoma, radiation therapy, perirectal abscess, inflammatory bowel disease, lymphogranuloma venereum, and trauma.

KEY POINTS, cont'd

- Postoperative fistulas between the rectum and vagina usually present 7 to 14 days after the procedure.

- After the diagnosis of a rectovaginal fistula has been made, the patient should be obstipated with a low-residue diet and diphenoxylate hydrochloride (Lomotil). Approximately one in four anatomic defects heals spontaneously before epithelialization of the tract.

- Most repairs of rectovaginal fistulas should not be undertaken until 8 to 12 weeks after the operation. The area surrounding the fistula should be free of edema, induration, and infection.

- Symptoms of wound infections occur most commonly between the fifth and tenth postoperative day, with the patient usually exhibiting tachycardia and fever.

- The incidence of wound dehiscence is approximately 1 in 200 gynecologic operations. Wound infection is found in approximately 50% of women with wound disruption.

- The classic symptom and sign of an impending wound disruption is the spontaneous passage of serosanguineous fluid from the abdominal incision.

- Granulation tissue at the vaginal vault apex often appears as friable, red, polypoid tissue at the 6-week postoperative check. This tissue may be treated with chemical cautery, cryocautery, or electrocautery.

- Ovarian abscesses arise from bacterial colonization of a disrupted ovarian capsule, usually by the presence of a corpus luteum or by surgical disruption during a procedure.

- Common causes of femoral neuropathy are continuous pressure from self-retaining retractors or exaggerated hip flexion or abduction from the lithotomy position in thin women.

- After the first 36 to 48 hours, postoperative pain may be successfully controlled with prostaglandin synthetase inhibitors.

BIBLIOGRAPHY

American College of Obstetricians and Gynecologists: Blood component therapy. ACOG Tech Bull 78:1,1984.

Arieff AI: Hyponatremia, convulsions, respiratory arrest, and permanent brain damage after elective surgery in healthy women. N Engl J Med 314:1529, 1986.

Bandy LC, Addison A, Parker RT: Surgical management of rectovaginal fistulas in Crohn's disease. Am J Obstet Gynecol 147:359, 1983.

Batres F, Barclay DL: Sciatic nerve injury during gynecologic procedures using the lithotomy position. Obstet Gynecol 62:92S, 1983.

Blinder RA, Coleman RE: Evaluation of pulmonary embolism. Radiol Clin North Am 23:391, 1985.

Bonnar J: Venous thromboembolism and gynecologic surgery. Clin Obstet Gynecol 28:432, 1985.

Bourke DL: Errors in intraoperative hematocrit determination. Anesthesiology 45:357, 1976.

Breitenbucher RB: Bacterial changes in the urine samples of patients with long-term indwelling catheters. Arch Intern Med 144:1585, 1984.

Brown SE, Allen HH, Robins RN: The use of delayed primary wound closure in preventing wound infections. Am J Obstet Gynecol 127:713, 1977.

Buchsbaum HJ, Walton LA, eds: Strategies in gynecologic surgery. New York, Springer-Verlag, 1986.

Choo YC, Wong LC, Wong KP, et al: The management of intractable lymphocyst following radical hysterectomy. Gynecol Oncol 24:309, 1986.

Clarke DB, Abrams LD: Pulmonary embolectomy: A 25 year experience. J Thorac Cardiovasc Surg 92:442, 1986.

Clarke-Pearson DL, DeLong ER, Synan IS, et al: Complications of low-dose heparin prophylaxis in gynecologic oncology surgery. Obstet Gynecol 64:689, 1984.

Clarke-Pearson DL, Synan IS, Colemen RE, et al: The natural history of postoperative venous thromboembli in gynecologic oncology: A prospective study of 382 patients. Am J Obstet Gynecol 148:1051, 1984.

Clarke-Pearson DL, Synan IS, Hinshaw WM, et al: Prevention of postoperative venous thromboembolism by external pneumatic calf compression in patients with gynecologic malignancy. Obstet Gynecol 63:92, 1984.

Condon RE, DeCosse J, eds: Surgical Care II. Philadelphia, Lea & Febiger, 1985.

Consensus Conference: Prevention of venous thrombosis and pulmonary embolism. JAMA 256:744, 1986.

Coon WW: Venous thromboembolism. Clin Chest Med 5:391, 1984.

Creasman WT, Henderson D, Hinshaw W, et al: Estrogen replacement therapy in the patient treated for endometrial cancer. Obstet Gynecol 67:326, 1986.

Cruse PJE, Foord R: A five year prospective study of 23,649 surgical wounds. Arch Surg 107:206, 1973.

Cruse PJE, Foord R: The epidemiology of wound infection. Surg Clin North Am 60:27, 1980.

Daifuku R, Stamm WE: Association of rectal and urethral colonization with urinary tract infection in patients with indwelling catheters. JAMA 252:2028, 1984.

Dalen JE, Paraskos JA, Ockene IS, et al: Venous thromboembolism. Chest 89:370S, 1986.

Dudrick SJ, Baue AE, Eiseman B, et al, eds: Manual of preoperative and postoperative care, 3rd ed. Philadelphia, W.B. Saunders Co., 1983.

Duff GW: Is fever beneficial to the host: A clinical perspective. Yale J Biol Med 59:125, 1986.

Dunn LJ, Van Voorhis LW: Enigmatic fever and pelvic thrombophlebitis. N Engl J Med 276:265, 1967.

Fry DE, Milholen L, Harbrecht PJ: Iatrogenic ureteral injury. Arch Surg 118:454, 1983.

Fulkerson WJ, Coleman E, Ravin CF, et al: Diagnosis of pulmonary embolism. Arch Intern Med 146:961, 1986.

Gallup DG: Modifications of celiotomy techniques to decrease morbidity in obese gynecologic patients. Am J Obstet Gynecol 150:171, 1984.

Garcia CR, Cutler WB: Preservation of the ovary: A reevaluation. Fertil Steril 42:510, 1984.

Garibaldi RA, Burke JP, Dickman ML, et al: Factors predisposing to bacteriuria during indwelling urethral catheterization. N Engl J Med 291:215, 1974.

Georgy FM: Femoral neuropathy following abdominal hysterectomy. Am J Obstet Gynecol 123:819, 1975.

Goldman DR, Brown FH, Levy WK, et al, eds: Medical care of the surgical patient. Philadelphia, J.B. Lippincott Co., 1982.

Gorman ES, Warfield CA: The use of opioids in the management of pain. Hosp Prac 20:48A, 1986.

Hall R: Difficulties in the treatment of acute pulmonary embolism. Thorax 40:729, 1985.

Hardy JD, ed: Complications in surgery and their management, 4th ed. Phildelphia, W.B. Saunders Co., 1981.

Hassan AA, Reiff RH, Fayez JA: Femoral neuropathy following microsurgical tuboplasty. Fertil Steril 45:889, 1986.

Helmkamp BF: Abdominal wound dehiscence. Am J Obstet Gynecol 128:803, 1977.

Hemsell DL, Reisch J, Nobles B, et al: Prevention of major infection after elective abdominal hysterectomy: Individual determination required. Am J Obstet Gynecol 147:520, 1983.

Henriksson C, Kihl B, Pettersson S: Urethrovaginal and vesicovaginal fistula. Acta Obstet Gynecol Scand 61:143, 1982.

Hershey CO, Tomford JW, McLaren CE, et al: The natural history of intravenous catheter–associated phlebitis. Arch Intern Med 144:1373, 1984.

Hibbard LT: Surgical management of rectovaginal fistulas and complete perineal tears. Am J Obstet Gynecol 130:139, 1978.

Howkins J, Williams DK: Vault granulations after total abdominal hysterectomy. J Obstet Gynaecol Br Comm 75:84, 1968.

Huisman MV, Buller HR, TenCate JW, et al: Serial impedance plethysmography for suspected deep venous thrombosis in outpatients. N Engl J Med 314:823, 1986.

Hull RD, Raskob GE, Hirsch J: The diagnosis of clinically suspected pulmonary embolism. Chest 89:417S, 1986.

Hunt TK, ed: Wound healing and wound infection. New York, Appleton-Century-Crofts, 1980.

Hyers TM, Hull RD, Web JG: Antithrombotic therapy for venous thromboembolic disease. Chest 89:26S, 1986.

Jorgensen BC, Schmidt JF, Risbo A, et al: Regular interval preventive pain relief compared with on demand treatment after hysterectomy. Pain 21:137, 1985.

Kakkar VV: Pathophysiologic characteristics of venous thrombosis. Am J Surg 150:1, 1985.

Krebs HB: Intestinal injury in gynecologic surgery: A ten-year experience. Am J Obstet Gynecol 155:509, 1986.

Lubin MF, Walker HK, Smith RB, eds: Medical management of the surgical patient. Woburn, Mass., Butterworth, 1982.

Malt RA: Abdominal incisions, sutures and sacrilege. N Engl J Med 297:722, 1977.

McBride K, LaMorte WW, Menzoian JO: Can ventilation-perfusion scans accurately diagnose acute pulmonary embolism? Arch Surg 121:754, 1986.

Principles of Radiation Therapy and Chemotherapy in Gynecologic Cancer

KEY TERMS AND DEFINITIONS

Adoptive Immunotherapy. The use of extracts derived from sensitized lymphocytes to transfer "immunologic memory" and induce an antitumor response.

Alkylating Agent. A class of antineoplastic agents that covalently link (alkylation) with DNA, which inhibits the growth of dividing cells.

Antimetabolites. Antineoplastic agents that resemble naturally occurring purines or pyrimidines and interfere with normal cell metabolism.

Antitumor Antibiotic. Antineoplastic agents derived from bacterial or fungal cultures.

Beta Rays. Low-energy electron radiation produced by radionuclide decay.

Betatron. A circular accelerator for electrons for production of high energy.

Brachytherapy. A form of radiation therapy in which the source is placed close to the tumor. The application may be in the form of needles implanted into the tumor (interstitial) or placed in the vagina or cervical canal (internal).

Cellular Immunity. Cell-mediated immunity in which lymphoid cells directly react with foreign cells or antigens.

Complete Remission. Total disappearance of the tumor for at least 1 month.

Curie (Ci). A measure of the rate of disintegration of radioisotopes. One curie is equivalent to 3.7×10^{10} disintegrations per second.

Depth Dose. The specific dose of irradiation absorbed at a given distance beneath the surface.

Electron Volt. A unit of measurement of electromagnetic energy equivalent to 1.6×10^{-12} ergs. MeV = 1 million eV; keV = 1000 eV.

Fractionation. The practice of dividing radiation therapy treatments into numerous small doses to reduce damage to normal tissues.

Gamma Rays. A form of photon energy produced by the decay of radioactive isotopes.

Gray. A measurement of the dosage of radiation absorbed by tissue. 1 gray = 1 joule per kilogram (100 rads).

Growth Fraction. The proportion of tumor cells in a replicating phase.

Humoral Immunity. Antibody-mediated immunity resulting from antibodies produced in response to a variety of foreign antigens.

Interferon. A cell mediator that can be produced by lymphocytes or fibroblasts and that has an antiproliferative effect on tumor cells.

Isodose Curve. A curve connecting points that receive equivalent doses of irradiation.

Linear Accelerator. A machine that accelerates electrons in a straight line to produce high energy.

Linear Energy Transfer (LET). The measurement of the amount of energy transferred by ionizing radiation per unit of distance traveled.

Log Cell Kill. The proportion of cells killed by a particular treatment: 90% equals a 1-log cell kill; 99% equals a 2-log cell kill.

Objective Response. A greater than 50% reduction in the size of the tumor for at least 1 month.

Passive Immunity. The transfer of specific antibodies to try to increase the immune response.

Photons. Quanta of radiation whose energy is proportional to their frequency and inversely proportional to their wavelength (gamma rays and x-rays).

Progression. Increase in size or spread of tumor in a patient receiving therapy.

Rad. A measurement of the dose of radiation absorbed in tissue equivalent to 100 ergs per gram.

Radiocurability. The ability to cure a malignant tumor with radiation.

Radiosensitivity. The relative response of tumor cells to radiation.

Source-to-Skin Distance (SSD). The distance from the external radiation source to the skin of the patient receiving external therapy.

Stabilization. A term occasionally used to indicate that a tumor has not changed in size while a patient has been receiving therapy.

Systemic-Active Nonspecific Immunotherapy. Use of adjuvant agents, usually of microbiologic origin, to increase cellular and humoral immunity. Examples are bacillus Calmette-Guerin (BCG) and *Corynebacterium parvum* (C-Parvum).

Teletherapy. A form of radiation therapy with the placement of the radioactive source at a distance from the patient (external therapy).

Vinca Alkaloids. Antineoplastic agents derived from periwinkle plant *(Vinca rosea)* extracts.

X-ray. Electromagnetic radiation formed by accelerated electrons in a vacuum striking a target.

This chapter presents the general principles of radiation therapy and chemotherapy, with particular attention to those concepts, procedures, and drugs used to treat gynecologic cancers. The details of treatment of individual cancers are described separately in the various chapters dealing with specific gynecologic malignancies.

Included with the basic concepts of radiation physics are the types and measurements of radiation energy, the biologic effects of radiation on cells, and the factors that alter these effects. Common radiation sources and their properties are illustrated as they relate specifically to the treatment of gynecologic cancers. Risks and complications are also presented.

Cell growth and division are affected by cancerous processes and by chemotherapeutic treatments. The physician must know the various classes of chemotherapeutic agents, their actions in gynecologic malignancies, and their toxicities. There are also general approaches to be followed in administering chemotherapy, specifically including monitoring of patients receiving these agents. Finally, some newer techniques involving immunology offer promise in treating gynecologic cancers.

RADIATION THERAPY

Basic Radiation Physics

Radiation physics deals with the measurement of energy that is transferred from the source of the radiation to the tissues or cells being irradiated. One form of ionizing radiation is electromagnetic, which refers to x-rays or gamma rays. These sources of energy have no mass and no electrical charge. They are produced in discrete quanta or photons, and their energy is proportional to their frequency; that is, higher energies are transmitted at a higher frequency of electromagnetic radiation. Since the frequency of a photon is inversely proportional to the wavelength, electromagnetic radiation with shorter wavelengths has a higher frequency and thus a higher energy. The energy that is produced is measured in electron volts (eV); 1 eV = 1.6 × 10^{-12} ergs. Various x-ray radiotherapy units can range from 30,000 eV (30 kV) to over 30,000,000 eV (30 MV).

A second source of photon radiation comes from the production of gamma rays (similar to x-rays), which result from the decay of radioactive isotopes. Such decay or disintegration is measured in curies (Ci). One curie is defined as 3.7 × 10^{10} disintegrations per second, which is equivalent to the disintegration of 1 g of radium.

Regardless of the source of electromagnetic or photon radiation, the transmitted energy from the source diverges as the distance it travels from the source increases. This divergence causes a decrease in energy, and the relationship is described by the *inverse square law,* which indicates that the energy dose of radiation per unit area decreases proportionately to the square of the distance from the site to the source (l/d^2). For example, the dose of radiation 2 cm from a point source is only one fourth of the value of the dose at 1 cm (Fig. 25-1).

In general, x-rays or photons can be generated as a result of rapidly accelerated electrons in a vacuum striking a target. Modern generators that accelerate these electrons at high speed may do so in a circular fashion (betatron) or linearly (linear accelerator). Another type of radiation energy is known as particulate radiation and is produced by subatomic particles with a discrete mass. These particles are usually released by the disintegration of radionuclides. Four common types are alpha particles (the same as a helium nucleus), neutrons, pro-

tons, and electrons. Alpha particles produce a large number of ions over a short distance, but they currently have little practical use in radiation therapy because of their short range in tissue. Neutrons are highly penetrating and have no charge but have a large mass, and for the purposes of cancer treatment they are usually produced by machines. They cause high-energy collisions with atomic nuclei, principally of hydrogen, in the tissues. The resultant recoil proton loses energy to the surrounding tissue by ionization, which leads to cell death. Protons are positively charged particles, and generators are available for the direct production of protons to yield very high energy beams, which have specialized uses such as in the treatment of pituitary tumors.

Electrons may also be referred to as beta rays, produced by radionuclide disintegration. Electrons can be produced at different energies by machines for various therapeutic applications.

Radiation Biology

Photons (gamma rays or x-rays) act by dislodging orbital electrons from the atoms of the medium or tissue through which they pass. This collision produces a fast electron (Compton effect), which then ionizes molecules along its path, producing secondary electrons and free hydroxyl radicals. The process continues until the electromagnetic beam (photon) loses all of its energy. The cells are damaged by the free hydroxyl radicals and the negatively charged electrons that affect the DNA of the cell. This effect may be lethal and kill the cell, or it can be sublethal, in which case the cell will subsequently undergo repair of the DNA. In addition, free hydroxyl radicals may react with molecular oxygen to form peroxide in the tissues. This adds to the lethal effects of radiation on the cells. As shown by Gray et al., oxygen is important for the tissue effects of photon irradiation. This has practical implications in tumor therapy insofar as cancers tend to have poor blood supplies, which decreases the oxygenation, particularly at the center of large tumors. The effects of photon radiation in these hypoxic areas is therefore diminished.

The rate of loss of energy of an ionizing particle as it traverses a unit length of medium is

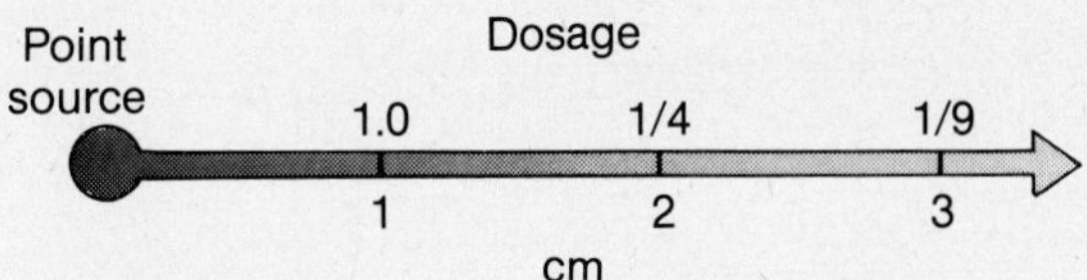

FIGURE 25-1
Radiation effects at various distances from point source of irradiation demonstrating the inverse square law.

known as linear energy transfer (LET). In the case of photon irradiation, the loss of energy per hit is small. This is described as low LET irradiation, which often causes a sublethal effect on a single cell and thus necessitates multiple hits to kill the cell as well as to produce toxic hydroxyl radicals. In the case of particulate radiation with heavy particles, the ionization is known as high LET. Thus neutrons, with their large mass, produce high-energy recoil protons that kill the cell directly on impact, independent of oxygenation. For this reason research has been directed toward the development of neutron generators to try to improve tumor therapy by overcoming the limitation of poor oxygenation of cancer cells.

An important principle is that a given dose of radiation kills a constant fraction of the number of cells irradiated. For example, if 90% of the cells of a tumor are killed with each fraction of radiation delivered, then 10% of the cells would survive. Thus if one were to begin to irradiate a tumor with 10 million cells, there would be 1 million cells surviving after the first fraction, 100,000 cells after the second fraction, 10,000 cells after the third fraction, etc. By the seventh fraction all of the cells would be killed.

As shown in Fig. 25-2 there are four phases of the cell cycle. Sinclair and Morton showed that during mitosis the cell is most sensitive to radiation. Thus rapidly dividing cells are the most radiosensitive. It has been demonstrated that dividing radiation treatment into a number of small doses (fractionation) allows for effective treatment of the tumor without increasing the complications of radiation to the normal tissues (bone marrow, intestine, and other rapidly dividing tissues) that would occur with single large doses. The more efficient repair of normal tissue occurring between treatment fractions affords a therapeutic advantage. The measurement of the amount of energy absorbed by tissue is the rad, which is defined as 100 ergs of energy absorbed per gram of tissue. Recently the term *gray* (1 joule per kilogram) has been introduced; 1 gray is equivalent to 100 rads.

Radiation Sources—External and Internal Therapy

In general two techniques are utilized in radiation treatment—brachytherapy (internal) and teletherapy (external). For brachytherapy the radiation source is placed within or adjacent to the target tissue. In the treatment of gynecologic malignant tumors radioactive needles may be implanted directly into the tissue to be irradiated (interstitial implant), or a tandem containing radioactive sources may be placed within the cervix and uterus accompanied by two vaginal ovoids on either side of the tandem that also contain radioactive sources

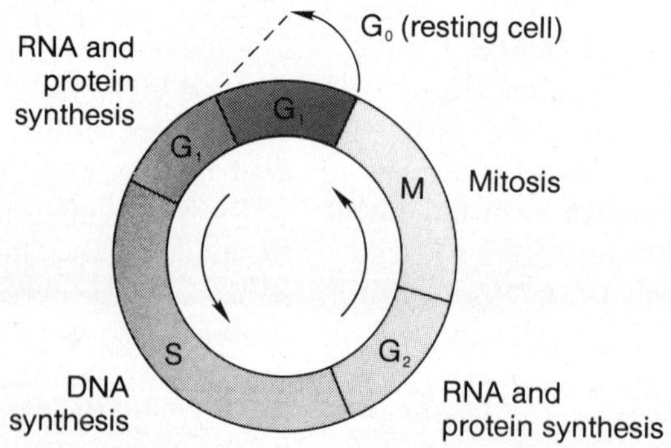

FIGURE 25-2

Phases of the cell. Following mitosis *(M)* there is an interval of variable duration during which there is RNA and protein synthesis and a diploid DNA content (gap$_1$, G$_1$). The cell may also enter a prolonged or resting phase *(G$_0$)* and then reenter the cycle during DNA synthesis, the *(S)* phase, in which DNA is duplicated. During gap$_2$ (G$_2$) there again is protein and RNA synthesis. During the *M* phase the cell divides into two cells, each of which receives a diploid DNA content.

(intracavitary therapy). Such an arrangement would be useful for treatment of a cervical tumor or a tumor located near the cervix (Fig. 25-3). In such an arrangement the dose delivered to the tissues is determined by the inverse square law. In practice the radioactive sources are placed in the devices after the apparatus has been properly placed within the endocervix and vagina. This "afterloading" technique reduces radiation exposure to the personnel treating the patient.

In brachytherapy various radioisotopes are used for treatment; which ones are chosen depends on the half-life of the radionuclide. In general those with a short half-life (such as gold 198) may be placed within the patient and left permanently, whereas those with a long half-life (cesium 137) are placed temporarily within the patient and then removed after a pre-

scribed dose of irradiation has been administered. Table 25-1 indicates the half-lives of some of the isotopes commonly used in treating gynecologic cancers. It is also important that a uniform distribution of radiation be achieved in the adjacent tissues to avoid "hot spots," which can lead to excess damage to normal tissue, as well as "cold spots," which can lead to undertreatment of the tumor.

Teletherapy refers to the placement of the radioactive source at a distance from the patient, in which case the machine delivers external radiation to the tumor. With external therapy the source of radiation is located at a distance 5 to 10 times greater than the depth of the tumor being irradiated in order to deliver a uniform dose to the tumor and thus avoid the large dose changes that result because of the inverse square law. This distance is referred to as the source-to-skin distance (SSD).

More recently, with the utilization of different angles and ports of treatment the concept of source axis distance (SAD) has been introduced; it denotes the distance from the radiation source to the central axis of machine rotation. The patient is positioned so that this axis passes through the center of the tumor, and treatment ports are arranged around this axis to optimize tumor dose and minimize the dose to vital structures.

To focus the beam from the external source, a collimator is used. The collimator prevents scatter and allows for a directed beam of a given field size (10 × 10 cm, for example) to be applied to the tissue being irradiated (Fig. 25-4). In general the higher the energy source of the radiation, the deeper the beam pene-

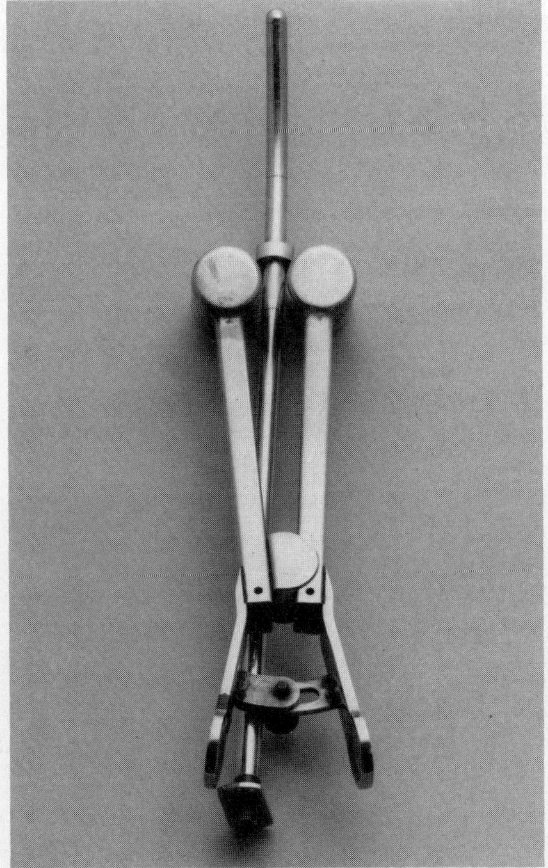

FIGURE 25-3
Fletcher-Suit applicator (tandem and ovoids) used for afterloading internal therapy.

TABLE 25-1
Half-Lives of Commonly Used Isotopes

Radionuclide	Half-Life
Gold 198	2.7 Days
Phosphorus 32	14.3 Days
Iodine 125	60 Days
Iridium 192	74.4 Days
Cobalt 60	5.3 Years
Cesium 137	30 Years
Radium 226	1620 Years

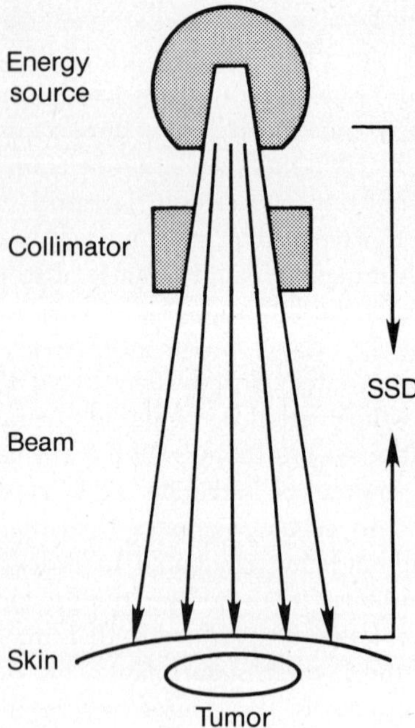

FIGURE 25-4
External therapy unit. Divergence of beam increases with distance from source. (Redrawn from Kase NG, Weingold AB: Principles and practice of clinical gynecology. New York, John Wiley & Sons, 1983.)

trates the tissue. Thus high-energy (short wavelength) radiation has its predominant effect in deeper tissues and spares the surface or the skin of radiation effect. The term *orthovoltage* refers to machines in the 125,000 to 400,000 electron volt (125 to 400 kV) range, whereas *supervoltage* or *megavoltage* refers to machines with 2 to 35 million electron volt (megavolt) range. Cobalt machines (equivalent to 1.25 MV) and 4 to 6 MV machines have similar properties and achieve their maximum dosage at about 0.5 cm beneath the skin; higher energy machines such as the 22 MV have their maximum effect at a depth of about 5 cm beneath the skin.

An isodose curve is a line that connects points in the tissue that receive equivalent dosages of irradiation. Fig. 25-5 contrasts the isodose curves for 6 and 22 MV machines. For the 6 MV machine the maximum dose is near the surface, with a more rapid falloff in the deeper tissues, in comparison to the 22 MV machine, which has its maximum dose well beneath the

surface. Thus at a given depth the higher dose of radiation can be achieved with 22 MV, sparing the effects of radiation on the skin. These high-energy machines are particularly useful for treating deep tumors and for obese patients. Achieving comparable large doses of irradiation in deep tissue with cobalt or 4 to 6 MV machines produces higher radiation levels on the surface, which can lead to increased skin reaction and eventually subcutaneous fibrosis.

In addition to the energy of the beam that is determined by the machine producing the radiation, the energy of radiation absorbed at various depths is affected by the size of the field being treated. Larger fields contain more scattered radiation, which leads to a greater dose at a given depth. Fig. 25-6 demonstrates the effect of increasing the size of the field with increasing dosage at a given depth for three different types of energy sources.

Thus the radiation dose delivered to the tumor is affected by the energy of the source, the depth of the tumor beneath the surface, and the size of the field undergoing irradiation. With external therapy usually 160 to 200 rads per day is given five times per week.

As previously noted, the effect of electromagnetic radiation also depends on the oxygenation of the tissue. Recently a number of pharmacologic agents such as hydroxyurea and metronidazole have been investigated for their abilities to potentiate the sensitivity to radiation. These radiation sensitizers are not yet used routinely in the treatment of gynecologic malignancies. Hyperthermia is also being explored to potentiate the therapeutic effectiveness of radiation. It appears to offer the most promise for tumors localized in an area that can effectively and safely tolerate increased temperatures (42° to 43° C). In some studies higher temperatures have been used locally.

Tissue Tolerance and Radiation Complications

Radiation acutely affects tissues undergoing continuous cell replacement, such as the skin, the intestinal mucosa, and the mucosa of the vagina and bladder. These tissues are undergoing rapid division, and radiation given in the fractions noted previously reduces the untoward effects of cell damage on normal tissue

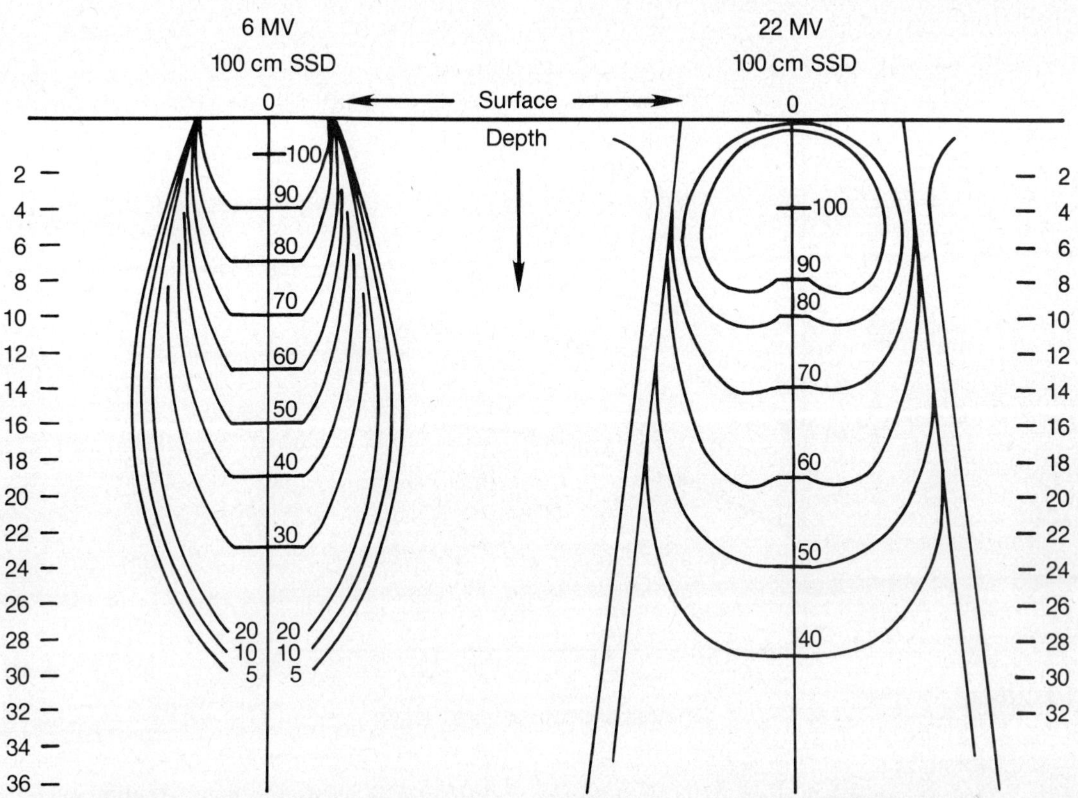

FIGURE 25-5

Comparison of isodose curves and depth-dose distribution for 6 MV and 22 MV betatrons. Note that the higher energy machine delivers radiation to greater depth for same surface dose, and there is considerable skin sparing. (Redrawn from DiSaia PJ, Creasman WT: Clinical gynecologic oncology, 2nd ed. St. Louis, The C.V. Mosby Co., 1984.)

and allows for normal healing to occur between treatment fractions. Side effects of radiation include depression of the quantity of circulating white cells as well as gastrointestinal effects such as nausea, anorexia, or diarrhea, which usually can be controlled with medication. The skin may be irritated with a "wet reaction," particularly if lower energy external sources are used; occasionally a treatment program may have to be temporarily discontinued.

Although the acute effects of radiation limit the rate at which the dosage is administered, late effects may occur many years later and can cause permanent damage. Late adverse effects include tissue necrosis and fibrosis as well as fistula formation, ulceration, and bleeding. These late-stage complications depend on the total dose of the radiation administered, the volume of tissue treated, and also, somewhat, on the size of the radiation fraction administered with each dose. It is thought that these late effects are due to radiation damage to the vascular tissue and connective tissue. An alternate explanation is that the radiation destroys the cells that are capable of regeneration, which eventually leads to tissue destruction.

It has been observed clinically that the response of the tumor to radiation treatment follows a sigmoid curve, with increasingly effective tumor control associated with increasing dosage (Fig. 25-7). A similar dosage effect exists for normal tissues, and the ability of radiation therapy to control tumors depends on the greater tolerance of normal tissues to radiation exposure. Thus if one were to use the level of radiation that causes no normal tissue damage,

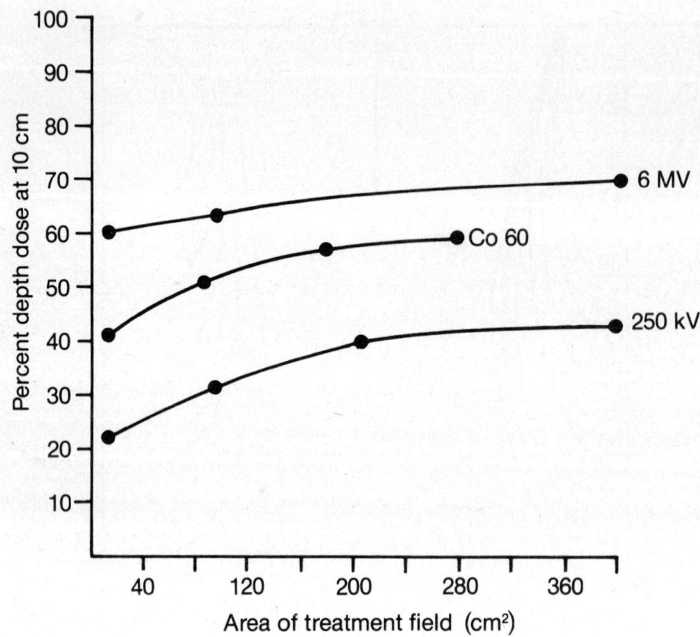

FIGURE 25-6

Variation of depth dose at 10 cm with energy and size of treatment field. (Redrawn from Joslin CAF: Basic parameters of radiotherapy. In Coppleson M, ed: Gynecologic oncology. Edinburgh, Churchill Livingstone, 1981. Reprinted by permission.)

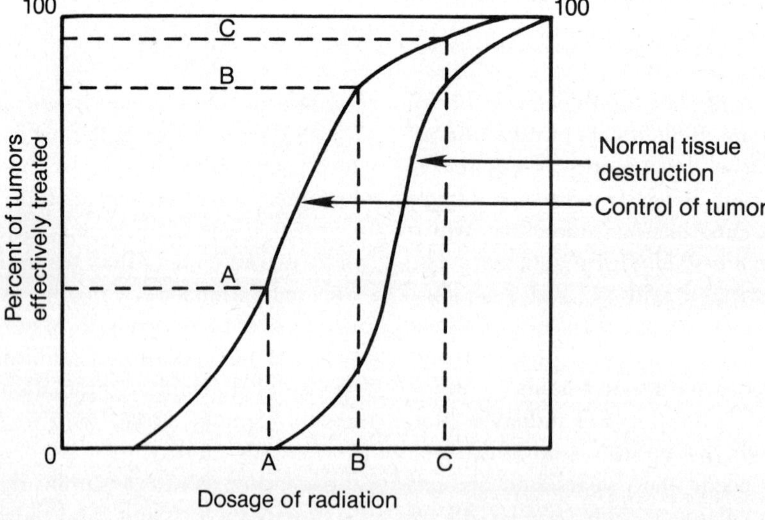

FIGURE 25-7

Concept of tumor control versus complications. At point *A* there are no complications but insufficient control. Point *C* has good control but excess complications. There is reasonable tumor control at *B* with a slight risk of complications.

only a small proportion of tumors would be controlled. Conversely, if one were to use a dosage that could control almost all tumors, massive damage to normal tissue would occur, and an unacceptable series of complications and even patient death could follow. The optimum goal is to achieve maximum tumor control with as little risk of damage to normal tissues as possible.

In the treatment of gynecologic malignancies the main sites of radiation damage are the bladder, rectum, and large and small bowel. As a rule, complications of the bladder can occur in the form of radiation cystitis, which can lead to complaints of dysuria and frequency. Hematuria may also occur, and therapy with sclerosing solutions or fulguration through a cystoscope may be necessary. In rare instances urinary diversion may be required. Fistulas between the vagina and bladder or between the vagina and rectum may develop when there has been extensive radiation damage to the intervening tissues. This usually takes place during therapy for large carcinomas of the cervix (see Chapter 27). As a general rule such complications will occur 6 months to 2 years after treatment, although they may occur many years after primary therapy.

Damage to the large bowel usually occurs in the form of inflammation (sigmoiditis), which may be associated with severe bleeding and pain. Less severe cases can often be controlled with a low-roughage diet and antispasmodic medication, while more severe cases may require bowel resection or permanent bowel diversion through a colostomy. The small bowel also receives irradiation during external therapy for pelvic tumors. In the acute phases of treatment this often leads to bowel irritability, and the patient complains of diarrhea. Long-term complications include fibrosis of the wall of the intestine, which can lead to permanent narrowing and even obstruction. Occasionally enteric fistulas also develop and bowel perforation may occur. In the latter cases surgical therapy is required, usually to bypass the affected area of the intestine. As a general rule extensive dissection of irradiated tissue is avoided. Small-bowel injuries are more frequent in patients who have had a previous operation, particularly pelvic surgery.

Spontaneous mobility of the bowel resulting

TABLE 25-2
Approximate Tolerance of Tissues to Radiation Therapy

Tissue	Approximate Tolerance Dose (rads)
Bladder	6,000-7,000
Rectum	6,000-7,000
Vaginal mucosa	7,000
Bowel	6,000
Cervix	>12,000
Kidney	2,000-2,300
Liver	2,500-3,500

from peristalsis may be decreased by adhesion formation. With reduction of bowel mobility, injury risks from radiation increase, since the loops of small bowel become fixed and are unable to have normal peristalsis, resulting in a higher radiation dose to the affected bowel segment. Table 25-2 presents the approximate tolerance of tissues to radiation therapy.

Generalizations regarding tissue tolerance in relation to total dosage must be regarded as only approximations. Multiple factors, as already discussed, influence late effects of radiation on normal tissue, such as dose fractionation, field size, port arrangement, extent of tumor damage to normal tissues, previous operations, concurrent chemotherapy, and other less well defined elements, including anemia, small-vessel pathology, and the patient's nutritional status.

CHEMOTHERAPY

The use of drugs to treat disseminated cancer has developed into an extensive clinical discipline, particularly since the 1950s. Numerous compounds have been tested to treat human tumors, and the first successful effort in gynecologic cancer was the demonstration by Li et al. that the antimetabolite methotrexate could cause permanent remission in cases of metastatic trophoblastic disease (Chapter 33). A number of general principles have been developed that provide guidelines for the use of chemotherapeutic agents to treat malignant disease. Many of these principles were developed

apeutic program that has the best chance of inducing tumor regression. The potential to treat simultaneously different cell lines within the tumor has led to the development in recent years of multiple-agent chemotherapy programs, which appear in many cases to be more effective than single agents in treating gynecologic cancers. Such combination therapy appears to enhance the cell kill, to provide broader coverage against multiple cell lines, and to help prevent the emergence of resistant cells. The recent introduction of in vitro chemosensitivity testing of tumor cells in soft agar offers the potential to identify the drugs that are most active against a given cancer. The technique is undergoing refinement and is not yet applicable to routine clinical situations.

Approaches to Treatment

The dosage of an anticancer agent is usually calculated in body surface area (square meters), which provides a better measure of potential toxicity than body weight in part because surface area more closely reflects cardiac output and blood flow. Chemotherapeutic agents have varying toxicities, which will be considered in the next section. A major problem with most agents is bone marrow toxicity, along with the resultant necessity to monitor carefully the hemopoietic system. Most gynecologic chemotherapy protocols are administered in cycles that frequently vary from 3- to 4-week intervals. If the blood elements (white cells and platelets) have not recovered adequately by the time the next cycle of chemotherapy is due to be administered, the dosage of the agent or agents must be reduced or the time interval between treatments extended. For example, the dosage of drugs that induce myelosuppression should be reduced about 50% if the white blood cell count is between 2500 and 4000/mm^3 or if the platelet count is between 50,000 and 100,000/mm^3.

An additional consideration in toxicity of chemotherapeutic agents relates to hepatic metabolism and/or renal excretion. It may be necessary to modify the dosage of the drug administered when either renal or hepatic function is compromised. For example, doxorubicin (Adriamycin) is metabolized in the liver, and dosage reductions must be made if the drug is administered to a patient with hepatic dysfunction; methotrexate effects are increased in patients with renal damage, necessitating dosage reduction in such patients; *cis*-platinum not only has its effects intensified in patients with renal damage but also is toxic to the kidney, requiring particular caution if it is administered to individuals with compromised renal function or patients receiving therapy with aminoglycosides, which are also toxic to the kidney.

Various chemotherapeutic agents can be differentially toxic to other organ systems of the body, including the intestine, nervous system, and lungs. The therapist must be aware of the individual adverse affects when administering these agents. The goal of treatment is to provide as high a dosage of the chemotherapeutic agent as possible to produce maximum therapeutic effectiveness without causing unacceptable toxicity and side effects.

In assessment of the effect of chemotherapeutic agents, a number of definitions are used to describe the response of the tumor being treated. A *complete remission* or *response* is total disappearance of the tumor for at least 1 month. An *objective response* is the reduction in the size of the tumor greater than 50% for at least 1 month. A *partial response* is the reduction in the size of the tumor of less than 50%. *Progression* indicates an increase in tumor size. Occasionally the term *stabilization* is used to indicate that the disease has not changed in size; however, clinically the possibility of confusion exists, insofar as stabilization of the disease may be assumed to be due to chemotherapy when the lack of observed increase in size may be related in part to a prolonged doubling time of the tumor.

Evaluation of New Agents

In the development of new drugs, serial evaluations are necessary to assess the effectiveness of the drug as well as to ascertain its toxicity. A number of trials are necessary to move a new agent from the point of evaluation to allow it to be used in regular medical practice. Such "phase trials" are defined as follows:

- *Phase I trial:* An initial trial to test new drugs at various doses to evaluate toxicity and determine tolerance to the drug. At the various doses tested some therapeutic effects may be observed.

- *Phase II trials:* Tests to determine the therapeutic effectiveness and extent of the toxicity of the drug at doses expected to be effective against the tumor.
- *Phase III trials:* Trials to compare the drug therapy to treatment currently in use to ascertain if the new therapy is superior.

Chemotherapeutic Agents Commonly Used in Gynecologic Cancer

A large number of drugs have been used in the therapy of cancer. In general the agents used in gynecologic oncology can be classified into six groups: alkylating agents, antitumor antibiotics, antimetabolites, vinca (plant) alkaloids, synthetic and miscellaneous compounds, and hormones.

Alkylating Agents

The primary action of these chemicals appears to be via direct interaction with DNA. The process of alkylation leads to the development of positively charged alkyl groups, which react with the negatively charged portion of DNA, leading to interference with DNA function. Cross-linking of DNA also occurs. The alkylating agents affect rapidly dividing cells and are particularly toxic to the bone marrow, leading to severe myelosuppression. They may be administered intravenously or orally and have been used extensively in gynecologic malignancies, particularly in ovarian cancers. The most commonly used agents are cyclophosphamide (Cytoxan), chlorambucil (Leukeran), and phenylalanine mustard (melphalan or Alkeran). In general the effectiveness of these agents appears similar, but there are some variations in toxicity. Phenylalanine mustard not only is acutely toxic to the bone marrow but also appears to have a cumulative effect on the marrow that may compromise marrow function after its use has been discontinued. Cyclophosphamide is associated with hemorrhagic cystitis. In addition, it has been noted that therapy with alkylating agents is associated with the subsequent risk of the patient's developing acute leukemia. This risk may range from 2% to 10% and appears to be related both to the dose

and to the duration of alkylating agent treatment.

Antitumor Antibiotics

Antitumor antibiotics are derived from products of bacterial or fungal cultures. Their mechanism of action is not clearly delineated, but it is thought that they directly attack DNA and appear to be able to produce DNA breaks and also interfere with DNA synthesis and transcription. The ones most commonly used in gynecologic cancer are actinomycin D (Cosmegen), doxorubicin (Adriamycin), and bleomycin (Blenoxane).

Actinomycin D is usually given intravenously often in 5-day courses every 4 weeks. The drug causes severe myelosuppression and can affect the gastrointestinal mucosa, leading to diarrhea and ulcers in the mouth. Alopecia and skin toxicity may also occur. The drug has a potentiating effect with radiation therapy, and this increased activity may be observed even when the drug is given after radiation treatment is completed. The drug is active in ovarian tumors and also widely used to treat trophoblastic disease. It is also sclerosing and has been used to treat malignant pleural effusions.

Doxorubicin must be carefully administered intravenously, since extravasation leads to soft tissue and skin necrosis and ulceration. It is metabolized in the liver, and dosages must be reduced in patients with compromised hepatic function. Myelosuppression occurs regularly with therapeutic doses. Complete alopecia is a common and almost constant side effect. The alopecia is reversible after cessation of the use of the drug, but it tends to be one of the greatest causes of patient distress. The drug also causes cardiomyopathy, which leads to congestive heart failure and can be life threatening. In general, doses are kept below 550 mg/m^2, and cardiac function is often monitored by ultrasound evaluation or radionuclide scans. The drug has widespread use in gynecologic cancers, particularly in sarcomas, ovarian tumors, and endometrial and cervical carcinomas.

Bleomycin may be administered intravenously, intramuscularly, or subcutaneously. It is excreted via the kidney, and some dosage reduction is made if renal function is markedly compromised. The drug does *not* have significant myelosuppressant properties, in contrast to most of the other cytotoxic agents. It is, however, highly toxic to the lungs, and pneumonitis and pulmonary fibrosis may occur. Thus particular care must be used in persons with compromised lung function. The drug is also toxic to skin and can produce erythema, peeling, and pigmentation. It has been used recently as part of combination therapy with particular effectiveness against ovarian germ cell tumors, and it has been tried for a variety of other gynecologic malignancies, particularly carcinoma of the cervix, but with limited success.

Antimetabolites

Antimetabolites interfere with cell metabolism by competing with naturally occurring purines or pyrimidines, whose chemical structure they resemble. In this way they interfere or prevent vital biochemical reactions.

5-Fluorouracil (5-FU) is a substitute pyrimidine that interferes with DNA synthesis and can also be incorporated into RNA. It is usually given intravenously and is also active orally. It is myelosuppressive, although less so than many other cytotoxic agents used in gynecologic cancer treatment. It causes gastrointestinal side effects (diarrhea) and ulceration of the oral mucosa. It is effectively metabolized in the liver, which has led to its use in hepatic artery infusions for liver metastasis. The clearing of 5-FU from the blood by the liver markedly reduces systemic toxicity in patients receiving these infusions. The drug is extensively used in gynecologic cancer, including ovarian carcinomas, endometrial adenocarcinomas, and some cases of cervical squamous cell carcinomas. It has also been used topically to treat intraepithelial neoplasia of the lower genital tract.

Methotrexate inhibits the enzyme dihydrofolate reductase, preventing the conversion of dihydrofolate to tetrahydrofolate. This prevents metabolic transfer of one carbon unit and inhibits the synthesis of thymidylic acid as well as different purine nucleotides. RNA and DNA syntheses are inhibited, and the drug works primarily in the S phase. Nondividing or resting cells are resistant. The effects of methotrexate can be overcome by the administration of folinic acid (citrovorum factor), which replenishes the tetrahydrofolate. Some chemotherapy protocols have used very high doses of methotrexate to treat the tumor, followed by citrovorum rescue to avoid severe toxic side effects. Fig. 25-10 illustrates schematically the action of the drug. Methotrexate is administered intravenously, intramuscularly, or orally. It is excreted in the urine, and dosage adjustments must be made if there is decreased renal function. Methotrexate is severely myelosuppressive and causes toxicity to the oral mucosa and intestines as well as the liver, and an increase in liver enzymes is seen after treatment. Blood levels of methotrexate can be monitored with radioimmunoassay. The predominant use of the drug in gynecologic cancer has been the effective treatment of trophoblastic disease; it has also been used in cervical and ovarian carcinomas.

Vinca (Plant) Alkaloids

A number of cytotoxic drugs have been isolated from plant extracts. Those in current use in gynecologic oncology include vinblastine, vincristine, and a more recently introduced agent termed VP-16 (etoposide). These drugs attack the cell during the M phase and cause toxic destruction of the mitotic spindle and thus arrest mitosis. This can result in synchro-

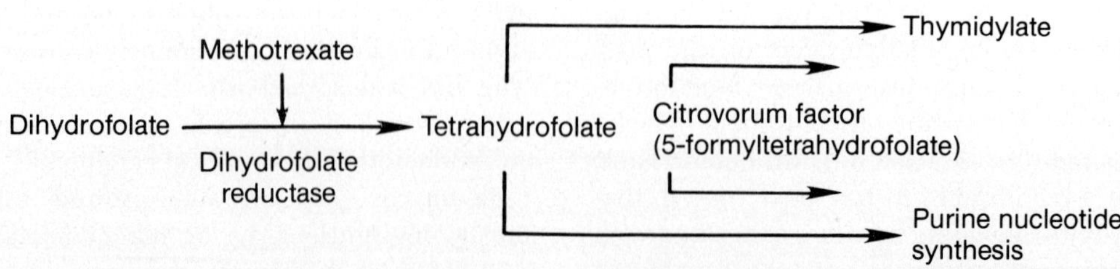

FIGURE 25-10
Schematic of action of methotrexate and reversal by citrovorum factor.

nization of the cell cycle for those cells surviving therapy. The drugs are given intravenously and have different side effects. Vincristine is severely neurotoxic and can produce numbness, motor weakness, and constipation as a result of its autonomic effects. There is little myelosuppression. Vinblastine is myelotoxic, and this tends to be a dose-limiting factor. However, it has less neurotoxicity than vincristine has. VP-16 appears to have fewer toxic side effects but is myelotoxic. These drugs have been used in ovarian germ cell tumors as well as in trophoblastic disease.

Synthetic and Miscellaneous Compounds

Recently synthetically produced drugs have been introduced that have antitumor activity. They do not have any single mode of action, and in some instances their mechanism of antitumor activity is unknown. Currently the two synthetic agents most commonly used in gynecologic cancers are *cis*-platinum and hexamethylmelamine.

Cis-platinum (*cis*-diaminedichloroplatinum, *cis*-DDP) has been found to have wide antitumor activity. It appears to bind to DNA and interfere with DNA synthesis, but its cell cycle specificity has not been clearly defined. It is administered intravenously and is very toxic to the kidney. A high urine output must be maintained during administration to try to reduce kidney toxicity, since the drug is excreted in the urine in its active form. It induces myelosuppression and also causes high-frequency ototoxicity, so that renal and auditory function must be monitored during treatment in addition to peripheral blood counts. *Cis*-platinum induces severe peripheral neuropathy, which may improve somewhat after cessation of therapy but tends to be permanent. One of the side effects most annoying to the patient is the production of severe nausea with vomiting, which may be controlled in part by antiemetic medication. The drug is widely used in the treatment of ovarian epithelial and germ cell tumors and is currently being tested for the treatment of all types of gynecologic cancers.

Hexamethylmelamine is orally active, but its mechanism of antitumor activity is unclear. It is thought to act somewhat similarly to alkylating agents, but it is structurally different from that class of compounds. It is myelosuppressive and causes nausea and vomiting. It is active in ovarian epithelial carcinomas and frequently is used as part of combination chemotherapy in the treatment of these tumors.

Hormones

Hormone therapy has been effectively developed in the treatment of breast cancer. Estrogen and progesterone receptors have been clearly identified in endometrial carcinomas and have been recently found in other types of gynecologic cancers, particularly ovarian epithelial carcinomas. Progestins such as megestrol (Megace), depo-medroxyprogesterone (Depo-Provera), and 17-OH progesterone caproate (Delalutin), as well as antiestrogens such as tamoxifen, have been used in the treatment of endometrial carcinomas and seem to have their best effects against well-differentiated tumors. Hormonal therapy is also being evaluated in the treatment of some ovarian epithelial carcinomas.

• • •

There are many other cytotoxic agents available to treat cancers. Table 25-3 summarizes the major side effects of those agents most commonly used currently in the treatment of gynecologic malignancies.

Immunotherapy

It has been shown that many experimental animal tumors are able to elicit an immune response, and the concept of tumor-specific antigens has gained wide acceptance. However, antigens specific for a given gynecologic tumor have not been identified. Nonetheless it is recognized that an immune response to human tumors does occur. It appears that tumor growth stimulates the major cells of the immune system: the T-lymphocyte, B-lymphocyte, and macrophage. T-lymphocytes are cells that confer cell-mediated immunity, while B-lymphocytes are cells associated with antibody production and humoral immunity. Macrophages also act directly on tumor cells. It has also been observed that immunosuppressed patients such as kidney transplant recipients are at greater risk

TABLE 25-3

Major Side Effects of Some Chemotherapeutic Agents Utilized in Gynecologic Cancer

Class/Drug	Marrow	G.I.	Nausea, Vomiting	Pulmonary	Cardiac	Renal	Neurologic	Hepatic	Alopecia
Alkylating agents									
Cyclophosphamide	Severe		Severe		Mild				Mild
Chlorambucil*	Severe	Severe	Mild	Mild			Mild		
Melphalan	Severe	Mild	Severe						
Antimetabolites									
5-FU	Severe	Severe	Mild				Mild		Mild
Methotrexate	Severe	Severe	Mild	Mild		Mild	Mild	Severe	Mild
Antibiotics									
Adriamycin†	Severe	Severe			Severe		Mild		Severe
Actinomycin D†	Severe	Severe							Severe
Bleomycin‡	Mild			Severe			Severe		
Vinca alkaloids									
Vincristine	Mild						Severe		Mild
Vinblastine	Severe								Mild
Miscellaneous synthetics									
Hexamethylmelamine	Severe	Severe	Severe				Mild		
Cis-platinum	Severe		Severe			Severe	Severe		

Modified from Tattersall MHN: Pharmacology and selections of cytologic drugs. In Coppleson M, ed: Gynecologic oncology. Edinburgh, Churchill Livingstone, 1981. Reprinted by permission.
*Toxic to bladder.
†Sclerosing.
‡Toxic to skin.

for the development of malignant disease. All of these considerations have led to efforts to utilize the immune system to treat human cancer. In the case of gynecologic malignancies a number of trials of immunotherapy have been conducted, but currently this modality of treatment is investigational.

Various approaches have been taken to augment the immune response to human tumors. One of the most common is active nonspecific immunotherapy, which involves the administration of adjuvant agents, usually of microbiologic origin, to stimulate cell-mediated and humoral immunity as well as to activate macrophages. Two examples are (bacillus Calmette-Guerin) (BCG) and *Corynebacterium parvum* (C-Parvum). Both of these produce marked proliferation of lymphocytes and have been tested in gynecologic malignancies, but no therapeutic role has been identified for their

routine use. It is thought that the benefits of BCG may be enhanced if it is administered in conjunction with other treatment modalities such as cytotoxic chemotherapy.

A second type of immunotherapy is active specific immunotherapy, which involves the use of tumor cells and their antigens to produce specific tumor immunities. The tumor cells may be modified with chemicals or irradiation and then placed into a growth medium to produce a vaccine to allow active immunization. Immunotherapy may also be given locally, such as BCG treatment of malignant melanoma or the use of dinitrochlorobenzene (DCNB) to treat skin cancers. Efforts are also underway to confer passive immunity. Transfer of specific immunity through extracts of lymphocytes sensitized to tumor antigens is being investigated. Extracts of such "transfer factor" may lead to a type of adoptive immunotherapy by transfer of "immunologic memory" to the patient's lymphocytes. Interferon is another substance being evaluated. It has been noted to prevent cancer cell division, perhaps through augumenting the action of natural killer (NK) cells. By preventing the replication of cancer cells, the treatment would gradually lead to tumor regression. Passive transfer of antibodies involves another method of potential immunotherapy involving the transfer of active antibodies against a given tumor. All of these approaches remain investigational at present.

KEY POINTS

- Electromagnetic radiation is a form of energy that has no mass or charge and travels at the speed of light.

- Particulate energy is a form of ionizing radiation consisting of subatomic particles (electrons, neutrons, and protons) whose energy is in part related to their mass and velocity.

- Inverse square law states that the energy measured from a radiation source is inversely proportional to the distance from the source.

- A given dose of radiation kills a constant fraction of tumor cells radiated. The tissue effects of electromagnetic radiation (x-rays and gamma rays) are dependent on oxygenation.

- The effect of photon radiation (low LET) on tissues is altered by tissue oxygenation, while neutron (high LET) radiation is independent of oxygenation.

- The cell replication cycle consists of M (mitosis), G_1 (Gap_1 = RNA and protein synthesis), S (DNA synthesis), and G_2 (Gap_2 = RNA and protein synthesis). When the cell is not in the replication cycle it is in the G_0 phase.

- The dose of radiation delivered to a tumor depends on the energy of the source, the size of the treatment field, and the depth of the tumor beneath the surface.

- Radiation acts on cells primarily in the M phase, making rapidly proliferating cells the most radiosensitive. Normal tissues recover from the effects of radiation therapy more efficiently than tumor tissue does.

- Cytotoxic chemotherapeutic agents act on various phases of the cell cycle, primarily affecting rapidly proliferating cells, and at a given dose destroy a constant fraction of tumor cells.

_______________ **KEY POINTS, cont'd** _______________________________

- Large tumors tend to have smaller growth fractions and a higher proportion of cells in the resting phase (G_0) of the cycle than small tumors. Tumors consist of a heterogeneous population of cells and have variable growth fractions.

- The major classes of cytotoxic chemotherapeutic agents used in gynecologic oncology are alkylating agents, antitumor antibiotics, antimetabolites, vinca (plant) alkaloids, and specially synthesized compounds.

- Systemic-active nonspecific immunotherapy results from the injection of agents derived from bacteriologic sources mixed with an adjuvant that cause a proliferation of lymphocytes leading to cellular and humoral immunity.

- Active specific immunotherapy is the use of tumor cells and their surface antigens to produce specific tumor immunity.

BIBLIOGRAPHY

Bruce WR, Meeker RE, Valeriote FA: Comparison of the sensitivity of normal hematopoietic and transplanted lymphoma colony-forming cells to chemotherapeutic agents administered in vivo. J Nat Cancer Inst 37:233, 1966.

Chabner BA, Myers CE: Clinical pharmacology of cancer chemotherapy. In DeVita VT Jr, Hellman S, eds: Cancer: Principles and practice of oncology. Philadelphia, J.B. Lippincott Co., 1982.

DeVita VT: Cell kinetic and the chemotherapy of cancer. Cancer Treat Rep 2:23, 1971.

Dickson JA: Hyperthermia in the treatment of cancer. Lancet 1:202, 1979.

Gray LH, Coger AD, Ebert M, et al: The concentration of oxygen dissolved in tissues at the time of radiation as a factor in radiotherapy. Br J Radiol 26:638, 1953.

Gutterman JU, Hirsh EM: Immunotherapy. In Holland JF, Frei A, eds: Cancer medicine, 2nd ed. Philadelphia, Lea & Febinger, 1982.

Hall EJ: Radiobiology for the radiologist, 2nd ed. Harper & Row, Publishers, 1978.

Hall EJ: Radiation dose rate: A factor of importance in radiobiology and radiotherapy. Br J Radiol 45:81, 1972.

Hellman S, DeVita VT Jr: Principles of cancer biology: Kinetics of cellular proliferation. In DeVita VT Jr, Hellman S, eds: Cancer: Principles and practice of oncology. Philadelphia, J.B. Lippincott Co., 1982.

Joslin CAF: Basic parameters of radiotherapy. In Coppleson M, ed: Gynecologic oncology. Edinburgh, Churchill Livingstone, 1981.

Lederer CM, Hollander J, Perlman I: Table of isotopes. New York, John Wiley & Sons, 1967.

Li MC, Hertz R, Spencer DB: Effect of methotrexate therapy upon choriocarcinoma and chorioadenoma. Proc Soc Exp Biol Med 93:361, 1956.

Sinclair WK: Cyclic x-ray responses in mammalian cells in vitro. Radiat Res 33:620, 1968.

Sinclair WK, Morton RA: X-ray sensitivity during cell generation cycle of cultured Chinese hamster cells. Radiat Res 29:450, 1966.

Skipper HE: Biochemical, pharmacologic, toxicological, kinetic, and chemical (subhuman and human) relationships. Cancer 21:600, 1968.

Skipper H, Schabel F, Wilcox WS: Experimental evaluation of potential anticancer agent XIII on the criterion and kinetics associated with "curability" of experimental leukemia. Cancer Chemother Rep 35:1, 1964.

Tattersall MHN: Pharmacology and selections of cytologic drugs. In Coppleson M, ed: Gynecologic oncology. Edinburgh, Churchill Livingstone, 1981.

Wilcox WS: The last surviving cancer cell—the chances of killing it. Cancer Chemother Rep 50:541, 1966.

Intraepithelial Neoplasia of the Cervix

Abnormal Transformation Zone. Area on the cervix or on the vagina that may contain columnar epithelium and squamous metaplasia and that often contains intraepithelial neoplasia that has an abnormal colposcopic pattern.

Acetowhite Epithelium. A colposcopic term to describe epithelium that initially looks normal but appears white after acetic acid application. The area is frequently found to have histologic evidence of human papillomavirus (HPV) infection, in which case the term *subclinical papilloma infection* (SPI) is used.

Carcinoma in Situ. A morphologic alteration of the epithelium that usually precedes, occasionally gives rise to, and is usually present in the vicinity of invasive carcinoma. The full thickness of the epithelium is replaced with dysplastic cells (CIN III).

Cervical Intraepithelial Neoplasia (CIN). A premalignant change in the cervical epithelium that can progress to the development of cervical carcinoma. The degree of change from mild to severe is described as CIN I, CIN II, or CIN III.

Colposcope. An instrument used to magnify and examine the epithelium of the transformation zone to identify abnormal areas in the lower genital tract that warrant biopsy.

Conization. A surgical technique to remove a cone-shaped central core of the cervix for diagnosis or treatment of intraepithelial neoplasia.

Cryotherapy. Freezing of the cervix to destroy abnormal epithelium.

Dysplasia. A term used to describe varying degrees of cervical intraepithelial neoplasia. It may be mild, involving approximately one third of the epithelium (CIN I); moderate, approximately two thirds of the epithelium (CIN II); or severe, full thickness of the epithelium (CIN III).

Endocervical Curettage (ECC). A biopsy procedure used to obtain endocervical tissue for histologic diagnosis.

Flat Wart. An alternate term to describe subclinical human papilloma virus (HPV) infection.

Koilocytosis. A cellular change associated with papillomavirus infection, which includes perinuclear cavitation and nuclear atypicality.

Laser. *L*ight *a*mplification by *s*timulated *e*mission of *r*adiation. A technique that uses energized light to vaporize tissue.

Leukoplakia. A colposcopic term to describe an area that appears white to the naked eye even before application of 3% acetic acid.

Mosaic Pattern. A colposcopic term to describe the rosette appearance of capillary vessels in an abnormal transformation zone.

Native Squamous Epithelium. The normal original squamous epithelium found in the vagina and on the portio of the cervix.

Normal Transformation Zone. Area of columnar epithelium and squamous metaplasia that has a normal colposcopic pattern.

Punctation. A colposcopic term to describe the stippled appearance of capillary vessels in the abnormal transformation zone.

Radiation Dysplasia. A term to describe abnormal cells in the cytologic smear of patients treated by ionizing irradiation for cervical cancer. These patients are at increased risk for recurrent disease.

Satisfactory Colposcopy. A colposcopic examination in which the entire transformation zone, including the squamocolumnar junction, is adequately visualized.

Squamocolumnar Junction. The junction of the squamous epithelium and columnar (glandular) epithelium usually located near the external cervical os.

Squamous Metaplasia. A physiologic process whereby squamous tissue replaces columnar tissue.

Subclinical Papilloma Infection (SPI). An area that looks normal to the naked eye but colposcopically appears white after acetic acid application. It often contains papillomavirus infection.

Because of the accessible location of the cervix and the upper vagina, intraepithelial neoplasia of the cervix has been investigated more than any other premalignant lesion of the female genital tract, and this process has resulted in improved detection and treatment. The development of cytology as a discipline to aid in the detection of neoplasia of the cervix and the colposcope as an instrument to localize the site of the most severe change and allow directed biopsy has contributed to improvement of the management of these disorders. This chapter will review the morphologic changes that characterize the intraepithelial neoplastic lesions of the cervix. The current concepts of the factors thought to lead to the development of cervical neoplasia, including a detailed consideration of human papillomavirus infection (HPV), will be reviewed and the methods of diagnosis and treatment described.

DEFINITIONS AND MORPHOLOGY

The *squamocolumnar junction* is an important landmark where neoplastic change develops in the cervix. In young adults this intersection between the cervical glandular (columnar) epithelium and the native squamous epithelium is usually located on the exocervix just distal to the external os. During pregnancy and after childbirth this area may enlarge and become more distally located on the portio of the cervix away from the os. After menopause the junction usually recedes and is frequently located in the endocervical canal. Thus in the normal adult female of reproductive age there are usually areas of columnar epithelium surrounding the exocervix. During puberty and throughout reproductive life, especially during pregnancy, this exposed columnar epithelium undergoes gradual replacement by squamous epithelium (squamous metaplasia). This process can be readily identified with the colposcope, and the areas of columnar epithelium and squamous metaplasia constitute the *normal transformation zone*. In contrast, abnormal or neoplastic squamous epithelium can also be found in the transformation zone, which leads to abnormal colposcopic patterns and characterizes the *abnormal transformation zone* (see colposcopy section).

Numerous terms have been used to describe the premalignant lesions of the cervix. It is important to emphasize that these changes are part of a continuum of slight to severe atypicality which can progress to invasive carcinoma (Fig. 26-1). Two terminologies are most commonly used to describe intraepithelial neoplasia. One relies on the term *dysplasia* (mild, moderate, or severe) to describe the early premalignant changes in the epithelium and the term *carcinoma in situ* to describe the most advanced premalignant change. An alternate nomenclature that describes the same histologic features utilizes the terminology of *cervical intraepithelial neoplasia (CIN)* of various grades of severity: CIN I (mild dysplasia), CIN II (moderate dysplasia), and CIN III (severe dysplasia to carcinoma in situ). The term *CIN* was introduced by Richart, who emphasized the concept of a single entity of intraepithelial neoplasia that has the potential to develop into invasive carcinoma.

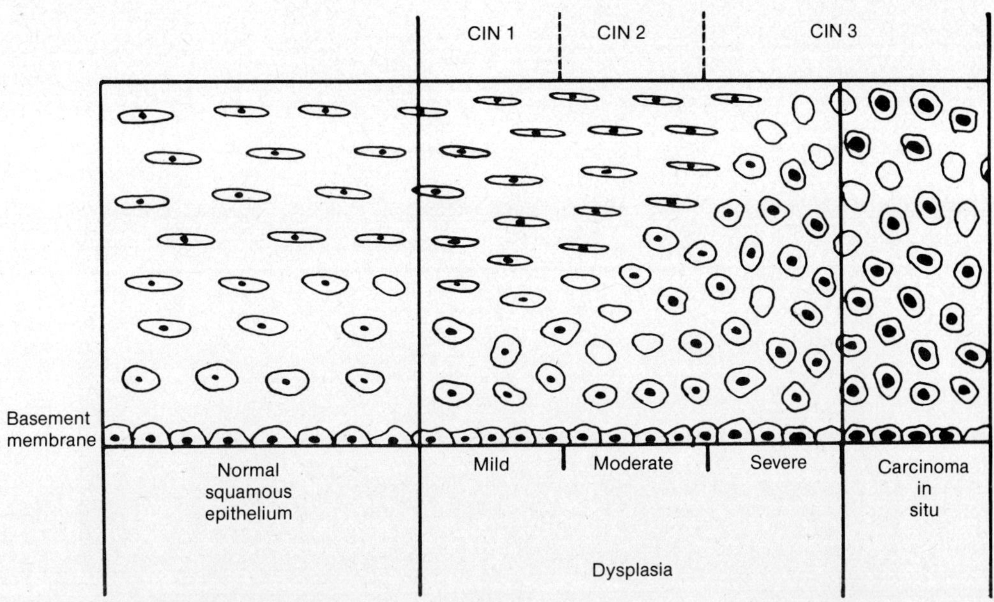

FIGURE 26-1
Diagram of cervical epithelium showing various terminology used to characterize progressive degrees of cervical neoplasia. (Modified from Richart RM: Can J Med Tech 38:177, 1976.)

The cytologic and histologic features of mild, moderate, and severe dysplasia and carcinoma in situ are illustrated in Figs. 26-2 to 26-5. The least disturbance of the squamous epithelium and the lowest proportion of abnormal cells occur in the lesion of mild dysplasia (CIN I). In the case of carcinoma in situ the entire thickness of the epithelium is replaced with abnormal cells but there is no invasion of the underlying stroma (CIN III). With progression, invasive carcinoma is diagnosed (Figs. 26-6 and 26-7). Unfortunately there is lack of agreement regarding the precise definition of each category of intraepithelial neoplasia, and there is no sharp morphologic boundary between them, a problem that often leads to disagreements in the diagnosis of the degree of severity of intraepithelial neoplasia. In addition, carcinoma in situ may develop in the crypts of the glands of the cervix as well as in the surface epithelium. Involvement of the glands leads to a diagnosis of "carcinoma in situ with gland involvement." For purposes of patient management this entity is the same as carcinoma in situ without gland involvement.

EPIDEMIOLOGY

Potential Factors in Carcinogenesis

Intraepithelial neoplasia of the cervix occurs mainly in young women. The Third National Cancer Survey, which was held in the decade 1960-1970, reports the incidence to be approximately twice as high in black women as in white. The peak in the age incidence of the disease appeared to be the early thirties, but recently it has been noted to be occurring more frequently in younger women. Furthermore it appears that the frequency of the diagnosis of carcinoma in situ has increased in the past 20 years, in part because of the effectiveness of cytologic screening (Pap smear). This has been accompanied by a concomitant decrease in the frequency of invasive carcinoma, as was documented by the studies of Devesa, who demonstrated a drop of approximately 50% in the frequency of cervical carcinoma from 1947 to 1977 in the United States. Fig. 26-8 shows the approximate age incidence curves for dysplasia, carcinoma in situ, and invasive cancer. First, it should be noted that dysplasia is the most com-

Text continued on p. 737.

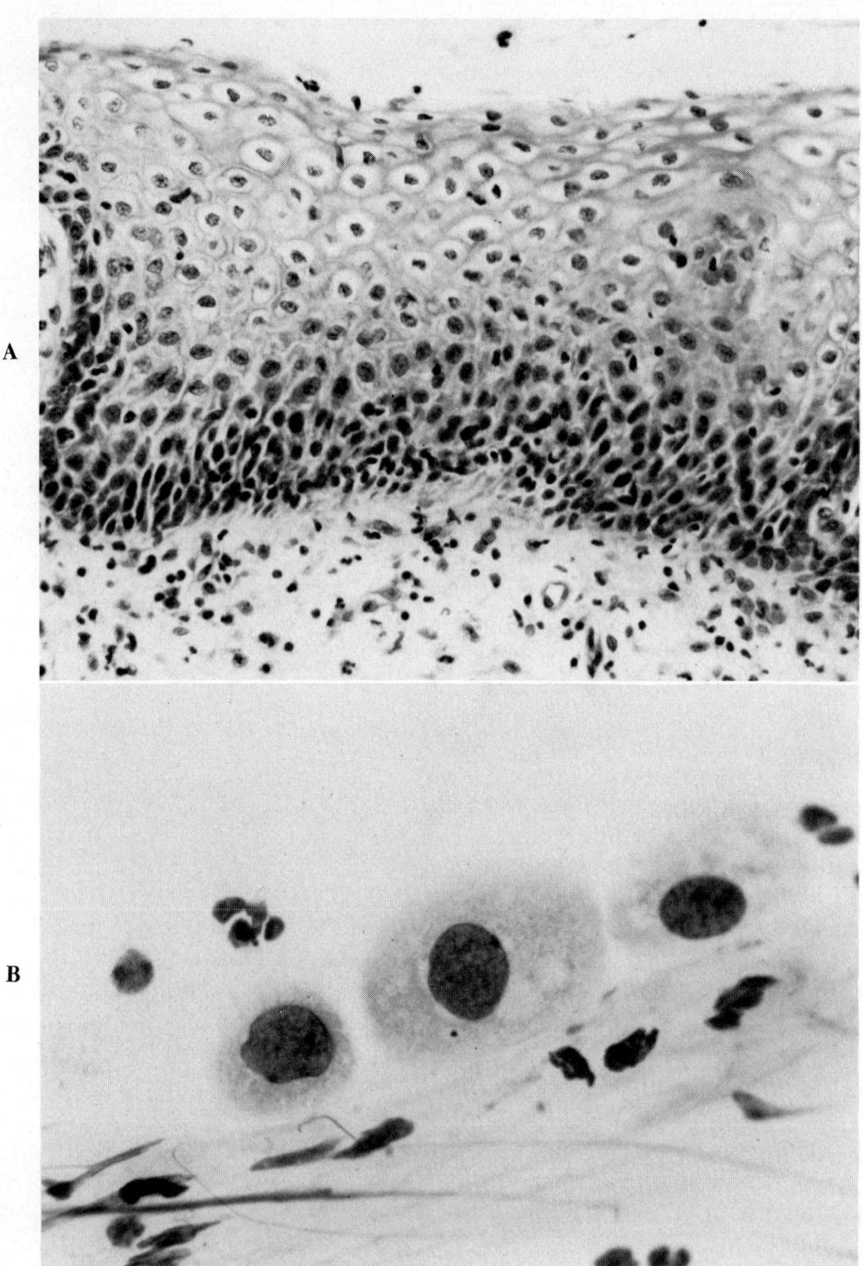

FIGURE 26-2

A, Mild dysplasia (histology). Undifferentiated cells are confined to lower two to four layers of epithelium. Cells of middle and upper thirds show nuclear enlargement and irregular nuclei. (H&E stain; ×250.) **B,** Mild dysplasia (cytology). Dysplastic cells have altered nuclear-cytoplasmic ratio, exhibit nuclear enlargement, and have finely granular chromatin structure. (Papanicolaou stain; ×800.)

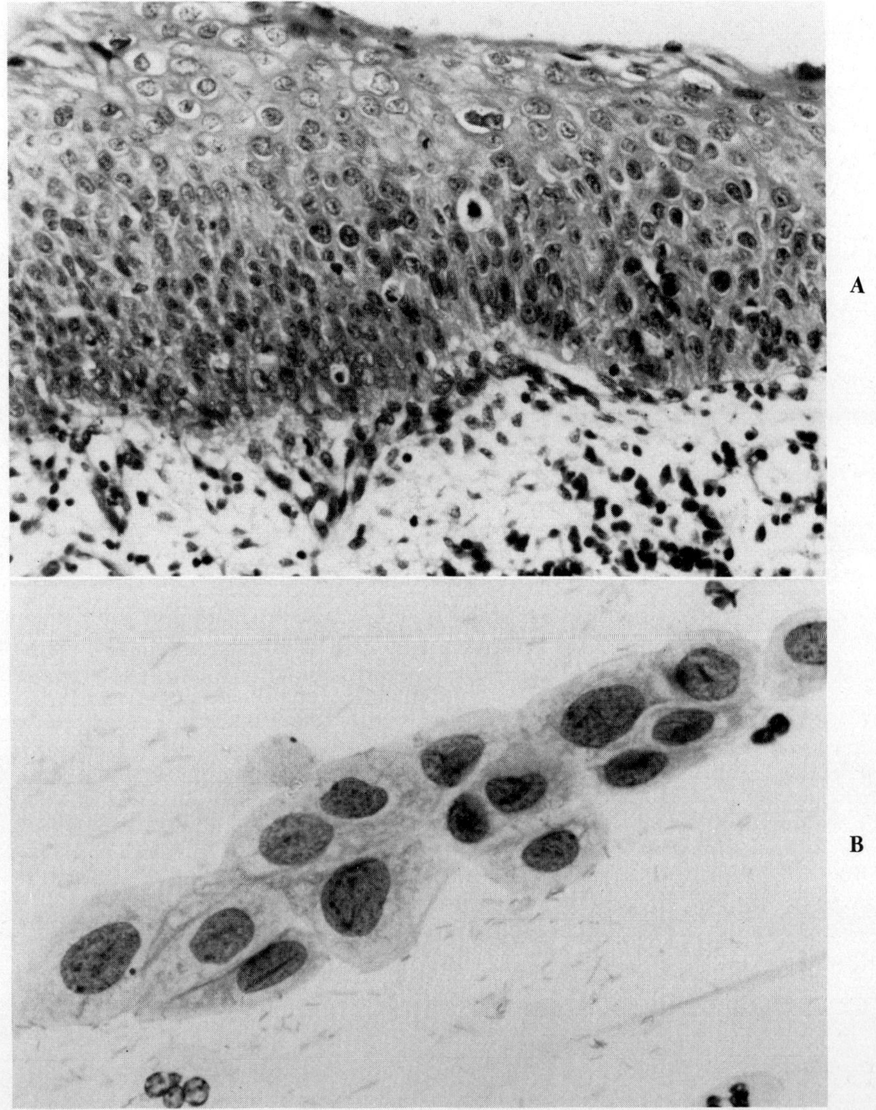

FIGURE 26-3
A, Moderate dysplasia (histology). Immature cells are confined to lower half of epithelium. Cells of upper half show well-defined cell borders and enlarged, pleomorphic nuclei. (H&E stain; ×300.) **B,** Moderate dysplasia (cytology). Cells derived from moderate dysplasia exhibit altered nuclear-cytoplasmic ratio with less cytoplasm than is seen in cells of mild dysplasia. There may be uniformly finely granular chromatin pattern with occasional chromocenter and (as cell at *right*) irregular nuclear envelope. (Papanicolaou stain; ×800.)

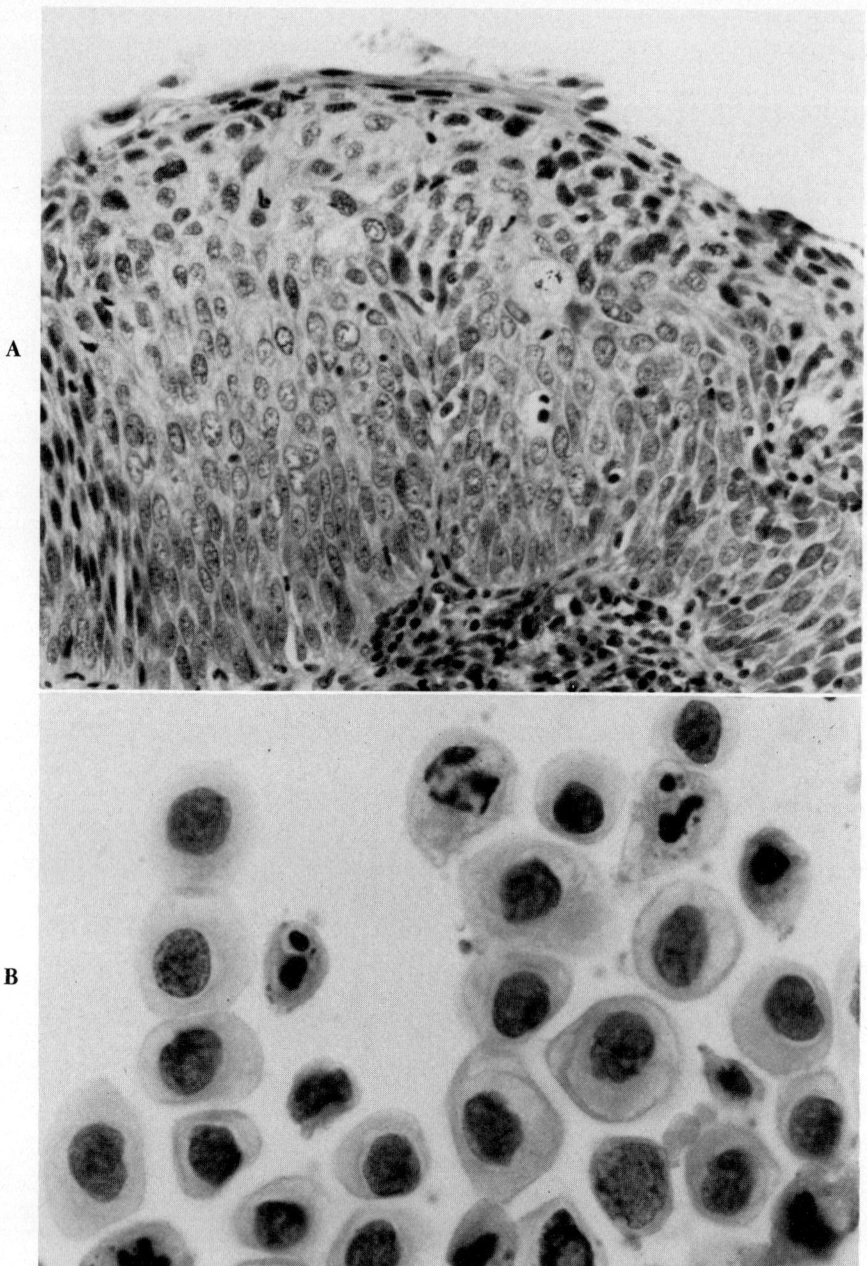

FIGURE 26-4

A, Severe dysplasia (histology). In this lesion, immature cells with spindle-shaped nuclei replace more than two thirds of the mucosal thickness. Upper layers show evidence of squamous cell differentiation (H&E stain; ×300.) **B,** Severe dysplasia (cytology). Cells derived from a severe dysplasia may exhibit enlarged hyperchromatic nuclei, an irregular nuclear envelope, a coarse chromatin structure, and less cytoplasm than less severe dysplastic reactions do. (Papanicolaou stain, ×1000.)

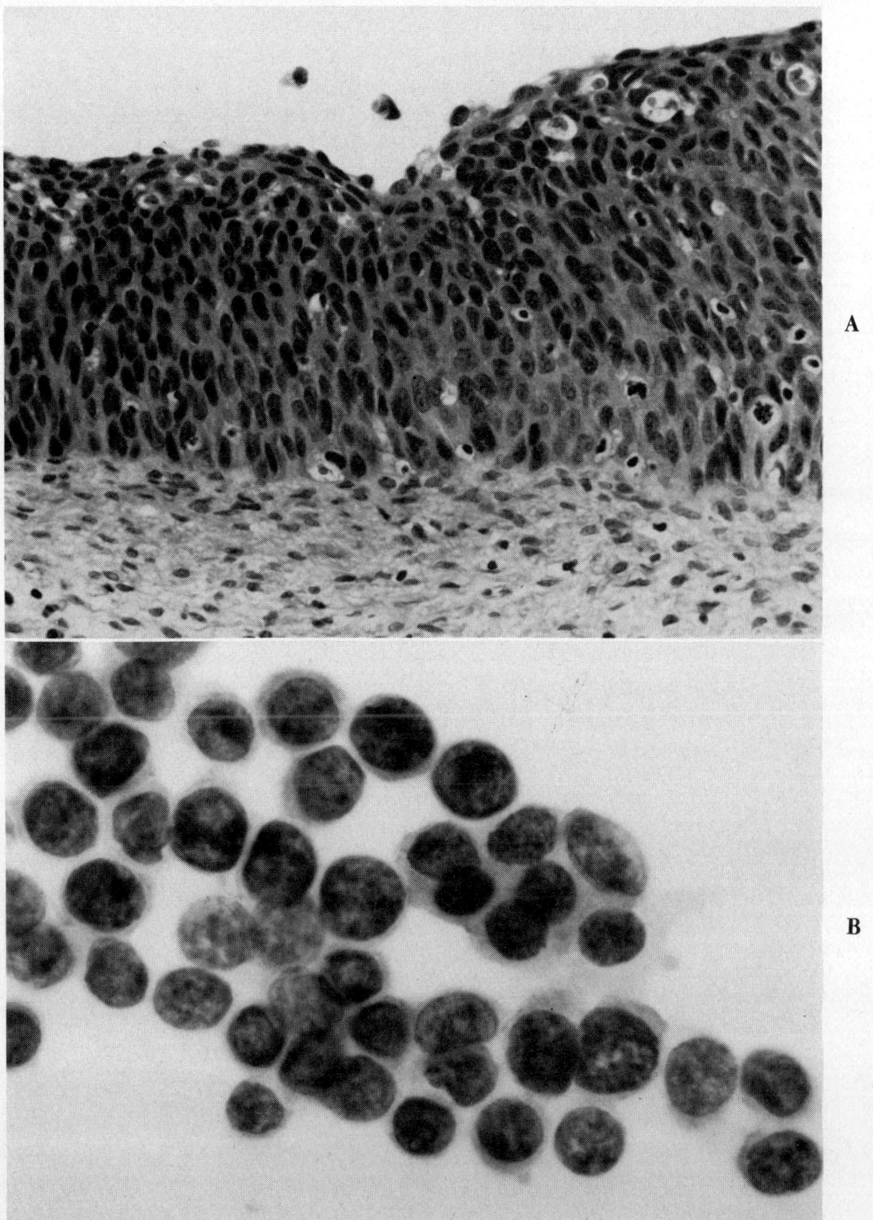

FIGURE 26-5
A, Carcinoma in situ (CIS) (histology). Basal-type cells with elongated nuclei and indistinct cytoplasmic boundaries occupy full thickness of mucosa. No maturation is present. (H&E stain; ×300.) **B,** Carcinoma in situ (CIS) (cytology). Carcinoma in situ in cytologic sample may reveal groups of primitive cells with scant, ill-defined cytoplasm, nuclei that are round or oval, and a coarsely granular chromatin pattern with distinct chromocenters. Nucleoli are usually absent. (Papanicolaou stain; ×800.)

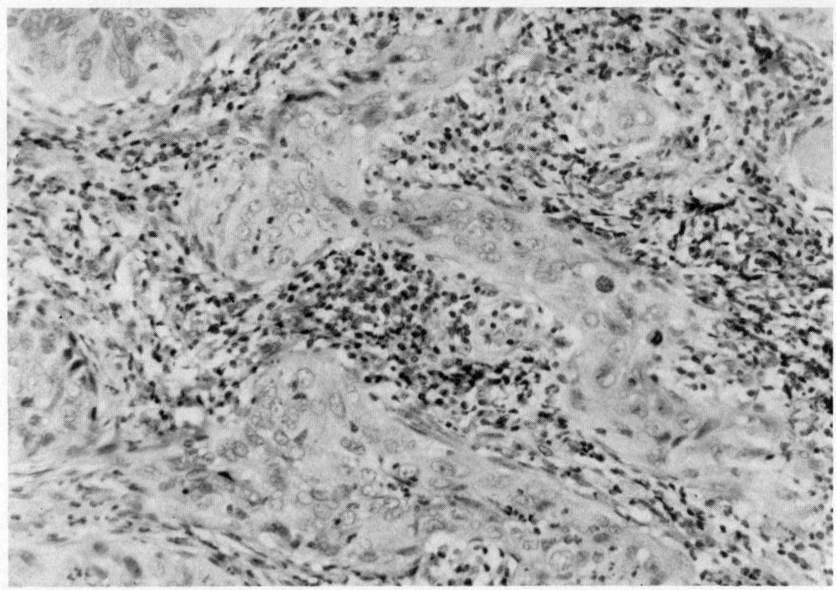

FIGURE 26-6
Invasive squamous carcinoma (histology). Irregular tumor nests infiltrate a stroma rich in inflammatory cells. Tumor cells are pleomorphic. A mitotic figure is seen at *left*. (H&E stain; ×200.)

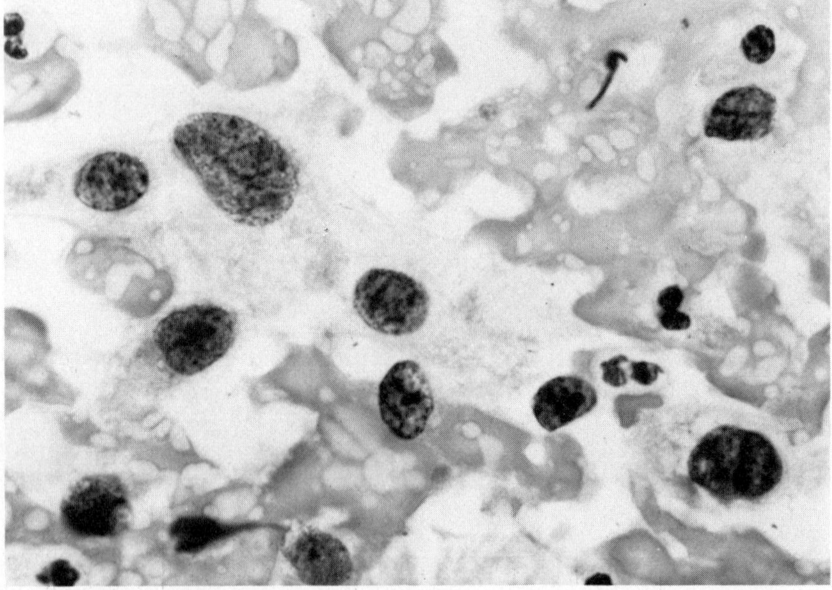

FIGURE 26-7
Invasive squamous cell carcinoma (cytology). Poorly differentiated squamous cell carcinoma may exhibit in the cytologic sample isolated malignant tumor cells with marked variation in nuclear size and shape. Because of the coarse and irregular chromatin pattern, nucleoli are not easily discerned here but are usually evident on direct microscopic examination. Background shows degenerated red blood cells and a few polymorphonuclear leukocytes. (Papanicolaou stain; ×1000.)

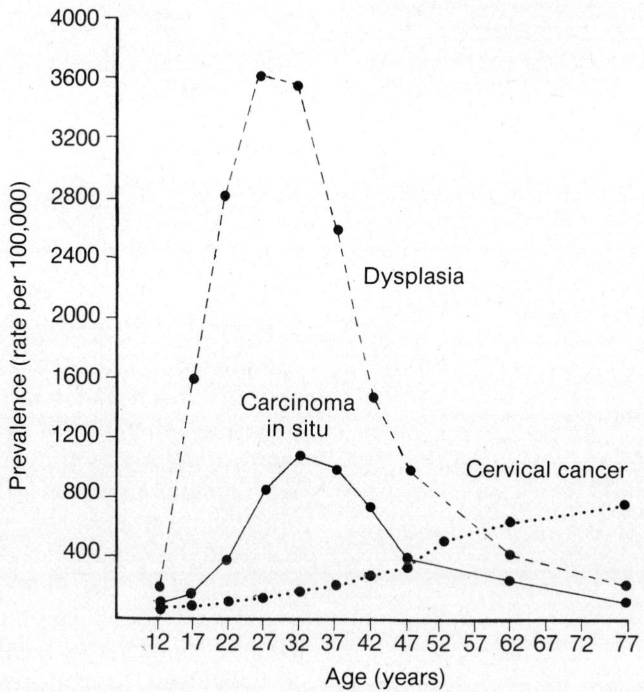

FIGURE 26-8

Graph of prevalence of minor precursors, major precursors, and invasive cancer. Precursors are much more common than invasive cancer. (From Reid R, Fu YS: In Peto R, ed: Banbury Report 21: Viral etiology of cervical cancer. Cold Spring Harbor, N.Y., 1986. Copyright © Cold Spring Harbor Laboratory, 1986.)

mon lesion, with a peak in the age incidence curve in the mid-twenties. Second, carcinoma in situ is much less frequent and peaks at a slightly later age. In contrast, the frequency of invasive cancer is a curve of different shape that appears to plateau in the late forties and then rises slowly with increasing age. As the individuals move into their sixties, invasive carcinoma becomes more common than carcinoma in situ. These age-incidence curves suggest that a large number of atypias (dysplasias) of the cervical epithelium develop during reproductive life yet do not progress to malignancy. On the other hand, data are available to indicate that some dysplasias can progress to cancer, and the risk of such progression increases with the more atypical lesions, such as carcinoma in situ.

The cause of cervical neoplasia is not known, but a number of factors have been studied regarding their potential role in carcinogenesis. The box on p. 738 outlines the major factors postulated to be related to the development of cervical neoplasia. Many of these have a venereal association. It is generally agreed that the atypical epithelium develops in the transformation zone of the cervix during the process of squamous metaplasia. Viruses (particularly HPV) are thought to have a major role in the genesis of premalignant lesions. In addition to this pathway of cervical carcinogenesis, it is recognized that some squamous cell cancers can arise de novo in areas outside of the transformation zone, as has been discussed by Burghardt. Some of these cancers may contribute to the continuing increased incidence of squamous cell carcinoma of the cervix that occurs in older women (see Fig. 26-8).

For many years it has been observed that carcinoma of the cervix occurs more frequently in persons who have sexual intercourse early in their lives as well as those who begin to have children at an early age. Women who have multiple sex partners are also at increased risk, and the disease is more frequent in young prostitutes. In contrast, squamous cell carcinoma of

POTENTIAL FACTORS IN CERVICAL NEOPLASIA

Epidemiologic Factors

Early intercourse
Multiple sex partners
Early marriage
Early childbearing
Prostitution
Male factors—"high-risk" consort
Socioeconomic status, race
Venereal infection

Other Potential Factors

Immune status
Prior radiation
Intrauterine DES exposure
Oral contraceptives
Cigarette smoking
Vitamins A and C

Viral Relations

Papillomavirus
Herpesvirus
Cytomegalovirus

the cervix is almost unknown in nuns. The disease is also rare among Jewish women, and this has led to speculation that circumcision might reduce the risk of development of the disease. Recent studies have failed to confirm that circumcision is a factor. Moreover, cervical carcinoma has been noted among Israeli Jews, especially if the usually associated venereal risk factors exist.

Recent studies have shown that the male consort can also be important in the development of the disease. For example, Kessler studied women who were married to men whose previous wives had developed cervical cancer. This cohort was compared with women who were married to men whose previous wives had not had cervical cancer. A threefold increased frequency of cervical cancer occurred among the former group.

The occurrence of venereal diseases such as gonorrhea have also been shown to be associated with the frequency of cervical carcinoma. Beral and colleagues noted that an increase in the frequency of gonorrhea in a given group was accompanied by a subsequent increase in cervical carcinoma. However, current data do not indicate a role for venereal diseases such as gonorrhea, *Trichomonas vaginalis,* or syphilis in the genesis of cervical carcinoma but suggest that the causative agent or agents may be transmitted as a result of sexual activity during which these diseases are also transmitted.

Other Potential Factors

As noted in the box at left other factors have potential involvement in the genesis of cervical neoplasia. Alteration in immune function could increase the risk. For example, patients receiving immunosuppressive therapy have been noted to be at increased risk for recurrent genital tract viral infection and recurrent papilloma wart infections. In addition Seski et al. have noted altered cellular immunity as measured by T-cell function in lymphocyte toxicity tests in individuals with recurrent papilloma infection. An increase in gynecologic malignancies and cervical carcinoma in immunosuppressed patients has been reported.

Radiation has also been considered as a potential factor in cervical neoplasia. Dysplasia of the cervix has been reported in cytologic (Pap) smears in patients following radiation therapy for carcinoma of the cervix. If these patients with so-called radiation dysplasia are carefully followed, they are found to be at increased risk for the development of recurrent disease in comparison to those who do not show radiation dysplasia changes. However, it is not clear if this radiation dysplasia is a result of the radiation or is an early morphologic cellular change that precedes the development of recurrent cancer. A definitive role for radiation in the development of cervical neoplasia has not been established.

Intrauterine diethylstilbestrol (DES) exposure is discussed in detail in Chapter 14. Because of the enlarged transformation zone that occurs in the cervix and occasionally the vagina of these females with concommitant larger areas of squamous metaplasia, there is concern that such patients may be at increased risk for squamous neoplasia. Although such patients require regular medical surveillance for the development of squamous neoplasia (see below), current evidence has not established that DES exposure is a risk factor for cervical squamous neoplasia.

Other potential hormonal effects in the genesis of cervical neoplasia have been evaluated with extensive studies of women ingesting oral contraceptives. Conflicting data exist on the potential role of these agents on cervical neoplasia, with some studies finding an increased risk and others demonstrating no increase in risk. Some of the studies are flawed by a lack of accurate sexual histories, which, as has been discussed, is itself an important factor in cervical neoplasia. The studies of Swan and Brown suggest that those who are already at high risk for cervical neoplasia because of sexual factors may have the risk increased even further by long-term oral contraceptive use. Such an increased risk did not occur in their study among oral contraceptive users who did not also have an elevated sexual factor risk. Other studies by Vessey et al. suggest that oral contraceptives may increase the risk of cervical neoplasia in comparison to controls with comparable sexual histories who used an IUD. The degree to which oral contraceptives promote or increase the risk of cervical neoplasia has not been established.

Cigarette smoking has also been implicated as a factor. Brinton et al. found a relative risk of 1.5 for the development of cervical neoplasia among women who smoke. This is similar to the observation of Trevathan et al., who noted an increased risk in persons who had a history of smoking 20 or more pack-years. In these studies a correction was made for the sexual histories.

Vitamins have also been evaluated as potential risk factors. Animal studies have suggested that deficiencies in vitamin A can promote neoplasia. Vitamin A deficiencies in humans have been associated with dysplastic-type changes in cytologic smears of the cervix, and these changes have been reversed by vitamin A administration. Some studies have been undertaken to evaluate vitamin A analogues (retinoids) in regard to their ability to prevent or reverse cervical neoplasia. Surwit et al. studied β-transretinoic acid in 18 patients with CIN II or III: one third improved, but half experienced severe vaginal burning, which in some cases required discontinuation of the drug. Recently Romney et al. noted a deficiency of vitamin C in patients who had an abnormal Pap smear in comparison to those who had normal smears, and they suggested that vitamin C deficiency might be a factor.

Viral Hypothesis (Herpes, Cytomegalic, Papilloma)

A number of studies have related genital tract infections with herpes simplex virus II (HSV II) to carcinoma of the cervix. The herpesvirus elicits antibody responses in humans, and elevated serum antibody titers to HSV II have been found more frequently among women with premalignant and malignant lesions of the cervix. Moreover, elevated antibody titers to this virus have also been observed in Jewish women with cervical carcinoma. The virus has been detected in tissues from cervical carcinoma, and viral antigens have also been detected in carcinoma tissues. Cervical carcinoma has also been found to contain antibodies to HSV II antigens. The virus has been found to be capable of transforming mammalian cells in vitro and has also been found to be able to produce tumors in experimental animals. Although HSV II is suspect in the etiology of cervical cancer, a definitive cause and effect relationship has not been established.

The cytomegalovirus is the largest member of the Herpesviridae family and also has been studied for its potential role in cervical carcinogenesis. It is transmitted by sexual contact, and a limited number of seroepidemiologic studies have shown elevated antibody titers in women with cervical cancer. The viral particles have been uncovered in cervical carcinoma biopsies, and in vitro malignant cellular transformation has been observed. Although it is a potential agent in the etiology of cervical carcinoma, it has not been as extensively studied as HSV II and is not currently thought to have a major role in cervical carcinogenesis.

Human Papillomavirus

Papillomaviruses belong to the Papovaviridae family. They are commonly associated with genital warts and have been extensively studied in the past few years for their potential role in the genesis of cervical neoplasia. Human papillomavirus (HPV) does not cause systemic

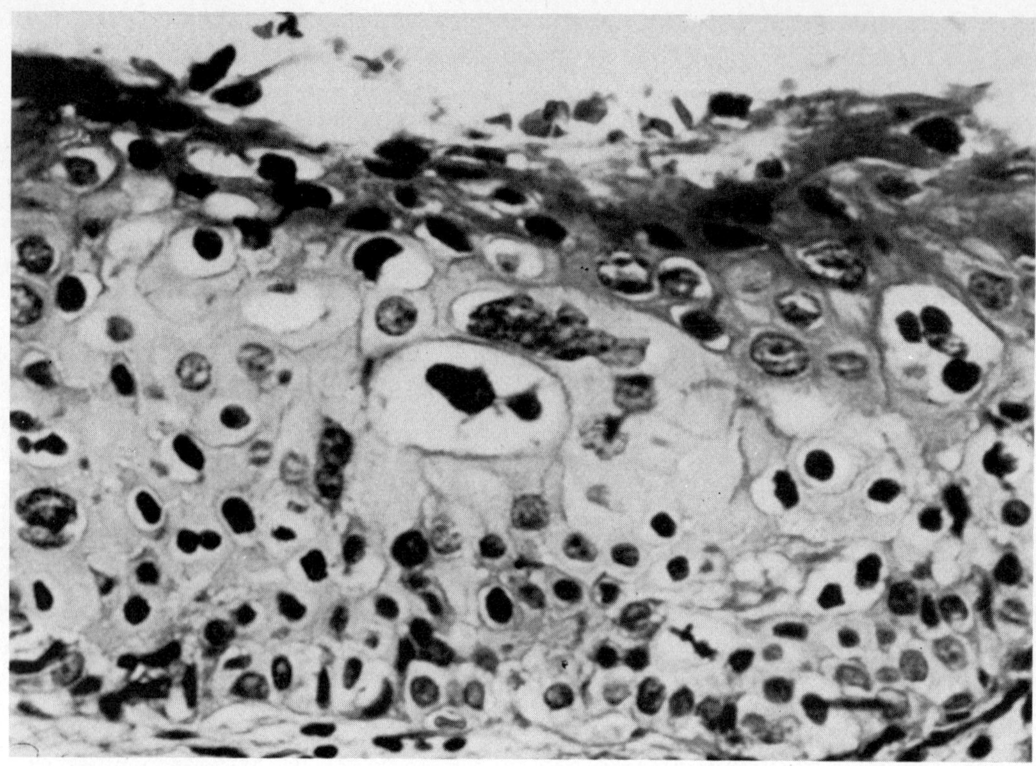

FIGURE 26-9
Human papillomavirus changes: koilocytosis, multinucleation, parakeratosis, and dyskeratosis. (Light microscopy; H&E stain.) (From Grunebaum AN, Sedlis A, Sillman F, et al: Obstet Gynecol 62:448, 1983. Reprinted with permission from The American College of Obstetricians and Gynecologists.)

infection, and serum antibodies to HPV have not been identified. Thus seroepidemiologic studies of the type conducted with herpes simplex virus II (HSV II) are not feasible. For many years there has been indirect evidence for a role of the papillomavirus in cervical neoplasia. Malignant transformation of papillomas in animals exposed to the papillomavirus have been observed, and human papilloma warts have also been noted to undergo malignant transformation. Like HSV II, papillomaviruses are sexually transmitted, and infections have been identified in the male partners of infected females; these females appear to be at increased risk for cervical neoplasia. In addition, papillomaviral infections have been noted by Meisels and Morin to precede invasive carcinoma of the cervix by 27.5 years.

In recent years evidence has accumulated linking HPV to cervical neoplasia more closely than HSV II or cytomegalovirus. HPV causes distinct cellular changes, the most common of which is koilocytosis (perinuclear cavitation) (Fig. 26-9). These cells are found in genital warts and are frequently identified in areas of intraepithelial neoplasia. Papillomaviral particles have been identified by electron microscopy in the nuclei of koilocytes (Fig. 26-10). Some of the morphologic changes of HPV infection mimic the changes of mild dyplasia (CIN I). The rapid increase in knowledge regarding HPV has affected both the diagnosis and the current management of atypias of the cervix.

Recently through the use of molecular hybridization of HPV DNA, a number of distinct types of HPV have been demonstrated. Some of these have been associated predominantly with wart infections, while others are associated more with neoplasia (Table 26-1). Newer types of HPV are under investigation, and it may be anticipated that other types will be

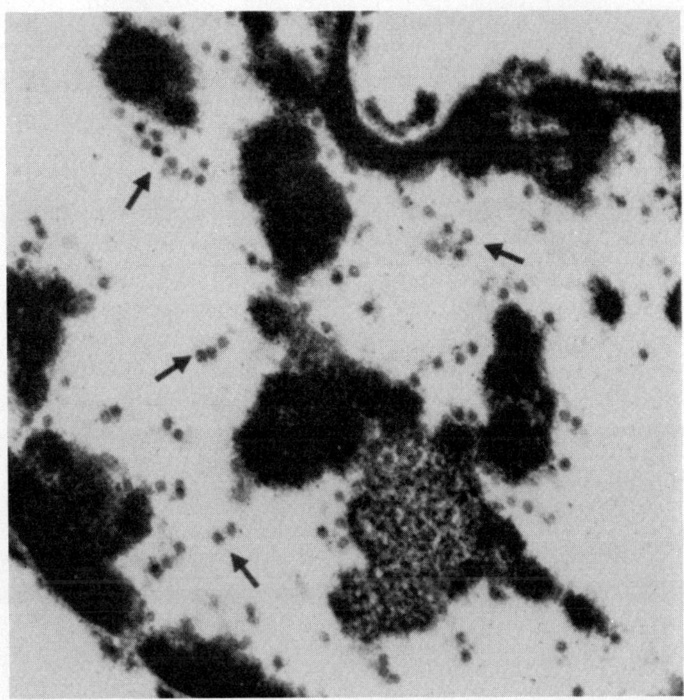

FIGURE 26-10
Higher magnification of Fig. 26-9. Human papillomavirus particles *(arrows)* measure 45 to 50 nm within nucleus. (TEM; ×39,900.) (From Grunebaum AN, Sedlis A, Sillman F, et al: Obstet Gynecol 62:448, 1983. Reprinted with permission from The American College of Obstetricians and Gynecologists.)

added in the future. The most extensively investigated are HPV types 6 and 11 (associated with benign condyloma) and HPV types 16, 18, and 31 (associated with neoplasia). The development of invasive cancer within 3 years of developing papilloma infection with types 16 and 18 has been reported by Syrjanen et al., and HPV 16 has been reported in as many as 90% of cervical cancers and 70% of intraepithelial neoplasias by McChance et al.

INTRAEPITHELIAL NEOPLASIA AND GENITAL PAPILLOMA INFECTION

As noted in the section on morphology, there is a continuum of premalignant change in the cervix ranging from mild dysplasia (CIN I) to severe dysplasia and carcinoma in situ (CIN III). In considering these changes it must be recognized that the morphology of the cervical epithelium is also altered by papillomavirus infection and that koilocytosis (see Fig. 26-9) can be accompanied by nuclear changes that on cytologic smear and biopsy resemble the alterations normally identified with intraepithelial neoplasia. Reid et al. have extensively studied papillomavirus infections and their role in neoplasia. He and others have used the term *subclinical papillomavirus infection* (SPI) to describe an entity that is not clinically visible to the naked eye but that can be recognized utilizing the colposcope and staining the vagina and cervix with acetic acid (see subsequent discussion on colposcopy). Subclinical papillomavirus infection and clinically evident condyloma

TABLE 26-1
Types of Human Papillomavirus

	HPV Type
Associated with condyloma	6, 11
Associated with neoplasia	16, 18, 31
Other types under investigation	33, 35

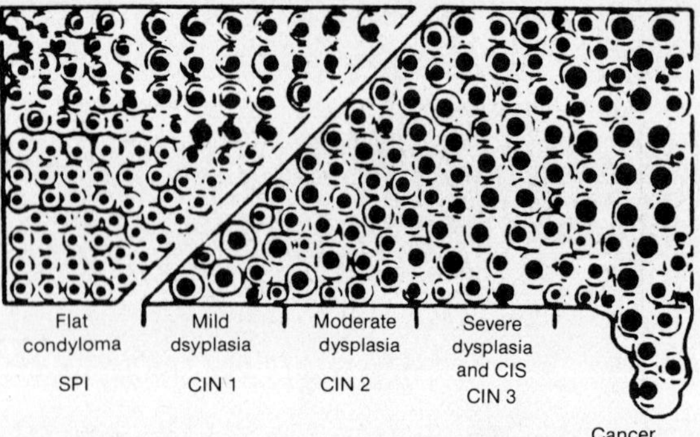

FIGURE 26-11
Schematic model explaining interrelationships between different grades of disorders and showing nomenclature division, according to the proportion of cells exhibiting morphologic features of either late viral expression *(left half)* or premalignant change *(right half)*. (From Reid R, Fu YS: In Peto R, ed: Banbury Report 21: Viral etiology of cervical cancer. Cold Spring Harbor, N.Y., 1986. Copyright © Cold Spring Harbor Laboratory, 1986.)

constitute important manifestations of papillomavirus infection of the lower genital tract; some of these infections may lead to malignant transformation. The spectrum of such changes, including subclinical papillomavirus, is shown in Fig. 26-11, which is a modification of the concept initially introduced by Richart (see Fig. 26-1). Moreover, it has been shown by Mitchell et al. that those with evidence of papillomavirus infection on Pap smear have 15 times the risk of developing carcinoma in situ or invasive cancer as that of controls, and the risk increases to 39-fold when such changes are found in those under the age of 21 years. The morphologic manifestations of papillomavirus infection, such as koilocytosis and papillomatosis, are most prominent in the early premalignant lesions such as mild dysplasia (CIN I) and decrease as the more severe alterations of the cervical epithelium occur. Moreover, it appears that some diagnoses reported as dysplasia in the past may in fact have been papillomavirus infection. The lesions related to papillomavirus infection types 6 and 11 do not carry important risk of premalignant change, while others, types 16 and 18 and possibly 31, are associated with an increased risk for the devel-

opment of neoplasia. Unfortunately, currently available clinical tools and morphologic techniques do not allow one readily to differentiate the types of papillomavirus infection that are seen in biopsy specimens and cytologic smears, although such techniques are available in research laboratories. For example, Wickenden et al. have shown it is possible by DNA hybridization techniques to ascertain the type of papillomavirus infection that is identified on the cytologic smear.

As noted previously, the rate of occurrence of mild cervical atypias is higher than the frequency of the more severe changes of carcinoma in situ. Currently available data are confusing in regard to the risk and duration of time required for progression from mild to severe dysplasia or to carcinoma in situ and invasive cancer. It appears that initial infection with an oncogenic virus, if accompanied by appropriate cofactors, will eventually lead to a progression of epithelial alterations that can develop into invasive cancer.

Risks of Progression and Natural History

What are the rates of progression of premalignant lesions of the cervix? Precise data are not available. However, Richart and Barron estimated transit times from mild, moderate, or severe dysplasia to carcinoma in situ to have a median duration of 44 months for all of the dysplasias. The shortest duration of progression was 12 months for severe dysplasia, while the longest was 86 months for mild dysplasia. Koss et al. studied 93 women with untreated CIS and observed that it did progress to invasive carcinoma. However, they also noted that cervical biopsy could occasionally eradicate the lesion, and in addition spontaneous disappearance of carcinoma in situ rarely occurred. In more recent studies of mild and moderate cervical dysplasia, Nasiell et al. used cervical cytology or biopsy to follow women in the Stockholm area from 1962 to 1983. Regression to normal from mild dysplasia occurred in 62% of the cases, while progression to more severe lesions of carcinoma in situ or severe dysplasia occurred in 16%, and two cases of invasive cancer were noted. The remaining 22% had persistence of mild dysplasia. In a similar study of moderate dysplasia, the same authors noted that regression occurred in 54% over 6 years, progression to severe dysplasia or carcinoma in situ in 30%, and persistence of severe dysplasia in 16%. While some have concern in regard to these studies, particularly with diagnoses based only on cytology findings, biopsies were done on many of the patients, and the results are consistent with the concept that the risk of progression of cervical neoplasia is higher for those with high-grade lesions but that spontaneous regression of these lesions can also occur. Current evidence suggests a slow progression to invasive cancer from intraepithelial neoplasia of the cervix, but the risk of such progression is small and usually it takes many months or years to occur. Current techniques do not allow accurate prediction concerning how fast any particular lesion will progress. Estimates of nuclear DNA content (see later discussion) appear to hold promise for identifying which lesions are at the greatest risk for progression.

Methods of Detection and Diagnosis

The Papanicolaou (Pap) smear has been used widely for about 50 years to screen large populations of women for malignant and premalignant cervical disease. Its usage has been effective to reduce the frequency of invasive carcinoma of the cervix. It is essential to realize that cervical cytology is only of use for screening, and its results do not establish definitive diagnosis. False negative and false positive results can also occur. For example, in the detection of cervical carcinoma it is estimated that approximately 5% to 10% of the cases will be missed by routine cytologic screening because of sampling variation or other technical difficulties that may contribute to a false negative result. Similarly, certain conditions can cause the cells on the smear to appear atypical and mimic neoplastic changes. Examples are severe cervical infection, *Trichomonas vaginalis* infection, herpesvirus infection (which can cause cellular nuclear change), and infections with the papillomavirus leading to koilocytosis (see Fig. 26-9). All these may cause confusion of interpretation of the Pap smear, especially for the less experienced cytologist. Once a Pap smear suggestive of cervical neoplasia is reported, the patient should be reexamined and the smear

repeated to verify the findings. Colposcopic evaluation is performed and a biopsy is obtained to establish the diagnosis.

Cytology

TECHNIQUE. The Pap smear is best obtained by taking a direct scrape (sample) from the tissue being studied. This is usually accomplished by exposing the cervix after introducing a speculum into the vagina and using a wood or plastic spatula to separately scrape the exocervix and endocervix (Fig. 26-12). Many centers obtain a separate smear initially from the vagina and from the cervix and endocervix (V, vaginal; C, cervical; E, endocervical), and these are placed on a glass slide. The cellular specimen is immediately fixed, either in 90% alcohol or sprayed with fixative. It is important to hold the fixative spray more than 12 inches from the smear and not to allow the smear to air dry before fixing in order to preserve the cellular architecture and not introduce artifacts.

INTERPRETATION OF THE SMEAR. Numerous classifications have been used to describe the Pap smear results. The most useful information is conveyed by describing the type of cellular changes observed by the cytology. One classification is demonstrated in the box below. It is very important that the smear be interpreted by laboratories with adequate volumes to maintain diagnostic skills. It is recommended that a cytopathologist annually supervise at least 25,000 cervical smears to achieve this. Cytologists also frequently indicate the type of inflammation or infection that may exist

---

CLASSIFICATION OF PAPANICOLAOU SMEAR

Normal
Metaplasia
Inflammation
Minimal atypia—koilocytosis
Mild dysplasia (CIN I)
Moderate dysplasia (CIN II)
Severe dysplasia—Carcinoma in situ (CIN III)
Invasive carcinoma

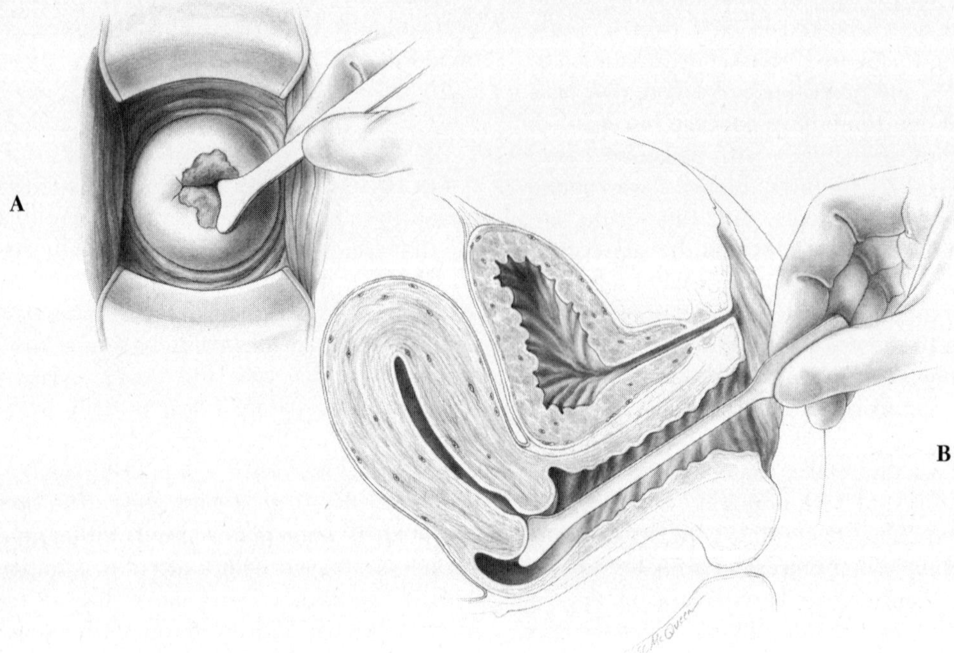

FIGURE 26-12
A, Scrape of endocervix. **B,** Scrape of exocervix.

if there are morphologic changes that allow the infectious agents such as herpesvirus, papillomavirus, *Chlamydia* or *Trichomonas vaginalis* to be identified. Figs. 26-2 to 26-7 illustrate the various cytologic changes that correspond to the various types of cervical neoplasia that are also demonstrated histologically.

In the past, cervical smears were classified in five categories: class I, benign; class II, inflammation; class III, mild to moderate atypia consistent with dysplasia; class IV, severe atypia consistent with severe dysplasia or carcinoma in situ; class V, suggestive of invasion of cancer. Current practice is not to utilize this classification for Pap smear results, but it is presented to the reader because many laboratories still use it. The more descriptive terminology identified on p. 743 is preferred. Based on this description the clinician can proceed with diagnosis and management.

If severe inflammation or infection is present, it should be treated as outlined in Chapter 21. In the case of nonspecific or so-called mild atypia it is often only necessary to repeat the smear in 4 to 6 months. If more severe changes are found, the cytologist may recommend to

the clinician that additional diagnostic procedures such as colposcopy or further biopsy are advisable. If the cytologic smear indicates mild or moderate dysplasia or a more atypical lesion, colposcopy is done and usually a biopsy is performed.

CYTOLOGIC SCREENING GUIDELINES. The ideal frequency for Pap smear screening is not established, and disagreement exists in regard to the interval between examinations for cytologic screening of the cervix. Much of the disagreement is in regard to the cost effectiveness of such screening and is based on studies of large populations. For example, the so-called Walton Report in Canada recommends annual smears when the individual becomes sexually active, to be repeated up to the age of 35. From the age of 36 years on, screening is done only once every 5 years after two negative tests and beyond the age of 60 it is discontinued after two negative tests. In contrast, the American College of Obstetricians and Gynecologists and the International Academy of Cytology recommend that cytologic screening start at age 18 or when the individual becomes sexually active and continue annually indefinitely. Development of cervical cancer has been reported to occur within 3 to 4 years after a negative Pap smear. In addition, even after hysterectomy the risk for neoplasia remains. Stuart et al., in a study of 29 cases of vaginal cancer, noted a 5.7-year interval for diagnosis of cancer after hysterectomy when the operation was performed for cervical intraepithelial neoplasia. When hysterectomy was performed for benign disease, the interval was 13.1 years. Table 26-2 shows a composite of recently recommended intervals for Pap smear screening.

An additional factor for the physician to consider is the importance of an annual pelvic examination, particularly for a woman over the age of 40 years, which allows for evaluation of ovarian size. In general, for women who are interested in an effective health maintenance program, an annual Pap smear and pelvic and physical examinations are indicated. For those who have had a hysterectomy for benign disease, and in whom the ovaries remain, an an-nual pelvic examination should be done and vaginal cytology performed every 3 to 5 years.

Biopsy

Instruments useful for biopsy of the cervix are shown in Fig. 26-13. The punch biopsy is capable of removing a small tissue sample 2 to 3 mm in size from the cervix. The colposcopically directed biopsy can easily be obtained in the office without anesthesia. Once the biopsy specimen is taken, it is usually fixed immediately either in Bouin's solution or in formalin. It is important that each specimen be placed in a separate container and appropriately labeled.

Current convention is to identify the location of the exocervix using the position of the 12 hours of the clock (Fig. 26-14). An endocervical curette is used to obtain an endocervical curettage (ECC) specimen. To obtain an adequate sample, the curette is introduced into the endocervix approximately 1 to 2 cm, and

---

TABLE 26-2
Recommendations on the Frequency of Pap Testing

	ACOG (1980)	American Cancer Society (1980)	Canadian Task Force (1982)	International Academy of Cytology (1980)	National Cancer Institute (1980)
Start	Age 18 or when sexually active	Age 20 or when sexually active	When sexually active	Age 18 or when sexually active	When sexually active
Age 18-35	Annually	Annually until two negative tests; then continue every 3 years	Annually if sexually active		After two negative tests, Continue every 1-3 years
Age 36-60	Annually	At least every 3 years; more frequently if high risk; pelvic examination should be done annually after age 40	After two negative tests, continue every 5 years	Annually	Every 1-3 years
Over age 60	Annually	At least every 3 years; more frequently if high risk; pelvic examination should be done annually	After two negative tests, testing may be stopped	Annually	After two negative tests, testing may be stopped

Modified from American College of Obstetricians and Gynecologists Newsletter, June 1984.

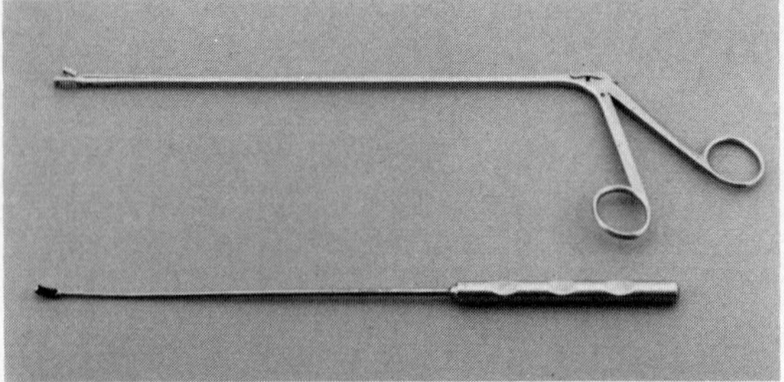

FIGURE 26-13
Cervical biopsy instruments. *Above,* Punch biopsy; *below,* endocervical curette.

firm pressure is applied to obtain a sample from the four quadrants of the endocervix. This part of the procedure often causes discomfort to the patient, and the administration of an oral analgesic is occasionally helpful. Usually the examination can be completed without analgesia. The endocervical curettage specimens are grouped together in one container and submitted to pathology, since it is important only to ascertain whether neoplasia exists in the cervical canal. It is not feasible to identify which portion of the canal contains abnormal epithelium.

Colposcopy

The colposcope is a magnifying instrument used to identify those abnormal cervical areas that require biopsy. The pertinent area is the transformation zone, which may be either normal or abnormal. A normal transformation zone, as previously noted, is the junction of normal columnar epithelium and squamous metaplasia, while the abnormal transformation zone contains patterns that may indicate the presence of neoplastic tissue or premalignant process.

Colposcopic examination is usually performed at ×10 to ×16 magnification. After excess mucus is gently wiped away from the cervix and the Pap smear has been taken, 3% acetic acid is applied. The colposcopic examination is usually performed using a green filter. Normal columnar epithelium will often produce a grapelike pattern, while squamous metaplasia appears as a smooth grey-white epithelium after the application of acetic acid (Fig. 26-15). The native squamous epithelium

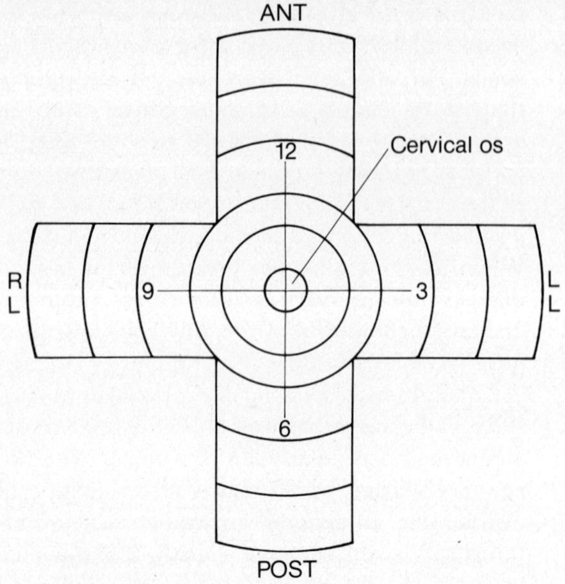

FIGURE 26-14
Diagram using the positions of the 12 hours of the clock; utilized during examination of cervix to record position of any abnormality.

outside the transformation zone has a smooth red-tan appearance.

An abnormal transformation zone may be marked by white areas with red stippling (punctation), sharp bordered lesions with vessels in a mosaic pattern (mosaic), white tissue with sharp borders (white epithelium), or atypical vessels. The white epithelium is seen best after acetic acid application and results from the piling up of cells with an increased nuclear-cytoplasmic ratio. A mosaic pattern results from neovascularization with capillaries running just beneath the surface epithelium, whereas punctation results from capillaries growing perpendicular to the surface. In addition, some areas may appear white before the application of acetic acid (leukoplakia).

The main criteria used by the colposcopist to establish the degree of atypicality and identify the sites for subsequent biopsies are (1) the vascular pattern (arrangement of the capillaries), (2) the distance between the capillaries, (3) the intensity of color tone after the addition of acetic acid, (4) the surface pattern—regular or irregular, and (5) the sharpness of the border of the suspected site in comparison to adjacent tissues. In general the more severe lesions

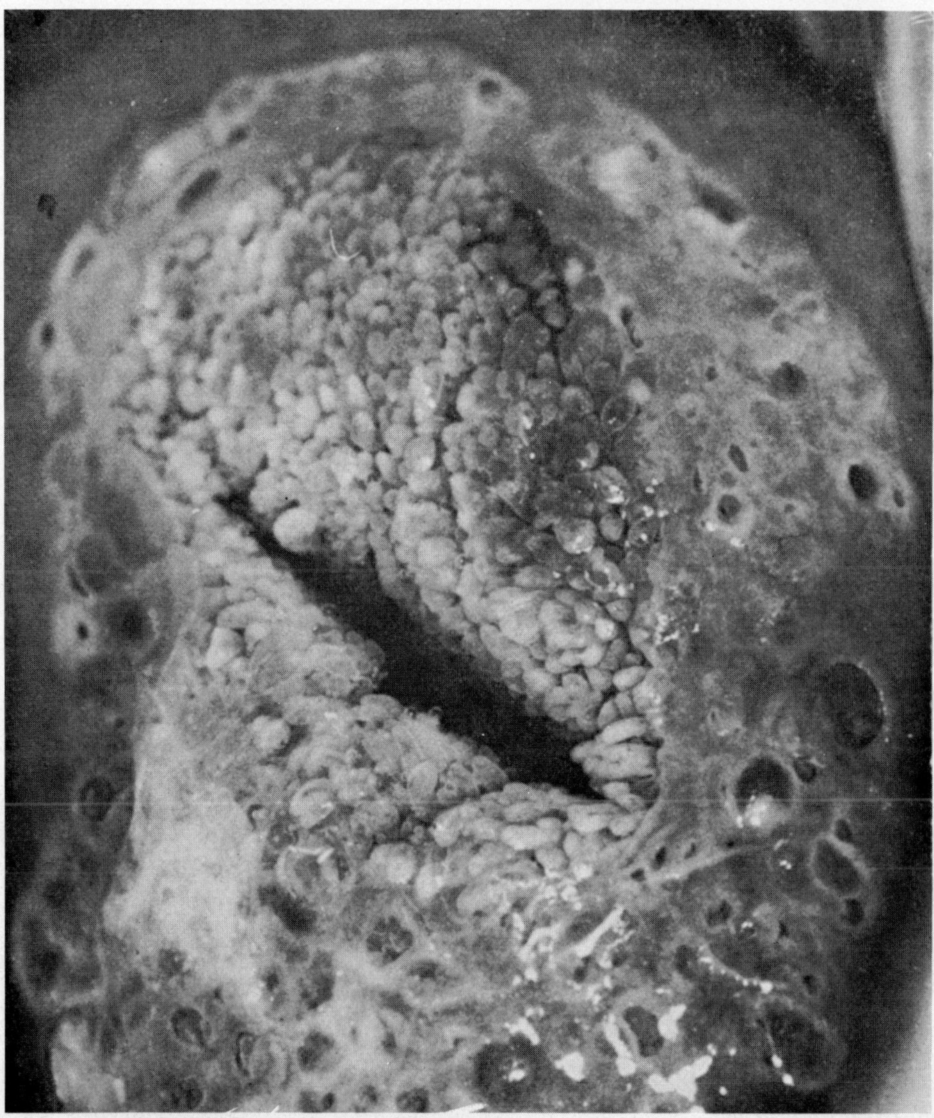

FIGURE 26-15
Typical transformation zone. The distal portion of columnar (grapelike) epithelium
is replaced by a crescentic sheet of metaplastic epithelium. At its outer edge it
adjoins native squamous epithelium at a clearly defined junction; at its inner edge
it adjoins columnar epithelium. (From Coppleson M, Pixley E, Reid B: Colposcopy—a scientific and practical approach to the cervix in health and disease.
Springfield, Ill., Charles C Thomas, Publisher, 1971.)

have a deeper whitish tone and greater width
and irregularity in the intracapillary distance.
Abnormal vessels may be present in advanced
lesions. In addition, the surface appears irregular and the vessels coarser.

As shown by Rome et al. the high-grade intraepithelial lesions are usually found in large
abnormal transformation zones (>63 mm^2),
whereas small abnormal transformation zones
(<46 mm^2) are associated with low-grade lesions. A large abnormal transformation zone
should heighten the examiner's suspicion of a
high-grade lesion and possibly a small invasive
carcinoma. Similarly atypical vessels usually in-

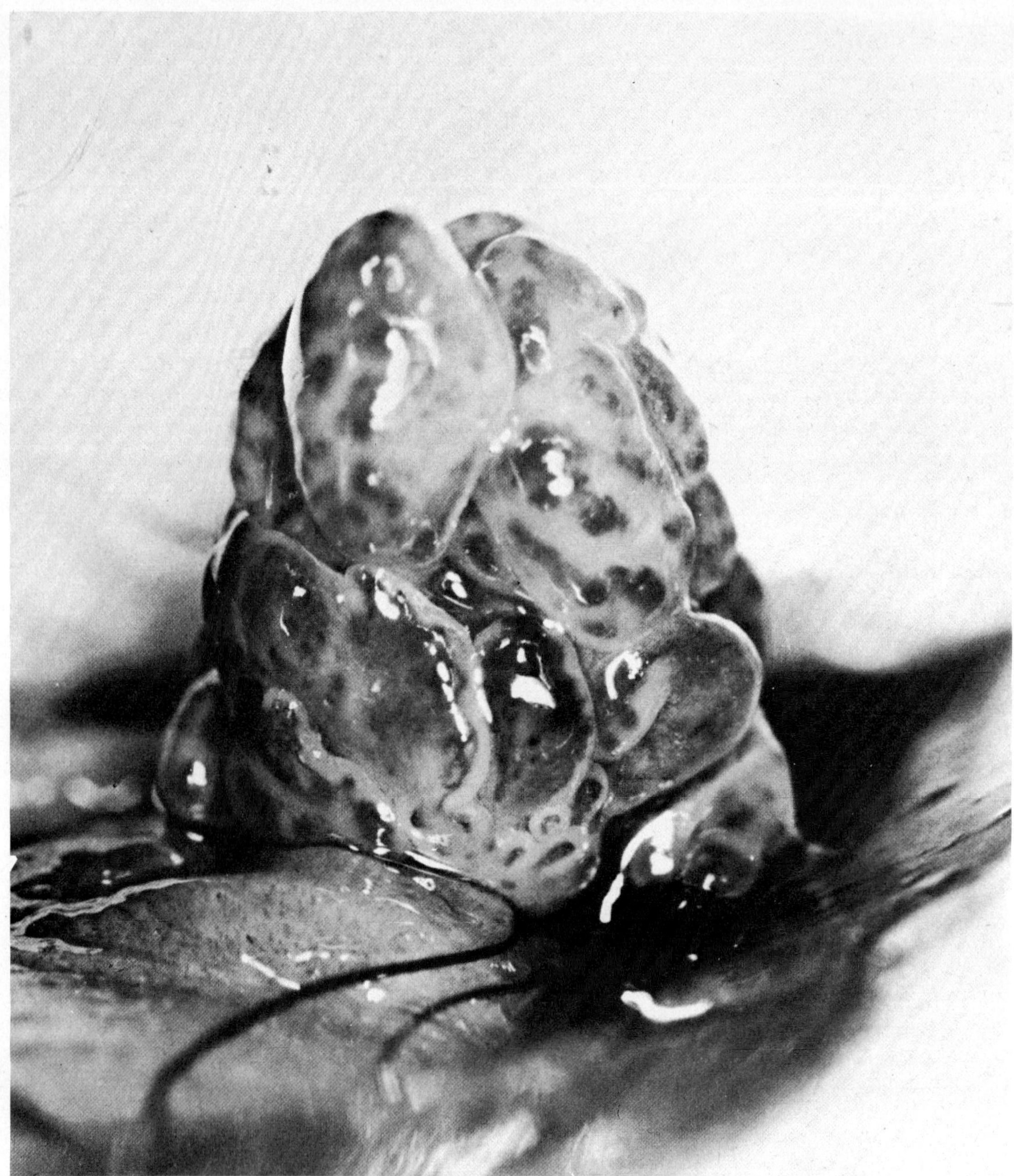

FIGURE 26-16
Condylomata acuminata of the vagina. These wartlike papillomata may be found on
the vulva, in the vagina, and on the ectocervix. The vessels appear as dark areas
surrounded by whitish epithelium. (×16.) (From Kolstad P, Stafl A: Atlas of colposcopy. Baltimore, University Park Press, 1972.)

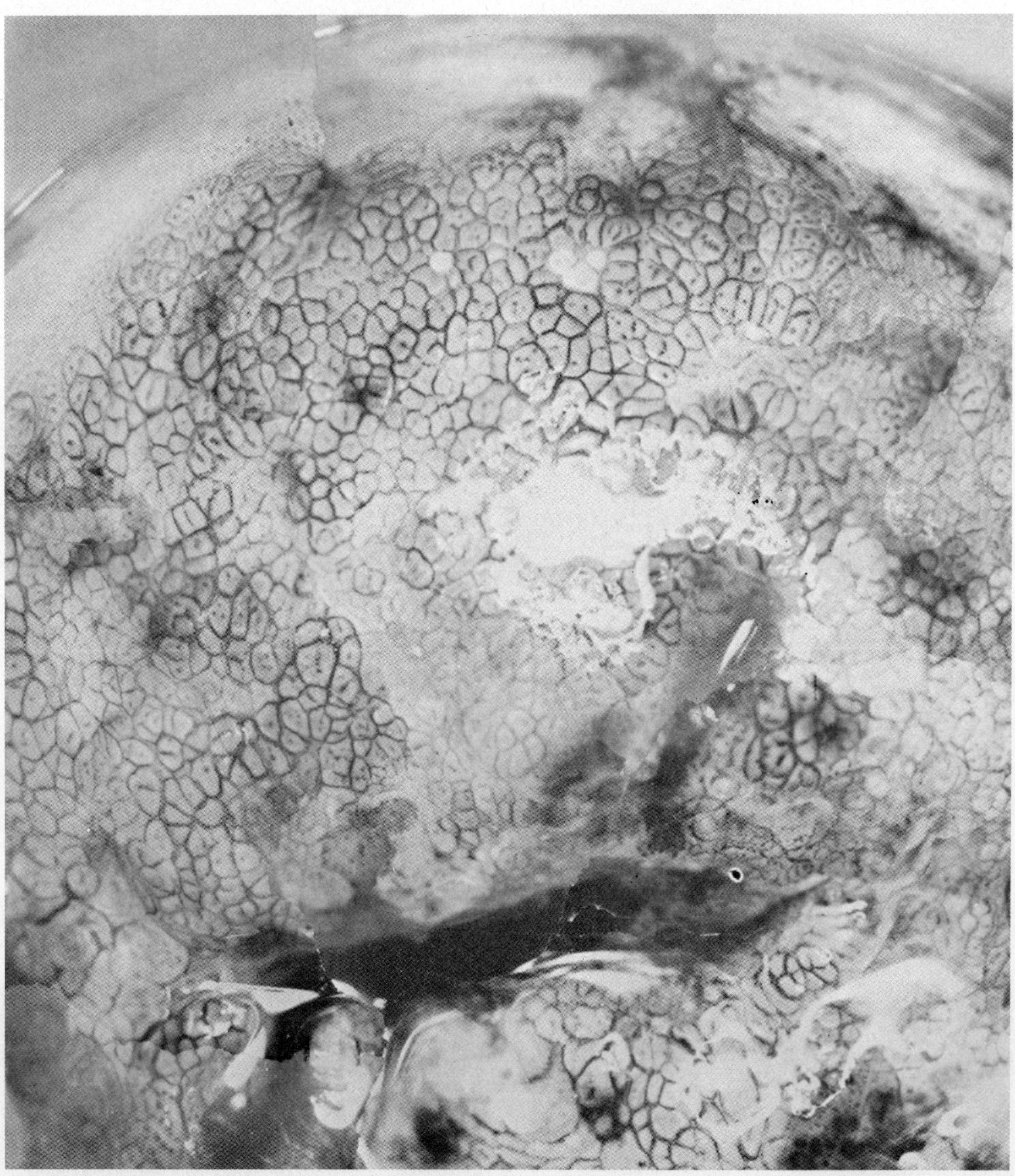

FIGURE 26-17
Extensive in situ carcinoma almost completely covers the visible part of ectocervix. The picture is dominated by coarse but regular mosaic vascular figures with greatly increased intercapillary distance. Atypical vessels are not to be seen. (×8.) (From Kolstad P, Stafl A: Atlas of colposcopy. Baltimore, University Park Press, 1972.)

dicate a high-grade intraepithelial lesion or invasive cancer.

An additional diagnostic criterion is the presence of "aceto-white epithelium." This is tissue that initially looks normal but takes a white color after acetic acid is applied. The areas are found outside the transformation zone and, as previously noted, frequently contain papillomavirus infection (subclinical papilloma infection, "flat warts" or "flat condyloma"). A clinically evident condyloma is illustrated in Fig. 26-16, and an example of intraepithelial neoplasia is shown in Fig. 26-17, which demonstrates punctation and variably sized mosaic structures. For a detailed description of the important colposcopic changes of the abnormal transformation zone and their interpretation, the reader should consult an atlas of colposcopy.

Only if the entire transformation zone can be seen colposcopically and if biopsies are obtained from the most abnormal areas is the examination considered technically satisfactory. If the transformation zone extends into the endocervical canal above the examiner's vision, the colposcopic examination is termed unsatisfactory, and diagnostic conization (see later discussion) is performed. If the colposcopic examination is technically satisfactory, multiple biopsy specimens are taken of the most abnormal areas. In addition, an endocervical curettage is usually performed even though the entire transformation zone can be seen. A scheme for the colposcopic evaluation of the abnormal Pap smear is shown in the box below, left. The results of biopsy of the abnormal areas are compared with the results of the cytologic examination to verify that the tissue samples appear to be representative of the abnormal cells identified cytologically. Precise agreement between the cytologic and histologic diagnoses is not necessary and often does not occur. However, it is vital that an invasive carcinoma not be missed, and the degree of atypicality found cytologically must be adequately explained by the tissue obtained on biopsy.

It is important to recognize that colposcopy does not establish a diagnosis and that the diagnosis is established only as a result of the evaluation of biopsy specimens. A good agreement may be obtained between the colposcopic impression and biopsy results, as shown by Stafl and Mattingly. In their study the biopsy results were usually only one grade of severity different than the colposcopic impression. However, it may occur that a microinvasive carcinoma is subsequently discovered on biopsy, although the colposcopic findings indicated only the presence of dysplasia. For this reason if a colposcopic evaluation of the transformation zone is not satisfactory or the biopsy and cytology results markedly disagree, diagnostic conization is indicated.

MANAGEMENT

General Principles

The general principle to be followed in the therapy of intraepithelial neoplasia is the eradication of the abnormal epithelium. In many instances this can be accomplished by procedures completed in the physician's office on an outpatient basis. A number of modalities are available to destroy the abnormal tissue, which is usually less than 1 mm to a few millimeters thick. Deeper destruction is required if the crypt of the glands is involved, since the glands usually lie approximately 5 mm below the surface, as shown by the studies of Anderson and Hartley. The size and extent of the lesion are also factors influencing therapy.

For outpatient therapy to be effective, a colposcopic examination must be satisfactory and the entire transformation zone visualized. The

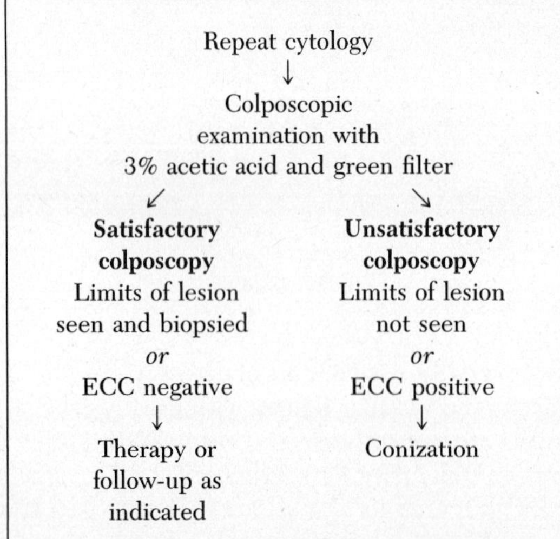

biopsy results should provide appropriate consistency with the abnormal cells seen cytologically, as well as with the colposcopic appearance of the transformation zone. Usually there is no more than one degree of severity in the differences of diagnoses (mild dysplasia versus moderate dysplasia). If the colposcopic examination is technically unsatisfactory, that is, the entire transformation zone cannot be seen, or if there is any suspicion of microinvasive disease, it is necessary to perform conization. Hysterectomy is considered only after it is ascertained that the patient does not have invasive cancer and no longer wishes to maintain childbearing function. Endocervical curettage is performed before outpatient therapy, and it is mandatory that the curettage results be negative before office therapy is undertaken.

In recommending various treatment modalities, the physician is often faced with the problem of whether or not the cellular atypicalities noted cytologically or on biopsy are potentially premalignant. Furthermore the differentiation of active squamous metaplasia, which is found at puberty and during pregnancy as well as in instances of tissue repair, can also produce a histomorphologic pattern that may be confused with neoplasia, as can papillomaviral infection (see later discussion). It may be difficult to make an accurate diagnosis using conventional histologic techniques, and marked differences of opinion regarding the correct diagnosis commonly occur. Therefore it is reemphasized that it is important for the therapist to be certain that the histologic biopsy findings appear to explain the morphologic abnormalities found on the cytologic smear and the colposcopic examination.

To help with the problems of morphologic interpretation, efforts have been made to identify authentic premalignant lesions. One laboratory aid is to estimate the ploidy of the lesion by microspectrophotometric measurement of nuclear DNA, as has been described by Richart, Fu, Reagan, and others. A Feulgen stain is used and the tissue is analyzed by measuring the ploidy of the lesion and comparing the cells under study to normal lymphocytes. The normal lymphocyte has a diploid (2N) distribution, while metaplastic lesions usually are tetraploid (4N); premalignant and malignant lesions have an aneuploid distribution. Fig. 26-18 demonstrates the analysis of a Pap smear and biopsy specimen. It should be noted that tetraploid lesions are occasionally also associated with low-grade neoplastic lesions as well. While this technique is primarily a laboratory investigative tool, recent refinements by Bibbo et al. suggest that it may be available in the near future for routine diagnostic utilization.

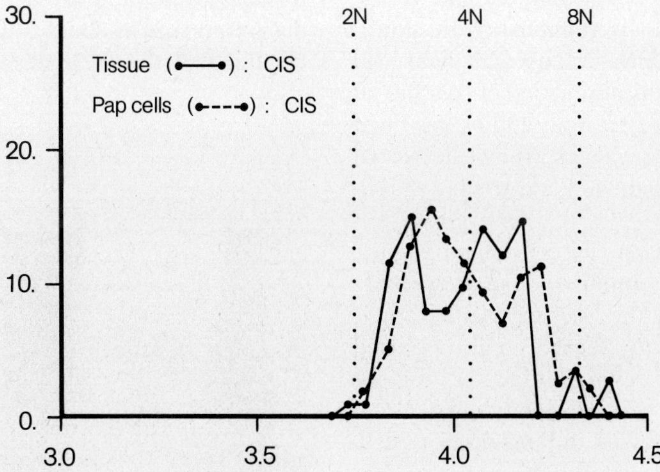

FIGURE 26-18
Histogram showing aneuploid distribution indicating neoplasia. In this case the tissue biopsy and cytology (Pap) results agree; *2N* corresponds to a normal diploid pattern.

Papillomavirus Infection

If koilocytic change is identified on biopsy, or a condyloma is identified (see Fig. 26-16), therapy of the affected area is usually undertaken. It is clear that not all papillomavirus infections have premalignant potential. Moreover, some of the infections regress spontaneously. A reliable histologic method to identify which lesions have neoplastic potential would be desirable but does not exist at the present time. Reid and Fu have noted that subclinical papillomaviral infection with a diploid pattern is seen with koilocytic atypia and metaplastic epithelium, while an aneuploid pattern is shown primarily with cervical intraepithelial neoplasia that demonstrates little histologic evidence of papillomavirus changes. Viral typing to distinguish HPV types 16, 18, and 31 from types 6 and 11 would also indicate which lesions are at greatest risk for premalignant change. However, such expensive, laborious techniques are specialized and cannot currently be applied routinely.

The current inability to differentiate possibly inconsequential from high-risk papillomavirus infections emphasizes the difficulty in choosing therapy of these lesions based on clinical findings. Current practice is to treat all of these disorders. This results in the treatment of many women with papillomavirus infection to prevent neoplasia in only a few. Insofar as malignant progression is uncommon and it appears to develop slowly, refinements in identifying the lesions which are premalignant will affect the current clinical practice of treating all lesions. The female is treated, and as has been emphasized by Levine et al., the male sexual partner should be evaluated and treated if condylomas are found.

For lesions involving the cervix and vagina, usually the laser is employed. For those only on the cervix, either the laser or cryotherapy is used. Cautery with anesthesia can also be used for cervicovaginal papilloma infection, and for isolated vaginal or cervical condylomata local application of podophyllin in benzoin or a resin has been tried (see Chapter 21) but occasionally can cause excess tissue slough. It is important that the patient douche 1 to 2 hours after the application to reduce normal tissue destruction. For cervical condyloma electrocautery is also effective but requires anesthesia for use in the vagina.

Outpatient Modalities

Cryotherapy

Cryotherapy is a popular technique used to treat intraepithelial neoplasia. It is also effective for subclinical papillomavirus infection of the cervix but is not appropriate to use in the vagina because of pain and difficulty in controlling the depth of freezing. The freezing process results from rapid expansion of fluid, usually carbon dioxide or nitrous oxide, into the probe (Fig. 26-19), which is placed against the cervix. The probe chosen depends on the size of the lesion to be treated, but the flat probes are commonly used, particularly since probes with long endocervical nipples can cause extensive destruction of the endocervix with resulting cervical stenosis. The contact is enhanced by putting water-soluble lubricating jelly on the tip of the probe, which is then applied closely against the cervix. While cryotherapy can be used in other areas such as the vulva, local anesthesia is usually required, but no anesthesia is required for cervical treatment. Once the gas is released into the probe an ice ball begins to form and is usually complete in a few minutes. It is important that the ice ball extend 3 to 4 mm beyond the edge of the lesion to ensure adequate freezing and destruction of abnormal epithelium. Usually the ball reaches its maximum size in about 3 to 5 minutes, and after the ball thaws, a second freeze is usually

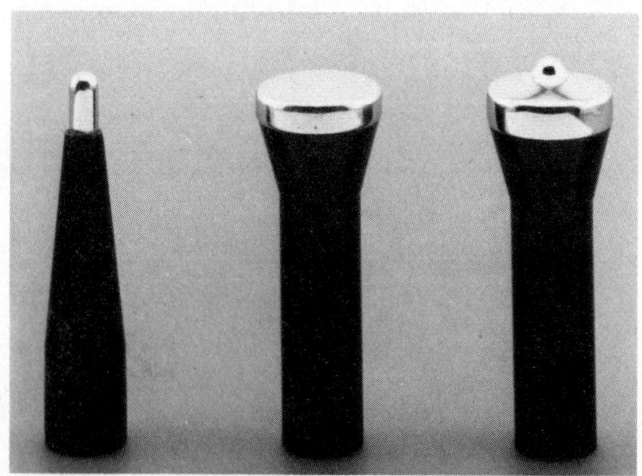

FIGURE 26-19
Three varieties of cryotherapy probes.

carried out, particularly with large lesions and when more extensive tissue necrosis is desired (double-freeze technique). It is sometimes necessary to reapply the probe to a different area to treat larger areas of intraepithelial neoplasia adequately.

Initial cure rates approximate 90% and averaged 89% for 4549 patients summarized from the literature in a review by Charles and Savage. Some have reported higher failure rates for carcinoma in situ (CIN III) using cryotherapy. This in part appears to be due to the extensive transformation zone usually seen with these lesions. There is also concern about the use of cryotherapy in lesions that involve the cervical crypts (gland involvement) on the grounds that such deep tissue might escape the effects of freezing. In theory the results of cryotherapy should be equivalent for all grades of cervical intraepithelial neoplasia, as recently reported by Bryson et al. Rates of cure with cryotherapy increase with the experience of the therapist as well as with the use of the double freeze technique. In addition, results can be improved if careful follow-up is carried out and the patient is treated a second time if needed.

After initial cryotherapy a follow-up examination is carried out in 4 months. Further evaluation is in accordance with the guidelines discussed subsequently for all cervical intraepithelial neoplasias, that is, a smear every 6 months for 1 year to 18 months, and after 3 or 4 successive negative smears, annual follow-up indefinitely. It is recommended that endocervical curettage be performed at least once after freezing to be certain there is no disease in the canal after freezing. A major concern after the use of cryosurgery is the potential for the future development of invasive carcinoma. A number of reports on the development of invasive carcinoma after cryotherapy have appeared and emphasize the importance of extreme care in being sure not only that intraepithelial neoplasia alone is being treated but also that all abnormal tissue is adequately destroyed and appropriate postcryosurgery follow-up occurs. Townsend et al. reviewed 66 cases of invasive cancer following outpatient cryotherapy and found errors in workup and diagnosis in most. Nonetheless it may be more hazardous to treat very large lesions with cryotherapy since many series report higher cryotherapy failure rates with large CIN III lesions. It is controversial whether these high-grade (CIN III) lesions, particularly those with gland involvement, can be treated with cryotherapy alone. Certainly any attempts at treatment of these high-grade lesions should be done only by an experienced colposcopist-cryotherapist. Many experts prefer laser or conization (see below) for such lesions. The best results with cryotherapy are obtained after the double-freeze technique as shown by Schantz and Thormann, and it is preferable for the lesion to occupy only two of the four cervical quandrants, as shown by Arof et al.

Possible complications in addition to recurrence of neoplasia following cryotherapy include infertility and cervical stenosis. Although both have been reported, there is no clear evidence of an increased risk of these adverse outcomes in patients treated with cryotherapy. Recurrent treatments or extensive therapy of the endocervical canal does increase the risk because of the more extensive destruction of the normal endocervix.

Laser Therapy

In recent years the laser has become widely used for the treatment of subclinical papillomavirus infection and intraepithelial neoplasia. The instrument is used in conjunction with the colposcope. The energy from the laser beam is absorbed by water with resultant vaporization of the target tissue. The laser beam is controlled by a small "joy" stick, and the spot size of the laser can be varied but is usually less than 1 mm. Different degrees of power are available, and for outpatient therapy of intraepithelial neoplasia approximately 25 to 35 watts are utilized. Most reports express the treatment mode as a power density, that is, watts per square centimeter. The laser is expensive (individual outpatient units cost from $15,000 to $30,000), but it allows precision in the depth and width of the area to be treated. Because therapy results in tissue vaporization, the resultant smoke must be evacuated with vacuum suction; thus a speculum with a special smoke evacuator is used to clear the operative field. This may be of particular importance to the therapist who is treating papillomaviral infections because of the risk of spread of these viruses to individuals who are exposed to the vaporized tissues. Graduated millimeter probes are often used to gauge the depth of the laser crater.

Reports have varied on the effectiveness of the laser to treat intraepithelial neoplasia. Current practice is to carry therapy to a depth of 5 to 7 mm and to use an approximate power density of over 600 W/cm^2. The treatment is more effective at higher power densities. However, the complications of pain and bleeding are also related to the power density and depth of treatment. This was recently shown by Caglar et al., who observed that pain and bleeding directly correlate with the power density and depth of destruction of tissue, while recurrence rates are inversely proportional to these parameters. If bleeding occurs during therapy, this can easily be controlled by coagulating the site by defocusing the laser beam and using a lower power density. Healing in the laser crater is usually complete in 4 to 6 weeks, and the site is covered with metaplastic squamous tissue in another 2 weeks. A particular advantage of the laser is that the transformation zone is more likely to remain visible colposcopically after treatment than is true with cryosurgery, following which the squamocolumnar junction is usually located in the endocervical canal.

Stanhope et al. treated lesions with the laser to a depth of 5 to 7 mm, as recommended earlier, and extended the treatment approximately 3 to 5 mm beyond the abnormal (non-iodine-staining) epithelium. These authors noted only a 9% failure rate of CIN III after such therapy. In a summary of reports from the literature of 1186 patients, Wetchler reported an 83% success rate for one laser treatment for CIN III and an 88% success rate for 1360 patients using single or multiple treatments. These figures are comparable to many reported overall results with cryotherapy. However, failure rates are reduced with higher power densities, treatment to greater depth (5 to 7 mm), with extension of the field beyond the abnormal epithelium for 3 to 5 mm, and with increasing experience of the therapist. It is likely that higher success rates will be reported in the future.

The laser is also used widely to treat papillomavirus infections, and it is important to treat not only the tissues infected with the pap-illomavirus but the adjacent normal tissues as well, as emphasized by Reid et al. Recently Ferenczy et al. demonstrated papillomavirus to be present in normal skin adjacent to condylomata caused by papillomavirus. These results indicate that the areas requiring therapy extend to normal adjacent tissue. This has led to the concept of "laser brushing," in which the laser beam is defocused to a larger spot, and lower power densities are used to treat the surrounding epithelium. A light brushing is used, causing only the whitened superficial layers to slough. Presumably this therapy eradicates latent virus in these tissues. The technique has been shown to reduce recurrence rates of papillomavirus infection.

Cautery

Electrocautery was the mainstay of outpatient therapy of intraepithelial neoplasia of the cervix before the advant of cryosurgery and more recently laser therapy. Cryotherapy became popular because it can be used for treatment in the office with less discomfort and also with less posttherapy vaginal discharge than cautery. Cervical stenosis can result from electrocautery if there is extensive treatment into the endocervical canal.

The treatment can be accomplished with a hot wire unit generating heat to the cervix or an electrodiathermy unit, which requires current to be passed through the tissues and electrical grounding of the patient. The treatment is carried out with sufficient depth to destroy cervical glands.

Chanen and Rome reported the results of cautery in 864 patients, 63% of whom had CIN III, with an overall success rate of 97.5%. In their treatment they used general anesthesia (day surgery) and colposcopically determined the areas to be treated. They also dilated the cervix during anesthesia to prevent subsequent stenosis. Only patients in whom the entire transformation zone can be visualized are treated. However, after therapy the squamocolumnar junction is usually located in the cervical canal, similar to the results after cryotherapy. According to Chanen and Rome, increased adverse effects of treatment on fertility or parturition are not observed. A disadvantage of this approach is the requirement for general anesthesia. However, effective outpatient therapy can be achieved without anesthesia, as recently noted by Deigan et al. from Canada, who treated 776 patients with electrocautery (hot wire pistol cautery) using colposcopic guidance. They achieved an overall initial eradication of intraepithelial neoplasia in approximately 90% of cases (92% for carcinoma in situ). Subsequent recurrences were usually treated with hot cautery. They required that the transformation zone be totally visualized, as is true for cryotherapy and laser therapy.

Electrocautery is much less expensive than the laser and appears to be able to yield comparable therapy results to cryosurgery. Kauraniemi et al. in Finland have utilized routine outpatient electrocautery to destroy the entire transformation zone in the cervices of a large population of women and have noted that these individuals have lower rates of invasive carcinoma and cervical intraepithelial neoplasia than those who did not have routine electrocautery.

Summary of Standard Outpatient Management

Outpatient therapy of intraepithelial neoplasia depends on adequate destruction of all abnormal tissues. Prerequisites for therapy are that the transformation zone should be completely visualized colposcopically with no neoplasia on ECC, that treatment should be carried out to a depth to reach the cervical crypts, and that it should also extend a few millimeters beyond the transformation zone to include normal-appearing tissue. Many authors have reported high failure rates with high-grade lesions and carcinoma in situ (CIN III) with cryotherapy, but this is in part due to the fact that these high-grade lesions cover larger areas of the cervix and extend more deeply into the cervical crypts. Success rates overall approximate 90%, and proven success has been obtained with the laser by treating to a depth of 5 to 7 mm at power densities above 600 watts per square centimeter and extending the treatment 3 to 4 mm beyond the abnormal epithelium. Similar area and depth requirements exist for electrocautery.

Results for cryotherapy are optimized providing the ice ball extends 3 to 4 mm beyond the transformation zone, and better results have also been reported using the so-called double-freeze technique. Ferenczy noted that lesions smaller than 3 cm could be equivalently treated by cryosurgery or laser but that larger lesions or those that extended up to 5 mm into the cervical canal faired better with laser treatment. Less vaginal discharge is usually noted after laser but it also is accompanied by higher rates of bleeding and risks of pelvic infection. Providing the entire transformation zone can be seen, the ECC results are negative, and a careful colposcopic protocol is followed, cryosurgery and electrocautery can be used as inexpensive and successful modalities for outpatient therapy of cervical intraepithelial neoplasia. Larger lesions, particularly those that begin to extend onto the vagina or into the cervical canal as well as those that obviously involve extensive areas of papillomavirus infection, are predominantly treated with the laser at present.

Other Outpatient Modalities

In some instances none of the previously described modalities are utilized and alternate forms of treatment may be tried. For example, this could arise in an elderly patient who has extensive intraepithelial neoplasia involving the vagina and cervix and in whom prolonged follow-up is difficult. Local radiation (tandem and ovoids, see Chapter 25) has been used in some circumstances as definitive treatment but is very rarely used today, particularly with the availability of the laser. Local chemotherapy with 5-fluorouracil (5-FU) is described in Chapter 25 and is also occasionally tried for patients with recurrent cervico-vaginal lesions. On an experimental basis, interferon gel has been used and has not been demonstrated to be efficacious.

Operative Therapy

Conization

Conization of the cervix is performed for diagnostic purposes if the colposcopic examination is unsatisfactory, if there is uncertainty regarding the presence of invasive disease, if the ECC results are positive, or if the cells seen on cytologic examination are not adequately explained by the biopsy specimens. If the biopsy suggests the possibility of microinvasion or if invasion cannot be confirmed, conization is performed for definitive diagnosis. A conization for treatment is carried out when childbearing function is to be maintained or when a patient prefers operative therapy less extensive than hysterectomy and is willing to adhere to a strict protocol for follow-up (see later discussion).

TECHNIQUE. The extent of the transformation zone on the exocervix is outlined by use of the colposcope. In addition, it is advisable to stain the cervix with iodine (Lugol's or Schiller's solution) to outline the limits of the resection margin of the cone. Since normal squamous epithelium contains glycogen and stains dark brown with iodine whereas neoplastic tissue fails to stain, care must be taken not to denude the normal epithelium with the blade of the speculum or an abrasive, since this will also lead to nonstaining. The degree to which the cone extends into the endocervical canal depends on the extent of the transformation zone. If the upper limits of the transformation zone cannot be seen, then the colposcopy is "unsatisfactory" and conization is performed in an attempt to have the upper margins of the cone include the transformation zone. If the upper limits cannot be seen in the endocervical canal or the ECC results are positive, the operation is adjusted so as to place the apex of the cone higher in the canal than in instances where the upper part of the transformation zone can be visualized as illustrated in Fig. 26-20.

Usually the procedure is done with a scalpel (cold knife cone). Recently therapists have utilized the laser to perform the conization, and this has become more popular since some believe it reduces blood loss in comparison to the cold knife conization as reported by Larsson et al. However, currently there is a much greater experience with cold knife conization and it is much more widely used.

After the resection limits of the conization specimen have been determined, absorbable sutures (Vicryl, catgut) are placed at the 3 and

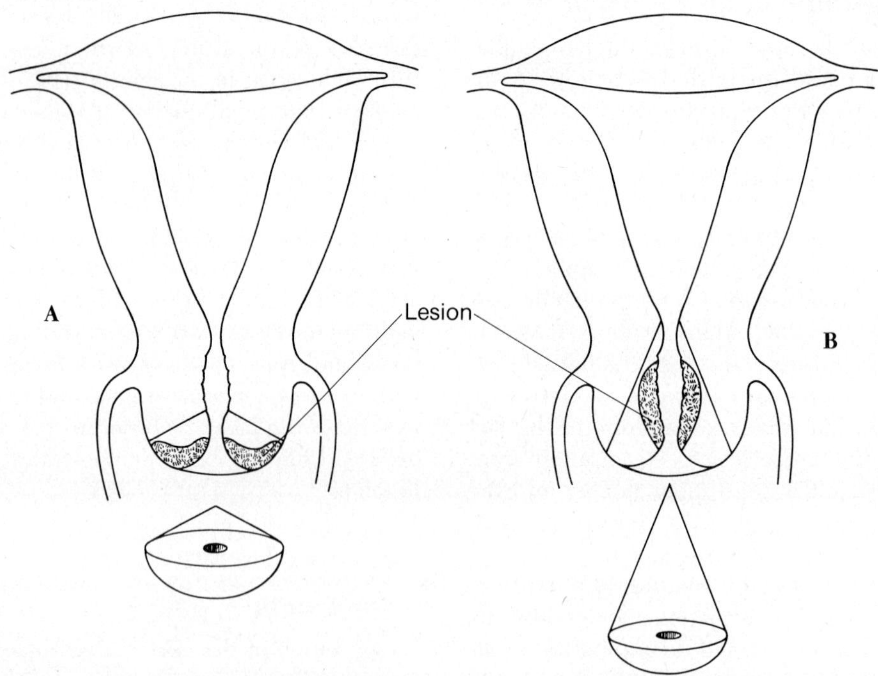

FIGURE 26-20
A, Cone biopsy for CIN of exocervix. Limits of lesion were identified colposcopically. **B,** Cone biopsy for endocervical disease. Limits of lesions were not seen colposcopically. (Redrawn from DiSaia PJ, Creasman WT: Clinical gynecologic oncology. St. Louis, The C.V. Mosby Co., 1984.)

9 o'clock positions on the cervix to reduce blood loss by ligating the descending cervical branches of the uterine artery. Some therapists use dilute vasopressin (1 ml in 100 ml sterile saline) and inject it into the stroma of the cervix to reduce bleeding from the bed of the cone. The endocervical canal is sounded and the cone cut so as to keep the apex below the internal os. It is sometimes helpful to leave the sound or cervical dilator in the canal during the procedure to serve as a guide. The posterior part of the cone (3 to 9 o'clock) is cut first so the resultant blood loss does not obscure the operative field. The upper margin of the cone is usually dissected free with scissors and the 12 o'clock position of the cone identified for the pathologists with a margin suture. An ECC is performed after the completion of the conization, and, if indicated, uterine curettage is done. It is advisable for one of the members of the operative team to examine the cone with the pathologist to ensure proper orientation. Individual arterial bleeding vessels are ligated, and the edge of the cone margin is repaired with interrupted figure of eight sutures. In the past the so-called Sturmdorf hemostatic suture, which turns the edge of the cervix into the canal, was widely used. This suture should not be used as it may bury abnormal cervical epithelium and also interferes with future colposcopic follow-up examination. It is advisable to sound the cervix at about 3 and 6 weeks after the procedure to help avoid stenosis. Recently Grundsell et al. reported a marked reduction in bleeding after laser conization using systemic antifibrinolytic agents (tranexamic acid), but this treatment is not widely practiced currently.

FOLLOW-UP. If the surgical margin of the conization specimen is free of neoplastic epithelium, the patient still requires long-term follow-up, since new lesions can develop. If the margins of the cone specimen are involved with neoplasia the patient should be considered for further treatment with hysterectomy, since there is an increased risk of failure in these cases. At the time of 5-year follow-up examination Ahlgren et al. noted 98% cure rates if the margin of the cervical conization was free, while the rate fell to 70% for those with positive margins. Kolstad and Klein followed 1128 patients for 15 to 25 years. Twenty-five of their patients had conization margins involved with neoplastic disease, and four of them eventually developed recurrence, some as long as 6 years after therapy. However, the remaining 21 were free of disease up to 15 years. These data emphasize that it is not always mandatory to perform hysterectomy if the margins of the cone are involved with intraepithelial neoplasia. This is particularly true if the ectocervical margins are involved, since subsequent outpatient therapy can usually eradicate any residual intraepithelial neoplasia at this site.

In the past it has been customary to perform the hysterectomy within 48 hours of conization or to wait more than 6 weeks to reduce the risk of postoperative infection at the time of the hysterectomy. Recent evidence from Webb and Symmonds as well as others suggests that it is not necessary to operate in these intervals. It is thought to be advisable to prescribe prophylactic antibiotics, such as cephalosporin, during the hysterectomy to reduce infections. Kolstad and Klein also noted that conization and hysterectomy were approximately equivalent in their effectiveness in treating carcinoma in situ. Conization was done in 795 patients and with 5 to 25 years of follow-up, recurrences of carcinoma in situ occurred in 2.3% whereas invasive cancer occurred in 0.9% (seven patients). For the 238 patients treated by hysterectomy, recurrence of carcinoma in situ occurred in 1.2% and invasive cancer in 2.1%. The recurrent carcinoma in situ or invasive cancer developed up to 10 years after primary treatment. These data indicate that conization is approximately as effective as hysterectomy for treatment of carcinoma in situ, particularly if the surgical margins are free. However, long-term follow-up is mandatory because of the risk of subsequent development of neoplasia. It should be emphasized that good results presented for conization are partly due to adequate pretherapy colposcopic evaluation.

Because of the apparent increased risk of invasive disease in older patients, Killackey et al. recommend that all patients over age 50 with a biopsy diagnosis of carcinoma in situ undergo conization to rule out invasive disease. In their series 3 of 16 patients (19%) so treated were found to have unsuspected invasive carcinoma despite adequate colposcopic evaluation with cytology and negative ECC results.

COMPLICATIONS. As previously noted, bleeding is the major short-term complication of conization. Long-term complications that have been of concern include cervical stenosis, infertility, loss of cervical mucus, and an increase in adverse pregnancy outcome (incompetent cervix). Definitive data are not available concerning the degree of risk of these adverse outcomes, but they are thought to be related in part to the height of the cone, that is, the degree to which the endocervical glands are removed. Buller and Jones evaluated infertility and pregnancy outcome in 166 patients and found no evidence of an increased rate of infertility or alteration of pregnancy outcome as a complication of the operation. In contrast a case control study from England of 66 matched patients found a statistically significant association with preterm delivery (17% versus 3%), and the risk of pregnancy loss was even more frequent among their patients with second pregnancies. Currently, no specific conclusions can be drawn regarding these risks. Patients desiring future childbearing function who need to undergo conization should be made aware of the potential risks of infertility, preterm labor, and cervical stenosis, but they can also be advised that the data are ambiguous concerning these risks.

Hysterectomy

Hysterectomy is performed for treatment of intraepithelial neoplasia if childbearing function is not to be preserved and if there is no evidence of invasive disease (in case of invasive carcinoma see Chapter 27). If neoplastic epithelium is found in the resection margin of the cervical cone, hysterectomy is sometimes performed. The need to perform hysterectomy following conization must be individualized depending on the clinicopathologic circumstances, including the patient's willingness to be followed and desire to preserve childbearing function. A vaginal hysterectomy is usually performed, or if the abdominal route is chosen, a class I hysterectomy (as described in Chapter 27) is done. The limits of the abnormal epithelium are defined before operation using the colposcope and iodine solution (Lugol's or Schiller's solution). If the vagina is involved with neoplasia, it is important to extend the surgical margins to include the abnormal vaginal tissue. It is important to remove the entire cervix, but resecting normal upper vagina does not improve therapeutic outcome. Follow-up is required after hysterectomy as after conization, since the patient is at risk for the development of lower genital tract intraepithelial neoplasia years later.

ABNORMAL PAP SMEAR IN PREGNANCY

When an abnormal Pap smear is discovered initially in a pregnant patient, evaluation is more complicated than in the nonpregnant patient because of the increased vascularity of the cervix, the presence of the fetus, and morphologic changes (edema, decidual reaction, etc.) in the cervix that develop as pregnancy progresses. Colposcopic evaluation in the pregnant patient is best performed by physicians with extensive experience. Intraepithelial neoplasia is not treated during pregnancy; therapy is postponed until the postpartum period. The prime objective in the pregnant patient with an abnormal Pap smear is to perform an adequate evaluation to rule out the presence of invasive carcinoma.

Many years ago DePetrillo et al. introduced a scheme (Fig. 26-21) for the evaluation of the abnormal Pap smear during pregnancy utilizing colposcopy. Insofar as the cervix everts during pregnancy, the squamocolumnar junction is more easily visible for evaluation. This circumstance also lessens the need for an ECC, which increases the risk of interrupting the pregnancy. When a patient has abnormal cytologic findings during pregnancy and the colposcopic examination is within normal limits, these examinations are repeated 4 to 6 weeks later. If there is neither evidence of neoplasia nor indication of a lesion requiring biopsy, the patient is followed and evaluated postpartum. If the colposcopic examination is abnormal, a biopsy is usually taken of the most abnormal area to confirm the cytologic and colposcopic findings, and the examination (including Pap smear) and colposcopy are repeated at 4- to 6-week intervals until the patient delivers. Then definitive evaluation is performed in the postpartum period. A major problem arises if the patient has an undetected invasive lesion. In all circum-

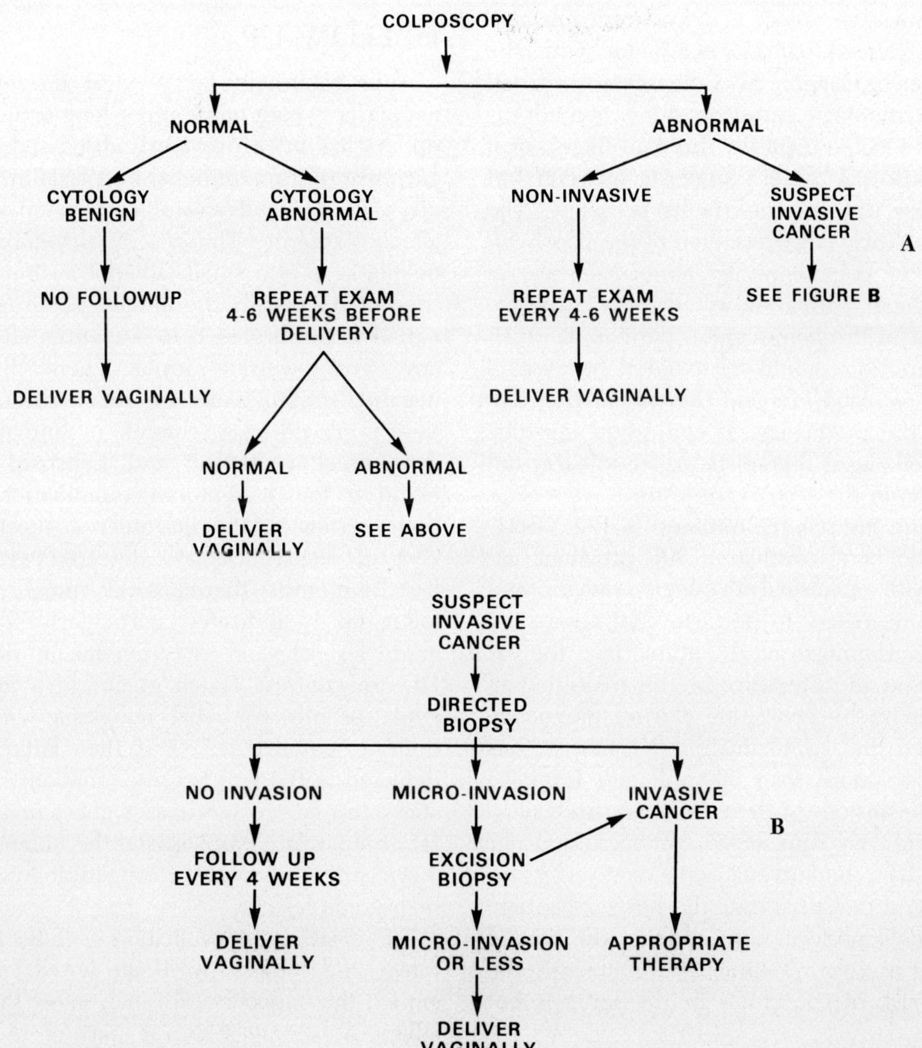

FIGURE 26-21
Scheme for evaluation of abnormal Pap smear during pregnancy utilizing colposcopy. **A,** Screening evaluation of abnormal Pap smear in pregnancy. **B,** Schematic of evaluation when an invasive lesion is suspected. (From DePetrillo AD, Townsend DE, Morrow CP, et al: Am J Obstet Gynecol 121:441, 1975.)

stances a directed biopsy is needed, and then the management is carried out as outlined in Fig. 26-21, *B*. If microinvasion is suspected, either conization or excision of the abnormal area is carried out. If following this procedure there is no evidence of invasive carcinoma, the patient may deliver vaginally and the necessary treatment is performed in the postpartum period. If invasive cancer is discovered, management is carried out in accordance with the guidelines in Chapter 27. Conization is needed if there is cytologic suspicion of invasion not explained by colposcopically directed biopsy or if the colposcopic pattern suggests invasion but the biopsy did not confirm its presence. The conization (or wedge resection of the poorly visualized or colposcopically abnormal area) in the pregnant patient is usually less extensive than that in the nonpregnant patient. If possible, conization should be avoided because of the risk of blood loss and the potential of disturbing the pregnancy. If conization must be performed, most therapists prefer to carry out conization in the second trimester.

Utilizing the scheme outlined in Fig. 26-21, DePetrillo et al. evaluated 300 pregnant patients with abnormal cytologic smears and found it necessary to perform conization only on three. Hannigan et al. summarized the experience in the literature of the treatment of 448 patients by conization during pregnancy and noted that approximately 9% had serious blood loss (more than 500 ml) and required blood transfusion. In their summary pregnancy losses did not appear to be increased for women who underwent conization. The authors noted that their data did not substantiate the need to perform conization in the second trimester as generally practiced. Currently the precise risk of conization to the fetus is not known.

There are studies, as reported by Kiguchi et al., to suggest that intraepithelial neoplasia has higher regression rates when detected in pregnant women than in nonpregnant individuals. The precise reason for this is not known, but two explanations are generally offered: (1) the low-grade intraepithelial changes, particularly those with mild dysplasia recorded during pregnancy, may represent cytologic changes that occur as a consequence of pregnancy itself, and (2) intraepithelial lesions may be removed during the trauma of vaginal delivery.

FOLLOW-UP

After treatment for cervical intraepithelial neoplasia a patient requires long-term follow-up. As has been previously discussed, the recurrence of intraepithelial neoplasia in the cervix, vagina, or vulva can take place many years after treatment. The risk of development of neoplasia is also small (about 3%) but is ever present. Generally the initial screening examination is performed 3 to 4 months after therapy. For low-grade lesions, generally three negative examinations are sufficient and a patient is placed on a schedule of annual follow-up thereafter. Berget and Lenstrup recommend a fourth 6-month examination, since their review of the literature suggested that 75% of recurrences are detected within the first 21 months; therefore this more extensive follow-up is indicated particularly for high-grade lesions such as carcinoma in situ (CIN III). In contrast Hatch et al., in a follow-up study of intraepithelial neoplasia with cryotherapy, noted that 90% of their failures were detected in the first two examinations. In their study the failure rate was highest in the CIN III group, again emphasizing the importance of more intensive and prolonged follow-up for high-grade lesions.

The posttherapy evaluation includes both cytology and colposcopy. If the initial lesion occupied the endocervical canal, many therapists advise a routine ECC as part of the initial posttherapy evaluation. However, biopsies are usually performed only when indicated as a result of the cytologic and colposcopic examinations.

KEY POINTS

- Intraepithelial neoplasia is a spectrum of premalignant changes in the epithelium of the cervix that histologically show varying degrees of cellular atypia. Numerous terms are used to describe the severity of the atypias, but there is no clearly defined boundary between them.

- During reproductive life the squamocolumnar junction is usually on the portio of the cervix near the external os. It may be found farther away from the os during and after pregnancy and usually recedes into the endocervical canal after menopause.

- Pap smear (cytology) screening appears to have decreased the frequency of invasive carcinoma of the cervix by 50% in the past two decades.

- Many cases of cervical intraepithelial neoplasia do not progress. Some spontaneously regress, but all have the potential for progression to malignancy.

- High-grade lesions (carcinoma in situ [CIN III]) are at greater risk for malignant progression and usually are found in larger abnormal transformation zones.

- Carcinoma in situ with gland involvement does not require hysterectomy for treatment.

- The cause of cervical neoplasia is not known but appears to be associated with sexual activity.

- Females with multiple sex partners are at increased risk for cervical intraepithelial neoplasia, and males with multiple sex partners increase the risk of neoplasia for a female sex partner.

- Cigarette smoking appears to increase the risk of cervical neoplasia. The effect of oral contraceptive use is uncertain, but it may increase the risk for those who have high-risk sexual factors.

- Herpes simplex virus II (HSV II) has been suspected to increase the risk of cervical neoplasia, but a definitive causative role has not been identified.

KEY POINTS, cont'd

- Papillomavirus infection is associated with an increased risk of cervical intraepithelial neoplasia. Types 6 and 11 are associated with benign condyloma, while types 16, 18, and possibly 31 are associated with neoplastic changes.

- Immunosuppressed patients are at an increased risk for genital papillomavirus infection and intraepithelial neoplasia.

- Papillomavirus infection can progress to intraepithelial neoplasia. Some papillomaviral infections spontaneously regress.

- The false negative rate for properly performed cytology smears is 5% to 10%.

- An adequate cytologic laboratory is supervised by a cytopathologist and processes at least 25,000 cervical smears annually.

- The colposcope is used to evaluate the cervix if an abnormal Pap smear is present. Usually multiple biopsy specimens of an abnormal transformation zone are needed for an adequate evaluation.

- Colposcopic and cytologic findings do not establish a diagnosis; biopsy is necessary.

- Endocervical curettage (ECC) should be performed before outpatient therapy is undertaken for intraepithelial neoplasia.

- Before outpatient therapy of cervical intraepithelial neoplasia the entire transformation zone must be seen, the ECC results must be negative, and the evaluation must be adequate to rule out the presence of invasive carcinoma.

- The crypts of the endocervical glands are located as deep as 5 mm beneath the surface.

- Atypical cells seen on the biopsy specimen should be of similar magnitude of abnormality as those seen on cytologic smears before therapy is begun.

- In the determination of the ploidy of a cell, those cells with an aneuploid content are neoplastic, cells with a tetraploid content may be metaplastic, and diploid cells are normal.

- Therapy of all papillomavirus infections results in treatment of many women to try to prevent a few cases of invasive carcinoma of the cervix.

- Conization of the cervix should be performed if colposcopy is unsatisfactory, if the biopsy results do not explain the cytologic findings, if the ECC sample has neoplastic cells, or if there is suspicion of invasive or microinvasive disease.

- Conization is done for therapy of carcinoma in situ if childbearing function is to be preserved.

- The goal of treatment in intraepithelial neoplasia is eradication of all abnormal tissue.

- Laser therapy, cryotherapy, and electrocautery have been reported to have equivalent results and lead to eradication of the lesions in about 90% of the patients with carcinoma in situ after initial therapy.

- Cryosurgery has been less effective than other modalities in treating large lesions as well as high-grade (carcinoma in situ [CIN III]) lesions. The effectiveness of cryotherapy is enhanced by treating for 3 to 4 mm beyond the abnormal epithelium and using a double-freeze technique.

- Cervical stenosis and infertility may result from outpatient therapy of intraepithelial neoplasia if large areas of the endocervix are destroyed.

- Laser therapy of intraepithelial neoplasia is usually done to a depth of 5 to 7 mm and extends 3 to 4 mm beyond the boundary of the abnormal epithelium. Higher power densities and greater depths of treatment increase the complications of bleeding and pain.

- Conization for the therapy of cervical intraepithelial neoplasia is as effective as hysterectomy if the margins are free of disease.

———————— KEY POINTS, cont'd ————————

- Hysterectomy is not always necessary if the margins of the conization specimen contain neoplastic tissue, especially low-grade lesions.

- Follow-up of patients treated for cervical intraepithelial neoplasia consists of colposcopy and cytology.

- Follow-up is done initially 3 to 4 months after initial therapy for cervical intraepithelial neoplasia and then every 6 months.

- When three consecutive examinations on patients with low-grade lesions or four consecutive examinations on patients with high-grade lesions are negative, annual follow-up is instituted and continued indefinitely.

- The risk of long-term development (up to 10 years) of neoplasia following initial therapy is about 3%.

- Most short-term recurrences of neoplasia occur within 1 to 2 years after initial treatment.

- Hysterectomy may be performed for therapy of intraepithelial neoplasia if childbearing function is not to be preserved and there is no evidence of invasive disease.

- Evaluation of the abnormal Pap smear in pregnancy is conducted primarily to rule out the presence of invasive carcinoma. Intraepithelial neoplasia is treated in the postpartum period.

BIBLIOGRAPHY

Ahlgren M, Ingemarsson I, Lindgerg LG, et al: Conization as treatment of carcinoma in situ of the uterine cervix. Obstet Gynecol 46:135, 1975.

American College of Obstetricians and Gynecologists Newsletter, June 1984.

Anderson MC, Hartley RB: Cervical crypt involvement by intraepithelial neoplasia. Obstet Gynecol 55:546, 1980.

Arof HM, Gerbie MV, Smeltzer J: Cryosurgical treatment of cervical intraepithelial neoplasia: Four-year experience. Am J Obstet Gynecol 150:865, 1984.

Beral V: Cancer of the cervix: A sexually transmitted infection? Lancet 1:1037, 1974.

Berget A, Lenstrup C: Cervical intraepithelial neoplasia. Examination, treatment and follow-up. Obstet Gynecol Surv 40:545, 1985.

Bibbo M, Alenghat E, Bahr GF, et al: A quality-control procedure on cervical lesions for the comparison of cytology and histology. J Reprod Med 28:811, 1983.

Brinton LA, Schairer C, Haenszel WB, et al: Cigarette smoking and invasive cervical cancer. JAMA 255:3265, 1986.

Bryson SCP, Lenehan P, Lickrish GM: The treatment of grade 3 cervical intraepithelial neoplasia with cryotherapy: An 11-year experience. Am J Obstet Gynecol 151:201, 1985.

Buller RE, Jones HW: Pregnancy following cervical conization. Am J Obstet Gynecol 142:506, 1982.

Burghardt E, Ostor AG: Site and origin of squamous cervical cancer: A histomorphologic study. Obstet Gynecol 62:117, 1983.

Caglar H, Ayhan A, Hreshchyshyn MM: CO_2 laser therapy for cervical intraephithelial neoplasia. Gynecol Oncol 22:46, 1985.

Campion MS, Singer A, Clarkson PK: Increased risk of cervical neoplasia in consorts of men with penile condyloma acuminata. Lancet 1:943, 1985.

Chanen W, Rome RM: Electrocoagulation diathermy for cervical dysplasia and carcinoma in situ: A 15-year survey. Obstet Gynecol 61:673, 1983.

Charles EW, Savage EW: Cryosurgical treatment of cervical intraepithelial neoplasia. Obstet Gynecol Surv 35:539, 1980.

Clarke EA, Anderson TW: Does screening by "Pap" smear help divert cervical cancer—a case control study. Lancet 2:1, 1979.

Coppleson M, Pixley E, Reid B: Colposcopy—a scientific and practical approach to the cervix in health and disease. Springfield, Ill., Charles C Thomas, Publisher, 1971.

Cramer DW: The role of cervical cytology in declining morbidity and mortality of cervical cancer. Cancer 34:2018, 1974.

Cramer DW, Cutler SJ: Incidence and histopathology of malignancies of the female genital organs in the United States. Am J Obstet Gynecol 118:443, 1974.

Crum CP, Levine RU: Review: Human papillomavirus infection and cervical neoplasia: New perspectives. Int J Gynecol Pathol 3:376, 1984.

Day NE: Effect of cervical cancer screening in Scandinavia. Obstet Gynecol 63:714, 1984.

Deigan EA, Carmichael JA, Ohlke ID, et al: Treatment of cervical intraepithelial neoplasia with electrocautery: A report of 776 cases. Am J Obstet Gynecol 154:255, 1986.

DePetrillo AD, Townsend DE, Morrow CP, et al: Colposcopic evaluation of the abnormal Papanicolaou test in pregnancy. Am J Obstet Gynecol 121:441, 1975.

Devesa SS: Descriptive epidemiology of cancer of the uterine cervix. Obstet Gynecol 63:605, 1984.

DiSaia PJ, Creasman WT: Clinical gynecologic oncology. St. Louis, The C.V. Mosby Co., 1984.

Fenoglio CM, Ferenczy A: Etiologic factors in cervical neoplasia. Semin Oncol 9:349, 1982.

Ferenczy A: Comparison of cryo- and carbon dioxide laser therapy for cervical intraepithelial neoplasia. Obstet Gynecol 66:793, 1985.

Ferenczy A, Mitao M, Nagai N, et al: Latent papillomavirus and recurring genital warts. N Engl J Med 313:784, 1985.

Grundsell H, Larsson G, Bekassy Z: Use of an antifibrinolytic agent (tranexamic acid) and lateral sutures with laser conization of the cervix. Obstet Gynecol 63:573, 1984.

Grunebaum AN, Sedlis A, Sillman F, et al: Association of human papillomavirus infection with cervical intraepithelial neoplasia. Obstet Gynecol 62:448, 1983.

Hannigan EV, Whitehouse HH III, Atkinson WD, et al: Cone biopsy during pregnancy. Obstet Gynecol 60:450, 1982.

Hatch KD, Shingleton HM, Austin JM Jr, et al: Cryosurgery of cervical intraepithelial neoplasia. Obstet Gynecol 57:692, 1981.

Hatch KD, Shingleton HM, Orr JW, et al: Role of endocervical curettage in colposcopy. Obstet Gynecol 65:403, 1985.

Hollyhock VE, Chanen W, Wein R: Cervical function following treatment of intraepithelial neoplasia by electrocoagulation diathermy. Obstet Gynecol 61:79, 1983.

Jones JM, Sweetnam P, Hibbard BM: The outcome of pregnancy after cone biopsy of the cervix: A case-control study. Br J Obstet Gynaecol 86:913, 1979.

Kauraniemi T, Rasanen-Virtanen U, Hakama M: Risk of cervical cancer among an electrocoagulated population. Am J Obstet Gynecol 131:533, 1978.

Kessler F: Etiologic concepts in cervical carcinogenesis. Gynecol Oncol 12:S7, 1981.

Kiguchi K, Bibbo M, Hasegawa T, et al: Dysplasia during pregnancy. A cytologic follow-up study. J Reprod Med 26:66, 1981.

Killackey MA, Jones WB, Lewis JL Jr: Diagnostic conization of the cervix: review of 460 consecutive cases. Obstet Gynecol 67:766, 1986.

Kolstad P, Klem V: Long-term followup of 1121 cases of carcinoma in situ. Obstet Gynecol 48:125, 1976.

Kolstad P, Stafl A: Atlas of colposcopy. Baltimore, University Park Press, 1972, p. 91.

Koss LG: Dysplasia. A real concept or misnomer? Obstet Gynecol 51:374, 1978.

Koss LG, Stewart FW, Foote FW, et al: Some histological aspects of behavior of epidermoid carcinoma in situ and related lesions of the uterine cervix. A long-term prospective study. Cancer 16:1160, 1963.

Kwikkel HJ, Bezemer PD, Helmerhorst ThJM, et al: Predictive value of a positive endocervical curettage in diagnosis and treatment of CIN. Gynecol Oncol 24:162, 1986.

Kwikkel HJ, Helmerhorst ThJM, Bezemer PD, et al: Laser or cryotherapy for cervical intraepithelial neoplasia: A randomized study to compare efficacy and side effects. Gynecol Oncol 22:23, 1985.

Larsson G, Gullberg B, Grundsell H: A comparison of complications of laser and cold knife conization. Obstet Gynecol 62:213, 1983.

Levine RU, Crum CP, Herman E, et al: Cervical papillomavirus infection and intraepithelial neoplasia: A study of male sexual partner. Obstet Gynecol 64:16, 1984.

McChance DJ, Campion MJ, Clarkson PK, et al: Prevalence of human papillomavirus type 16 DNA sequences in cervical intraepithelial neoplasia and invasive carcinoma of the cervix. Br J Obstet Gynaecol 92:1101, 1985.

Meisels A, Morin C: Human papillomavirus and cancer of the uterine cervix. Gynecol Oncol 12:S111, 1981.

Mitchell H, Drake N, Medley G: Prospective evaluation of risk of cervical cancer after cytological evidence of human papillomavirus infection. Lancet 1:573, 1986.

Moller BR, Johannesen P, Osther K, et al: Treatment of dysplasia of the cervical epithelium with an interferon gel. Obstet Gynecol 62:625, 1983.

Nasiell K, Nasiell M, Vaclavinkova V: Behavior of moderate cervical dysplasia during long-term follow-up. Obstet Gynecol 61:609, 1983.

Nasiell K, Roger V, Nasiell M: Behavior of mild cervical dysplasia during long-term follow-up. Obstet Gynecol 67:665, 1986.

Orr JW, Shingleton HM, Hatch KD, et al: Correlation of perioperative morbidity and conization to radical hysterectomy interval. Obstet Gynecol 59:726, 1982.

Piper JM: Oral contraceptives and cervical cancer. Gynecol Oncol 22:1, 1985.

Porreco R, Penn I, Droegemueller W, et al: Gynecologic malignancies in immunosuppressed organ transplant recipients. Obstet Gynecol 45:359, 1975.

Rapp F, Jenkins FJ: Genital cancer and viruses. Gynecol Oncol 12:S25, 1981.

Reid R, Fu YS: Is there a morphologic spectrum linking condyloma to cervical cancer? In Banbury Report 21: Viral etiology of cervical cancer. Cold Spring Harbor, NY, Cold Spring Harbor Laboratory, 1986.

Reid R, Stanhope R, Herschman BR, et al: Genital warts and cervical cancer. I. Evidence of an association between subclinical papillomavirus infection and cervical malignancy. Cancer 50:377, 1982.

Richart RM: Cervical intraepithelial neoplasia and the cervicologist. Can J Med Tech 38:177, 1976.

Richart RM, Barron BA: A follow-up study of patients with cervical dysplasia. Am J Obstet Gynecol 105:386, 1969.

Richart RM, Townsend DE: Outpatient therapy of cervical intraepithelial neoplasia with cryotherapy or CO_2 laser. In Advances in clinical obstetrics and gynecology. Baltimore, The Williams & Wilkins Co., 1982.

Rome RM, Urcuyo R, Nelson JH: Observations on the surface area of the abnormal transformation zone associated with intraepithelial and early invasive squamous cell lesions of the cervix. Am J Obstet Gynecol 129:565, 1977.

Romney SL, Dattagupta C, Basu J, et al: Plasma vitamin C and uterine cervical dysplasia. Am J Obstet Gynecol 151:976, 1985.

Sadeghi SB, Hsieh EW, Gunn SW: Prevalence of cervical intraepithelial neoplasia in sexually active teenagers and young adults. Am J Obstet Gynecol 148:726, 1984.

Savage EW, Matlock DL, Salem FA, et al: The effects of endocervical gland involvement on the cure rates of patients with cervical intraepithelial neoplasia undergoing cryosurgery. Gynecol Oncol 14:194, 1982.

Schantz A, Thormann L: Cryosurgery for dysplasia of the uterine ectocervix. A randomized study of the single- and double-freeze techniques. Acta Obstet Gynecol Scand 63:417, 1984.

Seski JC, Reinhalter ER, Silva JH: Abnormalities of lymphocyte transformations in women with condylomata acuminata. Obstet Gynecol 51:188, 1978.

Sillman F, Boyce J, Fruchter R: The significance of atypical vessels and neovascularization in cervical neoplasia. Am J Obstet Gynecol 139:154, 1981.

Singer A: The uterine cervix from adolescence to the menopause. Br J Obstet Gynecol 82:81, 1975.

Stafl A, Mattingly RF: Colposcopic diagnosis of cervical neoplasia. Obstet Gynecol 41:168, 1973.

Stanhope CR, Phibbs GD, Stuart GCE, et al: Carbon dioxide laser surgery. Obstet Gynecol 61:624, 1983.

Stuart GCE, Allen HH, Anderson RJ: Squamous cell carcinoma of the vagina following hysterectomy. Am J Obstet Gynecol 139:311, 1981.

Surwit EA, Graham V, Droegemueller W, et al: Evaluation of topically applied transretinoic acid in the treatment of cervical intraepithelial neoplasia. Am J Obstet Gynecol 143:821, 1982.

Swan SH, Brown WL: Oral contraceptive use, sexual activity and cervical carcinoma. Am J Obstet Gynecol 139:52, 1981.

Syrajanen K: Cervical papillomavirus infection progressing to invasive cancer in less than three years. Lancet 1:510, 1985.

Townsend DE, Richart RM, Marks E, et al: Invasive cancer following outpatient evaluation and therapy for cervical disease. Obstet Gynecol 57:145, 1981.

Trevathan E, Layde P, Webster LA, et al: Cigarette smoking and dysplasia and carcinoma-in-situ of the uterine cervix. JAMA 250:499, 1983.

Vessey MP, McPherson K, Lawless M, et al: Neoplasia of the cervix uteri and contraception: A possible adverse effect of the pill. Lancet 2:930, 1983.

Walton RJ: The Task Force on Cervical Cancer Screening Program. Can Med Assoc J, Oct 1, 1982.

Webb MJ, Symmonds RE: Radical hysterectomy: Influence of recent conization on morbidity and complications. Obstet Gynecol 53: 290, 1979.

Wentz WB, Reagan JW: Clinical significance of post irradiation dysplasia of the uterine cervix. Am J Obstet Gynecol 106:812, 1970.

Wetchler SJ: Treatment of cervical intraepithelial neoplasia with the CO_2 laser: Laser versus cryotherapy. A review of effectiveness and cost. Obstet Gynecol Surv 39:469, 1984.

Wickenden C, Malcolm A, Steele A, et al: Screening for wart virus infection in normal and abnormal cervices by DNA hybridisation of cervical scrapes. Lancet 1:65, 1985.

Malignant Diseases of the Cervix

KEY TERMS AND DEFINITIONS

Adenoma Malignum. A virulent adenocarcinoma of the cervix that histologically consists of glands that appear well differentiated.

Barrel-Shaped Cervix. A cervix containing a large carcinoma, usually of endocervical origin, that has replaced much of the cervix, causing it to widen (usually more than 6 cm).

Brachytherapy. A form of radiation therapy in which the source is placed close to the tumor. The application may be in the form of needles implanted into the tumor (interstitial therapy) or into the vagina or cervical canal (internal therapy). For cervical tumors an intracervical tandem and vaginal ovoids (colpostats) are usually used.

Cordotomy. A neurosurgical operation for relief of pain of the lower extremity in cases of recurrent cervical carcinoma. It interrupts the lateral spinothalamic tract.

Endophytic. A term used to describe a tumor that begins in the cervical canal and penetrates internally into the cervix.

Exophytic. A term used to describe a cervical tumor that grows on the outside surface of the cervix (exocervical part).

Extrafascial Hysterectomy. An operation that develops the pubocervical fascia to allow total removal of the cervix and uterus (class I hysterectomy).

Fletcher-Suit Applicator. A system that delivers brachytherapy to cervical carcinomas by use of a tandem in the cervical canal and ovoids (colpostats) in the vagina.

Glassy Cell Carcinoma. A virulent adenosquamous carcinoma that occurs in the cervix and metastasizes early in the course of the disease.

Microinvasive Carcinoma. A small (stage Ia) carcinoma of the cervix detected by microscopic examination that is confined to the cervix with little or no risk of spread to regional lymph nodes.

Modified Radical Hysterectomy. An operation that removes the uterus and cervix and some paracervical tissues but does not dissect the ureters distal to the uterine artery (class II hysterectomy).

Pelvic Exenteration. An extensive pelvic operation usually employed to treat a central pelvic recurrence of cervical carcinoma after radiation. A total exenteration involves removal of the bladder, uterus, cervix, and rectum. An anterior exenteration spares the rectum, while a posterior exenteration spares the bladder.

Persistent Tumor. The identification of invasive disease at the site of primary therapy less than 6 months after therapy.

Point A. A term used in radiation therapy of carcinoma of the cervix to identify a point 2 cm above the external os of the cervix and 2 cm lateral to the cervical canal.

Point B. A term used in the radiation treatment of carcinoma of the cervix to identify a point 3 cm lateral to point A or 5 cm from the cervical canal.

Radical Hysterectomy. An operation that removes the uterus, upper third of the vagina, cervix, and paracervical-parametrial tissues. The pelvic ureters are dissected to the uterovesical junction. It is usually combined with a pelvic lymph node dissection (class III hysterectomy).

Recurrent Tumor. The identification of invasive disease 6 months or more after therapy.

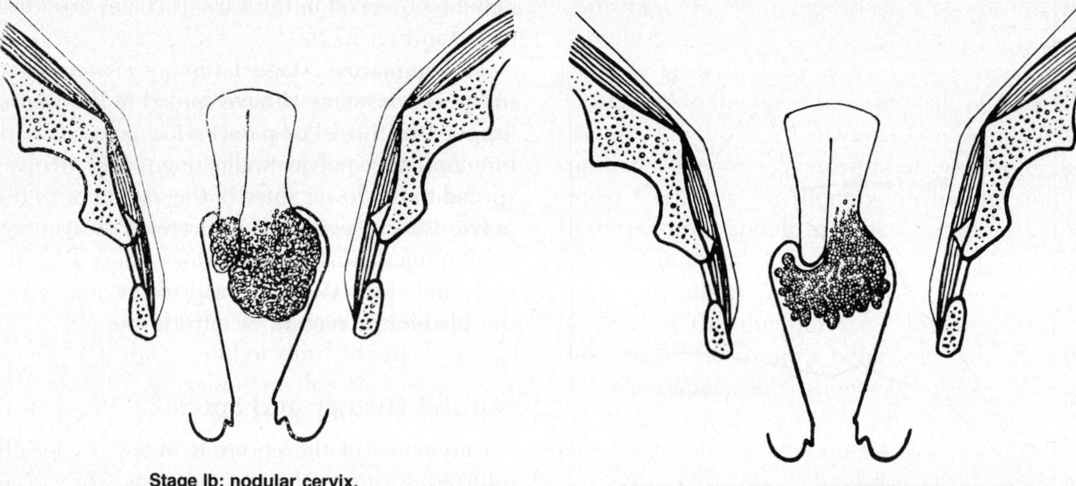

Stage Ib: nodular cervix.

Stage IIa: carcinoma extending into the left vault.

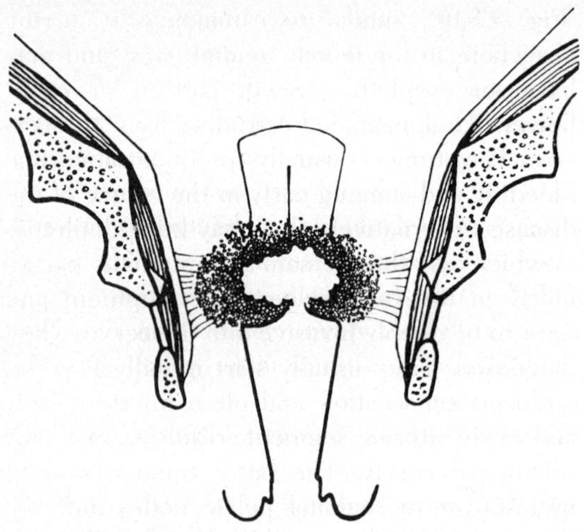

Stage IIb: parametrium involved on both sides, but the carcinoma has not invaded the pelvic wall; endocervical crater.

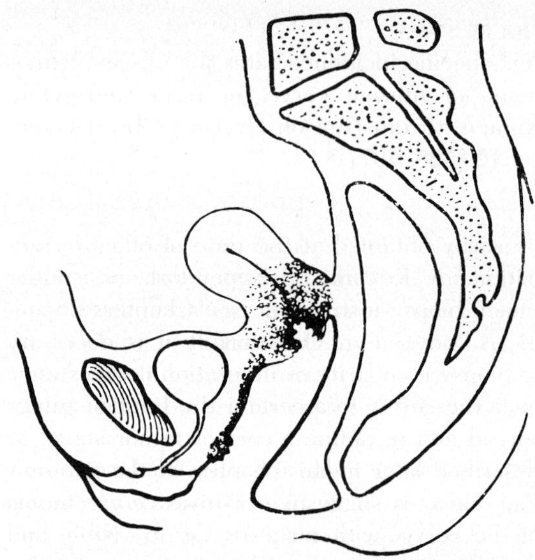

Stage IIIa: submucosa involvement of anterior vaginal wall and a small, papillomatous nodule in its lower third.

FIGURE 27-9

Staging of cervical carcinoma. (From Pettersson F: Semin Oncol 9:289, 1982.)

volved; the latter are particularly at risk for tumors that grow into the area of the rectum. The distribution of lymph node involvement was studied in detail for 26 cases of untreated carcinoma of the cervix by Henriksen (Fig. 27-11) (five stage I, six stage II, eight stage III, and seven stage IV). All were examined at autopsy, and the primary pelvic group had the

highest frequency of metastases with distal sites also involved, but less frequently. An important distal node that becomes involved after the paraaortic group is the left scalene node, that is, the left supraclavicular node. A clinical correlation is that biopsy of this node is frequently performed in the assessment of advance cervical carcinoma to clarify whether the

stage I
and II
and hi
   Wit
a very
has tl
stroma
(capill
nosis
studie
volver
Using
Boyce
culoca
major
correl;
218 p;
100 p;
lary-li
preser
size a
tant d
tumor
ter pr
and tl
diame
is also
evalua
vasion
than
nosis.
unifor
nifica1
entiat
nosis
but cu
Endor
cell ca
nosis.
fect tu
et al.
cervic

ADE
OF

   Cer
all ag
curs p
tumor
squan
as the

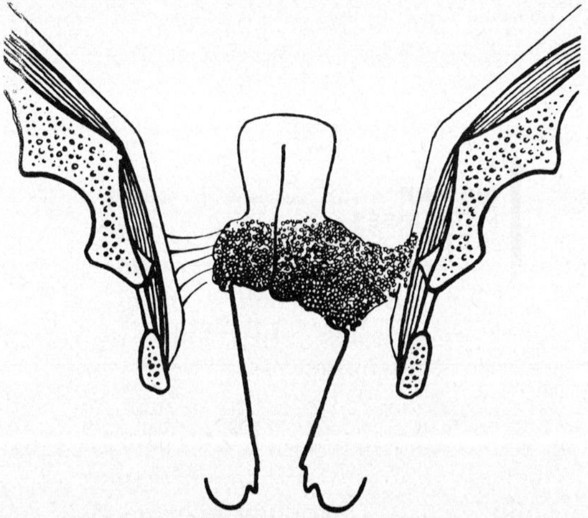

FIGURE 27-9, cont'd
Staging of cervical carcinoma.

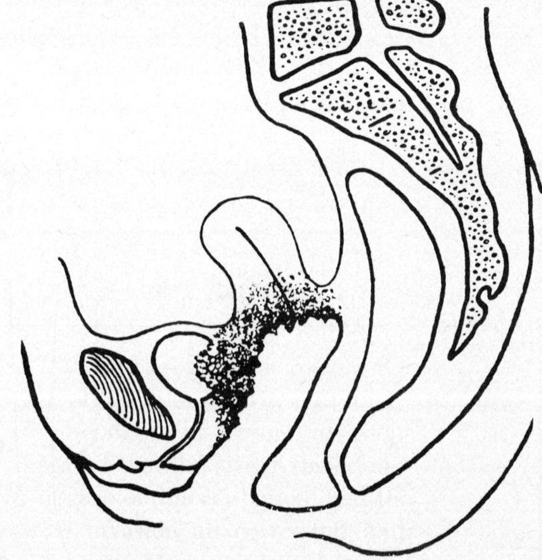

tumor has spread outside the abdomen. In addition to nodal spread, hematogenous spread of cervical carcinoma occurs primarily to the lung, liver, and less frequently bone (see recurrence section).

Prognostic Factors

Clinical stage is the most important determinant of prognosis for carcinoma of the cervix. Table 27-2 demonstrates the collated results for 17,843 cases treated worldwide between 1976 and 1978. Almost 70% of the tumors are in stage I or II, about 25% in stage III, and fewer than 5% in stage IV. Age appears to be a factor insofar as those under age 40 have a lower rate of survival than those between the ages of 40 and 69.

Numerous other factors have been evaluated to ascertain their importance in predicting the behavior of cervical carcinoma. These include tumor grade, depth of invasion, histologic type, presence of vasculolymphatic capillary space involvement, and status of regional pelvic nodes. Many of these factors, however, are interrelated; that is, the stage of the tumor closely correlates with the status of the regional pelvic nodes. For example, in a summary of 6560 cases Plentl and Friedman noted a frequency of 15% positive pelvic nodes in 3391 cases of stage I, 29% in 2952 cases of stage II, and 47% in 217 cases of stage III. Percentages based on a single series of patients are not available for paraaortic node involvement, but in a multi-institutional review of 290 patients by Lagasse et al. the proportion was 6% in

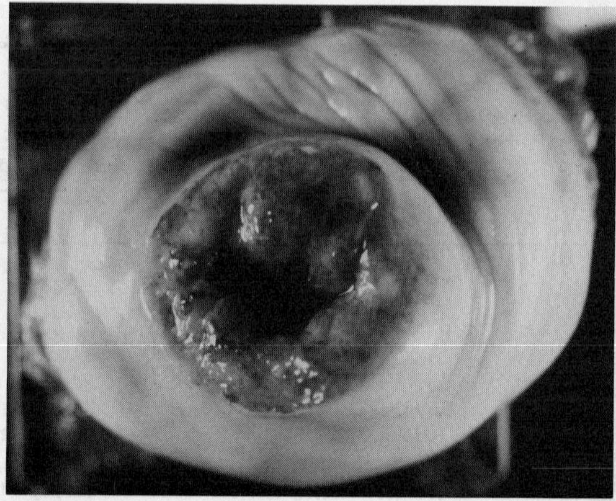

FIGURE 27-10
Carcinoma of cervix (gross specimen).

orrhage and also loss of the fetus. If it is necessary to perform a conization or a wedge resection of the cervix during pregnancy, it is probably best to perform this during the second trimester when the risks of fetal loss and hemorrhage are minimal. For patients in whom invasive cancer is diagnosed a therapeutic plan must be developed to deliver appropriate care with regard also for the outcome of the pregnancy.

The therapy of invasive carcinoma of the cervix during pregnancy is influenced by the stage of the disease, the time in pregnancy the cancer is diagnosed, and the beliefs and desires of the patient in terms of initiating therapy that can interrupt the pregnancy as opposed to postponing the therapy until fetal viability is achieved. If the carcinoma is diagnosed in the first trimester or early in the second trimester (before 20 weeks), treatment is preferably undertaken immediately because of the concern that a delay of over 4 months would lead to tumor progression or spread. If the patient has resectable tumor (stage Ib or early IIa), then effective treatment consists of radical hysterectomy and node dissection (class III). This procedure can usually be carried out without difficulty on a pregnant woman, especially before the twentieth week. Although an enlarged uterus can interfere with the operative field, increased uterine motility and edema of the pelvic tissue planes help to simplify the procedure for the experienced surgeon. Pregnancy does increase the risk of blood loss. For higher stage tumors therapy is begun with external beam radiation (teletherapy), and usually in 4 to 6 weeks this leads to spontaneous abortion. The dosage of external therapy prescribed varies depending on the stage of tumor, but approximately 40 to 50 Gy is given. Following abortion the uterus involutes, and an implant (brachytherapy) is performed. If the pregnancy does not spontaneously abort, dilation and curettage, prostaglandin-assisted delivery, or rarely hysterotomy may be necessary to empty the uterus before brachytherapy. Alternatively, if the initial tumor was small and has completely regressed, an extrafascial hysterectomy or modified radical hysterectomy (class I or II) may be performed.

For patients beyond the twentieth week of gestation a decision regarding initiating therapy immediately or delaying therapy until fetal viability must be made. If it is desired to continue the therapy, assessment must be made of the health of the fetus and its maturity. These are determined by appropriate ultrasound studies and amniotic fluid analysis to ensure fetal lung maturity. Delivery is usually accomplished by cesarean section, and after this, therapy is completed by operation or radiation with the same considerations of tumor stage and size for patients who are treated before the twentieth week of pregnancy. If immediate treatment is to be undertaken, hysterotomy is first performed and then operation or radiation therapy completed. Overall treatment results in pregnant patients are similar to those in nonpregnant patients, stage for stage. The reader should be aware that some published studies dealing with carcinoma of the cervix in pregnancy include cases treated as long as 1 year postpartum, which assumes the carcinoma was present during pregnancy. Hacker et al. summarized the results of 1249 cases reported in various series in the literature. Overall a 5-year survival rate of 49.2% was recorded for pregnant patients in comparison to 51% for nonpregnant patients treated during the same period of time. Their statistics included not only patients treated during pregnancy but also those treated up to 6 months after delivery, and the postpartum group had the poorest survival statistics. Survival was most closely related to stage, as expected, and persons diagnosed during the first trimester had a better prognosis than those diagnosed during the third trimester.

RECURRENCES

Approximately one third of patients treated for cancer of the cervix will experience tumor recurrence, which is defined as the reappearance of tumor 6 months or more after therapy. Earlier identification of tumor indicates persistent rather than recurrent disease. Metastases can occur anywhere, but most are in the pelvis (centrally in the vagina or cervix or laterally near the pelvic walls) or less frequently distally in the periaortic nodes, lung, liver, or bone. It should be noted that liver, lung, and distal bone metastases outside the pelvis likely result from hematogenous tumor spread.

The symptoms caused by recurrence depend on the site and extent of metastatic disease. Vaginal discharge and abnormal bleeding are often symptoms of an early central pelvic recurrence. Malaise, loss of appetite, and general symptoms associated with widespread metastatic disease are usually late manifestations of recurrence. Lateral pelvic recurrences often have a retroperitoneal component, which can lead to sciatic nerve irritation and cause severe pain around the distribution of the sciatic nerve in back of the leg as well as loss of muscle strength, causing the patient to walk with a limp. Unilateral leg edema frequently accompanies such metastases, or leg swelling may occur from fibrosis of lymphatics following operation or radiation. In addition, tumor recurrence can also cause ureteral obstruction, leading to unilateral or bilateral compromise of kidney function. Low back pain frequently occurs. Symptoms of pulmonary or hepatic disease will develop with progressive metastases in these areas. In addition, it should be remembered that the pattern of recurrence depends not only on the natural history of the tumor but also on the initial treatment utilized. For example, some tumors appear to be cured in the pelvis after radiation, only to recur later at a distant site as a result of blood-borne metastases.

Patients treated for carcinoma of the cervix are examined according to the same schedule as patients with other malignancies: every 3 months the first year, every 4 months the second year, every 6 months from years 3 to 5, and yearly thereafter. More frequent examinations are done if abnormal symptoms or signs develop. Examination consists of vaginal and cervical cytology (Pap smear) as well as complete physical and pelvic examinations. Generally chest x-ray films are obtained annually, and an IVP is also performed annually particularly during the first 3 years after treatment, when the majority of recurrences will develop. Special studies such as CT scans are ordered as indicated. A recently introduced blood test for squamous cell carcinoma (SCC) antigen has promise as an added modality to follow patients with squamous cell carcinoma who have detectable levels of the antigen in their blood. Once recurrent disease is suspected, verification is usually obtained by biopsy of an accessible mass or CT-directed thin needle aspiration depending on the location of the tumor recurrence.

Pelvic Recurrences

Approximately 50% of the recurrences of squamous cell carcinoma will develop in the pelvis. Other major sites are the abdomen and paraaortic nodes, liver, lung, and bone. Recurrences of adenocarcinoma are less frequent in the pelvis and are more likely to be at distant sites such as the lung or supraclavicular areas. For patients who were initially treated by operation, radiation is usually prescribed for pelvic recurrences, and approximately 50 Gy whole pelvic radiation is given. Supplemental interstitial or intracavitary radiation is also prescribed depending on the size and location of the recurrence in the pelvis. For patients who were initially treated with radiation who have developed a pelvic recurrence, surgical eradication of the tumor should be considered since further effective radiation is not possible and limited surgical resection of the pelvic recurrence will not lead to cure but will often cause severe complications of wound healing and intestinal and urinary fistulas.

Pelvic Exenteration

Exenterative therapy for central pelvic tumor recurrence is an extensive operative procedure that is used only if preoperative evaluation suggests that the patient's condition can be cured by this procedure. Exenteration is not performed for palliation. Three types of operation may be used. Anterior pelvic exenteration is the removal of the bladder, uterus, cervix, and part or all of the vagina. Posterior pelvic exenteration is the removal of the anus and rectum and resection of the uterus, cervix, and all or part of the vagina. Total exenteration is combined anteroposterior exenteration to remove all of the pelvic contents.

Before an exenterative operation is undertaken, the patient is thoroughly evaluated for any evidence of disease spread outside the pelvis. A CT scan is usually performed, and radiologic studies such as barium enema and IVP are done, particularly if a CT scan is not performed. Liver function tests are done, and, if indicated, radionuclide scan (including liver and bone scan) are performed. If there is suspicion of spread outside of the pelvis, a supraclavicular (scalene) node biopsy is undertaken. Assuming that the disease appears to be confined to the pelvis, operation is performed. Initially, a thorough abdominal exploration is carried out to be sure the tumor is resectable. Biopsy specimens of any enlarged lymph nodes or suspicious areas outside the pelvis are taken, and frozen section studies are performed including evaluation of the operative margins. Usually total exenteration is performed, and a colostomy is created for feces and an intestinal pouch (ileal bladder) for urine. Generally, the urinary stoma is located in the abdomen on the right side and the intestinal stoma on the left side.

Severe postoperative and intraoperative complications can occur with this extensive procedure, and perioperative mortalities as high as 10% to 20% have been reported in the past. Infection and bowel obstruction are the major risks. However, current surgical techniques of preoperative bowel preparation, use of antibiotics, careful intraoperative fluid and volume monitoring, and the use of parenteral nutrition have reduced the immediate postoperative mortality to less than 5%. The use of an omental flap created from the right or left side of the omentum and placed in the pelvis to protect the denuded pelvic floor can promote healing, help to avoid bowel obstruction, and reduce postoperative morbidity. Occasionally gracilis myocutaneous grafts are used both to create a new vagina and also to bring a new blood supply to the previously irradiated pelvis, which aids in wound healing. Recent series have reported 5-year survival rates of approximately 50%, in part as a result of careful selection of patients for this operation, but few patients are satisfactory candidates.

Nonpelvic Recurrences

Recurrences outside of the pelvis can be treated with radiation, operation, or chemotherapy. Localized recurrences in areas not previously irradiated are occasionally treated by means of radiation. Resection of the metastasis is rarely done, and it is usually restricted to a localized lesion that occurs 3 to 4 years after primary therapy on the assumption that such a solitary metastasis can be effectively treated with local resection. However, in general, distant metastases are usually manifestations of systemic disease and are not cured with local therapy.

Chemotherapy

Chemotherapy is usually prescribed for patients with unresectable pelvic recurrences following radiation therapy or for patients with disseminated metastatic disease. A variety of chemotherapeutic agents, either singly or in combination, have been used to treat recurrent squamous cell carcinoma of the vagina with generally poor results. Part of the problem is that in many of the cases there is compromise of renal function due to ureteral obstruction or loss of bone marrow reserve due to prior pelvic irradiation that reduces the dosage of chemotherapeutic agent that can be administered. In addition, squamous cell carcinomas in general have proven to be resistant to many chemotherapy programs.

Short-term responses of recurrent squamous cell carcinoma of the cervix have been reported with various multiple-agent protocols, and the best results appear to be obtained with protocols that contain *cis*-platinum. Bloch et al. reported on the use of bleomycin and *cis*-platinum in 17 patients and obtained an overall 53% response rate, only one case of which represented a complete response. The median survival time was 8 months. A more active program appears to be the use of *cis*-platinum with continuous infusion of 5-fluorouracil, which has been successfully employed in squamous cell carcinomas of the head and neck. Recently Rotmensch et al. utilized intravenous *cis*-platinum, 100 mg/m^2, followed by 5-fluorouracil, 1000 mg/m^2 per day for 3 to 5 days of continuous infusion, and the regimen was given every 3 to 4 weeks. Among the 25 patients so treated, the overall response rate was 52%, and complete response comprised 20% (5 patients). The median survival time was 40 weeks. The successful treatment of recurrent squamous cell carcinoma of the cervix will depend upon the introduction of new agents and different therapeutic approaches than are currently available.

Advanced Disease

As noted previously, pelvic pain can be a severe problem in patients with recurrent carcinoma of the cervix, especially when there is irritation or invasion of nerve trunks by tumor. This often becomes a particularly serious problem in patients with pelvic recurrence, where back pain and lower limb pain are often severe. Analgesics including narcotics are used as needed to control pain. Continuous intravenous infusion of narcotics such as morphine is occasionally very helpful. Local nerve blocks are also used and in selected cases neurosurgical procedures such as cordotomy (interruption of the lateral spinothalamic tract) provide the patient with excellent pain relief. Unfortunately, the operation also has potential severe side effects such as bladder atony.

In addition to pain, urinary or intestinal fistulas or obstruction may develop. In certain selected cases this is relieved with an operation to divert the feces or urine, although if possible an operation is avoided in patients with advanced disease. Urinary diversion is generally avoided since persons who undergo such a diversion frequently have prolonged periods of severe pain from metastatic disease in comparison to patients who do not have diversion and who succumb to uremia. The decision to use an operative approach to provide palliation to these patients depends on their activity status and near-term prognosis. The appropriate management of these difficult therapeutic problems requires sensitive and close interaction among the physician, allied health workers, and the patient and her family.

KEY POINTS

- Carcinomas of the cervix are predominantly squamous cell carcinomas (90% to 95%), and 5% to 10% are adenocarcinomas.

- Squamous cell carcinomas appear to have a viral and venereal association, whereas adenocarcinomas do not. The latter tend to occur in older and diabetic patients and those of low gravidity. In the United States squamous cell carcinoma is more frequent in blacks than in whites.

- Cervical carcinoma is the third most frequent malignancy of the lower female genital tract after endometrial and ovarian cancer and the second most frequent cause of death after ovarian cancer.

- The definitive diagnosis of microinvasive carcinoma is established by means of cervical conization, not biopsy.

- Microinvasive carcinoma of the cervix is effectively treated by total hysterectomy with a 5-year survival rate of almost 100%, but recurrent neoplasia can develop after 5 years.

added postoperatively, depending on the pathologic findings.

Radiation Therapy as the Sole Treatment of Stage I or II

Occasionally irradiation is used alone to treat stage I or II adenocarcinoma of the endometrium. Landgren et al. used Heyman packing with vaginal ovoids and two or three applications to treat stage I carcinomas. Either a dosage of 6000 mg-hours of radium was given to the uterus, or this dosage was reduced to 2500 mg-hours and supplemented later with 4000 rads of external radiation therapy. The best results were obtained with radium packing alone. This series was not randomized, but an improved result with the added external therapy was not demonstrated. The 5-year survival for stage I patients was approximately 75% in comparison with 55% for stage II patients. Later the same authors noted that treatment by uterine packing (6000 mg-hours) provided greater pelvic control of stage I disease than did 4000 rads of external irradiation in combination with only 2500 mg-hours of uterine packing.

Patanaphan et al. reported a 56% 5-year survival for 32 patients treated by irradiation in stage I and 40% for those in stage II. Tumor grade was not a significant factor in survival rate. Andersen et al. reported an overall 5-year survival rate of 49.6% for all stages, broken down to 65% for stage I and 42% for stage II. Irradiation can effectively control stage I or II disease locally, but eradication of the tumor through surgery, in combination with irradiation, remains the optimal mode of management when possible. The value of external radiotherapy in improving survival rates has not been clearly defined.

Stage III

In stage III carcinoma the disease has spread outside the uterus but remains confined to the pelvis. These tumors do not involve the mucosa of the rectum or bladder. They account for only 7% of all endometrial carcinomas and occur in patients who are older than those with lower stage tumors and often medically less able to undergo an operation. Aalders et al. reported on the results of 175 patients with stage III tumor, 52% of whom were over 60 years of age. These patients were divided into two groups: those with clinical evidence of extrauterine spread before therapy (usually to the vagina or parametrium, 108 cases) and those with subclinical evidence of spread to the adnexa (fallopian tube or ovary) discovered at the time of operation in a patient believed to have stage I or II carcinoma initially (67 cases). Operative eradication of microscopic tumor was of major prognostic importance in these cases; eradication was usually possible if the tumor involved only the uterine adnexa. The optimal therapy, when possible, was a total abdominal hysterectomy and bilateral salpingo-oophorectomy followed by external irradiation (40 to 50 Gy). If there was vaginal extension of cervical disease, the cervical field was shielded at 20 Gy and subsequent brachytherapy was administered to the vagina, bringing the vaginal surface dose to 60 Gy. For patients who could not undergo surgery, packing of the uterus was done as previously described (Fig. 28-12), followed by external irradiation therapy. Those with subclinical spread of tumor had a much better 5-year survival (40%) than those with overt clinical stage III disease (16%).

For intraperitoneal metastatic disease, Greer and Hamburger used whole abdominal irradiation in 31 patients. In 27 of the patients with residual tumor less than 2 cm, a 5-year survival of 63% was noted. These authors recommend that such salvage therapy could be effective for individuals with endometrial carcinoma, particularly stage III disease, providing tumor reduction surgery results in residual tumor under 2 cm in diameter, as shown in the data for ovarian epithelial carcinoma.

The patients with stage III endometrial carcinoma with the best prognosis have tumor spread only to the fallopian tubes or ovaries or both. If possible, therapy should include operative eradication of macroscopic tumor. This is combined with radiotherapy, the dosage and delivery system of which depend on the extent of tumor. If there is no extensive involvement of the cervix and paracervical areas, initial Heyman packing can be done before hysterectomy and external beam therapy. For tumor that extends into the vagina and paravaginal tissues, intracavitary irradiation is combined with external therapy, followed by hysterectomy if technically feasible. For tumor extending to the pelvic wall or patients in poor medical condition, usually only irradiation therapy is possible.

Stage IV

Approximately 3% of endometrial carcinomas are at stage IV, and many of these patients have tumor metastases outside the pelvis. In a series of 83 patients from the Norwegian Radium Hospital, Aalders et al. reported that the lung was the main site of extrauterine spread (36% of the cases), which is consistent with the generalized pattern of recurrent adenocarcinoma of the endometrium. They utilized hysterectomy to achieve local control of stage IV disease, usually followed by postoperative external irradiation therapy. Progestational therapy (17α-hydroxyprogesterone caproate, 1000 mg intramuscularly daily for 1 week, weekly for 3 months, and every other week for at least 1 year) was also prescribed for 17 patients, two of whom survived 3 and 13 years, respectively. Progestins were also used in 30 patients with pulmonary metastases, and eight had a complete remission (disappearance) of metastatic tumor. Complete remission occurred in seven patients with grade 2 tumors and in one patient with grade 3, but progression occurred in 11 of 13 patients with grade 3 carcinoma, a finding that is consistent with the observation that poorly differentiated adenocarcinomas are least responsive to progestational therapy. The 5-year survival was 10% for all 83 cases, similar to the general experience (see Table 28-6).

Individualization of therapy is necessary for the patient with stage IV endometrial carcinoma. If feasible, the uterus, tubes, and ovaries are removed to achieve local control. Irradiation therapy is administered as an adjunct or, if necessary, as the sole therapy for palliation to achieve pelvic control of disease. Progestational agents are particularly useful in the case of well-differentiated tumors.

Recurrent Adenocarcinoma of the Endometrium

Most recurrences of adenocarcinoma of the endometrium occur within 3 years of diagnosis, and 90% occur within 5 years of diagnosis.

Since 10% of recurrences will occur more than 5 years after initial diagnosis, patients with adenocarcinoma of the endometrium need prolonged follow-up. In the series of Aalders et al. involving 379 patients, half of the recurrences were in the pelvis and vagina; the most frequent sites of nonpelvic metastases were lung (17%), upper portion of the abdomen (10%), and bone (6%). Irradiation was the primary treatment of localized recurrent disease in patients who had an operation alone as the initial treatment, but operative excision of resectable nodules was also done when feasible. Progestational agents are added as initial treatment, particularly for disseminated disease. The 5-year survival rate for those patients who received progestins with other forms of treatment for grade 1 and grade 2 recurrences was 26%, in comparison with 14% for those who did not. For undifferentiated tumors the comparable survival was 9%.

CHEMOTHERAPY. Chemotherapy for endometrial carcinoma has primarily involved the use of progestins, as well as cytotoxic agents. Unfortunately, no clearly effective program of cytotoxic chemotherapy has emerged. Progestins have been used frequently, and responses of 10% to 30% have been reported. Responses are more likely in well-differentiated tumors, as well as those recurring at distant sites not previously treated, such as the lung.

Steroid hormone receptor content of tumor has been studied in relation to chemotherapeutic response. It has been shown that the well-differentiated tumors also have the highest content of estrogen and progestin steroid hormone receptors. Ehrlich et al. reported that progesterone and estrogen receptor levels correlate with grade of tumor—84% of grade 1 tumors were progesterone receptor positive, 55% of grade 2, and 22% of grade 3. The content of receptor correlated with response to progestin treatment; none of the 15 patients with receptor-negative tumors responded to progestational therapy, yet seven of eight with receptor-positive tumors responded. Numerous and various dosage schedules have been employed, including 17α-hydroxyprogesterone (Delalutin), discussed earlier; medroxyprogesterone (Depo-Provera), 400 mg intramuscularly weekly for 3 months, and then every 2 weeks; and oral megestrol acetate (Megace), 160 to 320 mg daily. Kohorn summarized many case reports from the literature and noted that responses were approximately 15% for poorly differentiated tumors and 32% for well-differentiated tumors. The results do not appear to depend on the type of progestin administered.

Recently antiestrogens such as tamoxifen have been added to treat recurrent endometrial carcinoma. A regimen of 5 days of therapy (10 mg orally twice daily) was associated with increased receptor content of endometrial carcinoma in the patients studied. Carlson et al. noted that only 13 of 25 tumors were progesterone receptor positive before tamoxifen therapy, whereas 21 of 25 tumors became positive after tamoxifen. These observations raise the possibility of combining tamoxifen and progestin therapy to improve the results of treatment. Swenerton et al. summarized recent results of tamoxifen therapy alone for 91 patients who had an overall response rate of 32%, similar to that with progestational agents alone.

Cytotoxic Chemotherapy. A number of cytotoxic agents have been used to treat endometrial carcinoma. No effective salvage therapy has emerged, however, and combinations of *cis*-platinum, doxorubicin (Adriamycin), and cyclophosphamide (Cytoxan) or 5-fluorouracil (5-FU) are usually employed. Turbow et al. used *cis*-platinum, 60 mg/m^2, doxorubicin, 50 mg/m^2, and cyclophosphamide, 600 mg/m^2 (CAP), administered intravenously every 4 weeks to 21 patients. Two complete clinical responses and seven partial responses were noted, and one complete clinical response was confirmed at second-look laparotomy. In a different study, Kauppila et al. treated 20 patients with a 3-day course of vincristine, 1.5 mg on day 1, with doxorubicin (40 mg/m^2) 4 hours later and then, in 2 hours, cyclophosphamide (500 mg/m^2). On days 2 and 3, 5-FU, 500 mg/m^2, was given intravenously over 2 hours. All patients had failed to respond to prior progestin administration. A complete response was achieved in 25% of the patients and a partial response in an additional 25%. Ten patients with either low estrogen or low progestin receptor values responded to the chemotherapy (70%), whereas those with high receptor values had only a 20% response rate, suggesting that endometrial carcinomas with low receptor con-

tent may be the most responsive to chemotherapy.

• • •

Newer approaches and agents are needed to deal with metastatic and recurrent adenocarcinoma of the endometrium. Even when progestational agents are combined with cytotoxic therapy, responses of 50% or less are achieved, and most of the regressions are temporary. Initially progestins should be used, particularly in tumors with high steroid hormone receptor content. Cytotoxic chemotherapy is more effective in tumors with low receptor content, and multiple-agent regimens utilizing cyclophosphamide, doxorubicin, and platinum and/or 5-FU currently offer occasionally effective results.

SARCOMAS

Uterine sarcomas are much less frequent than endometrial carcinomas, particularly in Western countries where carcinoma of the endometrium has become so common. Sarcomas comprise less than 5% of uterine malignancies. Numerous terms have been used to describe the many histologic types. One useful classification is based on determination of the resemblance of the sarcomatous elements to mesenchymal tissue normally found in the uterus (homologous sarcomas) in contrast to tissues foreign to the uterus (heterologous sarcomas). Homologous types include leiomyosarcomas, endometrial stromal sarcomas, and rarely angiosarcomas. Heterologous types include rhabdomyosarcomas, chondrosarcomas, osteosarcomas, and liposarcomas. These sarcomas may exist exclusively or may be admixed with epithelial adenocarcinoma, in which case the term *malignant müllerian mixed tumor* (MMMT) is applied. The box on p. 823 shows a morphologic classification for uterine sarcomas. No uniformly defined staging criteria exist for these tumors, and the most widely used definitions are similar to those for endometrial carcinoma, i.e., stage I confined to the corpus, stage II corpus and cervix involved, stage III spread outside the uterus but confined to the pelvis, and stage IV spread outside the true pelvis or into the mucosa of the bladder or rectum. Therapy for the more commonly occur-

MODIFIED CLASSIFICATION OF UTERINE SARCOMAS

I. Pure sarcoma
   A. Homologous
      1. Smooth muscle tumors
         a. Leiomyosarcoma
         b. Leiomyoblastoma
         c. Metastasizing tumors with benign histologic appearance
            (1) Intravenous leiomyomatosis
            (2) Metastasizing uterine leiomyoma
            (3) Leiomyomatosis peritonealis disseminata
      2. Endometrial stromal sarcomas
         a. Low grade: endolymphatic stromal myosis (ESM)
         b. High grade: endometrial stromal sarcoma (ESS)
   B. Heterologous
      1. Rhabdomyosarcoma
      2. Chondrosarcoma
      3. Osteosarcoma
      4. Liposarcoma
   C. Other sarcomas
II. Malignant müllerian mixed tumors (MMMT)
   A. Homologous (carcinosarcoma): Carcinoma + Homologous sarcoma
   B. Heterologous: Carcinoma + Heterologous sarcoma
III. Müllerian adenosarcoma
IV. Lymphoma

Modified from Clement P, and Scully RE: Pathology of uterine sarcomas. In Coppleson M, ed: Gynecologic oncology. New York, Churchill Livingstone, 1981, p. 591. Reprinted by permission.

ring types will be discussed, including leiomyosarcomas, endometrial stromal sarcomas, and malignant müllerian mixed tumors.

Homologous Sarcoma

Leiomyosarcoma

Among the uterine sarcomas, leiomyosarcomas are the most common, occurring somewhat more frequently than mixed malignant müllerian tumors. In summarizing 1089 uterine sarcomas from the literature, Piver and Lurain noted that leiomyosarcomas comprised 45% of the group. The determination of malignancy is made in part by ascertaining the number of mitoses in 10 high-power fields (hpf) as well as the presence of cytologic atypia (Fig. 28-13). Vascular invasion and extrauterine spread of tumor are associated with worse prognoses. A finding of more than 5 mitoses/10 hpf leads to a diagnosis of leiomyosarcoma; when there are 4 mitoses/10 hpf or less, the tumors usually have a benign clinical course. The worst prognosis is for tumors with over 10 mitoses/10 hpf; those with 5 to 9 mitoses/10 hpf are considered to be of low malignant potential. However, such tumors are usually classified as leiomyosarcoma if bizarre cells also exist. The presence of bizarre cells, however, does not necessarily establish the diagnosis (Fig. 28-14) because they can be seen in benign leiomyomas and in patients receiving progestational agents. Leiomyosarcomas tend to occur in patients in their 50s, occasionally in conjunction with leiomyomas, although leiomyosarcomas usually infiltrate diffusely into the myometrium. The development of leiomyosarcoma from leiomyoma is rare.

Premenopausal patients have been reported to have a better prognosis than postmenopausal patients. Usually the patient has an enlarged pelvic mass, occasionally accompanied by pain or vaginal bleeding. Leiomyosarcomas are suspected if the uterus undergoes rapid enlargement, particularly in patients in the perimenopausal or postmenopausal age group.

Treatment consists of surgical removal of all disease if possible. Mitotic rate is important in determining prognosis. With increasing mitotic rate the prognosis becomes worse. For patients with well-documented leiomyosarcoma the overall 5-year survival rate is about 20%; for those with stage I and II tumors it is approximately 40%.

The most important aspect of treatment is removal of the tumor, usually by total abdominal hysterectomy with bilateral salpingo-oophorectomy (TAH-BSO). Irradiation therapy has been used to treat residual pelvic disease but is of unproved value. Salazar et al. noted that irradiation therapy appeared to decrease the risk of pelvic recurrence of tumor but did not significantly improve survival rates.

In addition to local pelvic recurrences, distant metastases are frequent and most often oc-

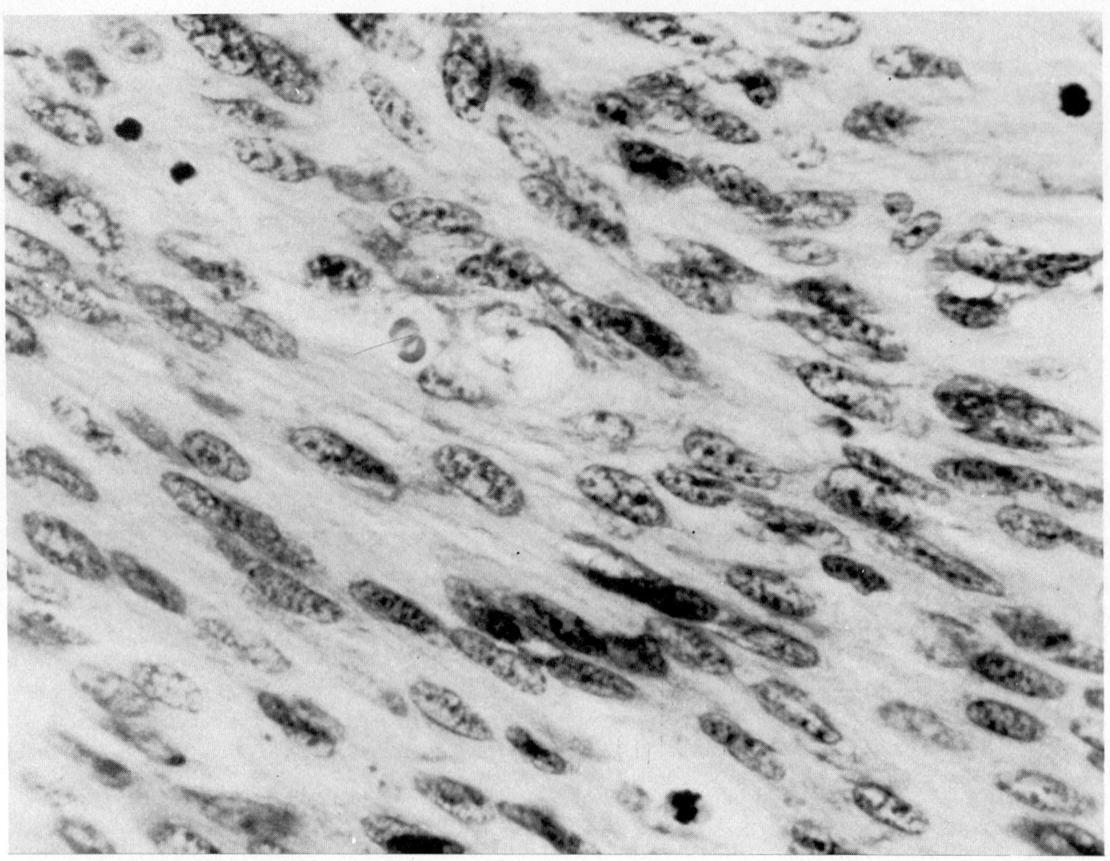

FIGURE 28-13
Leiomyosarcoma. Nuclear hyperchromatism and mitotic figures are present.
($\times$660.) (From Clement PB, Scully RE: Pathology of uterine sarcomas. In Coppleson M, ed: Gynecologic oncology. Edinburgh, Churchill-Livingstone, 1981. Reprinted by permission.)

cur in the lungs or intraabdominally. These are preferably treated by multiple-agent chemotherapy. Occasionally a patient of reproductive age has an unsuspected leiomyosarcoma diagnosed in a leiomyoma removed at myomectomy. Usually in such cases, hysterectomy is subsequently performed, but a few cures have been reported in individuals who have had no further treatment beyond myomectomy; a complete, accurate histologic assessment is vital to ascertain the risk. Pregnancy can increase the mitotic rate in smooth muscle tumors, which should be remembered when myomas are removed from pregnant or recently pregnant patients.

The clinician should be aware of variations of smooth muscle tumors that are not leiomyosarcomas or benign leiomyomas. These tumors include leiomyoblastoma, intravenous leiomyomatosis, metastasizing uterine leiomyoma, and leiomyomatosis peritonealis disseminata. Leiomyoblastomas are rare smooth muscle tumors that grossly resemble leiomyomas. They contain epithelial-like cells with spindle-shaped cells characteristic of smooth muscle tumors. Usually the mitotic rate is less than 5/10 hpf, and these tumors should be regarded as low-grade sarcomas for which operative removal is the preferred therapy. Intravenous leiomyomatosis is also rare and is usually a condition characterized by intravenous extension of smooth muscle tissue outside the uterus (Fig. 28-15). Wormlike projections of the tumor may be found in vascular spaces in the broad ligament or extending even into the vena cava. Occasionally smooth muscle nodules are found out-

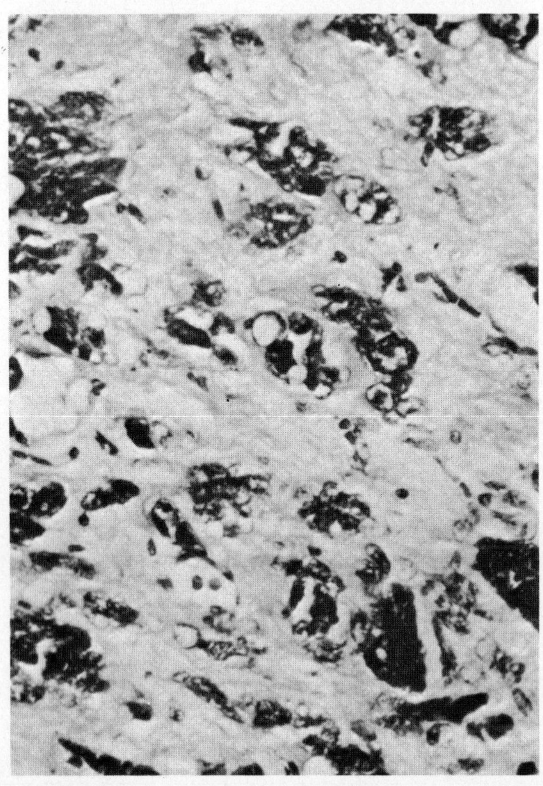

FIGURE 28-14
Leiomyoma with bizarre nuclei. No mitoses are present. (×256.) (From Clement PB, Scully RE: Pathology of uterine sarcomas. In Coppleson M, ed: Gynecologic oncology. Edinburgh, Churchill-Livingstone, 1981. Reprinted by permission.)

FIGURE 28-15
Intravenous leiomyomatosis replacing most of the uterus and extending into the broad ligaments and adjacent veins. (From Norris HJ, Zaloudek CJ: Mesenchymal tumors of the uterus. In Blaustein A, ed: Pathology of the female genital tract, 2nd ed. New York, Springer-Verlag, 1982.)

side the pelvis either in lymph nodes or in the lungs, in which case the term *metastasizing leiomyoma* is used. Removal of the uterus and the extrauterine lesion, if possible, is the treatment of choice, although leaving some tissue in cases of intravenous leiomyomatosis does not appear to lead to spread of the disease. Very rarely, small nodes of leiomyoma are found in the peritoneal cavity (leiomyomatosis peritonealis disseminata). The condition is found during pregnancy and usually regresses after delivery.

Endometrial Stromal Sarcoma

LOW GRADE—ENDOLYMPHATIC STROMAL MYOSIS. Endolymphatic stromal myosis is the least frequent among the uterine sarcomas, leiomyosarcomas, and malignant mixed müllerian tumors. The tumor consists of cells that resemble those of the uterine stroma, with a spindlelike appearance somewhat resembling fibrous sarcoma. Endolymphatic stromal myosis is diagnosed if the mitotic rate in the tumor is less than 10/10 hpf. Frequently these tumors have even fewer than 10 mitoses. Despite the comparatively innocuous appearance and prolonged clinical course, these tumors can be fatal.

Piver et al. recently summarized a comparative study of 152 cases of endolymphatic stromal myosis. The patients with this tumor were 20 to 70 years of age, but almost three

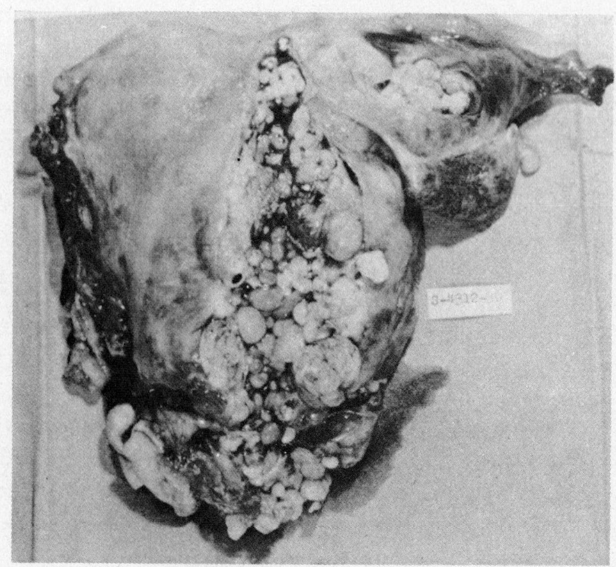

fourths were under age 50. Most had abnormal vaginal bleeding, and pelvic examination frequently revealed a large, irregularly shaped uterus. Occasionally the diagnosis is made on tissue obtained at diagnostic D&C. Press and Scully reported six cases associated with chronic estrogen stimulation and suggested that unopposed estrogen stimulation might increase the risk of these tumors.

The predominant mode of treatment is surgical and usually consists of total abdominal hysterectomy and bilateral salpingo-oophorectomy. Occasionally for tumors that spread to the cervix or paracervical areas a more radical procedure is performed, and a major effort is made to remove all gross disease. Long-term survivors are common, and 5-year survival of 100% was reported for the 15 patients originally described by Norris and Taylor; it was 88% in the collaborative series collected by Piver et al. for patients with tumors confined to the uterus.

Recurrence. Endolymphatic stromal myosis tends to recur locally in the pelvis or peritoneal cavity and frequently spreads to the lungs. In treating metastatic disease it should be remembered that these tumors contain estrogen and progestin steroid hormone receptors and are sensitive to progestational therapy. Megestrol acetate (Megace), medroxyprogesterone (Provera), and 17α-hydroxyprogesterone caproate (Delalutin) have been used. Complete resolution of the pulmonary lesions has been reported, and dosages of progestational drugs used are comparable to those for endometrial carcinoma. Nine patients reported by Thatcher and Woodruff were all living without evidence of disease 2 to 8 years after treatment, even though five had disease beyond the uterus at the time of initial operation. In view of the potential reappearance of disease, it is advisable to continue progestational therapy indefinitely after successful initial treatment of metastatic disease.

Irradiation has also been used to treat recurrences of these tumors, especially in the pelvis, with resolution of all residual tumor, but extensive experience with irradiation treatment is not available. Systemic chemotherapy with cytotoxic agents has not been reported generally to be effective, although complete response to doxorubicin (Adriamycin) has been reported.

HIGH GRADE—ENDOMETRIAL STROMAL SARCOMA. Endometrial stromal sarcomas are high-grade stromal tumors that behave aggressively and have a poor prognosis; microscopically more than 10 mitoses/10 hpf are present. Most series have reported 100% fatalities, although Vongtama et al. reported survival of over 60% for 24 patients with stage I and for one patient with stage II disease. All cases of endolymphatic stromal myosis were eliminated, and treatment consisted of either operation alone or operation plus irradiation.

Patients with endometrial stromal sarcoma have abnormal bleeding or a pelvic mass. The tumor can occur at any age during reproductive life but tends to be primarily diagnosed in women under age 50 years. Operative removal of the tumor is the treatment of choice, but in view of the frequently poor survival rate, adjuvant therapy should be considered even if all tumor has been removed. Kempson and Bari have advised adjuvant therapy if the mitotic index is more than 20 mitoses/10 hpf, even if the tumor is confined to the uterus and totally removed. In such a case, pelvic irradiation is given or systemic chemotherapy is prescribed for 6 to 12 months. Usually doxorubicin or a combination containing doxorubicin is prescribed. Current data have not established whether either irradiation or chemotherapy is effective in improving survival rates for patients with endometrial stromal sarcoma. Progestational agents are also administered, but there is no evidence of their efficacy in tumors with a high mitotic rate.

Recurrence. Recurrences are common in the pelvis, lung, and abdomen. If there has not been prior irradiation and the recurrence is confined to the pelvis, usually pelvic irradiation is prescribed. If there is disseminated disease, multiple-agent chemotherapy is then used.

Malignant Müllerian Mixed Tumors

Malignant müllerian mixed tumors (MMMTs) are aggressive malignancies that comprised 36% of 1089 cases reviewed by Piver and Lurain. As shown in the box on p. 823, these tumors consist of carcinomatous and sarcomatous elements native to the uterus that may resemble the endometrial stroma of smooth muscle (homologous tumor or carcinosarcoma) or of sarcomatous tissues foreign to the uterus (heterologous). Spanos et al. reviewed 188 patients with mixed mesodermal tumor and found both the prognosis and the pattern of survival similar for both homologous and heterologous tumors. Unlike patients with endometrial stromal sarcoma or leiomyosarcoma, those with MMMT tend to be older and primarily postmenopausal, usually beyond the age of 62 years. Prior pelvic irradiation has been identified as a predisposing factor and was experienced by 17 of the 136 patients reviewed by Norris and Taylor. The heterologous and homologous tumors occur with approximately equivalent frequency. These tumors spread into the myometrium and then to the pelvis, to the abdomen including the peritoneum, and frequently to the lungs and pleura, a pattern similar to the spread of endometrial carcinoma. A common symptom is postmenopausal bleeding, often accompanied by a large uterus. Occasionally the diagnosis is made in tissue removed with D&C, and the tumor may appear to be a polypoid excrescence from the cervix.

As is true for other sarcomas, the primary treatment for MMMT is operative removal of the uterus. An additional problem is the older age of these patients. The extent of the tumor and the depth of myometrial invasion are important prognostic factors. Those with deep myometrial invasion are more likely to have spread of MMMT to pelvic or paraaortic nodes, as in endometrial carcinomas. Patients with tumors confined to the uterus and little or no myometrial spread have the best prognosis. TAH and BSO are completed with stage I tumors; more extensive procedures are occasionally attempted for stage II tumors, as well as for those with early extrauterine spread. However, survival with operation alone is poor. Piver and Lurain summarized 610 cases collected from the literature and noted a 5-year survival rate of 21%. Stage is an important prognostic factor, and the reported survival rate varies from 30% to 50% for stage I cases to 0% for stage IV.

Because of the poor results with operation alone, supplemental treatment with irradiation or chemotherapy has been advocated. Perez et al. used preoperative intracavitary irradiation (5000 mg-hours) followed by TAH and BSO and then supplemented with full pelvic irradia-tion for stage I and stage II MMMT. The pelvic disease was eradicated, but distant metastases were common. Although irradiation may augment the beneficial effects of operation, particularly for the carcinomatous elements of MMMT, systemic dissemination of disease is common. Full control depends on the identification of an effective program of chemotherapy.

Müllerian Adenosarcoma

Müllerian adenosarcoma is a rare low-grade malignancy composed of both a sarcomatous stroma (homologous) and a proliferation of benign glandular elements that are intimately associated. It occurs predominantly in women older than 60 years. Ten cases were described initially by Clement and Scully. TAH with BSO is the treatment of choice.

Lymphoma

On rare occasions the uterus can be the original site for lymphoma, or, more commonly involvement of the uterus may be the initial presentation of disseminated lymphoma. About 40 cases of primary lymphoma of the uterus have been reported. They are usually treated by irradiation.

Chemotherapy

It is evident from available data that treatment beyond operative resection and irradiation therapy is needed to achieve control of uterine sarcomas. Once resection has been accomplished, cytotoxic chemotherapy is considered as an adjuvant to improve survival, particularly with high-grade tumors. Unfortunately, few data are available, and conflicting results have been reported. Marchese et al. studied 38 patients with sarcomas. Six with complete resection received adjuvant chemotherapy, primarily with vincristine, actinomycin D, and cyclophosphamide, and had a 5-year survival of 61%; survival was 15% for 23 patients with complete resections who did not receive chemotherapy. Confounding factors such as tumor histologic findings and stage were not controlled. In contrast, Hannigan et al. treated 34 patients with a variety of uterine sarcomas with either vincristine, 1.5 mg weekly, actinomycin D, 0.5 mg intravenously for 5 days, and cyclophosphamide, 300 mg intravenously for 5 days, or doxorubicin, 50 mg/m^2 alone, or doxorubicin with cyclophosphamide and vincristine. Sixty-seven patients did not receive adjuvant therapy, and there was no evidence of increased survival or a prolonged disease-free interval for the adjuvant chemotherapy group. Barter et al. found no benefit for adjuvant chemotherapy for patients with leiomyosarcomas.

No single program has proved superior for the treatment of endometrial stromal sarcoma, leiomyosarcoma, or mixed müllerian malignant tumor, with the exception of progestin therapy to treat low-grade endometrial stromal sarcoma (endolymphatic stromal myosis). Thus chemotherapy programs for these sarcomas can be considered together.

Azizi et al. treated six cases of metastatic leiomyosarcoma with vincristine, 1.2 mg/m^2 weekly for 7 to 8 weeks, doxorubicin, 20 to 25 mg/m^2 intravenously for 3 days, and dacarbazine (DTIC), 250 mg/m^2 for 5 days every 3 weeks. Three complete responses lasting up to 2 years and one partial response were observed. Hannigan et al. used vincristine, actinomycin D, and cyclophosphamide (Cytoxan) (VAC protocol, Chapter 29) and noted a 13% complete response rate and 16% partial response rate in 74 patients with advanced metastatic uterine sarcomas. A large collaborative trial was recently conducted by the Gynecologic Oncology Group and reported by Omura et al. The best responses were obtained for patients with lung metastases who received doxorubicin and DTIC. Current evidence suggests that a multidrug program that includes doxorubicin (Adriamycin) offers the greatest potential for inducing remission of uterine sarcomas. *Cis*-platinum also appears to have some effectiveness, but the optimal chemotherapy combination has not been identified. In view of the poor survival rate and the high likelihood of recurrence of uterine sarcomas, an effective program of chemotherapy is needed.

KEY POINTS

- Endometrial carcinoma is the most common malignancy of the lower female genital tract. In the United States about 1 woman in 100 will develop the disease.

- More deaths occur from ovarian and cervical cancer than from endometrial cancer.

- Most women who develop endometrial cancer are between 50 and 65 years of age.

- The primary symptom of endometrial carcinoma is postmenopausal bleeding.

- Chronic estrogen stimulation of the endometrium leads to endometrial hyperplasia and in some cases adenocarcinoma. Other important predisposing factors include obesity, nulliparity, late menopause, and diabetes.

- The risk of a woman's developing endometrial carcinoma is increased 3 times if she is 21 to 50 pounds overweight and 10 times if she is more than 50 pounds overweight. Nulliparous women have twice the risk of those with one child and three times the risk of those with five or more children. Menopause after 52 years of age increases the risk by 2.4 times in comparison with menopause before age 49 years. Diabetes raises the risk by a factor of 2.8.

- Prognosis in endometrial carcinoma is related to tumor grade, tumor stage, and histologic type.

- Endometrial carcinoma can develop without preexisting endometrial hyperplasia, particularly in older patients and those with less well differentiated tumors.

- Younger women with endometrial cancer have a better prognosis than older women.

- Cytologic atypia in endometrial hyperplasia is more important than architectural atypia in determining premalignant potential.

- Adenocarcinoma of the endometrium is detected only in about 50% of the cases by routine cervical-vaginal cytologic study (Papanicolaou smear).

- Initially, endometrial carcinoma spreads outside the uterus, to the retroperitoneal, pelvic, and paraaortic lymph nodes, to the adnexa, and then to the peritoneal cavity.

- Well-differentiated (grade 1) endometrial carcinomas usually contain measurable levels of steroid hormone receptors, whereas poorly differentiated (grade 3) tumors usually do not contain measurable levels of receptors.

- Receptor-positive endometrial carcinomas have a better prognosis than do those that are receptor negative.

- Ninety percent of recurrences of adenocarcinoma of the endometrium occur within 5 years.

- Overall survival rates for patients with adenocarcinoma of the endometrium by stage are as follows: stage I, 75%; stage II, 58%; stage III, 30%; and stage IV, 11%.

KEY POINTS, cont'd

- Histologic variants of endometrial carcinoma with a poor prognosis include adenosquamous carcinoma, papillary carcinoma, and clear cell carcinoma.

- The most frequent sites of distant metastasis of adenocarcinoma of the endometrium are the lung, retroperitoneal nodes, and abdomen.

- Progestin therapy results in responses of 10% to 30% in recurrent endometrial carcinoma. The highest response rates are in tumors with elevated sex steroid receptor levels, well-differentiated tumors, and recurrences at sites not previously irradiated.

- Uterine sarcomas comprise less than 5% of uterine malignancies.

- The optimal treatment of resectable endometrial carcinoma or uterine sarcoma is by operation that includes total abdominal hysterectomy and bilateral salpingo-oophorectomy. Supplemental irradiation or chemotherapy is prescribed depending on the extent of the disease and the histologic features of the tumor.

- Uterine sarcomas are treated primarily by removal of the uterus, tubes, and ovaries.

- Mitotic rate is an important prognostic factor in uterine leiomyosarcomas and is worse for those with more than 10 mitoses/10 hpf. Tumors with 5 to 9 mitoses/10 hpf have a low malignant potential.

- Endometrial stromal sarcomas are virulent sarcomas with 10 or more mitoses/10 hpf. For tumors with less than 10 mitoses/10 hpf, the prognosis is improved and a diagnosis of endolymphatic stromal myosis is made.

- Recurrences of uterine sarcomas are most frequent locally in the pelvis, the abdomen, and the lungs.

- Metastatic endolymphatic stromal myosis is treated with progestin therapy initially. More than half will resolve.

- Chemotherapeutic regimens that include doxorubicin (Adriamycin) are usually prescribed for metastatic sarcomas. Complete responses are rare, and overall responses are about 20% to 30%.

BIBLIOGRAPHY

Aalders JG, Abeler V, Kolstad P: Clinical (stage III) as compared to subclinical intrapelvic extrauterine tumor spread in endometrial carcinoma: A clinical and histopathological study of 175 patients. Gynecol Oncol 17:64, 1984.

Aalders JG, Abeler V, Kolstad P: Stage IV endometrial carcinoma: A clinical and histopathological study of 83 patients. Gynecol Oncol 17:75, 1984.

Aalders JG, Abelar V, Kolstad P: Recurrent adenocarcinoma of the endometrium: A clinical and histopathological study of 379 patients. Gynecol Oncol 17:85, 1984.

Andersen WA, Peters WA, Fechner RE, et al: Radioactive alternatives to standard management of adenocarcinoma of the endometrium. Gynecol Oncol 16:383, 1983.

Antoniades J, Brady LW, Lewis GC: The management of stage III carcinoma of the endometrium. Cancer 38:1838, 1976.

Azizi F, Bitran J, Javehari G, et al: Remission of uterine leiomyosarcomas treated with vincristine, adriamycin and dimethyl-triazeno-imidazole-carboxamide. Am J Obstet Gynecol 133:379, 1979.

Barter JF, Smith EB, Szpak CA, et al: Leiomyosarcoma of the uterus: Clinicopathologic study of 21 cases. Gynecol Oncol 21:220, 1985.

Bibbo M, Kluskens L, Azizi F, et al: Accuracy of three sampling technics for the diagnosis of endometrial cancer and hyperplasias. J Reprod Med 27:622, 1982.

Bickenbach W, Lochmuller H, Dirlich G, et al: Factor analysis of endometrial carcinoma in relation to treatment. Obstet Gynecol 29:632, 1967.

Blum RH, Corson JM, Wilson RE, et al: Successful treatment of metastatic sarcomas with cyclosphosphamide, Adriamycin, and DTIC (CAD). Cancer 46:1722, 1980.

Boronow RC, Morrow CP, Creasman WT, et al: Surgical staging in endometrial cancer: Clinical-pathologic findings of a prospective study. Obstet Gynecol 63:825, 1984.

Bruckman JE, Bloomer WD, Marck A, et al: Stage III adenocarcinoma of the endometrium: Two prognostic groups. Gynecol Oncol 9:12, 1980.

Carlson JA, Allegra JC, Day TG, et al: Tamoxifen and endometrial carcinoma: Alterations in estrogen and progesterone receptors in untreated patients and combination hormonal therapy in advanced neoplasia. Am J Obstet Gynecol 149:149, 1984.

Chen SS, Lee L: Retroperitoneal lymph node metastases in stage I carcinoma of the endometrium: Correlation with risk factors. Gynecol Oncol 16:319, 1983.

Christopherson WM, Alberhasky RC, Connelly PJ: Carcinoma of the endometrium. I. A clinicopathologic study of clear cell adenocarcinoma and secretory carcinoma. Cancer 49:1511, 1982.

Christopherson WM, Connelly PJ, Alberhasky RC: Carcinoma of the endometrium. V. An analysis of prognosticators in patients with favorable subtypes and stage I disease. Cancer 51:1705, 1983.

Christopherson WM, Gray LA: Premalignant lesions of the endometrium: Endometrial hyperplasia and adenocarcinoma in situ. In Coppleson M, ed: Gynecologic oncology. Edinburgh, Churchill Livingstone, 1981.

Clement PB, Scully RE: Müllerian adenosarcoma of the uterus. Cancer 34:1138, 1974.

Clement PB, Scully RE: Pathology of uterine sarcomas. In Coppleson M, ed: Gynecologic oncology. Edinburgh, Churchill Livingstone, 1981.

Cohen CJ, Bruckner HW, Deppe G, et al: Multidrug treatment of advanced and recurrent endometrial carcinoma: A Gynecologic Oncology Group study. Obstet Gynecol 63:719, 1984.

Connelly PJ, Alberhasky RC, Christopherson WM: Carcinoma of the endometrium. III. Analysis of 865 cases of adenocarcinoma and adenoacanthoma. Obstet Gynecol 59:569, 1982.

Cramer DW, Cutler SJ, Christine B: Trends in the incidence of endometrial cancer in the United States. Gynecol Oncol 2:130, 1974.

Creasman WT, McCarty KS, Barton TK, et al: Clinical correlates of estrogen- and progesterone-binding proteins in human endometrial adenocarcinoma. Obstet Gynecol 55:363, 1980.

Creasman WT, Soper JT, McCarty KS, et al: Influence of cytoplasmic steroid receptor content on prognosis of early stage endometrial carcinoma. Am J Obstet Gynecol 151:922, 1985.

Ehrlich CE, Young PCM, Cleary RE: Cytoplasmic progesterone and estradiol receptors in normal, hyperplastic and carcinomatous endometria: Therapeutic implications. Am J Obstet Gynecol 141:539, 1981.

Eifel PJ, Ross J, Hendrickson M, et al: Adenocarcinoma of the endometrium: Analysis of 256 cases with disease limited to the uterine corpus: Treatment comparison. Cancer 52:1026, 1983.

Elwood JM, Cole P, Rothman KJ, et al: Epidemiology of endometrial cancer. J Natl Cancer Inst 59:1055, 1977.

Gal D, Edman CD, Vellios F, et al: Long-term effect of megestrol acetate in the treatment of endometrial hyperplasia. Am J Obstet Gynecol 146:316, 1983.

Gompel C, Silverberg SG: Pathology in gynecology and obstetrics, 2nd ed. Philadelphia, J.B. Lippincott Co., 1977.

Greer BE, Hamburger AD: Treatment of intraperitoneal metastatic adenocarcinoma of the endometrium by the whole-abdomen moving-strip technique and pelvic boost irradiation. Gynecol Oncol 16:365, 1983.

Gusberg SB, Kaplan AL: Precursors of corpus cancer. IV. Adenomatous hyperplasia as stage 0 carcinoma of the endometrium. Am J Obstet Gynecol 87:662, 1963.

Hannigan EV, Freedman RS, Elder KW, et al: Treatment of advanced uterine sarcoma with vincristine, actinomycin D, and cyclophosphamide. Gynecol Oncol 15:224, 1983.

Hannigan EV, Freedman RS, Rutledge FN: Adjuvant chemotherapy in early uterine sarcoma. Gynecol Oncol 15:56, 1983.

Hendrickson M, Ross J, Eifel P, et al: Uterine papillary serous carcinoma: A highly malignant form of endometrial adenocarcinoma. Am J Surg Pathol 6:93, 1982.

Homesley HD, Boronow RC, Lewis JL: Stage II endometrial adenocarcinoma. Obstet Gynecol 49:604, 1977.

Kauppila A, Jänne O, Kujansuu E, Vihko R: Treatment of advanced endometrial adenocarcinoma with a combined cytotoxic therapy: Predictive value of cytosol estrogen and progestin receptor levels. Cancer 46:2162, 1980.

Kempson RL, Bari W: Uterine sarcomas. Hum Pathol 1:331, 1970.

Kohorn EI: Gestagens and endometrial carcinoma. Gynecol Oncol 4:398, 1976.

Koss LG, Schreiber K, Oberlander SG, et al: Screening of asymptomatic women for endometrial cancer. Obstet Gynecol 57:681, 1981.

Koss LG, Schreiber K, Oberlander SG, et al: Detection of endometrial carcinoma and hyperplasia in asymptomatic women. Obstet Gynecol 64:1, 1984.

Kurman RJ, Kaminski PF, Norris HJ: Behavior of endometrial hyperplasia: A long-term study of "untreated" hyperplasias in 170 patients. Cancer 56:403-412, 1985.

Kurman RJ, Norris HJ: Endometrial neoplasia: Hyperplasia and carcinoma. In Blaustein A, ed: Pathology of the female genital tract, 2nd ed. New York, Springer-Verlag, 1982.

Kurman RJ, Scully RE: Clear cell carcinoma of the endometrium. Cancer 37:872, 1976.

Landgren RC, Fletcher GH, Delclos L, et al: Irradiation of endometrial cancer in patients with medical contraindication to surgery or with unresectable lesions. Am J Roentgenol 126:148, 1976.

Landgren RD, Fletcher GH, Gallagher HS, et al: Treatment failure sites according to irradiation technique and histology in patients with endometrial cancer. Cancer 40:131, 1977.

MacMahon B: Risk factors for endometrial cancer. Gynecol Oncol 2:122, 1974.

Malkasian GD, Annegers JF, Fountain KS: Carcinoma of the endometrium: Stage I. Am J Obstet Gynecol 136:872, 1980.

Marchese MJ, Liskow AS, Crum CP, et al: Uterine sarcomas: A clinicopathologic study, 1965-1981. Gynecol Oncol 18:299, 1984.

Melin JR, Wanner L, Schulz DM, et al: Primary squamous cell carcinoma of the endometrium. Obstet Gynecol 53:115, 1979.

Muggia FM, Chia G, Reed LJ, et al: Doxorubicin, cyclophosphamide: Effective chemotherapy for advanced endometrial adenocarcinoma. Am J Obstet Gynecol 128:314, 1977.

Norris HJ, Parmley T: Mesenchymal tumors of the uterus. V. Intravenous leiomyomatosis: A clinical and pathologic study of 14 cases. Cancer 36:2164, 1975.

Norris HJ, Taylor HB: Postirradiation sarcomas of the uterus. Obstet Gynecol 26:689, 1965.

Norris HJ, Taylor HB: Mesenchymal tumors of the uterus. I. A clinical and pathological study of 53 endometrial stromal tumors. Cancer 19:755, 1966.

Norris HJ, Zaloudek CJ: Mesenchymal tumors of the uterus. In Blaustein A, ed: Pathology of the female genital tract, 2nd ed. New York, Springer-Verlag, 1982.

Omura GA, Major FJ, Blessing JA, et al: A randomized study of Adriamycin with and without dimethyl-triazeno-imidazole-carboxamide in advanced uterine sarcomas. Cancer 52:626, 1983.

Onsrud, M, Aalders J, Abeler V, et al: Endometrial carcinoma with cervical involvement (stage II): Prognostic factors and value of combined radiological-surgical treatment. Gynecol Oncol 13:76, 1982.

Onsrud M, Kolstad P, Normann T: Postoperative external pelvic irradiation in carcinoma of the corpus, stage I: A controlled clinical trial. Gynecol Oncol 4:222, 1976.

Patanaphan V, Salazar OM, Chougule P: What can be expected when radiation therapy becomes the curative alternative for endometrial cancer? Cancer 55:1462, 1985.

Perez CA, Askin F, Baglan RJ, et al: Effects of irradiation on mixed müllerian tumors of the uterus. Cancer 43:1274, 1979.

Petterson I, Kolstad P, Ludwig H, et al: Annual report on the results of treatment in gynecologic cancer, vol. 19. Stockholm, International Federation of Gynecology and Obstetrics, 1985.

Piver MS, Lurain JR: Uterine sarcomas: Clinical features and management. In Coppleson M, ed: Gynecologic oncology. Edinburgh, Churchill Livingstone, 1981, p. 608.

Piver MS, Rutledge FN, Copeland L, et al: Uterine endolymphatic stromal myosis: A collaborative study. Obstet Gynecol 64:173, 1984.

Piver MS, Yazigi R, Blumenson L, et al: A prospective trial comparing hysterectomy, hysterectomy plus vaginal radium, and uterine radium plus hysterectomy in stage I endometrial carcinoma. Obstet Gynecol 54:85, 1979.

Plentl AA, Friedman EA: Lymphatic system of the female genitalia. Philadelphia, W.B. Saunders Co., 1971.

Potish RA, Twiggs LB, Adcock LL, et al: Paraaortic lymph node radiotherapy in cancer of the uterine corpus. Obstet Gynecol 65:251, 1985.

Press MF, Scully RE: Endometrial "sarcomas" complicating ovarian thecoma, polycystic ovarian disease and estrogen therapy. Gynecol Oncol 21:135, 1985.

Procope BJ: Aetiology of postmenopausal bleeding. Obstet Gynaecol Scand 50:311, 1971.

Reagan JW: The changing nature of endometrial cancer. Gynecol Oncol 2:144, 1974.

Reagan JW, Fu YS: Pathology of endometrial carcinoma. In Coppleson M, ed: Gynecologic oncology. Edinburgh, Churchill Livingstone, 1981.

Salazar OM, Bonfiglio TA, Patten SF, et al: Uterine sarcomas: Natural history, treatment and prognosis. Cancer 42:1152, 1978.

Salazar OM, Bonfiglio TA, Patten SF, et al: Uterine sarcomas: Analysis of failures with special emphasis on the use of adjuvant radiation therapy. Cancer 42:1161, 1978.

Seski JC, Edwards CL, Herson J, et al: Cisplatin chemotherapy for disseminated endometrial cancer. Obstet Gynecol 59:225, 1982.

Spanos WJ, Wharton JT, Gomez L, et al: Malignant mixed müllerian tumors of the uterus. Cancer 53:311, 1984.

Surwit EA, Fowler WC, Rogoff EE: Stage II carcinoma of the endometrium. Obstet Gynecol 52:97, 1978.

Surwit EA, Joelsson I, Einhorn N: Adjunctive radiation therapy in the management of stage I cancer of the endometrium. Obstet Gynecol 58:590, 1981.

Swenerton KD, Chrumka K, Patterson AHG, et al: Efficacy of tamoxifen in endometrial cancer. Progr Cancer Res Ther 31:417, 1984.

Thatcher SS, Woodruff JD: Uterine stromatosis: A report of 33 cases. Obstet Gynecol 59:428, 1982.

Tiltman AJ: Mucinous carcinoma of the endometrium. Obstet Gynecol 55:244, 1980.

Tsukamoto N, Kamura T, Matsukuma K, et al: Endolymphatic stromal myosis: A case with positive estrogen and progesterone receptors and good response to progestins. Gynecol Oncol 20:120, 1985.

Turbow MM, Ballon SC, Sikic BI, et al: Cisplatin, doxorubicin and cyclophosphamide chemotherapy for advanced endometrial carcinoma. Cancer Treat Rep 69:465, 1985.

Vellios F: Endometrial hyperplasia, precursors of endometrial cancer. In Sommers SC, ed: Pathology annual. East Norwalk, Conn., Appleton-Century-Crofts, 1972, p. 201.

Vihko R, Isotalo H, Kauppila A, et al: Endocrine indicators of endometrial and ovarian tumor aggressiveness. In Bresciani F, et al, ed: Progr Cancer Res Ther 31:377, 1984.

Vongtama V, Karlen JR, Piver MS, et al: Treatment results and prognostic factors in stage I and II sarcomas of the corpus uteri. Am J Roentgenol Rad Ther Nucl Med 126:139, 1976.

Wallin TE, Malkasian GD, Gaffey TA, et al: Stage II cancer of the endometrium: A pathologic and clinical study. Gynecol Oncol 18:1, 1984.

Welch WR, Scully RE: Precancerous lesions of the endometrium. Hum Pathol 8:503, 1977.

Wentz WB: Progestin therapy in endometrial hyperplasia. Gynecol Oncol 2:362, 1974.

Wheeless CR: Atlas of pelvic surgery. Philadelphia, Lea & Febiger, 1981.

Wheelock JB, Krebs HB, Schneider V, et al: Uterine sarcoma: An analysis of prognostic variables in 71 cases. Am J Obstet Gynecol 151:1016, 1985.

White AJ, Buchsbaum HJ, Macasaet MA: Primary squamous cell carcinoma of the endometrium. Obstet Gynecol 41:912, 1973.

Yoonessi M, Hart WR: Endometrial stromal sarcomas. Cancer 40:898, 1977.

Neoplastic Diseases of the Ovary

KEY TERMS AND DEFINITIONS

Adenoma. A benign ovarian epithelial tumor consisting of glandular (adenomatous) elements.

Adenofibroma. An epithelial tumor that consists of glandular and large amounts of ovarian stromal (fibroblast) elements.

Alpha-fetoprotein. A secretory product from endodermal sinus tumors that can be measured in serum and serves as a specific tumor marker.

Borderline Tumors. A term used to describe an epithelial carcinoma of low malignant potential (grade 0).

Brenner Tumor. An epithelial neoplasm that consists of cells resembling urothelium and so-called Walthard nests of the ovary. These are mixed with ovarian stroma.

Carcinoid. A rare type of teratoma that histologically resembles the carcinoid tumors that arise in the gastrointestinal tract.

Clear Cell Tumor (Mesonephroma). An ovarian neoplasm that consists of clear cells (containing glycogen) or "hobnail" cells. Histologically they resemble clear cell tumors that arise in the endocervix, endometrium, and vagina.

Cyst. A descriptive term added as a prefix to the designation of epithelial tumors to indicate the presence of cystlike spaces, for example, cystadenoma.

Cytoreductive Surgery. The practice of reducing the bulk of carcinomatous tissue and removing, if possible, all gross disease.

Dermoid. A benign cystic germ cell tumor (cystic teratoma) that may contain elements of all three germ cell layers. It is the most common ovarian neoplasm in those under 30 years of age.

Dysgerminoma. The most common of ovarian malignant germ cell tumors. It consists of primitive germ cells.

Endodermal Sinus Tumor. A malignant germ cell tumor. It is derived from germ cells and recapitulates extraembryonic tissue and may resemble the yolk sac of the rodent placenta.

Endometrioid Tumor. An ovarian epithelial tumor whose cells resemble those of the uterine endometrium.

Epithelial Tumor. The most common type of ovarian neoplasms. It is derived from the surface (coelomic) epithelium and ovarian stroma.

Fibroma. The most common benign ovarian solid tumor composed of stromal cells (fibroblasts). In some cases it is associated with benign ascites and hydrothorax (Meigs' syndrome).

Germ Cell Tumor. The second most common type of ovarian neoplasm after epithelial tumors. Germ cell tumors contain cells that recapitulate embryonic tissues (ectoderm, mesoderm, or endoderm) or extraembryonic elements.

Gonadoblastoma. A rare tumor that arises in abnormal (dysgenetic) gonads and consists of sex-cord stromal elements and germ cells.

Granulosa-Thecal Cell Tumor. A sex-cord stromal tumor that often secretes estrogens and consists of granulosa cells (sex cord) and ovarian stromal cells (thecal cells or fibroblasts).

Immature Teratoma. A teratoma with malignant (immature) embryonic elements (ectoderm, mesoderm, or endoderm).

Krukenberg Tumor. A tumor consisting of signet-ring cells that have developed from metastases to the ovary and that usually originate from the gastrointestinal tract, most frequently the stomach, and then from the large intestine.

Mucinous Tumor. An ovarian epithelial tumor whose cells contain mucin and resemble those of the endocervix.

Ovarian Neoplasm. An ovarian tumor that is not physiologic and will not regress with time. It may be benign or malignant.

Papillary. A descriptive term added to the designation of epithelial tumors if papillary-like projections are present, for example, papillary cystadenocarcinoma.

Pseudomyxoma Peritonei. Intraperitoneal spread of mucin-secreting cells that originate from ovarian mucinous cystadenoma or cystadenocarcinoma or mucoceles of the appendix that lead to recurrent abdominal masses and bowel obstruction.

Second-Look Operation. A laparotomy with extensive biopsy sampling and cytologic sampling of the peritoneal cavity, as well as evaluation of the retroperitoneal nodes. It is usually performed after chemotherapy in a patient who is clinically in remission.

Serous Tumor. An ovarian epithelial tumor whose cells resemble those of the fallopian tube.

Sertoli-Leydig Cell Tumor. A rare sex-cord stromal tumor with male elements. It often causes virilization.

Sex-Cord Stromal Tumors. A class of ovarian tumors in which the constituents of the ovary or testes are recapitulated.

Stages of Ovarian Cancer
   Stage I. Confined to one or both ovaries.
   Stage II. Extension to pelvic structures.
   Stage III. Extension outside of pelvis or to retroperitoneal nodes.
   Stage IV. Outside of peritoneal cavity or to liver parenchyma—pleural effusion with malignant cells.

Stroma Ovarii. A specialized ovarian teratoma that consists of thyroid tissue as a major or exclusive component. It may rarely produce sufficient thyroid hormone to induce hyperthyroidism.

Teratoma. An ovarian germ cell tumor that recapitulates any one or all of tissues of the ectoderm, mesoderm, or endoderm. The tissues can be benign (mature) or malignant (immature).

Thecoma. A benign ovarian stromal tumor consisting of thecal cells.

Ovarian cancer is the second most common malignancy of the lower part of the female genital tract, occurring less frequently than cancers of the endometrium but more frequently than cancers of the cervix. However, it is the most frequent cause of death from gynecologic neoplasms. The data of the National Cancer Institute SEER Program suggest that approximately 18,500 new cases of ovarian cancer will be diagnosed yearly in the United States, and there will be 11,500 deaths. A major contributing factor to the high death rate from relatively few cases is the late detection of the disease because of the intraabdominal location of the ovary and the fact that these cancers often do not cause symptoms until the malignancy is widespread. The death rate from ovarian cancer (Fig. 29-1) rises with age, becoming most marked beyond 50 years, with a gradual increase continuing to age 70 years.

Despite numerous epidemiologic investigations, a clear-cut cause of ovarian cancer has not been defined. A number of theories have been advanced. It is thought that these malig-

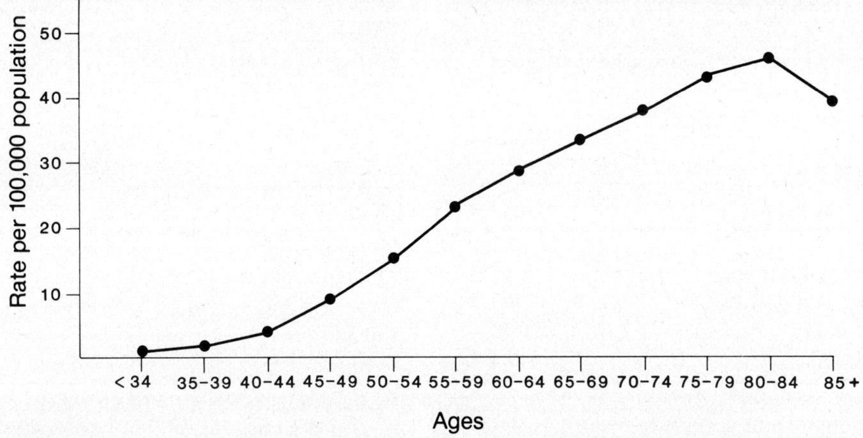

FIGURE 29-1
Death rate from cancer of the ovary by age, per 100,000 population in the United States, 1981.

nancies are related to frequent ovulation, and therefore women who ovulate regularly appear to be at higher risk. Included are those with a late menopause, a history of nulliparity, or late childbearing. Conversely, women who have had several pregnancies or who have used oral contraceptives appear to have some protection against ovarian cancer. Casagrande et al. related the development of ovarian cancer to "ovulatory age," that is, the number of years during which the patient has ovulated. This number would be reduced by pregnancy, breast feeding, or oral contraceptive use. In addition, talcum powder used on the perineum has been postulated to increase the risk, presumably by migration of the irritant powder through the vagina, cervix, and fallopian tubes to the peritoneal surface of the ovary. Subclinical mumps infection before menarche has been suggested as potentially increasing the risk of ovarian cancer. Cramer et al. recently found women with ovarian cancer to have a diet high in animal fat in comparison with control subjects.

There are geographic and racial differences in the distribution of ovarian cancers. These cancers occur most frequently in industrialized and affluent countries such as the United States and Western Europe and less frequently in Asia and Africa. The disease is more frequent among white than black women. Finally, patients with ovarian carcinoma have an increased risk of developing breast and endome-

trial cancer. The major factors, however, appear to be related to the frequency of ovulation and residence in an industrialized country.

There appears to be a familial association, and a familial occurrence of ovarian cancer has been reported. A few families have been identified that appear to have a genetically increased risk of ovarian cancer. Unfortunately, carcinomatosis throughout the abdomen has developed in some of these individuals despite prophylactic removal of the ovaries.

The following sections consider the classification and histologic types of the major ovarian neoplasms. Pertinent histologic findings, clinical behavior, and appropriate therapy are presented.

CLASSIFICATION OF OVARIAN NEOPLASMS

The most widely used classification of ovarian neoplasms is that of the World Health Organization. This classification, along with frequency of occurrence of the primary ovarian neoplasms, is shown in Table 29-1.

The common epithelial tumors are the most frequent ovarian neoplasms. They are believed to arise from the surface (coelomic) epithelium. Sex cord stromal tumors are the third most frequent and contain elements that recapitulate the constituents of the ovary or testis. These tumors may secrete sex steroid hormones or may be hormonally inactive. Lipid (lipoid) cell

TABLE 29-1

World Health Organization Classification of Ovarian Neoplasms

Class	Approximate Frequency (%)
Common epithelial tumors	65
Sex cord stromal tumors	6
Lipid (lipoid) cell tumors	<0.1
Germ cell tumors	20-25
Gonadoblastoma	<0.1

Soft tissue tumors (not specific to ovary)
Unclassified tumors
Secondary (metastatic) tumors
Tumorlike conditions (not true neoplasm)

Modified from Scully RE: Tumors of the ovary and maldeveloped gonads. In Atlas of tumor pathology, Fascicle 16, 2nd series. Washington, D.C., Armed Forces Institute of Pathology.

TABLE 29-2

Epithelial Ovarian Tumor Cell Types

	Approximate Frequency (%)	
	All Ovarian Neoplasms	Ovarian Cancers
Serous	20-50	35-40
Mucinous	15-25	6-10
Endometrioid	5	15-25
Clear cell (mesonephroid)	<5	5
Brenner	2-3	Rare

Modified from Scully RE: Tumors of the ovary and maldeveloped gonads. In Atlas of tumor pathology, Fascicle 16, 2nd series. Washington, D.C., Armed Forces Institute of Pathology, 1979.

tumors are extremely rare and histologically resemble the adrenal gland. Germ cell tumors are the second most frequent of the ovarian neoplasms and are the most common among young women. There are a large variety of histologic types. They may be composed of extraembryonic elements or may have features that resemble any or all of the three embryonic layers (ectoderm, mesoderm, or endoderm). These tumors are the main cause of ovarian malignancy in young women, particularly those in their teens and early twenties. Gonadoblastomas consist of germ cells and sex-cord stromal elements. They occur in individuals with dysgenetic gonads, particularly when a Y chromosome is present. All these ovarian neoplasms will be discussed in this chapter.

Soft tissue tumors not specific to the ovary, such as hemangioma or lipoma, are rare and are categorized according to the criteria for soft tissue tumors arising elsewhere in the body. Unclassified tumors, as the name implies, cannot be placed in any of the preceding categories. Metastatic tumors to the ovary arise elsewhere in the reproductive tract, as well as in distant sites. Tumorlike conditions refer to enlargements of the ovary, such as extensive edema, pregnancy luteoma, endometriomas, and follicular or luteal cysts, none of which are true neoplasms. With the exception of metastatic tumors, none of these latter conditions are considered further in this chapter.

EPITHELIAL OVARIAN NEOPLASMS

According to Scully, two thirds of ovarian neoplasms are epithelial tumors; malignant epithelial tumors account for about 85% of ovarian cancers. As stated earlier, it is believed that these tumors arise from the surface (coelomic) epithelium and adjacent ovarian stroma. Table 29-2 summarizes the five cell types that most commonly comprise epithelial ovarian tumors, indicating their relative frequency.

Epithelial tumors can be categorized as benign (adenoma), malignant (adenocarcinoma), or of an intermediate form, known as borderline malignant adenocarcinoma or tumor of low malignant potential. The term *papillary* or the prefix *cyst* (as in *cystadenoma*) is used when the tumor has, respectively, papillae or cystic structures. The suffix *fibroma* (as in *adenofibroma*) is added when the ovarian stroma predominates, with the exception of a Brenner tumor, which normally contains a large amount of ovarian stroma.

Well-differentiated serous tumors (Fig. 29-2, *A* and *B*) consist of ciliated epithelial cells that resemble those of the fallopian tube. Serous tumors (Fig. 29-2, *C*) are the most frequent ovarian epithelial tumors. The malignant forms account for up to 40% of ovarian cancer; the benign forms (serous cystadenomas) occur primarily during the reproductive years; the borderline tumors occur in women 30 to 50 years of age; and the carcinomas occur in women over 40 years of age.

Mucinous tumors (Fig. 29-3, *A* and *B*) consist of epithelial cells filled with mucin; most are benign. These cells resemble cells of the endocervix or may mimic intestinal cells, which can pose a problem in the differential diagnosis of tumors that appear to originate from the

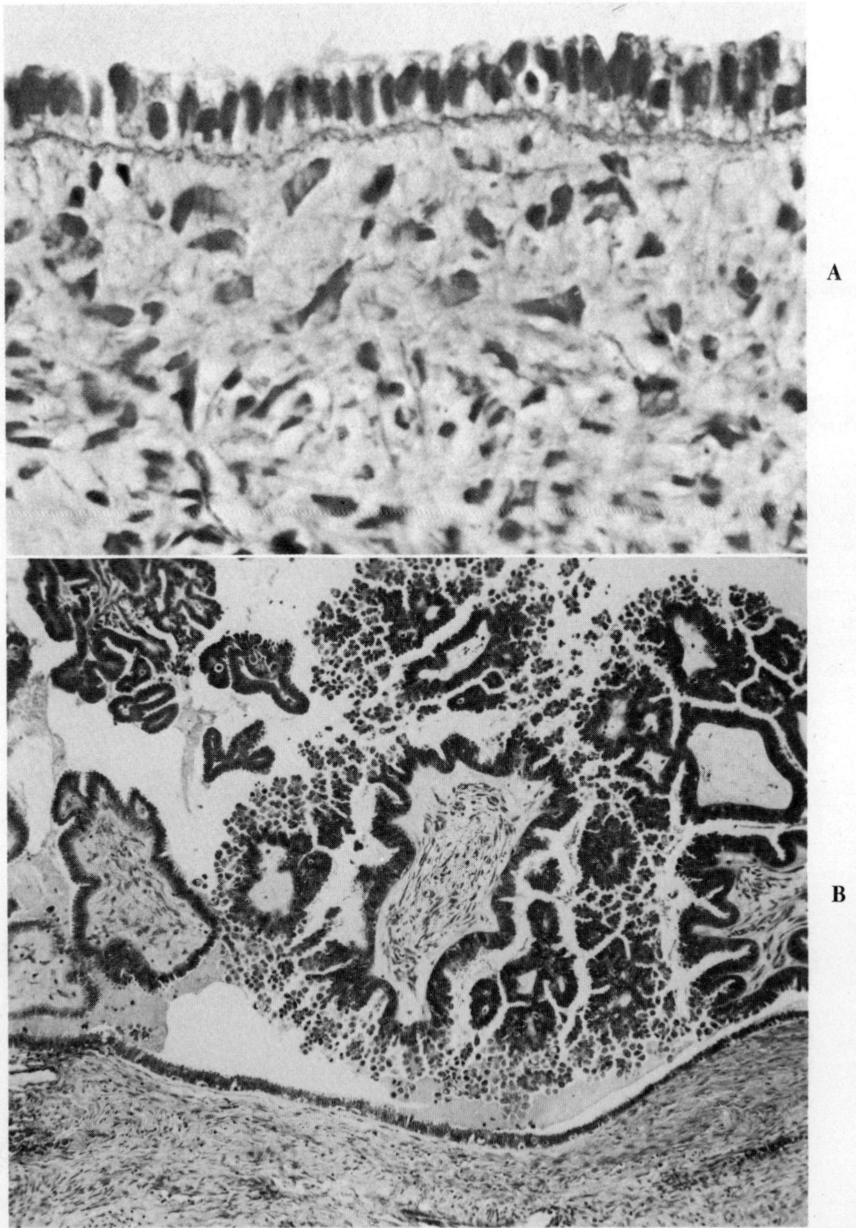

FIGURE 29-2

A, Ciliated epithelium of a well-differentiated serous tumor. (×800.) **B,** Serous papillary cystadenoma of borderline malignancy. The epithelium resembles that of the fallopian tube, and a well-developed papillary pattern is present. (×80.)

Continued.

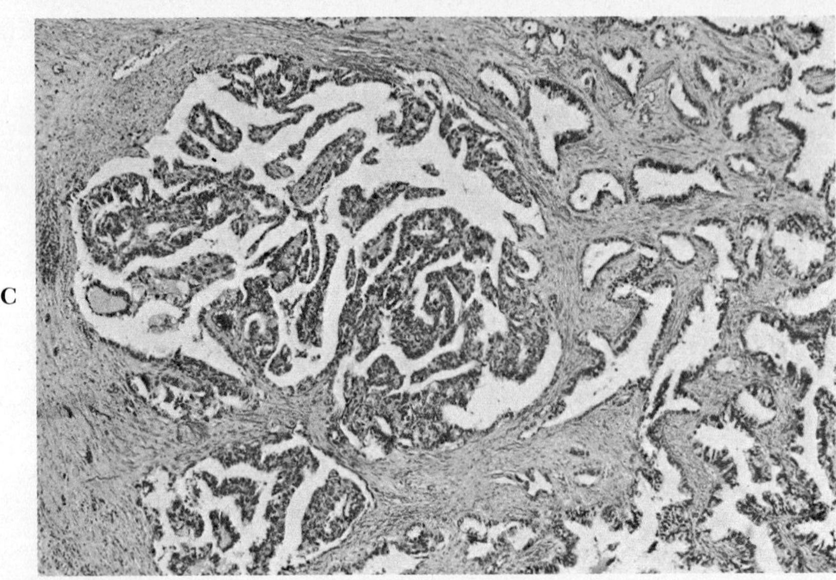

FIGURE 29-2, cont'd
C, Serous papillary adenocarcinoma. (×50.) The neoplastic epithelium invades the stroma. (**A** and **C** from Serov SF, Scully RE, Sobin LH: Histologic typing of ovarian tumors. Geneva, World Health Organization, 1973. **B** courtesy Robert E. Scully.)

ovary or intestine. Benign mucinous tumors are found primarily during the reproductive years, and mucinous carcinomas (Fig. 29-3, *C*) usually occur among those in the 30 to 60 year age range. Overall they can account for about one fourth of ovarian tumors and up to 10% of ovarian cancers.

Endometrioid tumors (Fig. 29-4), as the name implies, consist of epithelial cells resembling those of the endometrium. In the ovary

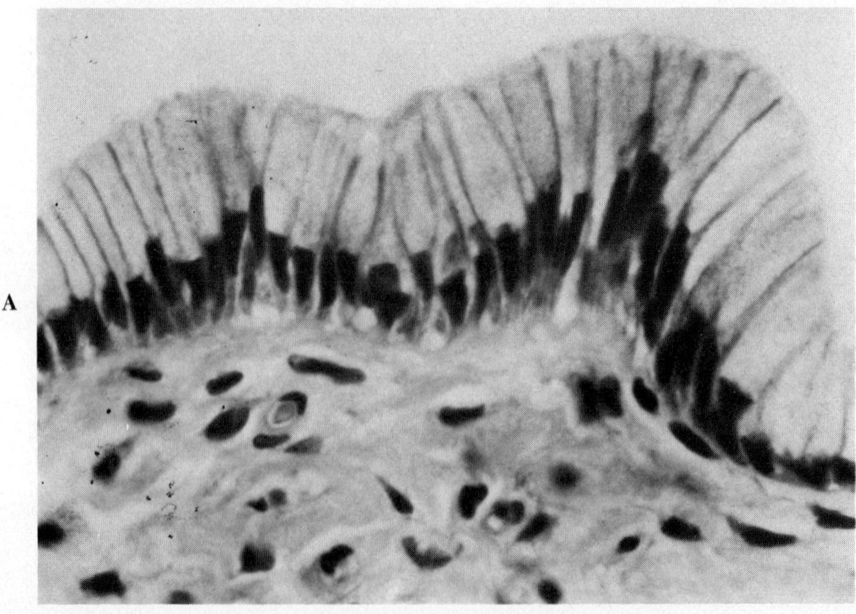

FIGURE 29-3
For legend see opposite page.

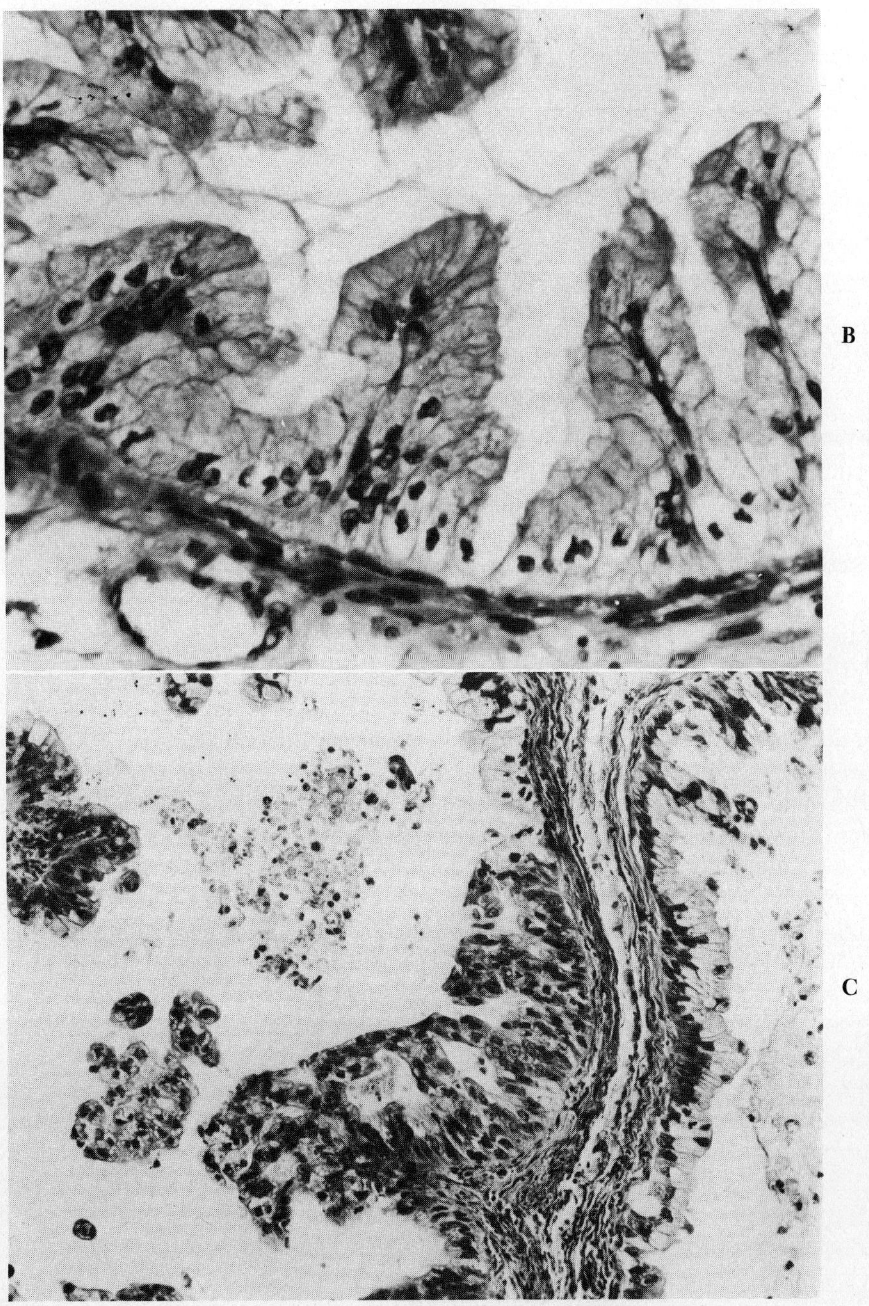

FIGURE 29-3

A, Mucinous cystadenoma. (×800.) **B,** Mucinous borderline tumor. Epithelium resembles that of the endocervix. **C,** Mucinous carcinoma. (×120.) Incomplete stratification of cells and atypicality is present. (**A** and **C** from Serov SF, Scully RE, Sobin LH: Histologic typing of ovarian tumors. Geneva, World Health Organization, 1973. **B** courtesy Robert E. Scully.)

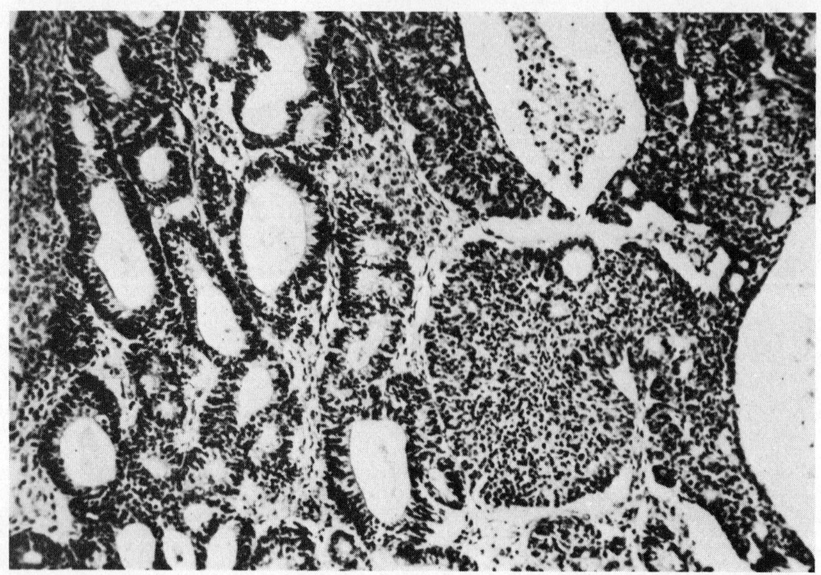

FIGURE 29-4
Endometrioid carcinoma. Tubular glands are lined by stratified endometrium.
(×80.) (From Meadowbrook Staff Journal 1:148-163, 1968. Courtesy Dr. R.E.
Scully.)

these neoplasms are less frequent (approximately 5%) than either the serous or mucinous tumors, but the malignant variety can account for about 20% of ovarian carcinomas. Endometrioid carcinomas usually occur in women in their forties and fifties. They may be seen in conjunction with endometriosis and ovarian endometriomas, although an origin from endometriosis is rarely demonstrated. Most endometrioid carcinomas arise directly from the surface epithelium of the ovary, as do the other epithelial tumors.

Clear cell (mesonephroid) tumors contain cells with abundant glycogen (Fig. 29-5, A) and so-called hobnail cells (Fig. 29-5, B), in which the nuclei of the cells protrude into the glandular lumen. Tumors with identical histologic features are found in the endometrium, cervix, and vagina, the latter two often associated with intrauterine diethylstilbestrol (DES) exposure. Clear cell ovarian tumors not related to DES exposure comprise about 5% of ovarian cancers and occur primarily in women 40 to 70 years of age.

It can be seen that the major cell types of ovarian epithelial tumors recapitulate the müllerian-derived epithelium of the female reproductive system (serous—fallopian tube; muci-nous—endocervix; endometrioid—endometrium). This differentiation occurs even though the ovary is not derived directly from the müllerian ducts (Chapter 2). The clear cell tumors also mimic this müllerian tendency, frequently being admixed with endometrioid carcinomas as well as with ovarian endometriomas.

Brenner tumors (Fig. 29-6) consist of cells that resemble the transitional epithelium of the bladder and Walthard nests of the ovary. There is abundant stroma. These tumors constitute only 2% to 3% of all ovarian tumors.

In addition to the cell types shown in Table 29-2, epithelial tumors may be classified as undifferentiated if the tumor consists of poorly differentiated epithelial cells not characteristic of any particular cell type. They may be considered unclassifiable if they cannot be placed in any of the categories shown in Table 29-2.

Many epithelial ovarian tumors can be bilateral, and the risk of bilaterality is an important consideration in therapy, particularly when an ovarian tumor is discovered in a young woman of reproductive age. Widely varying percentages have been reported for bilaterality in ovarian tumors, and the most widely quoted are summarized in Table 29-3. Malignant epithelial tumors tend to involve both ovaries more fre-

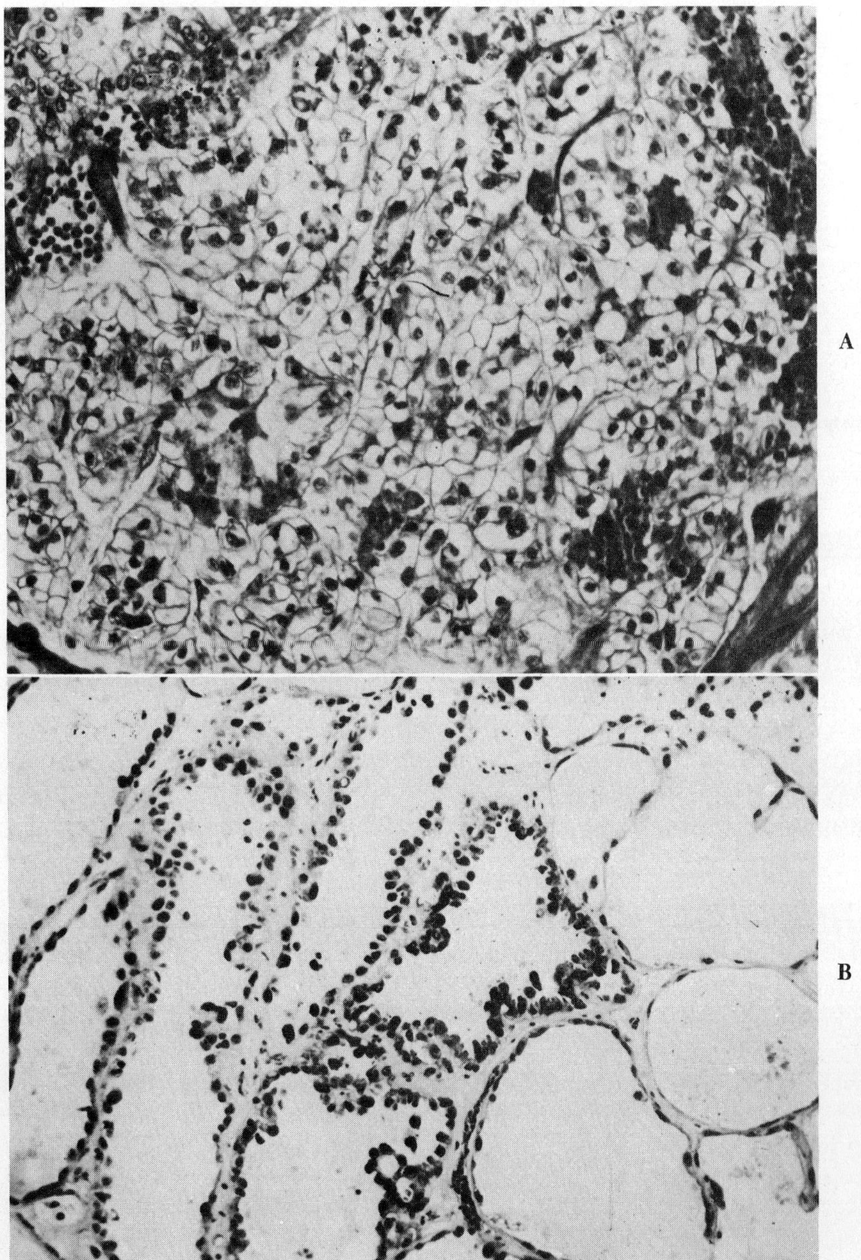

FIGURE 29-5

A, Clear cell adenocarcinoma. (×200.) Solid pattern of abundant polyhedral tumor cells containing abundant clear cytoplasm is present. **B,** Clear cell adenocarcinoma. (×200.) *Left:* Hobnail cells with scant cytoplasm; protruding nuclei line shows tubules. *Right:* Cysts lined by flattened tumor cells. (**A** from Barlow JF, Scully RE: Cancer 20:1405, 1967. **B** from Meadowbrook Staff Journal 1:148-163, 1968. Courtesy Dr. R.E. Scully.)

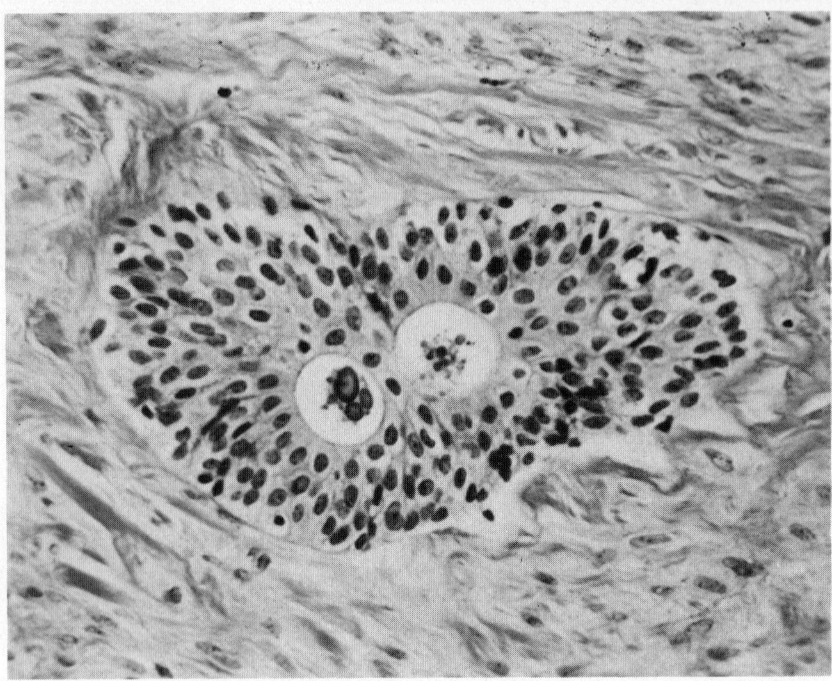

FIGURE 29-6
Brenner tumor. (×350.) Note nest of transition-like epithelium containing spaces
with eosinophilic material. (From Atlas of tumor pathology, Fascicle 16, 2nd series.
Washington, D.C., Armed Forces Institute of Pathology, 1979.)

quently than do benign epithelial tumors. Serous tumors also tend to be bilateral more frequently than do mucinous tumors.

Benign Epithelial Ovarian Tumors

As noted in Chapter 6, enlargement of the ovary beyond 5 cm is considered abnormal. However, age and menstrual status must also be considered before the appropriate course of action is chosen. A 5- to 8-cm ovarian mass in a woman with regular menses, even if she is in her early forties, is frequently a functioning ovarian cyst, such as a follicular or corpus luteum cyst. It will usually regress spontaneously during a subsequent menstrual cycle. Enlargements of this type do not automatically require immediate operative intervention and should be observed for two menstrual cycles. An exception would be a mass in a patient who is taking oral contraceptives, in which case exploration is indicated. Unilocular 5- to 8-cm cysts are likely to be functional (Chapter 16), whereas multilocular or partially solid tumors

are more likely to be neoplastic. An ultrasound examination helps to differentiate these lesions.

Beyond the age of 40 years the risk of malignancy rises sharply, and an operation is usually advised for all ovarian enlargements.

Since the ovary shrinks during menopause and usually recedes to less than 1.5 cm in greatest diameter, it is not normally palpable. A postmenopausal patient with a palpable ovary is at risk for an ovarian neoplasm because enlargement may signal malignancy. Thus a palpable ovary in a postmenopausal patient requires visualization by laparoscopy or laparotomy.

Most nonmalignant epithelial ovarian tumors are observed initially as asymptomatic unilateral adnexal masses that can be treated by oophorectomy or occasionally cystectomy (see section on benign cystic teratomas, later in this chapter). Some have recommended bisecting the opposite ovary to rule out bilaterality in the case of benign epithelial ovarian tumors (Table 29-3), but in view of the risk of adhesions and infertility in these young patients, wedge re-

TABLE 29-3
Bilaterality of Ovarian Tumors

Type of Tumor	Percent of Occurrence
Epithelial tumors	
Serous cystadenoma	10
Serous cystadenocarcinoma	33-66
Mucinous cystadenoma	5
Mucinous cystadenocarcinoma	10-20
Endometrioid carcinoma	13-30
Benign Brenner tumor	6
Germ cell tumors	
Benign cystic teratoma (dermoid)	12
Immature teratoma (malignant)	2-5
Dysgerminoma	5-10
Other malignant germ cell tumors	Rare
Sex-cord stromal tumors	
Thecoma	Rare
Sertoli-Leydig cell tumor	Rare
Granulosa-theca cell tumor	Rare

section of the contralateral ovary in the case of any benign epithelial ovarian neoplasm is not recommended if the contralateral ovary appears normal. In a woman beyond her reproductive years, especially when a serous cystadenoma, which tends to be bilateral, is present, abdominal hysterectomy and bilateral salpingo-oophorectomy are usually performed.

Mucinous tumors can become particularly large and reach sizes up to 30 cm. Possible complications of mucinous cystadenoma are perforation and rupture, which can lead to the deposit and growth of mucin-secreting epithelium in the peritoneal cavity (pseudomyxoma peritonei, discussed later under borderline mucinous tumors).

Adenofibromas consist of fibrous and epithelial elements. The epithelial component may be serous, mucinous, clear cell, or endometrioid—the architectural subtypes of these benign ovarian tumors. Their appearance will depend on the predominant histologic features—epithelial or fibrous. These tumors are also managed by simple excision. Endometriomas are considered in Chapter 18.

Brenner tumors (see Fig. 29-6) are rare and often incidental findings when oophorectomy is performed for an indication other than ovarian enlargement. Most often, these tumors occur in women in their forties and fifties, but both younger and older patients have been found to have them. Brenner tumors are almost always benign and can usually be managed by oophorectomy. When the ovary is palpably enlarged, approximately 5% of Brenner tumors will prove to be malignant. These tumors often occur in perimenopausal and postmenopausal women, in which case hysterectomy and bilateral salpingo-oophorectomy are indicated. Unfortunately, malignant Brenner tumors appear to have a poor prognosis despite this operative therapy, and an effective program of chemotherapy has not been developed.

The differential diagnosis for and approach to an adnexal mass in female patients of various ages are discussed in Chapter 6. Ovarian enlargement in the premenarchal female is usually the result of a germ cell tumor, which may be malignant but is usually benign (see later discussion of germ cell tumors). During the reproductive years ovarian neoplasms are usually benign. For the patient in her twenties or thirties most ovarian enlargements can be approached operatively through a lower abdominal transverse (Pfannenstiel) incision, unless there is a possibility of malignancy, such as a solid tumor or one with papillae viewed on ultrasound examination. In these cases, as well as in women over age 40 or those with a large mass extending out of the pelvis and into the abdomen, a low midline vertical incision is indicated. The tumor must be removed intact, and if malignancy is present, as is more likely in older patients, a thorough surgical evaluation is indicated (outlined in the section on epithelial carcinoma).

A frozen section should be obtained if gross examination of the ovarian tumor is at all suspicious for malignancy. For women of reproductive age, if the diagnosis of malignancy is suspected but uncertain even after a frozen section is obtained, the operation should be terminated after removal of the ovarian tumor. A second procedure can be performed if malignancy is confirmed after detailed histologic study of the permanent sections. This is preferable to risking an unnecessary hysterectomy or bilateral salpingo-oophorectomy in a patient who desires to preserve childbearing function.

TABLE 29-4a
Staging of Ovarian Carcinomas (FIGO)*

Stage	Characteristics
I	Growth limited to the ovaries
IA	Growth limited to one ovary; no ascites
	1. No tumor on external surface; capsule intact
	2. Tumor present on external surface or capsule ruptured or both
IB	Growth limited to both ovaries; no ascites
	1. No tumor on external surface; capsule intact
	2. Tumor present on external surface or capsule(s) ruptured or both
IC	Tumor either stage IA or IB, but with ascites† present or positive peritoneal washings
II	Growth involving one or both ovaries with pelvic extension
IIA	Extension or metastases to the uterus or tubes or both
IIB	Extension to other pelvic tissues
IIC	Tumor either stage IIA or IIB, but with ascites† present or positive peritoneal washings
III	Growth involving one or both ovaries with intraperitoneal metastases outside pelvis or positive retroperitoneal nodes or both
	Tumor limited to true pelvis with histologically proved malignant extension to small bowel or omentum
IV	Growth involving one or both ovaries with distant metastases (If pleural effusion is present, there must be positive cytologic findings to allot a case to stage IV. Parenchymal liver metastases equals stage IV.)
Special category	Unexplored cases that are thought to be ovarian carcinoma

*Based on findings at clinical examination and operative exploration. The final histologic picture after surgery is to be considered in the staging, as well as cytologic findings, as far as effusions are concerned.
†Ascites is peritoneal effusion that in the opinion of the surgeon is pathologic or clearly exceeds normal amounts.

Table 29-4b
Staging of Ovarian Carcinomas (FIGO)
Modified 1985

Stage	Characteristics
I	Growth limited to the ovaries.
IA	Growth limited to one ovary; no ascites. No tumor on the external surface; capsule intact.
IB	Growth limited to both ovaries; no ascites. No tumor on the external surfaces; capsules intact.
IC	Tumor either stage IA or IB but with tumor on surface of one or both ovaries; or with capsule ruptured; or with ascites present containing malignant cells or with positive peritoneal washings.
II	Growth involving one or both ovaries with pelvic extension.
IIA	Extension and/or metastases to the uterus and/or tubes.
IIB	Extension to other pelvic tissues.
IIC	Tumor either stage IIA or IIB, but with tumor on surface of one or both ovaries; or with capsule(s) ruptured; or with ascites present containing malignant cells or with positive peritoneal washings.
III	Tumor involving one or both ovaries with peritoneal implants outside the pelvis and/or positive retroperitoneal or inguinal nodes. Superficial liver metastasis equals stage III. Tumor is limited to the true pelvis but with histologically proven malignant extension to small bowel or omentum.
IIIA	Tumor grossly limited to the true pelvis with negative nodes but with histologically confirmed microscopic seeding of abdominal peritoneal surfaces.
IIIB	Tumor of one or both ovaries with histologically confirmed implants of abdominal peritoneal surfaces none exceeding 2 cm in diameter. Nodes are negative.
IIIC	Abdominal implants greater than 2 cm in diameter and/or positive retroperitoneal or inguinal nodes.
IV	Growth involving one or both ovaries with distant metastases. If pleural effusion is present, there must be positive cytology to allot a case to stage IV. Parenchymal liver metastasis equals stage IV.

Epithelial Carcinomas

Diagnosis, Staging, Spread, and Preoperative Evaluation

Ovarian carcinomas are usually diagnosed by detection of an adnexal mass on pelvic examination. Unfortunately the diagnosis is frequently made only after the disease has spread beyond the confines of the ovary. Scully states that the risk of malignancy in a primary ovarian tumor rises to about 33% in a woman over the age of 45 years, whereas it is less than 1 in 15 for women who are 20 to 45 years of age. In general, over half of ovarian carcinomas occur in women beyond the age of 50 years.

Patients with ovarian carcinoma frequently develop ascites, and a swollen abdomen may be their first symptom, either due to ascites or tumor spread. Vague lower abdominal discomfort is a frequent complaint, but severe pain is not a prominent symptom. Vaginal cytologic testing can detect ovarian carcinoma cells because of their transmigration through the tubes, uterus, and cervix into the vagina. However, an ovarian carcinoma is rarely initially detected from vaginal cytologic smears. The diagnosis is established by histologic examination of the tumor tissue removed at operation. Occasionally the initial diagnosis is suggested by examination of ascitic fluid obtained at paracentesis, which may reveal cells characteristic of ovarian epithelial malignancy.

The clinical staging of ovarian cancer (Tables 29-4a and 29-4b) is designed according to the criteria of the International Federation of Gynecology and Obstetrics (FIGO) and is based on the results of operative exploration, in contrast to the staging of cancers of the cervix, endometrium, and vulva, all of which are based on clinical evaluation and are not altered by operative findings. The system was modified in 1985, and the earlier classification, which has been widely quoted, is shown in Table 29-4a and the modified system in 29-4b.

Before operative exploration the patient with suspected ovarian carcinoma has the preoperative workup usual for a major abdominal operation (Chapter 23). Additional diagnostic studies include intravenous pyelography (IVP) and a barium enema. The latter is of particular importance for evaluation of the possibility of a primary colon carcinoma, which may be found initially as an adnexal mass in the older patient. A sigmoidoscopy is performed if there is evidence of gastrointestinal bleeding or the suggestion of rectosigmoid disease. An upper gastrointestinal tract series is also obtained if there are upper gastrointestinal symptoms or evidence of gastrointestinal bleeding. Preoperative screening tests can be performed, but there is no currently available specific screening test for ovarian carcinoma. Occasionally the level of the isoenzyme lactic acid dehydrogenase (LDH) is elevated, but this test is not specific. Bast et al. studied the ovarian antigen designated CA-125 in serum and found it to be elevated in approximately 80% of carcinoma cases. If the CA-125 level is elevated at the time of operation, the test is useful for following the progress of the patient with ovarian carcinoma after treatment and demonstrating the response to therapy or detecting tumor progression.

Preoperatively a program to cleanse the bowel is instituted in case intestinal resection is required. In one program the patient is given a liquid diet 48 hours preoperatively. Cathartic agents (one bottle of citrate of magnesia) is given morning and evening, with a cleansing enema given in the evening of the first day and 45 to 60 ml of castor oil given the afternoon of the second day. Neomycin, 1 g, is started 24 hours before surgery, although the important principle is mechanical cleansing of the bowel (see Chapter 23). Treatment with prophylactic low-dose heparin (mini-heparin) is advisable to reduce the risk of thromboembolism. The patient usually receives heparin, 5000 IU intramuscularly, 2 hours before surgery and every 12 hours thereafter.

In a consideration of therapy for ovarian epithelial carcinoma, knowledge of its natural path of spread is important. The tumors spread along the peritoneal surface to involve ovarian, parietal, and intestinal peritoneal surfaces, as well as the undersurface of the diaphragm, particularly on the right side (Fig. 29-7). This knowledge is particularly important because tumors that appear at operation to be confined to the ovary may have small areas of diaphragmatic involvement as the sole site of extraovarian spread. Such a tumor should be classified as a stage III ovarian carcinoma (see Table 29-4), rather than stage I. Lymphatic dissemina-

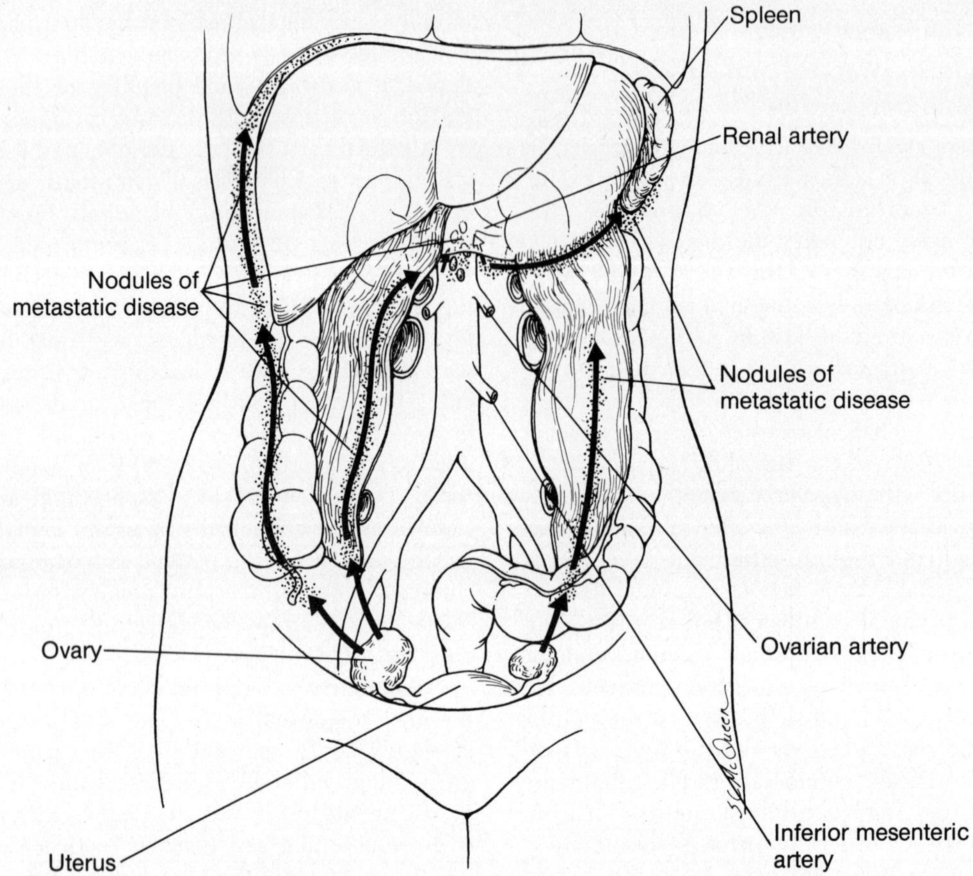

FIGURE 29-7

Peritoneal spread of ovarian cancer. Portions of omentum, small intestine, and transverse colon have been resected. (From Knapp RC, Berkowitz RS, Leavitt T Jr: Natural history and detection of ovarian cancer. Gynecology and obstetrics, vol. 4. Philadelphia, J.B. Lippincott Co., 1986.)

TABLE 29-5

Five-Year Survival in 5254 Cases of Ovarian Cancer (1973-1975)*

Stage	Proportion of Cases	5-Year Survival (%)
I	25.2	66.4
II	17.6	45.0
III	39.5	13.3
IV	17.8	4.1

Modified from Richardson GS, Scully RE, Nikrui N, et al: Common epithelial cancer of the ovary. N Engl J Med 312:415, 1985. Reprinted with permission of The New England Journal of Medicine.
*Overall 5-year survival is 30.6%.

tion is also a prominent part of disease spread (Fig. 29-8), and it is particularly important to note that the paraaortic nodes are at risk through lymphatics that run parallel to the ovarian vessels. Knapp and Friedman noted that of 26 patients with ovarian cancer apparently limited to the ovary, 19% had paraaortic involvement and all had poorly differentiated tumors. Piver et al. noted that approximately 10% of apparent stage I ovarian tumors had paraaortic node metastases; the risk was greatest for women with poorly differentiated tumors.

The prognosis for patients with ovarian carcinoma is related to tumor stage, tumor grade, cell type, and the amount of residual tumor af-

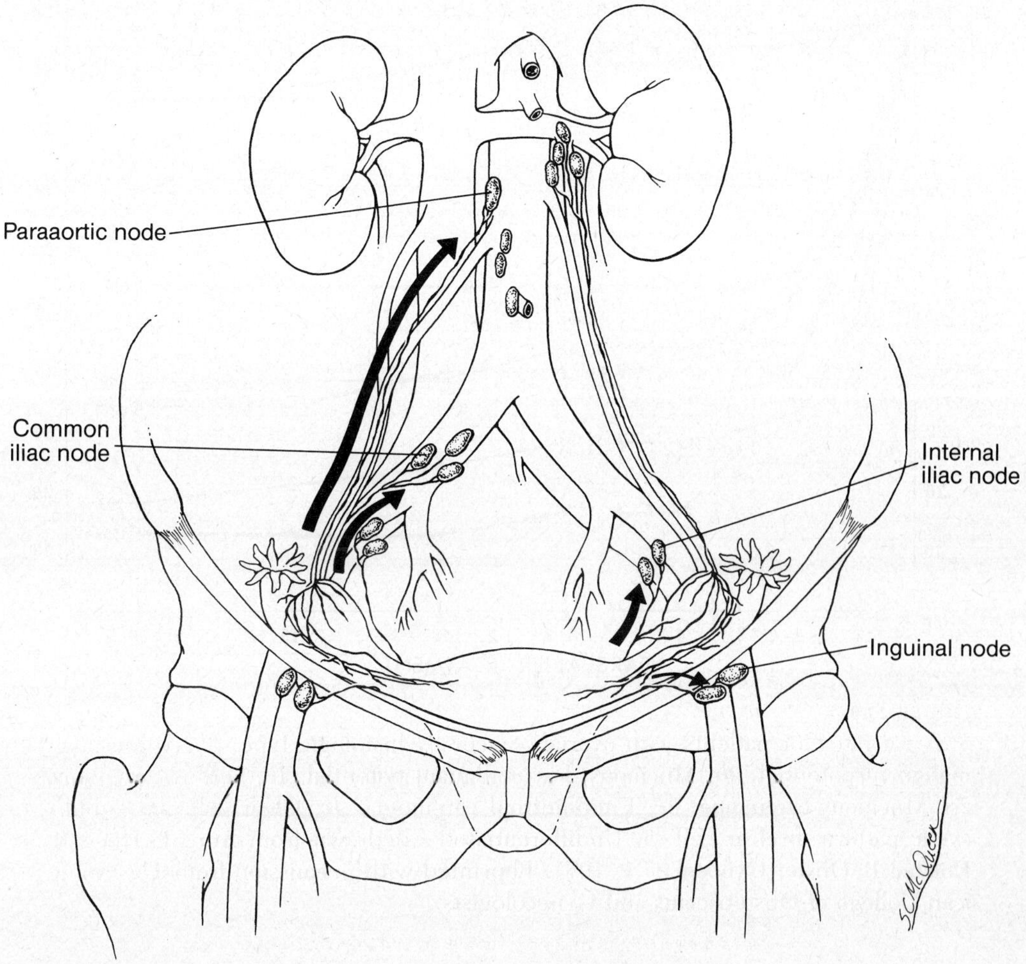

FIGURE 29-8
Lymph nodes draining ovaries. Primary routes of spread to the pelvic and paraaortic nodes are illustrated. (Redrawn from Musumeci, R.: Cancer **40:**1444, 1977.

ter resection. Richardson (Table 29-5) summarized the results of therapy for ovarian cancer from a number of institutions according to stage.

Cell type has been reported to be an important factor in prognosis, as shown in Fig. 29-9, which summarizes the 20-year survival rate of a group of patients. The most common invasive epithelial cancers, serous carcinomas, have the worst prognosis; prognosis is better for mucinous, endometrioid, and clear cell tumors. However, it should be noted that *stage* and *grade* affect these observations, insofar as serous tumors tend to be more poorly differen-

tiated and discovered at a higher stage than are mucinous tumors, which tend to be of lower grade and/or stage.

In addition to stage, the grade of the tumor is a major determinant of patient prognosis. Fig. 29-10 demonstrates the survival of 442 patients with ovarian carcinoma by grade, with a markedly worse prognosis for poorly differentiated tumors (grade 3). The relationship between grade and survival also exists when the results are examined separately for each stage of disease. Grade 0 (borderline) tumors have the best prognosis (Fig. 29-9).

The size of residual nodules and the pres-

particular agent did not appear to affect results, and complete response rates of 10% to 20% were reported, with overall responses (complete plus partial) on the order of 50%. In 1978 Young et al. reported a randomized clinical trial comparing melphalan with a four-drug combination of hexamethylmelamine, cyclophosphamide, methotrexate, and 5-fluorouracil. They noted a 75% response rate in patients treated with four drugs in comparison with 54% in those treated with melphalan alone. Median survival time was prolonged in the four-drug group (29 versus 17 months), and more complete remissions (33% versus 16%) were obtained. In a subsequent randomized trial, Neijt et al. noted that *cis*-platinum given with hexamethylmelamine, cyclophosphamide (Cytoxan), and doxorubicin (Adriamycin) (CHAP) resulted in response rates (91%) that were superior to those obtained with the four-drug nonplatinum combination used in the Young study. Decker et al. reported a 2-year survival of 62% in women who received a combination of *cis*-platinum and cyclophosphamide in comparison with only 19% for those who received cyclophosphamide alone. Thus multiple-agent, *cis*-platinum–containing programs appear to result in higher initial response rates and improved survival. A number of studies using two- to four-drug combinations containing *cis*-platinum for treating ovarian carcinoma have been reported; the results of a few are summarized in Table 29-7. As can be seen from this table, initial response rates are on the order of 90%, but by 4 to 5 years after treatment the survival has decreased to about 30%. Although a four-drug combination of oral hexamethylmelamine (150 mg/m^2 on days 1 to 7), intravenous cyclophosphamide (Cytoxan) (500 mg/m^2 on day 1), intravenous doxorubicin (Adriamycin) (30 mg/m^2 on day 1), and intravenous *cis*-platinum (50 mg/m^2 on day 1), given every 3 to 4 weeks, has been widely used in therapy for ovarian cancer, it should be noted that comparable results were obtained by Decker et al. in their 2-year study of 21 patients, with only intravenous cyclophosphamide (1000 mg/m^2) and intravenous *cis*-platinum (50 mg/m^2) given every 4 weeks. In addition to hematologic toxic effects, the multiple-drug combination also gives rise to renal and auditory toxic effects and peripheral neuropathy (*cis*-platinum) and cardiac toxic effects (doxorubicin).

All the studies indicate that the response rate is related to the amount of residual disease postoperatively, with the best results achieved for patients with minimal or no observable disease after resection, poorer results for those with masses less than 2 cm in diameter, and the worst results for those with residual masses greater than 2 cm in diameter. Some studies have suggested that the responses to the *cis*-platinum protocols in stage III ovarian carcinoma may not be related to tumor grade, and complete responses have been noted for poorly differentiated stage III cases. Moreover some

TABLE 29-7

Examples of Responses to Platinum-containing Regimens in Ovarian Epithelial Carcinoma

Study (First Author)	Drugs	Patients (No.)	% Initial Response (CR + PR)	% Survival	Duration of Study (Years)
Decker 1982	Cytox & Plat	21		62	2
Bruckner 1983	Hexa, Cytox, Plat, Adria	37		43	3
Wharton 1984	Melph, Plat	46		43	4
Cohen 1983	Cytox, Adria, Plat	64		56	2
	Hexa, Cytox, Plat, Adria	37		30	5
Neijt 1984	Hexa, Cytox, Plat, Adria	92	91	30 (approx)	4 (approx)
Vogl 1983	Cytox, Hexa, Plat, Adria	38	92	30 (approx)	4 (approx)
Greco 1981	Hexa, Cytox, Adria, Plat	46	95	NA	NA

CR = Complete response; PR = partial response; NA = not available; Cytox = cyclophosphamide (Cytoxan); Plat = *cis*-platinum; Hexa = hexamethylmelamine, Adria = doxorubicin (Adriamycin); Melph = melphalan.

patients with large residual tumors and stage III or IV disease have also achieved complete remission with multiple-agent programs containing platinum. As suggested in Table 29-7, the proportion of surviving patients unfortunately decreases with the passage of time, and it is not clear at present to what degree platinum-containing regimens will produce a long-term cure of ovarian carcinomas.

Evaluation of Chemotherapy Results: Second-Look Procedures

Chemotherapy is usually administered every 3 to 4 weeks for 1 year. The patient is monitored with careful physical examination; blood tests to measure hematologic, liver, and kidney functions; and radiologic studies such as chest x-ray examinations, ultrasound tests, or (usually) computed tomography (CT) scans of the abdomen and the pelvis. If tumor is suspected on CT scan, needle biopsy can frequently document the presence of persistent or recurrent disease. A negative CT scan, however, does not indicate complete clinical response. Goldhirsch et al. noted that 5 of 26 patients with tumor nodules larger than 1 cm had negative CT scans, and the examination was most effective (80%) for detecting metastasis in retroperitoneal nodes. CA-125 levels, if positive before therapy, are used to monitor the course of the patient with carcinoma. A value greater than 35 U/ml is positive and is found in approximately 80% of patients with ovarian cancer. It may be predictive of recurrent disease, but high false negative rates preclude its use exclusively for monitoring patients. Usually after 1 year of chemotherapy, second-look laparotomy is employed to evaluate the patient who appears to have had a complete response to chemotherapy.

Some therapists perform a laparoscopy before laparotomy. If gross tumor is not visualized and biopsy specimens and cytologic sampling through the laparoscope are negative, an exploration is then performed. Many prefer to use only the second-look laparotomy not only to confirm the presence or absence of tumor but also to perform cytoreduction of any residual tumor. The steps of an adequate second-look laparotomy are as follows:

1. Exploratory laparotomy is done with sampling of any free peritoneal fluid for cytologic study.
2. Saline washings for cytologic evaluation are taken from the pelvis and abdomen, usually separately from each hemidiaphragm, and from the gutters lateral to the ascending and descending colon. The hemidiaphragms can be effectively sampled by scraping with a tongue depressor and spreading the scrapings on a slide, fixing them in the operating room, and sending them for analysis.
3. Multiple biopsy specimens are taken of any adhesions and nodules suggestive of tumor, as well as areas that previously contained tumors, with particular attention to the areas of residual disease noted at initial laparotomy.
4. Biopsy specimens are taken from the cul-de-sac and bladder peritoneum, the areas of the infundibulopelvic ligament, and the upper part of the abdomen, including the omentum along the transverse colon.
5. Any residual omentum is removed.
6. The retroperitoneal paraaortic and pelvic nodes from which biopsy specimens had not previously been taken or that have become enlarged are sampled for histologic evaluation.

If all these studies show negative results for malignancy, the patient should be considered free of disease and therapy discontinued.

Berek et al. assessed 56 patients clinically free of disease after chemotherapy by second-look laparotomy. All had received platinum-containing, multiple-agent chemotherapy for 1 year for stage III disease. One third were confirmed to be free of disease, and an additional 15% had no gross tumor, only microscopic disease. In this study a negative second look was more likely in the patient who had low-grade tumor, had minimal residual tumor at initial surgery, and was under age 50 years. Negative second-look rates have been reported to range from 25% to 77%. The percentages varied, depending on the proportion of patients with favorable factors initially, as well as the duration of chemotherapy and the protocol used. Although therapy is discontinued after a negative second-look operation, close follow-up is needed, since tumors can recur. Podratz et al. studied 135 patients from the Mayo Clinic who

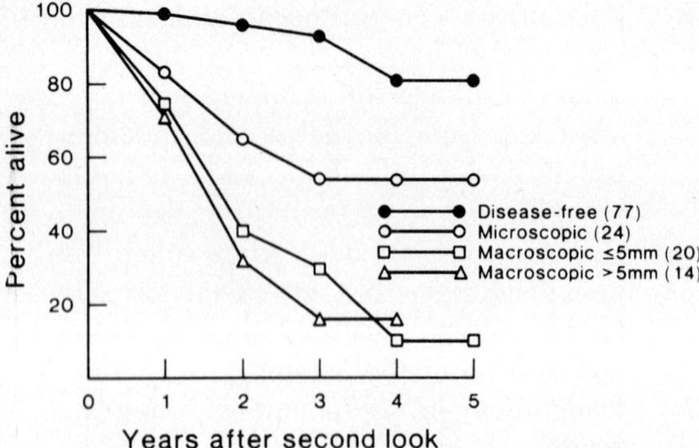

FIGURE 29-12

Survival rates for patients with ovarian carcinomas, second-look procedures. (From Podratz K, Malkasian GD, Hilton JF, et al: Am J Obstet Gynecol 152:230, 1985.)

had second-look procedures (Fig. 29-12). Of the 77 patients who had negative second-look procedures, 83% were alive 5 years after operation, and those who had only minimal disease had a 5-year survival of approximately 43%. For those with gross nodules greater than 2 cm in diameter after second-look procedure, the median survival time was under 24 months.

Both chemotherapy and radiotherapy have been prescribed for patients with residual disease after a second-look procedure. In general the most favorable group has only microscopic disease or minimal disease less than 5 mm in diameter. Hacker et al. administered pelvic and abdominal irradiation therapy to 15 patients with minimal disease, six of whom survived 19 to 41 months. Longer follow-up is necessary, but morbidity was serious, since 9 of the 30 patients subsequently required laparotomy for small bowel complications. Menczer et al. found no benefit for radiotherapy given to patients with limited or no disease after second-look laparotomy. A number of protocols with various chemotherapeutic agents have also been used as second- and third-line therapy, but no effective program has emerged.

Complications and Alternative Considerations

MALIGNANT EFFUSIONS. Patients with ovarian cancer frequently develop ascites or hydrothorax or both, requiring repeated drainage by paracentesis or thoracentesis. Occasion-

ally sclerosing solutions are used in the thoracic cavity to prevent reaccumulation of fluid, with resultant adherence of the pleural surfaces. Nitrogen mustard, tetracycline, and quinicrine have all been used successfully for this purpose.

INTRAPERITONEAL THERAPY. Intraperitoneal instillation of chemotherapeutic agents has been tried recently to increase the effect of cytotoxic drugs on the tumor within the abdominal cavity. *Cis*-platinum has been widely studied, and high intraperitoneal concentrations are achieved with instillation of the drug into the peritoneal cavity. Eventually serum levels comparable to those seen after intravenous therapy are obtained. The drug can be instilled with a catheter similar to that used for peritoneal dialysis. One modification is shown in Fig. 29-13, in which a needle is allowed subcutaneous access through the skin into the port to administer the chemotherapy intraperitoneally through the catheter. No large-scale clinical trials of intraperitoneal therapy in gynecologic tumors have been conducted. Preliminary results suggest that patients with small tumor nodules (under 5 mm in diameter) will have a good response. Intraperitoneal adhesions and bowel obstruction are potential complications. A valid comparison between intravenous and intraperitoneal therapy has not yet been done.

IMMUNOTHERAPY. Immunotherapy agents such as *Corynebacterium parvum* (C-Parvum), and bacillus Calmette-Guérin (BCG) have been administered to try to augment the immunologic response and promote tumor resistance in the host. These agents have also been used in combination with cytotoxic chemotherapy, and preliminary improved results have been reported. The Gynecologic Oncology Group recently reported responses for up to 6 months in 5 of 28 patients treated with interferon. Long-term studies are not available, and immunotherapy is not routinely advocated at present.

HORMONE RECEPTORS. Holt et al. have noted that about 50% of ovarian epithelial carcinomas have detectable levels of estrogen receptors. These receptors are similar physicochemically to those noted in breast and endometrial carcinomas. However, their presence in ovarian carcinomas does not, in general, appear to correlate with tumor differenti-

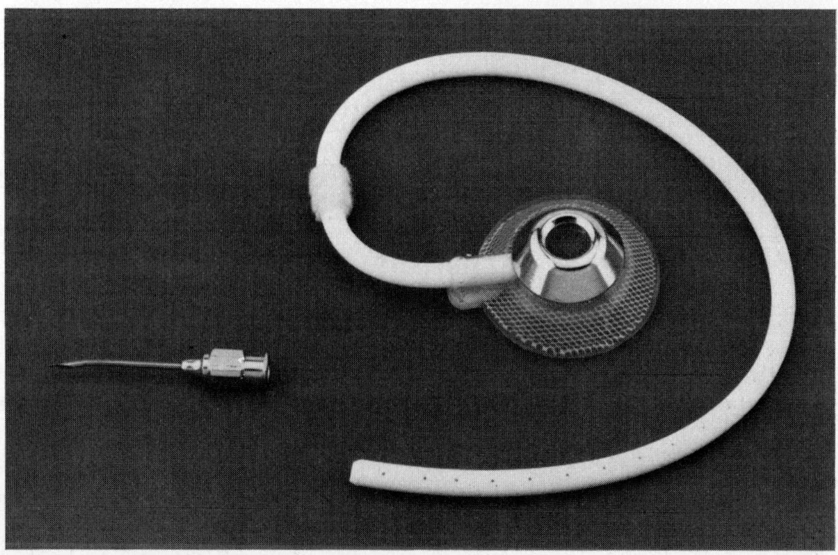

FIGURE 29-13
Peritoneal catheter with access port for infusion of drugs.

ation or clinical behavior. Hormone therapy with progestins and antiestrogens such as tamoxifen has been tried, and a few isolated reports of responses or stabilization of disease have been reported. However, response has been reported in only 5% to 10% of patients.

HUMAN TUMOR STEM CELL ASSAY. The in vitro method of human tumor stem cell assay was developed by Salmon et al. in 1978. The test is based on the growth of cultured cells in vitro, which are then tested against a variety of chemotherapeutic agents. Such clonogenic assays may someday provide useful clinical information regarding drug selection for chemotherapy in gynecologic malignancies, but at present they are not reliable for regular clinical use.

Summary

Therapy for epithelial ovarian carcinoma is based on removal of all gross disease and sampling of areas at high risk for spread in the peritoneal cavity and retroperitoneal nodes. Postoperative therapy is employed depending on the stage and grade of the primary tumor. For accurately staged cases, postoperative ^{32}P is used in low-stage tumors such as stage Ic carcinomas where there is a risk of intraperitoneal tumor seeding but no residual disease.

External irradiation is effective in tumor treatment, especially in accurately documented stage II cases, but its use usually compromises bone marrow function and interferes with the future use of chemotherapy. Single-agent alkylating therapy is often employed as adjunctive treatment for poorly differentiated tumors, such as stage I, grade 3, or for stage II cases without residual tumor, but such treatment carries with it a high risk of subsequent development of leukemia, which may reach 10% by 8 years after therapy.

Multiple-agent chemotherapy including platinum is used for treatment of high-stage tumors and for patients with residual disease after initial tumor resection. It is accompanied by multiple short- and long-term toxic side effects but results in initial response rates in advanced cases that may exceed 90%. Five-year survival rates drop to 30% or less. Long-term randomized trials will be needed to improve rates of salvage and to optimize therapy for epithelial ovarian carcinomas.

GERM CELL TUMORS

These tumors are derived from the germ cells of the ovary. As a group they are the second most common of ovarian neoplasms, and they account for about 20% to 25% of all ovarian tumors. The classification of germ cell tu-

WHO CLASSIFICATION OF GERM CELL TUMORS

Dysgerminoma
Endodermal sinus tumor
Embryonal carcinoma
Polyembryoma
Choriocarcinoma
Teratomas
  Immature
  Mature
    Solid
    Cystic
      Dermoid cyst (mature cystic teratoma)
      Dermoid cyst with malignant transformation
  Monodermal and highly specialized
    Struma ovarii
    Carcinoid
    Struma ovarii and carcinoid
    Others
Mixed forms

mors according to the World Health Organization (WHO) designation is shown in the box above.

The most frequent germ cell tumor is the benign cystic teratoma (dermoid); overall only 2% to 3% of germ cell tumors are malignant. Among the malignant germ cell tumors, the most frequent is the dysgerminoma, which accounts for 1% to 2% of ovarian cancers. Next in frequency are the immature teratomas and endodermal sinus tumors, each of which comprises less than 1% of ovarian malignancies. However, in female patients under age 21 years, germ cell tumors are the most frequent ovarian neoplasm, and about one third of the germ cell tumors encountered in those under age 21 years are malignant.

The histogenesis of germ cell tumors has been extensively studied and summarized by Talerman. Fig. 29-14 summarizes the theory of the histogenesis of these tumors—that they originate from the primitive germ cell and then gradually differentiate to mimic the developmental tissues of embryonic origin (ectoderm, mesoderm, or endoderm) and the extra embryonic tissues (yolk sac and trophoblast). Germ cell tumors that originate in the ovary have homologous counterparts in the testes, i.e., dysgerminoma and seminoma. These tumors are usually unilateral, with the exception of teratomas and dysgerminomas (Table 29-3). The morphologic and clinical aspects of each of the various types of germ cell tumors will be separately considered.

Teratomas

Teratomas consist of tissues that recapitulate the three layers of the developing embryo (ectoderm, mesoderm, and endoderm). One or more of the layers may be represented, and the tissues can be mature (benign) or immature (malignant). Chromosomal studies indicate that teratomas appear to arise from a single germ and have an XX karyotype. In the older literature, terms such as *malignant teratoma* and *teratocarcinoma* were used to denote the malignant variety of these tumors, but these terms have been replaced by the nomenclature shown in box at left.

Benign Cystic Teratomas (Dermoids)

Benign cystic teratomas are of the most common germ cell tumors and account for about 20% to 25% of all ovarian neoplasms. They primarily occur during the reproductive years but may occur in postmenopausal women and in children. The risk of malignant transformation (see later discussion) is markedly increased if these tumors are found in postmenopausal women. One of the interesting facets of teratomas is their ability to produce adult tissue, including skin, bone, teeth, hair, and dermal tissue. The presence of calcified bone or teeth allows the tumor to be diagnosed preoperatively with ultrasound or radiography, the latter having been reported to detect dermoids preoperatively in about one third of the cases (Fig. 29-15).

Dermoids are usually unilateral, but 10% to 15% are bilateral. The outside wall of the tumor tends to be smooth with a yellowish appearance caused by the sebaceous-fatty material that fills the tumor. Hair is also a prominent feature once the cyst is opened (Fig. 29-16). Usually the tumors are asymptomatic, but they can cause severe pain if there is torsion or if the sebaceous material perforates the

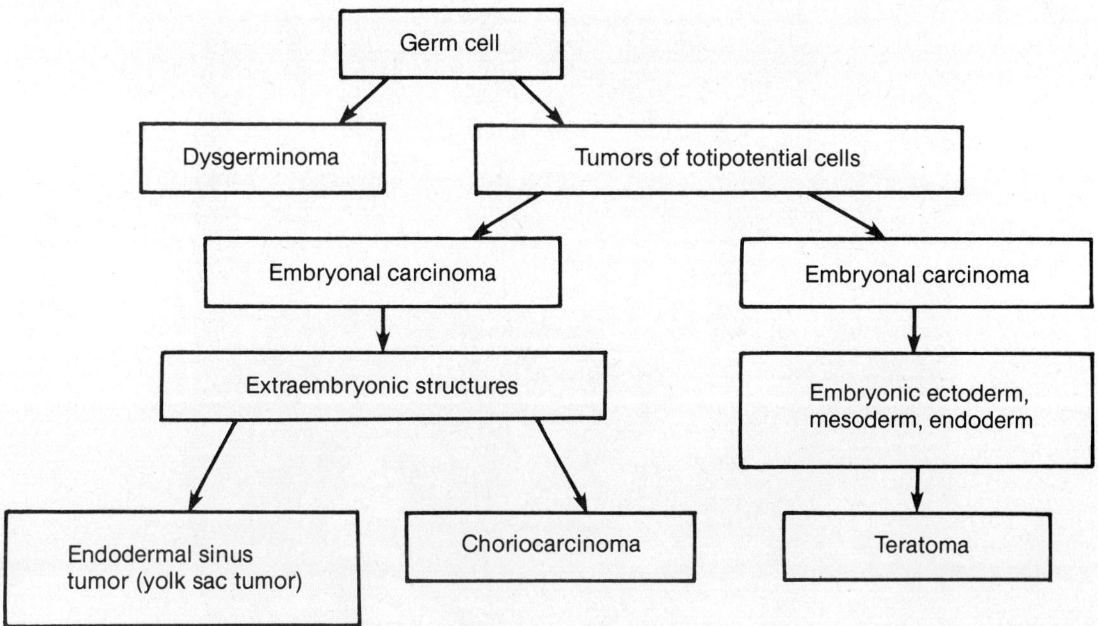

FIGURE 29-14

Histogenesis of germ cell tumors. (Modified from Talerman A: Germ cell tumors of the ovary. In Blaustein A, ed: Pathology of the female genital tract. New York, Springer-Verlag, 1982.)

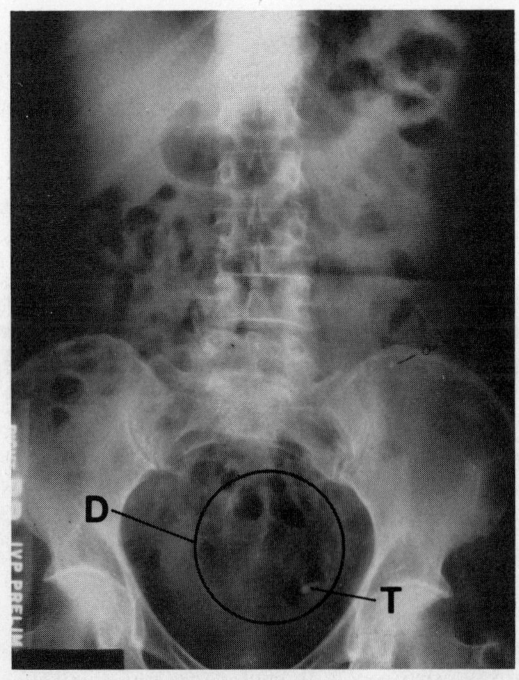

FIGURE 29-15

X-ray film of a dermoid. *D*, Dermoid; *T*, tooth. (Courtesy E.K. Senekjian.)

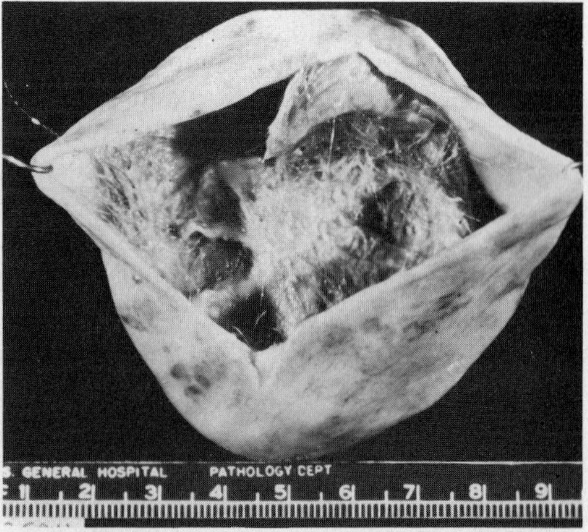

FIGURE 29-16

Gross specimen of a dermoid cyst that was filled with sebaceous material and hair. (Courtesy Robert E. Scully.)

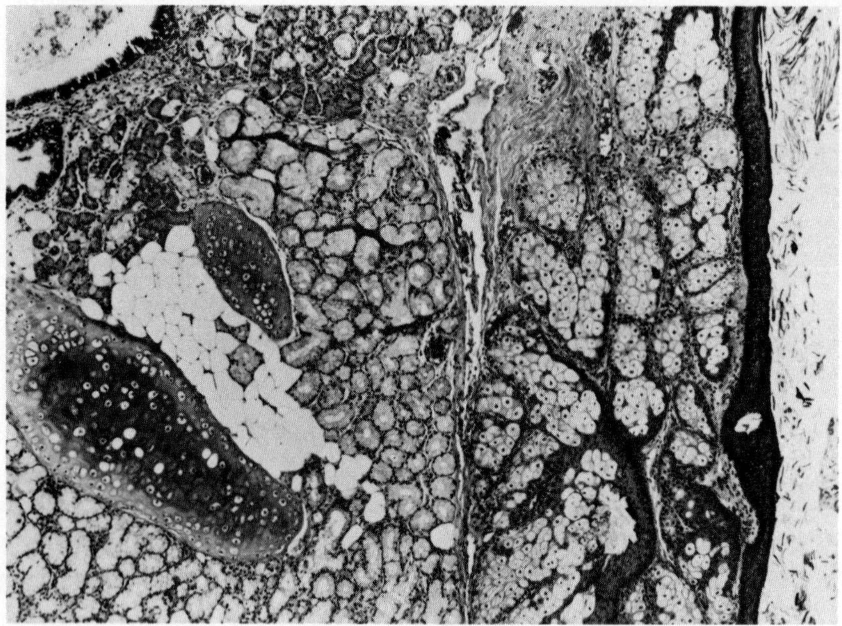

FIGURE 29-17

Photomicrograph of dermoid. Cartilage is shown *(right)* lined by epidermis and accompanying appendages *(left)*. (×50.) (From Serov SF, Scully RE, Sobin LH: Histologic typing of ovarian tumors. Geneva, Switzerland, World Health Organization, 1973.)

cyst wall, leading to a reactive peritonitis. This rare complication is severe and can occur during pregnancy. Microscopically a number of adult tissues are seen (Fig. 29-17).

Treatment of the reproductive-age female patient or of the child consists of either cystectomy or unilateral oophorectomy. In most cases it should be possible to remove only the cyst and preserve normal ovarian tissue. The technique is demonstrated in Fig. 29-18. The opposite ovary should be inspected. If it is grossly normal, nothing further need be done. In the past, bivalving of a normal-appearing ovary was suggested to rule out a contralateral dermoid, but this procedure results in a high risk of adhesions and subsequent infertility. Doss et al. studied 148 women with ovarian teratomas who had a grossly normal-appearing contralateral ovary. Ninety of them had a biopsy or tissue removed from the opposite normal-appearing contralateral ovary, and no dermoid was detected. The 58 other patients did not have a surgical procedure on the contralateral ovary,

and subsequently only one of these patients (0.6% of the total) required laparotomy for a dermoid. These data strongly reinforce the desirability of inspecting only the contralateral ovary if it appears grossly normal. In women beyond childbearing years, therapy for a dermoid usually consists of removal of the uterus, both tubes, and the ovaries.

Occasionally teratomas may be solid and may consist only of adult tissues, leading to the diagnosis of solid, mature teratoma. These benign germ cell tumors are rare.

A cystic teratoma can undergo malignant degeneration, which usually occurs in the squamous epithelial elements of the dermoid, producing a squamous cell carcinoma. It is a rare complication estimated to occur in fewer than 2% of these tumors, most frequently in postmenopausal women. If the malignant tissue has spread beyond the confines of the ovary, the prognosis is poor. In such cases additional therapy for squamous cell carcinoma with irradiation or chemotherapy or both are indicated.

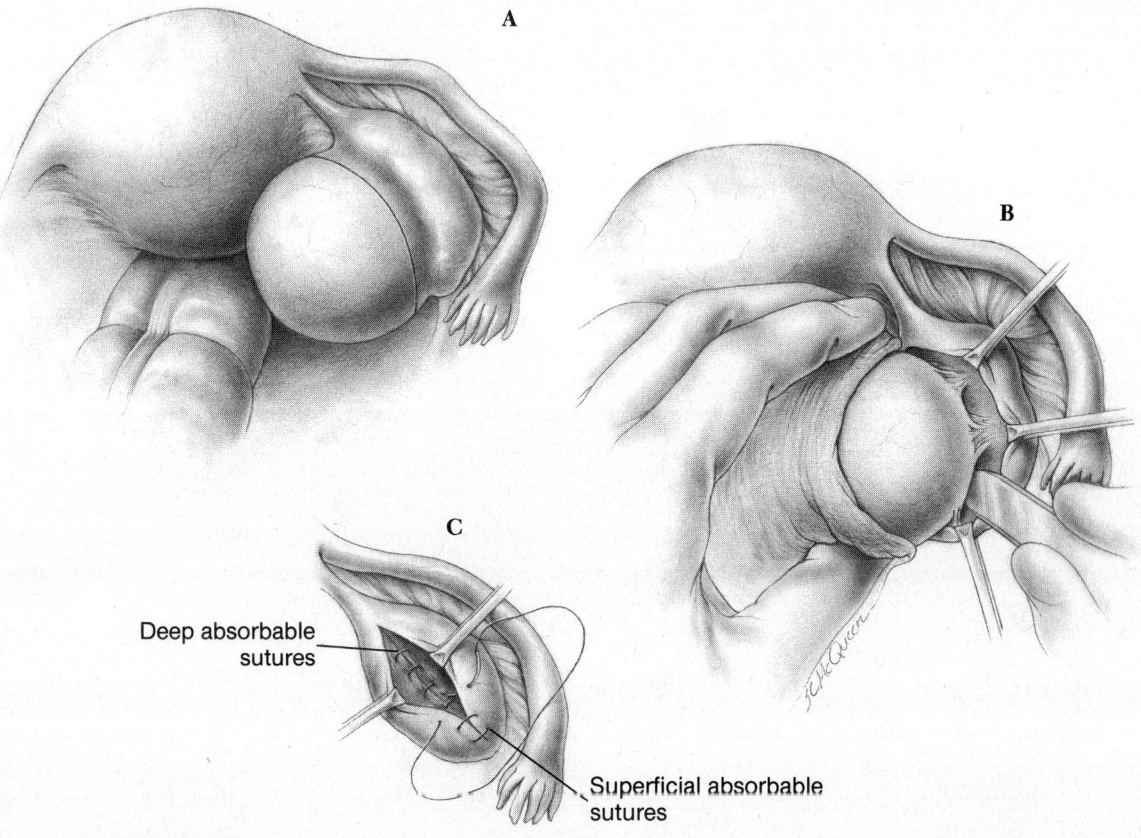

FIGURE 29-18
Shelling out of teratoma. **A,** Scalpel incision in ovary at intersection of dermoid and normal ovary. **B,** Dermoid being separated. Note how upper part peels away. **C,** Reconstruction of normal ovary.

Immature Teratomas

Immature teratomas are malignant and account for up to 20% of the malignant ovarian tumors found in women under the age of 20 years but less than 1% of all ovarian cancers. They have not been documented to occur in women after menopause. They consist of immature embryonic structures that can be admixed with mature elements.

The prognosis for patients with immature teratomas is related to the stage (FIGO) and grade of the tumor. The grade of the tumor is based on the degree of immaturity of the various tissues. Grade 3 tumors consist of the most immature tissues and often have a high proportion of immature neuroepithelium. Fig. 29-19 shows the survival of patients with immature teratomas by stage and grade. Because these tumors occur in young women, preservation of childbearing function is an important consideration. Kurman and Norris reported that patients with stage IA immature teratoma had a 10-year actuarial survival of 70% after unilateral salpingo-oophorectomy; this rate is comparable to that recorded after bilateral salpingo-oophorectomy. The opposite ovary is rarely involved by immature teratoma, although a benign cystic teratoma (dermoid) is present in 5% of cases. If the opposite ovary appears grossly normal, unilateral salpingo-oophorectomy alone is adequate. If there is extension of tumor outside the ovary, implants and metastases should be extensively sampled and graded histologically to decide on therapy.

Multiple-agent chemotherapy has improved the outlook for patients with immature tera-

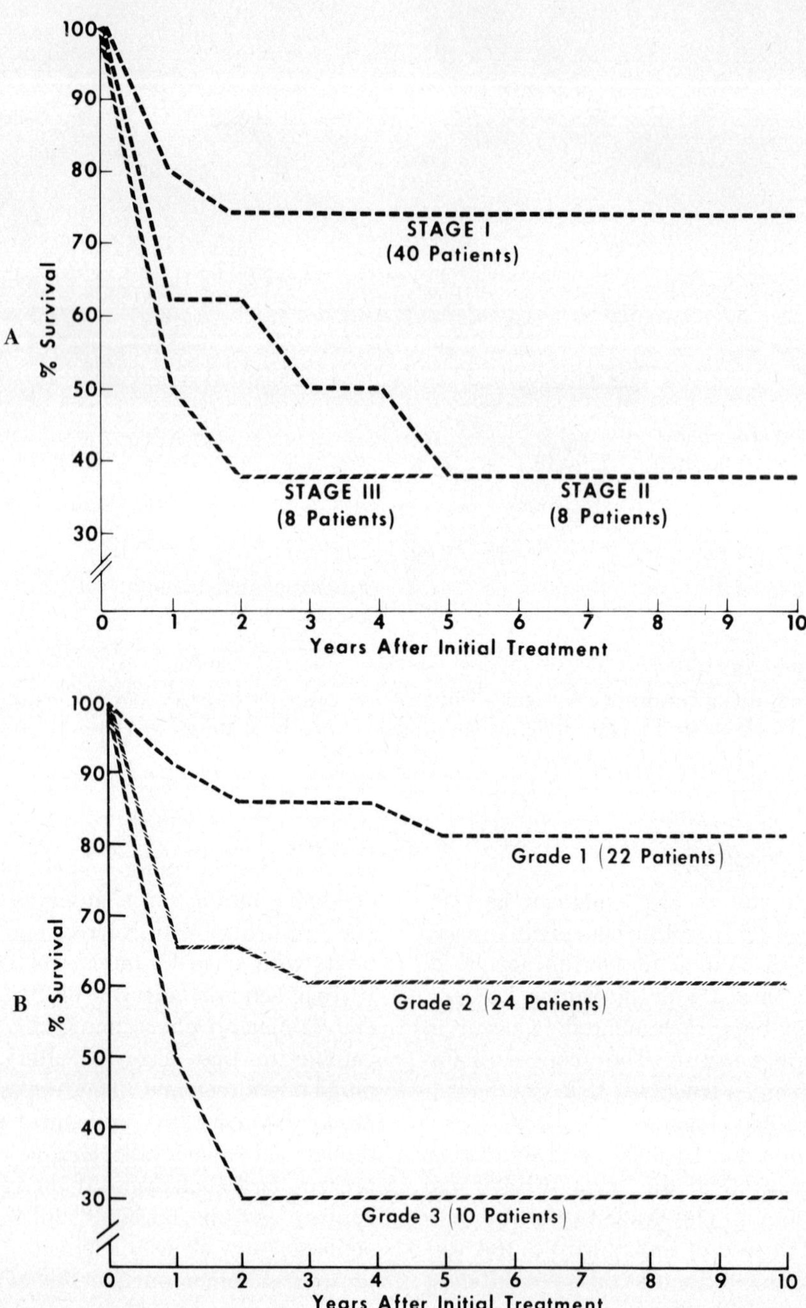

FIGURE 29-19

A, Actuarial survival of 56 patients with malignant teratoma by neoplasm stage. **B,** By neoplasm grade. (From Norris HJ, Zirkin H, Benson WL: Cancer 37:2359, 1976.)

toma. A widely used protocol is the so-called VAC regimen (vincristine, 1.5 mg/m² given intravenously weekly for 12 weeks and actinomycin D, 0.5 mg, with cyclophosphamide (Cytoxan) 5 to 7 mg/kg/day given intravenously daily for 5 days every 4 weeks). The treatment is usually continued for 1 year. Curry et al. noted that 10 of 12 patients so treated were surviving 1 to 5 years. Conversion of metastatic immature teratoma (grades 2 and 3) after chemotherapy to mature elements (grade 0) has been reported by DiSaia et al. Mature elements require no further therapy.

Chemotherapy is indicated for metastatic immature teratoma (other than grade 0). For stage IA tumors that are composed of grade 2 or 3 elements, adjunctive chemotherapy is indicated because of the associated poor prognosis for tumors of these grades (Fig. 29-19, *B*). If metastatic disease is noted at operation, a second-look procedure is performed after completion of chemotherapy. For patients with grade 1 primary tumors with or without grade 0 implants, no further therapy is needed.

Specialized Germ Cell Tumors— Struma Ovarii and Carcinoids

Specialized ovarian germ cell tumors are rare; two types are commonly recognized (see box on p. 858): the struma ovarii and carcinoids. Struma ovarii are dermoids with thyroid tissue exclusively or as a major component. The thyroid tissue can be functional, leading to clinical hyperthyroidism. Most of these tumors are benign, but malignant changes are possible. Metastatic disease, if present, has been reported to be effectively treated with iodine 131.

Carcinoids are ovarian teratomas that histologically resemble similar tumors in the gastrointestinal tract. Carcinoids are rare and are unilateral in the ovary. In about 30% of cases a true carcinoid syndrome will develop, and 5-hydroxyindoleacetic acid (5-HIAA) can be detected and used to monitor the tumor postoperatively. These tumors occur primarily in older women and tend to grow slowly; the prognosis after hysterectomy and bilateral salpingo-oophorectomy is excellent. For a young woman desiring preservation of childbearing function, a stage Ia carcinoid can be treated by unilateral salpingo-oophorectomy.

Dysgerminomas

Dysgerminomas are the most common type of malignant germ cell tumors. They consist of primitive germ cells with stroma infiltrated by lymphocytes (Fig. 29-20). They are analogous to seminoma in the male testis, and they comprise about 1% of ovarian malignancies. Dysgerminomas occur primarily in women under the age of 30 years. The tumor is often discovered during pregnancy. Some arise in dysgenetic gonads (see later discussion of gonadoblastomas). Unlike other malignant germ cell tumors, dysgerminomas are bilateral in about 10% of cases (see Table 29-3); therefore sampling of the contralateral ovary is indicated in cases of apparent stage Ia dysgerminoma. The prognosis is related to tumor size (improved if less than 15 cm), unilaterality, encapsulation (not ruptured), lack of spread to retroperitoneal nodes, and lack of ascites. If all these criteria are present, the prognosis in stage Ia cases is excellent (greater than 90% 5-year survival).

Insofar as patients with dysgerminoma are young, preservation of childbearing function is desirable, if possible. The tumor can spread within the peritoneal cavity and to retroperitoneal nodes, a more likely occurrence with larger dysgerminomas. If the tumor is confined to one ovary, a unilateral salpingo-oophorectomy should be performed and the abdomen thoroughly explored to determine the presence of intraperitoneal and retroperitoneal spread. Suspicious areas or pelvic or paraaortic nodes should be biopsied and any enlarged nodes excised. The contralateral ovary should have a wedge biopsy even if it appears normal. If frozen section indicates pure dysgerminoma and there is no evidence of spread outside the primary tumor, only a unilateral salpingo-oophorectomy is indicated. Patients so treated have a 5-year survival in excess of 90%. Assadourian and Taylor noted that unilateral salpingo-oophorectomy was as effective as more radical treatment for unilateral dysgerminoma. There can be a recurrence in as many as 20% of cases, primarily in tumors over 15 cm, but most of these tumors can be effectively treated by an

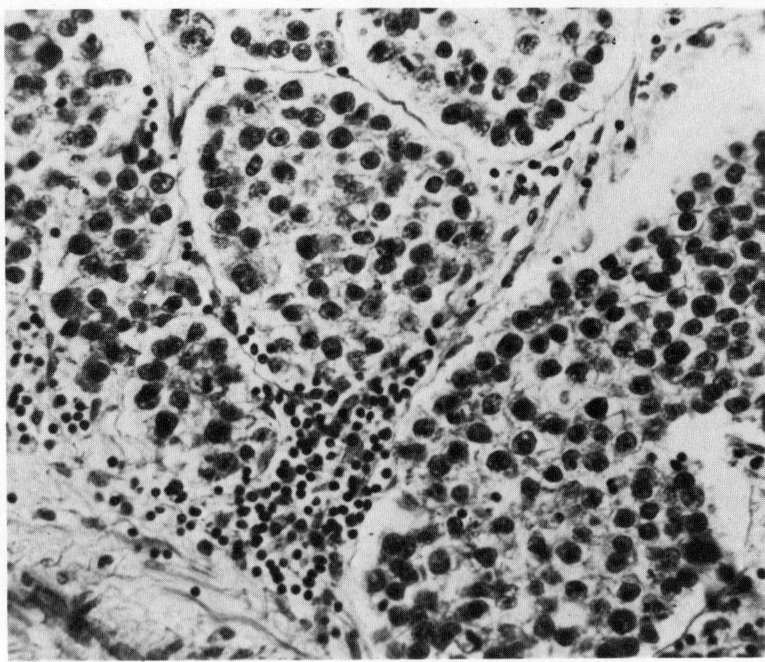

FIGURE 29-20
Dysgerminoma. (×300.) Dysgerminoma cells are demonstrated, as well as infiltration of stroma by lymphocytes. (From Scully RE: Germ cell tumors of the ovary and fallopian tube. In Meigs JV, Sturgis SH, eds: Progress in gynecology, vol. 4. New York, Grune & Stratton, 1963.)

additional operative procedure or irradiation or both. These tumors are extremely radiosensitive and can be cured with less than 3000 rads, a dosage used to treat extraovarian residual tumor after primary surgery or for recurrence. Patients treated conservatively should be closely followed up and periodic CT scans performed to monitor the abdominal cavity and retroperitoneal nodes. Lymphangiography has also been frequently employed to check on the status of the retroperitoneal nodes. In cases of radiation failure or when the patient cannot receive irradiation, multiple-agent chemotherapy such as VAC (see immature teratoma) or vinblastine, *cis*-platinum, and bleomycin (see discussion of endodermal sinus tumor, below) can be utilized.

It is important to emphasize that these considerations apply to pure dysgerminoma. Other germ cell elements may coexist with these tumors (mixed germ cell tumor), in which case the prognosis is markedly worse. Some of the reports in the earlier literature of poor prognosis with unilateral dysgerminoma were probably unrecognized cases of mixed germ cell tumors.

Endodermal Sinus Tumors (Yolk Sac Tumors)

The endodermal sinus tumor is a malignant germ cell tumor that accounts for less than 1% of ovarian cancers and in part resembles the yolk sac of the rodent placenta, thus recapitulating extraembryonic tissues (see Fig. 29-14). One typical histologic pattern is shown in Fig. 29-21. Other terms have been applied to this tumor, including *mesonephroma* and *embryonal carcinoma*, but these terms are no longer used. The tumor secretes alpha-fetoprotein as a specific marker that is useful in identifying and following these tumors clinically.

These rapidly growing tumors occur in females between 13 months and 45 years of age. A median age of 19 years at diagnosis was noted by Kurman and Norris. Stage Ia cases can be treated by unilateral adnexectomy. Before modern chemotherapy the tumor was usu-

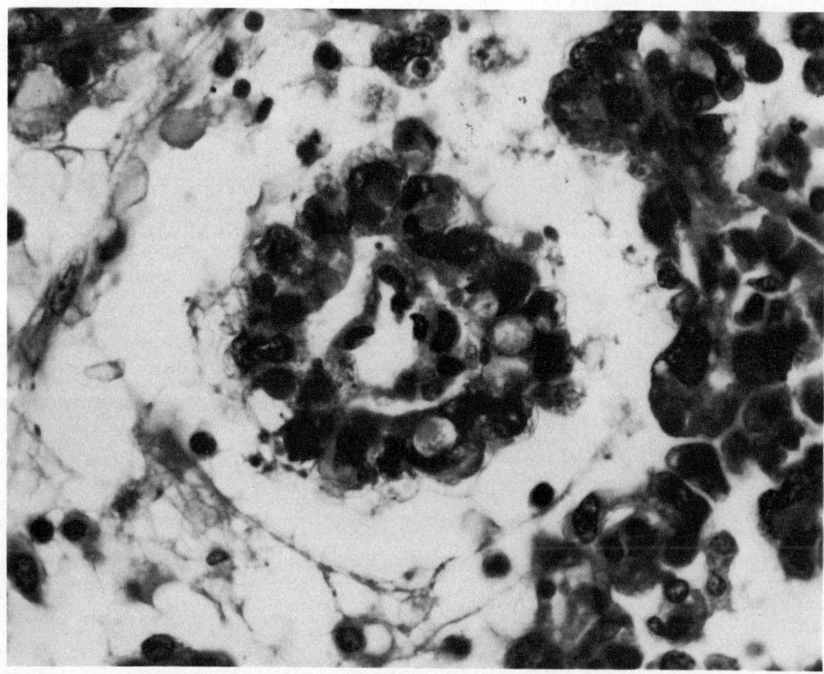

FIGURE 29-21
Schiller-Duvall body associated with numerous hyaline droplets in an endodermal sinus tumor. ($\times$ 350.) (From Kurman RJ, Norris HJ: Malignant germ cell tumors of the ovary. Hum Pathol 8:551, 1977. Reprinted with permission from W.B. Saunders Co., Philadelphia, 1977.)

ally fatal, even if it was confined to one ovary. Therefore patients with endodermal sinus tumor should undergo chemotherapy postoperatively. The VAC protocol (see immature teratoma) has been widely used, with remissions of more than 2 years noted in 68% of the 25 patients reported by Gallion et al. Another effective regimen has been a 5-day program: actinomycin D, 10 µg/kg/day, 5-fluorouracil (5-FU), 8 mg/kg/day up to 500 mg, and cyclophosphamide (Cytoxan), 7 mg/kg/day up to 450 mg (Act-FU-Cy). Forney noted regression of endodermal sinus tumor with this program and also reported subsequent pregnancy in a patient so treated. More recently, Einhorn and Donahue reported a potent combination of vinblastine, 12 mg/m^2 intravenously every 3 weeks for four doses, bleomycin, 20 units/m^2 (maximum dose, 30 units/m^2) intravenously given weekly for seven doses and an eighth course on week 10, and *cis*-platinum, 20 mg/m^2 daily for 5 days given every 3 weeks for up to four courses. This regimen has been found to be effective in treating patients with metastatic germ cell tumors of the testis and in inducing remissions in endodermal sinus tumors. Multiple-agent chemotherapy is needed, and of the 41 patients reported by Gershenson et al. all of the 21 who survived had received multiple-agent chemotherapy with one of these protocols.

Choriocarcinomas

Nongestational choriocarcinoma is a highly malignant rare germ cell tumor resembling extraembryonic tissues. Like gestational choriocarcinoma (Chapter 33) it consists of malignant cytotrophoblasts and syncytiotrophoblasts; human chorionic gonadotrophin (HCG) is a useful tumor marker. Most patients developing this tumor primarily in the ovary are under the age of 20 years. The disease was usually fatal in the past and does not appear to respond to single-agent chemotherapy such as methotrexate or actinomycin D with the same frequency as gestational trophoblastic disease. This lack of response may be due in part to the occurrence of these tumors in combination with other malignant germ cell tumors (mixed germ cell tumor), and on occasion the other germ cell elements may not be histologically recognized. Multiple-agent chemotherapy is advisable.

Embryonal Carcinomas

An embryonal carcinoma is a rare malignant germ cell tumor composed of primitive embryonal cells. It occurs in young females between the ages of 4 and 28 years. Kurman and Norris summarized 15 cases. Trophoblastic elements may be present, and both HCG and alpha-fetoprotein have been reported to be present.

Polyembryomas

Polyembryomas are exceedingly rare tumors that are usually found in the testes. They can occur in the ovary and consist of embryonal bodies that resemble early embryos. Trophoblastic elements with HCG and placental lactogen secretion have been reported.

Mixed Germ Cell Tumors

Mixed germ cell tumors are combinations of any of the previously described germ cell tumors of the ovary. They can be bilateral if dysgerminoma elements are involved; otherwise they are unilateral. Treatment of apparent stage IA mixed germ cell tumors consists of unilateral adnexectomy. A wedge biopsy of the opposite ovary is performed in women desiring to preserve reproductive function if dysgerminoma is present. Multiple-agent chemotherapy with VAC or with vinblastine, bleomycin, and *cis*-platinum, as previously described, is recommended. The most frequently found elements in mixed germ cell tumors are dysgerminomas and teratomas. Survival of patients with mixed germ cell tumors is related primarily to the immaturity of the constituent tissues; it can reach 100% for small mixed germ cell tumors. It is diminished for women with large tumors or with a predominance of endodermal sinus elements, choriocarcinoma, or grade 3 immature teratoma.

GONADOBLASTOMAS (GERM CELL SEX CORD–STROMAL TUMORS)

The term *gonadoblastoma* was introduced by Scully in 1953 to describe a tumor that consists of germ cell and sex cord–stromal elements. Approximately 100 cases have been reported. The germ cells usually resemble dysgerminoma, whereas the sex cord–stromal elements may consist of immature granulosa and Sertoli cells. Leydig cells and luteinized cells may be present. The tumor usually occurs in patients with abnormal (dysgenetic) gonads. Most patients have a female phenotype but may be virilized. These patients have a Y chromosome detected in their karyotype, and patients with gonadal dysgenesis and a Y chromosome are at risk for the development of gonadoblastoma or malignant germ cell tumors, predominantly dysgerminoma, which may occur in an individual as young as 6 months of age. Removal of these gonads is indicated when they are discovered. Both gonads should be removed, and if the presence of pure gonadoblastoma is confirmed, the prognosis is excellent, since these tumors have not been reported to metastasize.

SEX CORD STROMAL TUMORS

The sex cord stromal tumors are derived from the sex cords of the ovary and the specialized stroma of the developing gonad. The elements can have a male or female differentiation, and some of these tumors are hormonally active. The group accounts for about 6% of ovarian neoplasms and the majority of hormonally functioning ovarian tumors. For the female derivatives the sex cord component is the granulosa cell, and the stromal component is the theca cell or fibroblast. For the male counterpart the similar components are the Sertoli cell and the Leydig cell. Granulosa-theca cell tumors and Sertoli-Leydig tumors tend to behave as low-grade malignancies. Their clinical and morphologic aspects will be separately considered.

Granulosa-Theca Cell Tumors

Granulosa cell tumors consist primarily of granulosa cells and a varying proportion of

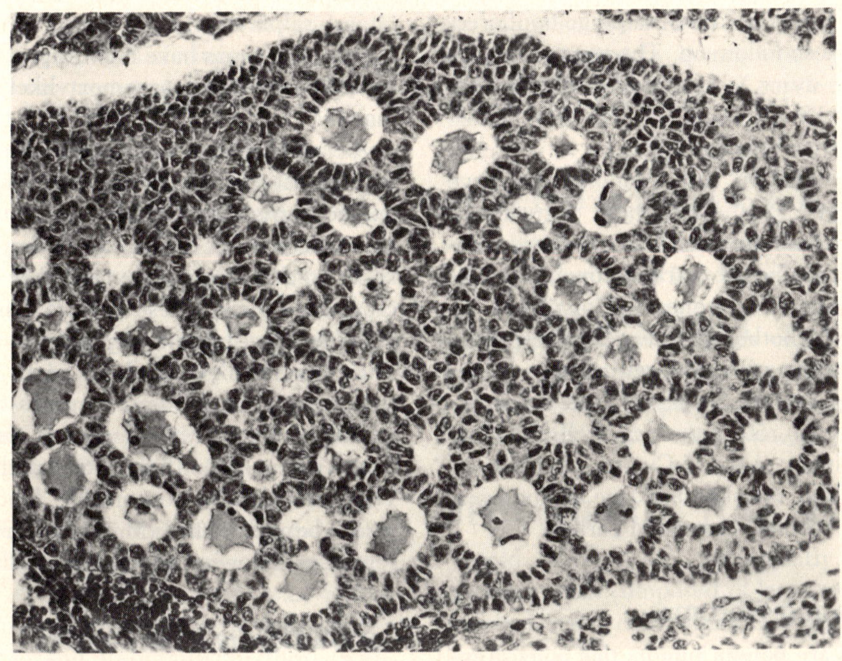

FIGURE 29-22
Granulosa cell tumor. (×460.) (From Scully RE, Morris J: Functioning ovarian tumors. In Meigs JV, Sturgis SH, eds: Progress in gynecology, vol. 3. New York, Grune & Stratton, 1957.)

theca cells or fibroblasts or both. One characteristic microscopic pattern is shown in Fig. 29-22, which demonstrates the so-called Call-Exner bodies, eosinophilic bodies surrounded by granulosa cells. Functional granulosa cell tumors are primarily estrogenic. About 5% occur before puberty, and they can be one of the causes of precocious puberty, but the tumors have been described in women of all ages. In postmenopausal women these tumors can produce elevated levels of blood estrogens, uterine bleeding, and occasionally endometrial carcinoma. It is estimated that about 5% of the granulosa cell tumors in adults are associated with endometrial neoplasia. In menstruating women the functional granulosa cell tumor can produce abnormal menstrual patterns, menorrhagia, and even amenorrhea.

These tumors can become large and may present as a ruptured mass, leading to laparotomy for an acute condition of the abdomen with hemoperitoneum. Because of the low-grade malignant character of these tumors, recurrences are frequent more than 5 years after primary therapy. In general, prognosis does not correlate with the histologic pattern of the tumor. However, advanced clinical stage, the presence of tumor rupture, a large primary tumor (greater than 15 cm), and a high mitotic rate have been associated with a poorer prognosis. Overall 10-year survival rates of 90% have been reported.

The primary therapeutic approach is the operative removal of the tumor. Since these tumors are rarely bilateral (less than 5%), stage IA tumors can be treated by unilateral adnexectomy with biopsy of the contralateral ovary to rule out bilaterality. Lack et al. reported 10 cases of granulosa cell tumors in premenarchal female patients, all of whom were treated by unilateral salpingo-oophorectomy. Two tumors were ruptured. All 10 of the patients were surviving with no evidence of disease 2 to 33 years after therapy. Evans et al. did note a higher recurrence rate among women who were treated by unilateral salpingo-oophorectomy for stage IA cases in comparison with those treated with bilateral salpingo-oophorectomy. This finding has led to the recommendation that women of reproductive age treated for granu-

Vulvar Intraepithelial Neoplasia

Once the diagnosis of VIN has been established by biopsy, therapy is performed to eradicate the area containing the neoplasia. The clinician must be aware that the progress of vulvar atypia (mild dysplasia—VIN I) to moderate dysplasia (VIN II) to severe dysplasia and carcinoma in situ (VIN III) and then to invasive carcinoma is not as well documented for vulvar neoplasia as it is for squamous cell neoplasia of the cervix. Moreover, vulvar neoplasia is frequently multifocal, requiring treatment of several areas. An additional complication is that some cases originally diagnosed as intraepithelial neoplasia have been reported to regress spontaneously. Finally, areas contiguous to the vulva are frequently involved in intraepithelial neoplasia (Fig. 30-12).

In 1972 Friedrich reported Bowenoid atypia (histologically similar to carcinoma in situ) in a pregnant patient that regressed spontaneously postpartum. Others also reported spontaneous regression of this lesion. These spontaneously regressing lesions tend to be discrete elevations in young women. Some may be explained by recent studies of nuclear DNA content of vulvar atypias that suggest not all lesions with this designation are premalignant. Fu et al. noted that only four of eight cases of vulvar atypia had an aneuploid (neoplastic) distribution. A polyploid distribution was noted in four of the cases, which is consistent with a benign process, while aneuploidy is consistent with intraepithelial neoplasia.

Most patients with vulvar epithelial neoplasia have been reported to be in their forties or older, but recently the disease has been diagnosed with increasing frequency in younger women, particularly in those with a papillomavirus infection (Fig. 30-13). The potential importance of papillomavirus in intraepithelial neoplasia is considered in greater detail in Chapter 26. Crum et al. found that older patients (over 45 years) with vulvar intraepithelial neoplasia (VIN) did not show the stigmas of

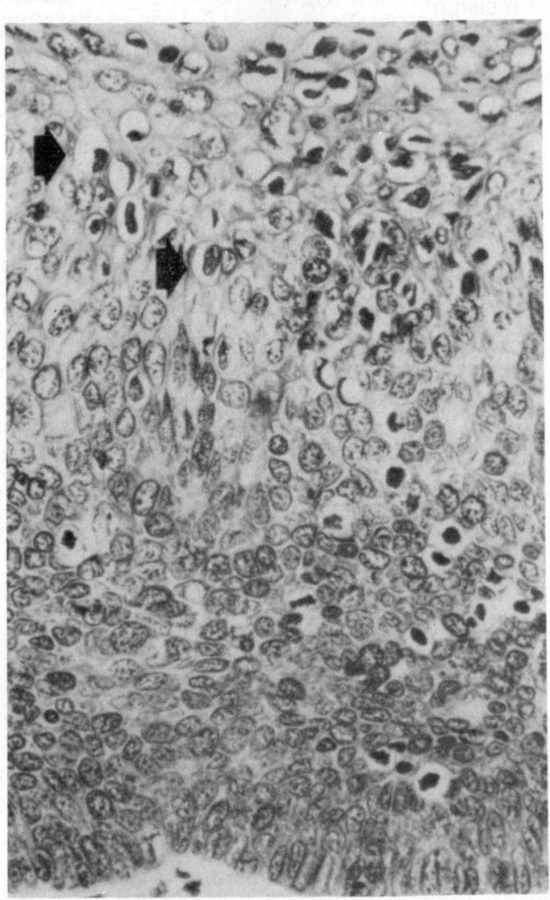

FIGURE 30-13
Vulvar intraepithelial neoplasia with koilocytosis. Lower half of lesion contains pleomorphism and abnormal mitoses. Upper half contains koilocytotic atypia with numerous halo cells (arrows). (From Crum PC, Liskow A, Petras P, et al: Cancer 54:1429, 1984.)

FIGURE 30-12
Frequency of involvement of contiguous structures by carcinoma in situ. (From Friedrich EG: Vulvar disease, 2nd ed. Philadelphia, W.B. Saunders Co., 1983.)

papillomavirus infection in vulvar biopsy specimens, whereas those with VIN accompanied by either koilocytosis or condyloma, produced by the papillomavirus, had a medium age of approximately 31 years. Invasive vulvar carcinoma occurred in five patients, all of whom were over the age of 45. This suggests that papillomavirus may be involved in the genesis of vulvar intraepithelial neoplasia, but the viral infection may not necessarily lead directly to vulvar carcinoma. The rates of progression from vulvar intraepithelial neoplasia to invasive carcinoma are not established. However, current evidence suggests that the potential of VIN to develop into invasive cancer is low. Buscema et al. followed 102 patients with vulvar carcinoma in situ for 1 to 15 years without treatment, and four patients developed invasive disease, two of whom were immunosuppressed. Unfortunately, current techniques do not allow prediction of which lesions of vulvar intraepithelial neoplasia are at the greatest risk for progression to invasive disease.

THERAPY. Current therapy involves eradication of all lesions of intraepithelial neoplasia of the vulva as well as venereal warts of the vulva (condyloma acuminata produced by the papillomavirus) once the diagnosis is established. Long-term follow-up is needed in view of the risk of recurrence of disease. As noted previously, the treatment is complicated by the fact that many lesions are multifocal, and wide and separate areas may be affected. Most lesions of intraepithelial neoplasia of the vulva tend to be posterior, predominantly in the perineal area. Surgical removal has been effectively used, but the type of operation has changed in recent years. In the past, simple vulvectomy was widely practiced to treat carcinoma in situ of the vulva, but this disfiguring operation is now infrequently used, particularly since the disease is occurring in younger women. To improve the cosmetic result and sexual function, Rutledge and Sinclair introduced the method of "skinning vulvectomy." This removes the superficial vulvar skin, preserving the clitoris, and replaces the removed skin with a split-thickness vulvar graft. In many cases, however, such extensive surgery is not needed, and the abnormal area of the vulva can often be removed with wide local excision. Sixty-two of the patients in the series reported by Buscema were treated with local excision; 68% showed no recurrence. For comparison, in 28 patients treated by vulvectomy, 70% showed no recurrence. The risk of recurrence is higher if neoplastic epithelium is found at the resection margin. Friedrich noted a 10% risk of recurrence if the surgical margins were free of disease in comparison to a 50% risk if the surgical margins were involved with neoplasia. However, since recurrence may develop even if the resection margins are negative, long-term follow-up is mandatory.

Alternatives to operations have been introduced. The carbon dioxide laser has recently been utilized to treat vulvar intraepithelial neoplasias. This results in eradication of the abnormal vulvar tissue and healing without scarring. Most patients require a single treatment, but some patients require two to four, particularly those with large or multiple lesions. A few patients can be treated on an outpatient basis with local anesthesia, but most require either general or regional anesthesia. Current evidence indicates that laser therapy is as effective as surgical excision in most situations, but some patients have needed an excision after laser treatment to control disease. It is essential to be certain that the patient does not have invasive disease before utilizing the laser. Therefore the therapist should be experienced in the diagnosis and treatment of vulvar disease before utilizing laser ablation. Treatment is usually carried out to a depth of 3 to 4 mm, and healing is usually complete within 2 to 3 weeks. Leuchter et al. treated 142 patients with carcinoma in situ of the vulva. Of the 42 treated by laser 17% had recurrence; 4 (25%) of the 16 treated with vulvectomy and 15 (33%) of 45 treated by local excision also had recurrence.

5-Fluorouracil (5-FU) cream has been used successfully to treat carcinoma in situ of the vulva. While such therapy has been reported to be successful in approximately 75% of the cases, the treatment causes severe vulvar edema and pain over a 6-week period; for that reason it is not usually prescribed.

Paget's Disease of the Vulva

Paget's disease is generally seen in postmenopausal women and appears grossly as a diffuse erythematous eczematoid lesion that has usually been present for a prolonged time. Itching is a common problem. The disease is primarily seen in whites, and the average age of the patient is approximately 65 years. The major importance of Paget's disease of the vulva is the frequent association with other invasive carcinomas. They may present as squamous carcinoma of the vulva or cervix or an adenocarcinoma of the sweat glands of the vulva or Bartholin's gland carcinoma. Cases of adenocarcinoma of the GI tract accompanying Paget's disease have also been reported. Once a diagnosis of Paget's disease of the vulva is made, it is important for the gynecologist to rule out the presence of malignancy at other sites, including the breast. In a review by Lee et al. a total of 75 cases of Paget's disease of the vulva were identified, and an underlying invasive carcinoma of the adnexal structures of the skin was reported in only 16 (22%) and a carcinoma in situ in 7 (9%). Twenty-two of the patients (29%) had cancer at distant sites, including adenocarcinoma of the rectum, carcinoma of the breast, carcinoma of the urethra, basal cell carcinoma of the skin, and carcinoma of the cervix.

If no primary malignancy is uncovered, a total vulvectomy is usually performed. It is important to remove the full thickness of the skin to the subcutaneous fat to be certain that all the skin adnexal structures are excised, as they may have a subclinical malignancy. As a rule, other forms of local therapy, such as the laser and 5-FU cream or local excision, have not been used for vulvar Paget's disease. However, insofar as the disease may recur and multiple surgical procedures can lead to extensive scarring, laser treatment or topical 5-FU has occasionally been tried. Even if resection margins are free of Paget's disease at the time of surgical excision, local recurrence remains a major risk. Those women who have been treated for Paget's disease of the vulva should have as part of their routine follow-up annual examination of the breast, cytologic evaluation of the cervix and vulva, and screening for gastrointestinal disease at least by testing for occult blood in the stool. Progression of Paget's disease of the vulva to invasive adenocarcinoma has been reported, but such cases are rare.

MALIGNANT CONDITIONS

Squamous Cell Carcinoma

Squamous cell carcinomas comprise approximately 90% of primary vulvar malignancies, but a variety of other vulvar cancers are encountered; the primary ones are listed in the box on p. 889. Melanomas account for about 4% to 5% and the other types for the remainder.

Morphology and Staging

Grossly, vulvar carcinomas usually appear as polypoid masses on the vulva (Fig. 30-14). Biopsy of the lesion reveals the characteristic histologic appearance of squamous cell carcinoma (Fig. 30-6, *C*).

Four clinical stages are defined for carcinoma of the vulva according to the International Federation of Gynecology and Obstetrics (FIGO), similar to the system used for other gynecologic malignancies. In addition, many centers use the T (tumor), N (nodes), M (metastases) classification; T denotes the size and extent of the tumor, N the clinical status of the nodes, and M the presence or absence of metastatic disease (see accompanying box, p. 890).

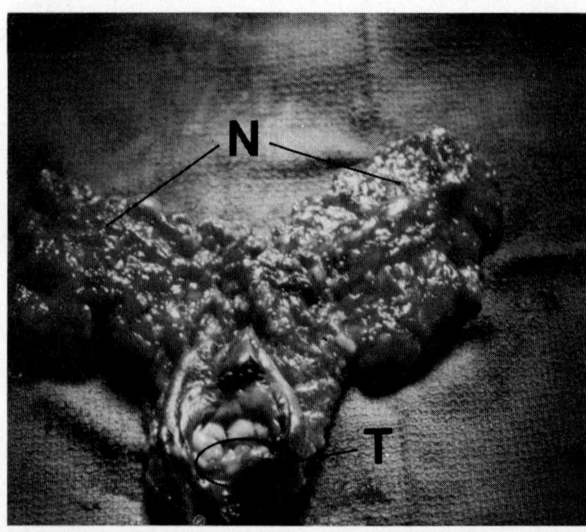

FIGURE 30-14
Radical vulvectomy specimen.

PRIMARY VULVAR MALIGNANCIES

Squamous cell carcinoma
Adenocarcinoma (including Bartholin's gland)
Verrucous carcinoma
Basal cell carcinoma
Melanoma
Sarcoma

Natural History, Spread, and Prognostic Factors

The vulvar area is rich in lymphatics with numerous cross connections. The main lymphatic pathways are illustrated in Fig. 30-15.

Tumors located in the middle of either labium tend to drain initially to the ipsilateral femoral-inguinal nodes, whereas perineal tumors can spread to either the left or the right side. Tumors in the clitoral or urethral areas can also spread to either side. From the inguinal-femoral nodes the lymphatic spread of tumor is cephalad to the deep pelvic iliac and obturator nodes. Although there has been concern in the past that tumors in the clitoral-urethral area would spread directly to the deep pelvic nodes, current evidence indicates that this rarely, if ever, occurs. The characteristics of lymph drainage of the vulva have recently been evaluated by Iverson and Aas, who injected ^{99m}Tc-colloid subcutaneously into the anterior and posterior labia majora, anterior and posterior labia minora, clitoral area, and perineum. They

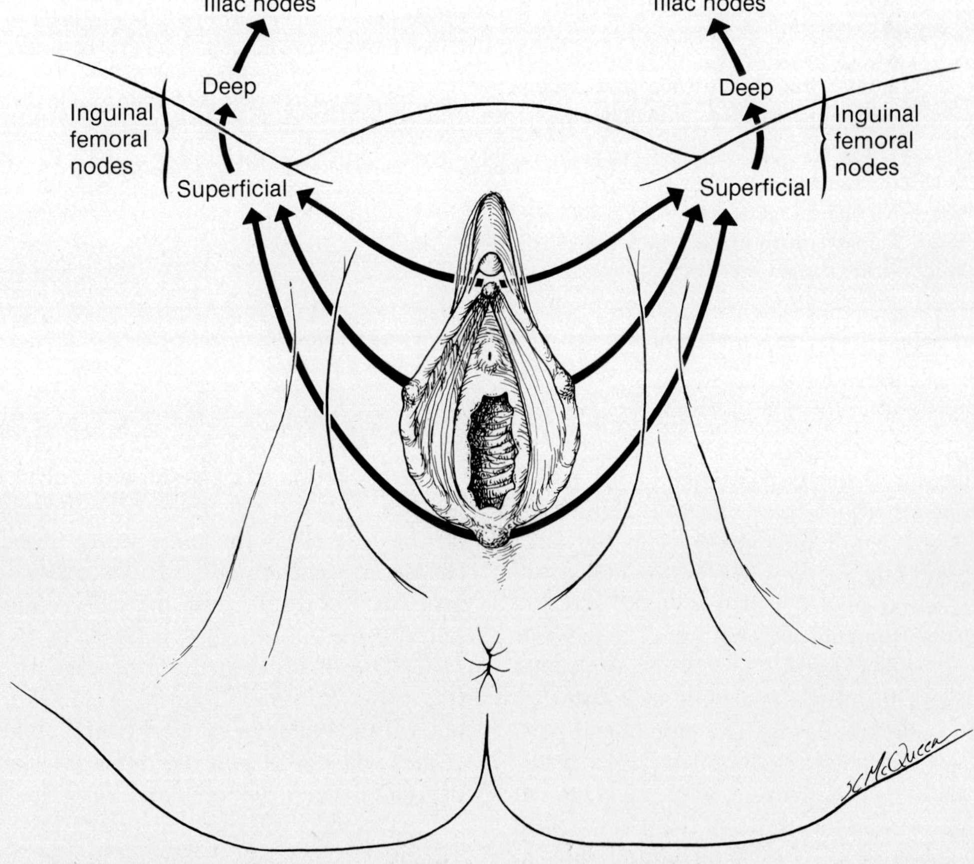

FIGURE 30-15
Vulva lymph drainage. General schematic representation of major drainage channels of vulva.

TNM AND STAGING CLASSIFICATIONS OF CARCINOMA OF THE VULVA

<table>
<tr><td valign="top">

TNM

T Primary tumor

Tis   Preinvasive carcinoma (carcinoma in situ)

T 1   Tumor confined to the vulva—2 cm or less in larger diameter

T 2   Tumor confined to the vulva—more than 2 cm in diameter

T 3   Tumor of any size with adjacent spread to the urethra, or vagina, or perineum, or anus or all of these

T 4   Tumor of any size infiltrating the bladder mucosa or the rectal mucosa or both including the upper part of the urethral mucosa or fixed to the anus

N Regional lymph nodes

N 0   No nodes palpable

N 1   Nodes palpable in either groin, not enlarged, mobile (not clinically suspicious of neoplasm)

N 2   Nodes palpable in either one or both groins, enlarged, firm, and mobile (clinically suspicious of neoplasm)

N 3   Fixed or ulcerated nodes

M Distant metastases

M 0   No clinical metastases

M 1a   Palpable deep pelvic lymph nodes

M 1b   Other distant metastases

</td><td valign="top">

Staging (FIGO)

Stage I:

All tumor confined to vulva with maximum diameter $\leq$2 cm. No nodes palpable ($T_1 \, N_0 \, M_0$) or nodes palpable not suspicious for neoplasm ($T_1N_1M_0$)

Stage II:

All tumor confined to vulva with maximum diameter >2 cm. Node status same as stage I ($T_2N_0M_0$ or $T_2N_1M_0$)

Stage III:

Tumor extending beyond limits of vulva to lower urethra or vagina or perineum or anus without suspicious nodes ($T_3N_1M_0$) or tumors with nodes suspicious for tumor ($T_1N_2M_0$), ($T_2N_2M_0$), ($T_3N_2M_0$)

Stage IV:

Tumor of any size invading mucosa of bladder or rectum or upper part of urethra or fixed to bone ($T_4N_0M_0$) or ($T_4N_1M_0$) or ($T_4N_2M_0$) or any tumor with fixed or ulcerated nodes (N_3) or with metastases (M_{1a}) or (M_{1b})

</td></tr>
</table>

then measured the radioactivity in the pelvic lymph nodes, which were surgically removed 5 hours later. From the injections in the labia majora and minora, over 98% of the radioactivity was found in the ipsilateral node and less than 2% on the contralateral side. The anterior labial injections resulted in 92% concentration of radioactivity in the ipsilateral side with 8% on the contralateral side. The clitoral and perineal injections developed a bilateral nodal distribution of radioactivity in all the patients. It is of interest that two thirds of the patients with labial injections had a small amount of detectable radioactivity in the contralateral nodes. Thus, anastomoses of the lymphatics do exist, but a direct connection from the clitoris to the deep nodes was not demonstrated.

The prognosis of a patient with vulvar carcinoma is related to the stage of the disease (Fig. 30-16), as well as the presence or absence of cancer in regional nodes. The worldwide five-year survival results from the *19th Annual Report on the Results of Treatment of Gynecologic Cancer* are stage I, 71%; stage II, 47%; stage III, 32%; and stage IV, 11%. The presence of carcinoma in regional lymph nodes correlates with the size of the primary lesion, the degree of tumor differentiation, and the extent of involvement of vascular spaces by tumor. Tumor size is usually estimated by the greatest tumor diameter; for example, $\leq$2 cm or >2 cm separates stage I from stage II disease. Moreover, in most series that record the depth of invasion, it has been noted that metastases to

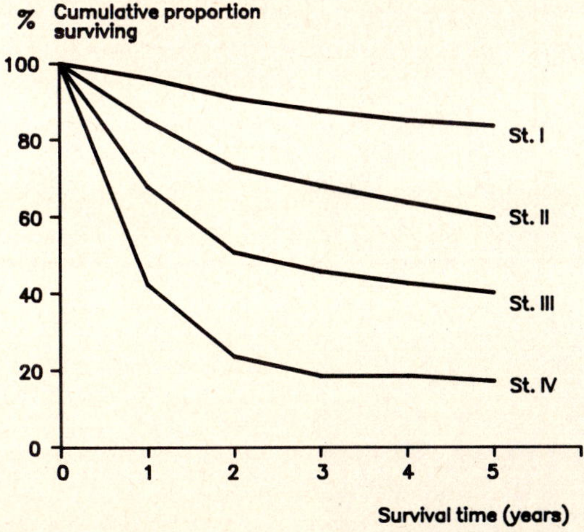

FIGURE 30-16
Stage and survival of carcinoma of vulva. (Adapted from the 19th Report on End Results of Therapy of Gynecologic Malignancies. Stockholm, International Federation of Gynecology and Obstetrics, 1985.)

TABLE 30-1
Correlation of Clinical and Pathologic Parameters in Vulvar Carcinoma—84 Cases

Factor	Cases	Positive Inguinal Nodes No.	%
Stage I	16	2	13
II	33	9	27
III	25	14	56
IV	5	5	100
Tumor diameter (cm)			
0-1.0	6	0	0
1.1-2.0	14	3	21
2.0-4.0	22	8	36
>4.0	29	16	55
Depth invasion (mm)			
1-3	15	0	0 ⎫ 8%
4-5	9	2	22 ⎭
6-10	28	13	46
>10	19	11	58
Vascular invasion			
Yes	9	7	77
No	65	22	34

Adapted from Boyce J, Fruchter RG, Kasombilides E, et al: Prognostic factors in carcinoma of the vulva. Gynecol Oncol 20:365, 1985.

regional nodes occur infrequently in tumors that invade to less than 5 mm. Both the smaller tumors and those that are well differentiated have the least tendency to spread to regional nodes. In a study of 153 patients, Figge et al. reported regional nodes to be involved by tumor in 13% of well-differentiated tumors, 20% of those of intermediate differentiation, and 35% of poorly differentiated tumors. Boyce et al. reported a direct correlation between tumor size (diameter), clinical stage, depth of invasion, and vascular invasion with involvement of regional nodes by tumor (Table 30-1). These factors also correlated with patient survival and the subsequent development of tumor recurrence.

In general, spread to regional nodes has been reported to vary from 0% to 10% in tumors with less than 5 mm invasion, but this statistic is affected by both tumor size and tumor grade. Depth of invasion, tumor diameter and differentiation, and involvement of vascular spaces are important considerations to define appropriate therapy for cancer of the vulva, particularly for "microinvasive" carcinoma (see below).

Stage IA: Carcinoma of the Vulva (Early or Microinvasive Carcinoma)

DEFINITION AND CLINICAL-PATHOLOGIC RELATIONSHIPS. The term *microinvasive carcinoma of the vulva* has no uniformly accepted definition. To identify early tumors unlikely to spread to regional nodes, many authorities have defined microinvasion as a small vulvar tumor less than 2 cm in diameter that invades less than 3 mm. However, varying clinicopathologic results are reported when this definition is used. For example, Hoffman et al. noted no nodal metastases among 43 patients whose tumors invaded less than 2 mm. They noted spread to regional nodes was less likely among tumors with individual tumor tongues spreading into the stroma rather than those that were confluent. In contrast Hacker et al. reported six of seven tumors with less than 3 mm invasion had spread to regional nodes.

Part of the confusion is due to different reference points from which the depth of invasion is measured, that is, from the surface or basement membrane. Dvoretsky et al. carefully an-

operation and treat the deep pelvic nodes only if the superficial nodes are involved with tumor. A frozen section is usually done at the time of operation to determine if there is tumor involvement of the high femoral nodes removed near the inguinal ligament.

Until recent times, radical vulvectomy and groin dissection were carried out through a single suprapubic incision that extended between the left and right anterior iliac spines and then an en bloc dissection in continuity with the radical vulvectomy. The operation removes the entire vulva, including the clitoris and subcutaneous tissues. For anteriorly located lesions the distal urethra must be removed occasionally, which can usually be accomplished without loss of urinary continence. However, wound breakdown and infection may affect up to 50% of patients undergoing radical vulvectomy. For that reason, modifications have been introduced to perform the inguinal-femoral node dissection through separate inguinal incisions and then complete the radical vulvectomy. Fig. 30-14 shows the type of specimen that can be obtained through separate groin incisions. It appears that an adequate surgical dissection with decreased wound complications can be accomplished by this technique. It is advisable to use suction drainage in the inguinal area until all drainage is complete, which usually takes 7 to 10 days, and drains are frequently also used in the vulvar area. Insofar as vulvar recurrences are the main problem, it is important that an adequate margin, usually 1 to 2 cm, be obtained around the primary tumor at the time of surgery. Tumor recurrence has occurred rarely in the skin bridge over the symphysis when separate groin incisions are used, without an en bloc dissection of the vulva and intervening lymph tissue.

In treating stage I and II tumors of the vulva, the results of histologic evaluation of the inguinal-femoral nodes are important. If these nodes do not contain metastatic tumor, no further therapy is given after the primary operation of radical vulvectomy and bilateral inguinal-femoral node dissection. If the lymph nodes, particularly the upper femoral group, are involved with tumor, then the deep pelvic nodes require treatment. This can be accomplished surgically by a retroperitoneal pelvic node dissection that is usually performed at the

time of primary surgery, if the patient's medical condition permits. Because these patients are often elderly, many therapists defer treatment of the pelvic nodes until after the primary incision has healed, at which time radiation therapy in the form of 4500 to 5000 rads to the deep pelvic nodes is prescribed, usually 4 to 6 weeks after operation.

The results of therapy in stage I and II disease relate not only to the stage of the disease but also to the status of the regional pelvic nodes. If the nodes do not contain metastatic tumor and the patient can be successfully treated by radical vulvectomy and bilateral node dissection, 5-year survivals of about 95% are reported. Recently Iverson et al. in a series of 424 patients with carcinoma of the vulva noted lymph node metastasis in 10.5% of stage I cases, 30% of stage II, 66% of stage III, and 100% of stage IV. The number of positive nodes in the radical vulvectomy specimen correlates with the size of the primary tumor and also with the patient's survival. In a study of 113 patients, Hacker et al. noted an actuarial 5-year survival of 96% for those with negative nodes, but there was a progressive fall in survival to 94% for those having one positive node; 80% for two positive nodes; and 12% for three or more positive nodes. In various cases that have been studied the deep pelvic nodes do not contain tumor unless the upper inguinal-femoral nodes contain metastatic disease. The number of nodes involved as well as the size of the metastasis are both important. Hoffman et al. noted that 14 of 15 patients with lymph node metastasis measuring less than 36 mm^2 survived free of disease 5 years in comparison to 12 of 29 whose lymph node metastases measured more than 100 mm^2. These results should be taken into consideration when planning additional therapy for patients with two positive nodes.

What form of therapy should be undertaken if the inguinal-femoral nodes contain tumor? A recent national cooperative randomized study of 118 patients suggests radiation is superior. Homesley et al. reported improved survival for those who received radiation (4500 to 5000 rads) to the deep pelvic nodes in comparison to those who had a pelvic node dissection.

The standard treatment for stage I and II carcinoma of the vulva and resectable stage III tumors that do not involve either the urethra or the anus is radical vulvectomy with bilateral inguinal-femoral lymphadenectomy. If the regional inguinal nodes are clinically positive for tumor and the patient is in good medical condition, a retroperitoneal node dissection may be added at the time of primary operation. If the nodes are not clinically involved, further therapy is dictated by the results of the final pathologic examination of the specimen. If only one node is microscopically involved with tumor, no further therapy is needed. However, if three or more nodes are involved, pelvic radiation as outlined is usually prescribed. For patients with only two nodes involved, the decision for further therapy will depend on the location of the node and the size of the metastatic deposit of tumor. However, 5-year survivals of 80% have been recorded for those with two positive nodes and 90% for those with one node, without further therapy beyond primary operation.

Advanced Vulvar Tumors

Large tumors of the vulva, particularly those that encroach on the anal-rectal area or the urethra, require more extensive treatment than radical vulvectomy to achieve effective tumor control. In such instances, removal of the anus or urethra is usually necessary as part of the primary procedure, in which case diversion of the urinary or fecal stream is required (see discussion of exenterative surgery for carcinoma of the cervix, Chapter 27). The best results are achieved by selecting patients with tumors that involve the urethra or anal areas that have not metastasized to regional nodes. Five-year survivals of approximately 50% have been reported. Because of the large defect created in the vulvar area, a gracilis myocutaneous flap from the leg is often applied to the vulvar area to aid in healing.

Alternative therapeutic approaches have been recently tried because of the morbidity associated with such extensive surgery in elderly patients and because of the necessity for diversion of the urine and feces. One effective regimen has been to initially treat the large vulvar tumor with external radiation and then, after the tumor has been reduced in size, remove it surgically, usually by radical vulvectomy with or without regional lymph node dissection. External radiation is used to deliver approximately 4000 rads to the tumor and 4500 rads to the pelvis and inguinal nodes. Operation is usually performed about 5 weeks after the completion of radiation therapy. Although a large series of patients have not been treated by this technique, a sufficient number have been treated to demonstrate that marked tumor regression does occur. The primary cancer can be eradicated by an operation that does not require diversion of the urine or feces. Boronow summarized the treatment of 26 patients with primary carcinoma of the vaginal vulvar area with this technique and noted a 5-year survival of 80%. Complications included stenosis of the introitus, urethral stenosis, and rectovaginal fistulas. This technique does appear to be an effective alternative to primary exenteration for large vulvar vaginal carcinomas.

Radiation Therapy and Recurrences

In a few instances the medical condition of the patient precludes operation, and radiation therapy may be employed as the sole treatment. However, the vulvar skin is prone to radiation dermatitis fibrosis and ulceration, making irradiation, as the sole form of therapy, a less desirable treatment of these tumors. Therefore irradiation is seldom used as the sole treatment of carcinoma of the vulva.

As may be expected, the risk of recurring carcinoma rises as the stage of the disease increases. Podratz et al. in an analysis of 224 patients with vulvar carcinoma noted a recurrence rate of 14% in stage I and 71% in stage IV. Local vulvar recurrences were the most common and occurred in 40 of 74 cases of recurrence (54%). The remaining recurrences were in the groin, pelvis, or distant sites. Radiation therapy or additional operations for local vulvar recurrences usually provide effective control and 5-year survivals of approximately 50%. The risk of recurrence of the disease in the vulva requires careful attention to the surgical resection margins at the time of initial operation. Treatment of patients with disseminated disease requires chemotherapy but, unfortunately, no chemotherapeutic regimen has been successful in this disease. Squamous cell carcinomas of the female genital tract have generally not been responsive to cytotoxic chemotherapy, and the protocols followed are similar to those described for recurrent squamous cell carcinomas of the cervix (Chapter 27).

Other Vulvar Malignancies

Bartholin's Gland Carcinoma

These are adenocarcinomas which compromise about 1% to 2% of vulvar carcinomas. An enlargement of Bartholin's gland in a postmenopausal patient should raise suspicion for this malignancy. These tumors are treated similarly to primary squamous cell carcinoma of the vulva, and radical vulvectomy with bilateral inguinal-femoral lymphadenectomy is the treatment of choice. If the regional lymph nodes are free of tumor, the prognosis is good.

Basal Cell Carcinoma

Basal cell carcinomas can arise in the vulva as they can arise in the skin elsewhere in the body. They are rare and comprise about 2% of vulvar carcinomas. Therapy consists of wide local excision of the lesion, which is generally ulcerated. If the surgical resection margins are free of tumor, the disease is cured.

Verrucous Carcinoma

Verrucous carcinomas of the vulva are also rare. They are a special variant of squamous cell cancer with distinctive histologic features. Clinically they appear as a large condylomatous mass on the vulva. Histologically they consist of mature squamous cells and extensive keratinization with nests that invade the underlying vulvar tissue. It is often necessary to perform multiple biopsies of the condylomatous lesion to establish a diagnosis of malignancy. Radiation therapy is ineffective, can worsen the prognosis, and is therefore contraindicated for these tumors. The treatment is surgical.

In 24 cases of verrucous carcinoma Japaze et al. noted no lymph node metastases. Some of the primary tumors were as large as 10 cm in diameter. Recurrences developed in nine of the patients, five of whom had prior irradiation. Wide local excision is usually effective

therapy. Depending on the size and location of the tumor, simple vulvectomy may be needed, but a radical vulvectomy or inguinal node dissection is not indicated. The 17 cases treated surgically and reported by Japaze et al. had a 5-year survival of 94%.

Melanoma

Melanoma is the most frequent nonsquamous cell malignancy of the vulva. It comprises about 5% of primary cancers of this area. As is true elsewhere in the body, melanomas arise from junctional or compound nevi. Pigmented lesions of the vulva are usually junctional nevi, and all such lesions should be removed by excision.

Patients with malignant melanoma of the vulva vary widely in age from their late teens to women in their eighties. The average age is approximately 50 years. Clinically, melanomas appear as brown, black, or blue-black masses on the vulva. The lesion can be flat or ulcerated. Occasionally it is nodular, and small darkly pigmented areas (satellite nodules) may surround the primary lesion. Occasionally the melanomas may be without pigment and can grossly resemble squamous cell carcinoma of

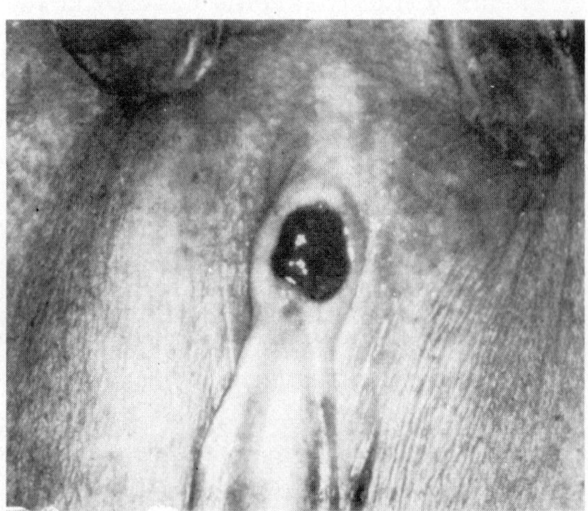

FIGURE 30-18
Nodular melanoma arising directly from glans clitoris. (Courtesy J. McL. Morris, M.D., John Slade Ely Professor of Gynecology, Yale University School of Medicine, New Haven, Connecticut.)

the vulva. Most melanomas of the vulva occur on the labia minora or the clitoris (Fig. 30-18).

The standard therapy for vulvar melanoma has been radical vulvectomy and bilateral inguinal-femoral node dissection. Since the tumors are rare, a single large clinical experience is not available. It has been previously believed that melanoma of the vulva can metastasize to pelvic nodes, bypassing the inguinal femoral nodes; recent series have not demonstrated pelvic node involvement without inguinal node involvement. A further therapeutic consideration is that patients with melanoma whose pelvic nodes are involved with tumor do not usually survive the disease. Thus current practice is to do radical vulvectomy and bilateral groin dissection with pelvic node dissection added only if there is evidence of inguinal femoral node involvement at primary operation.

Vulvar melanomas are staged using the FIGO classification employed for squamous carcinomas (Table 30-1). However, recent evidence indicates that staging is not as useful a prognostic indicator as is the depth of invasion. A system for vulvar melanoma analogous to that used by Clark for cutaneous melanomas have been adopted. Five levels (I to V) have been defined based on the Clark classification. Fig. 30-19 shows the depth of invasion for each level of superficial spreading melanoma and nodular melanoma, the two most common varieties of melanomas that occur on the vulva. Superficial spreading melanoma is more common and fortunately has a better prognosis, with a 5-year survival of 71% reported in the series by Podratz et al. The 5-year survival for nodular melanoma, which is more invasive, was only 38%. The level of invasion correlates with survival, which varies from 100% for level II, to 83% for level IV, to 28% for level V.

Tumor thickness is also useful to evaluate the tumor. Breslow et al. reported that overall prognosis is excellent and spread to regional node is not likely for melanomas whose thickness measured from the surface epithelium to the deepest point of penetration is less than

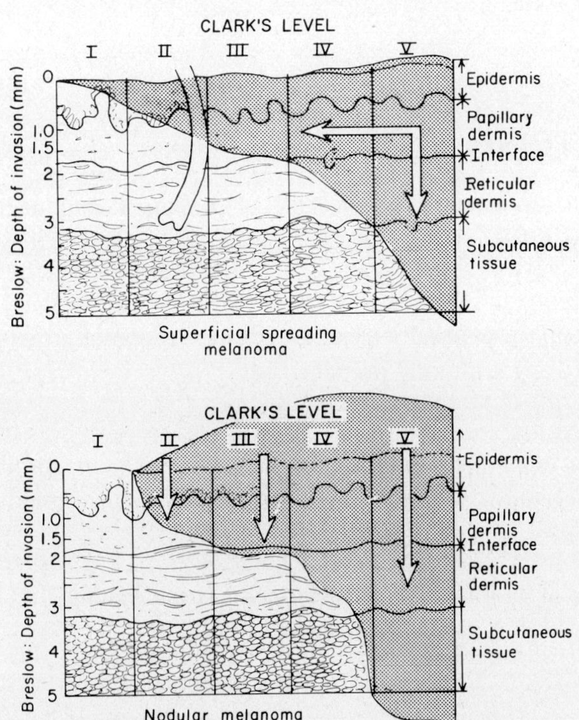

FIGURE 30-19
Level of invasion for superficial spreading melanoma and nodular melanoma. (From Podratz KC, Gaffey TA, Symmonds RE, et al: Gynecol Oncol 16:153, 1983.)

0.76 mm. Most of these lesions would correspond to level I or level II penetration by the modified Clark system. Such melanomas can probably be safely treated by wide local excision without inguinal-femoral node dissection. Although long-term results are not available, the 5-year survival has been reported to be 100% in tumors satisfying these criteria. Radical vulvectomy and inguinal node dissection are needed for more extensive tumors. The prognosis is poor for patients with melanomas more than 3 mm thick. If the regional lymph nodes are negative, survival will be greater than 60%, but it drops to less than 30% if they are involved with tumor. Most series of malignant melanoma report overall survivals of approximately 50%.

Distant metastases are frequently noted, and no effective program of chemotherapy has been described. Regressions (but not cures) have been reported with various multiagent cytotoxic programs. Current efforts are devoted to developing an effective program of immunotherapy, particularly in view of the occasional favorable responses reported with agents such as BCG.

Sarcoma

Sarcomas of the vulva are extremely rare. Twelve cases were reported by DiSaia et al., and surgical removal of the primary tumor is the treatment of choice. Chemotherapeutic considerations are the same as those for sarcomas of other sites in the female genital tract.

Granular Cell Myoblastomas

Granular cell myoblastoma is also an extremely rare tumor that is almost invariably benign but does morphologically show pleomorphism. Local excision is generally sufficient therapy. The tumor appears as a solitary, firm, nontender, slowly growing nodule in the subcutaneous tissue of the vulva.

KEY POINTS

- Squamous cell carcinoma comprise 90% of primary vulvar malignancies. More than half the patients are over 60 years of age at the time of diagnosis.

- Vulvar dystrophies are usually treated with medication after appropriate diagnosis on biopsy. They are rarely premalignant.

- Paget's disease generally occurs in postmenopausal women and is usually treated by simple vulvectomy. Invasive carcinomas at other sites should be ruled out.

- Prolonged use of fluorinated corticosteroids to treat itching accompanying vulvar dystrophy can lead to vulvar contraction.

- Topical testosterone is often beneficial to treat lichen sclerosus but is absorbed systemically and occasionally can produce masculinizing symptoms.

- Intraepithelial neoplasia of the vulva is usually treated by local excision or laser therapy of the atypical area.

- Unilateral vulvar tumors are more likely to metastasize to ipsilateral inguinal-femoral nodes, but contralateral metastases also occur.

- The deep pelvic nodes do not become involved with metastatic vulvar cancer unless the inguinal-femoral nodes are affected.

- Most patients with cancer of the vulva are treated by radical vulvectomy and bilateral inguinal-femoral node dissection. The 5-year survival of those with negative nodes is over 95%. With one positive node the 5-year survival is approximately the same, that is, 94%; with two nodes it decreases to 80%; with three or more, to 12%.

- The worldwide 5-year survival for carcinoma of the vulva by stage is I, 71%; II, 47%; III, 32%; and IV, 11%.

- Verrucous carcinomas are a variant of squamous cancer that does not metastasize to regional nodes. Radiation therapy is contraindicated, and local surgical extirpation is utilized.

- The overall 5-year survival of patients with vulvar melanoma is about 50%.

- Superficial spreading melanomas have a better prognosis than nodular melanomas.

- Prognosis of vulvar melanoma is related to tumor invasion (level) and to tumor thickness.

- Basal cell carcinoma of the vulva is treated by wide local excision.

BIBLIOGRAPHY

Boronow RC: Combined therapy as an alternative to exenteration of locally advanced vulvar vaginal cancer. Cancer 49:1085, 1982.

Boyce J, Fruchter RG, Kasambilides E, et al: Prognostic factors in carcinoma of the vulva. Gynecol Oncol 20:364, 1985.

Breslow A: Thickness, cross-sectional areas, and depth of invasion in the prognosis of cutaneous melanoma. Ann. Surg. 172:908, 1970.

Buscema J, Woodruff JD, Parmley TH, et al: Carcinoma in situ of the vulva. Obstet Gynecol 55:225, 1980.

Cavanagh D, Shephard JH: The place of pelvic exenteration and primary management of advanced carcinoma of the vulva. Gynecol Oncol 13:318, 1982.

Christopherson W, Buchsbaum HJ, Vort R, et al: Radical vulvectomy and bilateral groin lymphadenectomy utilizing separate groin incisions: Report of a case with recurrence in the intervening skin bridge. Gynecol Oncol 21:247, 1985.

Chu J, Tamimi HK, Ek M, et al: Stage I vulvar cancer: Criteria for microinvasion. Obstet Gynecol 59:716, 1982.

Crum PC, Liskow A, Petras P, et al: Vulvar intraepithelial neoplasia (severe atypia and carcinoma in situ). Cancer 54:1429, 1984.

DiSaia PJ, Rutledge F, Smith JP: Sarcoma of the vulva—report of 12 patients. Obstet Gynecol 38:180, 1971.

Donaldson ES, Powell DE, Hanson MB, et al: Prognostic parameters in invasive vulvar cancer. Gynecol Oncol 11:184, 1981.

Dvoretsky PM, Bonfiglio TA, Helkamp BF, et al: The pathology of superficially invasive thin vulva squamous cell carcinoma. Int J Gynecol Pathol 3:331, 1984.

Farey RN, McKay PA, Benedet JL: Radiation treatment of carcinoma of the vulva, 1950-1980. Am J Obstet Gynecol 151:591, 1985.

Figge DC, Tamimi HK, Greer BE: Lymphatic spread in carcinoma of the vulva. Am J Obstet Gynecol 152:387, 1985.

Franklin EW III, Rutledge F: Epidemiology of epidermoid carcinoma of the vulva. Obstet Gynecol 39:165, 1972.

Friedrich EG: Reversible vulvar atypia: A case report. Obstet Gynecol 39:173, 1972.

Friedrich EG: Vulvar disease, 2nd ed. Philadelphia, W.B. Saunders Co., 1983.

Friedrich EG, Wilkinson EJ, Steingraber PH, et al: Paget's disease of the vulva and carcinoma of the breast. Obstet Gynecol 46:130, 1975.

Friedrich EF, Wilkinson EJ, Fu YS: Carcinoma-in-situ of the vulva: A continuing challenge. Am J Obstet Gynecol 136:830, 1980.

Fu YS, Reagan JW, Townsend DE, et al: Nuclear DNA study of vulvar intraepithelial and invasive squamous neoplasms. Obstet Gynecol 57:643, 1981.

Hacker NF, Nieburg RK, Berek JS, et al: Superficially invasive vulvar cancer with nodal metastases. Gynecol Oncol 15:65, 1983.

Hacker NF, Berek JS, Lagasse LD, et al: Management of regional lymph nodes and their prognostic influence in vulvar cancer. Obstet Gynecol 61:408, 1983.

Hart WR, Norris HJ, Helwig ED: Relation of lichen sclerosus et atrophicus of the vulva to development of carcinoma. Obstet Gynecol 45:369, 1975.

Helwig EP, Graham JH: Anogenital (extramammary) Paget's disease. Cancer 16:387, 1963.

Hoffman JS, Kumar NB, Morley GW: Microinvasive squamous cell carcinoma of the vulva: A search for definition. Obstet Gynecol 61:615, 1983.

Hoffman JS, Kumar NB, Morley GW: Prognostic significance of groin lymph node metastases of squamous carcinoma of the vulva. Obstet Gynecol 66:402, 1985.

Homesley HD, Bundy BN, Sedlis A, Adcock L: A randomized study of radiation therapy versus pelvic node resection for patients with invasive squamous cell carcinoma of the vulva having positive groin nodes. (A Gynecologic Oncology Study Group). Obstet Gynecol 68:733, 1986.

Husseinzadeh N, Zaino R, Nahhas WA, et al: The significance of histologic findings in predicting nodal metastases in invasive squamous cell carcinoma of the vulva. Gynecol Oncol 16:105, 1983.

International Society for the Study of Vulvar Disease: New nomenclature for vulvar disease. Obstet Gynecol 47:122, 1976.

Iverson T, Aas M: Lymph drainage from the vulva. Gynecol Oncol 16:179, 1983.

Iverson T, Abler V, Aalder J: Individual treatment of stage I carcinoma of the vulva. Obstet Gynecol 57:85, 1981.

Iverson T, Elders JG, Christensen A, et al: Squamous cell carcinoma of the vulva: Review of 424 patients, 1957-1974. Gynecol Oncol 9:271, 1980.

Japaze H, Dinh TV, Woodruff JD: Verrucous carcinoma of the vulva: Study of 24 cases. Obstet Gynecol 60:462, 1982.

Jaramillo BA, Ganjei P, Averette HE, et al: Malignant melanoma of the vulva. Obstet Gynecol 66:398, 1985.

Kaufman RH, Gardner HJ, Merrill JA: Diseases of the vulva and vagina. In Romney SL, et al, eds: Gynecology and obstetrics. New York, McGraw-Hill Book Co., 1980.

Kneale BL, Cavanagh D, DiPaola GR, et al: Microinvasive cancer of the vulva: Report of the ISSVD task force. J Reprod Med 29:454, 1984.

Lee SC, Roth LM, Ehrlich C, et al: Extramammary Paget's disease of the vulva—a clinicopathologic study of 13 cases. Cancer 39:2540, 1977.

Leuchter RS, Hacker NF, Voet RL, et al: Primary carcinoma of the Bartholin gland: A report of 14 cases and review of the literature. Obstet Gynecol 60:361, 1982.

Leuchter RS, Townsend DE, Hacker NF, et al: Treatment of vulvar carcinoma in situ with the CO_2 laser. Gynecol Oncol 19:314, 1984.

Lieb SM, Gallousis S, Freedman H: Granular cell myoblastoma of the vulva. Gynecol Oncol 8:12, 1979.

Mabuchi K, Bross DS, Kessler II: Epidemiology of cancer of the vulva: A case-control study. Cancer 55:1843, 1985.

Menczer J, Voliovitch Y, Modan B, et al: Some epidemiologic aspects of carcinoma of the vulva in Israel. Am J Obstet Gynecol 143:893, 1982.

Morrow CP: Melanoma of the female genital tract. In Coppleson M, ed: Gynecologic oncology. Edinburgh, Churchill Livingstone, 1981.

Phillips GL, Twiggs LB, Okagaki T: Vulvar melanoma: A microstaging study. Gynecol Oncol 14:80, 1982.

Plentl AA, Friedman EA: Lymphatic system of the female genitalia. Philadelphia, W.B. Saunders Co., 1971.

Podratz KC, Gaffey TA, Symmonds RE, et al: Melanoma of the vulva: An update. Gynecol Oncol 16:153, 1983.

Podratz KC, Symmonds RE, Taylor WF: Carcinoma of the vulva and vagina. In Coppelson M, ed: Gynecologic oncology. New York, Churchill Livingstone, 1981.

Reid R: Superficial laser vulvectomy. III. A new surgical technique for appendage conserving ablation of refractory condylomas and vulvar intraepithelial neoplasia. Am J Obstet Gynecol 152:504, 1985.

Ridley JH: Gynecologic surgery: Errors, safeguards, salvage. Baltimore, Williams & Wilkins, 1974.

Rutledge F, Sinclair M: Treatment of intraepithelial neoplasia of the vulva by skin excision and graft. Obstet Gynecol 102:806, 1968.

Skinner MS, Sternberg WH, Ichinose H, et al: Spontaneous regression of Bowenoid atypia of the vulva. Obstet Gynecol 42:40, 1973.

Woodruff JD, Genadry R, Poliakoff S: Treatment of dyspareunia and vaginal outlet distortions by perineoplasty. Obstet Gynecol 57:750, 1981.

Woodruff JD, Julian CS: Surgery of the vulva. In Ridley JH: Gynecologic surgery: Errors, safeguards, salvage. Baltimore, The Williams & Wilkins Co., 1974.

Premalignant and Malignant Diseases of the Vagina

KEY TERMS AND DEFINITIONS

Clear Cell Adenocarcinoma. A vaginal or cervical malignancy occurring primarily after 14 years of age. It is often associated with prenatal exposure to diethylstilbestrol.

Endodermal Sinus Tumor. A rare adenocarcinoma of the vagina occurring in infants less than 2 years of age. It is usually fatal.

Field Defect. The propensity of squamous epithelium of the lower genital tract (cervix, vagina, and vulva) to undergo premalignant change.

Laser (Light Amplification by Stimulated Emission of Radiation). An energized source of light that can be used to vaporize tissue and to treat intraepithelial neoplasia.

Pelvic Exenteration. An extensive pelvic operation usually employed to treat a central pelvic recurrence of cervical carcinoma after radiation. A total exenteration involves removal of the bladder, uterus, cervix, and rectum. An anterior exenteration spares the rectum, while a posterior exenteration spares the bladder.

Pseudosarcoma Botryoides. A benign tumor occurring in the vagina of infants and pregnant women that has a polypoid shape. Mi-

croscopically it may be confused with sarcoma botryoides.

Sarcoma Botryoides. A rare, often fatal, malignancy of the vagina that occurs in infants and children.

Vaginal Tumor Stage. A clinical classification that describes the extent of spread of vaginal carcinoma:
Stage I. Limited to vaginal wall.
Stage II. Extends to subvaginal tissue.
Stage III. Reaches the pelvic wall.
Stage IV. Extends beyond the true pelvis or into mucosa of the bladder or rectum.

VAIN-1. Vaginal intraepithelial neoplasia of the least severe type (comparable to mild dysplasia), usually occupying the lower one third of the epithelium.

VAIN-2. Vaginal intraepithelial neoplasia of intermediate severity (comparable to moderate dysplasia), usually occupying the lower two thirds of the epithelium.

VAIN-3. Vaginal intraepithelial neoplasia of the most severe type (comparable to severe dysplasia and carcinoma in situ), usually replacing the full thickness of the epithelium.

Premalignant changes in the vagina appear as intraepithelial squamous atypicalities and occur less frequently than comparable lesions in the cervix and vulva. However, the histologic appearance of intraepithelial neoplasia of the vagina is similar to that described for the cervix (Chapter 26). These changes are also similarly designated as dysplasia (mild, moderate, or se-

vere) and carcinoma in situ. The term *VAIN* (vaginal, *VA*; intraepithelial, *I*; neoplasia, *N*) has been used to describe these histologic changes; the comparable categories are VAIN-1 (mild dysplasia), VAIN-2 (moderate dysplasia), and VAIN-3 (severe dysplasia to carcinoma in situ). The cytologic and histologic features of these changes are illustrated in Fig. 31-1.

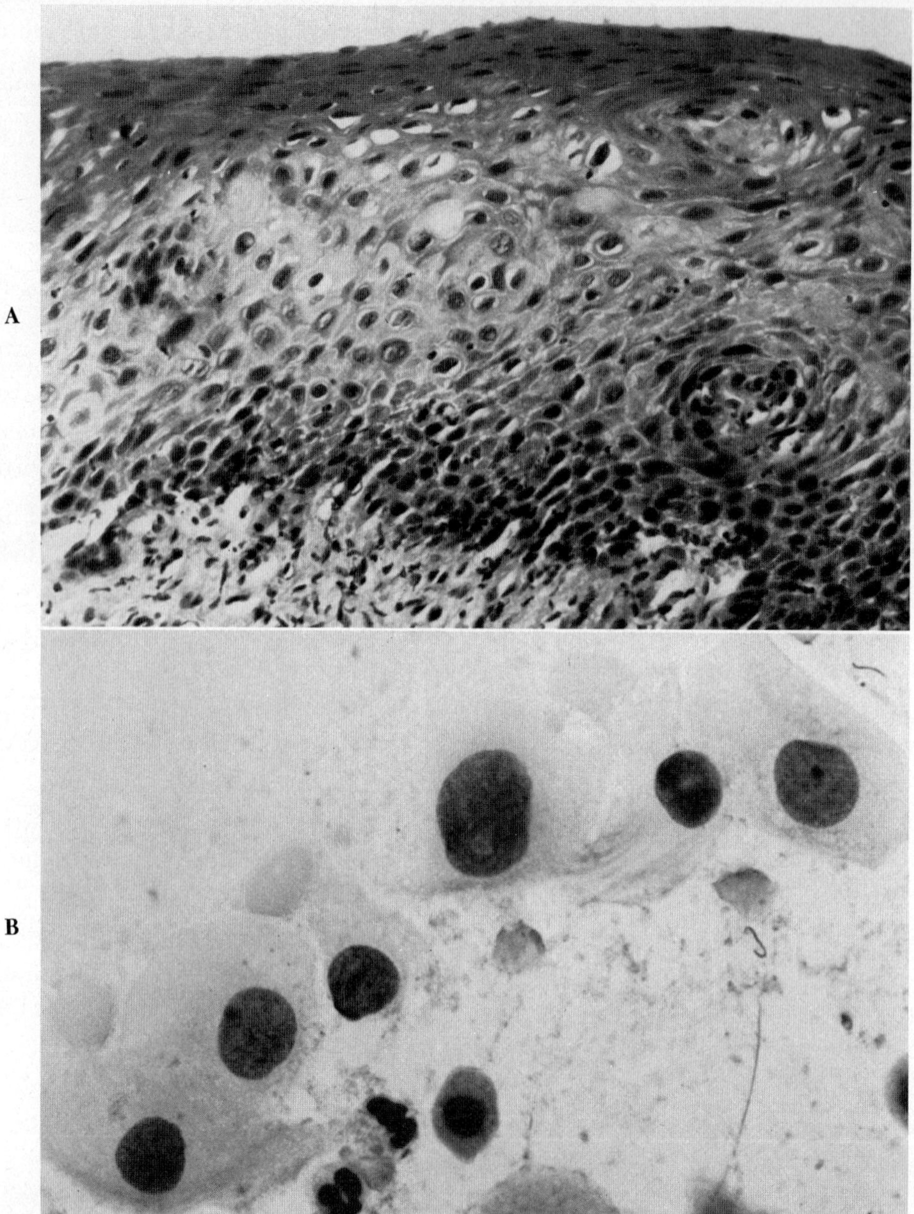

FIGURE 31-1

A, Section of vagina showing dysplasia. Epithelium appears thickened and shows abnormal maturation. Immature, hyperchromatic cells occupy lower two to four layers. Middle and upper third of mucosa show evidence of cytoplasmic differentiation with well-defined cellular borders. Nuclei in these areas are enlarged and pleomorphic. Parakeratosis is apparent on surface. Because immature cells are confined to lower third mucosa, dysplasia is classified as mild. (H&E stain; ×250.) **B,** Cytologic specimen showing mild dysplasia. Note sheet of dysplastic cells. Cells show well-defined cytoplasmic borders. Nuclei are enlarged, and nuclear contour is smooth. Chromatin is uniformly, finely granular. Focal condensations of chromatin (chromocenters) are present in some nuclei. Nucleoli are not present. (Papanicolaou stain; ×1000.)

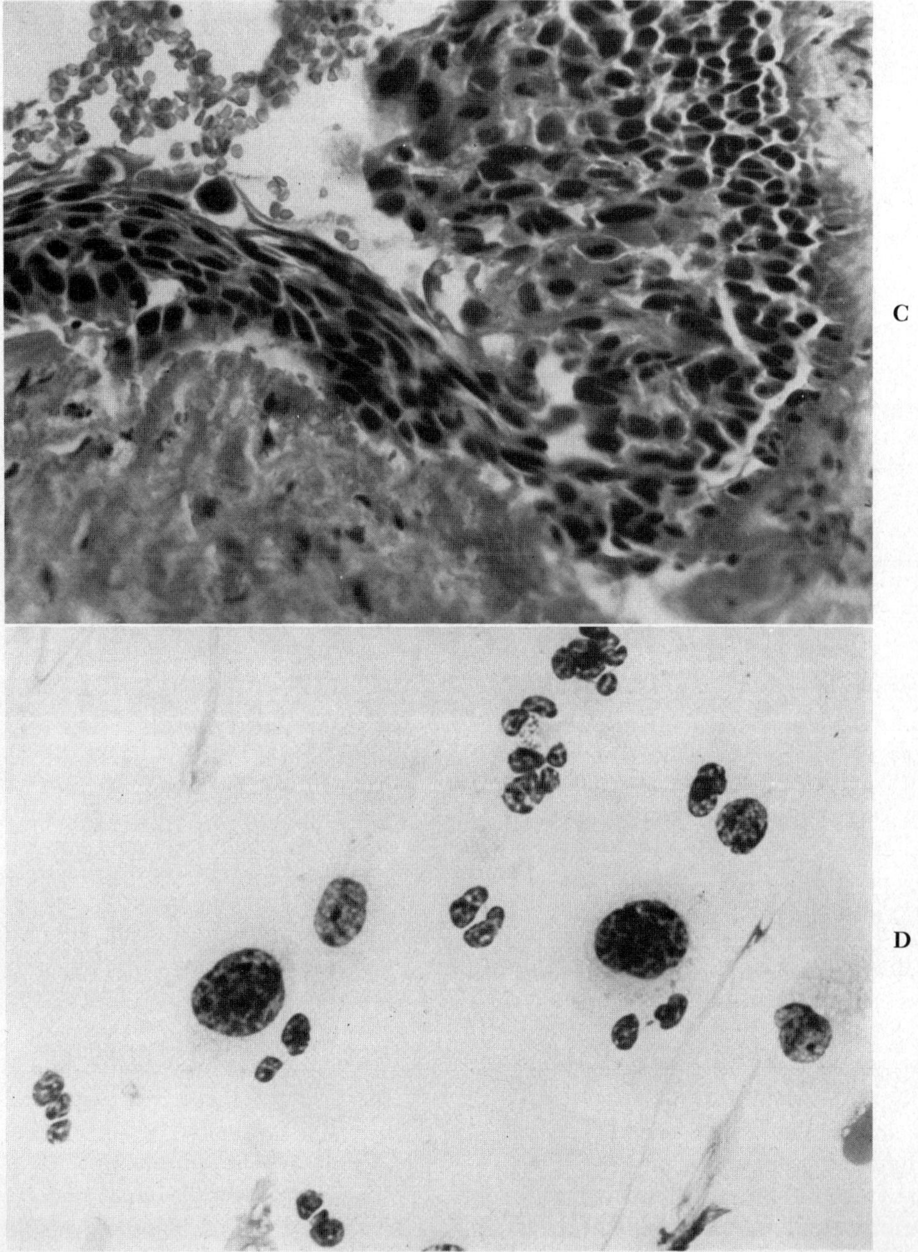

FIGURE 31-1, cont'd

C, Section showing severe dysplasia to carcinoma in situ. Entire epithelial thickness is occupied by hyperchromatic, dysplastic cells. Marked nuclear variation and mitoses are seen. Because of occasional cells with squamous differentiation (spindle-shaped cells, cells with well-defined cytoplasmic borders) in superficial layers this lesion is sometimes classified as severe dysplasia. In carcinoma in situ immature cells replace the full thickness, and there is no evidence of squamous differentiation on the surface. (H&E stain; ×400.) **D,** Cytologic specimen showing carcinoma in situ. Several isolated immature cells with high nuclear cytoplasmic ratio and poorly defined cytoplasmic borders can be seen. Chromatin is coarsely granular, and no nucleoli are present. In background are several polymorphonuclear leukocytes and strings of mucus. (Papanicolaou stain; ×1000.) *Continued.*

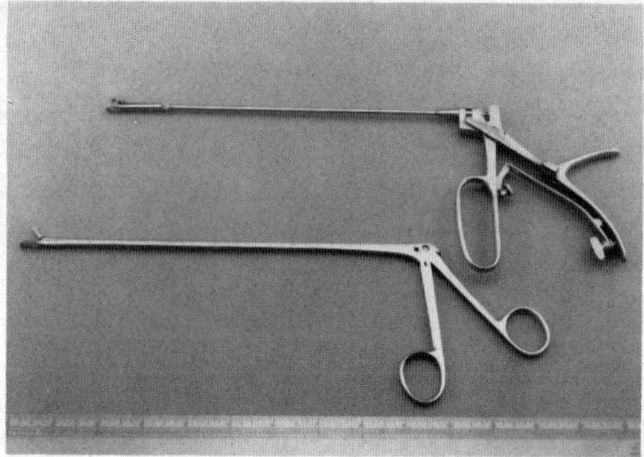

FIGURE 31-2
Eppendorf *(upper)* and Kevorkian *(lower)* punch biopsy instruments.

itself. A less precise method for identifying an area for biopsy is to stain the vaginal epithelium with half-strength Lugol's solution and to take a biopsy specimen from the nonstaining areas. The vaginal epithelium must be adequately estrogenized so that sufficient epithelial glycogen is present for the normal tissue to stain dark brown. Local estrogen cream used for 1 week before examination is frequently helpful in postmenopausal patients and in patients with severe atrophic vaginitis in which atypical cells are first detected on cytologic (Pap) smear.

It is important for the examiner to realize that vaginal neoplasia is often multifocal. While the process is frequently located in the vaginal apex, it can occur anywhere along the vaginal tube, necessitating examination of the vagina in its entirety.

Management

As in the case of the cervix, the abnormal epithelium must be completely eradicated. Small lesions, particularly those at the vaginal apex in patients who have undergone hysterectomy, usually are excised locally. However, excision of large areas may require skin grafting, and for that reason, other therapeutic modalities are often chosen.

Alternative nonsurgical treatment modalities are also directed toward destruction of all the abnormal epithelium. Radiation therapy, although used in the past, often leads to scarring and fibrosis and is generally not currently rec-

ommended for treatment of noninvasive disease. Because of the proximity of the bladder and rectum and the availability of newer modalities, cryotherapy is not used as frequently today as in the past. Widely used nonsurgical approaches include the laser, which is most commonly employed, or 5-fluorouracil (5-FU) cream for widespread lesions, particularly those with papillomavirus infection.

The carbon dioxide laser allows vaporization of the abnormal tissue. The beam is directed colposcopically. Iodine staining of the vagina can also outline those areas requiring therapy. Treatment is frequently performed on an outpatient basis with a local anesthetic or analgesic, or both. If the lesions are extensive, general or regional anesthesia may be required. The intensity of therapy is regulated by adjusting the wattage of the laser, most commonly 15 to 20 watts if carried to a depth of 2 to 4 mm. The patient will experience a discharge for a few days after therapy. Healing usually requires a few weeks. Although long-term experience and follow-up with laser treatment of vaginal neoplasia is not available, preliminary results reported by Petrilli et al. show success rates on the order of 90%. Regular follow-up every 4 months, including a Pap smear and colposcopy, is required during the first year and usually 6 to 12 months thereafter.

Five percent 5-FU cream should be used for approximately 7 days. One half of a vaginal applicator (approximately 5 g) is inserted into the vagina nightly. Because the cream is irritating, some protective ointment such as zinc oxide should be applied to the vulva. If excess leakage occurs, less than half of an applicator should be used. In addition, the treatment should be discontinued before 7 days if the patient notes excessive irritation. A cycle of therapy should be repeated in 3 to 4 weeks if the intraepithelial process persists. In some cases the application of 5-FU is continued for 10 to 14 days, in which case the nontherapy interval is increased to 2 or 3 months. Lesions with a thickened white crust (hyperkeratosis) appear to be less sensitive to this treatment. On the other hand, postmenopausal women tolerate only small doses of 5-FU, presumably because of the comparative thinness of the vaginal epithelium. Ballon et al. and Petrilli et al. reported success rates of 80% to 90% after multiple treatment cycles; the method appears particularly useful for patients with multifocal diffuse lesions. Follow-up includes repeat Pap smears and colposcopy every 3 to 4 months during the first year and 6 to 12 months thereafter. Depending on the location and extent of the lesions, recurrences can be treated with repeat laser therapy. If the patient cannot tolerate these repeated treatments or the lesion is not accessible by laser, local excision is usually done.

MALIGNANT DISEASE OF THE VAGINA

Symptoms and Diagnosis

Primary vaginal cancers are rare, constituting less than 2% of all gynecologic malignancies, and usually occur as squamous cell carcinomas in women over the age of 50 years. To be considered a primary vaginal tumor, the malignancy must arise in the vagina and not involve the external os of the cervix superiorly or the vulva inferiorly. Otherwise the tumor is classified as cervical or vulvar. This is also an important therapeutic consideration insofar as the same management techniques apply to small tumors of the upper one third of the vagina and cervical carcinomas. Tumors of the lower one-third of the vagina are treated similarly to vulvar cancers (Chapter 30). Table 31-2 lists the staging criteria for vaginal cancers according to the International Federation of Gynecology and Obstetrics.

Delay in the diagnosis of these cancers frequently occurs, in part because of their rarity as well as because of a lack of recognition that the abnormal symptoms may be due to a malignancy. The most common symptom of vaginal cancer is abnormal bleeding or discharge. Pain is usually a symptom of an advanced tumor. Urinary frequency is also reported occasionally, particularly in the case of anterior wall tumors, whereas constipation or tenesmus may be reported when the tumors involve the posterior vaginal wall. In general the longer the delay in diagnosis, the worse the prognosis and the more difficult the therapy. Vaginal cancer is usually diagnosed by direct biopsy of the tumor mass (Fig. 31-1, *E*). Abnormal cytologic findings (Fig. 31-1, *F*) may prompt a thorough pelvic examination that will lead to diagnosis of

TABLE 31-2

International Federation of Gynecology and Obstetrics (FIGO) Staging Classification for Vaginal Cancer

Stage	Characteristics
0	Carcinoma in situ
I	Carcinoma limited to vaginal wall
II	Carcinoma involves subvaginal tissue but has not extended to pelvic wall
III	Carcinoma extends to pelvic wall
IV	Carcinoma extends beyond true pelvis or involves mucosa of bladder or rectum (bullous edema as such does not assign a patient to stage IV)

vaginal cancer. It is important during the course of the pelvic examination to inspect and palpate the entire vaginal tube and to rotate the speculum carefully to visualize the entire vagina, since often a small tumor may occupy the anterior or posterior vaginal wall.

Tumors of Adult Vagina

Squamous Cell Carcinoma

Squamous cell carcinoma is the most common of the vaginal malignancies and accounts for 90% of primary vaginal cancers. Although reported in women in their 30s, the disease occurs primarily in those over 40 years of age. Most squamous cell carcinomas occur in the upper third of the vagina, but primary tumors in the middle third and lower third are also common. Grossly the tumor appears as a fungating, ulcerating mass, often accompanied by a foul smell and discharge related to a secondary infection. Microscopically (Fig. 31-1, *E*) the tumor demonstrates the classic findings of an invasive squamous cell carcinoma infiltrating the vaginal epithelium.

Treatment of these tumors is based on the size, stage, and location. Therapy is limited by the proximity of the bladder anteriorly and the rectum posteriorly. It is also influenced by the location of the tumor in the vagina, which determines the area of lymphatic spread (Fig. 31-3).

The lymphatics of the vagina envelop the mucosa and anastomose with lymphatic vessels

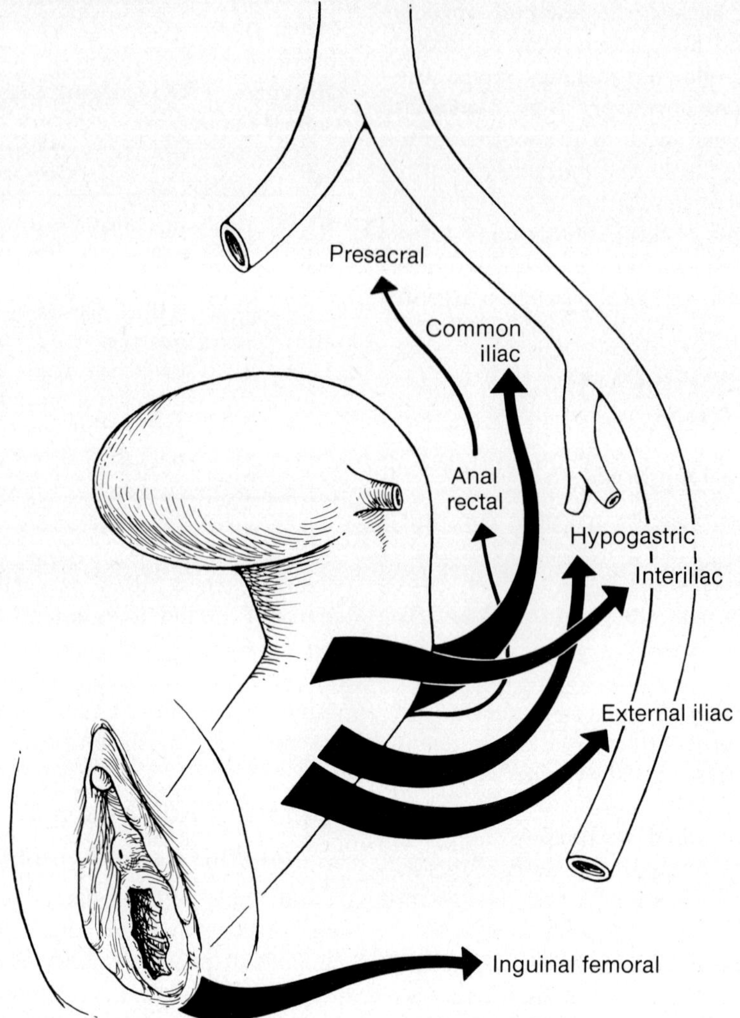

FIGURE 31-3
Lymphatic drainage of vagina. The predominant pathways from the various parts of
the vagina are demonstrated.

in the muscularis. Those of the middle to upper vagina communicate superiorly with the lymphatics of the cervix and drain into the pelvic nodes of the obturator and internal and external iliac chains. In contrast, the lymphatics of the distal third of the vagina drain to both the inguinal nodes as well as to the pelvic nodes, similar to the drainage of the vulva. The posterior wall lymphatics anastomose with the rectal lymphatic system and then to the nodes that drain the rectum, such as the inferior gluteal, sacral, and rectal nodes.

MANAGEMENT. Both surgery and irradiation therapy have been effective, considering the limits imposed by the proximity to the bladder and rectum and the risk of fistula formation from these organs to the vagina. Radiation therapy has been the most frequent mode of treatment in recent years. External radiation therapy with megavoltage equipment is initially utilized to shrink the tumor. This is then followed by a local cesium or radium implant placed interstitially with needles or by intracavitary radiation using a tandem or ovoids similar to the delivery systems used for cervical carcinoma (particularly in the case of a tumor in the upper one third of the vagina if the cervix is present) (Chapter 27). The treatment is

TABLE 31-3
Summary of Average Dosages* for Treatment of Vaginal Carcinoma

	External Therapy	Implant (Interstitial)
Stage I		
Small tumors (< 2 cm)	May omit	6000-7000 rads, 6-7 days
All others	4000 rads, whole pelvis	3000-4000 rads, 3-4 days
Stage II	4000-5000 rads, whole pelvis	3000-4000 rads, 3-4 days
Stage III, Stage IV	5000 rads, whole pelvis; an additional 1000-2000 rads through reduced field if implant not possible	2000 rads by implant if possible

Modified from Nori D, Hilaris BS, Stanimir G, Lewis JL: Radiation therapy of primary vaginal carcinoma. Int J Radiat Oncol Biol Phys 9:1471, 1983.
*100 rads = 1 gray (Gy).

individualized depending on tumor size and stage. Some therapists have advocated using only local sources of radiation if the primary carcinoma is small (under 2 cm) and accessible to needle implantation. For larger lesions the dosage of the external component of radiation therapy is increased, with a concomitant reduction in the local vaginal component of treatment of the primary tumor. Usually a total tumor dose of approximately 7000 rads (70 Gy) is administered. Implants cannot be done in some patients with stage III or IV carcinoma; in such cases only external therapy can be used and a central "boost" is given after an initial 5000 rads (50 Gy) whole-pelvic treatment (Table 31-3).

For localized tumors in the upper one third of the vagina, radical hysterectomy and vaginectomy can be effective, especially in younger patients. In most instances radical pelvic surgery, including removal of the bladder (anterior exenteration) or removal of the rectum (posterior exenteration) or both (total exenteration), is necessary only in patients with localized recurrence after radiation therapy. Initially the tumors recur locally, as in squamous cell carcinoma of the cervix and vulva, but distant metastases also occur as in vulvar and cervical cancers. An effective chemotherapy program for recurrent vaginal carcinoma has not been developed. A variety of regimens for squamous cell carcinoma utilizing multiple-agent chemotherapy is usually employed (Chapter 27).

SURVIVAL. Overall 5-year survival rates for patients with primary carcinoma of the vagina have been reported to be approximately 45%. Table 31-4 demonstrates that survival is related to stage.

Clear Cell Adenocarcinoma

Clear cell adenocarcinomas in young women have been seen more frequently since 1970 as a result of the association of many of these cancers with intrauterine exposure to diethylstil-

TABLE 31-4
Stage and Survival from Collated Series of Squamous Cell Carcinoma of Vagina

	Patient (n)	5-Year Survival	Percentage
Stage I	95	67	71
Stage II	174	81	47
Stage III	63	16	25
Stage IV	40	3	8
TOTAL	372	167	45

Adapted from Benedet JL, Murphy KS, Fairey RN, et al: Primary invasive carcinoma of the vagina. Obstet Gynecol 62:715, 1983. Reprinted with permission from The American College of Obstetricians and Gynecologists.

bestrol. The nonmalignant manifestations of this exposure are discussed in Chapter 14.

MANAGEMENT. Therapeutic considerations are similar to those for squamous cell carcinoma, taking into account the young age of the patients undergoing therapy. Cervical clear cell adenocarcinomas are treated like primary cervical carcinomas (Chapter 27). The results of therapy for both vaginal and cervical clear cell adenocarcinoma in young women will be discussed together in this section. These tumors are also staged according to the International Federation of Gynecology and Obstetrics (FIGO) (See Tables 27-3 and 31-2). The majority (80%) have been diagnosed as stage I or II. The overall results of therapy, based on the stage of the tumor at the time of treatment, are shown in Table 31-5. As can be seen, the survival rate is related directly to the stage of the tumor, similar to other gynecologic malignancies at these sites.

In general, operation is the primary treatment modality because of the young age of the patients. For stage I and early stage II tumors, radical hysterectomy with partial or complete vaginectomy, pelvic lymphadenectomy, and replacement of the vagina with split-thickness skin grafts has been the most common approach. In most cases, ovarian function was preserved. In addition, efforts have been made to preserve fertility in patients who have small tumors of the vagina by the use of local irradiation of the primary tumor and immediate adjacent tissues to spare the ovaries. Since metastases to regional pelvic nodes can occur even with small stage I tumors, retroperitoneal lymph node dissections have frequently been performed before local therapy. Usually local excision of the tumor has been performed before irradiation to facilitate local application. Senekjian et al. have noted that the survival of patients with small vaginal tumors treated by local excision and then local irradiation is comparable to those with conventional extensive therapy. Eight pregnancies have been recorded in 5 patients locally treated. Larger tumors, however, have been treated with full pelvic irradiation in addition to an intracavitary implant. In a few instances exenterative surgery has been performed. Local vaginal excision as the sole therapy is not usually adequate for small tumors since the tumor frequently recurs.

SURVIVAL. Three predominant histologic patterns are found in patients with clear cell adenocarcinoma (Fig. 31-4). In addition, a number of prognostic factors have been identified. The older patients (over 19 years of age) have been found to have a more favorable prognosis in comparison to younger subjects (under 15 year of age). This difference is associated with a more favorable outcome for those with the tubulocystic pattern of clear cell adenocarcinoma, which is the most frequent histologic pattern found in older patients. In addition, smaller tumor diameter and superficial depth of invasion correlate with improved patient survival. If the regional pelvic nodes are free of tumor, the prognosis is also more favorable. It is more likely that the regional pelvic lymph nodes will be free of tumor if other factors are favorable (see box below).

Clear cell adenocarcinomas can spread locally as well as by lymphatics and blood ves-

---

TABLE 31-5

Five-Year Survival for 500 Patients with Clear Cell Adenocarcinoma of the Vagina and Cervix

Stage	% Surviving*
I	91
II	78
III	36
IV	0

*The survival rate is 82% overall.

FAVORABLE FACTORS IN SURVIVAL OF PATIENTS WITH CLEAR CELL ADENOCARCINOMA

Low stage
Older age
Tubulocystic histologic pattern
Small tumor diameter
Reduced depth of invasion
Regional lymph nodes free of tumor

A

B

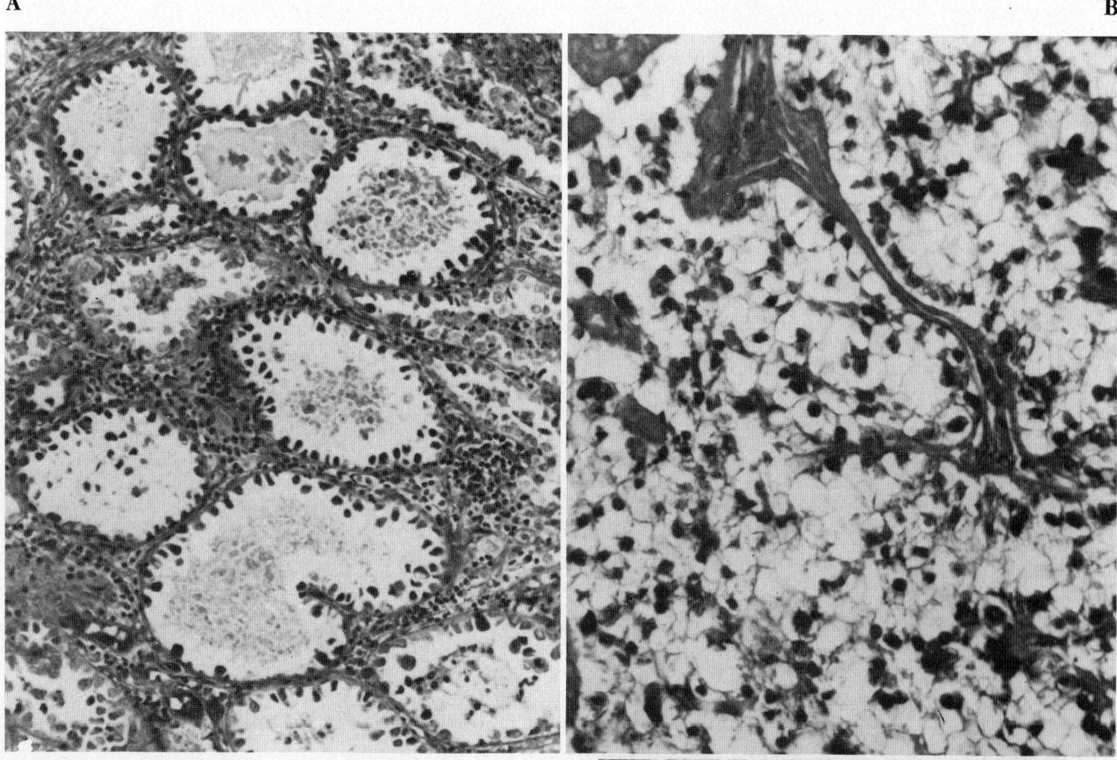

FIGURE 31-4

Clear cell adenocarcinoma. **A,** Tubulocystic cell pattern. Note hobnail cells extruding into lumina of tubular structures. (H and E stain; ×180.) **B,** Solid pattern. (H and E stain; ×300.) **C,** Papillary pattern. (H and E stain; ×50.) (**A** and **B** from Scully RE, Robboy SJ, Herbst AL: Ann Clin Lab Sci 4:222, 1974, Copyright 1974, Institute for Clinical Science; **C** from Scully RE, Robboy SJ, Welch WR: Pathology and pathogenesis of diethylstilbestrol-related disorders of the female genital tract. In Herbst AL, ed: Intrauterine exposure to diethylstilbestrol in the human. Washington, D.C., American College of Obstetricians and Gynecologists, 1978.)

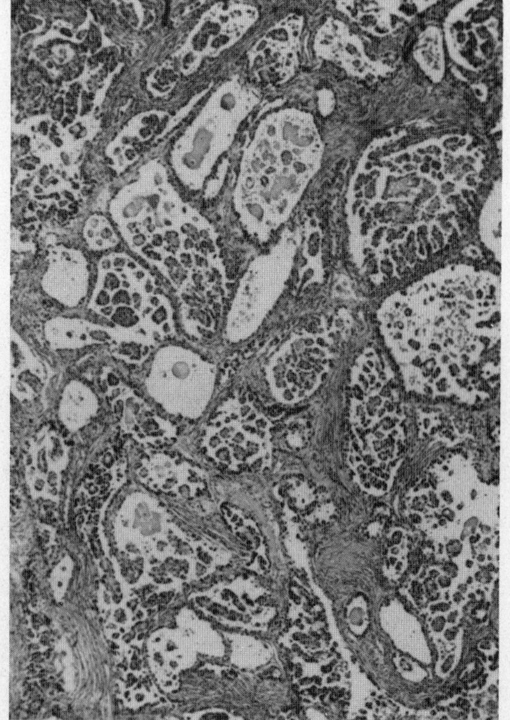

C

sels. Metastases to regional pelvic nodes are found in about one sixth of stage I cases. The spread to regional pelvic nodes becomes more frequent in higher-stage tumors. Depending on the location of the tumor recurrence, therapy has consisted of additional radical surgery or extensive radiation in localized pelvic disease and systemic chemotherapy in cases of metastatic disease. Multiple-agent cytotoxic chemotherapy is usually prescribed. Unfortunately no single agent or combination of chemotherapeutic agents has emerged as an effective therapy.

Malignant Melanoma

Vaginal melanomas are rare, with only approximately 100 cases reported to date. The tumors occur in adult patients predominantly (average age 60 years). They tend to be deeply invasive in the vagina, although histologically they may resemble other melanomas such as those of the vulva.

MANAGEMENT. Treatment usually consists of radical surgery with wide excision of the vagina and dissection of the regional nodes (pelvic or inguinal-femoral or both) depending on the location of the lesion. Adjunctive radiotherapy and chemotherapy have also been used.

SURVIVAL. Local recurrence is common, and the disease is usually fatal. Recently Chung et al. reported a 5-year survival of only 21% in a series of 19 patients.

Vaginal Tumors of Infants and Children

Endodermal Sinus Tumor (Yolk-Sac Tumor)

This type of adenocarcinoma is a rare germ cell tumor that usually occurs in the ovary (Chapter 29). The tumor secretes alpha-fetoprotein (AFP), which provides a useful tumor marker to monitor patients treated for these neoplasms. Approximately 20 cases of this unusual malignancy originating in the vagina of infants, predominantly those under 2 years of age, have been reported. The tumor is aggressive, and most of the patients have died. Some infants have survived longer than 3 years. These patients were treated by irradiation or radical surgery or a combination of both. Recently Young and Scully reported six patients

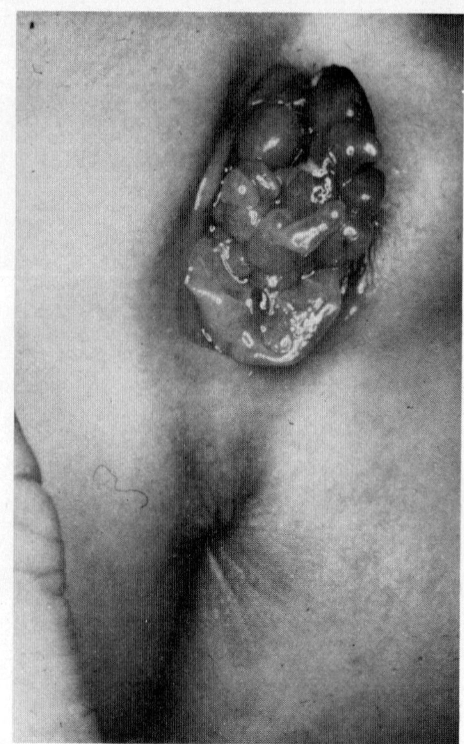

FIGURE 31-5
Sarcoma botryoides protruding through vaginal introitus. (From Herbst AL: Cancer of the vagina. In Gusberg SB, Frick HC, eds: Gynecologic cancer, 5th ed, Baltimore, Williams & Wilkins, 1978. © 1978 by The Williams & Wilkins Co., Baltimore.)

who were free of disease 2 to 9 years after operation or irradiation or both with vincristine, actinomycin-D, and cyclophosphamide (VAC; Chapter 29) chemotherapy.

Sarcoma Botryoides (Embryonal Rhabdomyosarcoma)

This rare sarcoma is usually diagnosed in the vagina of a young female, generally before the age of 2 years. Rarely does it occur in a young child over 8 years of age, although cases in adolescents have been reported. The most common symptom is abnormal vaginal bleeding with an occasional mass at the introitus (Fig. 31-5). The tumor grossly will resemble a cluster of grapes forming multiple polypoid masses.

The tumors are believed to begin in the subepithelial layers of the vagina and expand rapidly to fill the vagina. These sarcomas often are

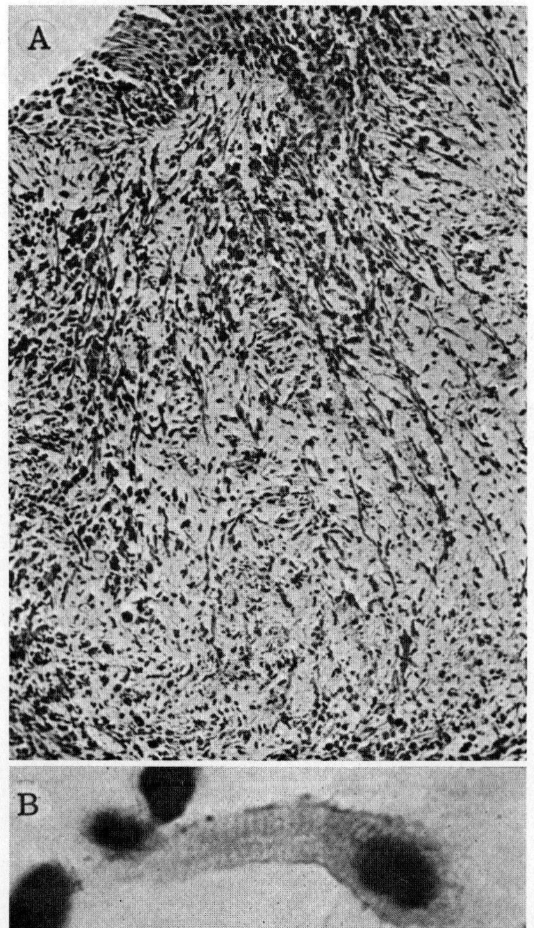

FIGURE 31-6
Section showing sarcoma botryoides. Note rhabdomyoblasts and strap cells. (From Hilgers RD, Malkasian GD, Soule EH: Am J Obstet Gynecol 107:484, 1970.)

multicentric. Histologically they have a loose myxomatous stroma with malignant pleomorphic cells and occasional eosinophilic rhabdomyoblasts that often contain characteristic cross striations (strap cells) (Fig. 31-6).

These virulent tumors have been treated in the past by radical surgery such as pelvic exenteration. Recently effective control with less radical surgery appears to have been achieved with a multimodality approach consisting of chemotherapy (vincristine, actinomycin D, and cyclophosphamide) or pelvic irradiation or both. The preliminary radiotherapy and chemotherapy is generally followed by hysterectomy and vaginectomy. Long-term survival data for a large number of patients are not available, but this combined approach appears to result in effective treatment with less mutilating surgery than primarily exenterative procedures. Dewhurst has reported six patients free of disease 2 to 6.5 years after this treatment.

Pseudosarcoma Botryoides

A rare benign vaginal polyp that resembles sarcoma botryoides is found in the vagina of infants or pregnant women. Although large atypical cells may be present microscopically, strap cells are absent. Grossly these polyps do not resemble the grapelike appearance of sarcoma botryoides. They are called *pseudosarcoma botryoides*. Treatment by local excision is effective.

KEY POINTS

- Predisposing factors associated with the development of vaginal intraepithelial neoplasia include infection with herpesvirus II and papillomavirus, prior radiation therapy to the vagina, and immunosuppression.

- The tendency of intraepithelial squamous neoplasia to develop anywhere in the lower female genital tract is termed *field defect* and describes the increased risk of premalignant changes occurring in the cervix, vagina, or vulva.

- The most common primary vaginal malignancy is squamous cell carcinoma (90%).

- Most cancers occurring in the vagina are metastatic.

- Vaginal cancers comprise less than 2% of gynecologic malignancies.

- Radiation therapy is the most frequently used modality for treatment of squamous cell carcinoma of the vagina.

- Overall 5-year survival of patients treated for squamous cell carcinoma of the vagina is approximately 45%.

- Clear cell adenocarcinoma is associated with prenatal DES exposure and has an improved prognosis if the patient is over the age of 19 years, has a predominant tubulocystic tumor pattern, and has low-stage disease.

- The overall 5-year survival of patients treated for clear cell adenocarcinoma is approximately 80%, in part due to the high proportion of low-stage cases.

- Sarcoma botryoides occurs primarily in children under the age of 8 years. It is treated by a multimodality approach using chemotherapy or irradiation or both and operative removal.

BIBLIOGRAPHY

Allyn DL, Silverberg SG, Salzberg AM: Endodermal sinus tumor of the vagina: Report of a case with 7-year survival and literature review of so-called "mesonephromas." Cancer 27:1231, 1971.

Ballon SC, Roberts JA, Lagasse LD: Topical 5-fluorouracil in the treatment of intraepithelial neoplasia of the vagina. Obstet Gynecol 54:163, 1979.

Benedet JL, Murphy KS, Fairey RN, et al: Primary invasive carcinoma of the vagina. Obstet Gynecol 62:715, 1983.

Chung AF, Casey MJ, Flannery JT, et al: Malignant melanoma of the vagina: Report of 19 cases. Obstet Gynecol 55:720, 1980.

Dewhurst J: Genital malignancies in the prepubertal child. In Coppleson M, ed: Gynecologic oncology. New York, Churchill Livingstone, 1981.

Elliott GB, Reynolds HA, Fidler HK: Pseudosarcoma botryoides of cervix and vagina in pregnancy. J Obstet Gynaecol Br Comm 74:728, 1967.

Frick HC, Jacox HW, Taylor HC: Primary carcinoma of the vagina. Am J Obstet Gynecol 101:695, 1968.

Gallup DG, Morley GW: Carcinoma in situ of the vagina. A study and review. Obstet Gynecol 46:334, 1975.

Herbst AL, Green TH, Ulfelder H: Primary carcinoma of the vagina: An analysis of 68 cases. Am J Obstet Gynecol 106:210, 1970.

Herbst AL, Norusis MJ, Rosenow PJ, et al: An analysis of 346 cases of clear cell adenocarcinoma of the vagina and cervix with emphasis on recurrence and survival. Gynecol Oncol 7:111, 1979.

Herbst AL, Scully RE: Adenocarcinoma of the vagina in adolescence. Cancer 25:745, 1970.

Herbst AL, Ulfelder H, Poskanzer DC: Adenocarcinoma of the vagina. N Engl J Med 284:878, 1971.

Hilgers RD: Pelvic exenteration for vaginal embryonal rhabdomyosarcoma: A review. Obstet Gynecol 45:175, 1975.

Miettinen M, Wahlstrom T, Vesterinen E, et al: Vaginal polyps with pseudosarcomatous features: A clinicopathologic study of seven cases. Cancer 51:1148, 1983.

Nori D, Hilaris BS, Stanimir G, et al: Radiation therapy of primary vaginal carcinoma. Int J Radiat Oncol Biol Phys 9:1471, 1983.

Perez CA, Arneson AN, Dehner LP, et al: Radiation therapy in carcinoma of the vagina. Obstet Gynecol 44:862, 1974.

Perticucci S: Diagnostic, prognostic, and therapeutic considerations in invasive carcinoma of the vagina. Obstet Gynecol 40:843, 1972.

Petrilli ES, Townsend DE, Morrow CP, et al: Vaginal intraepithelial neoplasm: Biologic aspects and treatment with topical 5-fluorouracil and the carbon dioxide laser. Am J Obstet Gynecol 38:321, 1980.

Plentl AA, Friedman EA: Lymphatic system of the female genitalia. Philadelphia, W.B. Saunders Co., 1971.

Prempree T, Viravathana T, Slawson RG, et al: Radiation management of primary carcinoma of the vagina. Cancer 40:109, 1977.

Pride GL, Schultz AE, Chuprevich TW, et al: Primary invasive squamous carcinoma of the vagina. Obstet Gynecol 53:218, 1979.

Scully RE, Robboy SJ, Herbst AL: Vaginal and cervical abnormalities, including clear cell adenocarcinoma related to prenatal exposure to stilbestrol. Ann Clin Lab Sci 4:222, 1974.

Scully RE, Welch WR: Pathology of the female genital tract after prenatal exposure to diethylstilbestrol. In Herbst AL, Bern HA, eds: Developmental effects of diethylstilbestrol (DES) in pregnancy. New York, Thieme-Stratton, 1981.

Senekjian EK, Frey KW, Anderson D, Herbst AL: Local therapy in stage I clear cell adenocarcinoma of the vagina (abst). 18th Annual Meeting of the Society of Gynecologic Oncologists. Gynecol Oncol (in press).

Townsend DE: Intraepithelial neoplasm of the vagina. In Coppleson M, ed: Gynecologic oncology. New York, Churchill Livingstone, 1981.

Wharton JT, Fletcher GH, Delclos L: Invasive tumors of the vagina. In Coppleson M, ed: Gynecologic oncology. New York, Churchill Livingstone, 1981.

Young RH, Scully RE: Endodermal sinus tumor of the vagina: A report of nine cases and review of the literature. Gynecol Oncol 18:380, 1984.

Malignant Disease of the Fallopian Tube

Primary cancers of the fallopian tube are the rarest of female genital tract malignancies and almost all of them are adenocarcinomas. This malignancy comprises approximately 0.3% to 1.1% of all gynecologic cancers. Approximately 80% to 90% of fallopian tube malignancies are metastatic from other sites, usually arising in the ovary or uterus and occasionally in the gastrointestinal tract. Metastatic carcinomas are approximately 10 times as frequent as primary tumors. Over 1000 cases of primary fallopian tube carcinoma have been reported, mostly from studies comprising individual cases or small series of patients treated at a single center. This heterogeneity of data combined with lack of a uniform staging system for these very rare cancers has made it difficult to provide precise information regarding their optimal management. This chapter reviews current information with particular emphasis on diagnosis, natural history, and management.

ETIOLOGY AND AGE DISTRIBUTION

The etiology of adenocarcinoma of the fallopian tube is unknown. It has been postulated that chronic salpingitis and prior pelvic inflammatory disease are associated factors. However, pelvic inflammatory disease is common,

and these carcinomas are extremely rare, suggesting that other factors are involved.

The disease primarily affects older women, the average age being the 50s with a range from 18 to 80 years. Podzcaski and Herbst recently summarized the age distribution of 188 cases reported in the literature since 1970 (Fig. 32-1) and noted an average age of 54.9 years.

DIAGNOSIS

These cancers are usually asymptomatic, and the diagnosis is most frequently made only after the patient has undergone surgical exploration. The most commonly reported sign is abnormal or excessive vaginal bleeding or discharge, which occurs in about 50% of the patients. Pain is less frequently reported. Occasionally an adnexal mass is noted. Abnormal vaginal discharge and bleeding combined with lower abdominal pain and an adnexal mass in the postmenopausal woman are considered pathognomonic for the diagnosis of tubal malignancy. Unfortunately, these three conditions rarely exist together, which is why the diagnosis is frequently made postoperatively. The term *hydrops tubae profluens* has been used to describe the abnormal discharge and pain that presumably result from blockage of the distal part of the fallopian tube. Subsequent peristal-

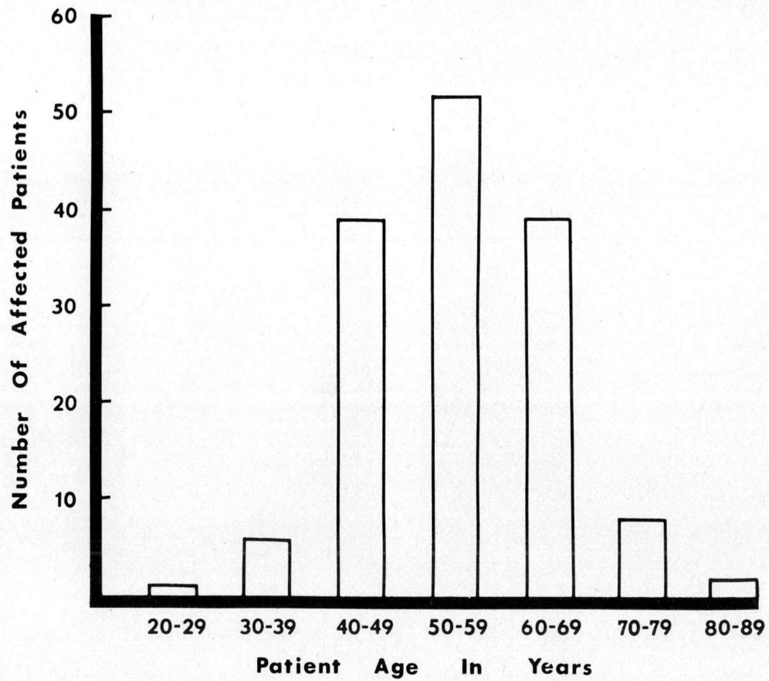

FIGURE 32-1
Histogram illustrating age distribution of patients with tubal carcinomas. (From Podczaski E, Herbst AL: Cancer of the vagina and fallopian tube. In Knapp RC, Berkowitz RS, eds: Gynecologic oncology. New York, Macmillan Publishing Co., 1983.)

sis produces the discharge occasionally accompanied by the disappearance of the mass secondary to the expulsion of fluid from the dilated tube. The disease should be strongly suspected in anyone with these findings. Vaginal cytology may show malignant adenocarcinoma cells in cases of tubal cancer. However, vaginal cytology is usually negative; Benedet et al. found it to be positive in only 10% of their 40 patients.

The diagnosis of tubal carcinoma should be considered in any patient with vaginal cytology positive for adenocarcinoma in whom the diagnosis of endometrial carcinoma has been excluded, although ovarian and endocervical adenocarcinomas are other possibilities. The diagnosis should also be suspected in patients with postmenopausal uterine bleeding for whom dilation and curettage fail to reveal the cause. Laparoscopy can be of benefit in establishing the diagnosis for such patients.

PATHOLOGY

On gross examination the fallopian tube containing primary adenocarcinoma often apears dilated and may resemble a hydrosalpinx until the tube is opened, revealing an infiltrating tumor (Figs. 32-2 and 32-3). Sometimes it is difficult to be certain that the tumor is of tubal origin, and confusion with metastatic carcinoma, particularly from the ovary, can be a diagnostic problem. In 1950 Hu, Taymor, and Hertig suggested the following criteria to allow the diagnosis of primary tubal carcinoma:

1. The primary tumor is grossly within the lumen of the tube.
2. The mucosa of the tube is involved with the tumor, which displays a papillary (or medullary) pattern.
3. A transition can be demonstrated between the malignant and nonmalignant tubal epithelium (if the tubal wall is involved to a great extent).

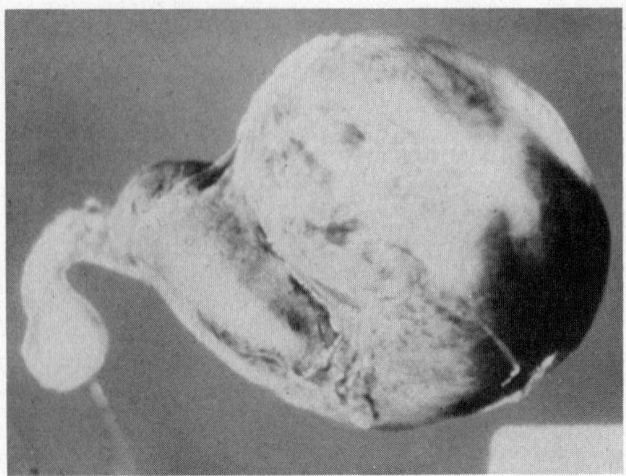

FIGURE 32-2
External appearance of fallopian tube with primary adenocarcinoma. (From Podczaski E, Herbst AL: Cancer of the vagina and fallopian tube. In Knapp RC, Berkowitz RS, eds: Gynecologic oncology. New York, Macmillan Publishing Co., 1983.)

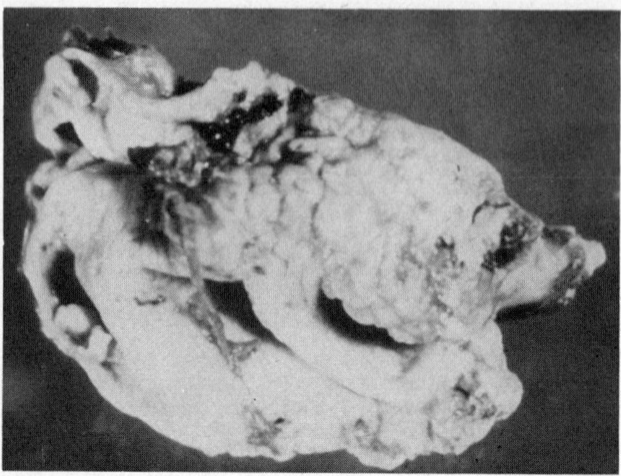

FIGURE 32-3
Cross section through fallopian tube demonstrating primary adenocarcinoma. (From Podczaski E, Herbst AL: Cancer of the vagina and fallopian tube. In Knapp RC, Berkowitz RS, eds: Gynecologic oncology. New York, Macmillan Publishing Co., 1983.)

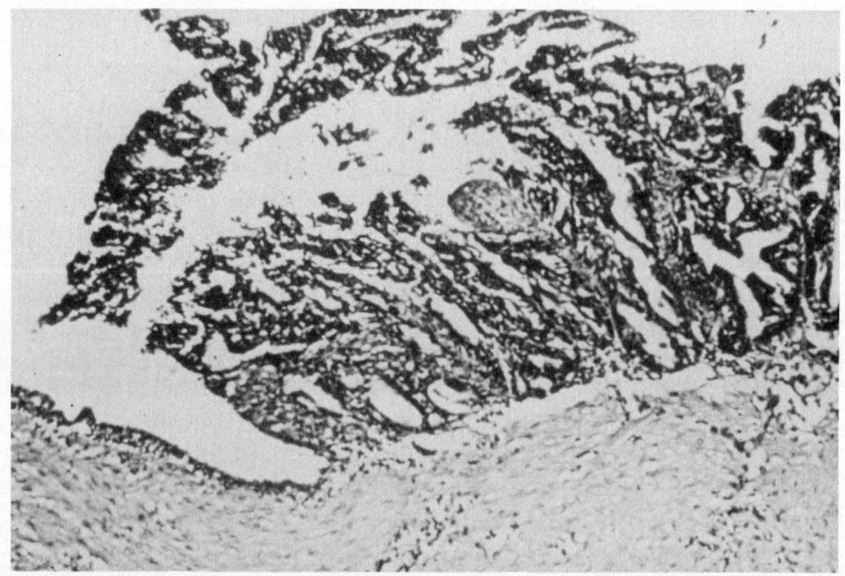

FIGURE 32-4
Microscopic appearance of well-differentiated papillary adenocarcinoma of fallopian tube. (From Podczaski E, Herbst AL: Cancer of the vagina and fallopian tube. In Knapp RC, Berkowitz RS, eds: Gynecologic oncology. New York, Macmillan Publishing Co., 1983.)

Figs. 32-4 and 32-5 demonstrate a primary tubal carcinoma showing a papillary-alveolar pattern. These tumors can arise in either tube with approximately equal frequency and occasionally may be bilateral.

CLINICAL STAGING

No widely accepted staging system exists for fallopian tube carcinoma. The tumor spreads in a manner similar to epithelial carcinoma of the ovary. Therefore many authors have suggested a staging system for fallopian tube carcinoma based on that used for primary ovarian carcinomas. A suggested system is shown in Table 32-1.

NATURAL HISTORY

The carcinoma is initially confined to the lumen of the tube but can penetrate to the serosa and then spread intraperitoneally to involve the surface of the bowel, the omentum, and the parietal peritoneum, similar to ovarian carcinoma. The peritoneum is the most frequent site of metastatic spread of tubal carcinoma. In addition, lymphatic spread occurs, particularly to the paraaortic nodes. Tamini and Figge noted metastases to the paraaortic nodes in 5 of 15 patients, and these nodes were the only site of metastatic disease in 2 patients. Thus the retroperitoneal nodes must also be considered as sites of common spread in the management of these cancers, similar to considerations for ovarian epithelial carcinomas.

MANAGEMENT

As noted previously, the diagnosis of primary tubal carcinoma is most frequently made at the time of surgical exploration. Once the diagnosis

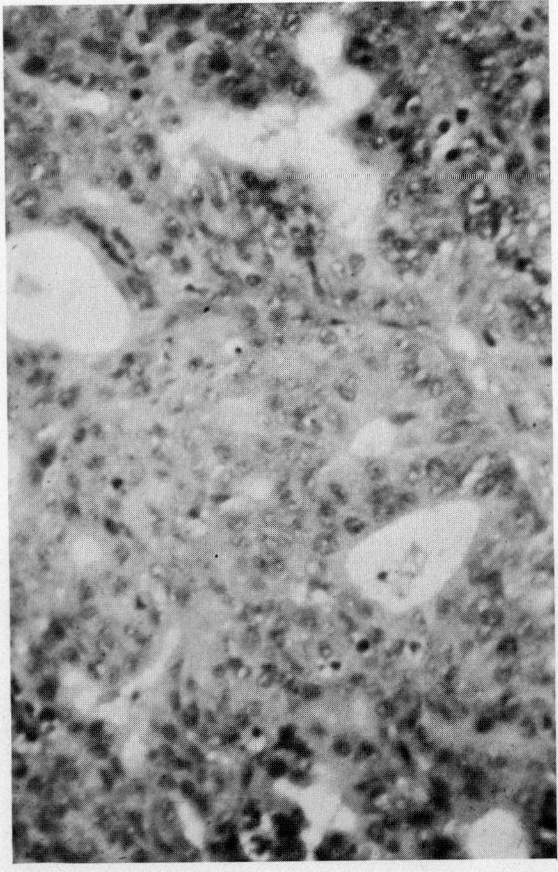

FIGURE 32-5
Poorly differentiated tubal carcinoma with a predominantly solid growth pattern. (From Azizi F, Johnston GA: Female Patient 7:42, 1982.)

TABLE 32-1
Suggested Staging System for Tubal Carcinoma*

Stage	Characteristics
I	Tumor confined to one or both tubes, not involving the serosa
Ia	One tube
Ib	Both tubes
Ic	Positive peritoneal washings or ascitic fluid positive for malignant cells
IIa	Tumor involving one or both tubes and spread to either the ovary or uterus
IIb	Tumor extends to other pelvic tissues
III	Tumor involves one or both tubes with intraperitoneal spread including retroperitoneal nodes
IV	Tumor involves one or both tubes with metastases outside the peritoneum or to the parenchyma of the liver (pleural fluid containing malignant cells allows assignment to stage IV)

*Not officially adopted by the International Federation of Gynecology and Obstetrics (FIGO).

is established, frequently by frozen section, a thorough operative staging procedure is carried out, including a total abdominal hysterectomy and bilateral salpingo-oophorectomy. Peritoneal cytology testing is performed using 200 to 300 ml of normal saline solution mixed with 0.5 ml (5000 IU) of heparin to prevent clotting of any blood present in the fluid. If there is no evidence of intraperitoneal spread, a paraaortic node biopsy should be performed to rule out extrapelvic spread. This is particularly important in cases of large or poorly differentiated tumors in view of the fact that these carcinomas can metastasize to the paraaortic nodes without evidence of intraperitoneal spread. An omentectomy should also be performed. As emphasized by Podratz et al., meticulous staging is important both for optimal effective treatment and to help decide if additional postoperative therapy is advisable.

Because of the varied experience in the treatment of these malignancies, a number of therapeutic approaches have been suggested. The value of postoperative radiation therapy or chemotherapy is not established at present, although those modalities have been reported to be effective. In the case of a stage I carcinoma in which the cancer is confined to the tubal lumen and peritoneal cytology is negative, therapy usually consists only of primary operation. If there is positive peritoneal cytology (stage Ic), postoperative intraperitoneal ^{32}P is advisable or whole abdominal radiation is used. If there is spread of tumor outside of the tube to the pelvis, postoperative radiation including the paraaortic nodes should also be considered, depending on the extent of disease discovered at surgery. Brown et al. recommend abdominopelvic radiation postoperatively providing there is no residual disease greater than 2 cm^2 after operation.

For widespread intraperitoneal disease or for recurrent metastatic carcinoma, chemotherapy usually is considered. Traditionally alkylating agents have been prescribed, since these were active against ovarian epithelial carcinomas and presumed effective in tubal carcinomas. Recently Deppe et al. reported two patients with widespread disseminated fallopian tube carcinoma who were treated with *cis*-diamminedichloroplatinum (*cis*-platinum 50 mg/m^2) and doxorubicin (Adriamycin 37.5 mg/m^2) as well as a progestin, megestrol acetate (Megace 160 mg daily). One patient also received cyclophosphamide (Cytoxan 400 mg/m^2). At a second-look procedure 10 to 13 months later both patients showed no evidence of disease. Because platinum combinations appear to be superior to single-agent alkylating therapy for ovarian carcinoma (see Chapter 29) they should also be utilized in disseminated fallopian tube carcinoma.

No definitive conclusions can yet be drawn regarding the results of therapy. Sedlis noted a 5-year survival of 38% for all stages of tubal carcinoma. Patients with tubal carcinoma confined to the tube have the best prognosis, expecting a 70% to 80% 5-year survival. High-grade tumors are thought to behave more aggressively, but definitive data relating tumor grade to survival are lacking.

OTHER TUMORS

Sarcomas of the fallopian tube are extremely rare. They may be mixed, containing carcinomatous elements (carcinosarcoma), or may have heterologous sarcomatous tissue, in which case the term *mixed mesodermal tumors* is used. These tumors' behavior is similar to that of other sarcomas and mixed müllerian tumors within the uterus (Chapter 28). Treatment consists of surgery, with removal of the uterus and tube, and follow-up chemotherapy, usually with a regimen including doxorubicin (Adriamycin). Choriocarcinoma of the tube has also been reported and is believed to result from trophoblastic disease associated with ectopic pregnancy. The same considerations of therapy apply to these lesions as for trophoblastic disease elsewhere (see Chapter 33).

—————————— KEY POINTS ——————————

- Ninety percent of tubal cancers are metastatic, mostly from the ovary, uterus, or gastrointestinal tract.

- Only 10% of patients with fallopian tube carcinoma have positive vaginal cytology.

- Primary tubal carcinoma is the rarest gynecologic malignancy (0.3% to 1.1%), with only approximately 1000 cases reported.

- The diagnosis of tubal carcinoma is usually made at operation.

- The average age of patients with tubal carcinoma is 55 years.

- The most common site of spread of tubal carcinoma is to the peritoneum and retroperitoneal lymph nodes.

- Overall 5-year survival for all stages of primary tubal carcinoma is approximately 40%.

- The diagnosis of tubal carcinoma should be considered for anyone with vaginal cytology positive for adenocarcinoma in whom the diagnosis of endometrial carcinoma has been excluded. It should also be considered for anyone with postmenopausal uterine bleeding in whom a D&C fails to reveal the cause.

- The triad of abnormal bleeding, adnexal mass, and watery discharge in a postmenopausal woman is suggestive of tubal carcinoma.

BIBLIOGRAPHY

Benedet JL, White GW, Fairey RN, Boyes DA: Adenocarcinoma of the fallopian tube. Obstet Gynecol 50: 654, 1977.

Brown MD, Kohorn EI, Kapp DS, et al: Fallopian tube carcinoma. Int J Radiat Oncol Biol Phys 11:583, 1985.

Deppe G, Bruckner HW, Cohen CJ: Combination chemotherapy for advanced carcinoma of the fallopian tube. Obstet Gynecol 56:530, 1980.

Erez S, Kaplan AL, Wall JA: Clinical staging of carcinoma of the uterine tube. Obstet Gynecol 30:547, 1967.

Hershey DW, Fennell RH, Major FJ: Primary carcinoma of the fallopian tube. Obstet Gynecol 57:367, 1981.

Hu CY, Taymor ML, Hertig AT: Primary carcinoma of the fallopian tube. Am J Obstet Gynecol 59:58, 1950.

Phelps HM, Chapman KE: Role of radiation therapy in treatment of primary carcinoma of the uterine tube. Obstet Gynecol 43:669, 1974.

Podczaski E, Herbst AL: Cancer of the vagina and fallopian tube. In Knapp RC, Berkowitz RS, eds: Gynecologic oncology. New York, Macmillan Publishing Co., 1983.

Podratz KC, Podczaski ES, Gaffey TA, et al: Primary carcinoma of the fallopian tube. Am J Obstet Gynecol 154:1319, 1986.

Schiller HM, Silverberg SG: Staging and prognosis in primary carcinoma of the fallopian tube. Cancer 28:389, 1971.

Sedlis A: Primary carcinoma of the fallopian tube. Obstet Gynecol Surv 16:209, 1961.

Sedlis A: Carcinoma of the fallopian tube. Surg Clin North Am 58:121, 1978.

Tamini HK, Figge DC: Adenocarcinoma of the uterine tube: Potential for lymph node metastases. Am J Obstet Gynecol 141:132, 1981.

Wu JP, Tanner WS, Fardal PM: Malignant mixed müllerian tumor of the uterine tube. Obstet Gynecol 41:707, 1981.

Yoonessi M: Carcinoma of the fallopian tube. Obstet Gynecol Surv 34:257, 1979.

Gestational Trophoblastic Disease

KEY TERMS AND DEFINITIONS

Androgenesis. Impregnation of an inactive egg by a paternal haploid sperm that duplicates its chromosomes to provide a diploid complement. This results in a complete mole.

Choriocarcinoma. A morphologic term applied to a type of trophoblastic neoplasia in which both the cytotrophoblast and syncytiotrophoblast grow in a malignant fashion.

Complete Mole. A molar pregnancy with swelling of all placental villi. Fetal tissues are absent.

Gestational Trophoblastic Disease (GTD). The spectrum of diseases resulting from the abnormal proliferation of trophoblast associated with pregnancy.

Gestational Trophoblastic Neoplasia (GTN). Malignant gestational trophoblastic disease or gestational trophoblastic tumor. It can be either nonmetastatic or metastatic.

Hydatidiform Mole. A placental abnormality involving swollen placental villi and trophoblastic hyperplasia with loss of fetal blood vessels. There are two types: partial and complete.

Partial Mole. A molar pregnancy with some normal and some swollen villi plus some fetal or cord or amniotic membrane elements.

Gestational trophoblastic disease (GTD) refers to the spectrum of proliferative abnormalities of the trophoblast associated with pregnancy. These neoplasias have been known for hundreds of years, and they are unique in that they secrete human chorionic gonadotrophin (HCG). The recent availability of extremely sensitive and specific radioimmunoassays (RIA) to measure HCG allows prediction of the status of the disease, permitting refinement of its classification and thus improving understanding of its pathophysiology. The initial use of methotrexate in 1956 by Li, Hertz, and Spencer to successfully treat malignant trophoblastic disease completely altered the prognosis of patients with these cancers and represents a milestone in the cure of human tumors by chemotherapeutic agents.

This chapter presents the current classification of GTDs and the factors that appear to be associated with their development. The methods of diagnosis, appropriate therapy, and necessary follow-up of these patients are reviewed.

CHARACTERISTICS

Trophoblastic tissue is unusual insofar as it shares certain characteristics with malignancies, such as the ability to divide rapidly, to invade locally, and occasionally to metastasize to distant sites such as the lung, yet these activities usually cease at the end of pregnancy, and the trophoblast disappears. However, in GTD, abnormal growth and development continue beyond the end of pregnancy.

MORPHOLOGY

Hydatidiform Mole

A hydatidiform mole has three morphologic characteristics: (1) a mass of vesicles (distended villi) that appear as large grapelike dilations

(Fig. 33-1), (2) a loss of fetal blood vessels, which are either diminished or absent from the villi, and (3) hyperplasia of the syncytiotrophoblast and cytotrophoblast.

The terms *complete mole* and *partial mole* have recently been used to describe the variations of molar pregnancies. Vassilakos et al. noted that these two conditions appear to have different morphologic presentations and are developmentally distinct. With a complete mole, all placental villi are swollen and the fetus, cord, and amniotic membrane are absent. In

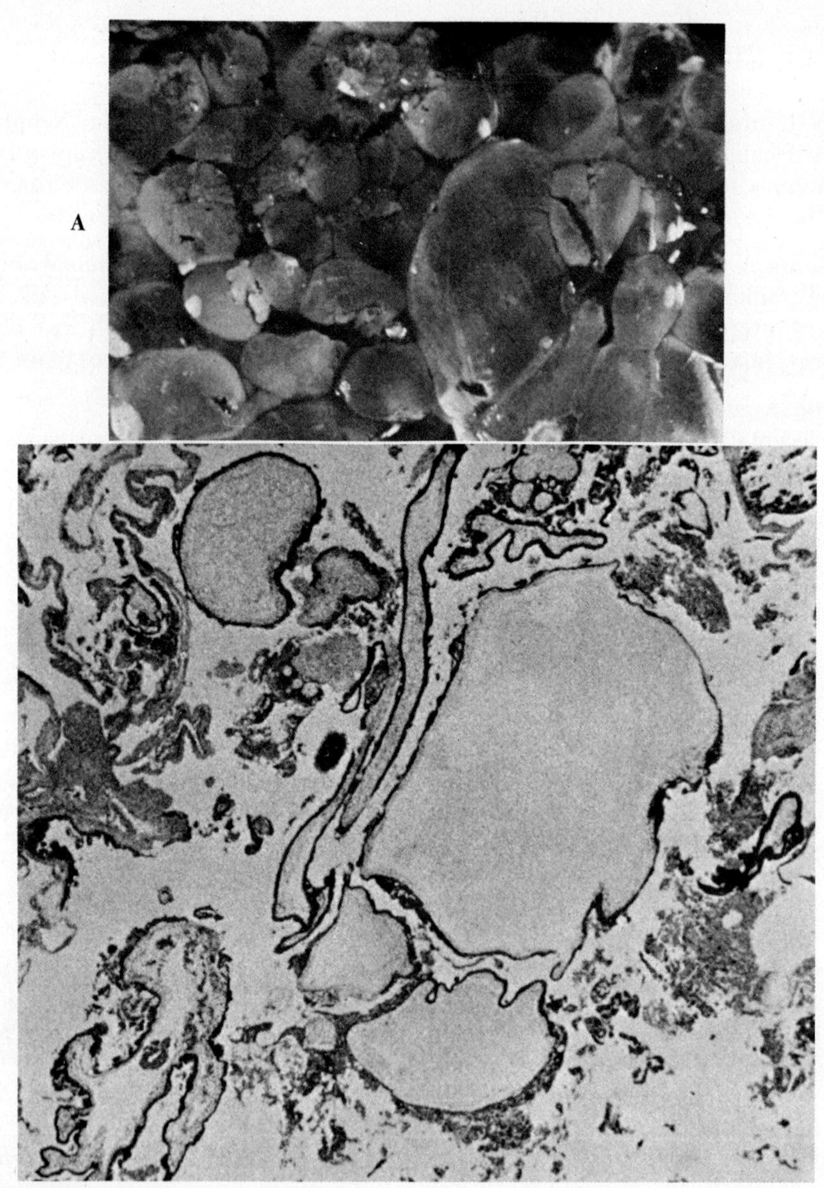

FIGURE 33-1

A, Hydatidiform mole. A few vesicles approach 1 cm in diameter. The background is formed by smaller vesicles. **B,** Hydatidiform mole aborted by suction curettage. A large intact vesicle is near the center. Many vesicles, however, have been ruptured and have collapsed. (From Bigelow B: Gestational trophoblast disease. In Blaustein A, ed: Pathology of the female genital tract, 2nd ed. New York, Springer-Verlag, 1982.)

partial molar pregnancy only some chorionic villi are swollen, whereas others appear normal, and a fetus, cord, or amniotic membrane is present. With a partial mole the trophoblastic hyperplasia is limited to the syncytiotrophoblast.

The genetics of molar pregnancy has been extensively studied. Chromosomal banding techniques have provided useful information regarding the development of these tumors. In normal pregnancy half the chromosomes of the conceptus are paternal and the other half maternal, resulting in a diploid content. In complete mole, only paternal chromosomes are present; there are 46 chromosomes and nearly always 46 XX, although a few moles with 46 XY karyotype have been reported. The development of complete mole appears to result from the fertilization of an "empty egg," one with an absent or inactive nucleus. The haploid paternal set of chromosomes from the sperm impregnate the inactive egg, and these paternal chromosomes then duplicate to give the diploid number, a process known as *androgenesis*, the development of an "embryo" due only to chromosomes from an X-bearing sperm (Fig. 33-2). In the rare case of complete mole with an XY

chromosomal content the "empty egg" is fertilized by two haploid sperm, one X bearing and one Y bearing. Thus a complete mole is entirely derived from paternal chromosomes.

Incomplete or partial moles are triploid and have 69 chromosomes of both maternal and paternal origin. The most common mechanism for the origin of partial mole (Fig. 33-3) is a haploid egg being fertilized by two sperm, resulting in three sets of chromosomes. Alternatively, triploidy could result when an abnormal diploid sperm fertilizes the haploid egg. It is also possible for an abnormal diploid egg to be fertilized by a haploid sperm, but this latter mechanism usually results in an abnormal conceptus with congenital abnormalities rather than a partial mole. Partial mole is often difficult to diagnose and may be present with a fetus as a missed abortion in the second trimester. In such cases the uterus is small for dates. Partial moles are rarely associated with the subsequent development of malignant trophoblastic disease, and Berkowitz et al. observed that 9.9% of their 81 patients with partial mole subsequently developed nonmetastatic gestational trophoblastic neoplasia.

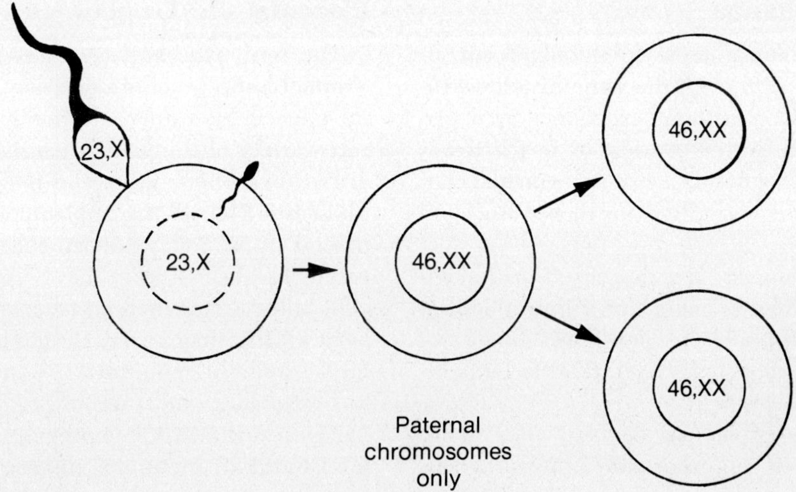

FIGURE 33-2
Paternal chromosomal origin of a complete classic mole (46,XX). Left to right, entry of normal sperm with haploid set of 23,X into egg whose 23,X haploid set is lost; egg is "taken over" by paternal chromosomes, which duplicate (without cell's division) to reach requisite complement of 46. Observe that virtually the same result can be obtained through a fertilization by two sperm gaining entry into an "empty egg" (dispermy). (From Szulman AE, Surti U: Clin Obstet Gynecol 27:172, 1984.)

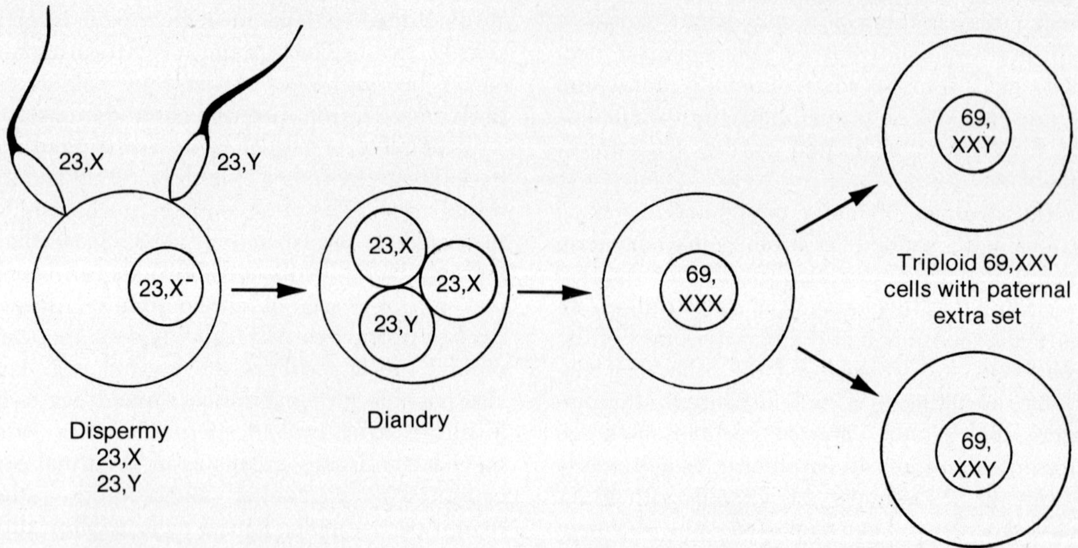

FIGURE 33-3
Triploid chromosomal origin of partial mole (69,XXY—dispermy). Fertilization of an egg equipped with a normal 23,X complement by two independently produced sperm (dispermy) to give total of 69 chromosomes. Observe that triploidy can also result through fertilization by sperm carrying father's total complement of 46,XY (paternal meiosis—I error). (From Szulman AE, Surti U: Clin Obstet Gynecol 27:172, 1984.)

Choriocarcinoma

Choriocarcinomas most commonly occur after pregnancy, although the same histologic tumor can develop without pregnancy as a primary neoplasm in the ovaries, or in the testes in men. The prognosis for primary gonadal choriocarcinomas is worse than for those associated with gestation.

Choriocarcinomas are diagnosed pathologically by finding a malignant cytotrophoblast and syncytiotrophoblast. Chorionic villi are absent. These tumors (Fig. 33-4) tend to be hemorrhagic and necrotic.

Most choriocarcinomas develop after molar pregnancies but can occur after other pregnancies. Trophoblastic tissue regresses within 2 to 3 weeks after normal delivery, including cells that have spread to the lung. The normal processes leading to this regression are unknown, but the finding of trophoblastic cells in the uterus more than 3 weeks after delivery should lead one to consider the possibility of choriocarcinoma.

Placental-site Trophoblastic Tumor

The term *placental-site trophoblastic tumor* (trophoblastic pseudotumor) has recently been introduced by Young and Scully to describe a rare variety of tumor that consists of excessive groups of mononucleate and multinucleate trophoblastic cells at the implantation site accompanied by an inflammatory cell reaction. Histocytochemical studies have shown that the cells of these tumors tend to stain more for prolactin (HPL) than for HCG, and both HCG and HPL should be monitored. The tumor can lead to hemorrhage and uterine perforation requiring hysterectomy. Chemotherapy is usually administered for metastatic disease but is less effective with these tumors than with other gestational trophoblastic tumors.

EPIDEMIOLOGY

Extensive investigation has been performed to ascertain the factors that enhance the occurrence of trophoblastic disease. The major areas evaluated are geographic distribution and so-

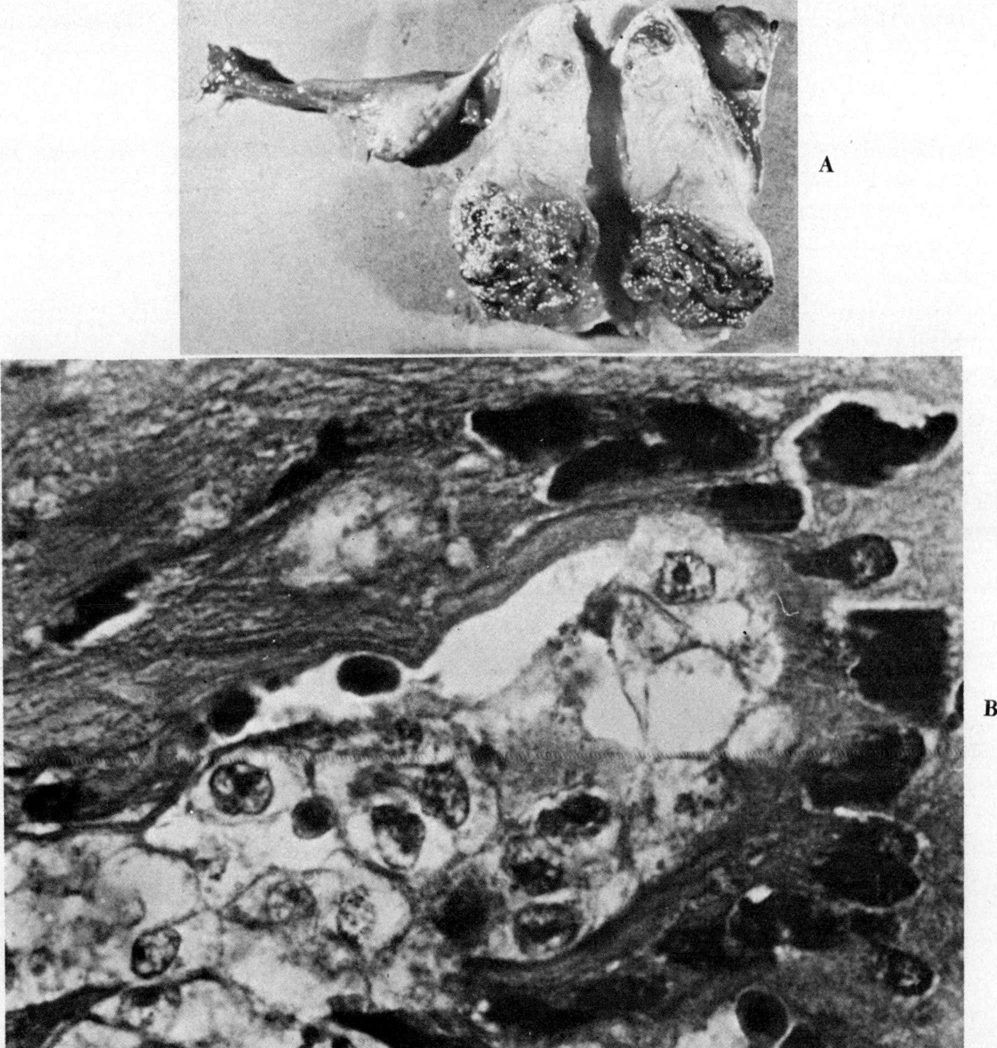

FIGURE 33-4
A, Choriocarcinoma. Hemorrhagic tumor occupies lower uterine segment and cervix. Smaller foci of choriocarcinoma can be seen in left and right fundal walls. **B,** Choriocarcinoma, high-power view. Central pale cytotrophoblast is surrounded by syncytiotrophoblasts. Nuclei are pleomorphic. (From Bigelow B: Gestational trophoblast disease. In Blaustein A, ed: Pathology of the female genital tract, 2nd ed. New York, Springer-Verlag, 1982.)

cioeconomic factors, maternal age, race, history of fetal wastage or prior hydatidiform mole, and ABO blood groupings.

INCIDENCE

Hydatidiform Mole

There is wide variation in the reported incidence of hydatidiform mole, with the most ac- curate statistics derived from population-based studies rather than from those based on hospital referral center data. The rates are usually expressed in terms of molar gestations per numbers of pregnancies. In the United States the rate is estimated to be approximately 0.75 per 1000. The rates from Southeast Asia are 1.5 to 2.5 times higher with much larger variations, and rates up to 8 per 1000 have been reported. The high rates reported in some studies are derived from hospital-based rather than population-based statistics. As already noted, hydatidiform mole develops because of abnormal fertilization. A few reports note molar pregnancies occurring among female siblings. An additional risk factor is a history of prior hydatidiform mole, which increases the risk of subsequent mole by 20 to 40 times. Spontaneous abortion is also common in women who have had moles, and there is a suggestion that they are associated with twins.

The increased frequency among those with lower socioeconomic status as well as in underdeveloped areas, particularly in Southeast Asia, has led to the suggestion that poor nutrition is a factor in the development of this disease. However, evidence is conflicting, and as noted by Grimes, a dietary etiology for hydatidiform mole is not supported by current data.

The risk appears to vary with race and ethnic origin. In Southeast Asia the rates are double for Eurasians as compared to those of Chinese, Malaysian, or Indian origin. A decreased rate has also been reported among blacks in the United States in comparison to whites, and rates are higher among those of Latin American origin. Mexicans and Filipinos appear to have elevated rates in comparison to Japanese and Chinese.

Maternal age is an extremely important risk factor. The lowest rates are among those in their twenties and thirties with a great increase in those over 40, after which the risk progressively increases with age. There is also an increase in risk among those under the age of 20 years, but the magnitude is not nearly so great as it is among older women. A summary of age risks for hydatidiform mole is shown in Table 33-1.

Choriocarcinoma

Choriocarcinoma primarily occurs in about 3% to 5% of those who have had a prior complete hydatidiform mole and the risk factors for molar pregnancy also apply to choriocarcinoma. In Western countries choriocarcinomas are reported at rates between 0.014 and 0.1 per 1000 pregnancies. The rate in the United States is about 1 per 20,000 pregnancies. Although most choriocarcinomas occur after complete molar pregnancies, occurrences have been reported after incomplete mole, and rare choriocarcinomas have developed after normal pregnancy (1 per 40,000 term pregnancies). The disease also follows incomplete abortion and ectopic pregnancy. The risk factors for complete mole, particularly maternal age and pregnancy loss, are indirectly associated with choriocarcinoma. An additional factor for choriocarcinoma has been found among ABO blood groups. Some studies, including those of Bagshawe, have shown that women with type A blood married to men with type O and vice versa are at higher risk for choriocarcinoma in comparison to matings of other blood groups. No differential in the risk for hydatidiform mole for ABO blood groups has been demonstrated.

CLINICAL CLASSIFICATION OF GTD

The histologic terminology previously used to describe trophoblastic disease is somewhat confusing, since the terms were based on the morphologic appearance of the abnormal tissue. Previously the term *hydatidiform mole* referred to a molar pregnancy; *invasive mole* or *chorioadenoma destruens* referred to a molar pregnancy that had invaded the uterus away from the implantation site; and *choriocarcinoma* referred to the malignant variation that metastasized and was often fatal. The diagnosis of invasive mole has been made primarily in

TABLE 33-1
Relationship of Age to Risk of Hydatidiform Mole

Age	Risk
Less than 20	1.53
20-24	1.17
25-29	1
30-34	1.04
35-39	1.33
40-44	2.66
45-49	24.89
Over 50	80.76

Adapted from Buckley JD: The epidemiology of molar pregnancy and choriocarcinoma. Clin Obstet Gynecol 27:153, 1984.

**CLASSIFICATION OF GESTATIONAL
TROPHOBLASTIC DISEASE**

Hydatidiform mole
1. Complete
2. Incomplete
Gestational trophoblastic neoplasia
1. Nonmetastatic
2. Metastatic
   a. Low risk
   b. High risk

**SYMPTOMS AND SIGNS OF
HYDATIDIFORM MOLE**

Abnormal bleeding in early pregnancy
Lower abdominal pain
Toxemia before 24 weeks of gestation
Hyperemesis gravidarum
Hyperthyroidism (rare)
Uterus large for dates (50%)
Enlargement of ovaries (20%)
Absent fetal heart tones and fetal parts
Expulsion of swollen villi

the cases requiring hysterectomy for bleeding or uterine perforation. With the use of sensitive and specific radioimmunoassays for β-HCG and modern diagnostic techniques, clinical terminology more useful in describing trophoblastic disease has been found, as shown in the box above. This terminology allows the physician to describe all forms of gestational trophoblastic disease and also offers an effective way of analyzing the treatment and the biologic behavior of these abnormal trophoblastic conditions.

CLINICAL ASPECTS OF GTD

Hydatidiform Mole

Symptoms and Signs

The most common presenting symptom is abnormal bleeding in a patient who has experienced delayed menses and seems to be pregnant. Abnormal bleeding is present in almost all patients with gestational trophoblastic disease, and associated symptoms often mimic an incomplete or threatened abortion. Occasionally the patient notices a swollen villus that has been passed from the uterus. The uterus is frequently large for dates; Curry et al. noted this change in about half of their patients with molar pregnancy. However, as many as one fourth of the patients may have a uterus small for dates. Malignant sequelae appear to be more common among those with an enlarged uterus. In about 20% of the patients an additional physical finding is enlargement of the ovaries, which is associated with a higher frequency of future malignant change (approximately 50%)

as compared to less than 15% for those without ovarian enlargement. The development of these theca-lutein cysts is secondary to the luteinizing hormone–like effect of excessive HCG stimulation on the ovary.

Nausea and vomiting are common complaints, as is true in normal pregnancy, and hyperemesis gravidarum has been reported. Additionally, preeclamptic toxemia may occur in as many as one fourth of the patients, although its frequency has been reported to be less in many series.

Insofar as molar pregnancies are frequently diagnosed in the latter part of the first trimester of pregnancy, gestational trophoblastic disease should be considered in any patient with signs of toxemia during this time or during the early part of the second trimester. In addition, laboratory manifestations of hyperthyroidism have been reported, but clinical manifestations of hyperthyroidism are rare. The changes are in part due to the production of thyrotrophin-like hormone by the abnormal trophoblastic tissue, although a weak thyroid-stimulating-hormone action for HCG has also been hypothesized. These changes are reversible and usually abate after treatment of trophoblastic disease. The signs and symptoms of hydatidiform moles are summarized in the box above.

Clinically the behaviors of partial and complete moles differ. Complete mole is the more common and also has a more serious prognosis, with increased risk for the subsequent development of gestational trophoblastic neoplasm. Szulman and Surti recently analyzed the characteristics of 200 moles, both complete and partial; their results are summarized in Table

TABLE 33-2
Complete Versus Partial Moles

	Complete Mole		Partial Mole	
Clinical presentation and average gestational age	Molar pregnancy 16 weeks	48%	Molar pregnancy 19.7 weeks	8%
	Spontaneous abortion 13.7 weeks	40%	Spontaneous abortion 14.4 weeks	49%
	Missed abortion 19.5 weeks	6%	Missed abortion 24.8 weeks	43%
Preeclampsia		6%		8%
Uterus large for dates		33%		11%

Adapted from Szulman AE, Surti U: The syndromes of partial and complete molar gestation. Clin Obstet Gynecol 27:172, 1984.

33-2. HCG levels tend to be lower in partial moles.

Diagnosis

In a patient suspected of having a molar pregnancy the most valuable diagnostic aid is ultrasound (Fig. 33-5). The examination usually reveals absence of a fetus (in the case of a complete mole) and characteristic swollen villi that produce a snow storm–like pattern. The examination may also demonstrate ovarian enlargement secondary to the development of a theca-lutein cyst. If a fetal sac is detected, the possibility of a partial mole still exists. However, beyond the seventh week a fetal heart should be detected by ultrasound; its absence may suggest a missed abortion. If hydropic villi are present, it is possible that a blood clot in the uterus has been mistaken for a fetal sac. If there is doubt concerning the presence of fetal tissue and the existence of a partial mole, follow-up sonographic examinations are indicated.

Other diagnostic techniques were once used to diagnose a molar pregnancy, including intraamniotic injection of radioopaque dye (amniogram) to visualize the abnormal villi and arteriograms. These techniques subjected a potentially normal pregnancy to radiation exposure and, because of the refinement of ultrasound, have now been completely replaced by sonographic diagnosis.

The measurement of HCG is an integral part of the diagnosis and evaluation of the patient suspected of having trophoblastic disease. Radioimmunoassay (RIA) allows the measurement of extremely small amounts of HCG in blood and urine, as little as 1 mIU/ml. These sensitive tests have also been able to detect LH, which cross reacts with HCG, causing inaccurate assays. Vaitukaitis et al. developed specific antibodies for the beta subunit of HCG, the unique unit that allows its differentiation from LH, and virtually eliminated its cross reactivity with LH in RIAs. The RIA of the beta subunit of HCG provides a specific and sensitive measurement of this hormone. The levels in normal pregnancy reach a peak at about 10 to 14 weeks and rarely exceed levels of 100,000 mIU/ml. They can be higher in twin gestation, are frequently elevated in trophoblastic disease and may appear elevated in patients whose

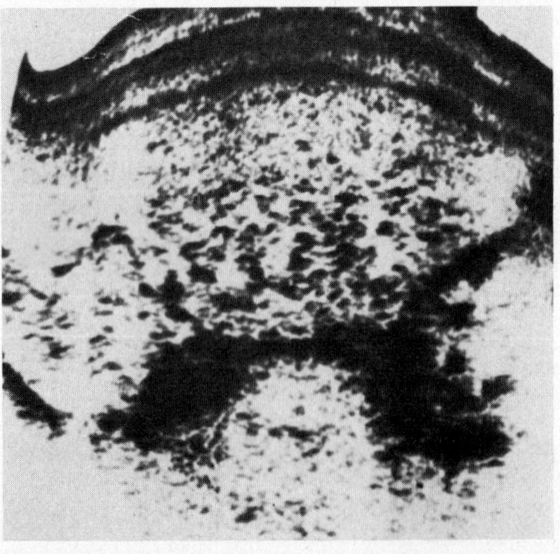

FIGURE 33-5
Ultrasound of uterus demonstrating "snow-storm" appearance of hydatidiform mole.

dates are not accurate. With molar pregnancy it is possible that the titer of HCG may not be elevated, so that a single determination is not diagnostic and will not necessarily differentiate normal pregnancy, multiple pregnancy, and trophoblastic disease. However, a titer in excess of 100,000 mIU/ml suggests trophoblastic disease. The HCG titers tend to be elevated above normal pregnancy values in complete mole, whereas partial mole tends to produce lower levels.

Management

Once the diagnosis of molar pregnancy is made, the uterus should be evacuated. Medical problems such as anemia due to blood loss, pregnancy-induced hypertension, pulmonary insufficiency, and hyperthyroidism should be evaluated and, when necessary, corrected. Occasionally disseminated intravascular coagulation (DIC) occurs, leading to a consumptive coagulopathy that requries correction as well as prompt uterine evacuation. Preevacuation chest x-ray examination is performed to rule out the spread of trophoblastic disease to the lungs and also for comparison in future follow-up. Unless a viable fetus is found, the pregnancy should be promptly terminated.

Acute pulmonary insufficiency may also occur. Acute dyspnea and cyanosis may develop, usually within 4 hours of evacuation. As noted by Cotton et al., this risk is greatest in patients whose uterus is more than 16 weeks' gestation size. Trophoblastic embolization and fluid overload with blood volume expansion appear to contribute to the picture of cardiac decompensation and pulmonary edema. If there are signs of pulmonary distress, arterial PO_2 should be monitored. In severely compromised patients ventilatory assistance, monitoring of pulmonary arterial pressure, and management in an intensive care unit may be needed.

Goldstein et al. have advocated the use of prophylactic cytotoxic chemotherapy to prevent the malignant sequelae of molar pregnancy. However, this practice has not gained widespread acceptance because giving chemotherapy at the time of evacuation of the mole exposes the patient to toxic and dangerous drugs even though most patients with hydatidiform mole do not require further treatment.

Approximately 80% of the patients require only uterine evacuation as definitive therapy. If malignant sequelae do develop, which is a risk for the remaining 20%, chemotherapy can then be used.

The most effective and widely used method of emptying the uterus of a molar pregnancy is suction curettage. A *Laminaria* tent is frequently inserted into the cervix the evening before D&C to facilitate cervical dilation. In many instances the molar pregnancy will have already begun to abort, and suction can complete the process. Intravenous oxytocic agents are used during the evacuation and immediately postoperatively to aid in uterine contraction and to help reduce blood loss. However, it is not advisable to use oxytocic drugs before evacuation of the molar pregnancy because of the risk of disseminating abnormal trophoblastic cells. If possible, a large suction curette (12 mm) should be used to aid in evacuation. The operator should begin the evacuation in the lower part of the uterus near the cervix and gradually extend it toward the fundus.

Previously for uterine enlargement beyond the size of a 16-week pregnancy hysterotomy was used to evacuate a hydatidiform mole. However, suction evacuation has proven to be safe and effective even with a larger uterus. After evacuation by suction curettage is complete, a gentle sharp curettage should be performed to ensure completion of the procedure.

If the patient has completed childbearing, hysterectomy may be considered as primary therapy for molar pregnancy. This is particularly desirable treatment in patients at greater risk for malignant sequelae following the molar pregnancy, especially older patients with ovarian lutein cysts or an enlarged uterus. The ovarian lutein cyst regresses after termination of the pregnancy, and oophorectomy should not be performed.

Follow-up

After evacuation of the uterus of a molar pregnancy (or in the rare case of therapy by hysterectomy), the patient should be carefully monitored for the potential development of malignant sequelae, specifically gestational trophoblastic neoplasia (GTN). The key to monitoring is the serial determination of β-HCG by

---

BASELINE DATA FOR PATIENT WITH MOLAR PREGNANCY

HCG serum titer (preevacuation)
Chest x-ray
Age
Uterine size
Presence or absence of ovarian lutein cysts
Presence or absence of fetal tissue
History of prior molar pregnancy
Assessment for medical complications
  Anemia
  Toxemia
  Pulmonary compromise
  Hyperthyroidism
  Coagulation defects

RIA in the patient's serum. While pregnancy tests can measure HCG, their lack of sensitivity and specificity requires an RIA specific for β-HCG. In most laboratories this assay has a sensitivity of 2 to 5 mIU/ml. Abnormal regression of the HCG titers following therapy for GTD is an early indication in the 20% of patients who will develop malignant sequelae.

Evaluation of the patient should include the data summarized in the box at left, which also allow identification of those at higher risk for malignant sequelae. The risk of trophoblastic neoplasia is increased in those with a large uterus, high HCG titer, lutein cysts, and a history of molar pregnancy and toxemia, as well as in older exposed patients, particularly individuals over 40. The risk of malignant sequelae is less in the absence of these factors and also if fetal tissue is present (partial mole).

To follow the course of the disease after evacuation of a molar pregnancy, the physician must carefully monitor the HCG titers. A normal regression curve is shown in Fig. 33-6. There is a gradual decline after evacuation of hydatidiform mole, reaching a normal range usually by the fourteenth week after evacuation. However, in some instances the titer returns to normal after a longer interval. Adequate monitoring consists of weekly HCG titers until the level reaches normal values. The patient must not become pregnant, and usually oral contraceptives are prescribed. There has been some suggestion in the literature that birth control pills might increase the risk of gestational trophoblastic neoplasia, but recent evidence from Morrow et al. suggests that birth control pills are safe and effective in this situation.

After the initial pelvic examination a repeat evaluation is performed usually every 2 weeks until the uterus and ovaries have returned to normal size. Theca-lutein cysts characteristically resolve within 2 months. However, patients with the high-risk factors listed earlier are approximately 10 times more likely to develop the sequelae of neoplasia in comparison to those without these factors. Once the HCG titers reach undetectable levels it is preferable to monitor them monthly for 1 year, after which the patient may be advised that she can safely attempt another pregnancy.

There may be an abnormal regression curve

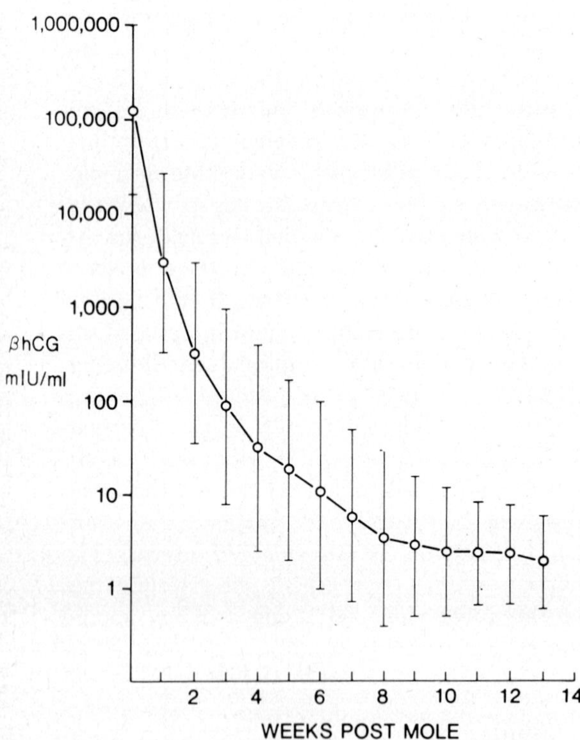

FIGURE 33-6
Mean value and 95% confidence limits describing normal postmolar β-HCG regression curve. (From Schlaerth JB, Morrow CP, Kletzky OA, et al: Obstet Gynecol 58:478, 1981. Reprinted with permission from The American College of Obstetricians and Gynecologists.)

after evacuation (Fig. 33-7), and in such instances the patient requires therapy for gestational trophoblastic neoplasia. A rise in titer (a doubling over a 2-week period) or a plateau in titer (failure to decrease over a 3-week interval) indicates the presence of postmolar trophoblastic neoplasia. The box below right outlines the management of hydatidiform mole, including the indications for chemotherapy.

Gestational Trophoblastic Neoplasia

Incidence and Diagnosis

As has been noted, malignancy (gestational trophoblastic neoplasia, GTN) develops after approximately 20% of complete hydatidiform moles. Conversely, about half the cases of trophoblastic neoplasia arise after molar pregnancy, while one fourth occur after normal pregnancy and one fourth after abortion or ectopic pregnancy. Therefore patients who continue to have abnormal bleeding after any pregnancy should have a β-HCG assay performed. Once GTN is diagnosed, chemotherapy is initiated unless complications such as uterine hemorrhage or perforation arise that require hysterectomy.

First a thorough evaluation must be done, including a complete physical examination, measurement of β-HCG titer, and extensive diagnostic tests to rule out metastatic disease. The physical examination includes pelvic and neurologic evaluations. These patients may have symptoms of metastatic disease such as hemoptysis (due to pulmonary lesions) or neurologic signs (secondary to brain metastases). Because of the fatal ramifications of brain and liver metastases, these areas must be thoroughly assessed with a computed tomography (CT) scan or radionuclide brain scan.

With the new generation of CT scanners, CT is usually preferred for evaluating both the brain and the liver. A pelvic ultrasound examination should be combined with the abdominal CT scan to complete the evaluation of the abdomen and pelvis. The most frequent site of metastatic GTN is the lungs (80% to 90% of cases), and less frequently the liver, brain, ovary, and vagina are involved. However, metastatic disease can occur at any site. Tests of renal and liver chemistries should also be performed in addition to a hematologic profile.

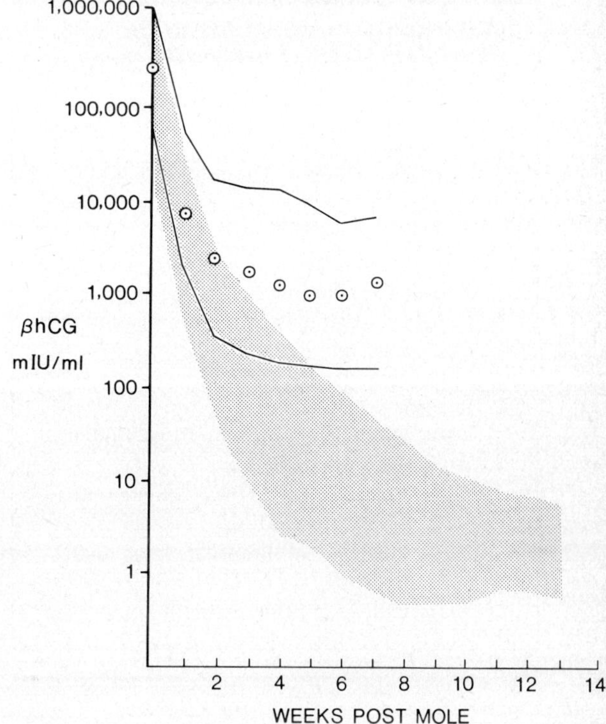

FIGURE 33-7
Mean value and 95% confidence limits for serum β-HCG titers obtained weekly after molar pregnancy in 38 patients whose regression curve deviated early in follow-up from normal regression curve represented by stippled area. (From Schlaerth JB, Morrow CP, Kletzky OA, et al: Obstet Gynecol 58:478, 1981. Reprinted with permission from The American College of Obstetricians and Gynecologists.)

MANAGEMENT OF HYDATIDIFORM MOLE

HCG: weekly serum determination until normal for two values, then monthly for 1 year

Chest x-ray examination initially and repeat if abnormal or if HCG plateaus or rises

Contraception for 1 year

Pelvic examination every 2 weeks until normal, then every 3 months

Initiate chemotherapy if—
  HCG titer increases or plateaus
  Metastatic disease is present
  Choriocarcinoma is diagnosed on tissue
  Elevated HCG is detected after normal levels are reached

PROGNOSTIC CLASSIFICATION OF GESTATIONAL TROPHOBLASTIC NEOPLASIA

1. Nonmetastatic GTN
2. Metastatic GTN: Disease outside the uterus
   A. Good prognosis:
      1. Disease present less than 4 months (short duration)
      2. Pretreatment HCG less than 40,000 mIU/ml
      3. No prior chemotherapy
   B. Poor prognosis:
      1. Disease present more than 4 months (long duration), or
      2. Pretreatment HCG greater than 40,000 mIU/ml, or
      3. Presence of brain or liver metastases, or
      4. Failure of prior chemotherapy

Depending on the location of the disease, the duration of symptoms, the level of the HCG titer, and a history of prior chemotherapy, it is possible to categorize the patient as having low-risk or high-risk GTN, as outlined in the box above. It has been stated that prior term pregnancy results in high-risk GTN, but recent evidence by Olive et al. from the John Brewer Trophoblastic Disease Center indicates that GTN after term pregnancy may be considered as low risk unless one of the poor prognosis factors listed is also present.

Management

NONMETASTATIC AND GOOD PROGNOSIS METASTATIC GTN. Single-agent chemotherapy is started for nonmetastatic GTN and good-prognosis (low-risk) metastatic GTN. Many programs of single-agent chemotherapy have been used, including methotrexate 0.3 mg/kg intravenously or intramuscularly daily for 5 days every 2 weeks; actinomycin D 10 to 12 µg/kg intravenously daily for 5 days every 2 weeks, or methotrexate 1 to 1.5 mg/kg intramuscularly or intravenously days 1, 3, 5, 7 followed by citrovorum factor rescue (leukovorin) 0.1 to 0.15 mg/kg intramuscularly on days 2, 4, 6, 8; and finally pulse actinomycin D 1.25 mg/m^2 intravenously once every 2 weeks. The latter regimen was introduced by Morrow et al. to treat low-risk nonmetastatic disease and has the advantage of being able to be given conveniently on an outpatient basis. It is used only for low-risk postmolar trophoblastic neoplasia, although few patients on this program have been studied. Preliminary evidence suggests that it is effective, although it may require a longer treatment time to attain regression of HCG to normal values. However, hospitalization is not required, and the treatment is more convenient and less expensive for the patient.

The 5-day actinomycin D and methotrexate courses have been found to be equally effective, but methotrexate appears to have more toxicity, particularly for the oral mucosa, and the severity of its toxicity increases with liver or renal compromise (see Chapter 25). High-dose methotrexate with citrovorum rescue has not proven to be more effective than the other single agents given alone. Some investigators have alternated the 5-day actinomycin D and methotrexate courses in the belief that this results in reduced toxicity and more rapid resolution of the disease. VP-16 (etoposide) has also been effectively used as single-agent therapy.

Patients are treated until a negative β-HCG level has been obtained; then one additional course of chemotherapy is usually given. Although recurrence rates of approximately 5% may be expected after therapy, recurrence more than 1 year after treatment is extremely unusual. Weekly serum determinations are made until three negative β-HCG titers are obtained. Then monthly titers are taken for at least 1 year, after which pregnancy may be attempted. Even with recurrence, chemotherapy can be expected to cure 100% of patients with low-risk nonmetastatic trophoblastic disease. Hysterectomy may be performed in good operative candidates with nonmetastatic GTN who desire no further children or who have uterine disease resistant to chemotherapy.

HIGH-RISK METASTATIC GTN. The treatment of poor-prognosis GTN requires multiple-agent chemotherapy. One frequently utilized protocol, designated MAC, consists of methotrexate (0.3 mg/kg), actinomycin D (8 to 10 µg/kg), and chlorambucil (0.2 mg/kg) or cyclophosphamide (3 to 5 mg/kg) given intravenously daily for 5 days. The cycle is repeated in 9 to 14 days as toxicity permits. To repeat the cycle, the white blood cell count must be greater than

3000, granulocytes over 1500, the platelet count more than 100,000, and the liver profile within normal limits.

More recently Surwit and Hammond have modified a multiple-agent treatment protocol introduced by Bagshawe (see below). This treatment has been used for those who have failed MAC therapy, but because of its success, some therapists have used this for primary treatment of poor-prognosis GTN. The therapy is highly toxic, and salvage rates in those undergoing primary therapy for high-risk GTN is over 70%, with some centers reporting even higher success rates. In a cooperative Gynecologic Oncology Group randomized study, Curry et al. recently reported superior results for MAC therapy with less toxicity than the Bagshawe regimen produces.

Vinblastine, bleomycin, and *cis*-platinum (Einhorm regimen) have also been used for high-risk GTN as for ovarian germ cell tumors (Chapter 29). The chemotherapy of poor-prognosis GTN is continued for three courses after

titers become negative, a practice that appears to decrease the rate of relapse.

If brain metastases are diagnosed, 2000 to 3000 rads are given immediately along with systemic chemotherapy. Liver metastases are usually treated by systemic chemotherapy, but 2000 rads to the liver is occasionally added to decrease the risk of hemorrhage.

As many as 20% of patients with poor-prognosis GTN who attain a negative HCG titer have a recurrence. In comparison the recurrence rate for those with good-prognosis GTN is 5%, while those with nonmetastatic GTN have recurrence rates of 1% to 2%.

After a negative titer is achieved for three cycles in patients with high-risk GTN, the titer is repeated every 2 weeks for 3 months and then monthly for 1 year. Some therapists continue the measurement of HCG titers every 6 months for as long as 5 years because of the slight risk of late recurrence of the disease. Chest x-ray examinations are also usually repeated every 3 months during the first year of follow-up, but the HCG titer is the crucial element in following the patient. A few isolated cases of choriocarcinomas have been reported in the absence of elevated levels of β-HCG. After 1 year of negative follow-up the patient may again attempt pregnancy.

MODIFIED BAGSHAWE CHEMOTHERAPY REGIMEN

Day 1	Hydroxyurea 500 mg PO q6h beginning 0600
	Actinomycin D 0.2 mg IV 1900
Day 2	Vincristine 1 mg/m^2 IV 0700
	Methotrexate 100 mg/m^2 IV-push 1900
	Methotrexate 200 mg/m^2 IV 12-hour infusion 1900
	Actinomycin D 0.2 mg IV 1900
Day 3	Actinomycin D 0.2 mg IV 1900
	Cyclophosphamide 500 mg/m^2 IV 1900
Day 4	Folinic acid 14 mg IM q6h beginning 0100
	Actinomycin D 0.5 mg IV 1900
Day 5	Folinic acid 14 mg IM 0100
	Actinomycin D 0.5 mg 1900
Day 6-7	No therapy
Day 8	Melphalan 6 mg/m^2 PO 1900 *or*
	Cyclophosphamide 500 mg/m^2 IV
	Doxorubicin (Adriamycin) 30 mg/m^2 IV 1900

Repeat cycle in 10 to 14 days with 25% reduction in dose if toxicity is severe.

Fertility After Treatment for GTN

There is concern, particularly among patients who have been treated for GTD, that a subsequent pregnancy will lead to repeat GTD or recrudescence of the disease. While repeat molar pregnancy is an increased risk (2% to 3%) among these patients, current evidence suggests that normal pregnancy usually results. Recent data from Rustin et al. indicate no increased frequency of congenital anomalies among infants whose mothers received chemotherapy. Goldstein reported that 67.4% of 929 individuals treated at various centers for GTD subsequently had a normal term delivery, while only 1.4% experienced a recurrent molar pregnancy. If pregnancy occurs following GTD, it is important to perform an ultrasound examination of the pelvis early to identify a gestational sac in the uterus as well as a fetal heart, which should be evident by the seventh week of pregnancy. HCG titers should be obtained after delivery to rule out any recurrence of GTD.

______________ **KEY POINTS** ______________

- The monitoring of trophoblastic disease and its follow-up is accomplished by the measurement of the beta-subunit of HCG by radioimmunoassay.

- The risk of hydatidiform mole is about 0.75 per 1000 pregnancies in the United States.

- Choriocarcinomas follow 1 in 40,000 term pregnancies and 3% to 5% of complete molar pregnancies.

- Risk factors for molar pregnancy include age (over 40 and under 20 years), geographic location (Southeast Asia and Mexico), and a history of prior molar pregnancy. Choriocarcinoma risk factors are similar, with an increased risk for women with blood type O impregnated by men of type A and those with type A impregnated by men of type O.

- The risk of developing a second molar pregnancy after a primary mole is about 20 to 40 times greater than the initial risk.

- About half the cases of GTN follow molar pregnancy, one fourth follow normal pregnancy, and one fourth follow abortion or ectopic pregnancy.

- Complete moles are of paternal origin, are diploid, and carry a 20% risk of malignant sequelae.

- Partial moles are of maternal and paternal origin, are triploid, and rarely are followed by GTN.

- Hydatidiform molar pregnancy should be suspected in a woman with persistent bleeding in the first half of pregnancy, toxemia before 24 weeks' gestation, or hyperemesis. The uterus is large for dates in about half the cases, and ovarian enlargement occurs in about 20%.

- An elevated serum level of β-HCG is not diagnostic of GTD but may indicate a multiple gestation or a normal pregnancy with incorrect dates.

- The diagnosis of a molar pregnancy (complete mole) can be established with ultrasound, which displays a "snowstorm" pattern.

- Hydatidiform moles are effectively and safely evacuated from the uterus using suction curettage.

- Low-risk GTN is gestational trophoblastic neoplasia in which the initial serum titer is <40,000 mIU/ml; the disease is present less than 4 months; and there has been no prior chemotherapy. It is usually treated by single-agent chemotherapy.

- High-risk GTN is gestational trophoblastic neoplasia in which one or more of the following are present: the initial serum titer is >40,000 mIU/ml; the disease has been present more than 4 months; brain or liver metastases are present; there is failure of prior chemotherapy. It is treated with multiple-agent chemotherapy.

- Recurrence rate for patients treated for GTN whose HCG titer reached normal is 5% for good-prognosis metastatic GTN and 1% to 2% for good-prognosis non-metastatic GTN. However, nonmetastatic GTN and low-risk GTN are 100% curable by chemotherapy.

- Patients with high-risk GTN are successfully treated with chemotherapy in more than 70% of the cases.

- Patients treated for GTN should not become pregnant for at least 1 year after treatment to allow accurate assessment of β-HCG titers.

- Infants born to mothers treated for GTD do not appear to have an increased frequency of congenital anomalies.

BIBLIOGRAPHY

Atrash HK, Hogue CJR, Grimes DA: Epidemiology of hydatidiform mole during early gestation. Am J Obstet Gynecol 154:906, 1986.

Bagshawe KD, Rawlings G, Pike MC, et al: The ABO blood groups in trophoblastic neoplasia. Lancet 1:553, 1971.

Bagshawe KD: Some facets of trophoblastic neoplasia in man. J Reprod Fertil Suppl 31, p. 175, 1982.

Bandy LC, Clarke-Pearson DL, Hammond C: Malignant potential of gestational trophoblastic disease at the extreme ages of reproductive life. Obstet Gynecol 64:395, 1984.

Berkowitz RS, Goldstein DP, Bernstein MR: Natural history of partial molar pregnancy. Obstet Gynecol 66:667, 1983.

Bigelow B: Gestational trophoblast disease. In Blaustein A, ed: Pathology of the female genital tract, 2nd ed. New York, Springer-Verlag, 1982.

Buckley JD: The epidemiology of molar pregnancy and choriocarcinoma. Clin Obstet Gynecol 27:153, 1984.

Cotton DB, Bernstein SG, Read SA, et al: Hemodynamic observations in evacuation of molar pregnancy. Am J Obstet Gynecol 138:6, 1980.

Curry SL, Blessing J, DiSaia P, et al: A prospective randomized comparison of methotrexate, actinomycin D, and chlorambucil (MAC) versus modified Bagshawe regimen in "poor prognosis" gestational trophoblastic disease (abst). Presented at 18th Annual Meeting of the Society of Gynecologic Oncology. Gynecol Oncol (in press).

Curry SL, Hammond CB, Tyrey L, et al: Hydatidiform

mole—diagnosis, management and long term follow-up of 347 patients. Obstet Gynecol 45:1, 1975.

Davis JR, Surwitt EA, Garay JP, et al: Sex assignment in gestational trophoblastic neoplasia. Am J Obstet Gynecol 148:722, 1984.

Dawook MY, Teoh ES, Ratnam SS: ABO blood group in trophoblastic disease. J Obstet Gynaecol Br Comm 78:918, 1971.

Goldstein DP, Berkowitz RS, Bernstein MR: Reproductive performance after molar pregnancy and gestational trophoblastic tumor. Clin Obstet Gynecol 27:221, 1984.

Grimes DA: Epidemiology of gestational trophoblastic disease. Am J Obstet Gynecol 150:309, 1984.

Hammond CB, Soper JT: Poor-prognostic metastatic gestational trophoblastic neoplasia. Clin Obstet Gynecol 27:228, 1984.

Lemonnier M-C, Glezerman V, Auclair R, et al: Choriocarcinoma associated with undetectable levels of human chorionic gonadotropin. Gynecol Oncol 25:48, 1986.

Li MC, Hertz R, Spencer DB: Effect of methotrexate therapy upon choriocarcinoma and chorioadenoma. Proc Soc Exp Biol Med 93:36, 1956.

Lurain JR, Brewer JI: Treatment of high-risk gestational trophoblastic disease with methotrexate, actinomycin D, and cyclophosphamide chemotherapy. Obstet Gynecol 65:830, 1985.

Morrow P, Nakamura R, Schlaerth JB, et al: The influence of oral contraceptives on the post molar HCG regression curve. Am J Obstet Gynecol (in press).

Olive DL, Lurain JR, Brewer JI: Choriocarcinoma associated with term gestation. Am J Obstet Gynecol 148:711, 1984.

Rustin GJS, Booth M, Dent J, et al: Pregnancy after cytotoxic chemotherapy for gestational trophoblastic tumors. Br Med J 288:103, 1984.

Schlaerth JB, Morrow CR, Kletzky OA, et al: Prognostic characteristics of serum human chorionic gonadotropin titer regression following molar pregnancy. Obstet Gynecol 58:478, 1981.

Schlaerth JB, Morrow CP, Nalick RH, et al: Single-dose actinomycin D in the treatment of post molar trophoblastic disease. Gynecol Oncol 19:53, 1984.

Smith EB, Szulman AE, Hinshaw W, et al: Human chorionic gonadotropin levels in complete and partial hydatidiform moles and in nonmolar abortuses. Am J Obstet Gynecol 149:129, 1984.

Surwit EA, Hammond CB: Treatment of metastatic trophoblastic disease with poor prognosis. Obstet Gynecol 55:565, 1980.

Szulman AE, Surti U: The syndromes of partial and complete molar gestation. Clin Obstet Gynecol 27:172, 1984.

Vaitukaitis JL, Braunstein GD, Ross GT: A radioimmunoassay which specifically measures human chorionic gonadtropin in the presence of human luteinizing hormone. Am J Obstet Gynecol 113:751, 1972.

Vassilakos P, Riotten G, Kajii T: Hydatidiform mole: Two entities. A morphologic and cytogenic study with some clinical considerations. Am J Obstet Gynecol 127:167, 1977.

WHO Scientific Group: Gestational trophoblastic diseases. Technical Report Series 692. Geneva, WHO, 1983.

Young RH, Scully RE: Placental-site trophoblastic tumor: current status. Clin Obstet Gynecol 27:248, 1984.

ENDOCRINOLOGY AND INFERTILITY

<table><tr><td>CHAPTER
34</td><td>

Dysmenorrhea and Premenstrual Syndrome

</td></tr></table>

Cervical Stenosis. Narrowing of the cervical canal, often at the level of the internal os, in such a way that menstrual flow is impeded and intrauterine pressure is increased at the time of menses.

Dysmenorrhea. Painful cramping sensation in the lower abdomen often accompanied by other symptoms such as sweating, tachycardia, headaches, nausea, vomiting, diarrhea, and tremulousness. These all occur just before or during the menses. Primary dysmenorrhea begins at or shortly after menarche and is usually not accompanied by pelvic pathologic conditions. Secondary dysmenorrhea arises later and usually is associated with other pelvic conditions.

Mittelschmerz. Midcycle pelvic pain usually related to ovulation. The actual mechanism is not clearly understood.

Pelvic Congestion Syndrome. Vascular engorgement of the uterus and the vessels of the broad ligament and lateral pelvic walls which may lead to chronic pelvic pain.

Premenstrual Syndrome (PMS). A group of symptoms, both physical and behavioral, that occur in the second half of the menstrual cycle and often interfere with work and personal relationships. They are followed by a period entirely free of symptoms.

Prostaglandin-Synthetase Inhibitors (PGSIs). Substances that block the activity of prostaglandin synthetase, thereby preventing the effect of prostaglandins on tissue. These basically consist of two chemical groups: the arylcarboxylic and the arylalkanoic acids.

Dysmenorrhea and premenstrual syndrome afflict a large percentage of women in the reproductive years. These conditions have a negative effect on the quality of the patients' lives and on the lives of their families, and they are also responsible for a huge economic loss as a result of decreased productivity. This chapter will discuss current thinking with respect to the etiology, pathophysiology, and management of these two conditions, which are not always related.

DYSMENORRHEA

Dysmenorrhea is defined as a severe, painful cramping sensation in the lower abdomen often accompanied by other biologic symptoms, including sweating, tachycardia, headaches, nausea, vomiting, diarrhea, and tremulousness, all occurring just before or during the menses. In the past the definition has been subdivided into primary and secondary dysmenorrhea. The term *primary dysmenorrhea* was reserved for women who had no obvious pathologic condition. We currently recognize that these patients are suffering from the effects of endogenous prostaglandins. *Secondary dysmenorrhea,* on the other hand, is associated with pelvic conditions or pathology that causes pelvic pain in conjunction with the menses. Primary dysmenorrhea almost always occurs in women younger than 20. Indeed, the patient will report pain as soon as she establishes ovulatory cycles. Secondary dysmenorrhea may, of course, occur in women under 20, but it is most often seen in women over 20.

Incidence

A number of studies have attempted to determine the prevalence of dysmenorrhea; a wide range (3% to 90%) has been reported. These studies have been performed on students, teenagers and their mothers, and individuals from various specific populations such as industrial workers or college students. The best estimate of the prevalence of primary dysmenorrhea is about 75%. Andersch and Milsom surveyed all the 19-year-old women in the city of Gothenburg, Sweden. A total of 90.9% of such women responded to a randomly distributed questionnaire, and 72.4% of these stated that they suffered from dysmenorrhea. In addition, 34.3% of the total population reported mild menstrual symptoms, 22.7% cited moderate symptoms that required analgesia, and 15.4% stated that they had severe dysmenorrhea that clearly inhibited their working ability and that could not be adequately assuaged by general analgesia (Table 34-1). This study verified the work of others who found that women who had vaginally delivered a child, who took birth control pills, or who were smokers were less likely to have dysmenorrhea. Pregnancy itself without actual birth did not seem to alleviate dysmenorrhea, as women who had ectopic pregnancies or spontaneous or voluntary terminations of pregnancy were not relieved of their symptoms, whereas women who delivered babies were.

Oral contraceptive use was noted by these investigators to reduce the prevalence and severity of dysmenorrhea significantly ($P \leq .01$). IUD use did not affect prevalence or severity in any measurable way.

Relationship to Menstruation and the Menstrual Cycle

Andersch and Milsom demonstrated a significant positive correlation between the severity of dysmenorrhea and the duration of menstrual flow, amount of menstrual flow, and early menarche. They showed no relationship with the actual duration of the menstrual cycle.

In their series, 38.3% of the patients reported that they had experienced dysmenorrhea for the first time during the first year after menarche, and only 20.8% reported that dysmenorrhea had not occurred until 4 years after menarche.

Family History

Dysmenorrhea has been reported to be significantly increased among mothers and sisters of women with dysmenorrhea.

Pathogenesis of Primary Dysmenorrhea

Although the pathogenesis of dysmenorrhea is still unknown, the fact that there is a close association between an elevated prostaglandin $F_{2\alpha}$ level in the secretory endometrium and the symptoms of dysmenorrhea, including uterine hypercontractility, complaints of severe cramping, and other prostaglandin-induced symptoms, have led to the theory that prostaglandin $F_{2\alpha}$ is associated with the pathogenesis of dysmenorrhea. Prostaglandin-synthetase inhibitors (PGSIs) have been demonstrated to alleviate these symptoms. These substances are nonsteroidal and antiinflammatory. They have been used as analgesics for a number of conditions,

TABLE 34-1
Severity of Primary Dysmenorrhea
in a Population of 586 Swedish,
19-year-old Women

Severity	No.	%
None	162	27.6
Mild*	201	34.3
Moderate†	133	22.7
Severe‡	90	15.4

Data from Andersch B, Milsom I: An epidemiologic study of young women with dysmenorrhea. Am J Obstet Gynecol 144:655, 1982.
*No systemic symptoms, medication rarely required, work rarely affected.
†Few systemic symptoms, medication required, work moderately affected.
‡Multiple symptoms, poor medication response, work inhibited.

including arthritis, and generally are divided into two chemical groups—the arylcarboxylic acids, which include acetyl salicylic acid (aspirin) and fenamates, and the arylalkanoic acids, including the arylpropionic acids (ibuprofen, naproxen, and ketoprofen) as well as the indoleacetic acids (indomethacin). The specific effect of these agents on the uterine musculature is reduction of contractility as measured by reduction of intrauterine pressure.

In 1984 Owen reviewed the effectiveness of PGSIs in the treatment of primary dysmenorrhea. She reviewed 51 trials carried out in 1649 women. More than 72% of the women suffering from dysmenorrhea reported significant pain relief with PGSIs; 18% reported minimal or no pain relief, and 15% showed a placebo response. Owen concluded that PGSI compounds were effective and safe for the majority of women with primary dysmenorrhea. The fenamates seemed to be more effective in providing pain relief than ibuprofen, indomethacin, or naproxen. All the compounds demonstrated minimal PGSI-associated side effects with the exception of indomethacin. In trials with indomethacin the dropout rate was higher primarily because of symptoms involving the central nervous system and gastrointestinal tract.

PGSIs should not be given to patients who have shown previous hypersensitivity to such drugs. It is also contraindicated for individuals who have had nasal polyps, angioedema, and bronchospasm related to aspirin or nonsteroidal antiinflammatory agents. In addition, these agents are contraindicated for individuals with a history of chronic ulceration or inflammatory reaction of the upper or lower gastrointestinal tract and for those with preexisting chronic renal disease. During the use of such agents, autoimmune hemolytic anemia, rash, edema and fluid retention, and central nervous system symptoms such as dizziness, headache, nervousness, and blurred vision occur. In up to 15% of users slight elevation of hepatic enzymes may also be found. Table 34-2 lists some of the PGSIs in common use for the treatment of dysmenorrhea.

Etiology and Management of Secondary Dysmenorrhea

A variety of other conditions cause or are associated with dysmenorrhea. These conditions may occur at any age, and in most cases the pain experienced is either secondary to the pathologic process of the condition or a specific result of the condition. These would constitute the so-called secondary dysmenorrhea group of problems and include cervical stenosis, ectopic endometrial tissue, pelvic inflammation, pelvic congestion, conditioned behavior, and stress and tension (see box below).

Cervical Stenosis

Severe narrowing of the cervical canal, particularly at the level of the internal os, may impede menstrual flow, causing an increase in intrauterine pressure at the time of menses. In addition, retrograde menstrual flow through the fallopian tubes into the peritoneal cavity may take place. Thus severe cervical stenosis may eventually be associated with pelvic endometriosis as well. The etiology of cervical stenosis may be congenital or may be secondary to cervical injury such as with electrocautery, cryocautery, or operative trauma (i.e.,

TABLE 34-2
Commonly Used Prostaglandin-Synthetase Inhibitors

Brand Name	Generic Name	Usual Regimen (mg q6h)
Motrin	Ibuprofen	400-800
Naprosyn	Naproxen	250-500
Anaprox	Naproxen sodium	275-550
Ponstel	Mefenamic acid	250-500

CAUSES OF SECONDARY DYSMENORRHEA

Cervical stenosis
Endometriosis and adenomyosis
Pelvic infection and adhesions
Pelvic congestion
Conditioned behavior
Stress and tension

conization). The condition may also be due to an inflammatory process caused by infection or by the application of caustic substances. Following any of these conditions the cervical canal may narrow because of the formation of scar tissue.

The possibility of cervical stenosis should be considered if there is a history of scant menstrual flow and if severe cramping continues throughout the menstrual period.

The diagnosis is suspected when the external os appears scarred or when it is impossible to pass the uterine sound through the internal os during the proliferative stage of the menstrual cycle. Diagnosis is generally documented by the inability to pass a thin probe of a few millimeters' diameter through the internal os or by hysterosalpingogram, which demonstrates a thin, stringy-appearing canal. If dilation and curettage (D&C) are performed, finding the passage through the internal os with a thin probe is often difficult but can frequently be accomplished with patience. The patient should be anesthetized.

Treatment consists of dilating the cervix; this may be accomplished by D&C with progressive dilators or by the use of progressive *Laminaria* tents. In the past the insertion of stem pessaries has been noted to be of some value in such cases. Unfortunately, cervical stenosis often recurs after therapy, necessitating repeat procedures. Pregnancy and vaginal delivery often afford more lasting cure.

Ectopic Endometrial Tissue (Endometriosis)

Ectopic endometrial tissue or endometriosis (including endometriosis and adenomyosis) should be considered when there is a history of pain becoming more severe during menses. Frequently dyspareunia and infertility are accompanying symptoms. Pertinent physical findings may include uterosacral ligament nodules or evidence for endometriosis in the vagina or cervix.

Specific diagnosis of endometriosis is made by direct visualization via laparoscopy or laparotomy or by direct biopsy of vaginal or cervical lesions.

Treatment of endometriosis is discussed in Chapter 18. Management should be designed for the patient's specific needs.

Pelvic Inflammation

Pelvic infections secondary to gonorrhea, chlamydia, or other infectious agents may cause pelvic inflammation or pelvic abscess and with healing may be associated with pelvic adhesions that cause pelvic pain. Often this may be aggravated at menses, causing dysmenorrhea. Infections secondary to other conditions such as appendicitis or IUD use may also create a similar response. The pain may be secondary to the congestion and edema that occur normally at menses, which may subsequently be aggravated by the healed inflammatory areas and adhesions.

Pelvic Congestion Syndrome

Pelvic congestion syndrome, which was first described by Taylor several years ago, is due to engorgement of pelvic vasculature. The pain is usually burning or throbbing in nature, worse at night, and worse after standing. Physical examination of the vagina and cervix usually reveals vasocongestion with evidence of some uterine enlargement and tenderness. Diagnosis is made by observation of the features noted and by laparoscopy, which not only rules out other causes of pelvic pain but also demonstrates congestion of the uterus and engorgement or varicosities of the broad ligament and pelvic side wall veins. If laparoscopy is used for diagnosis, it is important to observe the broad ligament vasculature as the pressure of the carbon dioxide or nitrous oxide is released. At full pressure during the procedure these vessels may be obliterated but will reappear as pressure is reduced.

The pathophysiology of pelvic congestion syndrome is probably related to tension and psychosomatic problems. Consequently, management relates to careful history of the patient's past and present social situation and, where appropriate, the use of counseling.

Severe cases of pelvic congestion syndrome that do not respond to counseling or other medical types of pain management may respond to hysterectomy, although such management should be considered a last resort.

Conditioned Behavior

In individuals with strong family histories of dysmenorrhea, or in situations where a careful history demonstrates a possibility for societal reward or control because of the symptoms of pain, a conditioned behavior should be considered. It is important to obtain a careful medical and social history and to rule out all other causes of acquired dysmenorrhea.

Diagnosis can often be verified by the use of a personality profile test such as the Minnesota Multiphasic Personality Index. This test has been used clinically on many different groups of patients and is well standardized. It is frequently necessary to use such a test to demonstrate to the patient that she does indeed fit into such a category.

Treatment of patients with conditioned behavior dysmenorrhea includes reeducation so that the pain is not looked on as a rewarding experience. Teaching the patient an understanding of the pathophysiology of the problem and applying reconditioning techniques are useful. Psychologists or other similarly trained mental health workers can be consulted for this purpose.

Stress and Tension

Dysmenorrhea due to stress and tension usually is accompanied by a history of gradual onset, and the pain is generally worse at times, particularly when stress is severe and when there may be a possibility for secondary gain. The pathophysiology is difficult to define; it may be a combination of prostaglandin activity and engorgement.

The treatment is centered on finding the means to relieve stress, which may include education, the teaching of relaxation techniques, counseling, and, on rare occasions, antidepression or tranquilizing medications for short periods of time.

Other Causes

At times dysmenorrhea may be related to unusual pathologic findings. These include small leiomyomas or polyps at the junction of the internal os and lower uterine segment. Such a condition may produce a valvelike effect at the os at the time of menses. Frequently myomas or polyps become engorged or edematous at the time of menses, accentuating the problem. Diagnosis is generally made by history and by hysterosalpingography, hysteros-

copy, or D&C. Therapy consists of excising the pathologic tissue. In the case of a myoma a hysterectomy may be necessary.

PREMENSTRUAL SYNDROME

The premenstrual syndrome (PMS) is defined as a group of symptoms, both physical and behavioral, that occur in the second half of the menstrual cycle and that often interfere with work and personal relationships. These are followed by a period entirely free of symptoms. The condition was first described by Frank in 1931. That author attempted to relate symptoms of then so-called premenstrual tension with hormonal changes of the menstrual cycle. The term *premenstrual syndrome* was first used by Dalton in 1953. The symptoms do vary from woman to woman, and more than 150 symptoms have been linked with the disorder.

Incidence

While various reports place the prevalence of PMS at 5% to 95% of menstruating women, it is generally agreed that about 40% of women are significantly affected at one time or another. Severe symptoms occur in only 2% or 3% of women between the ages of 18 and 48.

Symptoms

In a review by O'Brien a number of common somatic and psychological symptoms were enumerated. These are summarized in the box on p. 946. In general, somatic symptoms relate to fluid retention, breast tenderness, and various pain constellations such as headache or pelvic pain. Psychological symptoms vary from irritability and tension to anxiety, aggression, and depression. The personality changes that occur in the second half of the menstrual cycle are so severe in some patients that the term "Dr. Jekyl and Mr. Hyde" is frequently used. In a few instances PMS has been used as a defense in murder trials.

Etiology

When Frank first described the syndrome he attributed it to estrogen excess. Seven years later Israel theorized that it was due to an im-

SYMPTOMS OF PREMENSTRUAL SYNDROME

Somatic Symptoms

Bloated feeling
Feeling of weight increase
Breast pain or tenderness
Skin disorders
Hot flushes
Headache
Pelvic pain
Change in bowel habits

Psychological Symptoms

Irritability
Aggression
Tension
Anxiety
Depression
Lethargy
Insomnia
Change in appetite
Crying
Change in libido
Thirst
Loss of concentration
Poor coordination, clumsiness, accidents

From O'Brien PMS: The premenstrual syndrome: a review of the present status of therapy. Drugs 24:140, 1982.

balance of estrogen and progesterone. Others have offered theories that the disorder is related to endogenous hormone allergy, hypoglycemia, vitamin B_6 deficiency, prolactin excess, fluid retention, inappropriate prostaglandin activity, elevated monoamine oxidase (MAO), endorphin malfunction, and multiple psychological disturbances. In 1981, Reid and Yen reviewed the subject and concluded that PMS was a multifactorial psychoendocrine disorder. As yet, however, the specific etiology remains unclear. Nevertheless, it is still worthwhile to review some of the data related to the specific theories that have been considered in order to offer some insight for therapy.

Steroid Allergy

The first of these theories involved the thought that the condition might be related to an allergy to an endogenous hormone, specifically progesterone. It had been observed that many women did, indeed, have dermatitis during the luteal phase of the menstrual cycle. In 1962, Rogers reported that 80% of his PMS patients who were desensitized with small amounts of pregnanediol reported some improvement of their symptoms. However, there were no control subjects in his study, and no placebo studies were carried out.

Hypoglycemia and Vitamin Deficiency

One of the older theories of the etiology of PMS related this condition to hypoglycemia. In 1953, Morton et al. reported finding that results of the glucose tolerance test (GTT) revealed flattening, with a delayed hypoglycemia in many patients immediately before or during menses. In such individuals the glucose tolerance level was found to be normal after the menstrual period. Since many patients craved sweets and complained of headaches, he felt there was supportive evidence for a hypoglycemic etiology. He therefore treated 249 volunteers in a New York state prison with high-protein diets. Some individuals received a placebo, while others received medication consisting of a diuretic, caffeine, and vitamin B complex. None of those on the medication regimen required isolation for behavior problems during their premenstrual period even though several had required this before the treatment had begun. In addition, their efficiency at work activities was judged as superior; they performed almost a third more work than they had previously. While 15% of patients treated with placebo demonstrated an improvement in symptoms, 39% treated with placebo and high-protein diet noted improvement. Patients who were treated with the drug regimen reported a 61% improvement in symptoms, and those treated with drug plus high-protein diet showed a 79% improvement. All individuals reported the greatest improvement in those symptoms that were related to nervousness and other emotional symptoms.

About the same time that the hypoglycemia theory was postulated, it was suggested that there was a vitamin B_6 deficiency in PMS patients as well. Originally it was suggested that a deficiency of vitamins could lead to impaired liver function, thus causing an increase in circulating estrogen. However, groups of women on diets severely lacking in vitamin B during wartime were found to have normal estrogen metabolism. With the discovery that vitamin B_6 is a coenzyme in the biosynthesis of dopamine and serotonin, the possibility that this agent might be involved in the etiology of PMS was raised. Also, in 1973, Adams et al. noted that vitamin B_6 therapy seemed to be associated with improvement of depression in women taking oral contraceptives in a double-blind trial. It was believed that the oral contraceptives caused an abnormal tryptophan metabolism and that vitamin B_6 to some extent reversed this. One double-blind study by Abraham and Hargrov demonstrated that vitamin B_6 administered in 200 to 800 mg doses daily prevented some of the symptoms of PMS in women with this affliction significantly better than did a placebo. Abraham and Hargrov theorized that deficiencies of vitamin B_6 and magnesium could result in a lower threshold to stress and to a potential hormone imbalance. They also noted that giving vitamin B_6 to a patient raised serum progesterone levels at mid-luteal cycle. The requirements for pyridoxine may increase with increased estrogen levels partly because estrogen may increase the metabolism of tryptophan via the kynurenine-niacin pathway. In this reaction pyridoxine is required as a cofactor. Estrogen conjugates also competitively inhibit pyridoxine activity. This action may lower brain serotonin levels, which may be involved in causing a depression reaction. However, a previous double-blind study by Stokes and Mendels failed to show any improvement by pyridoxine over placebo in alleviating PMS symptoms. However, only 13 women were studied in this trial.

Prolactin Effect

Some investigators believe that elevated prolactin may induce PMS symptoms. Kullander and Svanberg and Halbreich et al. actually offered evidence that elevated prolactin levels stimulate PMS symptoms in certain patients. Prolactin is known to affect the breast, and it is suspected to affect the kidneys' ability to excrete water. In 1981, Ylöstalo et al. studied 36 women suffering from PMS using bromocrip-

tine versus a placebo and norethisterone and a placebo in a double-blind study. Bromocriptine decreased breast engorgement and irritability as well as all PMS symptoms in general. These authors noted weight gain during the luteal phase to be smaller in the group treated with either drug than in the placebo group. Norethisterone alleviated breast tenderness and caused a decrease in serum levels of luteinizing hormone (LH), follicle-stimulating hormone (FSH), and progesterone while increasing the serum level of prolactin. Ylöstalo et al. concluded that bromocriptine was more efficient in the treatment of PMS than was norethisterone.

In the same year, Andersch and Hahn studied 34 PMS patients in a double-blind experiment in which patients were given bromocriptine or placebo during the luteal phase of cycles at random, with each patient serving as her own control. Serum prolactin levels were within normal limits without treatment and were significantly reduced by bromocriptine. Serum progesterone levels did not change during any treatment. The administration of any medication (bromocriptine or placebo) considerably improved all the premenstrual symptoms, but results with bromocriptine were not significantly better than with the placebo. These authors concluded that prolactin alone does not seem to cause premenstrual symptoms.

In a review in 1983 by Andersch, 14 placebo control studies in which PMS was treated with bromocriptine were reviewed. Andersch concluded that there was no substantial support that bromocriptine is an effective drug in treating PMS as an entity. He noted that irritability, depression, and anxiety were not significantly improved during treatment with the drug when compared to placebo treatment. The drug, however, was effective in treating premenstrual breast tenderness if the dosage of bromocriptine was above 5 mg per day. He concluded that bromocriptine had a place in the management of PMS only if breast tenderness was a major concern of the patient.

Fluid Retention

For some years fluid retention has been believed to be the single mechanism most likely to be responsible for PMS because fluid retention in the brain could cause mood changes, fluid retention in the breast could cause tenderness, and gastrointestinal symptoms could be due to edema of the gastrointestinal tract. It has been difficult, however, to demonstrate relationships between specific symptoms of PMS and luteal phase weight gain. Perceived swelling of the body is difficult to prove with actual careful weight analysis. Recently Faratian et al. evaluated 148 menstrual cycles in 52 women, and in each cycle various parameters were measured to determine an objective means of assessing the syndrome. These included daily mood assessment and measurement of body weight, plasma 17β-estradiol levels, and plasma progesterone levels. The abdominal girth was measured carefully in two dimensions: at the level of the umbilicus and at 10 cm below the umbilicus. At the same time these dimensions were subjectively judged by the patient. Mood scores showed a marked shift during the premenstrual phase of each cycle. The symptom of bloatedness was most marked during the premenstrual phase of the cycle. Despite these elevated scores for bloatedness, there was no increase in body weight or measured body dimension changes in any plane during this period of time. The patient's perception of body size did increase, and a discrepancy between the perceived body size and actual body size was noted. The authors divided their patients into those with predominantly somatic symptoms and those with predominantly psychological symptoms and also studied a control group. No hormonal differences were noted in the three groups.

Sex Steroids

Although sex steroid concentrations in patients with PMS have been quite thoroughly investigated, there is no evidence that these women have impaired corpus luteal function. Estrogen can lead to increased aldosterone levels by stimulating synthesis of angiotensinogen. Progesterone, on the other hand, exerts a natriuretic effect on renal tubules. It is presumed that progesterone blocks aldosterone action at this site. However, if progesterone is given, it causes an increase in aldosterone levels after 48 to 72 hours. This is apparently a compensatory response to the progesterone-induced sodium

loss. Progesterone may be responsible for the observed luteal phase increase in aldosterone, and some authors believe that aldosterone levels are higher in PMS patients who complain of fluid retention. Abraham thinks that this is due to vitamin B_6 and magnesium deficiencies and attributes the therapeutic effect of progesterone to its natriuretic effect. If it is accepted that aldosterone levels do increase in PMS, then diuretic therapy may have a place.

In a double-blind study, Werch and Kane reported benefit to PMS patients who used a diuretic if the patients had complained of swelling. They suggested that failure of diuretics to relieve symptoms in some PMS patients might relate to patient selection. O'Brien noted that patients treated with the diuretic spironolactone demonstrated decreases in depression, sadness, tension, bloating, loss of libido, aggression, lethargy, and anxiety. Thus, although it is difficult to understand why diuretics alleviate symptoms in certain PMS patients, their success in many cases makes their selective use reasonable.

Prostaglandins

Although prostaglandin substances are definitely related to the symptoms of primary dysmenorrhea, their role in causing symptoms in PMS patients is unclear. In a double-blind placebo-controlled study, Budoff examined the therapeutic value of one PGSI, zomepirac sodium. The substance reduced by more than half the severity of nine symptoms—cramping, backache, systemic weakness, headache, nausea, leg pain, insomnia, dizziness, and vomiting. In her series there was a strong placebo effect, but the drug proved significantly better than the placebo in relief of all symptoms except insomnia. Eighty percent of the women in her series had reportedly missed at least 1 day from their usual activities monthly before therapy. The placebo reduced this loss by 53% and the zomepirac sodium by 77%. It seems likely that some of the symptoms of PMS may be due to prostaglandin activity or at least are relieved by a PGSI, making it likely that the inclusion of one of these compounds in a treatment regimen of patients with specific symptoms may be useful.

Elevated Monoamine Oxidase

One theory of depression is that it may be caused by elevated brain MAO activity and that this may be the result of a deficiency in catecholamines. MAO catalyzes the oxidation of primary amines to aldehydes. Progesterone increases plasma levels of MAO during the luteal phase. Dalton believes that the cause of PMS lies in a faulty progesterone feedback pathway. Placebo-controlled studies with synthetic progestins have demonstrated little effect in treating PMS symptoms. Dalton favors the use of naturally occurring progesterone for the treatment of PMS and states that the indications for treatment include recurrent symptoms severe enough to interfere with normal activities, risk of suicide, battering or alcoholism, domestic disharmony and stress, and cyclic symptoms after menopause or hysterectomy. She recommends 50 to 100 mg of progesterone daily intramuscularly or 200 to 400 mg daily by progesterone vaginal suppository. Others advocate twice daily vaginal suppositories containing 50 to 100 mg of progesterone each. Dalton begins patients on this regimen 5 days before symptoms are expected and continues until the onset of menses or until the symptoms cease. She notes that in nulliparous women progesterone may cause euphoria, restless energy, insomnia, faintness, and uterine cramps during menstruation. In her patients symptoms returned 3 months after discontinuation of therapy. She maintains that failure is due to improper diagnosis or improper dosage schedule. Such therapy is extremely expensive. Double-blind studies by Smith and by Sampson failed to show any improvement when progesterone was compared to placebo.

Endorphins

It has been suggested that increased endorphin levels during the luteal phase inhibit catecholamines and that their abrupt decrease during menses leads to an increase in catecholamine activity. A decrease in catecholamines can be associated with depression, whereas an excess may be associated with irritability, aggression, and even psychotic symptoms. In monkey studies endorphins peak during the luteal phase and fall to imperceptible levels during menses. Cohen et al. administered nal-oxone, an endorphin antagonist, to volunteers and produced symptoms of irritability, anxiety, tension, and aggressiveness. Progesterone therapy will maintain high levels of endorphin, and this could be a means by which progesterone might be useful in PMS patients.

Diagnosis

Since the etiology of PMS is still unknown, the diagnosis is made by history. The facts given by the patient may allow the physician to construct a specific treatment regimen for that patient. It is important that the physician have a clear understanding of the patient's symptoms before undertaking therapy. After a complete history and physical examination, the physician should rule out any medical problems that could be influencing the symptomatology. The physician should then ask the patient to keep a diary of her symptoms throughout two menstrual cycles. Although the patient and the physician may focus on the second half of the menstrual cycle, the patient should be encouraged to keep track of all symptoms regardless of the stage of the menstrual cycle. A number of commercial diary sheets and symptom checkoff lists are available, but it is probably better to have the patient write the symptoms she perceives in her own words rather than clue her to specific response patterns. At the end of two cycles the physician should review the symptom diary with the patient and discuss carefully those symptoms that seem to be causing her the most difficulty.

Management

Diet

The physician should review the patient's diet and initially suggest a high-protein, well-balanced diet. Supplemental vitamins may be used, and the physician may elect to suggest that the patient use a vitamin B_6 (pyridoxine) supplement at the rate of 50 to 200 mg per day. It is appropriate to begin with this therapy and add other medications if necessary.

Diuretics

The physician may elect to add a diuretic to the regimen if the patient's complaints involve bloating and perceived change in body habitus during the luteal phase of the cycle. A potassium-saving diuretic should be selected. The lowest dose possible to achieve symptomatic relief should be utilized.

Progesterone

Although Dalton advocates the use of naturally occurring progesterone, the fact that progesterone receptors will respond to both synthetic progestins and progesterone would imply that any reasonable progestational agent would be appropriate. A regimen of 10 to 30 mg per day of medroxyprogesterone acetate (Provera) or 50 to 100 mg twice a day of progesterone vaginal suppositories can be tried.

Psychotherapy

Studies in the 1950s by Rees and Fortin et al. showed that 50% of patients inproved with psychotherapy alone. However, this is similar to the response rate of many placebo therapies. Certainly if patients have obvious psychiatric problems as detected by history, psychotherapy should be added. It is less effective as a primary therapy.

Psychoactive Drugs

Although psychoactive drugs may be useful in controlling acute problems at specific times in a patient's life, they should not be used for long periods or as primary medications. Few control studies have demonstrated any long-standing benefits of such agents in this condition.

Bromocriptine

Bromocriptine may be used in patients with breast tenderness and may be helpful for some of the other symptoms of PMS, although its use in any individual case will need to be evaluated. A dose of 5 mg per day during the luteal phase is appropriate.

Prostaglandin-Synthetase Inhibitors

For patients who complain of cramping or other systemic symptoms such as diarrhea or heat intolerance, a trial with a PGSI may be useful. It should be noted, however, that a toxic complication of PGSI use is nonoliguric renal failure. Since it is more likely to occur with PGSI use associated with severe dehydration, the agent should be discontinued if severe diarrhea is present and should not be used with diuretics.

• • •

The physician should be cautious in building a treatment regimen for any individual patient and should attempt to verify the patient's symptoms and to add medications only when relief has not been achieved. Medications that do not seem to be helping should be stopped. Since most agents when scrutinized by double-blind control methods are less than utopian in the treatment of this condition, it is not surprising that individualization of treatment is essential.

KEY POINTS

- Primary dysmenorrhea almost always occurs before the age of 20. Secondary dysmenorrhea may occur at any time during the menstrual years.

- Approximately 75% of all women complain of primary dysmenorrhea. Roughly 15% have severe symptoms.

- Pregnancy without vaginal birth does not seem to alleviate primary dysmenorrhea, whereas childbirth does.

- Oral contraceptives reduce the prevalence and severity of dysmenorrhea.

- IUD use does not affect the prevalence or severity of primary dysmenorrhea.

- The severity of primary dysmenorrhea correlates directly with the duration of menstrual flow, amount of menstrual flow, and age of menarche but does not correlate with the duration of the menstrual cycle.

- Among patients who had primary dysmenorrhea 38% reported onset of symptoms within the first year following menarche.

- Prostaglandin-synthetase inhibitors (PGSIs) are the treatment of choice in primary dysmenorrhea, with 72% of women suffering from dysmenorrhea reporting significant pain relief.

- Approximately 40% of all women suffer considerably from premenstrual syndrome (PMS), with 2% to 3% demonstrating severe symptoms.

- Bromocriptine is effective primarily in relieving breast tenderness in PMS.

- Although fluid retention–related symptoms are prevalent in patients with PMS, it is difficult to document such retention.

- There is no evidence that women with symptoms of PMS have impaired corpus luteal function.

- The most useful diagnostic tool in caring for PMS patients is a symptom diary.

BIBLIOGRAPHY

Abraham GE, Hargrov JT: Effect of vitamin B_6 on premenstrual symptomatology in women with premenstrual tension syndrome: A double blind crossover study. Infertility 3:155, 1980.

Abramson M, Torghele JR: Weight, temperature changes and psychosomatic symptomatology in relation to the menstrual cycle. Am J Obstet Gynecol 81:223, 1961.

Adams PW, Rose DP, Folkard J, et al: Effect of pyridoxine hydrochloride (vitamin B_6) upon depression associated with oral contraception. Lancet 1:897, 1973.

Andersch B: Bromocriptine and premenstrual symptoms. A survey of double blind trials. Obstet Gynecol Surv 38:643, 1983.

Andersch B, Hahn L: Bromocriptine and premenstrual tension: A clinical and hormonal study. Pharmatherapeutica 3:107, 1982.

Andersch B, Milsom I: An epidemiologic study of young women with dysmenorrhea. Am J Obstet Gynecol 144:655, 1982.

Baumann E, Marynick SP, Winters SJ, et al: The effect of osmotic stimuli on prolactin secretion and renal water excretion in normal men and in chronic hyperprolactinemia. J Clin Endocrinol Metab 44:199, 1977.

Bruce J, Russell GFM: Premenstrual tension: A study of weight changes and balances of water, sodium and potassium. Lancet 2:267, 1962.

Budoff PW: Zomepirac sodium in the treatment of primary dysmenorrhea syndrome. N Engl J Med 307:714, 1982.

Cohen MR, Cohen RM, Pickar D, et al: Behavioral effect of high dose naloxone administration in normal volunteers. Lancet 1:1110, 1981.

Dalton K: The premenstrual syndrome and progesterone therapy. London, William Heinemann Medical Books, 1977.

Faratian B, Gaspar A, O'Brien PMS, et al: Premenstrual syndrome, weight, abdominal swelling and perceived body image. Am J Obstet Gynecol 150:200, 1984.

Frank RT: The hormonal causes of premenstrual tension. Arch Neurol Psychol 126:1052, 1931.

Green R, Dalton K: The premenstrual syndrome. Br Med J 1:1007, 1953.

Halbreich U, Assael M, Ben-David M, et al: Serum prolactin in women with premenstrual syndrome. Lancet 2:654, 1976.

Henzl MR, Ortega-Herrera E, Rodriguez C, Izu A: Anaprox in dysmenorrhea: Reduction of pain in intrauterine pressure. Am J Obstet Gynecol 135:455, 1979.

Herzberg BN: Body composition and premenstrual tension. J Psychosom Res 15:251, 1971.

Israel SL: Premenstrual tension. JAMA 110:172, 1938.

Janowsky DS, Berens SC, Davis JM: Correlations between mood, weight and electrolyte during the menstrual cycle. Renin-angiotensin hypothesis of premenstrual tension. Psychosom Med 35:143, 1973.

Kullander S, Svanberg L: Bromocriptine treatment of the premenstrual syndrome. Acta Obstet Gynecol Scand 58:375, 1979.

Mattes JA, Martin D: Pyridoxine in premenstrual depression. Hum Nutr Appl Nutr 36(2):131, 1982.

Morton JH, Additon H, Addison RG, et al: A clinical study of premenstrual tension. Am J Obstet Gynecol 65:1182, 1953.

O'Brien PMS: The premenstrual syndrome: A review of the present status of therapy. Drugs 24:140, 1982.

Owen PR: Prostaglandin synthetase inhibitors in the treatment of primary dysmenorrhea: Outcome trials reviewed. Am J Obstet Gynecol 148:96, 1984.

Reid RL, Yen SSC: Premenstrual syndrome. Am J Obstet Gynecol 139:85, 1981.

Rogers WC: The role of endocrine allergy in the production of premenstrual tension. West J Surg Obstet Gynecol 70:100, 1962.

Sampson GA: Premenstrual syndrome: A double blind control trial of progesterone and placebo. Br J Psychiatry 135:209, 1979.

Smith SL: Mood and the menstrual cycle. In Sacher EJ, ed: Topics in cycle endocrinology. New York, Grune & Stratton, 1975.

Speroff L, Ramwell P: Prostaglandins in reproductive physiology. Am J Obstet Gynecol 107:1111, 1970.

Stokes J, Mendels J: Pyridoxine and premenstrual tension. Lancet 1:1177, 1972.

Taylor HC: Vascular congestion and hyperemia, their effect on the structure and function in the female reproductive system. Am J Obstet Gynecol 57:211, 1949.

Taylor JW: The timing of menstruation-related symptoms assessed by a daily symptom rating scale. Acta Psychiatr Scand 60:87, 1979.

Werch A, Kane RE: Treatment of premenstrual tension with metolazone: A double blind evaluation of a new diuretic. Curr Ther Res 19:565, 1976.

Ylikorkala O, Dawood MY: New concepts in dysmenorrhea. Am J Obstet Gynecol 130:833, 1978.

Ylöstalo P, Kauppila A, Puolakka J, et al: Bromocriptine and norethisterone in the treatment of premenstrual syndrome. Obstet Gynecol 58:292, 1982.

Abnormal Uterine Bleeding

KEY TERMS AND DEFINITIONS

Dysfunctional Uterine Bleeding (DUB). Excessive uterine bleeding with no demonstrable organic cause (genital or extragenital). It is most frequently due to abnormalities of endocrine origin, particularly anovulation.

Intermenstrual Bleeding. Bleeding of variable amounts occurring between regular menstrual periods.

Menometrorrhagia. Prolonged uterine bleeding occurring at irregular intervals.

Menorrhagia. Prolonged (more than 7 days) or excessive (greater than 80 ml) uterine bleeding occurring at regular intervals. The term *hypermenorrhea* is synonymous.

Metrorrhagia. Uterine bleeding occurring at irregular but frequent intervals, the amount being variable.

Nonsteroidal Antiinflammatory Drugs (NSAID). Drugs that inhibit the synthesis of prostaglandins.

Polymenorrhea. Uterine bleeding occurring at regular intervals of less than 21 days.

Abnormal uterine bleeding can take many forms: infrequent episodes, excessive flow, or prolonged duration of menses and intermenstrual bleeding. Alterations in the pattern or volume of blood flow of menses are among the most common health concerns of women. Infrequent uterine bleeding, defined as *oligomenorrhea* if the intervals between bleeding episodes vary from 35 days to 6 months, and *amenorrhea,* defined as no menses for at least 6 months, are discussed fully in Chapter 36. Excessive or prolonged bleeding will be discussed in this chapter. Recently several new therapeutic modalities have been successfully utilized to treat excessive uterine bleeding, and they will be discussed in this chapter.

To define excessive abnormal uterine bleeding it is necessary to define normal menstrual flow. The mean interval between menses is 28 days (± 7 days). Thus if bleeding occurs at intervals of 21 days or less, it is abnormal. The mean duration of menstrual flow is 4 days.

Since few women with normal menses bleed more than 7 days, bleeding more than 7 days is considered to be abnormally prolonged (menorrhagia). It is useful to document the duration and frequency of menstrual flow with the use of menstrual diary cards; however, it is difficult to determine the amount of menstrual blood loss (MBL) by subjective means. Several studies have shown that there is poor correlation between subjective judgment and objective measurement of MBL. Hallberg et al. found that 40% of women with blood loss greater than 80 ml considered their menstrual flow to be small or moderate in amount, while other studies have found that some women with small amounts of blood loss consider their menses to be heavy. Determining the number of sanitary pads used is also an unreliable indication of MBL. Grimes found that there is great variability of absorption among different types of sanitary products as well as among different devices in the same package. Furthermore, women differ markedly in their fastidiousness in changing sanitary products. Thus queries about the passage of blood clots or the degree of inconvenience caused by the bleeding are more helpful than determining the number of pads used in ascertaining that menorrhagia exists.

Because of the unreliability of subjective assessment, objective methods have been developed to quantify MBL. One method involves radioisotopic labeling of the patient's red blood cells. The other, which is the most widely used technique, involves photometric measurement

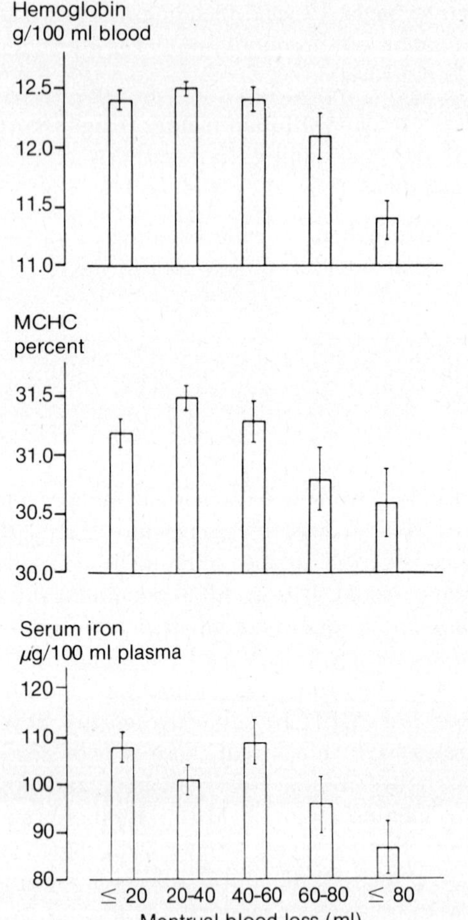

FIGURE 35-1
Mean values (± SEM) of hemoglobin concentration, menstrual cycle hematocrit (*MCHC*), and plasma iron concentration in different ranges of menstrual blood loss. (From Hallberg L, Högdahl AM, Nilsson L, Rybo G: Acta Obstet Gynecol Scand 45:320, 1966.)

to quantify hematin collected onto sanitary napkins. This alkaline hematin method, originated by Hallberg and Nilsson, has been modified by others and is accurate. Nevertheless the accuracy depends on complete collection of the sanitary napkins used by the patient. With these techniques it has been found in several studies that the mean amount of MBL in normal women (women with normal hemoglobin, hematocrit, and plasma iron) is about 35 ml, and 95% of normal women lose less than an average of 60 ml of blood during each menses. Hallberg et al. found that individuals with blood loss greater than 80 ml have significantly lower mean hemoglobin, hematocrit, and serum iron levels (Fig. 35-1). Therefore an MBL greater than 80 ml should be regarded as hypermenorrhea. For practical purposes if a patient experiences a change in duration of flow (i.e., from 3 to 6 days) it must be considered abnormal, even though by definition she does not have menorrhagia.

ETIOLOGY

The etiology of abnormal uterine bleeding is usually divided into two major categories—organic and dysfunctional (or endocrinologic). The organic causes of abnormal uterine bleeding are discussed in detail in other chapters of this book and will only be briefly outlined here.

Organic Causes

The organic causes can be subdivided into systemic disease and reproductive tract disease.

Systemic Disease

Systemic diseases, particularly disorders of blood coagulation such as von Willebrand's disease and prothrombin deficiency, may initially present as abnormal uterine bleeding. Other disorders that produce platelet deficiency such as leukemia, severe sepsis, idiopathic thrombocytopenic purpura, and hypersplenism can also cause excessive bleeding. Routine screening for coagulation defects is mainly indicated in the adolescent who has prolonged heavy menses beginning at menarche, unless otherwise indicated by clinical signs such as petechiae or ecchymoses. Coagulation disorders are found in about 20% of adolescent females who require hospitalization for abnormal uterine bleeding. Coagulation defects are present in about one fourth of those whose hemoglobin level falls below 10 g/100 ml and in approximately one third of those who require one or more transfusions.

Hypothyroidism is frequently associated with menometrorrhagia, so a thyroid-stimulating hormone (TSH) assay should be considered. Although hyperthyroidism is usually not associated with menstrual abnormalities, hypomenorrhea, oligomenorrhea, and amenorrhea have been reported.

Cirrhosis is associated with excessive bleeding secondary to the reduced capacity of the liver to metabolize estrogens. If the patient has hypoprothrombinemia, the tendency toward abnormal bleeding will be increased.

Reproductive Tract Disease

The most common causes of abnormal uterine bleeding during reproductive age are accidents of pregnancy such as threatened, incomplete, or missed abortion and ectopic pregnancy. In addition, trophoblastic disease must be considered in the differential diagnosis of abnormal bleeding in any woman who has had a recent pregnancy, so a sensitive beta–human chorionic gonadotrophin (β-HCG) assay should be performed as part of the diagnostic evaluation.

Malignancies of any portion of the genital tract may present as abnormal bleeding, particularly endometrial and cervical cancer. Less commonly, vaginal, vulvar, and oviductal cancer may produce abnormal bleeding. In addition, rare estrogen-producing ovarian tumors may become manifest by abnormal uterine bleeding. Thus granulosa-theca cell tumors may present with excessive uterine bleeding. Infection of the upper genital tract, particularly endometritis, may present as prolonged menses, although episodic intermenstrual spotting is a more common symptom.

Uterine organic lesions such as submucous myomas, endometrial polyps, and adenomyosis frequently produce symptoms of prolonged and excessive uterine bleeding as well. Cervical lesions such as erosions, polyps, and cervicitis may cause irregular bleeding, particularly postcoital spotting. These lesions can usually be diagnosed by visualization of the cervix. In addition, traumatic vaginal lesions, severe vaginal infections, and foreign bodies have been associated with abnormal bleeding.

Foreign bodies in the uterus, such as the IUD, frequently produce abnormal uterine bleeding. Other iatrogenic causes include oral and injectable steroids such as those used for estrogen replacement in the perimenopausal period or for the management of dysmenorrhea, hirsutism, acne, or endometriosis. Tranquilizers may interfere with the neurotransmitters responsible for releasing and inhibiting hypothalamic hormones, thus causing anovulation and abnormal bleeding.

Dysfunctional Causes

After organic, systemic, and iatrogenic causes for the abnormal bleeding are ruled out, the diagnosis of dysfunctional uterine bleeding (DUB) can be made. The predominant cause of DUB is anovulation secondary to alterations in neuroendocrinologic function. Anovulatory DUB most commonly occurs in the postmenarcheal and premenopausal years.

Other disorders that may cause DUB alter the life span of the corpus luteum. Prolonged life of the corpus luteum has been reported as a cause for abnormal bleeding (Halban's syndrome). This disorder is associated with a normal-appearing secretory endometrium. Its etiology is uncertain, and treatment is usually expectant. It should be differentiated from early pregnancy loss by means of a sensitive serum HCG assay. Irregular shedding of the endometrium can also produce menorrhagia. This diagnosis is made if a biopsy specimen obtained during the fourth day of flow reveals both proliferative and secretory endometrium.

In most patients with DUB, ovulation fails to occur. There is continuous estradiol production without corpus luteum formation and progesterone production. The steady state of estrogen stimulation leads to a continuously proliferating endometrium, which may outgrow its blood supply or lose nutrients with varying degrees of necrosis. In contrast to normal menstruation, uniform slough to the basalis does not occur, which produces excessive uterine blood flow.

In addition to anovulatory DUB, some individuals have DUB but apparently ovulate regularly. It is estimated that approximately 15% of individuals with DUB have regularly cyclic ovulation. It is more difficult to treat ovulatory DUB than anovulatory DUB.

DIAGNOSIS

After routine speculum examination and normal pelvic examination, the main methods used to diagnose these gynecologic causes of menorrhagia are endometrial biopsy and dilation and curettage (D&C). It is important to document the endometrial histology of patients with excessive uterine bleeding. It can easily be determined whether normal proliferative or secretory or pathologic endometrium is associated with the abnormal bleeding. An endometrial biopsy specimen is ideally obtained at the onset of the bleeding episode; otherwise, it should be deferred until a few days before the expected onset of the next bleeding episode to determine whether ovulation has occurred and secretory endometrium is present.

In patients who have evidence of ovulation as shown by secretory endometrium, even if the pelvic examination is normal, an additional diagnostic study is required to determine if there is an organic endometrial cavity defect such as a polyp or submucous leiomyoma. Curettage cannot always determine whether these lesions are present; therefore, the diagnosis is best made by either hysterosalpingography or hysteroscopy.

MANAGEMENT

In the absence of an organic cause for excessive uterine bleeding, it is preferable to use medical instead of surgical treatment, especially if the patient desires to retain her uterus for future childbearing or will be undergoing natural menopause within a short period of time. There are several acceptable medical methods for treatment of DUB. These include estrogens, progestins, nonsteroidal antiinflammatory agents, antifibrinolytic agents, and danazol.

Estrogens

The rationale for the therapeutic use of estrogen for the treatment of DUB is based on the fact that estrogen in pharmacologic doses causes rapid growth of the endometrium. Thus bleeding that results from most causes of DUB will respond to such therapy because a rapid growth of endometrial tissue occurs over the denuded and raw epithelial surfaces. The use of oral conjugated estrogen (CE) in a dose of 10 mg a day, administered in divided doses, is a good therapeutic regimen that has been found to be clinically useful. Acute bleeding from most causes is usually controlled by this method. If bleeding is not controlled within the first 24 hours with this dose of estrogen, higher doses of CE (20 mg) may be effective; however, consideration must be given to the fact that an organic cause such as an accident of pregnancy may be the cause of the bleeding, and curettage should usually be performed. Parenteral administration of estrogen has been shown to be effective in treating DUB. However, cessation of bleeding only occurs after repeated injections of estrogen and is, therefore, time related. At least several hours is required to induce mitotic activity and growth of the endometrium, whether the estrogen is administered orally or parenterally. Thus parenteral estrogen therapy accompanied by rapid metabolic clearance does not offer a distinct advantage over oral treatment. The latter is less costly, is easier to administer, and therefore is preferred. There is no reliable evidence that short-term estrogen therapy controls bleeding by altering the hemostatic process, despite evidence that long-term estrogen treatment may produce a hypercoagulable state.

Usually CE therapy reduces the amount of uterine bleeding within the first 24 hours after treatment is initiated. However, because most patients bleed because of anovulation, progestin treatment is also required. Therefore, after bleeding has ceased, CE therapy is continued at the same dosage, and a progestin, usually medroxyprogesterone acetate (MPA) 10 mg once a day, is added. Both hormones are administered for another 7 to 10 days, after which treatment is stopped to allow withdrawal bleeding, which may be increased in amount of flow but is rarely prolonged. Following the withdrawal bleeding episode several alternate treatment modalities may be used. Because estrogen therapy controls only the acute bleeding episode and is not curative, a definitive diagnosis is clearly warranted and should be made on the basis of endometrial histology, with definitive treatment based on this finding.

A more convenient regimen than the sequential high-dose estrogen-progestin regimen to stop acute bleeding is the use of a combination oral contraceptive containing both estrogen and progestin. Four tablets of an oral contraceptive containing 50 µg of estrogen taken every 24 hours in divided doses will usually provide sufficient estrogen to stop acute bleeding and simultaneously provide progestin. Treatment is continued for at least 1 week after the bleeding stops. This regimen is successful and convenient and is thus the preferred method of some clinicians. However, in one study it was found not to be as effective as the use of high doses of CE. A theoretical reason for this difference might be the fact that the combined use of estrogen and progestin does not afford as rapid endometrial growth as estrogen alone, because the progestin decreases the synthesis of estrogen receptors and increases estradiol dehydrogenase in the endometrial cell, thus inhibiting the growth-promoting action of estrogen. Natural estrogens are also preferred, since they do not produce the adverse effects on metabolic parameters to as great an extent as synthetic estrogens.

Progestins

Progestin therapy is ultimately the treatment of choice for the majority of patients with DUB because most of them are anovulatory. However, progestin therapy usually does not stop the acute bleeding episode as effectively as estrogen and is only warranted for long-term treatment of patients after the acute episode of bleeding has been controlled.

MPA in a dose of 10 mg daily for 10 days each month is a successful therapeutic regimen that produces regular withdrawal bleeding in patients with adequate amounts of endogenous estrogen to cause endometrial growth. Although other progestins have been used, MPA does not alter serum lipids as much as the 19-nortestosterone derivatives and thus may have fewer adverse long-term effects. Progestins are beneficial, since in pharmacologic doses they act as antiestrogens. They diminish the effect of estrogen on target cells by inhibiting estrogen receptor replenishment in the cell and induce the activation of 17-hydroxysteroid dehydrogenase, which converts estradiol to the less active estrone. These findings account for the antimitotic, antigrowth effect of the progestins and support the rationale for its use in the treatment of unopposed estrogen and endometrial hyperplasia.

Progestins, therefore, not only stop endometrial growth but also support and organize the endometrium in such a way that an organized slough occurs after its withdrawal. In the absence of progesterone, erratic unorganized breakdown of the endometrium occurs. With progesterone or progestin treatment, an organized slough to the basalis layer allows a rapid cessation of bleeding. Thus progestins do not stop the acute bleeding episode but produce a normal bleeding episode following their withdrawal.

Adolescent anovulatory patients represent an ideal model for the use of progestins in the treatment of DUB. These patients exhibit immaturity of the hypothalamic-pituitary axis, and progestin therapy for 10 days every month is a reasonable mode of treatment that is highly successful and produces regular cyclic withdrawal bleeding until maturity of the positive feedback system is achieved. This therapy does not interfere with the normal resumption of ovulatory cycles. Although controversial, it is probably best that these patients do not use oral contraceptives, since this therapy prolongs hypothalamic-pituitary inhibition and may delay the maturation of the hypothalamic-pituitary axis. In women of reproductive age who have DUB, long-term use of oral contraceptives is acceptable after the acute bleeding episode is controlled unless the patient wishes to conceive, in which case cyclic treatment with clomiphene citrate should be used.

The major therapeutic use of progestins is to treat anovulatory patients for 10 days each month. However, because progestins have a profound effect on inhibiting endometrial growth and inducing atrophic changes, a therapeutic trial with these agents may be used in patients with menorrhagia who also ovulate. These patients are difficult to treat; and a prolonged regimen of progestins may be administered for 14 to 21 days each month so that the amount of withdrawal bleeding will be reduced.

Some case reports have indicated that long-term suppression of hypermenorrhea can also be achieved by the use of progesterone-releasing IUDs, which deliver progesterone directly to the endometrial cavity. This mode of therapy is not suitable for all patients but can be considered as an alternative for patients who have contraindications to the use of oral contraceptives.

Nonsteroidal Antiinflammatory Drugs

Nonsteroidal antiinflammatory drugs (NSAIDs) are inhibitors of platelet aggregation and the platelet release reaction. Additionally, they block fatty acid cyclooxygenase, which catalyzes the conversion of arachidonic acid into prostaglandins and results in the production of the potent prostaglandin endoperoxide PGG_2. These drugs also block the formation of prostacyclin (PGI_2), an antagonist of thromboxane. PGI_2 relaxes vessel walls and reverses platelet aggregation. To decrease bleeding of the endometrium it would be ideal to selectively block the synthesis of prostacyclin alone, without decreasing thromboxane formation, as the latter increases platelet aggregation. Presently there are no NSAIDs that possess this ability. All NSAIDs are cyclooxygenase inhibitors and thus block the formation of both thromboxane and the prostacyclin pathway. Nevertheless, NSAIDs have been shown to reduce MBL, primarily in patients who ovulate. However, a complete understanding of the mechanisms whereby prostaglandin inhibitors reduce MBL is still undetermined, and their therapeutic action may take place through some yet undiscovered mechanism.

Anderson et al. used mefenamic acid, a potent NSAID, to treat unexplained menorrhagia. They reported an average reduction in blood loss of 30% with a dosage of mefenamic acid of 500 mg three times a day for a total of 3 days. The MBL was reduced to less than 80 ml in 17 of 22 patients. Additional studies confirmed the efficacy of this NSAID in reducing MBL in the majority of patients treated (Fig. 35-2). Other groups have investigated the role

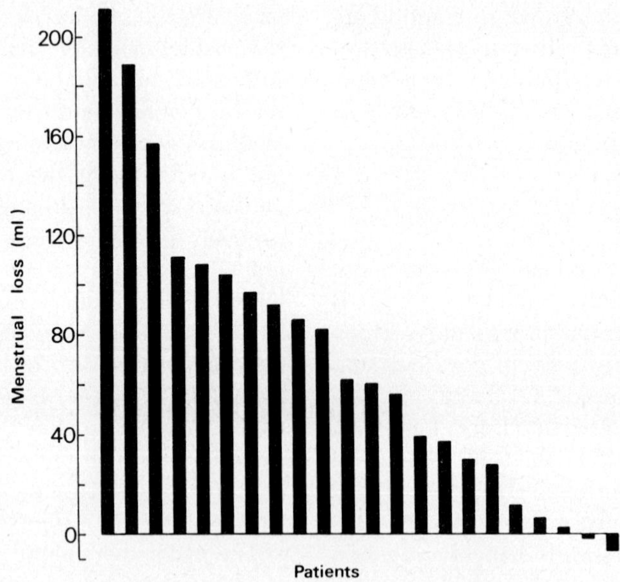

FIGURE 35-2
Mean reduction in menstrual blood loss during two menses in 22 patients taking mefanamic acid during menstruation as compared with blood loss during two pretreatment menses. Each histogram represents mean reduction in loss in one patient. (From Haynes PJ, Flint APF, Hodgson H, et al: Int J Gynaecol Obstet 17:567, 1980.)

of other NSAIDs in the treatment of unexplained menorrhagia. Naproxen, in a dosage of 750 mg daily for 3 days followed by 250 mg daily for 5 additional days, reduced MBL in 4 women by 24% as compared with controls in a double-blind study (Table 35-1).

To date, there have been very few studies comparing NSAIDs with other treatment modalities. It appears, however, that the beneficial reduction in MBL with NSAIDs occurs primarily in patients who ovulate. Furthermore the degree of reduction of MBL with NSAIDs is similar to that reported for the use of either antifibrinolytic agents or oral contraceptives alone.

Although NSAIDs are used to treat patients with DUB who ovulate, they are infrequently used alone but usually in combination with oral contraceptives or progestins. With this combined approach a greater therapeutic success rate has been achieved than with a single agent.

Antifibrinolytic Agents

Epsilon-aminocaproic acid (EACA), tranexamic acid (AMCA), and para-aminomethylbenzoic acid (PAMBA) are potent inhibitors of fibrinolysis and have, therefore, been used in the treatment of various hemorrhagic conditions. Nilsson and Rybo compared the effect on blood loss of EACA, AMCA, and oral contraceptives in 215 women with menorrhagia. EACA was given in a dose of 18 g per day for 3 days and then 12, 9, 6, and 3 g daily on successive days. The total dose was always at least 48 g. AMCA was administered in a dose of 6 g per day for 3 days followed by 4, 3, 2, and 1 g daily on successive days. The total dose of AMCA was at least 22 g. There was a significant reduction in blood loss after treatment with EACA, AMCA, and oral contraceptives, and use of each of these agents resulted in about a 50% reduction in MBL (Table 35-2). Of interest was the finding that the greatest reduction in blood loss with antifibrinolytic therapy occurred in women who exhibited the greatest MBL. The side effects of this class of drugs in decreasing order of frequency are nausea, dizziness, diarrhea, headaches, abdominal pain, and allergic manifestations. These side effects are much more common with EACA than with AMCA. Other investigators have compared use of AMCA to placebo in double-blind studies and have found no significant differences in the occurrence of side effects. Renal failure and

TABLE 35-1

Effects of Mefenamic Acid and Naproxen on Menstrual Blood Loss

	Mean Blood Loss (ml)	
	Before Treatment	During Treatment
Mefenamic acid	137	76
Naproxen	141	107

Data from Haynes PJ, Flint APF, Hodgson H, et al: Studies in menorrhagia: (a) mefenamic acid, (b) endometrial prostaglandin concentrations. Int J Gynaecol Obstet 17:567, 1980; and Nygren K-G, Rybo G: Prostaglandin and menorrhagia. Acta Obstet Gynecol Scand Suppl 113:101, 1983.

TABLE 35-2

Mean Menstrual Blood Loss and Reduction with Treatment with EACA, AMCA, Oral Contraceptives, and Methylergobaseimmaleate

	Mean Blood Loss (ml)		% Decrease
	Before Treatment	After Treatment	
EACA	164	87	47
AMCA	182	84	54
Oral contraceptives	158	75	52
Methylergobaseimmaleate	164	164	0

Adapted from Nilsson L, Rybo G: Treatment of menorrhagia. Am J Obstet Gynecol 110:713, 1971.

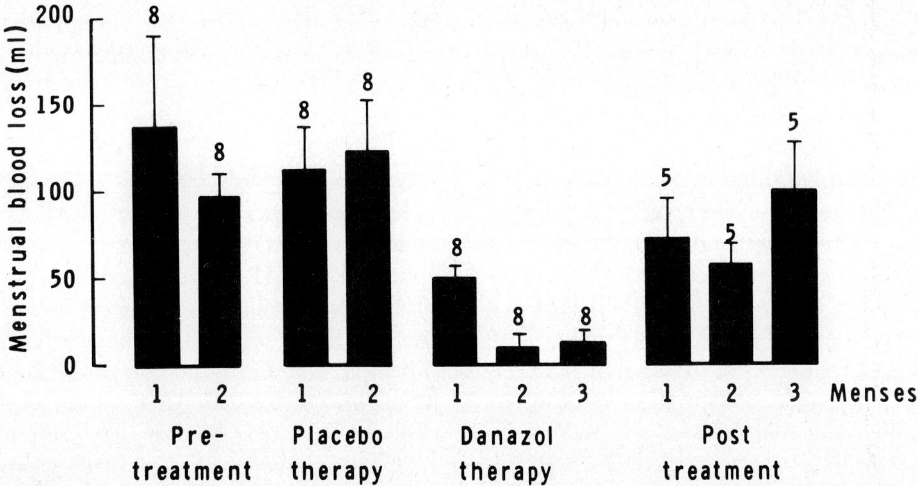

FIGURE 35-3

Mean ($\pm$ SEM) menstrual blood loss in eight patients with menorrhagia before treatment, with placebo therapy, with 200 mg danazol daily, and after treatment. Number of patients is shown above each histogram. (From Chimbria TH, Anderson ABM, Naish C, et al: Br J Obstet Gynaecol 87:1152, 1980.)

pregnancy are contraindications to the use of antifibrinolytic agents.

Antifibrinolytic agents clearly produce a reduction in blood loss and may be used as therapy for patients with menorrhagia who ovulate. However, their use is somewhat limited by the side effects. Furthermore, as with NSAIDs, they are best combined with another agent such as oral contraceptives for a greater effect on MBL reduction.

Ergot

Ergot derivatives are not recommended for therapy because they are rarely effective and have a high incidence of side effects (nausea, vertigo, abdominal cramps). Nilsson and Rybo demonstrated no reduction in blood loss among 82 women with menorrhagia who were treated with methylergobaseimmaleate (Table 35-2).

Androgenic Steroids (Danazol)

In recent years, the androgenic steroid that has proved most useful in the treatment of DUB is danazol. Danazol has been used by several investigators for the treatment of menorrhagia. Doses of 200 and 400 mg daily have been given over 12 weeks after careful pre-

treatment observation and evaluation. MBL was markedly reduced in these studies from more than 200 ml to less than 25 ml. Also, there was an increased interval between bleeding episodes (Fig. 35-3). The most common side effects of danazol treatment are weight gain and skin disorders such as acne. Reduction of dosage from 400 to 200 mg daily decreased the side effects but did not affect the reduction in blood loss (Fig. 35-4). Some patients may ovulate when receiving this dose of danazol. Further reduction to 100 mg daily did not effectively reduce MBL in most patients. Although danazol is effective, it is also expensive and has moderate side effects. Randomized studies are needed to compare the effectiveness of danazol with that of more conventional therapy.

Surgical Therapy

Dilation and Curettage

The performance of a D&C can be both diagnostic and therapeutic. For patients with severe menorrhagia who may be hypovolemic, the D&C is the quickest way to stop acute bleeding. Therefore it is the treatment of choice in women with DUB who suffer from hypovolemia. A D&C should also be utilized to

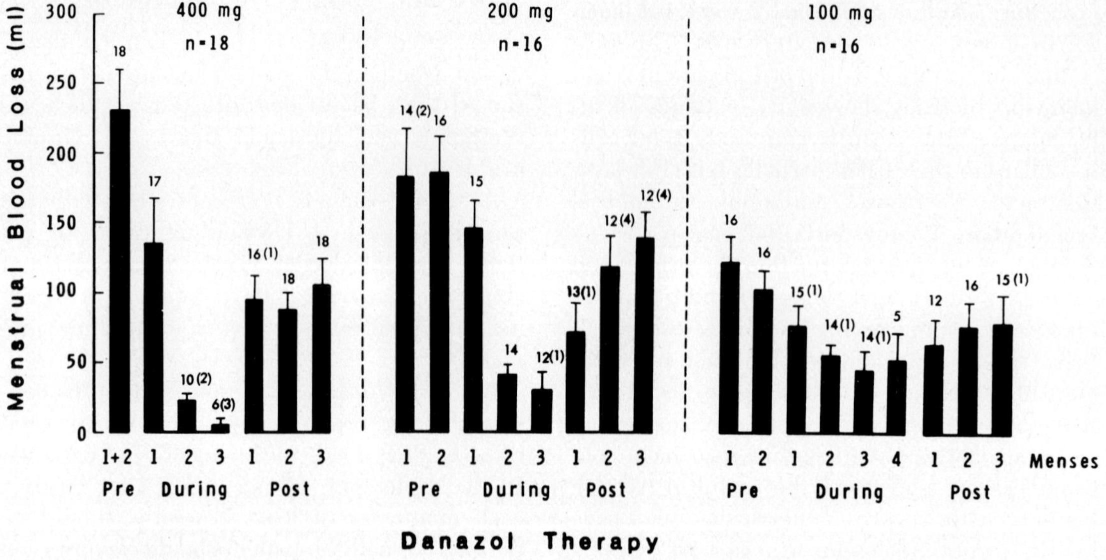

FIGURE 35-4

Mean ($\pm$ SEM) menstrual blood loss in three groups of patients with menorrhagia treated with 400, 200, or 100 mg danazol daily for 12 weeks. Menstrual blood loss measurements are shown for each group before, during, and after danazol therapy. Number of patients menstruating is shown above each histogram with number of missing menstrual loss collections in brackets. (Adapted from Chimbria TH, Anderson ABM, Naish C, et al: Br J Obstet Gynaecol 87:1152, 1980.)

stop the acute bleeding episode in patients over the age of 35 when the incidence of anatomic problems and pathologic findings increases.

The use of D&C for the treatment of DUB has been reported to be curative in a minority of patients. Temporary cure of the problem may occur in patients with chronic anovulation, as the curettage removes much of the hyperplastic endometrium; however, the underlying pathophysiologic cause is unchanged. A D&C has not proven useful for treatment of patients who ovulate and have menorrhagia. More than 1 month after the D&C, Nilsson and Rybo have shown that there is either no difference or an increase in MBL in patients who ovulate. However, in this instance a D&C may be useful in ruling out DUB by revealing an anatomic cavity defect. Therefore patients with menorrhagia, if they are perimenopausal or have other risk factors, may be treated initially by means of a D&C. However, if the histologic findings reveal a secretory endometrium and no cavity defect is found, consideration should

be given to treating the patient medically rather than waiting for the patient to benefit from the D&C alone.

D&C is therefore indicated for patients with acute bleeding resulting in hypovolemia, for older patients (who are at higher risk of having endometrial hyperplasia), and for patients for whom initial medical management is unsuccessful. Endometrial receptor studies have been carried out in the third group but have not proven useful. All other patients are best managed by means of endometrial biopsy and medical therapy as outlined above without a D&C.

Laser

Laser photovaporization of the endometrium for treatment of menorrhagia has been performed by Goldrath et al. Photovaporization of the endometrium was performed by use of a neodymium-YAG laser with hysteroscopic visualization. Patients were treated with danazol 800 mg per day for 2 to 3 weeks before the

procedure, and an additional 2 weeks of danazol treatment was given afterwards. This procedure was curative in 160 of 180 patients, and follow-up biopsies showed no evidence of inflammation other than foreign body giant cells secondary to the carbon particles left after laser treatment. There was minimum endometrial regeneration. Photovaporization causes varying degrees of uterine contraction, scarring, and adhesion formation, as demonstrated by follow-up hysterosalpingograms and hysteroscopy. If these results are confirmed by other researchers, this procedure may be used as an alternative to hysterectomy in patients for whom other modalities have failed or who have contraindications, and it may be useful in treating patients with severe menorrhagia who have medical contraindications against performing a hysterectomy. Obviously it should not be used in women who wish to maintain their reproductive capacity.

Cryotherapy

Cryotherapy has also been used in an attempt to destroy the endometrium. However, the results of this therapy have been disappointing because patients are either undertreated or overtreated. Chamberlain reported that patients treated with a cryoprobe had a similar rate of recurrence of menorrhagia as women who were treated by D&C.

Hysterectomy

Surgical removal of the uterus should be individualized and should usually be reserved for the patient with other indications for hysterectomy. However, when all available medical therapy has failed, hysterectomy may be necessary to treat the patient with persistent DUB. Not infrequently a histologic diagnosis of adenomyosis will be made after operation.

Short- and Long-Term Treatment

As stated earlier, it should first be determined whether the patient ovulates. Patients should then be divided into those with acute symptoms and signs and those with chronic problems.

Acute bleeding is best controlled with the use of estrogen. A D&C is indicated for patients over the age of 35 who have persistent abnormal bleeding or for patients with bleeding that is sufficiently severe to produce anemia.

After the diagnosis of anovulation is confirmed, long-term therapy should be directed by individual needs in the majority of patients. In the adolescent, 10 mg of MPA for 10 days each month for at least 3 months should be prescribed, and the patient should be observed carefully thereafter. In this group of patients additional diagnostic studies should be performed to detect possible defects in the coagulation process, particularly if bleeding is severe. For the woman of reproductive age, long-term therapy depends on whether the patient requires contraception, induction of ovulation, or treatment of DUB alone. In the last circumstance, MPA is administered, as stated above, monthly for at least 6 months, while oral contraceptives and clomiphene citrate are used for the other indications. In the perimenopausal patient who characteristically has lower amounts of circulating estrogen, use of cyclic MPA alone is frequently not curative. In these patients abnormal bleeding may be treated by the cyclic use of CE (0.625 to 1.25 mg) given for 25 days, with 10 mg of MPA added to the CE from days 15 to 25 after abnormal endometrial histologic findings have been ruled out.

Chronic treatment for ovulatory patients with menorrhagia constitutes the most difficult problem of DUB. In patients for whom cavity defects have been ruled out, long-term treatment is directed at a reduction in MBL. For these patients NSAIDs, prolonged progestin use, oral contraceptives, and danazol are part of the therapeutic armamentarium. A combination of two or more of these agents is often required to obviate the need for hysterectomy.

KEY POINTS

- The mean amount of menstrual blood loss (MBL) per cycle is 35 ml, with 95% of women losing less than 60 ml.

- An MBL greater than 80 ml is considered abnormal (hypermenorrhea), as it will produce iron deficiency anemia if untreated.

- Coagulation disorders are found in about 20% of adolescent females who require hospitalization for abnormal uterine bleeding.

- About 15% of individuals with dysfunctional uterine bleeding (DUB) ovulate, and 85% do not ovulate.

- Acute episodes of menorrhagia are best treated by high doses of estrogens or oral contraceptives. Dilation and curettage are indicated if the patient is over 35 or if the bleeding produces anemia.

- Nonsteroidal antiinflammatory drugs (NSAIDs) inhibit platelet aggregation and the platelet release reaction; they have been shown to reduce MBL, primarily in patients who ovulate.

- Ergot derivatives do not reduce MBL and should not be used as therapy.

- Anovulatory DUB can be treated by cyclic use of progestins, oral contraceptives, or intermittent clomiphene citrate.

- Patients with ovulatory DUB are best treated with oral contraceptives, NSAIDs (antiprostaglandins), danazol, or progestins during the luteal phase.

BIBLIOGRAPHY

Anderson ABM, Haynes PJ, Guillebaud J, et al: Reduction of menstrual blood loss by prostaglandin synthetase inhibitors. Lancet 1:774, 1976.

Callender ST, Warner GT, Cope E: Treatment of menorrhagia with tranexamic acid: A double-blind trial. Br Med J 4:214, 1970.

Chamberlain G: Dysfunctional uterine bleeding. Clin Obstet Gynaecol 8(1):93, 1981.

Chimbria TH, Anderson ABM, Naish C, et al: Reduction of menstrual blood loss by danazol in unexplained menorrhagia: Lack of effect of placebo. Br J Obstet Gynaecol 87:1152, 1980.

Chimbria TH, Cope E, Anderson ABM, et al: The effect of danazol on menorrhagia, coagulation mechanisms, haematological indices and body weight. Br J Obstet Gynaecol 86:46, 1979.

Claessens EA, Cowell CL: Acute adolescent menorrhagia. Am J Obstet Gynecol 139:277, 1981.

Cope E: Danazol in the treatment of menorrhagia. Drugs 19:342, 1980.

DeVore GR, Owens O, Kase N: Use of intravenous Premarin in the treatment of dysfunctional uterine bleeding: A double-blind randomized control study. Obstet Gynecol 59:285, 1982.

Goldrath MH, Fuller TA, Segal S: Laser photovaporization of endometrium for the treatment of menorrhagia. Am J Obstet Gynecol 140:14, 1981.

Granstrom E, Swahn ML, Lundstrom V: The possible roles of prostaglandins and related compounds in endometrial bleeding. Acta Obstet Gynecol Scand Suppl 113:91, 1983.

Grimes DA: Estimating vaginal blood loss. J Reprod Med 22:190, 1979.

Hallberg L, Högdahl A-M, Nilsson L, Rybo G: Menstrual blood loss—a population study: Variation at different ages and attempts to define normality. Acta Obstet Gynecol Scand 45:320, 1966.

Hallberg L, Nilsson L: Determination of menstrual blood loss. Scand J Clin Lab Invest 16:244, 1964.

Haynes PJ, Flint APF, Hodgson H, et al: Studies in menorrhagia: (a) mefenamic acid, (b) endometrial prostaglandin concentrations. Int J Gynaecol Obstet 17:567, 1980.

Jakubowitz DL, Wood C: The use of the prostaglandin synthetase inhibitor mefenamic acid in the treatment of menorrhagia. Aust NZ J Obstet Gynaecol 18:135, 1978.

Newton J, Barnard G, Collins W: A rapid method for measuring menstrual blood loss using automatic extraction. Contraception 16:269, 1977.

Nilsson L, Rybo G: Treatment of menorrhagia with an antifibrinolytic agent, tranexamic acid (AMCA). A double-blind investigation. Acta Obstet Gynecol Scand 46:572, 1967.

Nilsson L, Rybo G: Treatment of menorrhagia. Am J Obstet Gynecol 110:713, 1971.

Nygren K-G, Rybo G: Prostaglandins and menorrhagia. Acta Obstet Gynecol Scand Suppl 113:101, 1983.

Reynair JV: Dysfunctional uterine bleeding. J Reprod Med 17:293, 1976.

Shaw ST Jr, Aaronson DE, Moyer DL: Quantitation of menstrual blood loss: Further evaluation of the alkaline hematin method. Contraception 5:497, 1972.

Shaw ST Jr, Roche PC: Menstruation. In Roche CA, ed: Oxford reviews of reproduction and endocrinology, vol. 2. London, Oxford University Press, 1980, p. 41.

Whitehead MI, Townsend PT, Pryse-Davies J, et al: The effect of estrogens and progestins on the biochemistry and morphology of the postmenopausal endometrium. N Engl J Med 305:1599, 1981.

Willman EA, Collins WP, Clayton SG: Studies in the involvement of prostaglandins in uterine symptomatology and pathology. Br J Obstet Gynaecol 83:337, 1976.

Amenorrhea

_________________ KEY TERMS AND DEFINITIONS _________________

Amenorrhea. Absence of menses during the reproductive years. It can be either physiologic (pregnancy) or pathologic.

Androgen Insensitivity Syndrome. A genetically transmitted androgen receptor defect in a 46,XY individual with testes and normal male testosterone levels. These individuals have absent uterus, normal female phenotype, and scanty body hair.

Anorexia Nervosa. A psychiatric disease associated with a fear of weight gain or obesity, food aversion, and a distorted body image in which the individual limits caloric intake to starvation levels. In addition to severe weight loss, there is a decreased metabolic rate and amenorrhea.

Chromophobe Adenoma. A non-hormone-secreting pituitary tumor that can disrupt normal pituitary function and thus produce low gonadotrophin levels.

Congenital Absence of Uterus and Vagina. A malformation in a 46,XX individual with normal ovarian function resulting in failure of the uterus and vagina to form. It is also called uterovaginal agenesis and Rokitansky-Kuster-Hauser syndrome.

Cryptomenorrhea. Menstruation without egress of menses through the introitus.

Delayed Menarche. Onset of menses in women older than 16.5 years who have no reproductive abnormalities.

Gonadal Failure. Failure of the gonads to develop. It is also called gonadal dysgenesis if the karyotype is abnormal and gonadal agenesis if the karyotype is normal.

Gonadal Streaks. Streaks of fibrous tissue in the normal position of the ovaries.

Gonadotrophin-Resistant Ovary Syndrome. Premature ovarian failure in which the ovary contains normal-appearing primordial follicles but no follicular development. It is also called ovarian hypofolliculogenesis.

Hypogonadotrophic Hypogonadism. Failure of the ovaries to develop as a result of low amounts of circulatory gonadotrophins. When anosmia is present, the term _Kallmann's syndrome_ is used.

Hypothalamic Dysfunction. Secondary amenorrhea with undefined etiology. This is associated with an abnormal pattern of luteinizing hormone pulsatility and circulatory estradiol levels above 40 pg/ml.

Hypothalamic Failure. Secondary amenorrhea with undefined etiology. There is an abnormal pattern of luteinizing hormone pulsatility, and estradiol levels are below 40 pg/ml.

Insulin Tolerance Test. A test of adrenocorticotropic hormone function in which hypoglycemia is produced and cortisol measured.

Intrauterine Adhesions or Synechiae. A condition in which fibrous tissue partially or completely obliterates the uterine cavity. It is also called Asherman's syndrome.

Isolated Gonadotrophin Deficiency. The presence of hypogonadotrophic hypogonadism in individuals who do not produce gonadotrophins after prolonged administration of gonadotrophin releasing hormone.

Pituitary Destruction. Damage or necrosis of the pituitary gland caused by anoxia, thrombosis, or hemorrhage. It is called Sheehan's syndrome when related to pregnancy and Symmond's disease when unrelated to pregnancy.

Polycystic Ovary Syndrome. An endocrinologic disorder characterized by excessive androgen production, inappropriate gonadotrophin secretion, and chronic anovulation. It begins perimenarcheally, and its clinical manifestations include hirsutism, menstrual irregularity (oligomenorrhea or amenorrhea).

Premature Ovarian Failure. Cessation of menstruation due to depletion of ovarian follicles prior to the age of 40. It is also called premature menopause.

Primary Amenorrhea. Absence of any spontaneous menses in an individual older than 16.5 years of age.

Pure Gonadal Dysgenesis. Absence of the gonads in an individual with a normal 46,XX or 46,XY karyotype. It is also called gonadal agenesis.

Secondary Amenorrhea. Absence of menses for a variable period of time (for at least 3 to 12 months, usually 6 months or longer) in an individual who has previously had spontaneous menstrual periods.

Amenorrhea can be either physiologic, when it occurs during pregnancy and the postpartum period (particularly when nursing), or pathologic, when it is produced by a variety of endocrinologic and anatomic disorders. In the latter circumstance the failure to menstruate is a symptom of these various pathologic conditions. Thus amenorrhea itself is not a pathologic entity and should not be used as a final diagnosis.

Although the absence of menses causes no harm to the body, in a nonpregnant or postpartum woman it is abnormal and thus is a source of concern. For this reason women usually seek medical assistance when the condition occurs. Therefore the clinician needs to know the various etiologies of amenorrhea, how to diagnose the etiology, and how to treat the underlying pathologic condition. This chapter will present the etiology, diagnostic evaluation, and treatment of the various causes of both primary and secondary amenorrhea.

Many individuals with ambiguous external genitalia resulting from various intersex problems are raised as females and never menstruate. The etiology of the intersex problem is usually determined at birth or soon thereafter. Since such disorders are discussed in Chapter 3, they will not be discussed in this chapter. Although women with cryptomenorrhea caused by anatomic disorders interfering with the outflow of menses, such as an imperforate hymen or transverse vaginal septum, have the symptom of amenorrhea, they are actually menstruating. These conditions are discussed in Chapter 9. Severe systemic diseases such as metastatic carcinoma and chronic renal failure can also cause amenorrhea; however, since amenorrhea is not the presenting symptom of these disorders, they will not be discussed in this chapter.

Primary amenorrhea is defined as the absence of menses in a woman who has never menstruated by the age of 16½ years. The incidence of primary amenorrhea is less than 0.1%. Secondary amenorrhea is defined as the absence of menses for an arbitrary time period, usually longer than 6 to 12 months. The incidence of secondary amenorrhea of more than 6 months' duration in a survey of a general population of Swedish women of reproductive age was found by Pettersson et al. to be 0.7%. The incidence was significantly higher in women younger than 25 years of age and those with a prior history of menstrual irregularity.

DELAYED MENARCHE

Before the onset of menses the normal female goes through a progressive series of morphologic changes produced by the pubertal increase in estrogen and androgen production. In 1969 Marshall and Tanner defined five stages of breast development and pubic hair development (Fig. 36-1, Table 36-1). These changes sometimes are combined and called Tanner or pubertal stages 1 through 5. The first sign of puberty is usually the appearance of breast

TABLE 36-1

Classifications of Breast Growth and Pubic Hair Growth

Classification	Description
Breast Growth	
B1	Prepubertal: elevation of papilla only
B2	Breast budding
B3	Enlargement of breasts with glandular tissue, without separation of breast contours
B4	Secondary mound formed by areola
B5	Single contour of breast and areola
Pubic Hair Growth	
PH1	Prepubertal: no pubic hair
PH2	Labial hair present
PH3	Labial hair spreads over mons pubis
PH4	Slight lateral spread
PH5	Further lateral spread to form inverse triangle and reach medial thighs

Adapted from Roy S, Brenner PF: Puberty. Reproduced with permission from Infertility, contraception and reproductive endocrinology, 2nd ed, by Daniel R. Mishell, Jr., M.D., and Val Davajan, M.D. Copyright © 1986 Medical Economics Books, Oradell, N.J. 07649. All rights reserved.

TABLE 36-2

Mean Ages of Girls at the Onset of Pubertal Events (United States)

Event	Mean Age ± SD (Years)
Initiation of breast development (B2)	10.8 ± 1.10
Appearance of pubic hair (PH2)	11.0 ± 1.21
Menarche	12.9 ± 1.20

Adapted from Frisch RE, Revelle R: Height and weight at menarche and a hypothesis of menarche. Arch Dis Child 46:695, 1971.

TABLE 36-3

Pubertal Intervals

Interval	Mean Age ± SD (Years)
B2-peak height velocity	1.0 ± 0.77
B2-menarche	2.3 ± 1.03
B2-PH5	3.1 ± 1.04
B2-B5 (average duration of puberty)	4.5 ± 2.04

Adapted from Frisch RE, Revelle R: Height and weight at menarche and a hypothesis of menarche. Arch Dis Child 46:695, 1971.

budding followed within a few months by the appearance of pubic hair.

Thereafter the breasts enlarge, the external pelvic contour becomes rounder, and the most rapid rate of growth occurs (peak height velocity). Thus breast budding is the earliest sign of puberty and menarche the latest. The mean ages of occurrence of these events in American women are shown in Table 36-2, and the mean intervals (with standard deviation) between initiation of breast budding and other pubertal events are shown in Table 36-3. The mean interval between breast budding and menarche is 2.3 years, with a standard deviation of about 1 year. Some individuals can progress from breast budding to menarche in 18 months, while others may take 5 years. Thus although the arbitrary age of primary amenorrhea is 16½ years, if a woman 14 years of age or older presents to the clinician with absence of breast budding, diagnostic evaluation should be performed at this time, as it is highly unlikely she will menstruate within the next 2 years.

The mean time of onset of menarche was previously thought to occur when a critical body weight of about 48 kg or 106 lb was reached. However, it is now believed that body composition is more important than total body weight in determining the time of onset of puberty and menstruation. Thus the ratio of fat to both total body weight and lean body weight is probably the determining factor in the time of onset of puberty and menstruation. Individuals who are moderately obese, between 20% and 30% above the ideal body weight, will have an early onset of menarche. Malnutrition is known to delay the onset of puberty, and well-nourished individuals with pre-

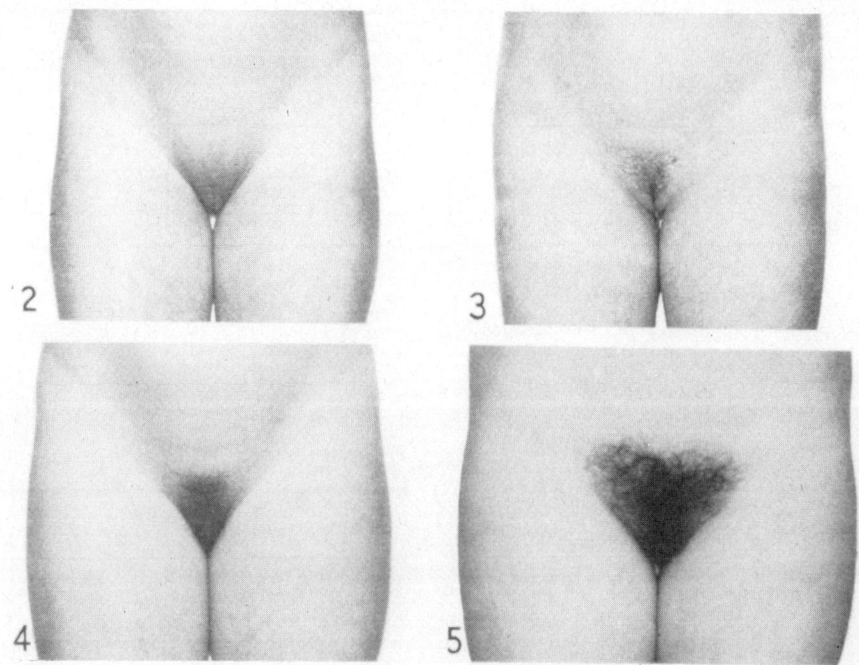

FIGURE 36-1

Standards for pubic hair ratings. (Modified from Tanner JM: Growth and endocrinology of the adolescent. In Gardner L, ed: Endocrine and genetic diseases of childhood, 2nd ed. Philadelphia, W.B. Saunders Co., 1975.)

pubertal strenuous exercise programs resulting in less total body fat have also been shown to have a delayed onset of puberty. Warren et al. reported that ballet dancers, swimmers, and runners had menarche delayed to about age 15 if they began exercising strenuously before menarche (Fig. 36-2). These investigators also determined that stress is not the cause of the delayed menarche in these exercising girls, as girls of the same age with stressful musical careers did not have a delayed onset of menarche. The girls with strenuous exercise programs have sufficient estrogen to produce some breast development and thus do not need extensive endocrinologic evaluation if concern arises about lack of onset of menses. Frisch et al. reported that for girls engaged in premenarcheal athletic training, menarche was delayed 0.4 years for each year of athletic training. An endocrinologic diagnostic evaluation is not necessary for these individuals. They should be counseled that they will have a delayed onset of menses, but it is not a health problem; they will have regular ovulatory cycles when

they either stop exercising or become older.

Before puberty, circulating levels of luteinizing hormone (LH) and follicle-stimulating hormone (FSH) are low (FSH/LH ratio being greater than 1) because the central nervous system (CNS)-hypothalamic axis is extremely sensitive to the negative feedback effects of low levels of circulating estrogen. As the critical weight or body composition is approached, the CNS-hypothalamic axis becomes less sensitive to the negative effect of estrogen, and gonadotrophin-releasing hormone (GnRH) is secreted in greater amounts, causing an increase in both LH and to a lesser extent FSH. The initial endocrinologic change associated with the onset of puberty is the occurrence of episodic pulses of LH occurring during sleep (Fig. 36-3). These pulses are absent before the onset of puberty. After menarche the episodic secretions of LH occur both during sleep and while awake. The last endocrinologic event of puberty is activation of the positive gonadotrophin response to increasing levels of estradiol, which results in the midcycle gonadotrophic response.

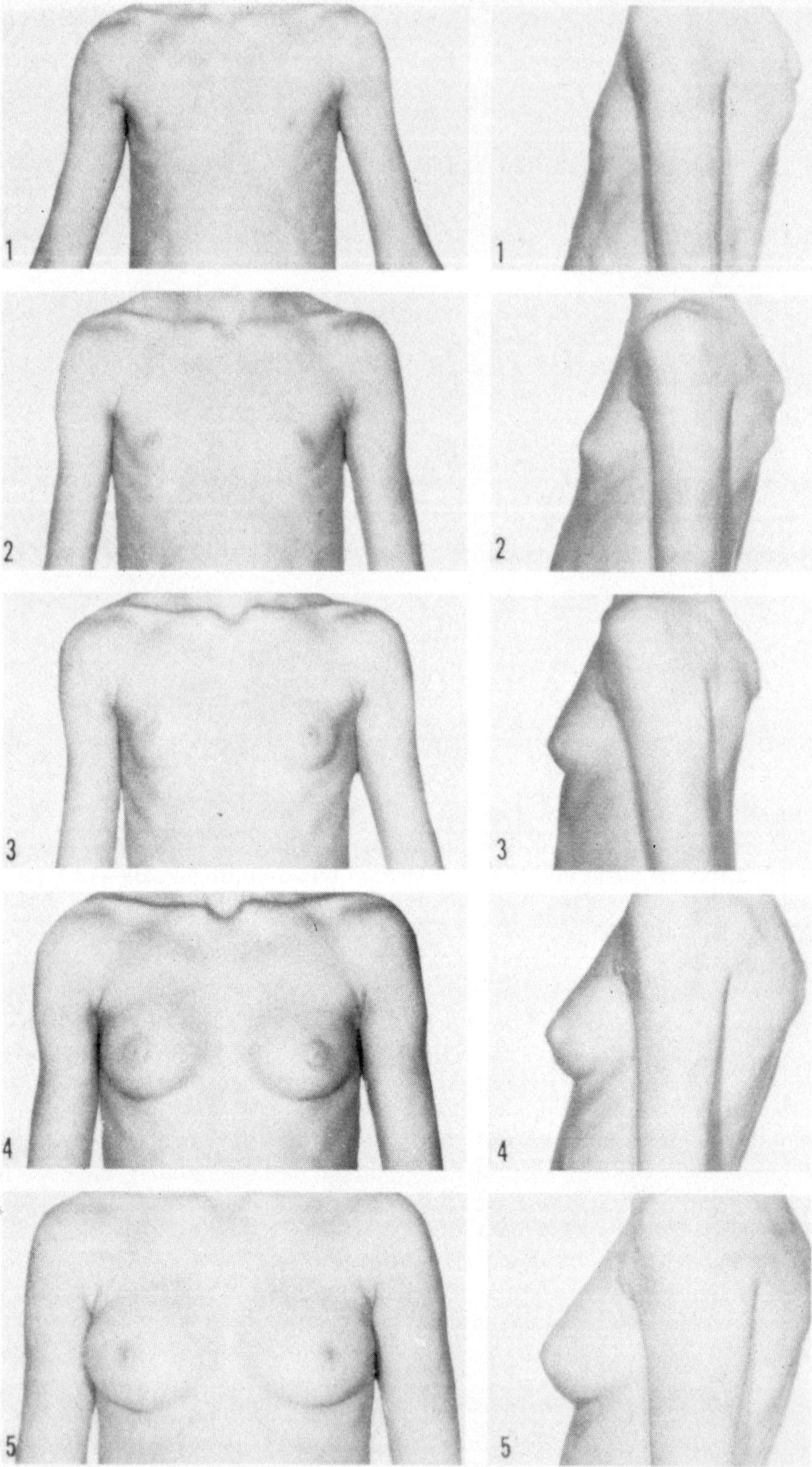

FIGURE 36-1, cont'd
Standards for breast ratings.

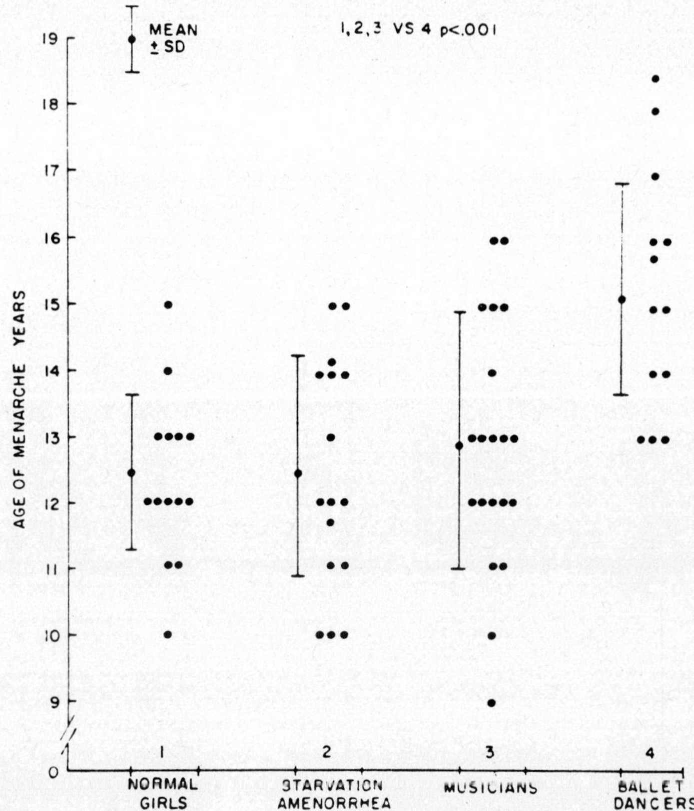

FIGURE 36-2

Ages of menarche in ballet dancers as compared with those of three other groups. (From Warren MP: The effects of exercise on pubertal progression and reproductive function in girls. J Clin Endocrinol Metab 51:1150, 1980. Copyright © by The Endocrine Society 1980.)

PRIMARY AMENORRHEA

It is important that the clinician understand both the sequential endocrinologic and the morphologic chronologic changes taking place during normal puberty in order to make the differential diagnosis between delayed menarche and primary amenorrhea. Although the former condition requires only reassurance, the latter requires an endocrinologic evaluation to establish the etiology of this symptom.

Etiology

Although numerous classifications have been used for the various etiologies of primary amenorrhea, it has been found most clinically useful to group them on the basis of whether secondary sexual characteristics (breasts) and female internal genitalia (uterus) are present or absent (see box, p. 971). Thus the findings of a physical examination can alert the clinician to possible causes and indicate which laboratory tests should be performed. In a series of 62 patients reported by Maschchak et al. the largest subgroup of individuals with primary amenorrhea (29) were those with absent breasts and a uterus present; the second largest subgroup (22) had both breasts and uterus; an absent uterus together with breast development accounted for the third largest category (9); and absent breasts and uterus were the least common (2).

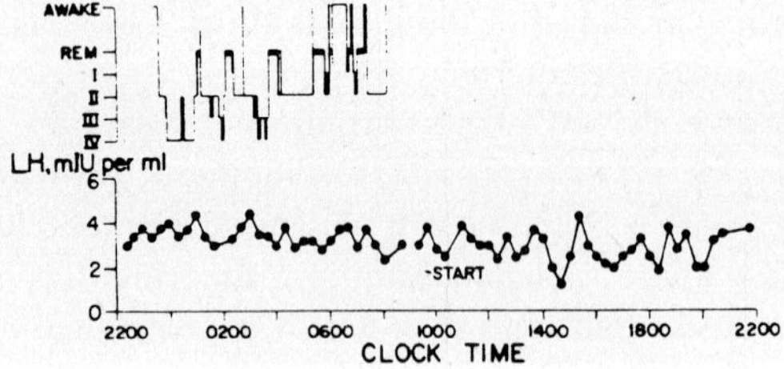

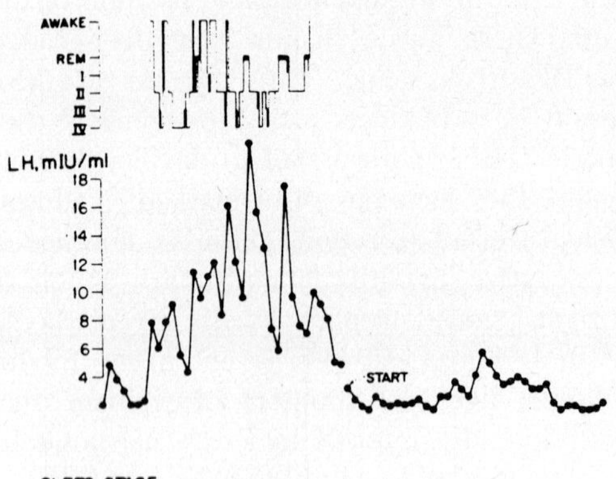

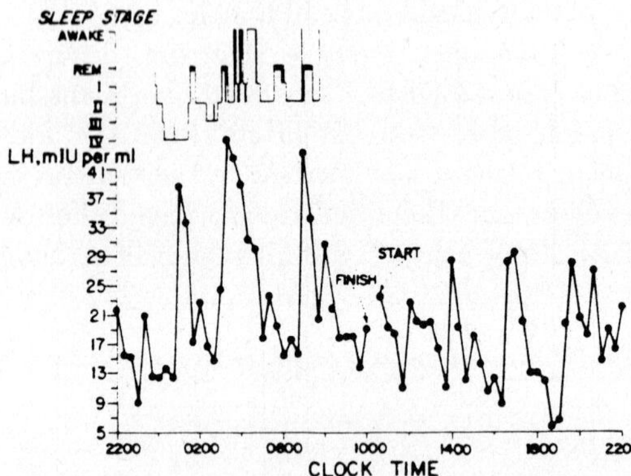

FIGURE 36-3

Plasma LH concentration measured every 20 minutes for 24 hours in normal prepubertal girl *(upper panel)*, early pubertal girl *(center panel)*, and normal late pubertal girl *(lower panel)*. In top and center panels sleep histogram is shown above period of nocturnal sleep. Sleep stages are awake, rapid eye movement (REM), and stages I to IV by depth of line graph. Plasma LH concentrations are expressed as milli–international units per milliliter of Second International Reference Preparation of Human Menopausal Gonadotropin. (Modified from Boyar RM, Katz J, Finkelstein JW, et al: N Engl J Med 291:861, 1974. Reprinted by permission of The New England Journal of Medicine.)

DIFFERENTIAL DIAGNOSIS OF PRIMARY AMENORRHEA WITH NORMAL FEMALE EXTERNAL GENITALIA

I. Primary amenorrhea without breast development and uterus present
  A. Gonadal failure
    1. 45,X
    2. 46,X, abnormal X (e.g., short-arm or long-arm deletion)
    3. Mosaicism (e.g., X/XX, X/XX/XXX)
    4. Pure XX and XY gonadal dysgenesis
    5. 17α-Hydroxylase deficiency (with 46,XX karyotype)
  B. CNS-hypothalamic-pituitary disorders
    1. CNS lesion
    2. Hypothalamic failure secondary to inadequate GnRH release
    3. Isolated gonadotrophin insufficiency

II. Primary amenorrhea with breast development and absent uterus
  A. Congenital absence of uterus (uterovaginal agenesis)
  B. Androgen insensitivity (testicular feminization)

III. Primary amenorrhea with no breast development and absent uterus
  A. 17,20-Desmolase deficiency
  B. Agonadism
  C. 17α-Hydroxylase deficiency (with 46,XY karyotype)

IV. Primary amenorrhea with breast development and uterus present
  A. Hypothalamic causes
  B. Pituitary causes
  C. Ovarian causes
  D. Uterine causes

Breasts Absent and Uterus Present

All individuals with no breast development and a uterus present have no ovarian estrogen production as a result of either a CNS hypothalamic-pituitary abnormality or a gonadal disorder. Although the phenotype of these individuals is similar, the etiology and prognosis for fertility of these disorders differ; therefore it is important to establish the exact diagnosis.

GONADAL FAILURE (HYPERGONADOTROPHIC HYPOGONADISM). Failure of gonadal development is the most common cause of primary amenorrhea, occurring in almost half the patients with this symptom. Gonadal failure is most frequently due to a chromosomal disorder or deletion of all or part of an X chromosome, but it is sometimes due to a genetic defect. The chromosome disorders are usually due to a random meiotic or mitotic abnormality (such as nondisjunction or anaphase lag) and thus are not inherited. However, if absent gonadal development occurs in the presence of a 46,XX or 46,XY karyotype, called pure gonadal dysgenesis, a gene disorder may be present, as it has been reported to occur in siblings. Rein dollar et al., in the largest single series of patients with primary amenorrhea, reported that all individuals with gonadal failure and an X chromosome abnormality were less than 63 inches in height. About one third had major cardiovascular or renal anomalies.

Since at least two X chromosomes are necessary for normal ovarian development, individuals with a 45,X karyotype, mosaicism involving a single X chromosome, or abnormalities of the X chromosome may fail to develop ovaries and usually only have a mass of fibrous tissue present in the normal anatomic position of the ovary. These fibrous bands have been called gonadal streaks (Fig. 36-4). Streaks are also present in individuals with pure gonadal dysgenesis. These persons fail to develop breasts because they have absent or markedly reduced gonadal steroid secretion. With the absence of the negative hypothalamic-pituitary action of estrogen, gonadotrophin levels are markedly elevated. Since estrogen is not necessary for müllerian duct development or wolffian duct regression, the internal and external genitalia are phenotypically normal female.

45,X Anomalies. *Turner's syndrome* occurs in about 1 per 2000 to 1 per 3000 live births but is much more frequent in abortuses. In addition to primary amenorrhea and absent breast development, these individuals have other somatic abnormalities, the most prevalent being

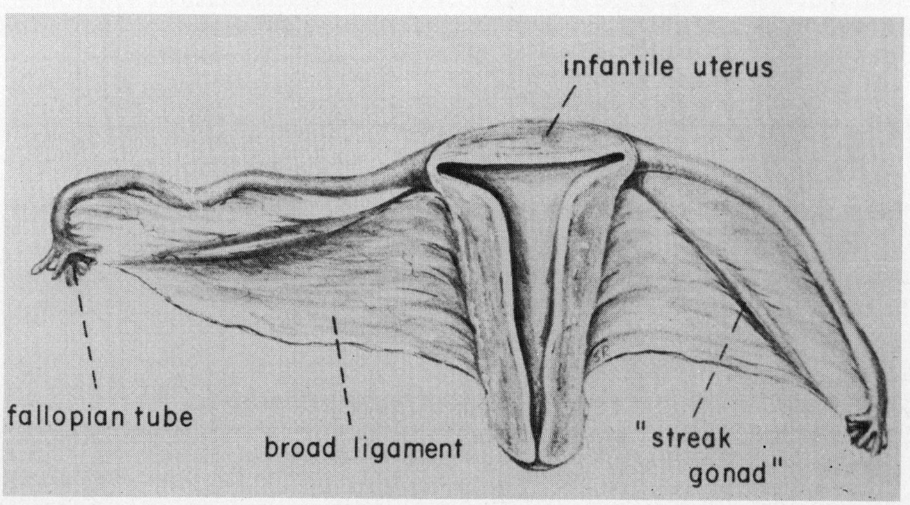

FIGURE 36-4
Internal genitalia of patient with gonadal dysgenesis (Turner's syndrome), featuring normal but infantile uterus, normal fallopian tubes, and pale, glistening "streak" gonads in both broad ligaments. (From Federman DD, ed: Disorders of gonadal development: Gonadal dysgenesis [Turner's syndrome]. In Abnormal sexual development. Philadelphia, W.B. Saunders Co., 1967.)

short stature (less than 60 inches in height), a web neck, a short fourth metacarpal, and cubitus valgus. Thus the diagnosis is usually made before puberty (see Chapter 3).

A wide variety of chromosomal mosaics are associated with primary amenorrhea and normal female external genitalia, the most common being X/XX. In addition, individuals with X/XXX and X/XX/XXX mosaicism have primary amenorrhea. These individuals are generally taller and have fewer anatomic abnormalities than individuals with a 45,X karyotype. In addition, some of them may have a few gonadal follicles, and about 20% have sufficient estrogen production to menstruate. Occasionally ovulation may occur.

Structurally Abnormal X Chromosome. Although individuals with this disorder have a 46,XX karyotype, part of one X chromosome is structurally abnormal. If there is deletion of the long arm of the X chromosome, normal height has been reported to occur, but in Reindollar's series such individuals were all short. These individuals have no somatic abnormalities. However, if there is deletion of the short arm of the X chromosome, the individual phenotypically resembles those with a 45,X karyotype (Turner's syndrome). A similar phenotype occurs in persons with isochrome of the long arm of the X chromosome. Other X chromosome abnormalities include a ring X and minute fragmentation of the X chromosome.

Pure Gonadal Dysgenesis (46,XX and 46,XY with Gonad Streaks; Gonadal Agenesis). As mentioned above, this abnormality is probably a genetic disorder, as it has been reported in siblings. These individuals have normal stature and phenotype, absence of secondary sexual characteristics, and primary amenorrhea. Some of these individuals have a few ovarian follicles, develop breasts, and may even menstruate spontaneously for a few years. In Reindollar's series nearly all such individuals were taller than 63 inches.

17α-Hydroxylase Deficiency with 46,XX Karyotype. A rare gonadal cause of primary amenorrhea without breast development and normal female internal genitalia is deficiency of the enzyme 17α-hydroxylase in an individual with a 46,XX karyotype. Only a few such individuals have been described in the literature, but it is important for the clinician to be aware of this entity because these individuals, in contrast to those described above, have hypernatremia and hypokalemia. Because of decreased cortisol, adrenocorticotropic hormone (ACTH) levels are elevated. The mineralocorticoid levels are also elevated, as 17α-hydroxylase is not necessary for the conversion of progesterone to deoxycortisol or corticosterone. Thus there is excessive sodium retention and potassium excretion, leading to hypertension and hypokalemia. Serum progesterone levels are also elevated because progesterone is not converted to cortisol. In addition to sex steroid replacement, these individuals need cortisol administration.

CNS-HYPOTHALAMIC-PITUITARY DISORDERS. In contrast to individuals with absent secondary sex characteristics and normal female internal genitalia caused by gonad disorders described above, these individuals have low gonadotrophin and estrogen levels. The etiology of low gonadotrophin production can be morphologic or endocrinologic.

Lesions. Any anatomic lesion of the hypothalamus or pituitary can be a cause of low gonadotrophin production. Many of these lesions, particularly pituitary adenomas, result in elevated prolactin levels (Chapter 37).

However, non-prolactin-secreting pituitary tumors (chromophobe adenomas) as well as craniopharyngiomas may not be associated with hyperprolactinemia and can rarely be the cause of primary amenorrhea with low gonadotrophin levels.

Inadequate GnRH Release (Hypogonadotrophic Hypogonadism). Individuals without a demonstrable lesion and a low gonadotrophin level were previously thought to have primary pituitary failure (hypogonadotrophic hypogonadism). However, when they are stimulated with GnRH, there is an increase in FSH and LH, indicating that the basic defect is either hypothalamic with insufficient GnRH or a CNS neurotransmitter defect resulting in inadequate GnRH synthesis or release or both. Although a single bolus of GnRH may not initially cause a rise in gonadotrophin level in these individuals, after 4 days of GnRH administration they will have a rise in gonadotrophins after a single GnRH bolus. Some of these individuals also have anosmia (Kallmann's syndrome), and they should be tested for olfaction with coffee, orange, and cocoa. Kallmann's syndrome is a ge-

netically transmitted disorder and is frequently associated with other anatomic and functional abnormalities.

Isolated Gonadotrophin Deficiency. Rarely individuals with primary amenorrhea and low gonadotrophin levels do not respond to GnRH even after 4 days of administration. These individuals nearly always have an associated disorder such as thalassemia major or retinitis pigmentosa.

Breast Development Present and Uterus Absent

In patients with breast development and absent uterus, two disorders can produce primary amenorrhea—androgen insensitivity and congenital absence of the uterus. The former is a genetic inherited disorder, whereas the latter is an accident of development and is only rarely genetically inherited.

ANDROGEN INSENSITIVITY. Androgen insensitivity, originally termed testicular feminization, is a genetically transmitted disorder in which there is an absence of androgen receptor synthesis or action. The syndrome is due to absence of an X-chromosomal gene responsible for the cytoplasmic or nuclear testosterone receptor. It is either an X-linked recessive or sex-limited autosomal dominant disorder with transmission through the mother. These individuals have an XY karyotype and normally functioning male gonads that produce normal male levels of testosterone and dihydrotestosterone. However, because of a lack of receptors in the target organs, there is a lack of male differentation of the external and internal genitalia. As occurs in the absence of sex steroids, the former remain feminine. Wolffian duct development, which normally occurs as a result of testosterone stimulation, fails to take place; however, müllerian duct regression, which is produced by the peptide elaborated by the fetal testes, müllerian inhibiting factor (MIF), occurs normally since steroid receptors are not necessary for its action. Thus individuals with this condition have no female or male internal genitalia, normal female external genitalia, and either a short or absent vagina. Pubic and axillary hair is absent or scanty as a result of a lack of androgenic receptors, but breast development is normal or enlarged due to the fact that there is no androgenic opposition to the stimulation of breast tissue by the small circulating levels of estrogen secreted by the gonads and adrenals as well as the estrogen produced by peripheral conversion of androstenedione. The abnormal gonads are at increased risk of developing a malignancy (gonadoblastoma or dysgerminoma), with an incidence reported to be about 20%. However, these malignancies rarely occur before age 20. Therefore it is usually recommended that the gonads be left in place until after puberty is completed to allow normal sexual maturity. After such time they should be removed. It is probably best that the patient not be informed that the gonads are testes and that they are male because these individuals are phenotypically female and have been raised as such. Instead they should be informed that they are sterile as a result of a missing piece of the X chromosome, and the gonad (not testes) needs to be removed because it has a high malignant potential.

CONGENITAL ABSENCE OF THE UTERUS (UTERINE AGENESIS; UTEROVAGINAL AGENESIS; ROKITANSKY KUSTER-HAUSER SYNDROME). This disorder is the second most frequent cause of primary amenorrhea. It occurs in 1 in 4000 to 5000 female births and accounts for about 15% of individuals with primary amenorrhea. Individuals with complete uterine agenesis have no underlying endocrine abnormality but are amenorrheic because of absence of the end organ. They have normal breast and pubic and axillary hair development but have a shortened or absent vagina in addition to absence of the uterus (Fig. 36-5). Congenital renal abnormalities occur in about one third of these individuals and skeletal abnormalities in about 12%. Cardiac and other congenital abnormalities also occur with increased frequency. The overwhelming majority of these disorders are due to an isolated developmental defect, but on occasion the condition is genetically inherited. Endocrinologically the ovaries are present and function normally, so that ovulation occurs cyclically. It is usually easy to differentiate these individuals from those with androgen insensitivity by the presence of normal pubic hair, but some individuals with incomplete androgen insensitivity have some pubic hair. However, women with congenital absence of the uterus are endocrinologically

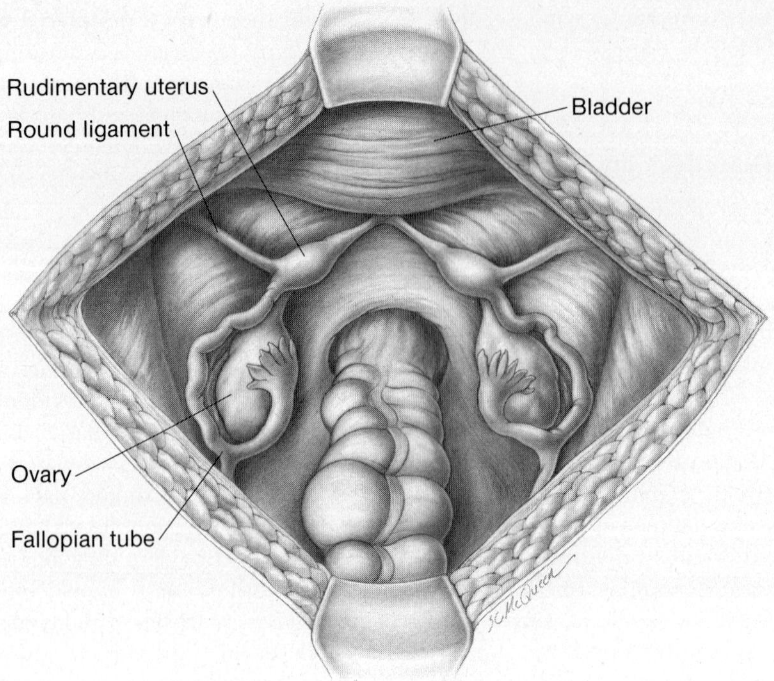

FIGURE 36-5
Congenital absence of vagina. Laparotomy revealed rudimentary uterus that showed evidence of failure of fusion of the müllerian ducts. This is a common finding in this condition and indicates that the disorder is more extensive than a simple anomaly of the vagina. (Redrawn from Jones HW Jr, Scott WW, eds: Hermaphroditism, genital anomalies and related endocrine disorders, 2nd ed. Baltimore, Williams & Wilkins Co., 1971.)

normal females, whereas those with androgen insensitivity are endocrinologically male with male testosterone levels and an XY karyotype, so the differential diagnosis is easily made.

Absent Breast and Uterine Development

Persons with no breast or uterine development are rare and have a male karyotype, elevated gonadotrophin levels, and testosterone levels in the normal or below normal female range. Etiologies for this phenotype include 17α-hydroxylase deficiency, 17,20-desmolase deficiency, and agonadism. Individuals with the first disorder have testes present but lack the enzyme necessary to synthesize sex steroids and thus have female external genitalia. Because they have testes, MIF is produced and the female internal genitalia regress; with low testosterone levels the male internal genitalia

do not develop. Insufficient estrogen is synthesized for breast development. A similar lack of sex steroid synthesis occurs in males with a 17,20-desmolase deficiency. Individuals with agonadism, sometimes called the vanishing testes syndrome, have no gonads present, but since the female internal genitalia are also absent it has been postulated that testicular MIF production occurred during fetal life, but the gonadal tissue subsequently regressed.

Secondary Sex Characteristics and Female Internal Genitalia Present

This is the second largest category of patients with primary amenorrhea. In the series reported by Maschchak et al., about 25% of these individuals had hyperprolactinemia and prolactinomas. The remaining patients had etiologies similar to those women with secondary amenorrhea and thus should be subcategorized and

treated similarly to patients with secondary amenorrhea, which is discussed in the latter half of this chapter.

Differential Diagnosis and Management

After a history is obtained and a physical examination performed, including measurement of height, span, and weight, such patients are placed into the four general categories listed above, depending on the presence or absence of secondary sex characteristics and female internal genitalia.

If breast development is absent and a uterus is present, the diagnostic evaluation should differentiate between CNS-hypothalamic-pituitary disorders and failure of normal gonadal development. Although individuals with both these disorders have similar phenotypes because of low estradiol levels, a single serum FSH assay can differentiate between these two major etiologic categories (Fig. 36-6). Only those individuals with an elevated FSH level should then have a peripheral white blood cell karyotype performed to determine if a Y chromosome is present. If a Y chromosome is present, the streak gonads should be excised, as the incidence of malignancy occurring subsequently, mainly gonadoblastomas, is relatively high. If a Y chromosome is absent, it is not necessary to perform laparoscopy or laparotomy or to remove the gonads; such surgical procedures should not be performed. It is also unnecessary to perform a karyotype on the gonadal tissue to detect mosaicism in the gonad unless there is physical evidence of excessive androgen production, that is, hirsutism.

All patients with an elevated FSH level and an XX karyotype should have electrolyte and serum progesterone levels measured to rule out 17 α-hydroxylase deficiency. In addition to hypernatremia and hypokalemia, individuals with 17 α-hydroxylase deficiency have an elevated serum progesterone level (>3 ng/ml), a low 17 α-hydroxyprogesterone level (<0.2 ng/ml), and an elevated serum deoxycorticoste-

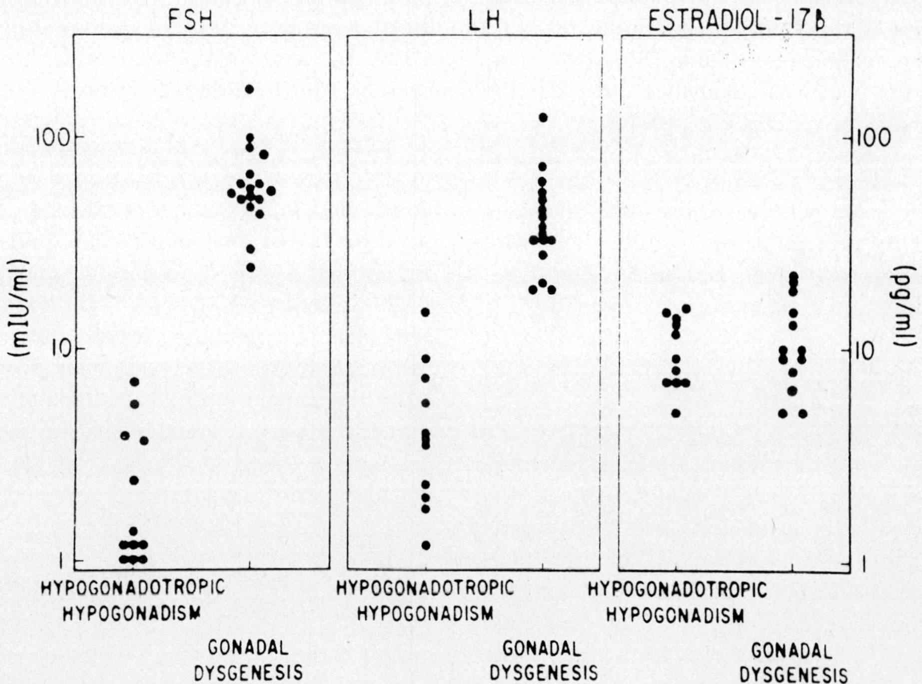

FIGURE 36-6

Levels of serum FSH, LH, and estradiol in patients with primary amenorrhea who have an intact uterus and no breast development. (From Maschchak CA, Kletzky OA, Davajan V, et al: Obstet Gynecol 57:715, 1981. Reprinted with permission from The American College of Obstetricians and Gynecologists.)

rone level (>17 ng/100 ml), so the diagnosis is easily established.

All individuals in this category are sterile but need estrogen-progestogen replacement therapy to develop breast tissue and prevent osteoporosis. The progestogen is necessary to decrease the risk of endometrial carcinoma, which may be increased by long-term unopposed estrogen administration. Ingestion of 0.625 mg conjugated estrogen daily for 25 days per month and 10 mg medroxyprogesterone acetate daily for the last 12 days of estrogen therapy is sufficient to achieve maximum breast growth and prevent osteoporosis. Larger doses of estrogen will not result in larger breasts. Those rare individuals with 17 α-hydroxylase deficiency need to have adequate cortisol replacement in addition to sex steroid treatment.

If the FSH level is low, the underlying disorder is in the CNS-hypothalamic-pituitary region and a serum prolactin measurement should be obtained. Even if the prolactin level is not elevated, all such individuals should have a cranial computerized tomography (CT) scan obtained to rule out a lesion in this area. If no tumor is found, it is not necessary to perform a karyotype, as all these individuals are 46,XX. The use of GnRH testing is optional but is expensive and is clinically unnecessary unless GnRH is going to be used for ovulation induction. Such individuals are potentially fertile because their ovaries are normal. Initially they should receive estrogen-progestogen treatment to promote breast growth. When fertility is desired, treatment with human menopausal gonadotrophins or pulsatile GnRH should be administered to induce ovulation.

The differential diagnosis of androgen insensitivity from uterine agenesis can be made by the presence in the latter condition of normal body hair, ovulatory and premenstrual type symptoms, a biphasic basal temperature, and a normal female testosterone level. Such individuals are sterile but are endocrinologically normal females, and they do not need hormonal therapy or karyotyping. An intravenous urogram should be performed because of the high incidence of renal abnormalities. They may need surgical reconstruction of an absent vagina (McIndoe procedure), but progressive mechanical dilation with plastic dilators as described by Frank should be tried first.

Individuals with androgen insensitivity have an XY karyotype and male levels of testosterone. After full breast development is obtained and epiphyseal closure occurs, the gonads should be removed because of their malignant potential. Thereafter estrogen-progestogen replacement therapy, as outlined above, should be administered.

Those rare individuals with absent breast development and absent internal genitalia should be referred to an endocrine center for the sophisticated type of testing necessary to establish the diagnosis. If gonads are present, they should be removed, because a Y chromosome is present, and replacement female sex steroid therapy should be administered.

SECONDARY AMENORRHEA

Etiology

The symptom of amenorrhea associated with hyperprolactinemia or excessive androgen or cortisol production will not be considered in this chapter as these disorders are discussed in Chapters 37 and 38. If amenorrhea is present without galactorrhea, hyperprolactinemia, or hirsutism, the symptom can be due to disorders in the CNS-hypothalamic-pituitary axis, ovary, or uterus. The uterine cause of amenorrhea is the only one with normal endocrinologic function and will be discussed first.

Uterine Cause

Intrauterine adhesions (IUAs) or synechiae (Asherman's syndrome) can obliterate the endometrial cavity and produce secondary amenorrhea. Rarely, a missed abortion or endometrial tuberculosis can also cause endometrial destruction. The most frequent antecedent factor of IUAs is endometrial curettage associated with pregnancy—either evacuation of a normal-gestation fetus by mechanical means or postpartum or postabortal curettage. Curettage for a missed abortion results in a high (30%) incidence of IUA formation. IUAs may also occur after diagnostic dilation and curettage (D&C) in a nonpregnant individual, so this procedure should only be performed when indicated and not routinely at the time of other surgical procedures such as diagnostic laparoscopy. A less common cause of IUA is severe

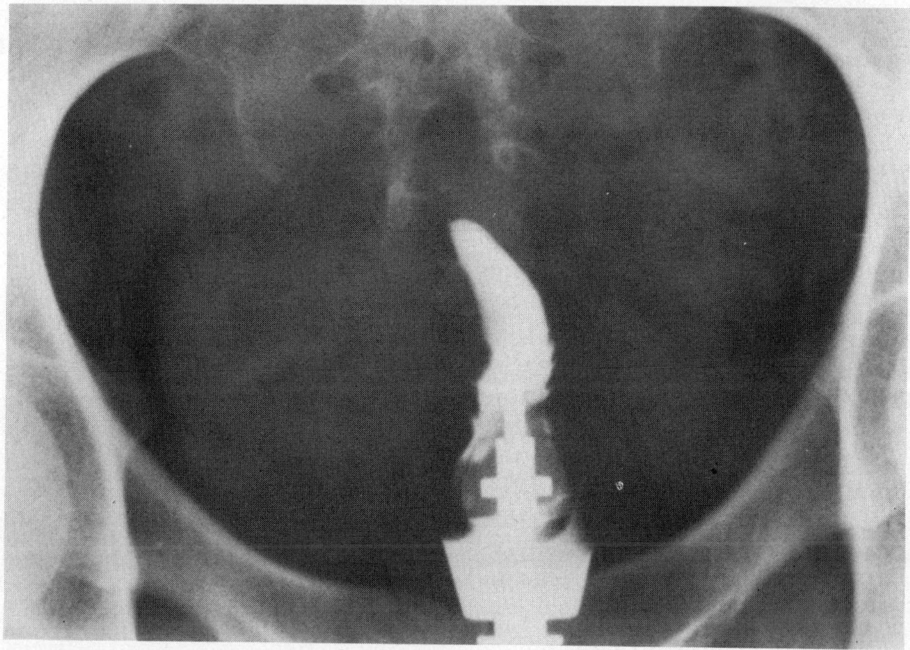

FIGURE 36-7

X-ray film of patient with Asherman's syndrome. Patient (33 years, gravida 3, para O, abortus 3) had been amenorrheic for 6 months after D&C for most recent therapeutic abortion (TAB). Filling of endocervical canal and nonvisualization of endometrial cavity are consistent with complete obliteration of the cavity by adhesions or with obstruction at internal os level by adhesions in lower endometrial cavity. This appearance may also be seen with advanced endometrial tuberculosis. (From Richmond JA: Hysterosalpingography. Reproduced with permission from Infertility, contraception and reproductive endocrinology, 2nd ed, by Daniel R. Mishell, Jr., M.D., and Val Davajan, M.D. Copyright © 1986 by Medical Economics Books, Oradell, N.J. 07649. All rights reserved.)

endometritis or fibrosis following a myomectomy, metroplasty, or cesarean section. The etiology should be suspected if there is difficulty or inability to pass a sound into the uterine cavity; this can be confirmed by means of a hysterogram (Fig. 36-7) or hysteroscopy. Although some researchers have advocated that sequential administration of estrogen-progestogen be used as the initial diagnostic procedure when IUA is suspected, withdrawal bleeding occurs following administration of the steroids in most patients with IUA, and therefore this test is not definitive for establishing the diagnosis and is unnecessary.

CNS-Hypothalamic Causes

LESIONS. The same anatomic lesions in the brain stem or hypothalamus that can produce primary amenorrhea by interfering with GnRH release can also cause secondary amenorrhea. Hypothalamic lesions include craniopharyngiomas, granulomatous disease (tuberculosis and sarcoidosis), and sequelae of encephalitis. When such uncommon lesions are present, circulating gonadotrophin levels and estradiol levels are low; as a result, uterine bleeding will not occur after progesterone administration.

DRUGS. Phenothiazine derivatives, certain antihypertensive agents, and other drugs listed in Chapter 37 can also produce amenorrhea without galactorrhea, although usually the prolactin levels are elevated. Therefore, every individual with secondary amenorrhea should have a detailed medication history obtained even if galactorrhea is not present. Oral contraceptive steroids inhibit ovulation by acting both on the hypothalamus to suppress GnRH

and directly on the pituitary to suppress FSH and LH. Sometimes this hypothalamic-pituitary suppression persists for several months after oral contraceptives are discontinued, producing the syndrome termed "postpill amenorrhea." This oral contraceptive–induced suppression does not last more than 6 months, as it has been reported that the incidence of amenorrhea persisting more than 6 months after discontinuation of oral contraceptives (0.8%) is about the same as the incidence of secondary amenorrhea in the general population (0.7%). Thus the etiology of amenorrhea persisting more than 6 months after discontinuation of oral contraceptives is unrelated to their use, except that the regular withdrawal bleeding produced by oral contraceptives masks the development of this syndrome.

STRESS AND EXERCISE. Stressful situations including a sudden change in environment (e.g., going away to school), a death in the family, or divorce can produce amenorrhea. A high percentage of women who had been placed in concentration camps or those sentenced for execution also became amenorrheic as a result of stress.

It is also now believed that the amenorrhea associated with strenuous exercise is also related to stress. Feicht et al. reported that the incidence of secondary amenorrhea in runners had a positive correlation with the number of miles run per week (Fig. 36-8). In a comparison of amenorrheic and eumenorrheic athletes, this group of investigators showed that physical parameters such as age, weight, lean body mass, and body fat were similar. The only significant difference between the two groups was the fact that the amenorrheic athletes ran more miles per week. McArthur et al. reported there was no significant difference in the percentage of body fat in amenorrheic runners compared with runners who were menstruating. In a longitudinal study of competitive swimmers, Russell et al. found that when the training became more strenuous, their LH and FSH levels fell significantly, while levels of beta-endorphin and catechol estrogens rose significantly as compared with levels of these hormones when the swimmers were exercising to a moderate degree (Tables 36-4 and 36-5). Individuals with a low percentage of adipose tissue have a shift in the pathway of estrogen metabolism from 16-hydroxylation, which forms estriol, to 2-hy-

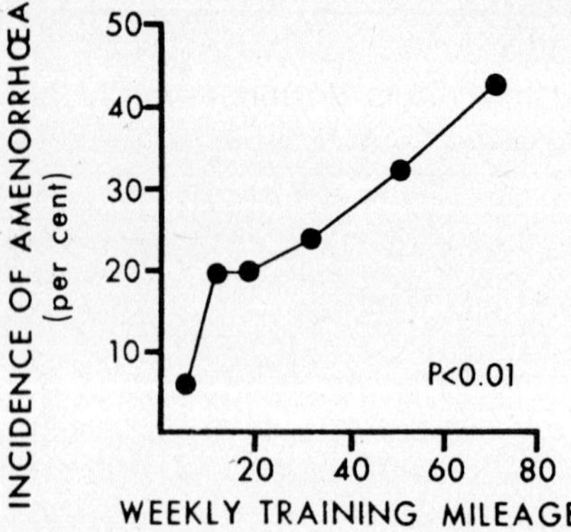

FIGURE 36-8
Correlation between training mileage and amenorrhea. Each point represents average of 21 respondents. Statistical significance of relationship was obtained from point-biserial correlation (1 mile [1.6 km]). (From Feicht CB, Johnson TS, Matrin BJ: Lancet 2:1145, 1978.)

droxylation, which forms catechol estrogens. It has been postulated that the decreased fatty tissue in individuals who exercise is the reason for the increased levels of catechol estrogens. However, when the swimmers were only exercising moderately, levels of catechol estrogens as well as beta-endorphin were not significantly different from those of a control group of similar body weight and percentage body fat who were not participating in organized physical activity. This group of investigators also reported that another group of swimmers and runners had significantly higher levels of catechol estrogens than a control group of normally menstruating women with a similar weight and low percentage of body fat. Whether catechol estrogens are increased as a result of less fatty tissue, the stress of training, or a combination of both, the increase may be the cause of the amenorrhea. Adashi et al. showed that infusion or injection of catechol estrogens decreased LH levels in humans.

Carr et al. also reported that physical conditioning facilitates the exercise-induced secretion of beta-endorphin and its precursor beta-lipoprotein in women. Reid et al. showed that infusion of beta-endorphin into women caused a significant decrease in LH. Beta-endorphin and its analogues inhibit GnRH release, possibly by inhibiting the stimulating effect of norepinephrine on GnRH.

TABLE 36-4

Analysis* of Protein Hormones for Swimmers During Moderate and Strenuous Exercise and for Nonexercising Control Subjects

| | | Swimmers | | Group Comparison (Median Values) | | |
Hormone	Control Subjects	Moderate (60,000 yards)	Strenuous (100,000 yards)	C vs. 60	C vs. 100	100 vs. 60
No.	6	5	5			
LH (mIU/ ml)	23.1[21.4] ± 10.5 (12.3-13.3)	22.9[22.2] ± 5.7 (15.9-30.7)	10.9[11.3] ± 2.8 (7.4-13.6)	$P = 0.66$	$P = 0.02$	$P = 0.02$
FSH (mIU/ ml)	10.9[9.6] ± 3.5 (7.1-15.7)	20.2[18.2] ± 5.1 (15.3-27.7)	6.54[6.8] ± 2.1 (4.0-9.5)	$P = 0.05$	$P = 0.04$	$P \leq 0.001$
Prolactin (ng/ml)	20.8[13.5] ± 15.0 (9.0-47.2)	10.6[10.5] ± 3.6 (5.9-16.1)	1.36[1.0] ± 0.9 (0.7-3.0)	$P = 0.18$	$P = 0.004$	$P = 0.006$

Adapted from Russel JB, Mitchell DE, Musey PI, et al: The role of β-endorphins and catechol estrogens on the hypothalamic-pituitary axis in female athletes. Fertil Steril 42:690, 1984. Reproduced with permission of the publisher, The American Fertility Society.
*Mean (median) value ± SD with range in parentheses.

TABLE 36-5

Analysis* of Beta-Endorphin Immunoreactivity, Estradiol, and Catechol Estrogens for Swimmers During Moderate and Strenuous Exercise and for Nonexercising Control Subjects

| | | Swimmers | | Group Comparisons | | |
Hormone	Control Subjects	Moderate (60,000 yards)	Strenuous (100,000 yards)	C vs. 60	C vs. 100	100 vs. 60
No.	6	5	5			
Estradiol (pg/ml)	264[193] ± 253 (78-759)	61.8[65] ± 16.8 (36-79)	76.8[52] ± 61.9 (36-185)	$P = 0.009$	$P = 0.003$	$P = 0.68$
Catecholestrogens (pg/ml)	35.3[35] ± 7.5 (25-46)	28.6[28] ± 1.2 (26-29)	92.4[88] ± 12.8 (83-115)	$P = 0.08$	$P \leq 0.001$	$P \leq 0.001$
Beta-endorphin immunoreactivity (pmol/L)	8.50[2] ± 15.4 (2-40)	4.40[4] ± 2.2 (2-8)	31.2[24] ± 14.3 (18-52)	$P = 0.25$	$P = 0.03$	$P = 0.01$

Adapted from Russel JB, Mitchell DE, Musey PI, et al: The role of β-endorphins and catechol estrogens on the hypothalamic-pituitary axis on female athletes. Fertil Steril 42:690, 1984. Reproduced with permission of the publisher, The American Fertility Society.
*Mean (median) value ± SD with range in parentheses.

Thus the increase in both catechol estrogens and beta-endorphins associated with strenuous exercise appears to be the mechanism whereby LH and probably FSH release is inhibited, most likely by acting on the neurotransmitters responsible for release of GnRH. The decreased gonadotrophin levels produce amenorrhea by failing to stimulate sex steroid production.

It is probable that emotionally stressful situations such as divorce or a sudden change in environment can also cause alterations in beta-endorphin and catechol estrogens. When the stressful situation (whether emotional in origin

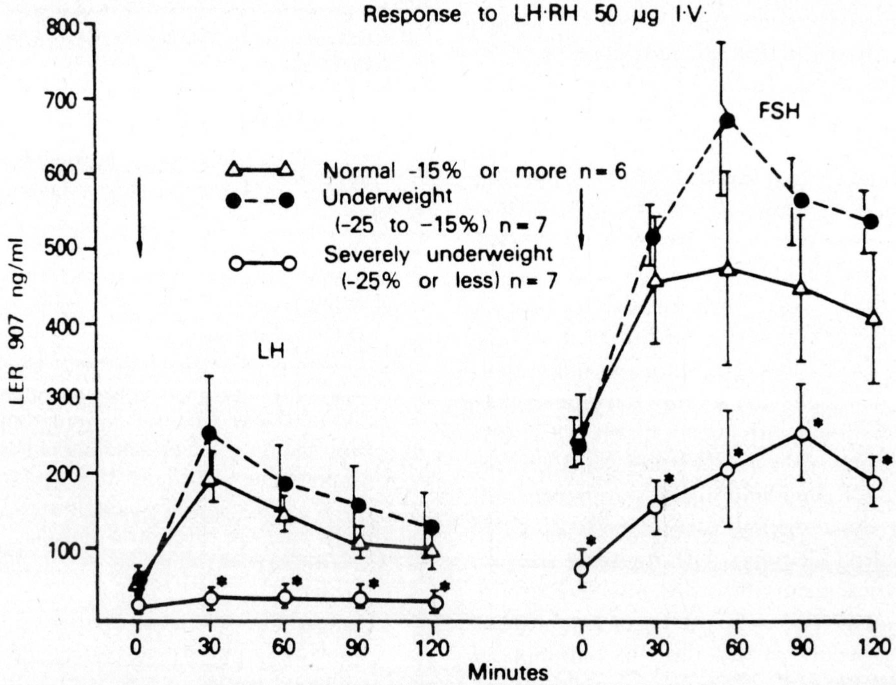

FIGURE 36-9

Effect of 50 µg LH-releasing hormone (LH-RH) in 20 women with amenorrhea and weight loss (vertical bars represent SEM). *Values significantly different from two other groups P = .05 — .001. (From Warren MP, Jewelwicz R, Dyrenfurth I, et al: The significance of weight loss in the evaluation of pituitary response to LH-RH in women with secondary amenorrhea. J Clin Endocrinol Metab 40:601, 1975. Copyright © by The Endocrine Society 1975.)

or related to strenuous exercise) abates, menstruation usually resumes promptly.

WEIGHT LOSS. Both male and female animals who are malnourished have decreased reproductive capacity. Weight loss is also associated with amenorrhea in women and has been classified into two groups: the moderately underweight group includes individuals whose weight is 15% to 25% below ideal body weight; severely underweight women are those whose weight loss is greater than 25% of ideal body weight. Weight loss can occur from excessive dietary restrictions as well as malnutrition. Vigersky et al. have demonstrated that women with amenorrhea associated with simple weight loss have both direct and indirect evidence of hypothalamic dysfunction, while pituitary and end-organ function is normal. However, Warren et al. showed that when women were severely underweight, in addition to hypothalamic dysfunction, pituitary gonadotrophin function was also altered because there was no increase in LH and a decreased response of FSH following GnRH administration (Fig. 36-9). However, these responses could be due to a lack of prolonged GnRH secretion, because the studies were not performed after several days of GnRH priming. Thus the amenorrhea associated with weight loss appears to be due mainly to failure of normal GnRH release, with a possible pituitary disorder also occurring when the weight loss is severe.

A severe psychiatric disorder called anorexia nervosa is also associated with severe weight loss and amenorrhea. Anorexia nervosa is not rare, and it is estimated to occur in about 1 in 1000 white women in the United States. It is uncommon in men and rare in blacks and Orientals. This disorder is most frequent in teenagers and is uncommon after the age of 25. It is one of the most important and probably the most common causes of secondary amenorrhea in adolescent women. This disorder is associated with other physical changes, including dry skin, bradycardia, hypotension, constipation, and hypothermia (see box at right). Individuals with anorexia nervosa usually have a normal thyroxine level (T_4) and an abnormally low serum triiodothyronine (T_3) level. If the clinician cannot make the differential diagnosis between amenorrhea caused by simple weight loss and that caused by anorexia nervosa on clinical findings alone, measurement of the serum T_3 level is most helpful, as individuals with simple weight loss usually have normal T_3 levels. In patients with anorexia nervosa T_4 levels are normal, T_3 levels are low, and reverse T_3 (an inactive metabolite) levels are increased, indicating that peripheral conversion of T_4 to T_3 is impaired. Patients with anorexia nervosa have a hypothalamic disorder interfering with normal GnRH release, and their amenorrhea frequently occurs at the time of initiation of food restriction before they lose weight. However, after severe weight loss occurs in these individuals and they are less than 65% of ideal body weight, an abnormal gonadotrophin response to GnRH takes place similar to those seen in individuals with severe weight loss caused by dieting. This indicates that pituitary dysfunction also occurs in persons with anorexia nervosa when the weight loss becomes severe. Boyer et al. have shown that patients with anorexia nervosa have an LH secretion pattern similar to that observed in prepubertal children (absent LH pulses) (Fig. 36-10) or pubertal premenarcheal girls (nocturnal LH pulses only). When these individuals gain weight, the normal 24-hour LH pulsatile patterns return. Weight gain in either individuals with anorexia nervosa or those with severe simple weight loss results in their gonadotrophin response to GnRH infusion becoming normal or even exaggerated, with the FSH response resuming in proportion to the weight gain and the LH responsiveness returning only after the individual reaches about 85% of ideal body weight. These progressive endocrine responses are also similar to those occurring during puberty, indicating the importance of body weight in causing maturation of the CNS-hypothalamic-pituitary axis and providing additional information as to why girls who exercise strenuously before menarche and have less

---

CRITERIA FOR DIAGNOSIS OF ANOREXIA NERVOSA

Onset before 25 years of age

Anorexia with accompanying weight loss of at least 25% of original body weight

Distorted, implacable attitude toward eating, food, or weight that overrides hunger, admonitions, reassurance, and threats—for example

  Denial of illness

  Failure to recognize nutritional needs

  Apparent enjoyment in losing weight

  Desired body image of extreme thinness

  Unusual hoarding or handling of food

No known medical illness that could account for the anorexia and weight loss

No other known psychiatric disorder

At least two of the following manifestations:

  Amenorrhea

  Lanugo

  Bradycardia (persistent resting pulse of 60 bpm or less)

  Periods of overactivity

  Episodes of bulimia

  Vomiting (may be self-induced)

From Sherman BM, Halmi KA, Zamudio R: LH and FSH response to gonadotropin-releasing hormone in anorexia nervosa: Effect of nutritional rehabilitation. J Clin Endocrinol Metab 41:135, 1975. Copyright © by the Endocrine Society, 1975.

---

body fat also have a delayed onset of menstruation. Frisch and Revelle reported that undernourished girls reach menarche at an older age but at the same mean weight as well-nourished girls.

Anorexia nervosa is a psychiatric disorder and patients with this disease should receive appropriate psychiatric treatment. These individuals as well as those with dietary weight loss usually resume ovulatory menstrual cycles when they gain weight and approach their ideal body weight.

POLYCYSTIC OVARY SYNDROME. It is now believed that polycystic ovary syndrome (PCO) is a CNS-hypothalamic disorder that produces tonically elevated LH levels. Most of the women with these disorders have elevated androgen levels, but not all have clinical evidence of androgen excess (hirsutism). Thus the presence of PCO must be considered in the differ-

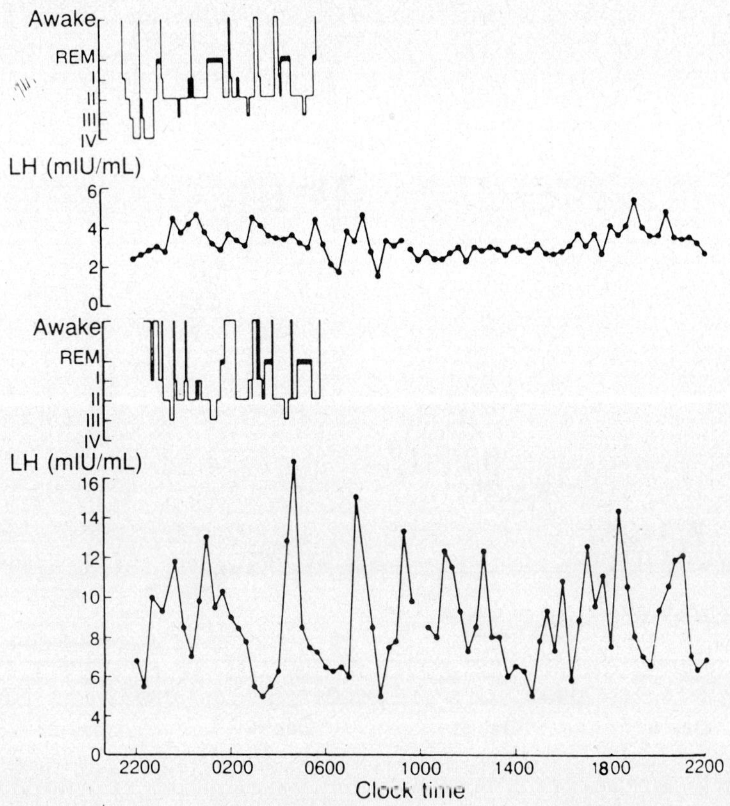

FIGURE 36-10

Plasma LH concentrations every 20 minutes for 24 hours during acute exacerbation of anorexia nervosa *(upper panel)* and after clinical remission with return of body weight to normal *(lower panel)*. (From Boyar RM, Katz J, Finkelstein JW, et al: N Engl J Med 291:861, 1974. Reprinted by permission of The New England Journal of Medicine.)

ential diagnosis of both primary and secondary amenorrhea even if hirsutism is absent. Because most individuals with PCO have signs of androgen excess, this subject is discussed in detail in Chapter 38.

HYPOTHALAMIC DYSFUNCTION AND HYPOTHALAMIC FAILURE. There is a group of individuals with secondary amenorrhea who do not ingest drugs, do not engage in strenuous exercise, are not under severe environmental stress, and have not lost weight. No pituitary, ovarian, or uterine abnormalities are present in these individuals. The general term *hypothalamic dysfunction* has been used to characterize this disorder, as there is an exaggerated pituitary gonadotrophin response when GnRH is administered to these individuals. Recently Reame et al. and Crowley et al., utilizing fre-

quent blood sampling, have shown that LH is secreted in a pulsatile manner that varies in frequency and amplitude throughout the normal ovulatory menstrual cycle, being more rapid in the follicular phase than the luteal phase (Fig. 36-11). These investigators have shown that women with amenorrhea due to hypothalamic dysfunction do not exhibit these characteristic cyclic alterations in LH pulsatility. They either have no pulses (Fig. 36-12) or have a persistent pattern of pulsatility that is normally found in only one portion of the ovulatory cycle, usually the slow frequency found in the luteal phase, despite having a steroid milieu similar to the follicular phase (Fig. 36-13). Since each LH pulse represents a response to a pulse of GnRH, it appears that these individuals have an abnormality in the normal cyclic

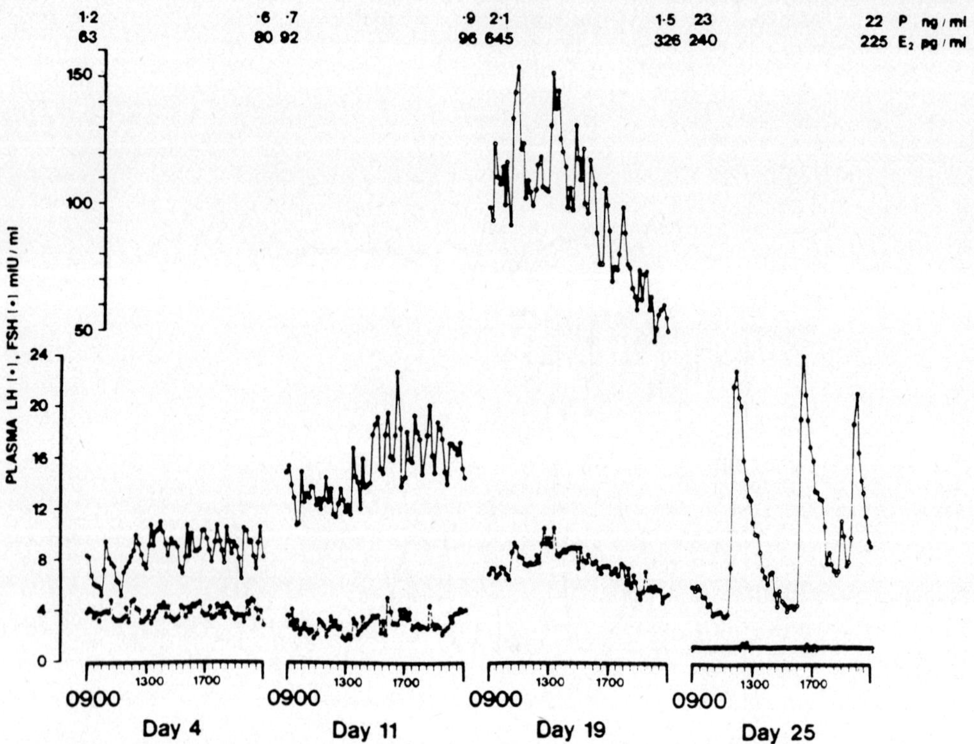

FIGURE 36-11

Serial measurements of plasma LH and FSH in two subjects sampled every 10 minutes at weekly intervals during cycles in which LH surge was observed on one of sampling days. (From Reame NE, Sauder SE, Kelch RP, et al: Pulsatile gonadotropin secretion during the human menstrual cycle: Evidence for altered frequency of gonadotropin-releasing hormone secretion. J Clin Endocrinol Metab 59:328, 1984. Copyright © by The Endocrine Society 1984.)

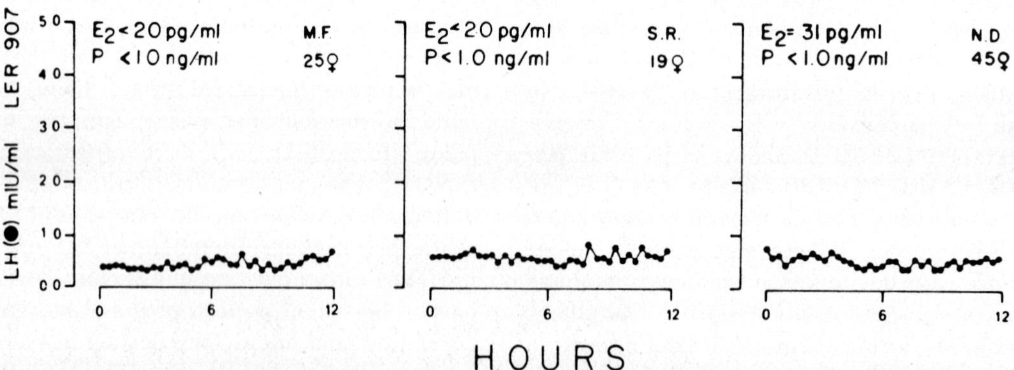

FIGURE 36-12

Apulsatile pattern of LH secretion in women with hypogonadotrophic hypogonadism and hypothalamic amenorrhea. (From Crowley WF Jr, Filicori M, Spratt DI, et al: Rec Prog Hormone Res 41:473, 1985.)

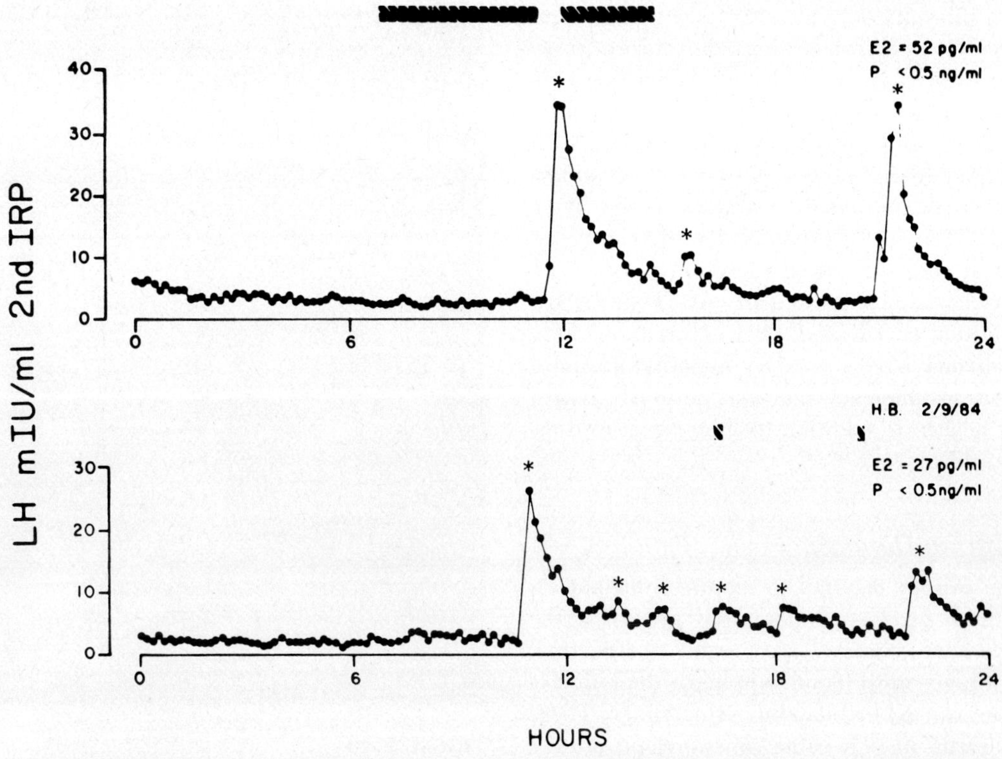

FIGURE 36-13
Defects in frequency of LH secretion episodes in subjects with hypothalamic amenorrhea. (From Crowley WF Jr, Filicori M, Spratt DI, et al: Rec Prog Hormone Res 41:473, 1985.)

variations of GnRH pulsatility, probably due to an abnormality in the CNS neurotransmitters and possibly produced by increased opioid activity. When sufficient GnRH is produced to stimulate sufficient gonadotrophin production to maintain circulating estradiol levels above 40 pg/ml, the term *hypothalamic-pituitary dysfunction* is used to characterize this disorder. However, when the estradiol levels fall below 40 pg/ml, the term *hypothalamic-pituitary failure* has been used, indicating a more serious disorder. Serum estradiol levels above 40 pg/ml are usually sufficient to stimulate endometrial growth to an extent that sloughing occurs when progesterone levels fall several days after an injection of progesterone in oil is given. The withdrawal bleeding response to progesterone administration has also been used to differentiate between these two diagnostic categories.

Pituitary Causes

NEOPLASMS. Although most pituitary tumors secrete prolactin, some do not and may be associated with the onset of secondary amenorrhea without galactorrhea. Chromophobe adenomas are the most common non-prolactin-secreting pituitary tumors; however, both basophilic (ACTH secreting) and acidophilic (growth hormone [GH] secreting) adenomas may be incapable of secreting prolactin. Individuals with the latter types of tumor, although having secondary amenorrhea, frequently have other symptoms produced by these lesions and present to the clinician with symptoms of acromegaly or Cushing's syndrome.

NONNEOPLASTIC LESIONS. Pituitary cells can also become damaged or necrotic as a result of anoxia, thrombosis, or hemorrhage

When pituitary cell destruction occurs as a result of a hypotensive episode during pregnancy, the disorder is called Sheehan's syndrome. When the disorder is unrelated to pregnancy, it is called Simmond's disease. It is important to diagnose this cause of secondary amenorrhea, because in contrast to the hypothalamic disorders, pituitary damage can be associated with decreased secretion of other pituitary hormones, particularly ACTH and TSH, in addition to LH and FSH. Thus these individuals may have secondary hypothyroidism or adrenal insufficiency that may seriously impair their health, in addition to their decreased estrogen levels.

Ovarian Damage

The ovaries may fail to secrete sufficient estrogen to produce endometrial growth if the follicles are damaged as a result of infection, interference with blood supply, or depletion of follicles caused by bilateral cystectomies. These individuals may become amenorrheic after a variable period of time has elapsed following medical treatment of bilateral tuboovarian abscess, after bilateral cystectomy for benign ovarian neoplasm, or sometimes after a hysterectomy during which the vascular supply to the ovaries is compromised (sometimes called cystic degeneration of the ovaries).

Occasionally the ovaries cease to produce sufficient estrogen to stimulate endometrial growth several years before the age of the physiologic menopause. When this condition occurs before the age of 40, the term *premature ovarian failure* (POF) instead of premature menopause is best used to describe the clinical entity. Histologically, individuals with POF have two types of ovarian pathologic findings. In one there is generalized sclerosis similar to the findings of a normal postmenopausal ovary, while in the other only primordial follicles with no progression past the antrum stage are seen (Fig. 36-14). The latter condition has been called the gonadotrophin-resistant ovary syndrome or ovarian hypofolliculogenesis and is histologically different from the gonadal streak, in which no follicles are seen. Women with this condition may have primary amenorrhea, but usually sufficient estrogen is produced so that they menstruate for several

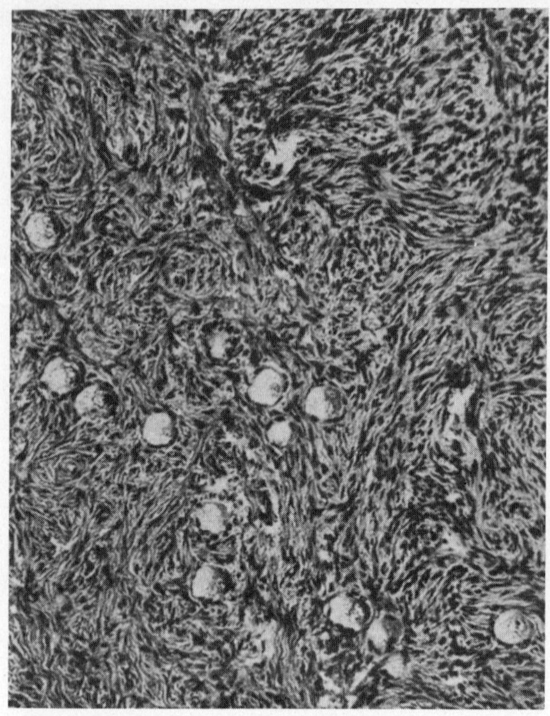

FIGURE 36-14
Microscopic view of ovaries in 21-year-old patient with questionable history of one or two spontaneous periods at age 14 years. Ovarian biopsy showed numerous primordial follicles but none up to antrum stage. (From Jones GS, Moraes-Ruehsen M de: Am J Obstet Gynecol 104:597, 1969.)

months or even years. POF has also been reported in individuals with steroid hormonal enzyme deficiencies who menstruate temporarily and then have secondary amenorrhea. Many individuals with POF, particularly those with primordial follicles that appear normal, also have an autoimmune disease such as hypoparathyroidism, Hashimoto's thyroiditis, or Addison's disease. Many individuals with POF have antibodies to gonadotrophins as well as to several other endocrine organs such as the thyroid and adrenal glands, suggesting an autoimmune etiology. POF can also occur after gonadal irradiation or systemic chemotherapy. In some instances the condition may be transient before permanent ovarian failure; occasionally these individuals may ovulate and conceive.

Diagnostic Evaluation and Management

For any patient consulting a clinician for the symptom of secondary amenorrhea, a diagnostic evaluation should be initiated at that visit, even though 6 months may not have elapsed since the last menstrual period. Amenorrhea is a source of concern to the patient, and it will relieve her concern if attempts are made to find the cause of the symptom. The clinician first should perform a detailed history and physical examination to rule out pregnancy as a cause of the amenorrhea. In addition, he should determine whether there is the possibility of IUA. Any instrumentation of the endometrial cavity, particularly temporally related to pregnancy, should alert the clinician to the possibility that a IUA is present. The next steps in the evaluation include placing a uterine sound into the uterine cavity and obtaining a hysterogram. The diagnosis can also be confirmed by detecting presumptive evidence of ovulation by means of either a biphasic basal temperature or an elevated serum progesterone level. If an IUA is ruled out, the history should disclose whether medications are currently being used or if oral contraceptives have been recently discontinued. In addition, questions regarding diet, weight loss, stress, and strenuous exercise are pertinent. A history of decreasing breast size or vaginal dryness and physical examination of these organs are helpful in estimating the degree of estrogen deficiency. If the history and physical examination fail to reveal the cause of the amenorrhea, measurement of thyroid function should be performed (T_3, T_4, and TSH) to rule out the uncommon asymptomatic thyroid disorders that produce secondary amenorrhea. A complete blood count, urinalysis, and serum chemistries should be measured to rule out systemic disease.

If the initial examination fails to reveal the cause of the amenorrhea, progesterone should be administered to determine if sufficient estrogen is present to produce endometrial growth that will slough after the progesterone levels fall (progesterone challenge test). As mentioned above, withdrawal bleeding after an intramuscular injection of 100 to 200 mg of progesterone in oil (depending on body weight)

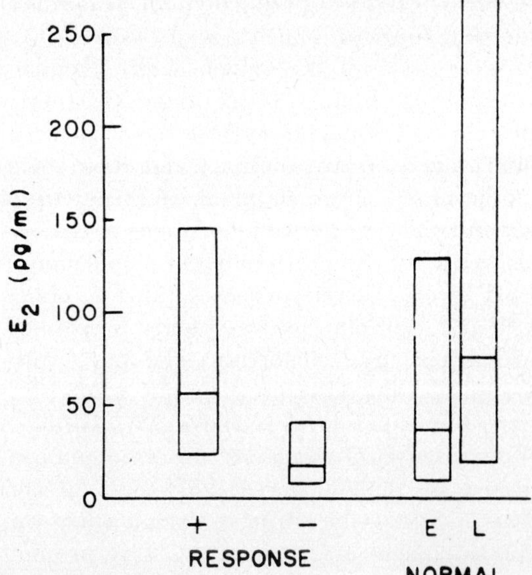

FIGURE 36-15
Estradiol levels in secondary amenorrhea in positive and negative categories. Mean values and 95% confidence limits in both groups are compared with estradiol levels in early and late follicular phase of normal ovulatory cycles. (From Kletzky OA, Davajan V, Nakamura RM, et al: Am J Obstet Gynecol 121:695, 1975.)

usually occurs if the circulating estradiol level is 40 pg/ml or greater (Fig. 36-15). Alternatively, oral progestogen (10 mg of medroxyprogesterone acetate [MPA] daily for 5 days) can be administered, but if oral MPA is prescribed, compliance may be a problem. Any type of clinically observed uterine bleeding, even spotting, occurring within 2 weeks after the injection should be considered a positive response. In addition to reassuring the patient that she can menstruate, the observation of withdrawal bleeding after progesterone indicates that estradiol secretion is not markedly decreased and the cause of the amenorrhea is not as serious as if bleeding had not occurred. Individuals with pituitary tumors, ovarian failure, severe dietary weight loss or anorexia nervosa, severe stress, or the rare hypothalamic lesions will usually not have withdrawal bleeding after progesterone administration. Patients with PCO, moderate stress, exercise weight loss, or hypothalamic-pituitary dysfunction will usually have sufficient estradiol production for withdrawal bleeding to occur.

In a study of 60 women with secondary amenorrhea, Kletzky et al. found that about two thirds had withdrawal bleeding after administration of progesterone, and their estradiol level was above 40 pg/ml. In this group of patients there were two populations of LH levels, high and low, with only one population of FSH levels. Therefore it is of value to obtain LH and prolactin measurements in patients with secondary amenorrhea who have withdrawal bleeding after progesterone administration. If the LH level is above 25 mIU/ml, a diagnosis of PCO should be suspected and confirmed by finding an LH/FSH ratio greater than 3. Even if hirsutism is absent, when this endocrinologic evidence of PCO is present, serum testosterone and DHEA-S should then be measured to determine if either or both are elevated.

If withdrawal bleeding occurs, LH and prolactin levels are in the normal range, and a history of drug ingestion, stress, weight loss, or strenuous exercise is not obtained, the patient should be told that hypothalamic-pituitary dysfunction is present and the exact etiology cannot be determined with current technology, as frequent LH sampling is costly and impractical. Hypothalamic-pituitary dysfunction is usually a self-limiting disorder and not a serious threat to health or a cause of untreatable infertility.

If withdrawal bleeding occurs and the prolactin level is elevated, further evaluation to detect the etiology of the hyperprolactinemia should be performed (Chapter 37).

If the patient with secondary amenorrhea fails to bleed after progesterone administration, Kletzky et al. found that the LH values belonged to a single population but the FSH values identified two populations, low and high. Those with low FSH levels had either a pituitary lesion or hypothalamic-pituitary failure, while those with elevated FSH levels (>30 mIU/ml) had POF.

Thus patients who fail to bleed after progesterone administration should have FSH and estradiol measured. Measurement of the actual estradiol level is useful in determining whether exogenous estrogen replacement is necessary. If the patient fails to bleed after progesterone and FSH is not elevated, prolactin should be measured. If severe weight loss, strenuous exercise, or severe stress is not present, a CT scan of the hypothalamic-pituitary region should be performed to rule out a lesion, even if the prolactin level is normal. If a lesion is seen or if there is a history compatible with possible pituitary destruction (hypotension during pregnancy), a test of ACTH reserve should be performed. An insulin tolerance test in which hypoglycemia is induced should normally cause an increase of 6 µg/100 ml of cortisol within 120 minutes and is a satisfactory test of ACTH function. If no lesion is identified, the term *hypothalamic-pituitary failure* may be used as a nonspecific diagnosis. Not frequently these individuals resume normal ovarian function without treatment.

If POF is diagnosed because of an elevated FSH level and no cause of ovarian destruction is elicited, the possibility of autoimmune disease should be considered if the patient is less than 35 years of age. In these individuals antithyroid antibodies and antinuclear antibodies should be measured and a 24-hour urine-free cortisol level measured to detect possible Addison's disease. To rule out mosaicism, a karyotype should be measured in women with POF who are 25 or younger, but not older. Biopsy of the gonads by laparoscopy or laparotomy is not indicated, because these individuals are usually sterile, although occasionally a follicle may ovulate. This systematic evaluation is shown schematically in the box on p. 989.

The appropriate treatment depends on the diagnosis and on whether conception is desired. Non-prolactin-secreting pituitary tumors should be surgically excised if possible. Individuals with weight loss should be advised to gain weight. If strenuous exercise results in low estrogen levels (<30 pg/ml), the amount of exercise should be reduced or estrogen supplementation advised to prevent possible development of osteoporosis. However, Schlechte et al. recently reported that amenorrheic women with estradiol levels lower than 25 pg/ml did not have decreased bone density of the radius unless their serum prolactin level was also elevated. Thus sufficient calcium intake may be all that is necessary to prevent osteoporosis in these exercising women. If women with PCO or hypothalamic-pituitary dysfunction desire conception, clomiphene citrate administration

DIAGNOSTIC EVALUATION OF SECONDARY AMENORRHEA

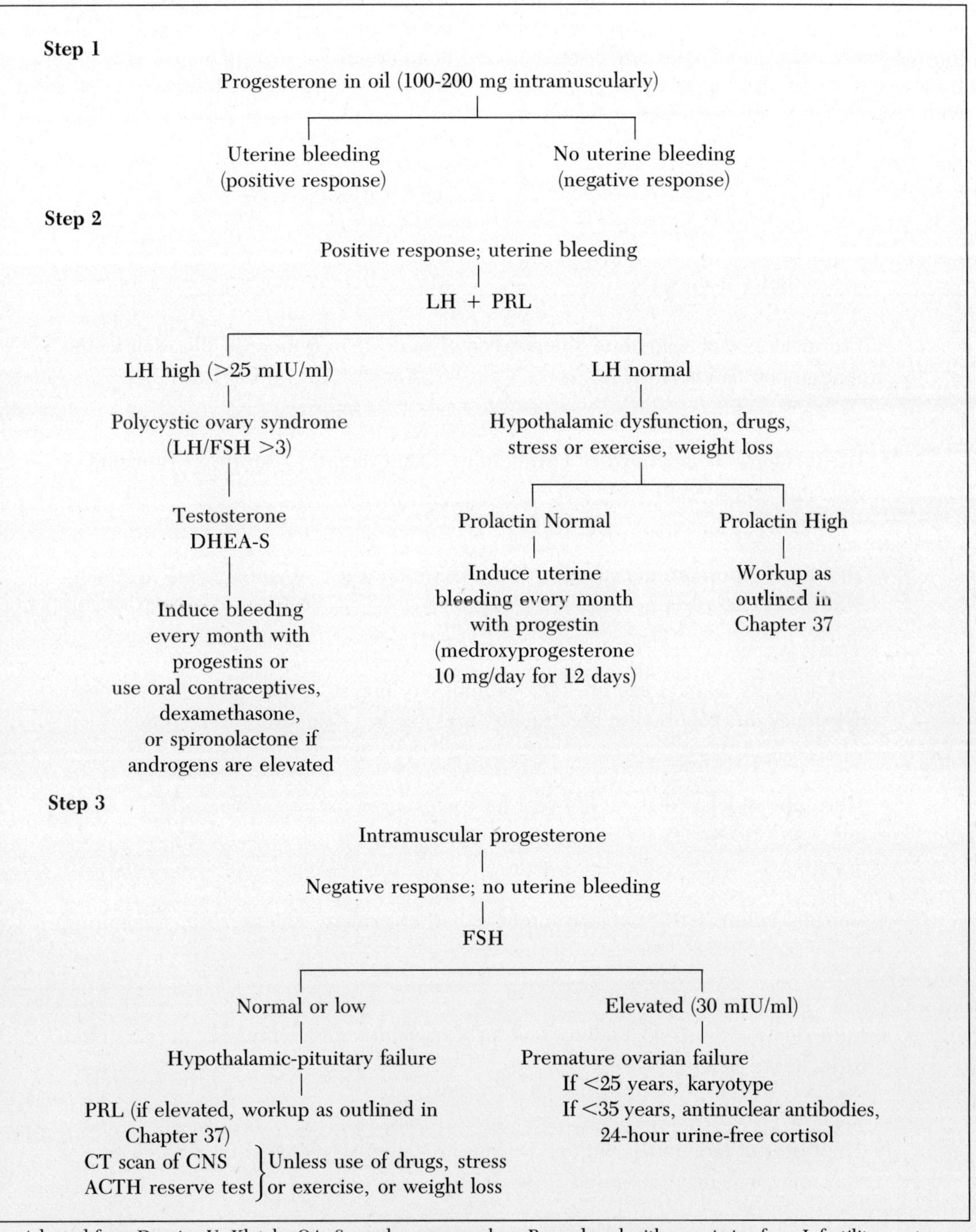

is very successful in inducing ovulation. If pregnancy is not desired, progesterone withdrawal bleeding with medroxyprogesterone acetate (10 mg/day for the first 12 days of each month) will reduce the increased risk of endometrial cancer associated with unopposed estrogen and should be prescribed. If patients with hypothalamic-pituitary failure desire fertility, ovulation can be induced with human menopausal gonadotrophin (HMG) or intermittent GnRH. Clomiphene is not successful if the estrogen levels are low. If pregnancy is not desired, then estrogen-progestogen replacement is indicated for such patients, as well as all individuals with POF, to reduce the risk of osteoporosis and atherosclerosis.

KEY POINTS

- The incidence of secondary amenorrhea of more than 6 months' duration in the general population is 0.7%.

- The incidence of amenorrhea lasting more than 6 months after discontinuation of oral contraceptives in 0.8%.

- The most important and probably most common cause of amenorrhea in adolescent girls is anorexia nervosa.

- A woman 13 years of age or older without any breast development has estrogen deficiency due to a severe abnormality and needs a diagnostic evaluation.

- Menarche is delayed about 0.4 year for each year of premenarcheal athletic training.

- Gonadal failure is the most common cause of primary amenorrhea, accounting for nearly half the patients with this syndrome.

- Individuals with gonadal failure and an X chromosome abnormality are less than 63 inches in height.

- The testes of individuals with androgen insensitivity have about a 20% chance of becoming malignant after age 20 years.

- Uterovaginal agenesis is the second most common cause of primary amenorrhea, with an incidence of about 15% of individuals with this symptom.

- About one third of individuals with gonadal failure have major cardiovascular or renal abnormalities.

- Congenital renal abnormalities occur in about one third of women with uterovaginal agenesis.

- The differential diagnosis between estrogen deficiency caused by gonadal failure and hypogonadotrophin hypogonadism is best made with measurement of serum follicle-stimulating hormone (FSH).

- Individuals with gonadal failure should have a peripheral karyotype performed to determine if a Y chromosome is present. If it is present, the gonads should be excised to prevent development of malignancy, mainly a gonadoblastoma.

- It is unnecessary to perform laparoscopy or laparotomy on an individual with gonadal failure if no Y chromosome is present in the peripheral karyotype unless the individual has hirsutism.

- Individuals with primary amenorrhea and hypogonatrophic hypogonadism do not need karyotyping but need a cranial computerized tomography (CT) scan to rule out a central nervous system (CNS) tumor.

- The most frequent cause of intrauterine adhesion (IUA) is curettage performed during pregnancy or shortly thereafter.

- The amenorrhea associated with strenuous exercise is related to stress, not weight loss, and is most probably caused by an increase in CNS opioids (beta-endorphin) and catechol estrogens, both of which interfere with gonadotrophin-releasing hormone (GnRH) release.

- When women lose weight 15% below ideal body weight, amenorrhea can occur due to CNS-hypothalamic dysfunction. When weight loss drops below 25% of ideal body weight, pituitary gonadotrophin function can also become abnormal.

- Anorexia nervosa occurs in about 1 in 1000 white women. It is uncommon in men and women older than 25 and rare in blacks and Orientals.

- Individuals with anorexia nervosa have impaired peripheral conversion of thyroxine (T_4) to triiodothyronine (T_3), resulting in normal T_4 levels, decreased T_3 levels, and increased reverse T_3 levels.

__________ **KEY POINTS, cont'd** __________

- The normal cyclic pattern of luteinizing hormone (LH) pulsatility is not present in individuals with hypothalamic dysfunction. Either no pulse or pulses of slow frequency, similar to those in the normal luteal phase, are usually observed.

- The GnRH alterations as reflected in LH pulsatility in persons with severe weight loss and anorexia nervosa are similar to those seen in normal prepubertal girls. When such individuals gain weight, GnRH changes similar to those occurring during puberty take place.

- When uterine bleeding fails to occur after progestin is administered, estradiol levels are usually lower than 40 pg/ml.

- In contrast to hypothalamic disorders, pituitary causes of amenorrhea can be associated with ACTH and TSH deficiency.

- Individuals with premature ovarian failure have two different histologic findings: generalized sclerosis or primordial follicles scattered through the stroma.

- Individuals with premature ovarian failure frequently have antibodies to gonadotrophins and other endocrine organs, indicating an autoimmune etiology.

- A karyotype should be obtained in women with premature ovarian failure younger than 25 but not in those who are older.

BIBLIOGRAPHY

Adashi EY, Casper RF, Fishman J, et al: Stimulatory effect of 2-hydroxyestradiol on prolactin release in hypogonadal women. J Clin Endocrinol Metab 51:413, 1980.

Adashi EY, Rakoff J, Divers W, et al: The effect of acutely administered 2-hydroxyestrone on the release of gonadotropins and prolactin before and after estrogen priming in hypogonadal women. Obstet Gynecol Surv 35:363, 1980.

Beumont PJV, George GCW, Pimstone BL, et al: Body weight and the pituitary response to hypothalamic releasing hormones in patients with anorexia nervosa. J Clin Endocrinol Metab 43:487, 1976.

Boyar RM, Katz J, Finkelstein JW, et al: Anorexia nervosa: Immaturity of the 24-hour luteinizing hormone secretory pattern. N Engl J Med 291:861, 1974.

Carr DB, Bullen BA, Skrinar GS, et al: Physical conditioning facilitates the exercise-induced secretion of beta-endorphin and beta-lipotropin in women. N Engl J Med 305:560, 1981.

Crowley WF Jr, Filicori M, Spratt DI, et al: The physiology of gonadotropin-releasing hormone (GnRH) secretion in men and women. Rec Prog Hormone Res 41:473, 1985.

Federman DD, ed: Abnormal sexual development. Philadelphia, W.B. Saunders Co., 1967.

Feicht CB, Johnson TS, Matrin BJ: Secondary amenorrhea in athletes. Lancet 1:1145, 1978.

Fries H, Nillius SJ, Pettersson F: Epidemiology of secondary amenorrhea. Am J Obstet Gynecol 118:473, 1974.

Frisch RE, Gotz-Welbergen AV, McArthur JW, et al: Delayed menarche and amenorrhea of college athletes in relation to onset of training. JAMA 246:1559, 1981.

Frisch RE, Revelle R: Height and weight at menarche and a hypothesis of critical body weights and adolescent events. Science 169:397, 1970.

Frisch RE, Revelle R: Height and weight at menarche and a hypothesis of menarche. Arch Dis Child 46:695, 1971.

Frisch RE, Rose E, Wyshak G, et al: Delayed menarche and amenorrhea in ballet dancers. N Engl J Med 303:17, 1980.

Griffin JE, Edwards C, Madden JD, et al: Congenital absence of the vagina. Ann Intern Med 85:224, 1976.

Kletzky OA, Davajan V, Nakamura RM, et al: Clinical categorization of patients with secondary amenorrhea using progesterone-induced uterine bleeding and measurement of serum gonadotropin levels. Am J Obstet Gynecol 121:695, 1975.

Lieblich JM, Rogol AD, White BJ, et al: Syndrome of anosmia with hypogonadotropic hypogonadism (Kallmann syndrome): Clinical laboratory studies in 23 cases. Am J Med 73:506, 1982.

Marshall WA, Tanner JM: Variations in pattern of pubertal changes in girls. Arch Dis Child 44:291, 1969.

Maschchak CA, Kletzky OA, Davajan V, et al: Clinical and laboratory evaluation of patients with primary amenorrhea. Obstet Gynecol 57:715, 1981.

McArthur JW, Bullen BA, Beitins IZ, et al: Hypothalamic amenorrhea in runners of normal body composition. Endocr Res Commun 7:13, 1980.

Moraes-Ruehsen M de, Blizzard RM, Garcia-Bunuel R, et al: Autoimmunity and ovarian failure. Am J Obstet Gynecol 112:693, 1972.

Penny R, Goldstein IP, Frasier SD: Gonadotropin excretion and body composition. Pediatrics 61:294, 1978.

Pettersson F, Fries H, Nillius SJ: Epidemiology of secondary amenorrhea. Am J Obstet Gynecol 117:80, 1973.

Reame NE, Sauder SE, Case GD, et al: Pulsatile gonadotropin secretion in women with hypothalamic amenorrhea: Evidence that reduced frequency of gonadotropin-releasing hormone secretion is the mechanism of persistent anovulation. J Clin Endocrinol Metab 61:851, 1985.

Reame NE, Sauder SE, Kelch RP, et al: Pulsatile gonadotropin secretion during the human menstrual cycle: Evidence for altered frequency of gonadotropin-releasing hormone secretion. J Clin Endocrinol Metab 59:328, 1984.

Reid RL, Hoff JD, Yen SSC, et al: Effects of exogenous β-endorphin on pituitary hormone secretion and its disappearance rate in normal human subjects. J Clin Endocrinol Metab 52:1179, 1981.

Reindollar RH, Byrd JR, McDonough PG: Delayed sexual development: A study of 252 patients. Am J Obstet Gynecol 140:371, 1981.

Richmond J: Hysterosalpingography. In Mishell DR Jr, Davajan V, eds: Infertility, reproductive endocrinology and contraception, 2nd ed. Oradell, N.J., Medical Economics Books, 1986.

Russell JB, Mitchell D, Musey PI, et al: The relationship of exercise to anovulatory cycles in female athletes: Hormonal and physical characteristics. Obstet Gynecol 63:452, 1984.

Russell JB, Mitchell DE, Musey PI, et al: The role of β-endorphins and catechol estrogens on the hypothalamic-pituitary axis in female athletes. Fertil Steril 42:690, 1984.

Schlechte JA, Sherman B, Martin R: Bone density in amenorrheic women with and without hyperprolactinemia. J Clin Endocrinol Metab 56:1120, 1983.

Sherman BM, Halmi KA, Zamudio R: LH and FSH response to gonadotropin-releasing hormone in anorexia nervosa: Effect of nutritional rehabilitation. J Clin Endocrinol Metab 41:135, 1975.

Vigersky RA, Andersen AE, Thompson RG, et al: Hypothalamic dysfunction in secondary amenorrhea associated with simple weight loss. N Engl J Med 297:1141, 1977.

Vigersky RA, Loriaux DL, Andersen AE, et al: Delayed pituitary hormone response to LRF and TRF in patients with secondary amenorrhea associated with simple weight loss. J Clin Endocrinol Metab 43:893, 1976.

Warren MP: The effects of exercise on pubertal progression and reproductive function in girls. J Clin Endocrinol Metab 51:1150, 1980.

Warren MP, Jewelwicz R, Dyrenfurth I, et al: The significance of weight loss in the evaluation of pituitary response to LH-RH in women with secondary amenorrhea. J Clin Endocrinol Metab 40:601, 1975.

Hyperprolactinemia, Galactorrhea, and Pituitary Adenomas

KEY TERMS

Bromoergocryptine (2-Br-Alpha-Ergocryptine Mesylate). Semisynthetic ergot alkaloid that is a dopamine receptor agonist and is used to treat hyperprolactinemia.

Computerized Tomography. An imaging technique to detect soft tissue abnormalities that uses a computer to integrate differences in x-ray beam attenuation resulting from varying densities in adjacent tissue.

Craniopharyngioma. A rare hypothalamic tumor that can produce hyperprolactinemia.

Empty Sella Syndrome. An intrasellar extension of the subarachnoid space resulting in compression of the pituitary gland and an enlarged sella turcica that may be associated with galactorrhea and hyperprolactinemia.

Galactorrhea. Nonpuerperal secretion from the breast of watery or milky fluid that contains neither pus nor blood.

Hyperprolactinemia. Levels of circulating prolactin above normal (greater than 20 to 25 ng/ml) that can cause galactorrhea or amenorrhea or both.

Hypocycloidal Tomography. Multiple radiographs of the sella turcica at intervals of 2 to 3 mm with a hypocycloidal movement.

Macroadenoma. An uncommon type of prolactin-secreting pituitary adenoma (prolactinoma) greater than 1 cm in diameter, usually with extrasellar extension.

Magnetic Resonance Imaging (MRI) (previously Nuclear Magnetic Resonance [NMR]). Technique of soft tissue imagery using resonance of hydrogen nuclei in static magnetic field exposed to low-frequency radiowaves.

Microadenoma. The more common type of prolactinoma less than 1 cm in diameter.

Prolactin. Polypeptide hormone secreted by anterior pituitary lactotrophs that has mammotrophic and lactogenic functions.

Prolactin-Inhibiting Factor. The neurotransmitter (believed to be dopamine) that inhibits prolactin synthesis and release.

Prolactinoma. The most common pituitary tumor arising from chromophobic cells that secrete prolactin.

Thyrotropin-Releasing Hormone (TRH) Stimulation Test. Provocative response of prolactin following TRH infusion. The normal response is greater than three times the baseline of prolactin after infusion of 500 μg of TRH.

Prolactin is a polypeptide hormone containing 198 amino acids and having a molecular weight of 22,000 daltons. It circulates in different molecular sizes—a monomeric (small) form (mol wt 22,000), a polymeric (big) form (mol wt 50,000), and an even larger polymeric (big-big) form (mol wt >100,000). Big prolactin is presumed to be a dimer, and big-big prolactin may represent an aggregation of monomeric molecules. The small form is biologically active, and about 80% of the hormone secreted is in this form. Most immunoassayable prolactin is also in this form; however, the larger forms are also immunoreactive and thus are measurable in prolactin radioimmunoassays. The biologic effects of the polymeric forms are unclear, but in some bioassays the forms are inactive, as they have reduced binding to mammary tissue membranes. Prolactin is synthesized and stored in the pituitary gland in chromophobe cells called lactotrophs, which are located mainly in the lateral areas of the gland. In addition, prolactin is synthesized in decidual and endometrial tissue. From these tissues prolactin is secreted into the circulation and, in the event of pregnancy, into the amniotic fluid. Prolactin is normally present in measurable amounts in serum, with mean levels of about 8 ng/ml in adult women. It circulates in an unbound form, has a 20-minute half-life, and is cleared by the liver and kidney. The main function of prolactin is to stimulate the growth of mammary tissue as well as to produce and secrete milk into the alveoli. Thus it has both mammogenic and lactogenic functions. Specific receptors for prolactin are present in the plasma membrane of mammary cells as well as many other tissues.

PHYSIOLOGY

Prolactin synthesis and release from the lactotrophs are controlled by central nervous system neurotransmitters, which act on the pituitary via the hypothalamus. The major control mechanism is inhibition, as pituitary stalk section results in increased prolactin secretion. It appears that the major physiologic inhibitor of prolactin release is the neurotransmitter dopamine, which acts directly on the pituitary gland. There are specific dopamine receptors on the lactotrophs, and dopamine inhibits prolactin synthesis and release in pituitary cell cultures. Thus dopamine appears to be the prolactin-inhibiting factor (PIF), also called prolactin release–inhibiting factor. Although a hypothalamic prolactin release factor (PRF) has not been isolated, it is known that both the neurotransmitter serotonin and thyrotropin-releasing factor stimulate prolactin release. Since the latter stimulates prolactin release only minimally unless infused, it appears that serotonin is PRF or is responsible for its secretion. The rise in prolactin levels during sleep appears to be controlled by serotonin.

Prolactin is secreted episodically, and serum levels fluctuate throughout the day and throughout the menstrual cycle, with peak levels occurring at midcycle. Although changes in prolactin levels are not as marked as the pulsatile episodes of luteinizing hormone (LH), Backstrom et al. reported a decline in both basal concentration and pulse frequency of prolactin in the luteal phase of the cycle. Estrogen stimulates prolactin production and release. Under the influence of estrogen, prolactin levels increase in females at the time of puberty.

During pregnancy, as estrogen levels increase, there is a concomitant hypertrophy and hyperplasia of the lactotrophs. The maternal increase in prolactin occurs soon after implantation, concomitant with the increase in circulating estrogen. Circulating levels of prolactin steadily increase throughout pregnancy, reaching about 200 ng/ml in the third trimester, and the rise is directly related to the increase in circulating levels of estrogen. Despite the elevated prolactin levels during pregnancy, lactation does not occur because estrogen inhibits the action of prolactin on the breast, most likely blocking prolactin's interaction with its receptor. A day or two following delivery of the placenta, both estrogen levels and prolactin levels decline rapidly and lactation is initiated. Prolactin levels reach basal levels in nonnursing women in 2 to 3 weeks. Although basal levels of circulating prolactin decline to the nonpregnant range about 6 months after parturition in nursing women, following each act of suckling, prolactin levels increase markedly and stimulate milk production for the next feeding.

Nipple and breast stimulation also increase prolactin levels in the nonpregnant female. Other physiologic stimuli that increase prolactin release are exercise, sleep, and stress. In addition, prolactin levels normally rise following ingestion of the noonday meal. For these reasons prolactin levels normally fluctuate throughout the day, with maximum levels observed during nighttime while asleep and a smaller increase occurring in the early afternoon (Fig. 37-1). When the amount measured in the circulation in the nonpregnant woman exceeds a certain level, usually 20 to 25 ng/ml, the condition is called hyperprolactinemia. The optimum time to obtain a blood sample for as-

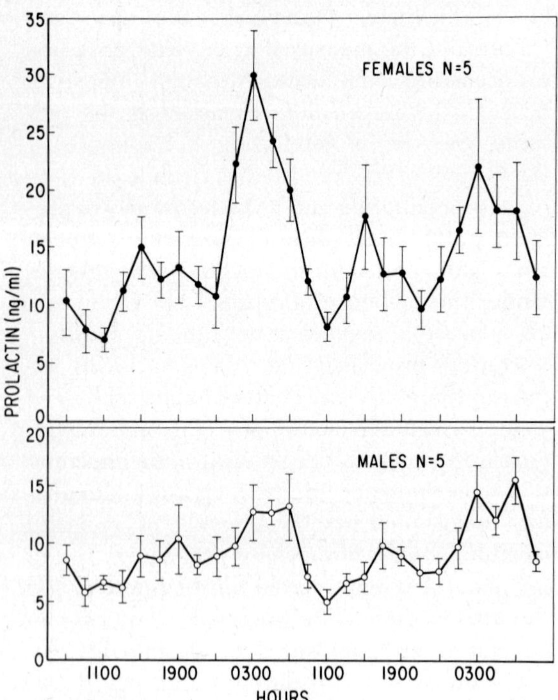

FIGURE 37-1

Hour-to-hour variation of serum prolactin concentration in normal women and men studied throughout 48 consecutive hours. (From Kletzky OA, Davajan V: Hyperprolactinemia: Diagnosis and treatment. Reproduced with permission from Infertility, contraception and reproductive endocrinology, 2nd ed, by Daniel R. Mishell, Jr., M.D., and Val Davajan, M.D. Copyright © 1986 Medical Economics Books, Oradell, N.J. 07649. All rights reserved.)

say to diagnose hyperprolactinemia is during the morning hours. Increases in prolactin levels above the normal range can occur without a pathologic condition if the serum sample is drawn from a patient who has recently awakened, has exercised, or has had recent breast stimulation such as breast palpation during a physical examination.

Hyperprolactinemia can produce disorders of gonadotrophin–sex steroid function, resulting in menstrual cycle derangement (oligomenorrhea and amenorrhea) and anovulation as well as inappropriate lactation or galactorrhea. The mechanism whereby elevated prolactin levels interfere with gonadotrophin release has not

been completely elucidated, but the major factor appears to be alterations in normal gonadotrophin-releasing hormone (GnRH) release. Women with hyperprolactinemia have abnormalities in the frequency and amplitude of LH pulsations, with a normal or increased gonadotrophin response following GnRH infusion.

This abnormality of normal GnRH cyclicity thus inhibits gonadotrophin release but not synthesis. The reason for the abnormal secretion of GnRH has not been completely elucidated, but it is hypothesized that the elevated prolactin levels produce a rise in hypothalamic dopamine levels by a short-loop feedback that fails to suppress prolactin but interferes with normal GnRH release, perhaps by altering norepinephrine secretion. In addition, elevated prolactin levels have been shown to interfere with the positive estrogen effect on midcycle LH release. It has also been shown that elevated levels of prolactin directly inhibit basal as well as gonadotrophin-stimulated ovarian secretion of both estradiol and progesterone. However, this mechanism is probably not the primary cause of anovulation, because women with hyperprolactinemia can have ovulation induced with various agents, including pulsatile GnRH. Some patients with moderate hyperprolactinemia as determined by radioimmunoassay have a greater than normal proportion of the big-big forms. Because of this form of prolactin's reduced bioactivity, these individuals can have normal pituitary and ovarian function.

The clinician should measure serum prolactin levels in all patients with galactorrhea, as well as those with oligomenorrhea and amenorrhea without the presence of an elevated level of follicle-stimulating hormone (FSH). Hyperprolactinemia has been reported to be present in 15% of all anovulatory women and 20% of women with amenorrhea of undetermined cause. Galactorrhea is defined as the nonpuerperal secretion from the breast of watery or milky fluid that contains neither pus nor blood. The fluid may appear spontaneously or after palpation. To determine if galactorrhea is present the clinician should palpate the breast, moving from the periphery toward the nipple in an attempt to express any secretion. The diagnosis of galactorrhea can be confirmed by observing multiple fat droplets in the fluid when

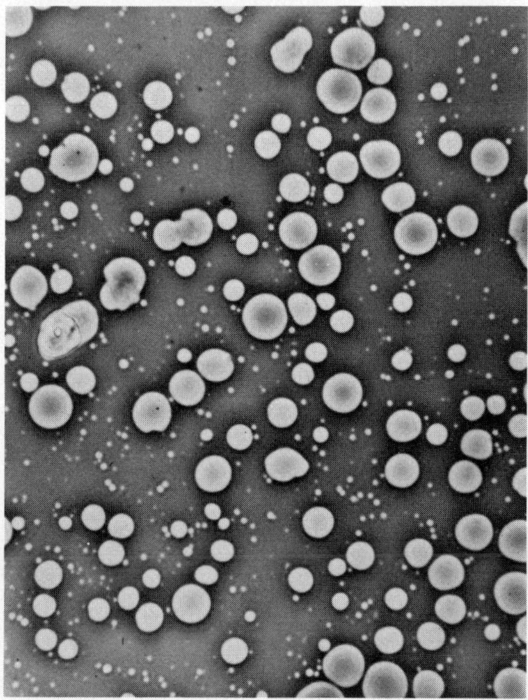

FIGURE 37-2
Fat droplets seen under the microscope from a patient with galactorrhea. (From Kletzky OA, Davajan V: Hyperprolactinemia: Diagnosis and treatment. Reproduced with permission from Infertility, contraception and reproductive endocrinology, 2nd ed, by Daniel R. Mishell, Jr., M.D., and Val Davajan, M.D. Copyright © 1986 Medical Economics Books, Oradell, N.J. 07649. All rights reserved.)

it is examined under low-power magnification (Fig. 37-2). The incidence of galactorrhea in women with hyperprolactinemia has been reported to range from 30% to 80%, and these differences probably reflect variations in the techniques used to detect mammary excretion. Unless there has been continued breast stimulation after a pregnancy, the presence of galactorrhea serves as a biologic indicator that the prolactin level is abnormally elevated. Davajan et al. reported that 62% of women with galactorrhea have hyperprolactinemia, and some individuals with galactorrhea have normal immunoassayable prolactin levels, indicating they may have elevated levels of biologically active prolactin. The incidence of hyperprolactinemia is higher (88%) in those women with galactor-

rhea who have amenorrhea and low estrogen levels than in those women with galactorrhea and normal menses, oligomenorrhea, or amenorrhea with normal estrogen levels (49%).

ETIOLOGY

Pathologic causes of hyperprolactinemia, in addition to a prolactin-secreting pituitary adenoma (prolactinoma) and other pituitary tumors that produce acromegaly and Cushing's disease, include hypothalamic disease, various pharmacologic agents, hypothyroidism, chronic renal disease, or any chronic type of breast nerve stimulation, such as may occur with thoracic operation, herpes zoster, or chest trauma.

One of the most frequent causes of galactorrhea and hyperprolactinemia is the ingestion of pharmacologic agents, particularly tranquilizers, narcotics, and antihypertensive agents. Of the tranquilizers, the phenothiazines and diazepam can produce hyperprolactinemia either by depleting the hypothalamic circulation of dopamine or by blocking its binding sites and thus decreasing dopamine action (Fig. 37-3). The tricyclic antidepressants block dopamine uptake, and propranolol, haloperidol, phentolamine, and cyproheptadine block hypothalamic dopamine receptors. The antihypertensive agent reserpine depletes catecholamines, and methyldopa blocks the conversion of tyrosine to dihydroxyphenylalanine (dopa). Ingestion of oral contraceptive steroids can also increase prolactin levels, with a greater incidence of hyperprolactinemia occurring with higher estrogen formulations. Nevertheless, galactorrhea does not usually occur during oral contraceptive ingestion because the exogenous estrogen blocks the binding of prolactin to its receptors.

Patients developing galactorrhea while ingesting oral contraceptives or any of the other drugs just listed should ideally discontinue the medication, and prolactin should be measured 1 month thereafter to determine if the level has returned to normal. If the medication cannot be discontinued, then the prolactin level should be measured, and if it is elevated above 100 ng/ml, visualization of the sella turcica should be performed by one of the techniques described below.

Primary hypothyroidism can also produce hyperprolactinemia and galactorrhea because of

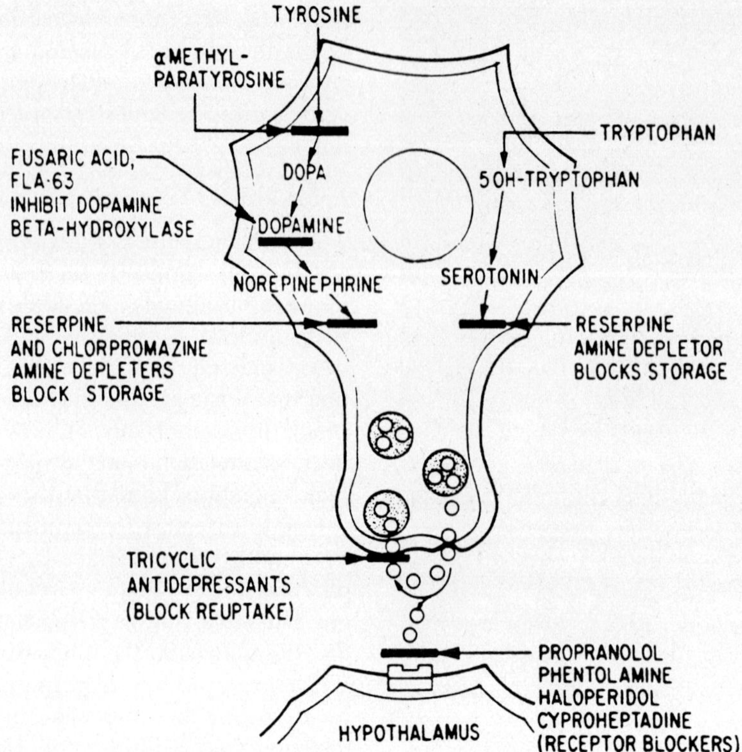

FIGURE 37-3
Schematic representation of inhibitory effects of drugs on synthesis and release of neurotransmitters. (From Kletzky OA, Davajan V: Hyperprolactinemia: Diagnosis and treatment. Reproduced with permission from Infertility, contraception and reproductive endocrinology, 2nd ed, by Daniel R. Mishell, Jr., M.D., and Val Davajan, M.D. Copyright © 1986 Medical Economics Books, Oradell, N.J. 07649. All rights reserved.)

decreased negative feedback of thyroxine (T_4) on the hypothalamic-pituitary axis. The resulting increase in thyrotropin-releasing hormone (TRH) stimulates prolactin secretion as well as thyroid-stimulating hormone (TSH) secretion from the pituitary. About 3% to 5% of individuals with hyperprolactinemia have hypothyroidism, and thus a TSH assay, the most sensitive indicator of hypothyroidism, should be obtained for all individuals with hyperprolactinemia. If the TSH level is elevated, triiodothyronine (T_3) and T_4 should be measured to confirm the diagnosis of primary hypothyroidism, as occasionally a TSH-secreting pituitary adenoma will be present. Treatment with appropriate thyroid replacement usually returns the TSH and prolactin levels to normal within a short time.

Hyperprolactinemia can occur in patients with abnormal renal disease resulting from decreased metabolic clearance as well as increased production rate. The cause of the latter is not known.

Central Nervous System Disorders

Hypothalamic Causes

Diseases of the hypothalamus that produce alterations in the normal portal circulation of dopamine can result in hyperprolactinemia. Such diseases include craniopharyngioma and infiltration of the hypothalamus by sarcoidosis, histiocytosis, leukemia, or carcinoma. All these conditions are rare, with craniopharyngioma being the most common. These tumors arise from remnants of Rathke's pouch along the pituitary stalk. Grossly they can be cystic, solid, or mixed, and calcification is usually visible on x-ray examination. They are most frequently diagnosed during the second and third decades of life and usually result in impairment of secretion of several pituitary hormones.

Pituitary Causes

Various types of pituitary tumors, lactotroph hyperplasia, and the empty sella syndrome can be associated with hyperprolactinemia. It has been estimated that as many as 80% of all pituitary adenomas secrete prolactin. The most common pituitary tumor associated with hyperprolactinemia is the prolactinoma, arbitrarily defined as a microadenoma if its diameter is less than 1 cm and as a macroadenoma if it is larger. Hyperprolactinemia has been reported to occur in about 25% of patients with acromegaly and 10% of those with Cushing's disease, indicating that the pituitary adenomas, which mainly secrete growth hormones and adrenocorticotropic hormone (ACTH), frequently also secrete prolactin. Hyperplasia of lactotrophs has been reported to occur in about 8% of pituitary glands examined at autopsy.

Another cause of hyperprolactinemia is the primary empty sella syndrome. The term *primary empty sella syndrome* describes a clinical situation in which an intrasellar extension of the subarachnoid space results in compression of the pituitary gland and an enlarged sella turcica. It is usually associated with normal pituitary function except for hyperprolactinemia. Although some patients with primary empty sella syndrome have a coexistent prolactinoma, Gharib et al. reported a series of 11 patients with an empty sella and hyperprolactinemia who had no histologic evidence of a prolactinoma or hyperplasia of the lactotrophs. They stated that about 5% of individuals with the empty sella have hyperprolactinemia or amenorrhea-galactorrhea or both. It is theorized that in these patients distortion of the infundibular stalk results in decreased levels of dopamine reaching the pituitary to inhibit prolactin. Serum prolactin levels are usually less than 100 ng/ml in patients with this syndrome, and some patients with this syndrome have galactorrhea with normal prolactin levels. Kleinberg et al. reported that about 10% of all patients with an enlarged sella turcica have the empty sella syndrome. Therefore, in patients with radiologic evidence of an enlarged sella a computerized tomography (CT) scan or pneumoencephalogram should be obtained to establish or rule out the presence of this entity.

Prolactinomas

In an unselected series of 120 autopsies of persons who had had no clinical evidence of pituitary disease, Burrow et al. found pituitary microadenomas to be present in 32 (27%). Of these, 41% stained for prolactin, indicating that more than 1 in 10 persons in the general population has a prolactinoma.

Overall about 50% of women with hyperprolactinemia have a prolactinoma. The incidence is higher when the prolactin levels exceed 100 ng/ml, and nearly all individuals with prolactin levels greater than 200 ng/ml harbor a prolactinoma. The vast majority of prolactinomas in women are microadenomas. Kleinberg et al. reported that overall 20% of individuals with galactorrhea and 35% of women with amenorrhea-galactorrhea had radiologic evidence of pituitary tumors. Tumors are also present in about 20% of women with hyperprolactinemia and menstrual irregularities without galactorrhea. The incidence of prolactinoma is greater in those individuals with a more profound disturbance of normal hypothalamic-pituitary-ovarian function. Davajan et al. reported that 70% of women with hyperprolactinemia, galactorrhea, and secondary amenorrhea with low estrogen levels had radiologic evidence of a pituitary adenoma. Evidence of a tumor occurred in only 20% to 30% of those with hyperprolactinemia and normal menses, oligomenorrhea, or secondary amenorrhea who had sufficient estrogen to undergo withdrawal bleeding after progesterone administration. In both these studies no evidence of tumor was found in individuals with normal menses, galactorrhea, and normal prolactin levels. Therefore radiologic studies do not need to be performed in such women.

Because prolactinomas develop in the lateral areas of the pituitary gland, it was originally hypothesized that decreased blood supply to these regions resulted in less dopamine being delivered and resultant increased size and number of lactotrophs. Recently studies of dopamine response by a variety of tests indicate that in patients with prolactinomas there is a defect in dopamine regulation of prolactin secretion that persists even after surgical removal of the adenoma. This loss of dopaminergenic inhibition of prolactin that persists for years after tumor removal is thought to explain the high rate of recurrence of tumors in the long-term follow-up of patients.

DIAGNOSIS

Because most prolactinomas are microadenomas that do not cause enlargement of the sella turcica, the diagnosis usually cannot be made by ordinary anteroposterior and lateral coned x-ray examination of the sella turcica. With the development of more precise radiologic methods of detecting soft tissue pituitary abnormalities, it is now possible to detect even small adenomas.

Initially detection of microadenomas was accomplished by obtaining tomographic radiographic examination of the sella turcica at intervals of 2 to 3 mm in the anteroposterior and lateral projections with a hypocycloidal movement. These are called hypocycloidal tomograms. Sometimes additional tomograms in the basal projection are obtained to more accurately assess the anterior sellar wall. With this technique, even though sellar enlargement is not evident, when a microadenoma is at least 4 mm in diameter, it may be diagnosed by observing localized bulging of the interolateral wall on only one side of the sella. If this asymmetry exceeds 2 mm with associated erosion of the lamina dura, the tomogram is considered abnormal; if it is less than 2 mm without laminar erosion, it is considered equivocal. Comparing the results of tomograms with the findings of microadenoma at autopsy, Burrow et al. found that the incidence of both false positive and false negative tomographic findings was about 20% each, with an overall accuracy rate of 61%. Furthermore, radiation exposure with polytomography may be in excess of 20 rads.

Since about 1980 a more accurate diagnostic technique, computerized tomography (CT) imagery, has been available. After infusion of at least 200 ml of 30% iodinated contrast medium, CT imagery is performed in coronal sec-

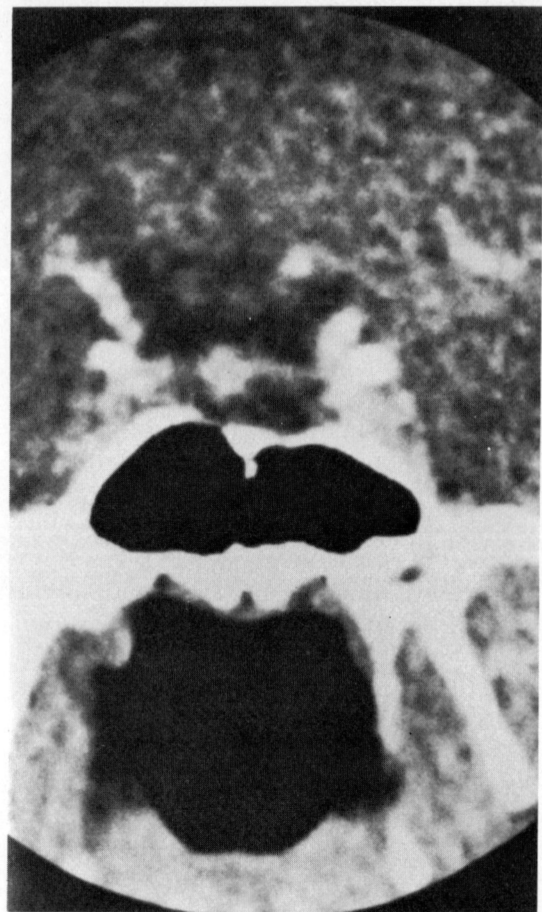

FIGURE 37-4
Coronal CT section of 24-year-old woman with amenorrhea, galactorrhea, and hyperprolactinemia, showing left hypodensity of pituitary gland and erosive changes of sellar floor. (From Bonneville J-F, Poulignot D, Cattin F, et al: Computed tomographic demonstration of the effects of bromocriptine on pituitary microadenoma size. Radiology 143:451-455, 1982.)

tions of 1.5 mm. The typical appearance of an adenoma is a region of diminished enhancement in the pituitary gland with a convex upper surface and an abnormal height of 8 mm or greater (Fig. 37-4). With this technique it is possible to accurately assess the presence of a microadenoma 2 mm in diameter or larger as well as the suprasellar and other extrasellar extensions. This technique also will indicate the presence of an empty sella. Radiation exposure in a CT scan is about 3 rads, significantly less than with polytomography.

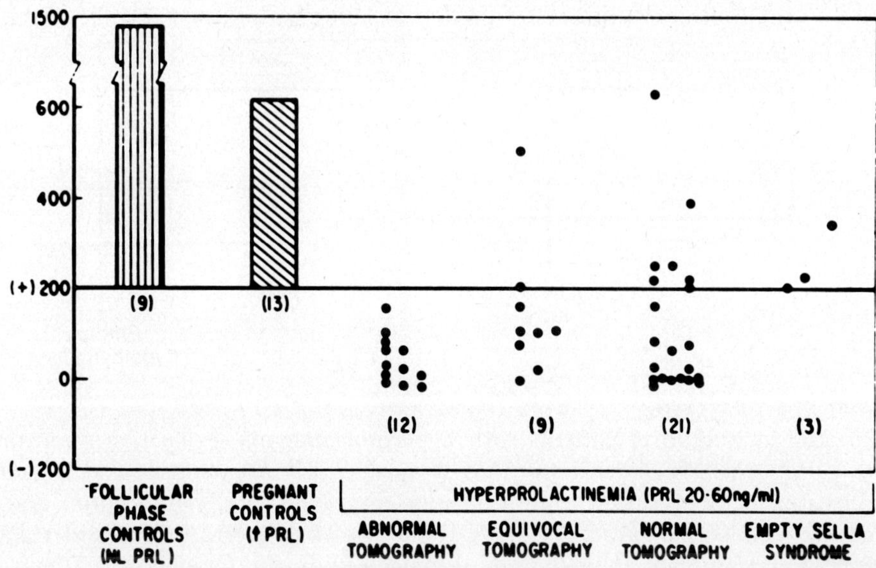

FIGURE 37-5
Individual prolactin responses to TRH stimulation in nonpregnant women with mild hyperprolactinemia in relation to tomographic findings. Bars represent 95% confidence limits for follicular phase and pregnancy controls. (From Shangold GA, Kletzky OA, Marrs RP, et al: Obstet Gynecol 63:771, 1984. Reprinted with permission from The American College of Obstetricians and Gynecologists.)

Recently the technique of nuclear magnetic resonance (NMR), which is now called magnetic resonance imagery (MRI), has been developed. With this technique accurate soft tissue imagery is obtained without radiation. Instead, hydrogen nuclei in static magnetic fields exposed to radiowaves of specific frequency resonate and depict tissue hydrogen density. This technique provides 1 mm resolution and thus should be able to detect all significant microadenomas. However, the number of centers with access to MRI is limited, so at present CT scan is the most commonly used method of diagnosis. If available, MRI may be used as an alternative.

Since provocative stimuli of dopamine release such as insulin-induced hypoglycogenemia and infusion of either chlorpromazine or TRH are abnormal in most individuals with prolactinomas, studies of the use of such stimuli as diagnostic tests to determine whether a tumor is present have been undertaken. Of these tests it appears that administration of TRH in individuals with mild hyperprolactinemia (less than 60 ng/ml) may be beneficial. Shangold et al. found that if prolactin is measured before and 20 minutes after administration of an intravenous bolus of 500 µg of TRH, normal individuals have at least a 200% increase (three times baseline) of prolactin.

All patients with hyperprolactinemia greater than 60 ng/ml as well as those with prolactin levels of 20 to 60 µg/ml and CT evidence of tumor had less than a three-fold increase in prolactin (Fig. 37-5). Thus if a normal response to TRH is found in individuals with mild hyperprolactinemia, there is no need to perform a CT scan.

Visual field determination and tests of adrenocorticotropic hormone (ACTH) and thyroid function are not necessary in patients with microadenomas, as these small tumors do not interfere with overall pituitary function and do not extend beyond the sella. However, these evaluations should be performed in individuals with macroadenomas because suprasellar extension of the tumor may exert pressure on the optic chiasm, resulting in bitemporal visual field defects and interference with vision. The size of these tumors may also affect other aspects of pituitary function. Thus a test of ACTH reserve such as insulin-induced hypo-

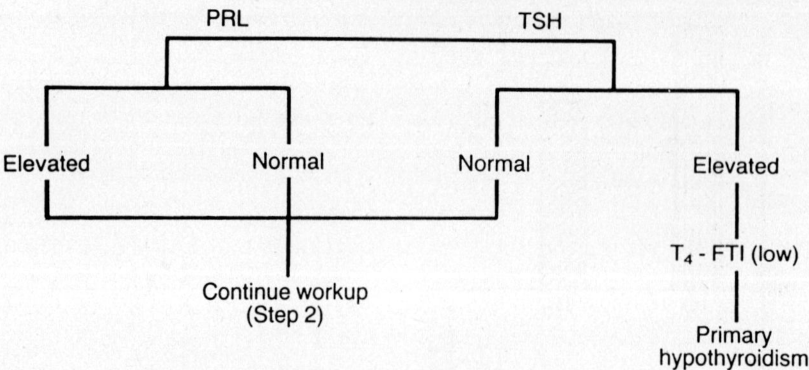

FIGURE 37-6

First step in workup of patients with hyperprolactinemia, evaluation of all those with galactorrhea. (From Kletzky OA, Davajan V: Hyperprolactinemia: Diagnosis and treatment. Reproduced with permission from Infertility, contraception and reproductive endocrinology, 2nd ed, by Daniel R. Mishell, Jr., M.D., and Val Davajan, M.D. Copyright © 1986 Medical Economics Books, Oradell, N.J. 07649. All rights reserved.)

glycemia (insulin tolerance test), as well as tests of thyroid function, should be performed on all individuals with a macroadenoma.

Recommended Diagnostic Evaluation

It is currently recommended that prolactin levels be measured in all patients with galactorrhea, oligomenorrhea, or amenorrhea who do not have an elevated FSH level. If prolactin is elevated, a TSH assay should be performed to rule out the presence of primary hypothyroidism. If TSH is elevated, T₃ and T₄ should be measured to rule out the rare possibility of a TSH-secreting pituitary adenoma (Fig. 37-6). If TSH is elevated, appropriate thyroid replacement should begin, and the prolactin level will usually return to normal. If TSH is normal and the patient has a normal prolactin level with galactorrhea, no further tests are necessary if she has regular menses (Fig. 37-7). Because some patients with galactorrhea, abnormal menstrual function, and normal prolactin levels have been found to have the empty sella syndrome, anteroposterior and lateral coned-down views of the sella should be obtained in such cases (Fig. 37-8). If these findings are abnormal, a CT scan should be obtained to establish the diagnosis.

In patients with a normal TSH level, a CT scan should be obtained if prolactin is elevated

above 60 ng/ml (Fig. 37-6). If the prolactin level is between 20 and 60 ng/ml, TRH should be administered as a bolus intravenously. Prolactin should be measured immediately before and 20 minutes after TRH administration. If a normal (three-fold) response of prolactin to TRH is obtained, a repeat test should be performed annually; CT scans are not necessary. However, anteroposterior and lateral coned-down views of the sella should be obtained to rule out the possibility of an empty sella. If the TRH test results are abnormal, a CT scan should be performed; not all individuals with an abnormal TRH response have radiologic evidence of a microadenoma.

Natural History of Prolactinomas

In a series of 84 women with surgically treated prolactinomas, Randall et al. reported that all had some form of menstrual abnormality. Eighty-four percent had secondary amenorrhea, 6% had primary amenorrhea, and 10% had oligomenorrhea. Of the total group, 87% had galactorrhea; therefore about 13% of patients with a prolactinoma may not have galactorrhea as a presenting symptom. Galactorrhea may occur before, after, or simultaneously with the onset of amenorrhea. Davajan et al. reported that in a large series of unselected patients with radiologic evidence of prolactinomas

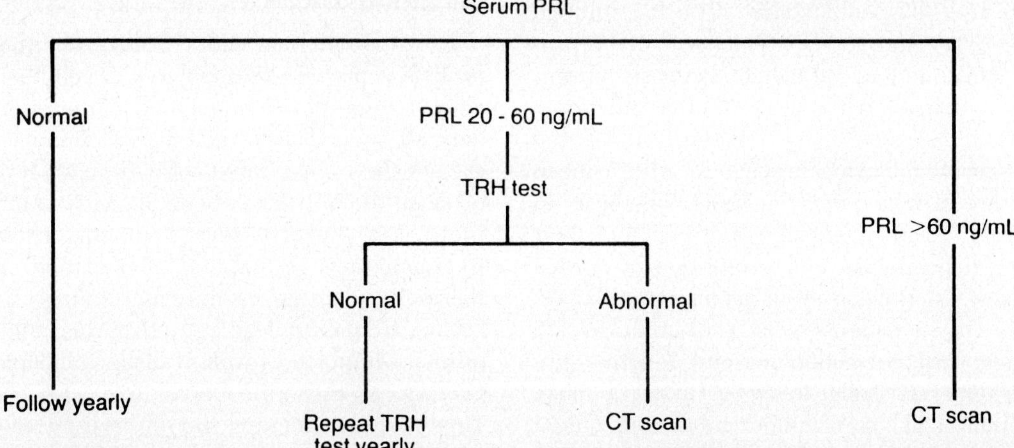

FIGURE 37-7

Second step in workup of patients with hyperprolactinemia. (From Kletzky OA, Davajan V: Hyperprolactinemia: Diagnosis and treatment. Reproduced with permission from Infertility, contraception and reproductive endocrinology, 2nd ed, by Daniel R. Mishell, Jr., M.D., and Val Davajan, M.D. Copyright © 1986 Medical Economics Books, Oradell, N.J. 07649. All rights reserved.)

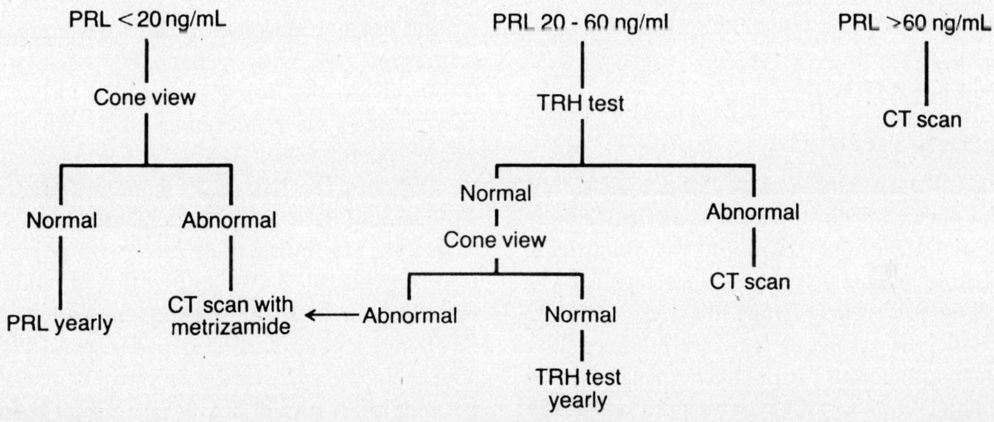

FIGURE 37-8

Third step in evaluation of women with oligomenorrhea and galactorrhea. (From Kletzky OA: Semin Reprod Endocrinol 2:23, 1984.)

the most common clinical findings were galactorrhea and secondary amenorrhea with low estrogen status. Therefore, the clinician should suspect that a prolactinoma is present in patients with galactorrhea and amenorrhea who fail to experience withdrawal bleeding after progesterone administration. The diagnosis becomes more likely if the prolactin levels exceed 100 ng/ml. Macroadenomas can enlarge and cause visual field distortion or disturbance of pituitary function. Thus even if these findings are not present when the diagnosis of macroadenoma is made, treatment should be initiated to prevent further enlargement of the macroadenoma.

Long-term studies of patients with microadenomas demonstrate that enlargement is uncommon and that some of these tumors can actually regress spontaneously. In a longitudinal study of 43 untreated patients with hyperprolactinemia and a radiologic diagnosis of microadenoma, March et al. found that only 2 patients had evidence of enlargement of the adenoma (1 following pregnancy) with a mean duration of follow-up of 5 years. Of these 43 patients, 3 had spontaneous regression of their hyperprolactinemia and resumption of normal menses. Koppelman et al. reported similar results. Of 25 patients with prolactinomas (18 women with microadenoma and 7 with minimally enlarged sella) followed up for a mean duration of 11 years without treatment, only 1 patient had slight progression of a sella abnormality. No patient had visual field or other pituitary function changes, 7 resumed normal menses spontaneously, and galactorrhea spontaneously resolved in 6. These studies demonstrate the benign course of untreated microadenomas. Therefore, treatment may not be necessary if the patient is not bothered by the amenorrhea or galactorrhea unless she appears to be at risk for developing osteoporosis.

MANAGEMENT

Expectant Treatment

Patients with radiologic evidence of a microadenoma who do not wish to conceive may be followed without treatment by measuring prolactin levels once yearly and performing CT scans every 2 years. Many of these patients have deficient estrogen, and low estrogen levels in combination with hyperprolactinemia have been shown to be associated with the early onset of osteoporosis. If the individual has low estrogen levels, treatment involves replacement estrogen-progestin therapy (as is used for postmenopausal women) or bromocriptine. Individuals with hyperprolactinemia with or without microadenomas who have adequate estrogen levels as evidenced by the presence of oligomenorrhea or amenorrhea with progesterone-induced withdrawal bleeding and who do not wish to conceive should be treated with periodic progestin withdrawal (medroxyprogesterone acetate 10 mg per day for 10 days each month) to prevent endometrial hyperplasia. Barrier types of contraception are advised.

Radiation Therapy

External radiation with cobalt, proton beam, or heavy particle therapy and brachytherapy with yttrium-90 rods implanted in the pituitary have all been used to treat macroadenomas but are not the primary mode of treatment. Results of such therapy have been inconsistent, and there is a delay of several months between treatment and resumption of ovulation. Furthermore, damage to normal pituitary tissue occurs, frequently leading to abnormal anterior pituitary function as well as diabetes insipidus. Damage to the optic nerves may also occur. Thus radiation therapy should be used only as adjunctive management following incomplete operative removal of large tumors.

Operative Approaches

Transsphenoidal microsurgical resection of prolactinoma has been widely used for therapy, and numerous reports of large series of patients treated by this technique have been published. In a review of these studies Randall et al. concluded that transsphenoidal operations have minimum risk with a mortality of less than 0.5%, all deaths being reported to occur after treatment of macroadenomas. The risk of temporary postoperative diabetes insipidus is 10% to 40%, but the risk of permanent diabetes insipidus and iatrogenic hypopituitarism is less than 2%. The initial cure rate, with normalization of prolactin levels and return of ovulation, is relatively high for microadenomas (65% to 85%) and less so with macroadenomas (20% to 40%). Vision can return to normal in 85% of patients with loss of acuity and visual field defects.

The initial cure rate is related to the pretreatment prolactin levels. Those tumors with levels less than 100 ng/ml have an excellent prognosis (85%), and those with levels greater than 200 ng/ml have a poor prognosis (35%). Operative treatment of tumors in patients older than 26 with amenorrhea for more than 6 months carries a poorer prognosis than tumors in younger patients with a shorter duration of amenorrhea. Nevertheless, long-term follow-up of patients after operation indicates that late recurrence of hyperprolactinemia is common. Serri et al. followed 28 patients with microadenomas and 16 with macroadenomas for 6 years

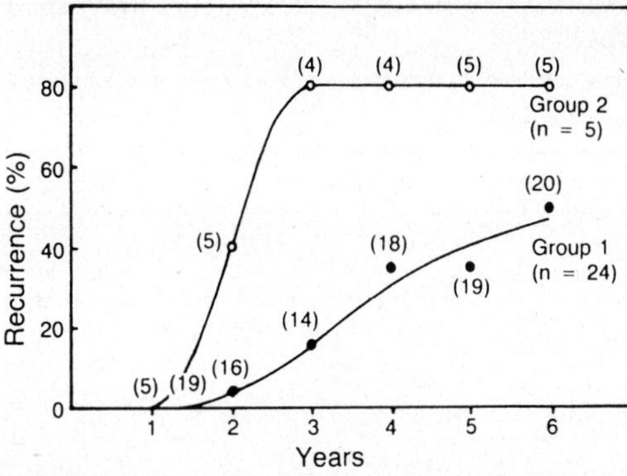

FIGURE 37-9
Cumulative recurrence rate in patients with microprolactinoma (group 1) or macroprolactinoma (group 2) after initially successful operation. Figures in parentheses indicate numbers of patients who were seen at each yearly interval. (From Serri O, Rasio E, Beauregard H, et al: N Engl J Med 309:280, 1983. Reprinted by permission of The New England Journal of Medicine.)

after operation. Although prolactin levels normalized and menses resumed in 24 (85%) of those with microadenomas and 5 (31%) of those with macroadenomas who had a good initial postoperative response, hyperprolactinemia recurred in half of those with microadenoma and 4 of the 5 with macroadenomas after a mean period of 4 and 2.5 years, respectively (Fig. 37-9). There was no significant difference in recurrence rates for those who conceived and those

who did not. Rodman et al. reported a lower postoperative recurrence rate (about 20% for both microadenomas and macroadenomas) following initial cure rates of 85% and 37%, respectively. The risk of recurrence in both series appeared to be related to the immediate postoperative prolactin levels, being greater in persons with a prolactin level greater than 10 ng/ml.

The relatively high rates of late recurrence indicate that these patients have an underlying hypothalamic defect in dopamine regulation that continues after operative removal of the adenoma.

Medical Therapy

Currently the treatment of choice for microadenomas as well as the initial treatment for macroadenomas is oral ingestion of a potent dopamine receptor agonist. Bromoergocryptine, methysergide, and metergoline have been used with success, but only bromoergocryptine (2-Br-alpha-ergocryptine mesylate) is approved for use in the United States (Fig. 37-10). The greatest amount of clinical experience has been with use of this agent. This semisynthetic ergot alkaloid was developed in 1967 to inhibit prolactin secretion. It directly stimulates dopamine receptors, and as a dopamine receptor agonist it inhibits prolactin secretion both in vitro and in vivo. After ingestion, bromoergocryptine is rapidly absorbed, with peak blood levels reached 1 to 3 hours later. Serum prolactin lev-

FIGURE 37-10
Formula of bromocriptine.

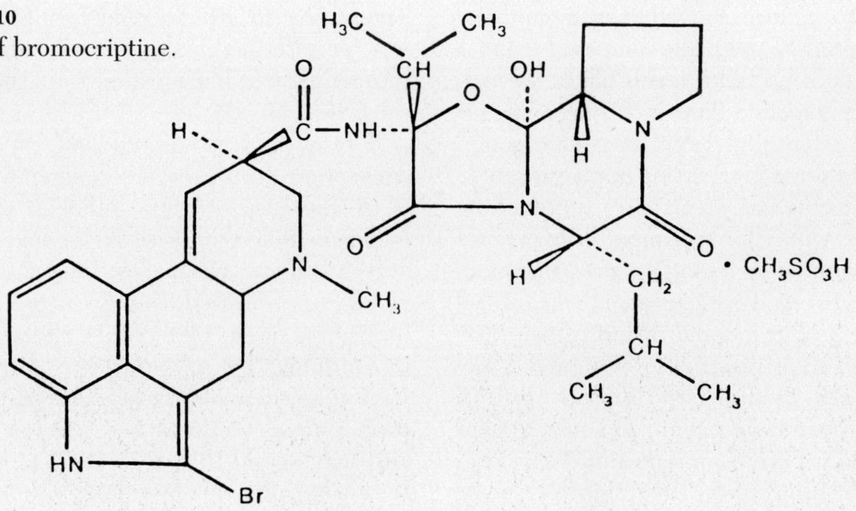

TABLE 37-1

Effective Dose of Bromocriptine to Normalize Prolactin or Achieve Pregnancy

Daily Dose (mg)	Adenoma (No. = 19)	No Adenoma (No. = 21)
5.0	9 (47%)	20* (95%)
7.5	5 (47%)	1
10.0	2 (47%)	0
15.0	1 (47%)	0
20.0	2 (47%)	0

From Kletzky OA, Marrs RP, Davajan V: Management of patients with hyperprolactinemia and normal or abnormal tomograms. Am J Obstet Gynecol 147:528, 1983.
*$P < 0.005$.

TABLE 37-2

Duration of Treatment (Weeks) to Correct Symptoms

	Adenoma	No Adenoma
Galactorrhea	11.3* ± 2.1 (No. = 17)	5.6 ± 1.1 (No. = 19)
Amenorrhea	8.7† ± 1.2 (No. = 17)	5.7 ± 0.6 (No. = 15)
Infertility	16.2‡ ± 2.1 (No. = 17)	9.8 ± 1.5 (No. = 12)

From Kletzky OA, Marrs RP, Davajan V: Management of patients with hyperprolactinemia and normal or abnormal tomograms. Am. J Obstet Gynecol 147:528, 1983.
*$P < 0.001$.
†$P < 0.01$.
‡$P < 0.02$.

els remain depressed for about 14 hours after ingestion of a single dose, after which time the drug is not detectable in the circulation. For this reason the drug is usually given at least twice daily, with initial therapy being started at one half of the 2.5 mg tablet to minimize side effects. The most frequent side effects are orthostatic hypotension (with an incidence of 15%), which can produce fainting and dizziness as well as nausea and vomiting. To minimize these symptoms the initial dose should be taken in bed and with food at nighttime. Less frequent adverse symptoms include headache, nasal congestion, fatigue, constipation, and diarrhea. Most of these reactions are mild, occur early in the course of treatment, and are transient. To reduce the adverse symptoms, the dose should be gradually increased every 1 to 2 weeks until prolactin levels fall to normal. The usual therapeutic dose is 2.5 mg twice or three times a day, but larger doses are sometimes used when a macroadenoma is present.

Bromoergocryptine is currently approved by the U.S. FDA only for treatment of hyperprolactinemia with and without the presence of an adenoma. In women without adenomas prolactin levels return to normal in more than 90% of cases, fertility is restored in 80%, and galactorrhea is eradicated in 60%. In patients with hyperprolactinemia and microadenoma, similar rates of success have been reported. Therefore, bromoergocryptine is the treatment of choice in patients with microadenoma who desire return of menses and ovulation and disappearance of galactorrhea.

Kletzky et al. reported that patients with hyperprolactinemia without radiologic evidence of tumor required a lower dose of bromoergocryptine than patients with adenomas to reduce prolactin levels to normal (Table 37-1) and less duration of therapy to resume ovulatory cycles, establish pregnancy, and end galactorrhea (Table 37-2).

Despite administration of up to 20 mg of bromoergocryptine per day, about 10% of patients with microadenomas fail to have prolactin levels return to normal, probably because of individual differences in the sensitivity of lactotrophs to bromoergocryptine. Nevertheless, despite the persistently elevated prolactin levels, many of these patients ovulate and conceive (Fig. 37-11).

If pregnancy is desired and effected, after conception occurs bromoergocryptine therapy is usually discontinued, although there is no evidence that the drug is teratogenic or adversely affects pregnancy outcome. If pregnancy is not desired, therapy is usually continued for at least 12 months, after which it is discontinued for a few weeks. Most patients with microadenomas have recurrence of hyperprolactinemia, amenorrhea, and galactorrhea, although about 10% to 20% have permanent remission after discontinuing bromoergocryp-

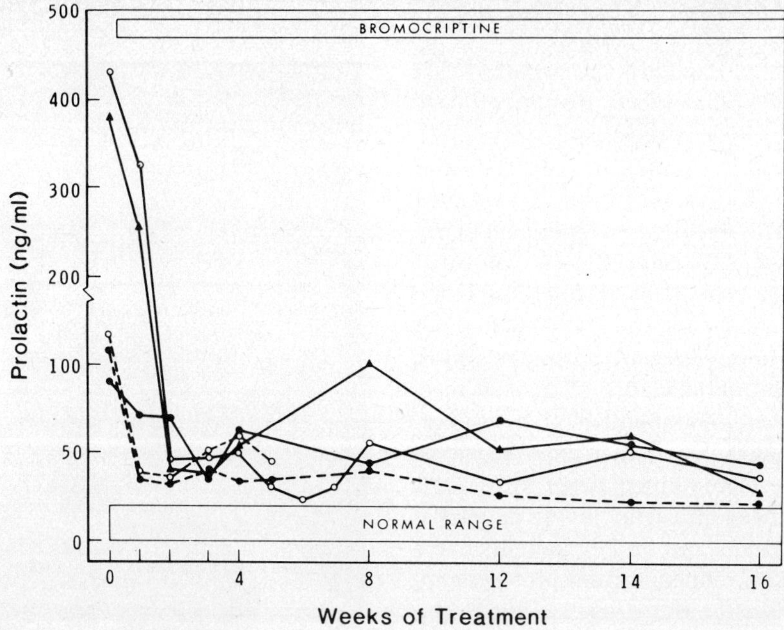

FIGURE 37-11

Mean serum prolactin response to bromocriptine therapy in five patients with radiographic evidence of pituitary adenoma and residual hyperprolactinemia. All five ovulated, and four conceived. (From Kletzky OA, Marrs RP, Davajan V: Am J Obstet Gynecol 147:528, 1983.)

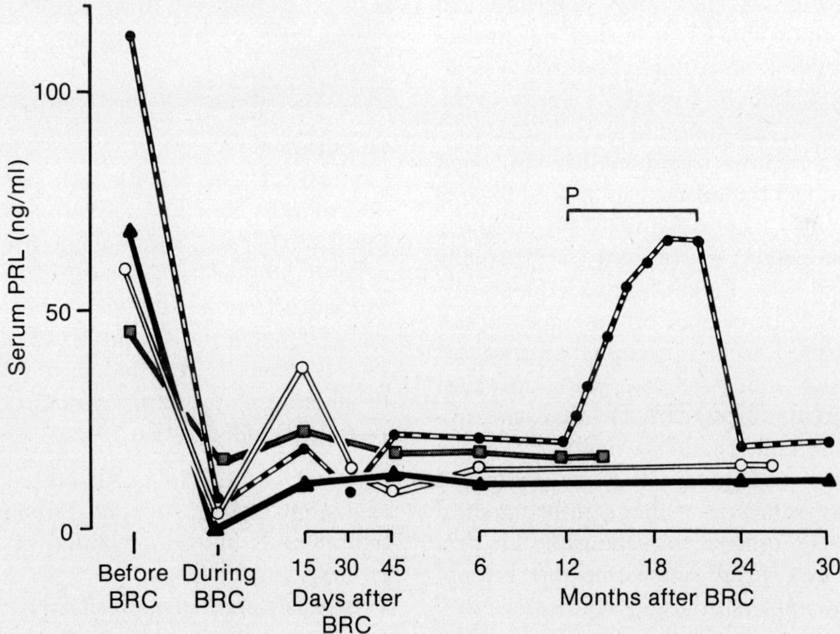

FIGURE 37-12

Serum prolactin levels in four patients who had persistently normal prolactin levels after bromocriptine *(BRC)* treatment for 12 months. *P,* pregnancy. (From Moriondo P, Travaglini P, Nissim M, et al: Bromocriptine treatment of microprolactinomas: evidence of stable prolactin decrease after drug withdrawal. J Clin Endocrinol Metab 60:764-772, 1985. Copyright © by The Endocrine Society 1985.)

tine treatment. Moriondo et al. reported that after 1 year of bromoergocryptine treatment, 11% of women with microadenomas had persistent normalization of prolactin, with return of regular menses after the drug was discontinued (Fig. 37-12). This incidence of permanent remission reached 22% after 2 years of treatment. A higher rate of permanent remission occurred in patients treated with 10 mg per day than with lower dosages, but higher doses of drug increase the incidence of adverse reactions and cause discontinuation of treatment. These investigators found that after bromoergocryptine was discontinued there was a 40% reduction in mean prolactin levels in all patients treated, and about 60% of patients had a greater than 30% reduction from pretreatment prolactin levels after the drug was discontinued. These data indicate that the remissions were drug related and not spontaneous. Using CT scans before and during bromoergocryptine therapy, Bonneville et al. found that about 75% of patients with microadenomas had reduction in tumor size during bromoergocryptine treatment, and in 40% the tumor had disappeared (Fig. 37-13). To determine if permanent remission has occurred the prolactin level should be measured about 6 weeks after discontinuation of treatment because the levels plateau at this time.

Bromoergocryptine treatment has also been shown to reduce tumor mass in 80% to 90% of individuals with macroadenomas. In addition, visual disturbances, if present, are usually promptly relieved. Following subsequent surgical removal of these bromoergocryptine-treated tumors, histologic examination revealed a reduction of tumor cell size, with shrinkage of the cytoplasm being greater than the nucleus. In addition, there are modifications of cell structure and morphology as compared with tumors removed without prior medical treatment. The organelles responsible for prolactin synthesis shrink, indicating that bromoergocryptine impairs prolactin synthesis as well as release. The reduction in size of macroadenomas usually occurs rapidly, within a few weeks after starting treatment, but following withdrawal of drug the tumor size may increase just as rapidly; thus the drug should be withdrawn cautiously. In contrast to the frequent occurrence of pituitary insufficiency, including diabetes insipidus, after surgical or radiologic

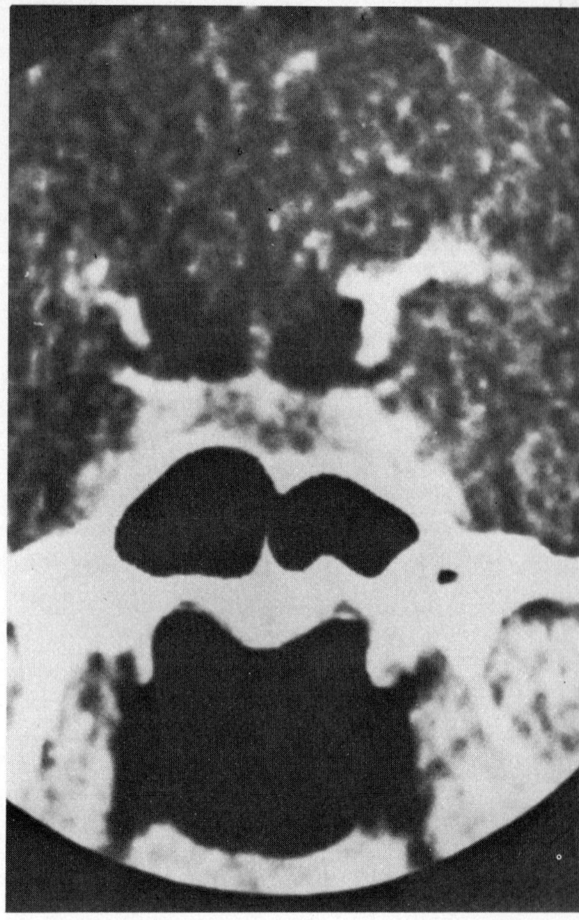

FIGURE 37-13
Coronal CT scan of same woman as in Fig. 37-4, 4 months after bromocriptine therapy (5 mg per day). Clinical and biologic results were excellent; pituitary gland is nearly normal, with reconstruction of sellar floor. (From Bonneville J-F, Poulignot D, Cattin F, et al: Computed tomographic demonstration of the effects of bromocriptine on pituitary microadenoma size. Radiology 143:451-455, 1982.)

treatment of large tumors, bromoergocryptine treatment is not accompanied by any type of pituitary insufficiency.

Because permanent remission rarely occurs following withdrawal of bromoergocryptine treatment from individuals with large tumors, long-term treatment is usually necessary. The drug has been administered for up to 12 years in some patients without problems, and once biochemical, radiologic, and clinical responses to treatment are established, they are generally maintained over a long-term period. Bromoergocryptine has also been successfully used to treat patients with failure of, or recurrence after, operation or irradiation therapy.

Molitch et al. reported the results of a recent 1-year prospective multicenter study of the use of bromoergocryptine as primary therapy for prolactin-secreting macroadenomas in 27 patients. Bromoergocryptine dosage ranged from 5 to 12.5 mg daily, with 7.5 mg being the most frequent dose. Prolactin levels fell in all patients, and to 11% or less of pretreatment values in all but one. Of this group, two thirds had prolactin levels decrease to normal during treatment. Tumor shrinkage was observed in all patients, being reduced by more than 50% in half the patients and by about 50% in an additional 20% of the study group. Visual field impairment disappeared in 9 of the 10 patients with abnormalities. In two thirds of the patients reduction in tumor size occurred by 6 weeks, but in one third it was not evident until 6 months, indicating there were both rapid and slow responses of tumor to drug treatment. Therefore at least a 6-month trial of medical therapy is warranted in patients with a macroadenoma.

Because of these excellent results, the poor initial results of operation, and the high recurrence rates, these investigators concluded that bromoergocryptine should be used as the initial management of patients with prolactin-secreting macroadenomas. After maximum shrinkage of tumor, medical therapy can be continued or operative treatment used. The cost of continuing bromoergocryptine treatment is considerable; it is inconvenient to take medication several times a day, and some patients have unpleasant side effects with the higher dosages that may be necessary. Therefore, some patients prefer operative treatment. In patients who elect to have an operation, the drug should be continued until the time of operation to prevent tumor expansion. The rates of success after operation are no different in patients who received or did not receive bromoergocryptine before the operation.

Pregnancy

Many women with hyperprolactinemia with or without adenomas wish to become pregnant. A small percentage conceive spontaneously, while most require treatment to induce ovula-

tion. Barbieri and Ryan recently compiled a literature review of the pregnancy courses of 275 women with adenomas, the majority of whose conceptions had been induced by bromoergocryptine. They reported that of 215 patients with microprolactinomas, less than 1% had changes in visual fields, radiologic evidence of tumor enlargement, or neurologic signs. About 5% developed headaches during pregnancy. Of 60 patients with macroprolactinomas, 20% developed adverse changes in visual fields and polytomographic or neurologic signs during pregnancy, and some of them required bromoergocryptine or operative treatment during pregnancy or shortly postpartum. For this reason some authorities recommend excision of macroprolactinomas before pregnancy is attempted. Nevertheless, because pituitary function is usually diminished after operation, induction of ovulation must be performed with complicated and expensive gonadotrophin treatment. Bromoergocryptine treatment does not interfere with pituitary function and is thus the therapy of choice for patients with macroadenomas who wish to conceive. Some authors advise continuous bromoergocryptine treatment throughout pregnancy in patients with macroadenomas, because with this therapy visual disturbances are rare. Despite a lowering of prolactin levels, there is no effect on placental hormone production, and pregnancy outcome does not appear to be affected.

Nevertheless, since the drug crosses the placenta and suppresses fetal prolactin levels, its long-term effects on the newborn are unknown. Therefore it is advised that patients with macroadenomas discontinue the drug after conception, as do patients with microadenomas, and have therapy reinitiated if and when symptoms of visual disturbance or severe headaches occur. Most patients who conceive after bromoergocryptine treatment have ingested the drug for a few weeks after conception. In a review of 1410 such pregnancies compiled by Turkalj et al. there was a spontaneous abortion rate of 11%, ectopic pregnancy rate of 0.7%, and twin pregnancy rate of 1.8%. The incidence of minor (2.5%) and major (1%) congenital defects was similar to pregnancy outcomes in untreated populations of women. The mean amount of drug ingested and duration of postconception treatment were similar in mothers who had normal children and those with defects. Thus ingestion of bromoergocryptine during pregnancy does not appear to increase the risk of congenital abnormalities, spontaneous abortion, or multiple gestation. Postnatal surveillance of more than 200 children born in this series has revealed no adverse effects to date.

Ruiz-Velasco and Tolis compiled the obstetric histories of nearly 2000 pregnancies occurring in hyperprolactinemic women that have been reported in the literature. Most of these pregnancies were induced with bromoergocryptine. There was a term delivery rate of 85%, an abortion rate of 11%, a prematurity rate of 2%, and a multiple pregnancy rate of 1.2%. Although prolactin levels increased during pregnancy, after delivery the levels returned to pretreatment values in about 85%. A postpartum increase over pretreatment levels was uncommon (3%), while prolactin levels returned to normal in 13%. Likewise, in patients who had postpartum radiologic sellar examination, 84% showed no change, 9% improved, and 7% worsened. Thus stopping treatment during pregnancy only occasionally results in tumor growth. It is advised that patients with macroadenoma have monthly visual field examination and neurologic testing during pregnancy, but this is probably unnecessary for patients with microadenoma unless they develop symptoms.

Following delivery, breast feeding may be initiated without adverse effects on the tumors. Following completion of nursing, as well as for women who do not breastfeed at all, bromoergocryptine should be ingested for 2 to 3 weeks and then discontinued. At that time serum prolactin measurement and repeat CT scan should be performed and treatment reinstituted according to the findings.

Patients with Hyperprolactinemia Who Do Not Wish to Conceive

For patients who do not wish to conceive and for whom galactorrhea is not a problem, no therapy is necessary unless estrogen levels are low. Thus to prevent osteoporosis in this clinical situation, bromoergocryptine should be given, regardless of whether an adenoma is present, and a mechanical type of contraceptive should be used. Long-term evaluation of all patients with hyperprolactinemia is important. Unless a macroadenoma is present, measurement of prolactin levels every 6 months and CT examination every 2 years are advised. If bromoergocryptine therapy is used, temporary discontinuation of medication every 1 to 2 years is advisable, with prolactin measurement 6 weeks later. If the level is normal, repeat prolactin measurements should be made semiannually. If the level is increased, therapy should be restarted, and if a microadenoma is present, the option of operation should be offered. During medical treatment of macroadenomas, CT and visual field examination should be performed every 6 months to determine the effect of medication on the tumor. At these intervals a decision about whether to continue long-term bromoergocryptine treatment or perform an operation can be made.

__________ **KEY POINTS** __________

- Estrogen stimulates prolactin release but blocks its action at the receptor in the breast.

- Physiologic stimuli for prolactin release include breast and nipple palpation, exercise, stress, sleep, and the noonday meal.

- The main symptoms of hyperprolactinemia are galactorrhea and amenorrhea, the latter caused by alterations in normal gonadotrophin-releasing hormone (GnRH) release.

- Hyperprolactinemia is present in 15% of all anovulatory women and 20% of women with amenorrhea of undetermined cause.

- About 60% of all women with galactorrhea have hyperprolactinemia, but almost 90% of women with galactorrhea, amenorrhea, and low estrogen levels have hyperprolactinemia.

- Pathologic causes of hyperprolactinemia include pharmacologic agents (tranquilizers, narcotics, and antihypertensive drugs), hypothyroidism, chronic renal disease, chronic neurostimulation of the breast, hypothalamic disease, and pituitary tumors (prolactinoma, acromegaly, Cushing's disease).

- About 3% to 5% of individuals with hyperprolactinemia have hypothyroidism.

- About 80% of all pituitary tumors secrete prolactin.

- About 25% of patients with acromegaly and 10% of those with Cushing's disease have hyperprolactinemia.

- About 10% of patients with an enlarged sella have the empty sella syndrome.

- Autopsy studies reveal that prolactinomas are present in about 10% of the population.

- About 50% of women with hyperprolactinemia will have a prolactinoma, as will nearly all of those with prolactin levels greater than 200 ng/ml.

- About 20% of women with galactorrhea and 35% of those with amenorrhea and galactorrhea have prolactinomas.

- About 70% of women with hyperprolactinemia, galactorrhea, and amenorrhea with low estrogen levels will have a prolactinoma.

———————— **KEY POINTS, cont'd** ————————

- Women with regular menses, galactorrhea, and normal prolactin levels do not have prolactinomas.

- About 13% of women with prolactinomas do not have galactorrhea.

- Most macroadenomas enlarge with time; most microadenomas do not.

- The initial operative cure rate for microadenomas is about 80% and for macroadenomas 30%, but the long-term recurrence rate is at least 20% for each.

- Most frequent side effects of bromoergocryptine are orthostatic hypotension, nausea, and vomiting.

- In patients with hyperprolactinemia and no macroadenoma, bromoergocryptine treatment returns prolactin levels to normal in 90%, induces ovulatory cycles in 80%, and eradicates galactorrhea in 60%.

- After 1 year of bromoergocryptine treatment, prolactin levels remain normal in 11% of women with macroadenomas; after 2 years permanent remission reaches 22%.

- Bromoergocryptine shrinks 80% to 90% of macroadenomas.

- When pregnancy occurs in women with microadenomas, less than 1% have visual field changes, tumor enlargement, or neurologic signs; about 20% of women with macroadenomas have such adverse changes.

- Bromoergocryptine induction of pregnancy is not associated with an increased risk of congenital abnormalities, spontaneous abortion, or multiple gestation.

- About 85% of patients with prolactinomas have no change in prolactin levels or tumor size after delivery, 10% improve, and 5% worsen.

BIBLIOGRAPHY

Bäckström CT, McNeilly AS, Leash RM, et al: Pulsatile secretion of LH, FSH, prolactin oestradiol and progesterone during the human menstrual cycle. Clin Endocrinol 17:29, 1982.

Barbieri RL, Ryan KJ: Bromocriptine: Endocrine pharmacology and therapeutic applications. Fertil Steril 39:727, 1983.

Bonneville J-F, Poulignot D, Cattin F, et al: Computed tomographic demonstration of the effects of bromocriptine on pituitary microadenoma size. Radiology 143:451, 1982.

Burrow GN, Wortzman G, Rewcastle NB, et al: Microadenomas of the pituitary and abnormal sellar tomograms in an unselected autopsy series. N Engl J Med 304:156, 1981.

Chapler FK: Hyperprolactinemia. In Pitkin RM, Zlatnik FJ: Year Book of obstetrics and gynecology. Chicago, Year Book Medical Publishers, 1985.

Davajan V, Kletzky O, March CM, et al: The significance of galactorrhea in patients with normal menses, oligomenorrhea, and secondary amenorrhea. Am J Obstet Gynecol 130:894, 1978.

Gharib H, Frey HM, Laws ER Jr, et al: Coexistent primary empty sella syndrome and hyperprolactinemia: Report of 11 cases. Arch Intern Med 143:1383, 1983.

Kleinberg DL, Noel GL, Frantz AG: Galactorrhea: A study of 235 cases, including 48 with pituitary tumors. N Engl J Med 296:589, 1977.

Kletzky OA: Diagnostic approaches to hyperprolactinemic states. Semin Reprod Endocrinol 2:23, 1984.

Kletzky OA, Davajan V: Hyperprolactinemia: Diagnosis and treatment. In Mishell DR Jr, Davajan V, eds: Infertility, reproductive endocrinology and contraception, 2nd ed. Oradell, N.J., Medical Economics Books, 1986.

Kletzky OA, Marrs RP, Davajan V: Management of patients with hyperprolactinemia and normal or abnormal tomograms. Am J Obstet Gynecol 147:528, 1983.

Koppelman MCS, Jaffe MJ, Rieth KG, et al: Hyperprolactinemia, amenorrhea, and galactorrhea: A retrospective assessment of 25 cases. Ann Intern Med 100:115, 1984.

March CM, Kletzky OA, Davajan V, et al: Longitudinal evaluation of patients with untreated prolactin-secreting pituitary adenomas. Am J Obstet Gynecol 139:835, 1981.

Molitch ME, Elton RL, Blackwell RE, et al: Bromocriptine as primary therapy for prolactin-secreting macroadenomas: Results of a prospective multicenter study. J Clin Endocrinol Metab 60:698, 1985.

Moriondo P, Travaglini P, Nissim M, et al: Bromocriptine treatment of microprolactinomas: Evidence of stable prolactin decrease after drug withdrawal. J Clin Endocrinol Metab 60:764, 1985.

Randall RV, Laws ER Jr, Abboud CF, et al: Transsphenoidal microsurgical treatment of prolactin-producing pituitary adenomas. Mayo Clin Proc 58:108, 1983.

Rodman EF, Molitch ME, Post KD, et al: Long-term follow-up of transsphenoidal selective adenomectomy for prolactinoma. JAMA 252:921, 1984.

Ruiz-Velasco V, Tolis G: Pregnancy in hyperprolactinemic women. Fertil Steril 41:793, 1984.

Serri O, Rasio E, Beauregard H, et al: Recurrence of hyperprolactinemia after selective transsphenoidal adenomectomy in women with prolactinoma. N Engl J Med 309:280, 1983.

Shangold GA, Kletzky OA, Marrs RP, et al: Hyperprolactinemia: comparison of thyrotropic-releasing hormone and tomography. Obstet Gynecol 63:771, 1984.

Turkalj I, Braun P, Krupp P: Surveillance of bromocriptine in pregnancy. JAMA 247:1589, 1982.

Hyperandrogenism

KEY TERMS AND DEFINITIONS

5α-Androstane-3α,17β-diol Glucuronide (A-diol-G). A metabolite of Adiol-G that can be measured in serum and is the most accurate indicator of peripheral androgen metabolism.

Congenital Adrenal Hyperplasia with Adult Onset. Mild degree of enzymatic deficiency of cortisol biosynthesis (usually 11β-hydroxylase or 21-hydroxylase) that produces signs of androgen excess after puberty without external sexual ambiguity being present at birth.

Dehydroepiandrosterone Sulfate (DHEA-S). An androgen secreted nearly exclusively by the adrenal gland. Serum levels are used as a marker of adrenal androgen activity.

Hilus Cell Tumor. Small testosterone-secreting ovarian tumors that most frequently develop after menopause.

Hirsutism. Presence of hair in locations where it is not normally found in a woman, specifically in the midline of the body.

Idiopathic Hirsutism (Constitutional or Familial Hirsutism). The most common disorder associated with androgen excess. It is due to increased peripheral androgen metabolism and is associated with normal circulating levels of testosterone and DHEA-S but increased levels of Adiol-G.

17-Ketosteroids. Urinary metabolites of DHEA, DHEA-S, androstenedione, and testosterone. They consist of DHEA, androsterone, and etiocholanolone.

Polycystic Ovarian Syndrome (PCOS). An endocrinologic disorder characterized by excessive androgen production, inappropriate gonadotrophin secretion, and chronic anovulation. It begins perimenarcheally, and its clinical manifestations include hirsutism, menstrual irregularity (oligomenorrhea or amenorrhea), and obesity.

5α-Reductase. The enzyme that converts testosterone to its more active metabolite, dihydrotestosterone (DHT).

Sertoli-Leydig Cell Tumors. Testosterone-secreting ovarian tumors that usually are unilateral and palpably enlarged. They occur most frequently in the second to fourth decades of life.

Spironolactone. Drug that decreases the rate of metabolism of testosterone in the end organ, thus acting as an antiandrogen.

Stromal Hyperthecosis. An ovarian disorder characterized by nests of luteinized theca cells within the stroma of bilaterally enlarged ovaries. Clinically this condition is associated with slowly but progressively increasing signs of virilization.

Virilization. Presence of signs of masculinization in a woman. These signs include temporal balding, voice deepening, clitoral enlargement, and increased muscle mass.

The clinical signs associated with excessive androgen production in women are hirsutism and virilization, with hirsutism being much more common. The presence of hirsutism without other signs of virilization is associated with relatively mild disorders of androgen production, and circulating testosterone levels are either normal or mildly to moderately elevated (less than 1.5 ng/ml). Hirsutism usually has a gradual onset and if unaccompanied by signs of virilization is not caused by a severe enzymatic defect or a neoplasm. The amount and location of the central hair growth found in women with hirsutism vary. Generally in the milder forms hair is found only on the upper lip and chin, whereas with increasing severity it appears on the cheeks, chest (intermammary), abdomen (superior to the umbilicus), inner aspects of thighs, and lower back and intergluteal areas. The severity of the hirsutism can be roughly quantified by means of the scoring system of Ferriman and Gallwey (Fig. 38-1 and Table 38-

1). Increased hair growth only on the extremities should not be considered hirsutism, as hair is normally found in this location in women. Women with hirsutism can have normal ovulatory menstrual cycles, oligomenorrhea, or amenorrhea.

Virilization is a relatively uncommon clinical finding, and its presence is usually associated with markedly elevated levels of circulating testosterone (2 ng/ml or greater). In contrast to the gradual development of hirsutism, signs of virilization usually occur over a relatively short period of time. These signs are due to both the masculinizing and the defeminizing (antiestrogenic) action of testosterone and include temporal balding, clitoral hypertrophy, decreased breast size, dryness of the vagina, and increased muscle mass. Women with virilization are nearly always amenorrheic. The presence of androgen-secreting neoplasms should always be suspected in any woman who develops signs of virilization, particularly if the onset is rapid.

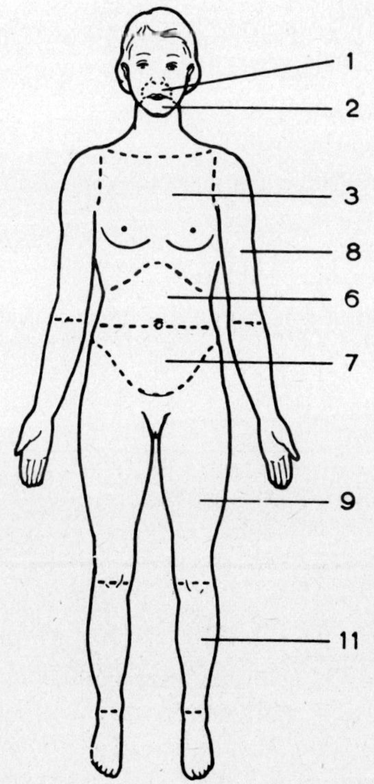
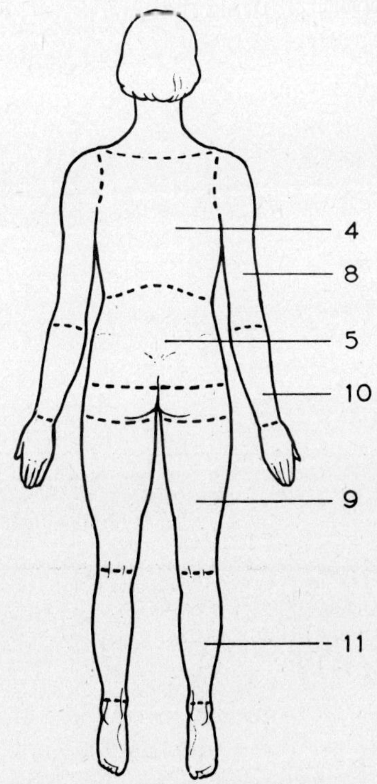

FIGURE 38-1

Demarcation of 11 sites used for numerically grading amount of hair growth—anterior and posterior views. (From Ferriman D, Gallwey JD: J Clin Endocrinol Metab 21:1440, 1961. © by The Endocrine Society, 1961.)

TABLE 38-1
Definition of Hair Gradings at 11 Sites*

Site	Grade	Definition
Upper lip	1	Few hairs at outer margin
	2	Small moustache at outer margin
	3	Moustache extending halfway from outer margin
	4	Moustache extending to midline
Chin	1	Few scattered hairs
	2	Scattered hairs with small concentrations
	3 & 4	Complete cover, light and heavy
Chest	1	Circumareolar hairs
	2	With midline hair in addition
	3	Fusion of these areas, with three-quarters cover
	4	Complete cover
Upper back	1	Few scattered hairs
	2	Rather more, still scattered
	3 & 4	Complete cover, light and heavy
Lower back	1	Sacral tuft of hair
	2	With some lateral extension
	3	Three-quarters cover
	4	Complete cover
Upper abdomen	1	Few midline hairs
	2	Rather more, still midline
	3 & 4	Half and full cover
Lower abdomen	1	Few midline hairs
	2	Midline streak of hair
	3	Midline band of hair
	4	Inverted V-shaped growth
Arm	1	Sparse growth affecting not more than one quarter of limb surface
	2	More than this; cover still incomplete
	3 & 4	Complete cover, light and heavy
Forearm	1,2,3,4	Complete cover of dorsal surface; 2 grades of light and 2 of heavy growth
Thigh	1,2,3,4	As for arm
Leg	1,2,3,4	As for arm

From Ferriman D, Gallwey JD: Clinical assessment of body hair growth in women. J Clin Endocrinol Metab 21:1440, 1961. © by The Endocrine Society, 1961.
*Grade 0 at all sites indicates absence of terminal hair.

PHYSIOLOGY

The sources of androgen production in the human female are the ovaries and the adrenal glands. The major androgen produced by the ovaries is testosterone and that of the adrenal glands is dehydroepiandrosterone sulfate (DHEA-S). Measurement of the amount of these two steroids in the circulation provides clinically relevant information regarding the presence and source of increased androgen production. In addition to glandular production of androgens, conversion of estrone to androstenedione and DHEA-S to testosterone occurs in peripheral tissue.

The ovaries secrete only about 0.1 mg of testosterone each day, mainly from the theca-

TABLE 38-2

Plasma Concentrations of Androgens During Menstrual Cycle

Steroid Hormone	Phase of Cycle	Plasma Concentration	
		Mean	Range
Androstenedione (ng/ml)	*	1.4	0.7-3.1
Testosterone (ng/ml)	*	0.35	0.15-0.55
Dehydroepiandrosterone (ng/ml)	*	4.2	2.7-7.8
Dehydroepiandrosterone sulfate (μg/ml)	*	1.6	0.8-3.4

From Goebelsmann U: Steroid hormones. Reproduced with permission from Infertility, contraception and reproductive endocrinology, 2nd ed, by Daniel R. Mishell, Jr., M.D., and Val Davajan, M.D. Copyright © 1986 Medical Economics Books, Oradell, N.J. 07649. All rights reserved.
*Unspecified; no major changes during menstrual cycle.

stroma cells. Other androgens secreted by the ovary are androstenedione (1 to 2 mg/day) and DHEA (<1 mg/day). The adrenal glands, in addition to secreting large quantities of DHEA-S (6 to 24 mg/day), secrete about the same daily amount of androstenedione (1 mg/day) as the ovaries and less than 1 mg of DHEA per day. The normal adrenal gland secretes little testosterone, although some uncommon adrenal tumors may secrete testosterone directly.

Androstenedione and DHEA do not have androgenic activity but are peripherally converted at a slow rate to a biologically active androgen, testosterone. Only about 5% of androstenedione and a smaller percentage of DHEA are converted to testosterone. The total daily production of testosterone in women is normally about 0.35 mg. Of this, 0.1 mg comes from direct ovarian secretion, 0.2 mg from peripheral conversion of androstenedione, and 0.05 mg from peripheral conversion of DHEA. Since the ovary and adrenal gland secrete about equal amounts of androstenedione and DHEA, about two thirds (0.22 mg) of the daily testosterone produced in a woman originates from the ovaries. Thus increased circulating levels of testosterone usually indicate abnormal ovarian androgen production. Normal circulating levels of these androgens in women of reproductive age are shown in (Table 38-2). Only a small amount of testosterone is metabolized to testosterone glucuronide and then excreted in the urine. Testosterone, which is not a 17-ketosteroid (17-KS), is mainly metabolized to androstenedione and then excreted as andro-

sterone and etiocholanolone, both of which are 17-KS. DHEA, DHEA-S, and androstenedione are excreted as DHEA, androsterone, and etiocholanolone, all of which are 17-KS. The origin of the major amount of urinary 17-KS is the precursor androgen produced in the greatest amounts, DHEA-S. Because DHEA-S has a long half life in serum, serum levels of DHEA-S correlate well with 17-KS excretion (Fig. 38-2). It is much better to measure serum DHEA-S than urinary 17-KS to assess adrenal androgen production. Because some glucocorticoid metabolites are also measured as 17-KS, the amount of creatinine in the urine needs to be determined, and it is difficult to collect a 24-hour urine specimen.

Most testosterone in the circulation (about 85%) is tightly bound to sex hormone–binding globulin (SHBG) and is believed to be biologically inactive. An additional 10% to 15% is loosely bound to albumin, with only about 1% to 2% not bound to any protein (free testosterone). Both the free and albumin-bound fractions are biologically active. Serum testosterone can be measured as the total amount, the amount that is believed to be biologically active (non-SHBG bound), and as the free form.

To exert a biologic effect, testosterone is metabolized peripherally in target tissues to the more potent androgen 5α-dihydrotestosterone (DHT) by the enzyme 5α-reductase, and its distal metabolite 5α-androstane-3α,17β-diol (A-diol) after further 3-keto reduction. Adiol is conjugated to 5α-androstane-3α,17β-diol glucuronide (Adiol-G), which is a stable, irrevers-

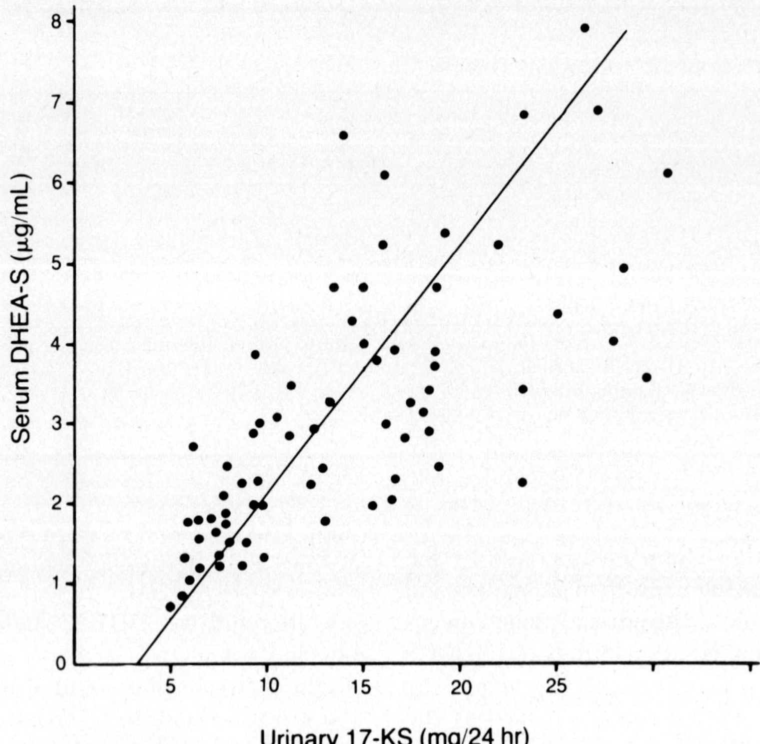

FIGURE 38-2

Correlation between serum dehydroepiandrosterone sulfate *(DHEA-S)* and urinary 17-ketosteroids *(17-KS)* in 71 patients ($r = 0.7$, $P < 0.0005$). (From Lobo RA, Paul WL, Goebelsmann U: Obstet Gynecol 57:69, 1981. Reprinted with permission from The American College of Obstetricians and Gynecologists.)

ible product of intracellular 5α-reductase activity (Fig. 38-3).

It is possible to measure this metabolite in serum, and Lobo et al. have shown it to be the most accurate indicator of the degree of peripheral androgen metabolism in women. Horton et al. have shown that although serum levels of total testosterone are similar in normal and hirsute women, there are significant differences in the amounts of non-SHBG bound testosterone as well as Adiol-G (Fig. 38-4). Non-SHBG bound testosterone is elevated in about 60% to 70% of hirsute women, but Adiol-G is elevated in more than 80% of such individuals. Thus increased levels of non-SHBG bound testosterone indicate increased ovarian production. If levels of non-SHBG bound testosterone are normal and Adiol-G are elevated, ovarian testosterone production is not increased but peripheral conversion of testosterone to its active metabolite is increased above normal. Either of

these processes can cause symptoms and signs of androgen excess.

ETIOLOGY

There are 10 currently recognized causes of androgen excess in women (see box on p. 1020). One main iatrogenic cause is administration of androgenic medication. In addition to testosterone itself, various anabolic steroids, 19-norprogestins, and danazol have androgenic effects. Thus a careful history of medication intake is important for all women with hirsutism.

Hirsutism or virilization can also be associated with some forms of abnormal gonad development. These individuals have signs of either external sexual ambiguity or primary amenorrhea in addition to findings of androgen excess and a Y chromosome present in the gonad. These conditions are discussed in Chapter 36

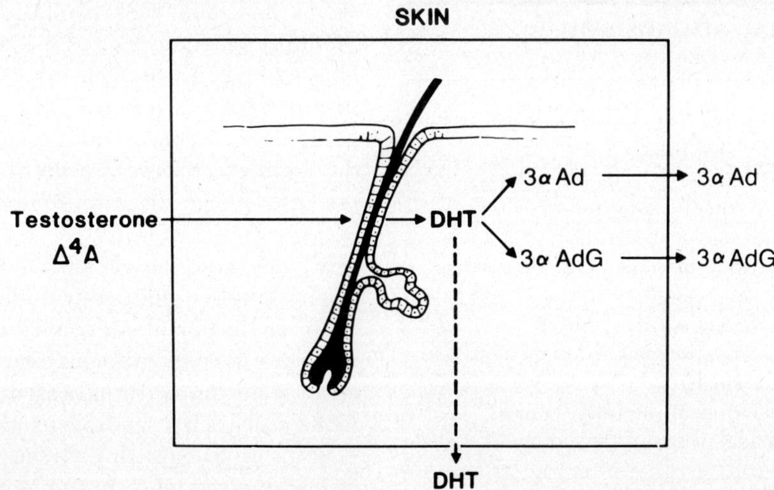

FIGURE 38-3

Current model for peripheral androgen metabolism. Although 5α-dihydrotestosterone *(DHT)* is the nuclear androgen in sexual tissue including skin, most of peripheral DHT is locally metabolized, and only small amounts *(dotted line)* enter the circulation. This explains why plasma DHT does not reflect peripheral production. DHT is metabolized separately by unconjugated and conjugated pathways. *3αAd*, 5α-androstane-3α,17β-diol; *3αAdG*, 5α-androstane-3α,17β-diol glucuronide. (From Horton R, Lobo RA: Clin Endocrinol Metab 15:293, 1986. © W.B. Saunders Co., Inc.

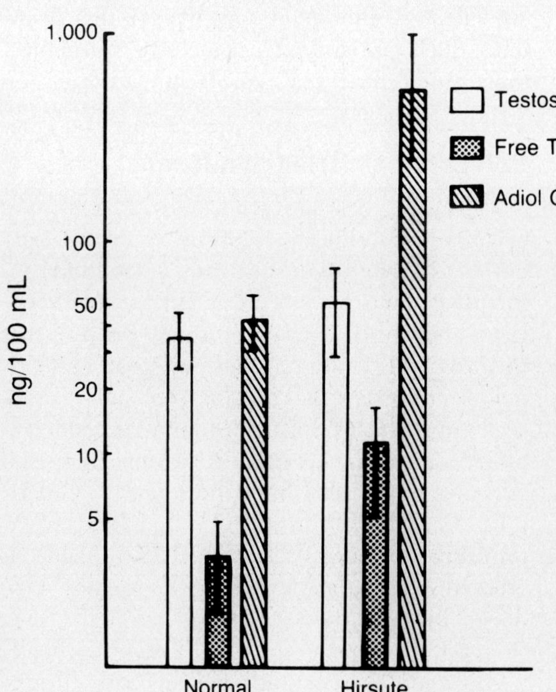

FIGURE 38-4

Plasma total testosterone, unbound testosterone *(free T)* and 5α-androstane-3α,17β-diol glucuronide *(Adiol Gluc)* in normal and hirsute women. Note insignificant elevation with overlap for testosterone and free T testosterone and highly significant increase in *Adiol Gluc* without overlap between two groups of women. (Reproduced from Horton R, Hawks D, Lobo RA: J Clin Invest 69:1203, 1982. By Copyright permission of The American Society for Clinical Investigation.)

DIFFERENTIAL DIAGNOSIS OF ANDROGEN EXCESS

Idiopathic hirsutism
Polycystic ovary syndrome
Stromal hyperthecosis
Androgen-producing ovarian tumors
Cushing's syndrome or disease
Adult manifestation of congenital adrenal hyperplasia
Androgen-producing adrenal tumors
Androgen excess in pregnancy: luteoma or hyperreactio luteinalis
Exogenous or iatrogenic androgen excess
Abnormal gonadal or sexual development

From Goebelsmann U: Androgen excess. Reproduced with permission from Infertility, contraception and reproductive endocrinology, 2nd ed, by Daniel R. Mishell, Jr., M.D., and Val Davajan, M.D. Copyright © 1986 Medical Economics Books, Oradell, N.J. 07649. All rights reserved.

and will not be further considered in the discussion of the differential diagnosis of androgen excess.

Signs of androgen excess during pregnancy can be caused by increased ovarian testosterone production. This is usually caused by either a luteoma of pregnancy or hyperreactio luteinalis. The former is a unilateral or bilateral solid ovarian enlargement, whereas the latter is bilateral cystic ovarian enlargement. After pregnancy the androgenic characteristics regress.

A diagnosis of these three causes of androgen excess can usually be easily made by means of a careful history and physical examination. The remaining causes of androgen excess will be discussed according to their approximate frequency.

Idiopathic Hirsutism (Peripheral Disorder of Androgen Metabolism)

The most common cause of androgen excess in women is manifested by signs of hirsutism and regular menstrual cycles in conjunction with normal circulatory levels of androgens (both testosterone and DHEA-S) as well as urinary 17-KS excretion. Because this type of disorder is frequently present in several individu-

als in the same family, particularly those of Mediterranean descent, it has also been called *familial* or *constitutional hirsutism*. Since neither ovarian nor adrenal androgen production is increased in these individuals, the cause of the androgen excess was not determined until recently, hence the term *idiopathic hirsutism*. Studies by Horton et al. have shown that nearly all those individuals have increased levels of Adiol-G, indirectly indicating that the cause of the hirsutism could be increased 5α-reductase activity, which converts normal levels of testosterone to increased amounts of the biologically active androgens DHT and Adiol. Paulsen et al. have directly measured the percent conversion of testosterone to DHT in genital skin as an assessment of 5α-reductase activity in the skin of women with idiopathic hirsutism. The amount of 5α-reductase activity was increased in hirsute women as compared with normal women and correlated well with both the degree of hirsutism and serum levels of Adiol-G (Fig. 38-5). Thus idiopathic hirsutism is in fact a disorder of peripheral androgen metabolism in the pilosebaceous apparatus of the skin and is possibly genetically determined. The condition should probably be renamed *abnormal peripheral androgen metabolism*. Antiandrogens that block peripheral testosterone action or interfere with 5α-reductase activity are effective therapeutic agents for this disorder. Such antiandrogens include spironolactone, cimetidine, and cyproterone acetate.

Polycystic Ovarian Syndrome

Polycystic ovarian syndrome (PCOS) was originally described in 1905 by Stein and Leventhal as a syndrome consisting of amenorrhea, hirsutism, and obesity in association with enlarged polycystic ovaries. It is now realized that this relatively common syndrome is an endocrinologic disorder that begins soon after menarche and consists of inappropriate gonadotrophin secretion associated with increased gonadotrophin-releasing hormone (GnRH) pulse frequency, tonically elevated levels of luteinizing hormone (LH) (Fig. 38-6), and increased circulatory levels of androgens produced by both the ovaries and adrenal glands (Fig. 38-7). Thus, as stated by Lobo, it is really a syndrome of hyperandrogenism with chronic

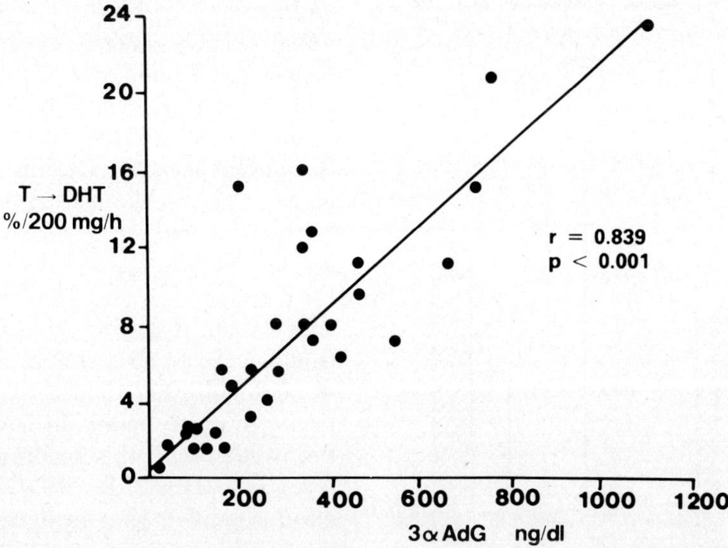

FIGURE 38-5

5α-reductase expressed as percent conversion of testosterone *(T)* to DHT per 200 mg genital skin per hour, correlated with 5α-androstane-3α,17β-diol glucuronide *(3αAdG)*. Correlation is highly significant: (r = 0.839, P < 0.001). (From Paulson RJ, Serafini PC, Catalino JA, et al: Fertil Steril 46:222, 1986. Reproduced with permission of the publisher, The American Fertility Society.)

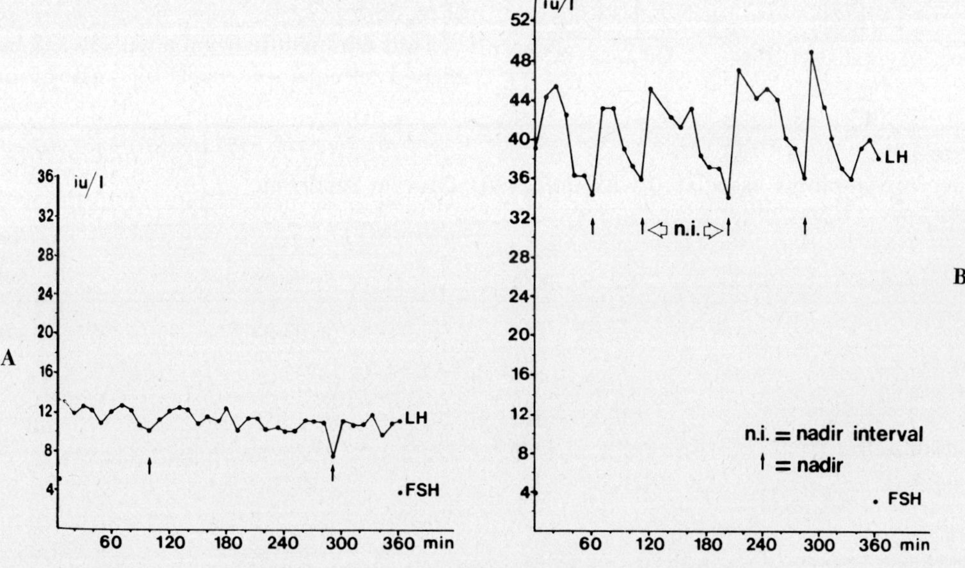

FIGURE 38-6

A, A normal subject sampled during follicular phase of cycle. **B,** Patient with polycystic ovarian syndrome *(PCOD)*. Sampling interval, 10 minutes. (From Burger CW, Korsen T, van Kessel H, et al: J Clin Endocrinol Metab 61:1126, 1985. © by The Endocrine Society, 1985.)

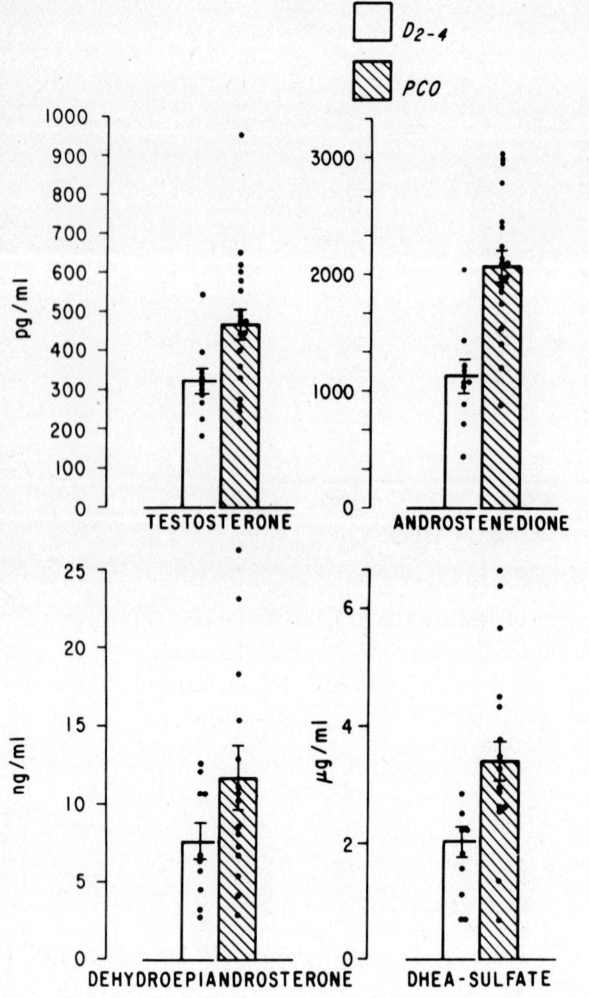

FIGURE 38-7
Mean ($\pm$SE) concentrations of testosterone, Δ^4androstenedione, DHEA, and DHEA-S in 19 patients with PCOS and 10 normal subjects between days 2 and 4 of their menstrual cycles. (From DeVane GW, Czekala NM, Judd HL, et al: Am J Obstet Gynecol 121:496, 1975.)

anovulation. If they are elevated, serum testostrone levels are usually between 70 and 120 ng/dl, and androstenedione levels are usually between 3 and 5 ng/ml. In addition, about half the women with this syndrome have elevated levels of DHEA-S. In 1963 Goldzieher and Axelrod compiled the incidence of the various symptoms associated with PCOS that had been reported in the literature (Table 38-3). From these and other data it has been estimated that about 30% of women with PCOS do not have hirsutism even though DeVane et al., as well as others, have reported that nearly all of them have elevated levels of circulating androgens. Lobo et al. found that the presence or absence of hirsutism depends on whether those androgens are converted peripherally by 5α-reductase to the more potent androgen DHT and A-diol as reflected by increased levels of Adiol-G (Fig. 38-8).

Thus nonhirsutic women with PCOS have elevated circulatory levels of testosterone or

TABLE 38-3
Incidence of Symptoms Associated with Polycystic Ovarian Syndrome*

Symptom	Incidence (%) Mean	Incidence (%) Range	No. of Usable Cases†
Infertility	74	35-95	596
Hirsutism	69	17-83	819
Amenorrhea	51	15-77	640
Obesity	41	16-49	600
Functional bleeding	29	6-65	547
Dysmenorrhea	23	—	75
Corpus luteum at operation	22	0-71	391
Virilization	21	0-28	431
Biphasic body temperature	15	12-40	288
Cyclic menses	12	7-28	395

From Goldzieher JW, Axelrod LR: Clinical and biochemical features of polycystic ovarian disease. Fertil Steril 14:631, 1963. Reproduced with permission of the publisher, The American Fertility Society.
*Tabulated from 187 references with a total of 1079 cases.
†Indicates how many of the 1079 total cases could be evaluated for the presence or absence of a particular symptom.

DHEA-S or of both but not of Adiol-G. The tonically elevated levels of LH are usually above 20 mIU/ml. Because FSH levels in PCOS patients are normal or low, it has been found that an LH-FSH ratio greater than 3, provided the LH level is not lower than 8 mIU/ml, may be used to suggest the diagnosis in women with clinical features of PCOS. Lobo et al. reported that about 70% of women with PCOS had either an elevated level of immunologic LH or an immunologic LH-FSH ratio greater than 3 but that all but one woman with PCOS had elevated serum levels of biologically active LH (Fig. 38-9).

Hoffman and Lobo reported that about half the women with PCOS have elevated levels of DHEA-S, with one third of them having levels

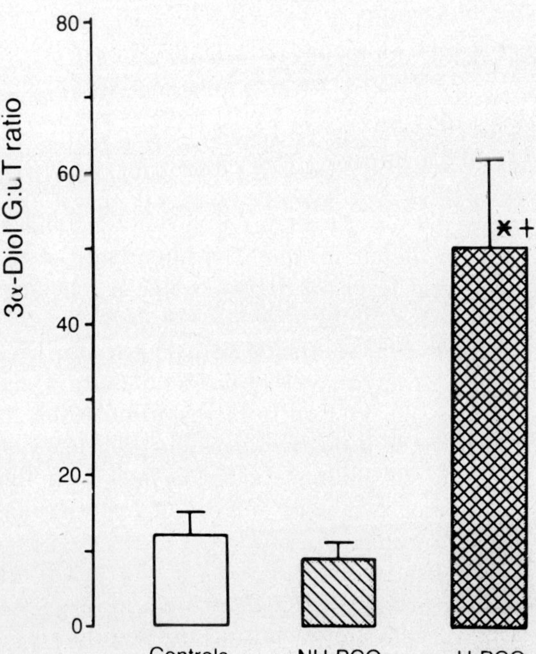

FIGURE 38-8

Ratios of serum 5α-androstane-3α,17β-diol glucuronide *(3α-DiolG)* to unbound testosterone *(uT)* in controls, nonhirsute PCOS patients *(NH-PCO)*, and hirsute PCOS patients *(H-PCO)*. *, Significantly higher level as compared with controls; +, significantly higher level in hirsute PCOS patients as compared with nonhirsute ones. (From Lobo RA, Goebelsmann U, Horton R: J Clin Endocrinol Metab 57:393, 1983. © by The Endocrine Society, 1983.)

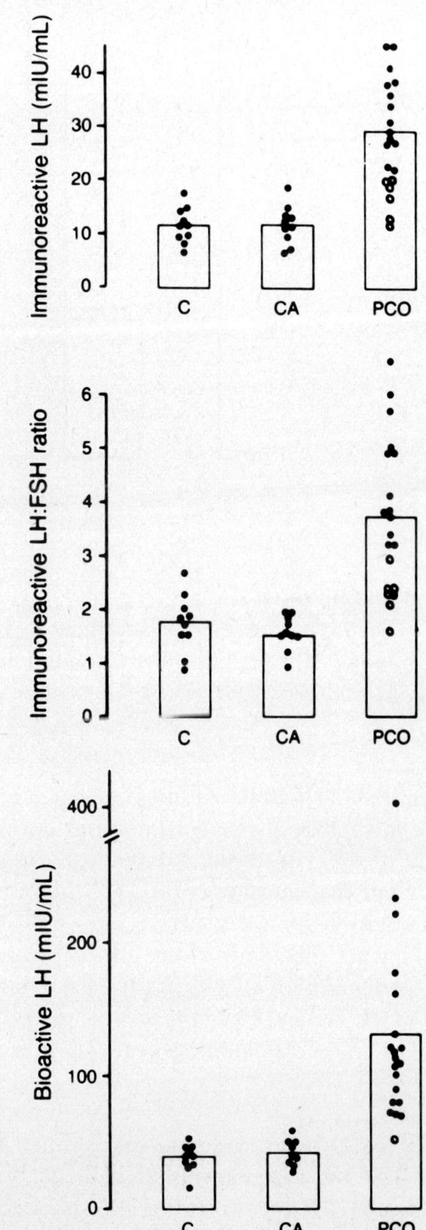

FIGURE 38-9

Serum measurements of immunoreactive LH, immunoreactive LH:FSH ratios, and bioactive LH in control subjects *(C)*, women with chronic anovulation *(CA)*, and women with PCOS *(PCO)*. Solid circles for women with PCOS indicate values exceeding 3±SD of mean control levels. (From Lobo RA, Kletzky OA, Campeau JD, et al: Fertil Steril 39:674, 1983. Reproduced with permission of the publisher, The American Fertility Society.)

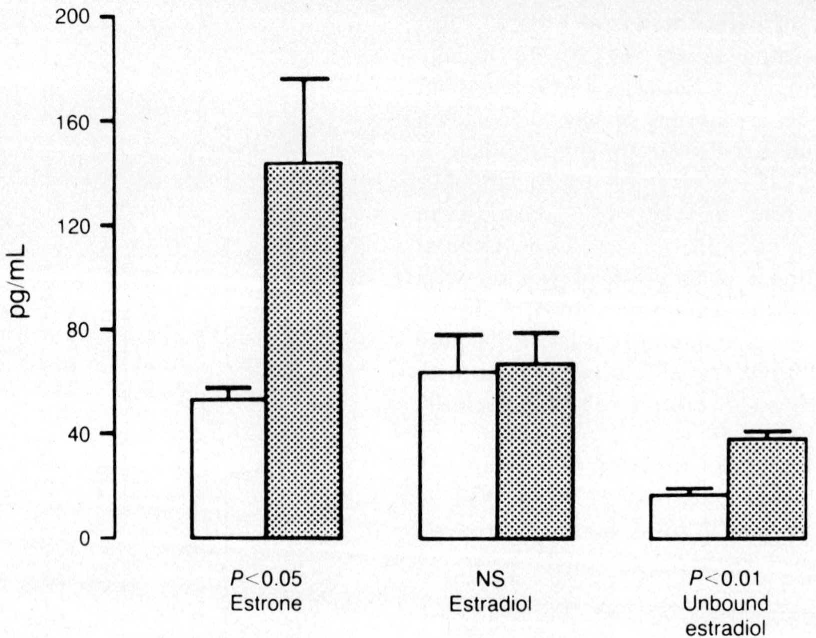

FIGURE 38-10

Serum estrogen concentrations in 13 normal women and 22 PCOS patients *(shaded areas)*. (From Lobo RA, Granger L, Goebelsmann U, et al: J Clin Endocrinol Metab 52:156, 1981. © by The Endocrine Society, 1981.)

greater than 4 ng/ml. Although Chang et al. have shown that adrenocorticotropic hormone (ACTH) levels in these women are normal, they found that infusions of ACTH produce an exaggerated response of DHEA-S, indicating that the zona reticularis of the adrenal gland in some patients with PCOS has increased sensitivity to ACTH and that the adrenal gland may be involved in the pathogenesis of this syndrome.

In addition to increased levels of circulatory androgens, Lobo et al. found that women with PCOS had increased levels of biologically active (non-SHBG bound) estradiol, although total circulating levels of estradiol were not increased (Fig. 38-10). The increased amount of non-SHBG bound estradiol is caused by a decrease in SHBG levels, which is produced primarily by the increased levels of androgens and secondarily by the obesity present in many of these women. The tonically increased levels of biologically active estradiol may stimulate increased GnRH pulsatility and produce tonically elevated LH levels and anovulation. In addition, the lowered SHBG level increases the bi-

ologically active fractions of the elevated androgens in the circulation. The importance of the decreased levels of SHBG is shown schematically in Fig. 38-11.

About 20% of women with PCOS also have mildly elevated levels of prolactin (20 to 30 ng/ml), possibly related to increased pulsatility of GnRH or to a relative dopamine deficiency or to both. In addition, many women with this syndrome have mild degrees of hyperinsulinism and insulin resistance.

The ovaries of most women with PCOS are enlarged, being as much as 5 cm in diameter. The capsules are smooth, white, and thickened (Fig. 38-12). Beneath the capsules are numerous small cysts (Fig. 38-13). These anatomic findings are not pathognomonic for PCOS, because they also have been noted in some women with Cushing's syndrome or congenital adrenal hyperplasia and in association with certain adrenal tumors. Although the ovaries of women with PCOS produce excessive amounts of androgen, particularly androstenedione, there is no inherent endocrinologic abnormality in the ovaries. The tonically elevated levels

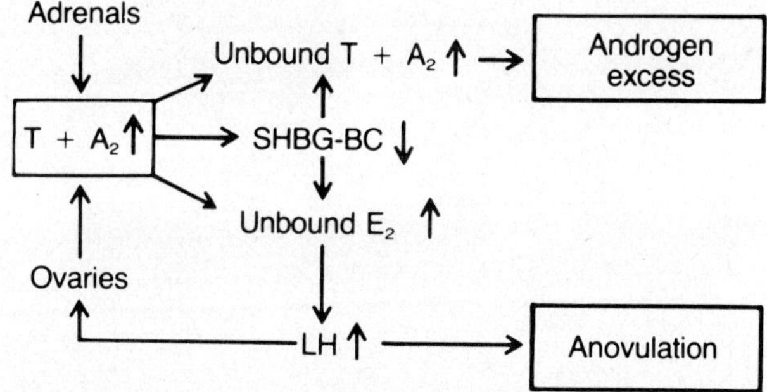

FIGURE 38-11

Scheme depicting the possible role of adrenal-derived androgen (T, testosterone; A_2, androstanediol) in initiating androgen excess and anovulation. (From Lobo RA, Goebelsmann U: Am J Obstet Gynecol 142:394, 1982.)

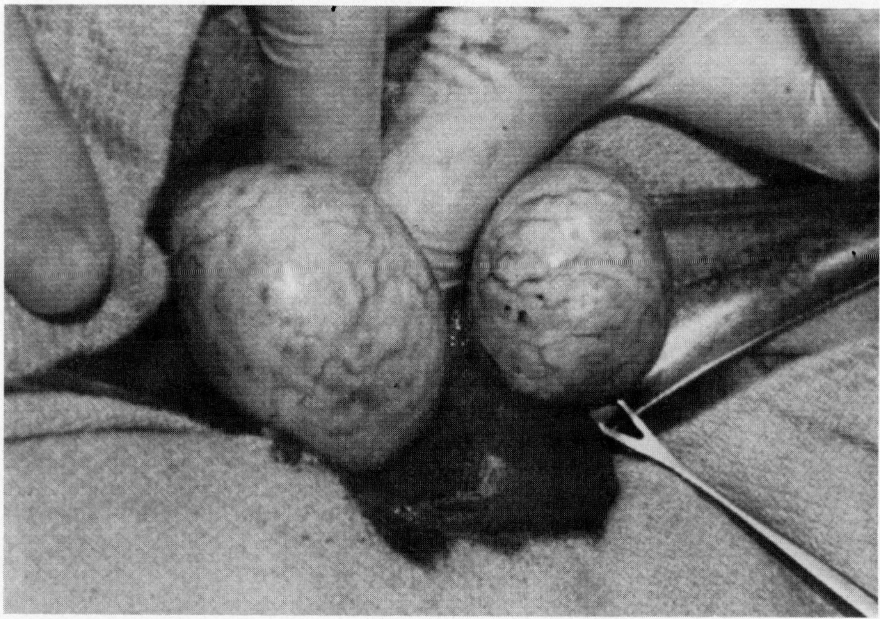

FIGURE 38-12

Gross characteristics of polycystic ovaries. Bilateral enlarged ovaries with smooth and thickened capsule. (From Yen SSC: Chronic anovulation caused by peripheral endocrine disorders. In Yen SSC, Jaffe RB, eds: Reproductive endocrinology, 2nd ed. Philadelphia, W.B. Saunders Co., 1986.)

of LH cause the stromal tissue to produce more androstenedione and other androgens, which in turn produces premature follicular atresia. Furthermore, the ovaries are deficient in aromatase, probably because of the low FSH levels, and this deficiency results in less conversion of androstenedione to estrogen in the ovary. The polycystic ovary does not secrete increased amounts of estrogen or estradiol, but the increased levels of androstenedione are peripherally converted to estrone, causing increased circulating estrone levels.

The etiology of this endocrinologic abnormality has not been determined. It has been suggested that heredity, central catecholamine abnormalities, psychological stress, and obesity

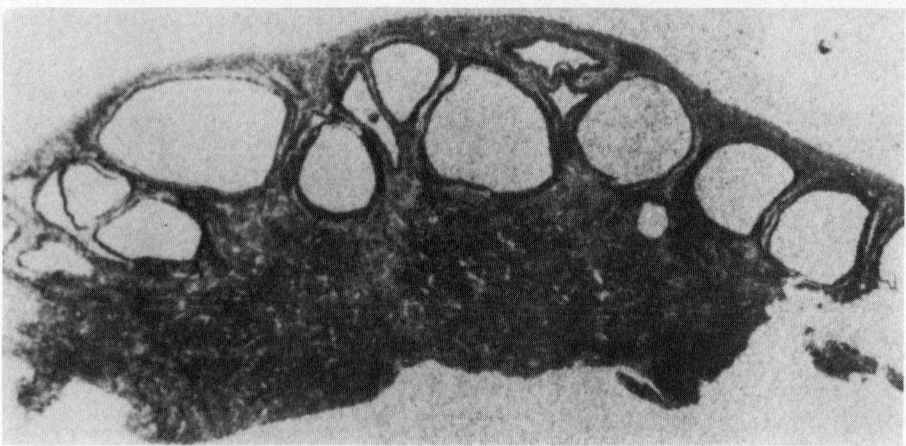

FIGURE 38-13

Sagittal section of typical Stein-Leventhal type of polycystic ovary illustrating large number of follicular cysts. (From Wilroy RS Jr, Givens JR, Wiser WL, Coleman SA, Anderson RN, Summitt RL: Hyperthecosis: An inheritable form of polycystic ovarian disease. In Bergsma D (ed): "Genetic Forms of Hypogonadism." Miami: Symposia Specialists for the National Foundation-March of Dimes, BD:OAS XI(4):81, 1975, with permission.

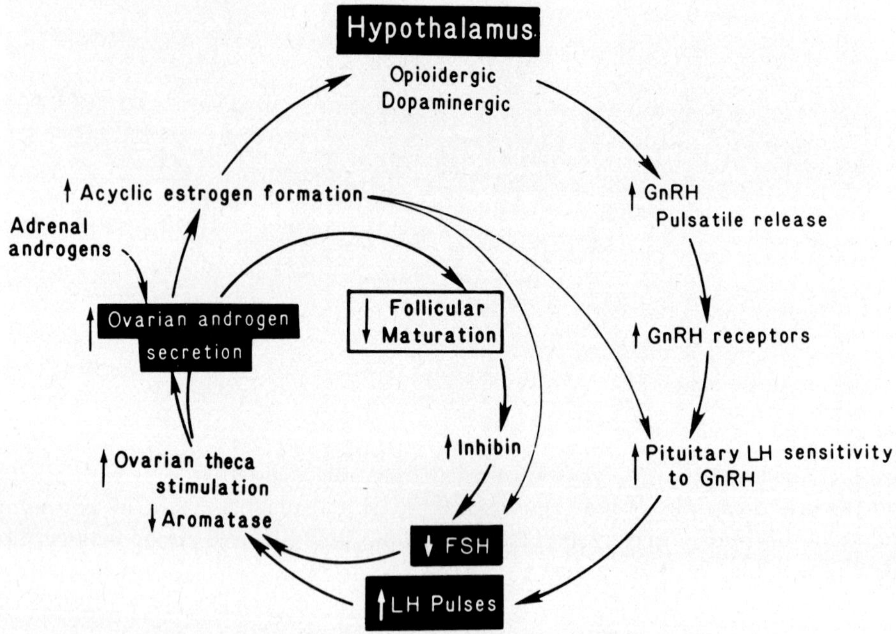

FIGURE 38-14

The interdependent event of high LH-FSH ratio occasioned by an increased GnRH secretion as a consequence of reduced hypothalamic inhibition. This setting induces an increased ovarian androgen production by the theca cells and acyclic estrogen feedback system in maintenance of chronic anovulation in PCOS. (Modified from Yen SSC, Chaney C, Judd HL: Functional aberrations of the hypothalamic-pituitary system in polycystic ovary syndrome: A consideration of the pathogenesis. In James VHT, Serio M, Guisti G, eds: The endocrine function of the human ovary. New York, Academic Press, 1976, pp. 373-385.)

may be involved. The evidence for a genetic cause is suggestive but not clearly established. Data suggesting an abnormality in central nervous system catecholamine metabolism are more convincing but not yet conclusive. Although women with PCOS have more psychological stress than do control subjects, the stress may be a result, not the cause, of the syndrome. Obesity probably enhances the syndrome because of the decrease in SHBG but is probably not important in its pathogenesis, because the syndrome occurs in some thin women and because many obese women do not have PCOS.

Whatever the etiology, the endocrinologic effects of PCOS produce a vicious cycle of events, as shown by Yen (Fig. 38-14). The increased pulsatility of GnRh produces tonically elevated LH levels and increased ovarian androgen production. Peripheral conversion of androstenedione to estrone in conjunction with the decreased SHBG levels causes tonic hyperestrogenism, which increases the pituitary sensitivity to GnRh and leads to increased LH release.

Stromal Hyperthecosis

Stromal hyperthecosis is an uncommon benign ovarian disorder in which the ovaries are bilaterally enlarged, being about 5 to 7 cm in diameter, and histologically have nests of lu-

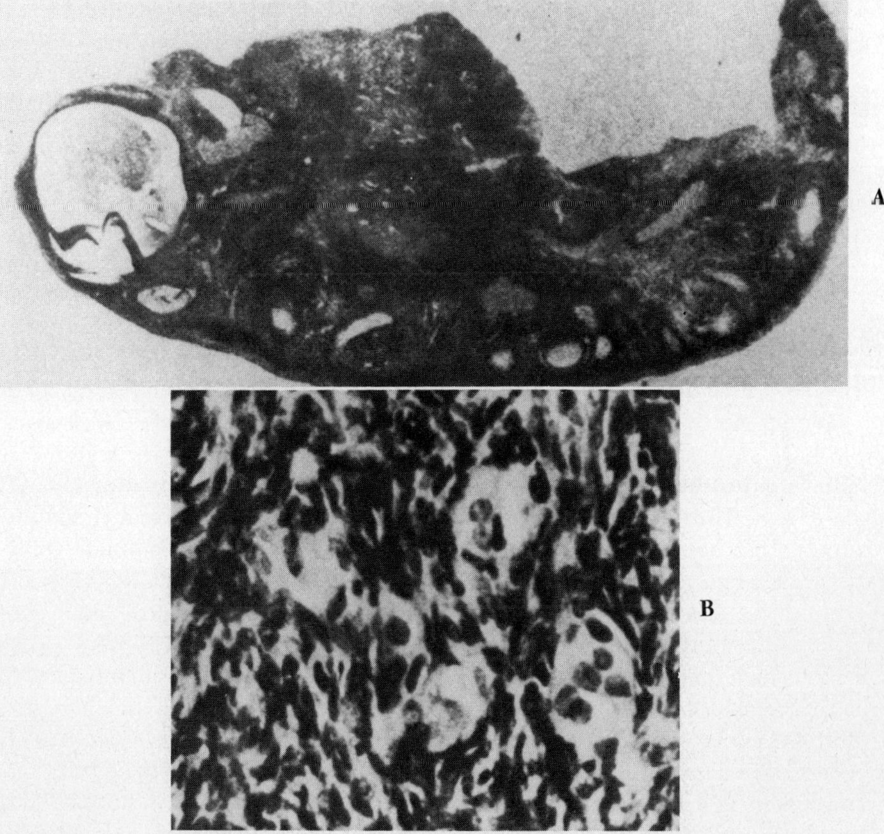

FIGURE 38-15
A, Sagittal section of typical hyperthecotic ovary illustrating small number of follicular cysts and massive amount of stromal hyperplasia. **B,** Islands of luteinized thecalike cells deep in stroma of ovary in hyperthecosis. (From Wilroy RS Jr, Givens JR, Wiser WL, Coleman SA, Anderson RN, Summitt RL: Hyperthecosis: An inheritable form of polycystic ovarian disease. In Bergsma D (ed): "Genetic Forms of Hypogonadism." Miami: Symposia Specialists for the National Foundation-March of Dimes, BD:OAS XI(4):81, 1975, with permission.)

teinized theca cells within the stroma (Fig. 38-15). The capsules of these ovaries are thick and similar to those found in women with PCOS, but unlike PCOS, subcapsular cysts are uncommon. The theca cells produce large amounts of testosterone as determined by retrograde ovarian vein catheterization. Like PCOS, this disorder has a gradual onset and is initially associated with anovulation or amenorrhea and hirsutism. However, unlike PCOS, with increasing age the ovaries secrete steadily increasing amounts of testosterone. Thus when women with this disorder reach the fourth decade of life, the severity of the hirsutism increases and signs of virilization such as temporal balding, clitoral enlargement, deepening of the voice, and decreased breast size appear and gradually increase in severity. By this time serum testosterone levels are usually in excess of 2 ng/ml, similar to levels found in ovarian and adrenal testosterone-producing tumors. However, with the latter conditions the symptoms of virilization appear and progress much more rapidly than with ovarian hyperthecosis, whose symptoms progress gradually over many years.

Androgen-Producing Tumors

Ovarian Neoplasms

It is possible for nearly every type of ovarian neoplasm to have stromal cells that secrete excessive amounts of testosterone and cause signs of androgen excess. Thus on rare occasions excess testosterone produced by both benign and malignant cystadenomas, Brenner tumors, and Krukenberg tumors has caused hirsutism or virilization or both. Certain germ cell tumors contain many testosterone-producing cells. The testosterone produced by two of these neoplasms—Sertoli-Leydig cell tumors and hilus cell tumors—nearly always causes virilization. In addition, lipoid cell (adrenal rest) tumors can produce increased amounts of testosterone or DHEA-S or both. Rarely granulosa-theca cell tumors can also produce testosterone in addition to increased levels of estradiol.

Androgen-producing ovarian tumors usually produce rapidly progressive signs of virilization. Sertoli-Leydig cell tumors usually develop during the reproductive age (second to fourth decades), and by the time they produce detectable signs of androgen excess the tumor is nearly always (more than 85% of the time) palpable during bimanual examination. These tumors are uncommon. Less than 1% of solid ovarian neoplasms are Sertoli-Leydig cell tumors. Hilus cell tumors most often occur after menopause. They are usually small and not palpable during bimanual examination; however, the history of rapid development of signs of virilization and the presence of markedly elevated levels of testosterone with normal levels of DHEA-S usually facilitate the diagnosis.

Congenital Adrenal Hyperplasia (Adult Onset)

Congenital adrenal hyperplasia (CAH) is due to an enzymatic defect (either 21-hydroxylase or 11β-hydroxylase) resulting in decreased cortisol biosynthesis. As a consequence, ACTH secretion is increased and adrenal production of cortisol precursors proximal to the enzymatic block is also increased. These precursors include both 17-hydroxypregnenolone and 17-hydroxyprogesterone (Fig. 38-16). Because of the enzymatic block these steroids are mainly converted to DHEA and androstenedione. These C_{19} steroids are in turn peripherally converted to testosterone, and the resultant elevated testosterone levels produce signs of androgen excess. Because the enzymatic defects are congenital, the complete block usually becomes manifest in fetal life through masculinization of the female external genitalia. CAH is the most common cause of sexual ambiguity in the newborn. However, incomplete mild defects may not produce physical signs associated with increased androgen production until after puberty. Thus this entity may be associated with the development of hirsutism or virilization or both in a woman in the late second or early third decade of life. Lobo and Goebelsmann have estimated that this entity may be present in as many as 5% of women with hirsutism. This entity is also usually associated with menstrual irregularity. It has been hypothesized that the mechanism for anovulation is similar to that occurring with PCOS. The increased levels of androgen lower SHBG levels, thus increasing the amount of biologically active circulating estradiol. The increased estradiol stimulates tonic LH release, which increases ovarian androgen production and locally inhib-

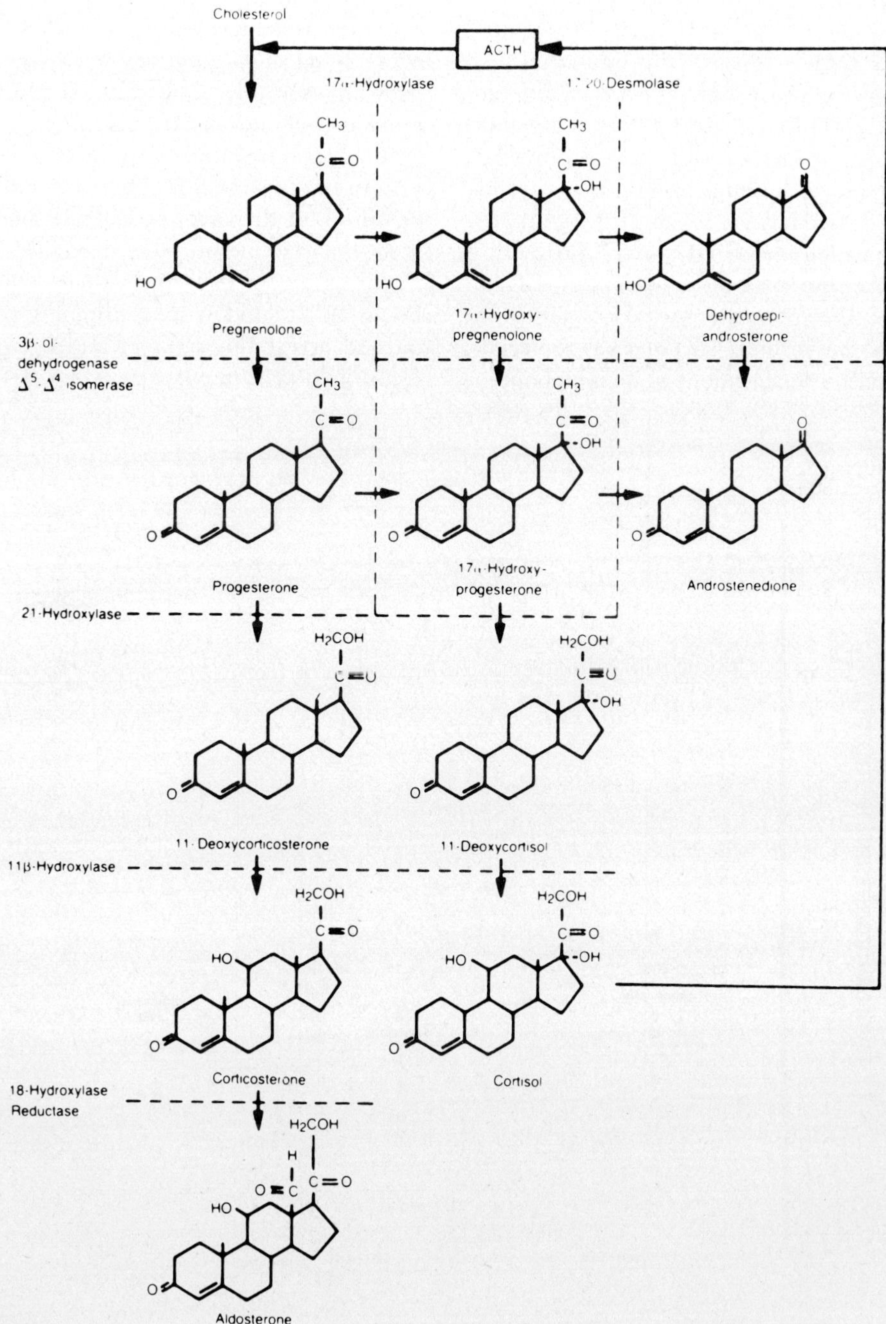

FIGURE 38-16

Adrenal steroid biosynthesis depicting mineralocorticoid, glucocorticoid, and C_{19} steroid ("androgen") pathways and corresponding enzymes. (From Goebelsmann U: Steroid hormones. Reproduced with permission from Infertility, contraception and reproductive endocrinology, 2nd ed, by Daniel R. Mishell, Jr., M.D., and Val Davajan, M.D. Copyright © 1986 Medical Economics Book, Oradell, N.J. 07649. All rights reserved.)

its follicular growth and ovulation. Thus women with this disorder present with postpubertal onset of hirsutism and oligomenorrhea or amenorrhea similar to women with PCOS. However, women with CAH, unlike those with PCOS, may have a history of prepubertal accelerated growth (ages 6 to 8 years) with later decreased growth and a short ultimate height. Such a history, a family history of postpubertal onset of hirsutism, findings of mild evidence of virilization, and DHEA-S levels > 5 μg/ml are each an indication that CAH may be present.

To confirm the diagnosis measurement of serum 17-hydroxyprogesterone (17-OHP) levels should be performed. This test has replaced the less precise measurement of its metabolite, pregnanetriol. If levels of 17-OHP are greater than 8 ng/ml, the diagnosis of CAH is established. If 17-OHP is above normal (3 ng/ml) but less than 8 ng/ml, an ACTH stimulation test should be performed. The patient should ingest 1 mg of dexamethasone at 11 P.M. The following morning a baseline 17-OHP should be measured and 25 IU of synthetic ACTH infused as a single bolus. One hour later another serum sample should be obtained and 17-OHP measured. If the level of 17-OHP increases to more than 20 ng/ml, the diagnosis is established (Fig. 38-17). Individuals with CAH should be treated with continuous corticosteroids to arrest the signs of androgenicity and restore ovulatory menstrual cycles.

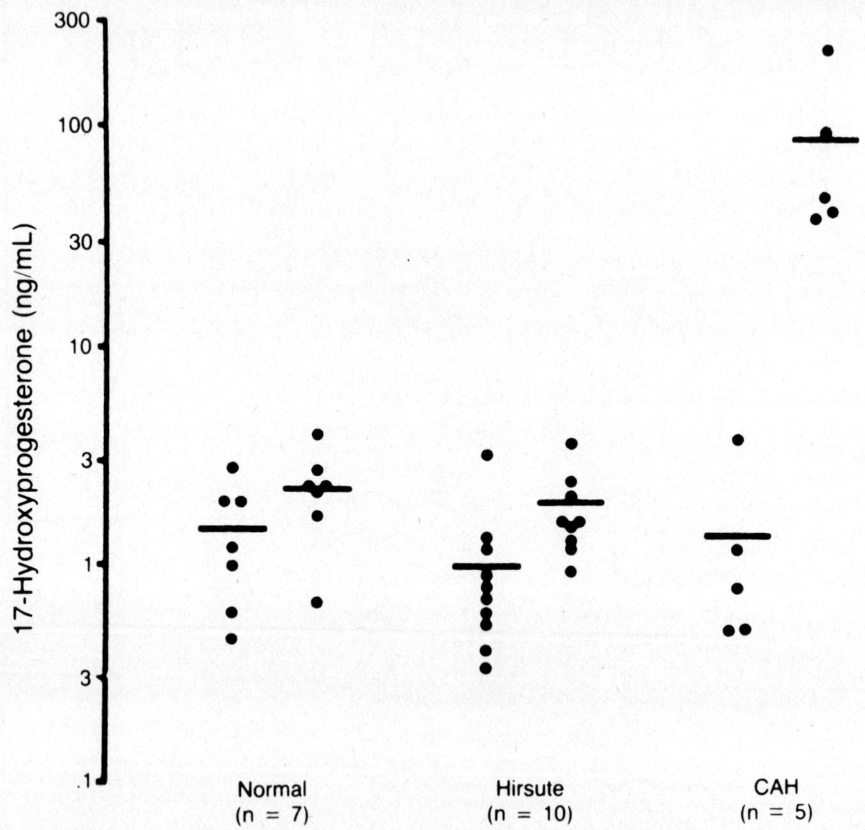

FIGURE 38-17

Serum 17-hydroxyprogesterone before and 60 minutes after a single intravenous bolus of 0.25 mg ACTH in normal women, hirsute patients, and patients with adult manifestation of congenital adrenal hyperplasia *(CAH)* after 1 mg of dexamethasone at 11 P.M. Note markedly increased response (log scale) only in patients with adult manifestation of congenital adrenal hyperplasia. (From Lobo RA, Goebelsmann U: Am J Obstet Gynecol 138:720, 1980.)

Cushing's Syndrome

Excessive adrenal production of glucocorticoids due to increased ACTH secretion (Cushing's disease) or adrenal tumors produces the signs and symptoms of Cushing's syndrome. These findings include hirsutism and menstrual irregularity in addition to the classic findings of centripetal obesity, dorsal neck fat pads, abdominal striae, and muscle wasting and weakness. The latter catabolic effect of glucocorticoid excess differs from the anabolic effects of testosterone excess, but some patients with PCOS may have other clinical findings that are similar to those found with Cushing's syndrome. In such instances Cushing's syndrome can be easily excluded by performing an overnight dexamethasone suppression test. Dexamethasone, 1 mg, is ingested at 11 P.M., and plasma cortisol is measured the following morning at 8 A.M. (Fig. 38-18). If the cortisol level is less than 5 µg/100 ml, Cushing's syndrome is ruled out. If the cortisol level fails to suppress to this degree, the diagnosis of Cushing's syndrome is not established. It is necessary to perform a complete dexamethasone suppression test (Liddle's test) to determine whether Cushing's syndrome exists.

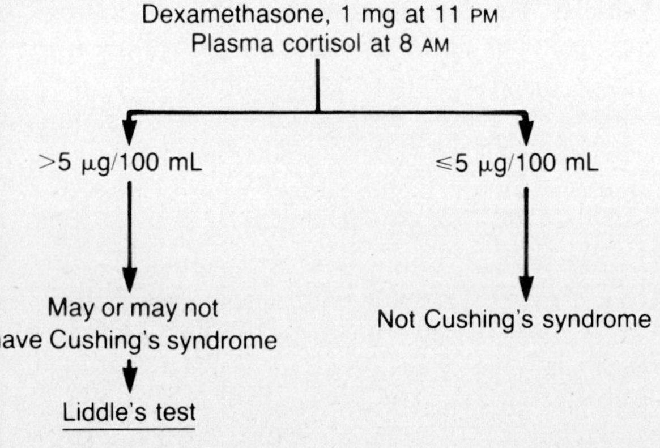

FIGURE 38-18
Outline of overnight dexamethasone suppression test. (From Goebelsmann U, Lobo RA: Androgen excess. Reproduced with permission from Infertility, contraception and reproductive endocrinology, 2nd ed, by Daniel R. Mishell, Jr., M.D., and Val Davajan, M.D. Copyright © 1986 Medical Economics Books, Oradell, N.J. 07649. All rights reserved.)

Adrenal Tumors

Nearly all the androgen-producing adrenal tumors are adenomas or carcinomas that generate large amounts of the C_{19} steroids normally produced by the adrenal gland: DHEA-S, DHEA, and androstenedione. Although these tumors do not usually directly secrete testosterone, testosterone is produced by extraglandular conversion of DHEA and androstenedione. Patients with these tumors usually have markedly elevated serum levels of DHEA-S (>8 µg/ml) as well as urinary excretion of 17-KS. Patients with these laboratory findings and a history of rapid onset of signs of androgen excess should undergo a computerized tomography (CT) scan of the adrenal glands to confirm the diagnosis. In addition to patients with these uncommon tumors a few patients with testosterone-producing adrenal adenomas have been reported. The cellular patterns of these tumors resemble those of ovarian hilus cells, and the tumors secrete large amounts of testosterone. Because adrenal adenomas also secrete DHEA-S, the presence of such tumors should be considered in patients with DHEA-S levels greater than 8 ng/ml and a testosterone level greater than 1.5 ng/ml.

DIFFERENTIAL DIAGNOSIS

The differential diagnosis of the causes of androgen excess presented above can usually be made without difficulty by means of a complete history, a careful physical examination, and measurement of serum levels of testosterone and DHEA-S to determine if there is an ovarian or adrenal source of excess androgen production. As mentioned above, androgen excess due to iatrogenic causes, sexual ambiguity, or pregnancy-associated ovarian tumors can usually be easily determined by the history and physical examination. Masculinizing ovarian or adrenal tumors are associated with rapidly progressive signs of hirsutism and virilization. Serum testosterone levels greater than 2 ng/ml with normal DHEA-S levels are consistent with ovarian tumors, and the diagnosis can be confirmed by bimanual pelvic examination or CT scans. Patients with rapid progression of virilization and DHEA-S levels greater than 8 µg/ml are most likely to have an androgen-producing adrenal adenoma, and the diagnosis can be confirmed by CT scan. A long history of gradually increasing hirsutism, even if accompanied by virilization, is not consistent with the diagnosis of adrenal or ovarian tumors. The diagnosis of ovarian stromal thecosis should be suspected for individuals with these signs and testosterone levels greater than 1.5 ng/ml. Patients with physical findings consistent with Cushing's syndrome should have the diagnosis ruled out or confirmed by an overnight dexamethasone suppression test followed by Liddle's test if necessary. The remaining three diagnoses—PCOS, adult-onset CAH and idiopathic hirsutism—may be associated with a similar history and findings at physical examination, although menstrual irregularity is an uncommon finding in women with idiopathic hirsutism. Patients with CAH may have a family history of androgen excess, early onset of rapid growth, and short stature as well as signs of mild virilization. The diagnosis can be established by measurement of 17-OHP either by a random serum sample or following ACTH stimulation. Most patients with PCOS have elevated LH levels and mildly increased testosterone or DHEA-S levels, whereas women with idiopathic hirsutism have normal levels of these hormones. Treatment of hirsutism depends on whether the source of the androgen excess is ovarian, adrenal, or peripheral.

MANAGEMENT

Ovarian and Adrenal Tumors

Nearly all Sertoli-Leydig cell tumors are unilateral. If the woman desires further reproduction and these tumors are well differentiated and confined to the ovary, the tumors may be treated by unilateral salpingo-oophorectomy. Since most hilus cell tumors occur after menopause, they are best treated by bilateral salpingo-oophorectomy and total abdominal hysterectomy. Adrenal adenomas and carcinomas also should be treated by operative removal. Adrenal carcinomas frequently have metastasized to the liver by the time the androgenic signs have developed. Despite chemotherapy the prognosis is poor after metastases have occurred. Stromal hyperthecosis is also best treated by bilateral salpingo-oophorectomy to-

gether with total abdominal hysterectomy. After removal of the ovaries of patients with stromal hyperthecosis or any of the androgen-producing tumors, the acne and oiliness of the skin disappear, breast size increases, and clitoral size decreases. The excess central hair becomes finer and grows less rapidly but does not disappear. Electrolysis can remove the facial hair, and depilatories, bleaches, or shaving can be used to treat the body hair.

Congenital Adrenal Hyperplasia

Patients with adult-onset of CAH should be treated daily with glucocorticoids such as hydrocortisone (20 to 25 mg), prednisone (5 to 7.5 mg), or dexamethasone (0.5 to 0.75 mg) in divided doses. Sometimes lower doses of these agents may be sufficient to suppress ACTH and decrease adrenal androgen production. Signs of androgen excess gradually lessen, and ovulation usually resumes within a few weeks.

Polycystic Ovarian Syndrome

The treatment of PCOS depends on which aspect of the disorder—hirsutism, infertility, or irregular prolonged menses (dysfunctional uterine bleeding)—is of greatest concern to the patient. The best treatment for PCOS, unless pregnancy is desired, is oral steroid contraceptives, because these agents inhibit LH, decrease circulating testosterone levels, and increase levels of SHBG and thus bind and inactivate more of the testosterone in the circulation (Fig. 38-19). It is best to use an oral contraceptive formulation that contains less than 50 µg estrogen and a progestin other than norgestrel, because norgestrel is the most androgenic progestin in current use. As reported by Wild et al. and Klove et al., oral contraceptives also decrease serum DHEA-S. If the levels are only mildly elevated, oral contraceptives alone will reduce them to normal. If DHEA-S levels are moderately elevated (>4 µg/ml), dexamethasone (0.25 to 0.5 mg at bedtime) should be given together with the oral contraceptive to reduce DHEA-S to normal. Silver et al. have shown that if hirsutism continues to be a problem, spironolactone (50 to 100 mg twice daily) causes regression of the

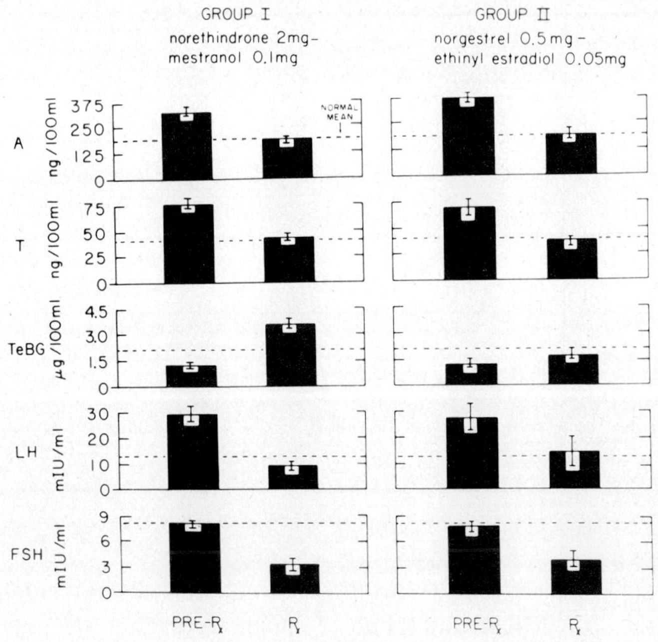

FIGURE 38-19

Mean pretreatment *(Pre-*R$_x$*)* and treatment (R$_x$) plasma levels of Δ^4-androstenedione *(A)*, testosterone *(T)*, testosterone-estrogen-binding globulin *(TeBG)* capacity, LH, and FSH of hirsute women. Bars define standard errors of means. (From Givens JR, Andersen RN, Wiser WL, et al: Am J Obstet Gynecol 124:333, 1976.)

hirsutism in women with PCOS by decreasing androgenic action in the target organs.

Although ovarian wedge resection was advocated in the past for treatment of androgen excess, the decrease in circulating androgens occurred for only a short period of time, and thus this therapy should no longer be used. However, for the woman over 35 who does not desire future childbearing and who has excess ovarian androgen production due to PCOS, bilateral salpingo-oophorectomy and hysterectomy may be a desirable method of alleviating the problem.

Women with PCOS who desire fertility should be treated with agents that stimulate ovulation, starting with clomiphene citrate and, if the condition is unresponsive, proceeding to human menopausal gonadotrophin (HMG) or GnRH. If women with PCOS do not have hirsutism but have dysfunctional bleeding or oligomenorrhea, regular withdrawal bleeding should be induced with monthly progestins such as oral medroxyprogesterone acetate 10 mg daily for the first 10 days of the month. Pro-

gestins should be administered to prevent development of endometrial hyperplasia due to unopposed menopausal estrogen.

Idiopathic Hirsutism

Although hirsutism is a benign condition, it is frequently of great concern to the patient. Women with idiopathic hirsutism have normal circulating levels of testosterone and DHEA-S. Nearly all those individuals with symptomatic hirsutism who have normal testosterone and DHEA-S levels have elevated levels of Adiol-G indicative of increased peripheral androgen activity. It is not necessary to measure Adiol-G in patients with hirsutism without elevated circulating androgen levels, because the presence of hirsutism is itself evidence of increased peripheral androgen activity. An agent that inhibits peripheral androgen activity should be administered to women with these findings. These antiandrogens include spironolactone, cimetidine, and cyproterone acetate. The last drug is available in Europe but not in the

TABLE 38-4

Treatment of Hirsutism According to Source of Androgen Excess

Androgen	Treatment
↑ T	Oral contraceptives
↑ DHEA-S (<4 μg/ml)	Oral contraceptives
↑ DHEA-S (>4 μg/ml), normal T	Dexamethasone
↑ T, ↑ DHEA-S (>4 μg/ml)	Oral contraceptives + dexamethasone
Normal T, normal DHEA-S, ↑ Adiol-G	Spironolactone*

From Goebelsmann U, Lobo RA: Androgen excess. Reproduced with permission from Infertility, contraception and reproductive endocrinology, 2nd ed, by Daniel R. Mishell, Jr., M.D., and Val Davajan, M.D. Copyright © 1986 Medical Economics Books, Oradell, N.J. 07649. All rights reserved.

T, testosterone.

*Spironolactone may also be substituted for any of the above regimens if no improvement is noted after 3 months of treatment.

United States. Spironolactone has been used and studied more extensively than cimetidine and should be considered the treatment of choice in the United States for women with idiopathic hirsutism (as well as some with PCOS). Cummings et al. have reported that hair shaft density and rate of hair growth decreased after 2 months of spironolactone therapy. Lobo et al. found that a dose of 200 mg/per day of spironolactone is more effective than 100 mg per day. With the higher dose, liver function tests and plasma electrolytes are unchanged, and side effects, primarily irregular bleeding, are uncommon.

In summary, the treatment of hirsutism should depend on the source of the excess androgens. If testosterone levels are elevated, indicating excess ovarian androgen production, then oral contraceptive therapy should be instituted. If DHEA-S levels are increased, indicating excess adrenal androgen secretion, then dexamethasone therapy should be used. If neither is elevated, then spironolactone should be administered. Lobo has developed an outline for the treatment of hirsutism according to the source of the androgen excess (Table 38-4). It can be used as a guide for therapy.

• • •

KEY POINTS

- Testosterone levels in women with hirsutism without virilization are lower than 1.5 ng/ml.

- Circulating testosterone levels in the presence of virilization are usually greater than 2 ng/ml.

- The major androgen provided by the ovaries is testosterone and that of the adrenal glands, DHEA-S.

- Total daily testosterone production is 0.35 mg: 0.1 mg from ovarian secretion, 0.2 mg from peripheral conversion of androstenedione, and 0.05 mg from peripheral conversion of DHEA.

- About two thirds of the daily testosterone production in a woman originates in the ovaries.

- Serum levels of DHEA-S correlate well with daily urinary 17-KS excretion.

- About 85% of testosterone is bound to SHBG and is biologically inactive, 10% to 15% is bound to albumin, and 1% to 2% is not bound. Both of the latter fractions are biologically active.

- Non-SHBG bound testosterone is elevated in about 60% to 70% of women with hirsutism, and Adiol-G is elevated in about 98%.

- Women with idiopathic hirsutism have increased peripheral 5α-reductase activity as well as circulating levels of Adiol-G.

- Women with PCOS have testosterone levels between 70 and 120 ng/dl and androstenedione levels of 3 to 5 ng/ml; about half have elevated levels of DHEA-S.

- About 30% of women with PCOS do not have hirsutism.

- About 70% of women with PCOS have elevated levels of immunologic LH or an immunologic LH-FSH ratio greater than 3, and nearly all have elevated levels of biologically active LH and biologically active estradiol.

- Women with adult onset of CAH have a block in cortisol biosynthesis of 11β-hydroxylase or 21-hydroxylase resulting in increased circulating levels of 17-OHP.

- If after an overnight dexamethasone suppression test serum cortisol levels are lower than 5 μg/100 ml, Cushing's syndrome is ruled out.

- The best treatment for hirsutism due to increased peripheral androgen metabolism is the antiandrogen spironolactone.

________________ **KEY POINTS, cont'd** ______________________________________

- Women with PCOS who desire fertility should be treated with agents that stimulate ovulation, starting with clomiphene citrate and, if the condition is unresponsive, proceeding to HMG or GnRH.

- The treatment of hirsutism should depend on the source of the excess androgens. If testosterone levels are elevated, indicating excess ovarian androgen production, then oral contraceptive therapy should be instituted. If DHEA-S is increased, indicating excess adrenal androgen secretion, then dexamethasone therapy should be used. If neither is elevated, then spironolactone should be administered.

BIBLIOGRAPHY

Anderson DC: Sex hormone-binding globulin. Clin Endocrinol 3:69, 1981.

Behrman SJ, Scully RE: Case records of the Massachusetts General Hospital: infertility and irregular menses in a 27-year-old woman. N Engl J Med 287:1192, 1972.

Boyers P, Buster JE, Marshall JR: Hypothalamic-pituitary-adrenocortical function during long-term low-dose dexamethasone therapy in hyperandrogenized women. Am J Obstet Gynecol 142:330, 1982.

Burger CW, Korsen T, van Kessel H, et al: Pulsatile luteinizing hormone patterns in the follicular phase of the menstrual cycle, polycystic ovarian disease (PCOD) and non-PCOD secondary amenorrhea. J Clin Endocrinol Metab 61:1126, 1985.

Casey J: Chronic treatment regimens for hirsutism in women: Effect on blood production rates of testosterone and on hair growth. Clin Endocrinol 4:313, 1975.

Chang RJ, Mandel FP, Wolfsen AR, et al: Circulating levels of plasma adrenocorticotropin in polycystic ovary disease. J Clin Endocrinol Metab 54:1265, 1982.

Cumming D, Yang JC, Rebar RW, et al: Treatment of hirsutism with spironolactone. JAMA 247:1295, 1982.

DeVane GW, Czekala NM, Judd HL, et al: Circulating gonadotropins, estrogens, and androgens in polycystic ovarian disease. Am J Obstet Gynecol 121:496, 1975.

Ferriman D, Gallwey JD: Clinical assessment of body hair growth in women. J Clin Endocrinol Metab 21:1440, 1961.

Givens JR, Andersen RN, Wiser WL, et al: The effectiveness of two oral contraceptives in suppressing plasma androstanedione, testosterone, LH and FSH, and stimulating plasma testosterone-binding capacity in hirsute women. Am J Obstet Gynecol 124:333, 1976.

Givens JR, Andersen RN, Wiser WL, et al: A gonadotropin responsive adrenocortical adenoma. J Clin Endocrinol Metab 38:126, 1974.

Goebelsmann U: Steroid hormones. In Mishell DR, Davajan V, eds: Infertility, contraception and reproductive endocrinology, 2nd ed. Oradell, N.J., Medical Economics Books, 1986.

Goebelsmann U, Lobo RA: Androgen excess. In Mishell DR, Davajan V, eds: Infertility, contraception, and reproductive endocrinology, 2nd ed. Oradell, N.J., Medical Economics Books, 1986.

Goldzieher JW: Polycystic ovarian syndrome. Fertil Steril 35:371, 1981.

Goldzieher JW, Axelrod LR: Clinical and biochemical features of polycystic ovarian disease. Fertil Steril 14:631, 1963.

Hensleigh PA, Woodruff JD: Differential maternal-fetal response to androgenizing luteoma or hyperreactio luteinalis. Obstet Gynecol Surv 33:262, 1978.

Hoffman D, Klove K, Lobo RA: The prevalence and significance of elevated dehydroepiandrone sulfate levels in anovulatory women. Fertil Steril 42:76, 1984.

Horton R, Hawks D, Lobo RA: 3α,17β-androstanediol glucuronide in plasma. A marker of androgen action in idiopathic hirsutism. J Clin Invest 69:1203, 1982.

Horton R, Lobo RA: Peripheral androgens and the role of androstanediol glucuronide. Clin Endocrinol Metab 15:293, 1986.

Ireland K, Woodruff JD: Masculinizing ovarian tumors. Obstet Gynecol Surv 31:83, 1976.

Judd HL, Rigg LA, Anderson DC, et al: The effects of ovarian wedge resection on circulating gonadotropin and ovarian steroid levels in patients with polycystic ovary syndrome. J Clin Endocrinol Metab 43:347, 1976.

Judd HL, Scully RE, Herbst AL, et al: Familial hyperthecosis: Comparison of endocrinologic and histologic findings with polycystic ovarian disease. Am J Obstet Gynecol 117:976, 1973.

Klove KL, Roy S, Lobo RA: The effect of different contraceptive treatments on the serum concentration of dehydroepiandrosterone sulfate. Contraception 29:319, 1984.

Lobo RA, Goebelsmann U: Adult manifestation of congenital adrenal hyperplasia due to incomplete 21-hydroxylase deficiency mimicking polycystic ovarian disease. Am J Obstet Gynecol 138:720, 1980.

Lobo RA, Goebelsmann U: Effect of androgen excess on inappropriate gonadotropin secretion as found in polycystic ovary syndrome. Am J Obstet Gynecol 142:394, 1982.

Lobo RA, Goebelsmann U: Evidence for reduced 3β-ol-hydroxysteroid dehydrogenase activity in some hirsute women thought to have polycystic ovary syndrome. J Clin Endocrinol Metab 53:394, 1981.

Lobo RA, Goebelsmann U, Horton R: Evidence for the importance of peripheral tissue events in the development of hirsutism in polycystic ovary syndrome. J Clin Endocrinol Metab 57:393, 1983.

Lobo RA, Granger L, Goebelsmann U, et al: Elevation in unbound serum estradiol as a possible mechanism for inappropriate gonadotropin secretion in women with PCO. J Clin Endocrinol Metab 52:156, 1981.

Lobo RA, Granger LR, Paul WL, et al: Psychological stress and increases in urinary norepinephrine metabolites, platelet serotonin and adrenal androgens in women with polycystic ovary syndrome. Am J Obstet Gynecol 145:496, 1983.

Lobo RA, Kletzky OA, Campeau JD, et al: Elevated bioactive luteinizing hormone in women with the polycystic ovary syndrome. Fertil Steril 39:674, 1983.

Lobo RA, Paul WL, Goebelsmann U: Dehydroepiandrosterone sulfate as an indicator of adrenal androgen function. Obstet Gynecol 57:69, 1981.

Lobo RA, Paul WL, Goebelsmann U: Serum levels of DHEA-S in gynecologic endocrinopathy and infertility. Obstet Gynecol 57:607, 1981.

Lobo RA, Shoupe D, Serafini P, et al: The effect of two doses of spironolactone on serum androgens and anagen hair in hirsute women. Fertil Steril 43:200, 1985.

Luciano AA, Chapler FK, Sherman BM: Hyperprolactinemia in polycystic ovary syndrome. Fertil Steril 41:719, 1984.

Mandel FP, Chang RJ, Dupont B, et al: HLA genotyping in family members and patients with familial polycystic ovarian disease. J Clin Endocrinol Metab 56:862, 1983.

Milewicz A, Silber D, Kirschner MA: Therapeutic effects of spironolactone in polycystic ovary syndrome. Obstet Gynecol 61:429, 1983.

Paulson RJ, Serafini PC, Catalino JA, et al: Measurements of $3\alpha,17\beta$-androstanediol glucuronide in serum and urine and the correlation with skin 5α-reductase activity. Fertil Steril 46:222, 1986.

Plymate SR, Fariss BL, Bassett ML, et al: Obesity and its role in polycystic ovary syndrome. J Clin Endocrinol Metab 52:1246, 1981.

Raj SG, Thompson IE, Berger MJ, et al: Clinical aspects of the polycystic ovary syndrome. Obstet Gynecol 49:552, 1977.

Rebar R, Judd HL, Yen SSC, et al: Characterization of the inappropriate gonadotropin secretion in polycystic ovary syndrome. J Clin Invest 57:1320, 1976.

Serafini P, Aflan R, Lobo RA: 5α-Reductase activity in the genital skin of hirsute women. J Clin Endocrinol Metab 60:349, 1985.

Shoupe D, Lobo RA: Prolactin responses after gonadotropin releasing hormone in polycystic ovary syndrome. Fertil Steril 43:549, 1985.

Vigersky RA, Mehlman I, Glass AR, et al: Treatment of hirsute women with cimetidine. N Engl J Med 303:1042, 1980.

Wild RA, Umstot ES, Andersen RN, et al: Adrenal function in hirsutism. II. Effect of an oral contraceptive. J Clin Endocrinol Metab 54:676, 1981.

Wilroy RS Jr, Givens JR, Wiser WL, et al: Genetic forms of hypogonadism. Birth Defects 11(4), 1975.

Yen SSC: Chronic anovulation caused by peripheral endocrine disorders. In Yen SSC, Jaffe RB, eds: Reproductive endocrinology, 2nd ed. Philadelphia, W.B. Saunders Co., 1986.

Yen SSC, Chaney C, Judd HL: Functional aberrations of the hypothalamic-pituitary system in polycystic ovary syndrome: a consideration of the pathogenesis. In James VHT, Serio M, Guisti G, eds: The endocrine function of the human ovary. New York, Academic Press, 1976.

Infertility

KEY TERMS AND DEFINITIONS

Artificial Insemination. Method to place sperm in the female reproductive tract by means other than sexual intercourse. If the sperm are from the husband, the technique is called *artificial insemination husband* (AIH). If the sperm are from another man, the method has been called *artificial insemination donor* (AID). Other terms are donor insemination and therapeutic donor insemination (TDI).

Azoospermia. Absence of sperm in the semen.

Clomiphene Citrate. Weak estrogenic compound given orally to induce ovulation in anovulatory women with a sufficient amount of circulating estrogen (>40 pg/ml).

Fecundability. Monthly conception rate among a group of couples attempting to conceive.

Fimbrioplasty. Surgical technique of removing adhesions between fimbrial fronds of the partially occluded distal end of the oviduct.

Gamete Intrafallopian Transfer (GIFT). Placement of human ova and sperm into the distal end of the oviduct.

Hamster Egg Penetration Assay (Sperm Penetration Assay). Test of the fertilizing ability of human sperm based on penetration of zona-free hamster ova by the sperm.

Hysterosalpingogram (HSG). Fluoroscopic and x-ray visualization of the interior of the female upper genital tract after instillation of radiopaque dye.

Human Menopausal Gonadotrophin (HMG). Formulation made up of follicle-stimulating hormone (FSH) and luteinizing hormone (LH) derived from urine obtained from menopausal women. The injectable agent is used to stimulate follicular development.

Infertility. Inability of couples of reproductive age to establish a pregnancy by having sexual intercourse within a certain period of time, usually 1 year. Infertility is considered primary if the woman has never been pregnant and secondary if it occurs after one or more pregnancies.

In Vitro Fertilization. Fertilization of human ova by sperm in a laboratory environment.

Luteal Phase Deficiency (Inadequate Luteal Phase). Deficient progesterone secretion or action resulting in a lag of normal endometrial development.

Microsurgery. Operative technique using magnification and fine, nonreactive suture material. Fine electrocoagulation and saline irrigation are also used.

Oligozoospermia (Oligospermia). Presence of fewer than 20 million sperm per milliliter of semen.

Ovarian Hyperstimulation. Enlargement of many ovarian follicles causing gross enlargement of the ovary. It is sometimes accompanied by ascites and hemoconcentration.

Postcoital Test. Microscopic examination of the sperm present in a cervical mucus specimen obtained from a woman several hours after sexual intercourse.

Salpingitis Isthmica Nodosa. Diverticula of the endosalpinx in the muscularis of the isthmic portion of the oviduct.

Salpingolysis. Removal of adhesions attached to an oviduct that appears normal on gross inspection.

Salpingostomy. Surgical creation of a new opening of a completely occluded distal end of the oviduct.

Semen Analysis. Quantitation of various parameters of a semen specimen analyzed after liquefaction has occurred.

Spinnbarkeit. Property of elasticity (distensibility) of cervical mucus.

Washed Intrauterine Insemination. Technique of separating sperm from the semen in an electrolyte solution and then placing the sperm directly into the uterine cavity.

It has been estimated that about 10% to 15% of all married couples in the United States are infertile. The inability of couples to conceive is one of the most common problems for which women seek gynecologic consultation. In 1985 Hull et al. estimated that as many as 10% of initial office visits and one fifth of all office visits for gynecologic problems are related to the diagnosis or treatment of infertility.

The incidence of infertility increases with increasing age of the woman. Earlier data from populations not practicing contraception as well as surveys in the United States indicated that the incidence of infertility gradually increases after the woman reaches age 25 (Table 39-1). In a study of conception rates after 12 cycles of artificial insemination of fertile women whose husbands were azoospermic, Schwartz and Mayaux found that the rate decreased from about 75% when the women were younger than 30, to 61.8% when they were 30 to 35, and to only 54% when they were older than 35. Recent data from an Oxford Family Planning Association study of married women older than 25 who stopped using various types of contraception in order to conceive are consistent with these findings (Table 39-2). Another finding of the Oxford study was that women who smoked more than 15 cigarettes per day had a higher incidence of infertility than nonsmoking women had (Table 39-3). Thus gynecologists should counsel women who wish to bear children to attempt conception as young as possible (preferably before age 30) and to stop smoking.

With currently available diagnostic techniques the etiology of the infertility can be determined for about 85% to 90% of couples. Although the incidence of the various causes of infertility varies among different populations, in the United States approximately 10% to 15% of cases of infertility are due to anovulation, 30% to 40% to an abnormality of semen production, 30% to 40% to pelvic disease interfering with normal tubal motility (adhesions, tubal blockage, or endometriosis), 10% to 15% to abnormalities of sperm transport through the cervical canal, and about 5% to various uncommon causes.

DIAGNOSTIC EVALUATION

During the initial visit a comprehensive history should be elicited and a thorough physical examination performed. The couple should receive complete information about the proposed diagnostic evaluation. This information should include the type of diagnostic procedures, the sequence of their performance, and the appropriate time in the cycle and approximate date when they will be accomplished. In addition, the degree of inconvenience and discomfort, as well as the cost engendered by each step in the evaluation process, should be discussed. The couple should be given information about normal fecundity patterns among fertile as well as

TABLE 39-1

Expected Percentages of Nonsterile Married Women Who Will Conceive in 12 Months of Unprotected Intercourse

Age Group	Conceiving in 12 Months (%)
20-24	86
25-29	78
30-34	63
35-39	52

From Hendershot GE, Mosher WD, Pratt WF: Infertility and age: An unresolved issue. Reprinted with permission from *Family Planning Perspectives* 14:287, 1982.

TABLE 39-2

Age as a Factor in Relative Fertility Rates (Oxford Family Planning Association Contraceptive Study)

Age, Nulliparous Women	No. of Episodes of Attempting Pregnancy	Months of Follow-up	Relative Fertility Rate (95% Confidence Interval)
25-27	1076	130	1.0
28-29	691	128	0.92 (0.83-1.01)
30-31	377	91	0.79 (0.70-0.90)
32-33	181	58	0.75 (0.64-0.89)
34-35	102	51	0.55 (0.43-0.71)
36-37	43	23	0.48 (0.31-0.73)

From Howe G, Westhoff C, Vessey M, et al: Effects of age, cigarette smoking, and other factors on fertility: Findings in a large prospective study. Br Med J 290:1697, 1985.

TABLE 39-3

Cigarette Smoking as a Factor in Relative Fertility Rates (Oxford Family Planning Association Contraceptive Study)

Cigarette Smoking (No./Day)	No. of Episodes of Attempting Pregnancy	Months of Follow-up	Relative Fertility Rate (95% Confidence Interval)
Never smoked	3672	134	1.0
Exsmoker	843	111	0.99 (0.92-1.11)
1-5	389	54	1.00 (0.90-1.11)
6-10	485	94	0.97 (0.88-1.07)
11-15	374	105	0.93 (0.84-1.04)
16-20	334	93	0.79 (0.70-0.89)
$\geq$21	97	29	0.78 (0.62-0.97)
			P (trend) <0.0001

From Howe G, Westhoff C, Vessey M, et al: Effects of age, cigarette smoking, and other factors on fertility: Findings in a large prospective study. Br Med J 290:1697, 1985.

infertile couples to help alleviate their impatience and frustration. They should be told that among fertile couples who have coitus shortly before ovulation there is only about a 25% chance of developing a clinical pregnancy in each ovulatory cycle. Studies of fecundity patterns of fertile couples attempting to conceive indicate that about half will become pregnant by 3 months, 75% by 6 months, and 90% by the end of 1 year (Fig. 39-1).

The mechanism of sperm and ovum transport as well as the anatomic location of fertilization and implantation should also be discussed. The couple should be informed that the optimal time to have sexual intercourse is a few hours before ovulation, because sperm are capable of fertilization for about 1 to 2 days after coitus, but that the egg probably begins to degenerate a few hours after it reaches the ampulla of the oviduct if fertilization does not occur.

The woman's basal body temperature (BBT) increases when circulating levels of progesterone increase, and the sustained increase of BBT occurs following ovulation. Therefore the time of ovulation cannot be predicted in advance by measuring BBT. Newill and Katz correlated the conception rate following a single episode of artificial insemination with the changes in BBT. They reported that the high-

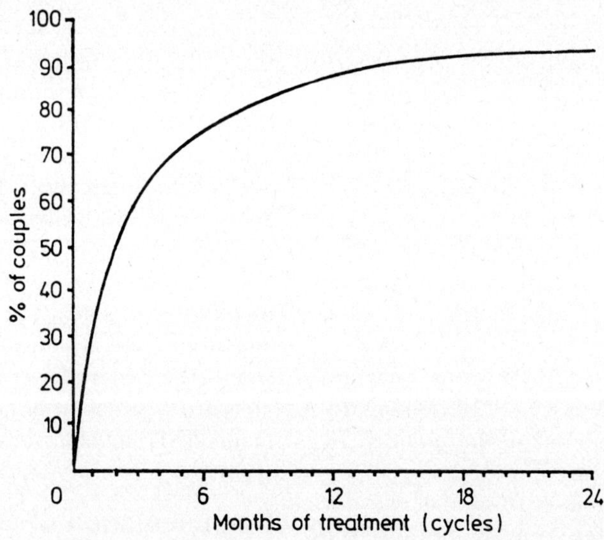

FIGURE 39-1

Cumulative monthly pregnancy rates reported for couples of proved fertility attempting to conceive. (From Hull MGR, Glazener CMA, Kelly NJ, et al: Br Med J 291:1693, 1985.)

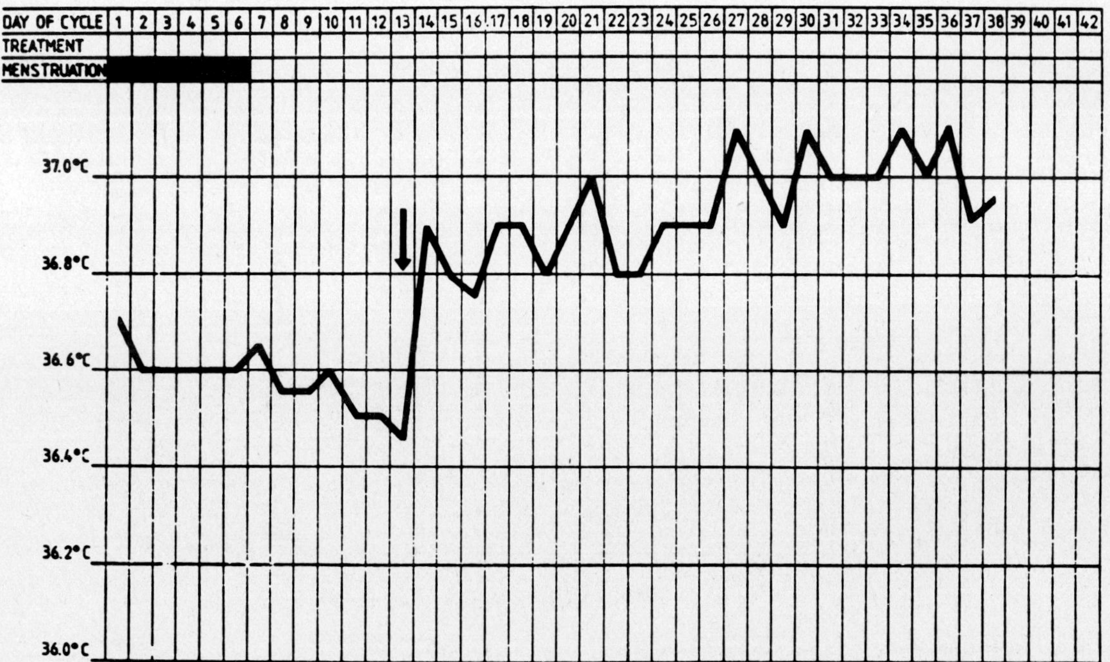

FIGURE 39-2

Pregnancy chart showing insemination *(arrow)* timed to occur on day before expected steep rise in BBT. (From Newill RG, Katz M: Fertil Steril 39:431, 1982. Reproduced with permission of the publisher, The American Fertility Society.)

est incidence of conception occurred when insemination was performed on the day before the rise of the BBT (Fig. 39-2). When insemination occurred more than 1 day after the luteal rise in BBT, conception did not take place. Since the BBT cannot be used to predict the day of ovulation, the couple should be instructed to have intercourse about every other day in the late follicular phase of the menstrual cycle and, if possible, daily in the estimated midcycle.

With the development of various enzyme-linked immunosorbent assays (ELISAs) for detection of a urinary luteinizing hormone (LH) peak that can be performed in the home, it has become possible for women to predict the day of ovulation with greater accuracy, because the urinary LH peak usually occurs 1 day before ovulation. Thus a more precise estimate of the optimal time to have coitus is now clinically available. At present these tests are time con-suming, expensive, and unnecessary until after the diagnostic evaluation has been completed. They assist in determining the optimal time for a postcoital test (PCT), however, as well as for insemination procedures. The couple should be advised to avoid the use of any vaginal lubricants (including saliva) during coitus, because these can interfere with sperm transport.

At the time of the initial visit a complete blood count, urinalysis, cervical cytologic examination, and 2-hour postprandial glucose test should be ordered. It is not cost effective to measure a prolactin or thyroid-stimulating hormone (TSH) level at the time of the initial visit.

Documentation of Ovulation

The first diagnostic step in the infertility evaluation is to obtain presumptive evidence that the woman is ovulating. Preliminary information that the woman is ovulating is provided

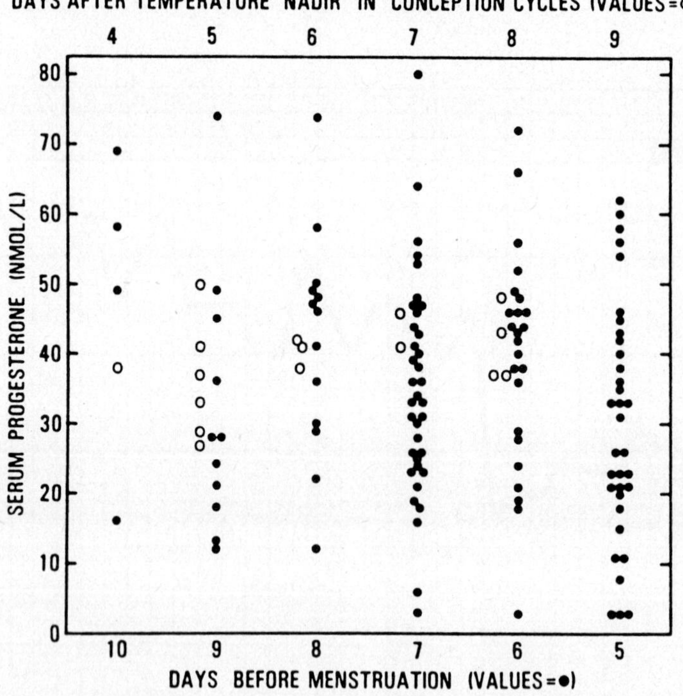

FIGURE 39-3
Midluteal serum progesterone concentration in untreated conception (open circles) and nonconception (closed circles) cycles related, respectively, to time elapsed since presumed ovulation or to time before the following menses. (1 ng/ml = 3.18 nmol/L.) (From Hull MGR, Savage PE, Bromham DR, et al: Fertil Steril 37:355, 1982. Reproduced with permission of the publisher, The American Fertility Society.)

by a history of regular menstrual cycles. If the woman is having regular menstrual cycles, a serum progesterone level should be measured in the midluteal phase to provide indirect evidence of ovulation as well as normal luteal function. Although in the normal luteal phase progesterone levels in blood vary in a pulsatile manner, a serum progesterone level above 10 ng/ml indicates adequate luteal function. Progesterone levels of 10 ng/ml or higher have been measured during at least 1 day of the luteal phase of normal ovulatory cycles in which conception occurred (Fig. 39-3). Measurement of daily BBT also provides indirect evidence that ovulation has taken place. The BBT graph also provides information concerning the approximate day of ovulation and duration of the luteal phase.

Women with oligomenorrhea (menses at intervals of 35 days or longer) or amenorrhea who wish to conceive should be treated with agents that induce ovulation regardless of whether they have occasional ovulatory cycles. Therefore for such women direct or indirect measurement of progesterone is unnecessary until after therapy is initiated.

Semen Analysis

While information about ovulation is being obtained, the male partner's reproductive system should be evaluated by means of semen analysis. The male partner should be advised to abstain from coitus for 2 to 3 days before collection of the semen sample, because frequent ejaculation lowers the sperm count in some individuals. It is best to collect the specimen in a clear (not necessarily sterile), wide-mouthed jar after masturbation. It is important that the entire specimen be collected, because the initial fraction contains the greatest density of sperm. Ideally, collection should take place in the location where the analysis will be performed. The degree of sperm motility should be determined as soon as possible after liquefaction, which usually occurs 15 to 20 minutes after ejaculation. Sperm motility begins to decline 2 hours after ejaculation, and it is best to examine the specimen within this period. Semen should not be exposed to marked changes in temperature, and if collected at home during cold weather, the specimen should be kept warm during the trip to the laboratory.

TABLE 39-4
Recommended Standards for Semen Analysis

Parameter	Recommended Normal Value
Volume	2-6 ml
Viscosity	Full liquefaction within 60 minutes
Sperm density	20-250 million/ml*
Sperm motility	
Progressive	Good to very good†
Quantitation	First hour ≥60%, 2-3 h ≥50%
Vital staining	≤35% dead cells
Sperm morphology	≥60% within normal configuration

Modified from Eliasson R: Parameters of male fertility. In Hafez ESE, Evans TN, eds: Human reproduction. New York, Harper & Row, Publishers, 1973.
*20 million/ml is low normal, in contrast to 40 million/ml, International Society of Andrology.
†3 to 4+ quality.

Parameters of semen that should be evaluated include volume, viscosity, sperm density, sperm morphology, and sperm motility. The last parameter should be evaluated in terms of percent of total motile sperm as well as quality of motility (rapidity of movement and amount of progressive motility). There are no absolute standards for determining the normality of a semen sample, but recommended guidelines are shown in Table 39-4. Because it is common for men to have great variabilities in sperm count over time, if the count in the initial specimen is low, it is best to obtain at least three semen sample analyses at monthly intervals to evaluate the male reproductive system more completely. It is beyond the scope of this text to fully discuss the etiology and diagnostic evaluation of men with semen abnormalities. The various etiologies of semen abnormalities are cited in Table 39-5, and the indications for performing the various types of additional diagnostic tests are listed in Table 39-6.

Postcoital Test

Although there are various in vitro tests to evaluate sperm–cervical mucus interaction, it is best to perform an in vivo postcoital test (PCT), as this is the only in vivo test that provides information from both partners. The

TABLE 39-5
Causes of Semen Abnormalities

Finding	Etiology
Abnormal count	
Azoospermia	Klinefelter's syndrome or other genetic disorders
	Sertoli-cell-only syndrome
	Seminiferous tubule or Leydig cell failure
	Hypogonadotrophic hypogonadism
	Ductal obstruction, including Young's syndrome
	Varicocele
	Exogenous factors
Oligozoospermia	Genetic disorder
	Endocrinopathies, including androgen receptor defects
	Varicocele and other anatomic disorders
	Maturation arrest
	Hypospermatogenesis
	Exogenous factors
Abnormal volume	
No ejaculate	Ductal obstruction
	Retrograde ejaculation
	Ejaculatory failure
	Hypogonadism
Low volume	Obstruction of ejaculatory ducts
	Absence of seminal vesicles and vas deferens
	Partial retrograde ejaculation
	Infection
High volume	Unknown factors
Abnormal motility	Immunologic factors
	Infection
	Varicocele
	Defects in sperm structure
	Metabolic or anatomic abnormalities of sperm
	Poor liquefaction or semen
Abnormal viscosity	Etiology unknown
Abnormal morphology	Varicocele
	Stress
	Infection
	Exogenous factors
	Unknown factors
Extraneous cells	Infection or inflammation
	Shedding of immature sperm

quality and quantity of cervical mucus are optimal when there is maximal estrogen stimulation unopposed by any progesterone, and this hormone profile occurs on the day before ovulation. Therefore during the cycle in which the PCT is scheduled, the woman should measure her BBT daily to determine the approximate day of ovulation and ensure that the test is performed at the optimal time of the cycle. If the mucus is scanty or viscid, the test should

TABLE 39-6
Indications for Various Types
of Diagnostic Tests

Findings	Recommended Tests
Most patients	General laboratory evaluation
Sperm count <40 × 10⁶/ml	Endocrine evaluation
Sperm count <20 × 10⁶/ml	Genetic studies
Teratozoospermia	
Partner has recurrent abortion	
Sperm agglutination	Immunologic studies
Poor motility	Microbiologic studies
Poor cervical mucus penetration	
Inflammatory or red blood cells in semen	Bacteriologic studies

Modified from Eliasson R: Semen analysis and laboratory
work-up. In Cockett ATK, Urry RL, eds: Male infertility:
Work-up, treatment, and research New York, Grune &
Stratton, 1977.

be repeated every 2 days until there is a shift
in the BBT. It is best to perform the PCT 2 to
3 hours after coitus, because as Tredway has
shown, the number of sperm in the mucus is
maximal at this time.

Although various techniques have been described for performing postovulatory testing,
the fractional PCT as described by Davajan is

FIGURE 39-4
Syringe attached to polyethylene suction catheter is used in aspiration of cervical mucus.
Tubing is stabilized by grasping it 2.5 cm from
the distal end with a clamp. Handle of clamp
should be adjusted so that when clamp is set at
first ratchet, tube is partially but not totally occluded. Aspiration must be initiated just as tip
of catheter is inserted into external os. (From
Davajan V: Postcoital testing: The cervical factor as a cause of infertility. Reproduced with
permission from Infertility, contraception and
reproductive endocrinology, 2nd ed, by Daniel
R. Mishell, Jr., M.D., and Val Davajan, M.D.
Copyright © 1986 Medical Economics Books,
Oradell, N.J. 07649. All rights reserved.)

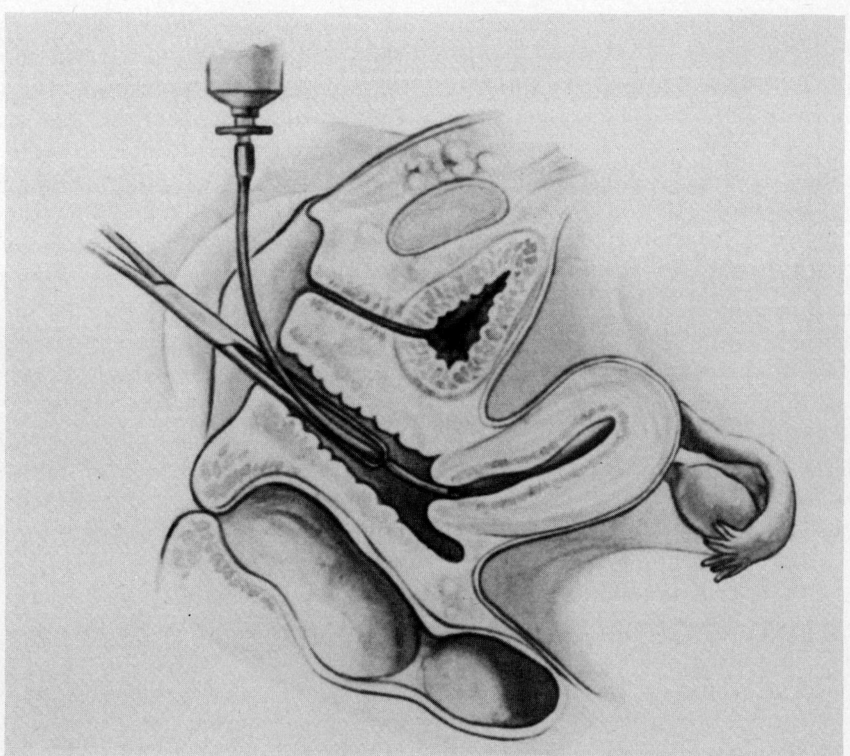

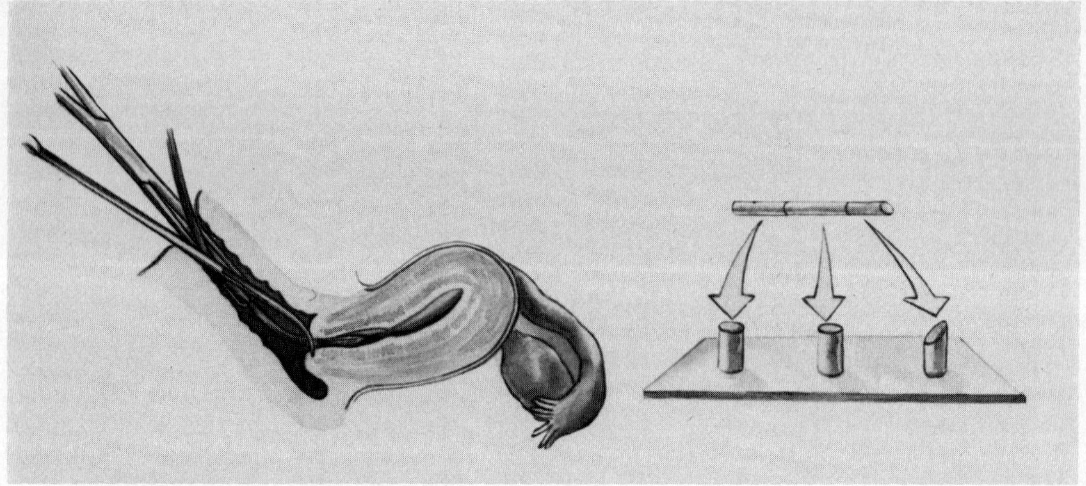

FIGURE 39-5
Catheter should be gently withdrawn and trailing mucus cut away with scissors. Catheter segment is then cut into three smaller segments. Distal segment (beveled end) contains mucus collected from internal os level, and most proximal segment contains mucus collected from level of external os. (From Davajan V: Postcoital testing: The cervical factor as a cause of infertility. Reproduced with permission from Infertility, contraception and reproductive endocrinology, 2nd ed, by Daniel R. Mishell, Jr., M.D., and Val Davajan, M.D. Copyright © 1986 Medical Economics Books, Oradell, N.J. 07649. All rights reserved.)

easily performed and interpreted. After the cervix has been cleansed with a saline-moistened sponge, the cervical mucus is aspirated through a portion of polyethylene tubing attached to a syringe. The tubing size should allow easy passage into the cervical canal, and the distal end should be beveled with scissors. The tubing should be stabilized by grasping it with an incompletely closed, large Allis clamp about 2.5 cm from the tip. As the tubing is advanced into the cervical canal, maintaining a constant negative pressure allows the mucus to be withdrawn into the tubing (Fig. 39-4). After the level of the internal os is reached, the clamp is closed and the tubing slowly withdrawn from the cervical canal. The trailing edge of mucus is cut at the level of the external os, and the mucus in the tubing is taken for examination (Fig. 39-5). The tubing is then cut into three segments, and the mucus within the distal segment, representing the mucus at the internal os level, is placed on a slide, covered with a coverslip, and examined under low- and high-power ($\times 400$) magnification. A portion of

the vaginal fluid should also be placed on a slide and examined to be certain that sperm were deposited in the vagina. The mucus from the proximal segment can be evaluated for spinnbarkeit and then dried to observe whether a fern leaf pattern is present.

Normal midcycle cervical mucus is clear and watery with a spinnbarkeit of at least 6 cm and a normal fern pattern. For a PCT result to be considered normal at least five motile sperm should be observed per high-power field in the mucus obtained from the level of the internal os. An abnormal PCT result can be due to anatomic defects of the cervix, abnormal cervical mucus, and abnormalities of the sperm in normal cervical mucus. The etiologies of these types of abnormal PCT results are listed in the box on p. 1047.

Hysterosalpingogram

It is best to schedule the hysterosalpingogram (HSG) during the week following the end of menses to avoid irradiating a possible preg-

CAUSES OF ABNORMAL POSTCOITAL TEST RESULTS

Anatomic Defects

Cervical stenosis
Varicosities of hypoplastic endocervical canal

Abnormal Cervical Mucus

Poor quality
Low quality

Abnormal PCT with Normal Cervical Mucus

Faulty coital technique
Vaginal factor or weak sperm factor
Oligospermia or low motility or both
Low semen volume
Immobilized sperm in endocervical canal
Large semen volume
Highly viscous semen

From Davajan V: Postcoital testing. Reproduced with permission from Infertility, contraception and reproductive endocrinology, 2nd ed, by Daniel R. Mishell, Jr., M.D., and Val Davajan, M.D. Copyright © 1986 Medical Economics Books, Oradell, N.J. 07649. All rights reserved.

nancy. Before the procedure a bimanual pelvic examination should be performed, and if adnexal tenderness is present the procedure should be postponed until antibiotic therapy has been administered and the tenderness has resolved. This technique reduces the risk of causing an episode of acute recurrent salpingitis. Some authorities recommend that antibiotic prophylaxis (such as doxycycline 100 mg twice a day for 5 days starting 2 days before the procedure) be given to all women who have an HSG. The examination should be performed with use of a water-soluble contrast medium and image-intensified fluoroscopy. A water-soluble contrast medium enables better visualization of the tubal mucosal folds and vaginal markings than does an oil-based medium. It is important to be able to evaluate the appearance of the intratubal architecture to determine the extent of damage to the oviduct. Although some studies have shown an increased pregnancy rate after use of an oil-based contrast medium, a recent randomized prospective study by Alper et al. has not confirmed this finding. The HSG not only will determine whether the tubes are patent but also, if dis-

ease is present, will help to determine the magnitude of the disease process as well as give information about the lining of the oviduct and uterine cavity that cannot be obtained by laparoscopic visualization. It can also determine whether salpingitis isthmica nodosa is present in the interstitial portion of the oviduct. The finding of a normal endometrial cavity at the time of HSG obviates the need for hysteroscopy. March reported that of 500 patients with infertility and a normal HSG, none had abnormalities of the uterine cavity when subsequently examined by hysteroscopy.

If severe tubal disease such as a large hydrosalpinx is found at the time of HSG, then it is not essential to perform diagnostic laparoscopy if the couple wishes to attempt in vitro fertilization. However, if the disease process is not too extensive, surgical tubal reconstruction may be advised, and then a diagnostic laparoscopic examination should precede the scheduled tubal operation to determine the extent of the disease process throughout the pelvis. Laparoscopy may be performed immediately before laparotomy, or the two procedures can be performed separately to allow time to explain the prognosis of tubal surgery to the patient.

Diagnostic Laparoscopy

If the HSG reveals no abnormalities, the fifth step in the infertility evaluation—diagnostic laparoscopy—should be scheduled to take place in the follicular phase of a menstrual cycle to determine whether peritoneal or peritubal pelvic disease, such as endometriosis or pelvic adhesions, is present. At the time of laparoscopy following a normal HSG neither a D&C (dilation and curettage) nor a hysteroscopy should be routinely performed. Neither procedure will provide additional information or therapy and the curettage may further impede future fertility by producing intrauterine adhesions. At the time of laparoscopy indigo carmine should be introduced through the cervix into the peritoneal cavity to confirm tubal patency. Performing the laparoscopy in the follicular phase of the cycle before maximal endometrial growth enables the dye to pass into the oviducts with less chance of obstruction.

• • •

If the first five steps of the infertility investigation produce normal results, an additional five investigative steps may be performed. These second five tests include (6) measurement of serum prolactin and TSH, (7) a late luteal phase endometrial biopsy, (8) immunologic tests to detect the presence of sperm antibodies, (9) bacteriologic cultures of the cervical mucus and semen, and (10) a zona-free hamster egg penetration test of the husband's sperm.

The value of performing the primary five steps of the infertility investigation has been documented by studies showing that when an abnormality is found, such as anovulation or tubal obstruction, treatment of that abnormality significantly increases the incidence of pregnancy as compared with withholding therapy. Similar data do not exist for the secondary five steps of the infertility investigation. Even if an abnormality is found in one of these tests, treatment of that abnormality has not been shown to be more effective than withholding therapy.

Rousseau et al. studied 47 couples who had evidence of regular ovulatory cycles and normal results of semen analysis, PCT, HSG, and laparoscopy. They had no further evaluation or treatment following laparoscopy, yet 65% conceived within 3 years (Fig. 39-6). Although numerous studies have stated that treatment of abnormalities in the secondary five steps of the infertility evaluation resulted in pregnancies in previously infertile couples, none of these studies have compared the results of therapy with either placebo or no treatment. Such studies must be performed before one can conclude that diagnosis and treatment of these abnormalities have validity.

MANAGEMENT OF THE CAUSES OF INFERTILITY

The management of the various causes of infertility will be presented in the order generally followed in an infertility investigation. Management of primary infertility factors are presented first, followed by management of secondary factors.

Anovulation

Therapeutic agents currently available to induce ovulation are clomiphene citrate, human menopausal gonadotrophin (HMG), and gonadotrophin-releasing hormone (GnRH). In addition, as discussed in Chapter 37, if anovulation is due to hyperprolactinemia, bromocriptine is an effective means to induce ovulation. Also, as noted in Chapter 38, women with congenital adrenal hyperplasia or anovulation accompanied by excessive production of adrenal androgens resulting from other causes can have ovulation induced by corticosteroid therapy.

Clomiphene Citrate

Clomiphene citrate is the pharmacologic agent of choice for women with oligomenorrhea as well as those with amenorrhea and evidence of sufficient ovarian follicular function to raise circulating estradiol levels above 40 pg/ml and thus have uterine withdrawal bleeding induced after progesterone administration. This synthetic, weak estrogen acts by competing with endogenous circulating estrogens for estrogen binding sites in the hypothalamus and blocking the negative feedback of endogenous estrogen. Thus GnRH is then released in a normal manner, stimulating FSH and LH, which in turn cause oocyte maturation with increased estradiol production. The drug is usually given daily

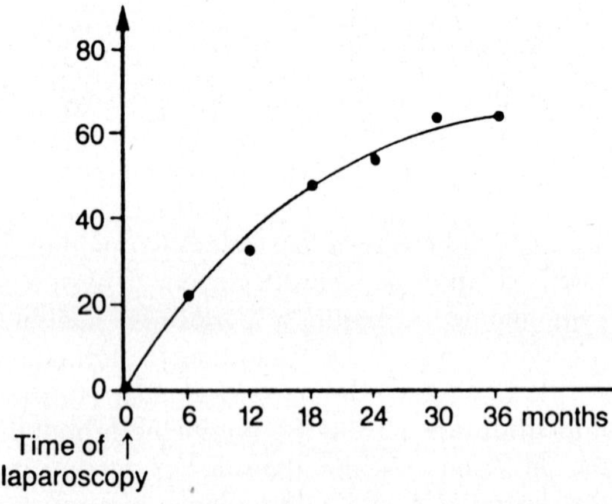

FIGURE 39-6
Cumulative pregnancy rate of all patients in study population from day of laparoscopy. (From Rousseau S, Lord J, Lepage Y, et al: Fertil Steril 40:768, 1983. Reproduced with permission of the publisher, The American Fertility Society.)

for 5 days beginning 5 days after the onset of spontaneous menses or withdrawal bleeding induced with progesterone in oil or an oral progestin.

During the days the drug is ingested, serum levels of LH and FSH rise, accompanied by a steady increase in serum estradiol (Fig. 39-7). Following ingestion of clomiphene, estradiol levels continue to increase, and the negative feedback on the hypothalamic-pituitary axis causes a decrease in FSH and LH, similar to the change seen in the late follicular phase of a normal ovulatory cycle. About 5 to 9 days (mean 7 days) after the last clomiphene tablet has been ingested, the exponentially rising level of estradiol from the dominant follicle has a positive feedback effect on the hypothalamus, producing a surge in LH and FSH, which usually results in ovulation and luteinization of the follicle.

Presumptive evidence of ovulation can be obtained by observation of a sustained rise in BBT or measurement of an elevation of serum progesterone. It is best to obtain the serum sample for progesterone measurement about 2 weeks after the last clomiphene tablet has been ingested, because this will usually be in the middle of the luteal phase, about 1 week after ovulation. A rise in serum progesterone level above 3 ng/ml correlates well with the finding of secretory endometrium on an endometrial biopsy sample, but Hull et al. have reported that maximal midluteal progesterone levels in clomiphene-induced ovulatory conception cycles are consistently above 15 ng/ml (Fig. 39-8). These levels are higher than the 10 ng/ml found in spontaneous ovulatory conception cycles because following artificial ovulation induction, more than one follicle usually matures and undergoes luteinization.

Various treatment regimens have been advocated for the use of clomiphene citrate. Most start with an initial dosage of 50 mg per day for 5 days beginning on the fifth day of sponta-

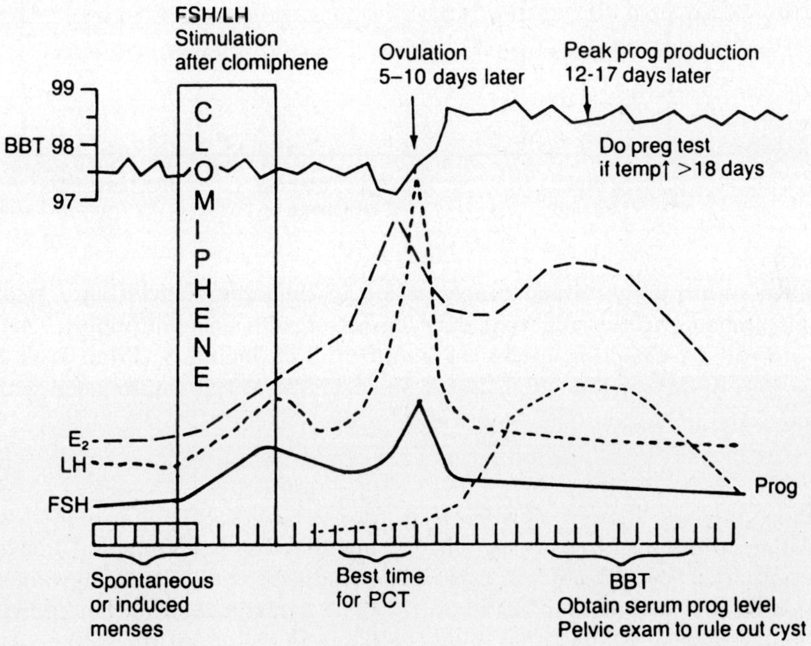

FIGURE 39-7

LH, FSH, estradiol (*E₂*), and progesterone *(prog)* levels before, during, and after successful treatment with clomiphene citrate. (From March CM, Mishell DR Jr: Induction of ovulation. Reproduced with permission from Infertility, contraception and reproductive endocrinology, 2nd ed, by Daniel R. Mishell, Jr., M.D., and Val Davajan, M.D. Copyright © 1986 Medical Economics Books, Oradell, N.J. 07649. All rights reserved.)

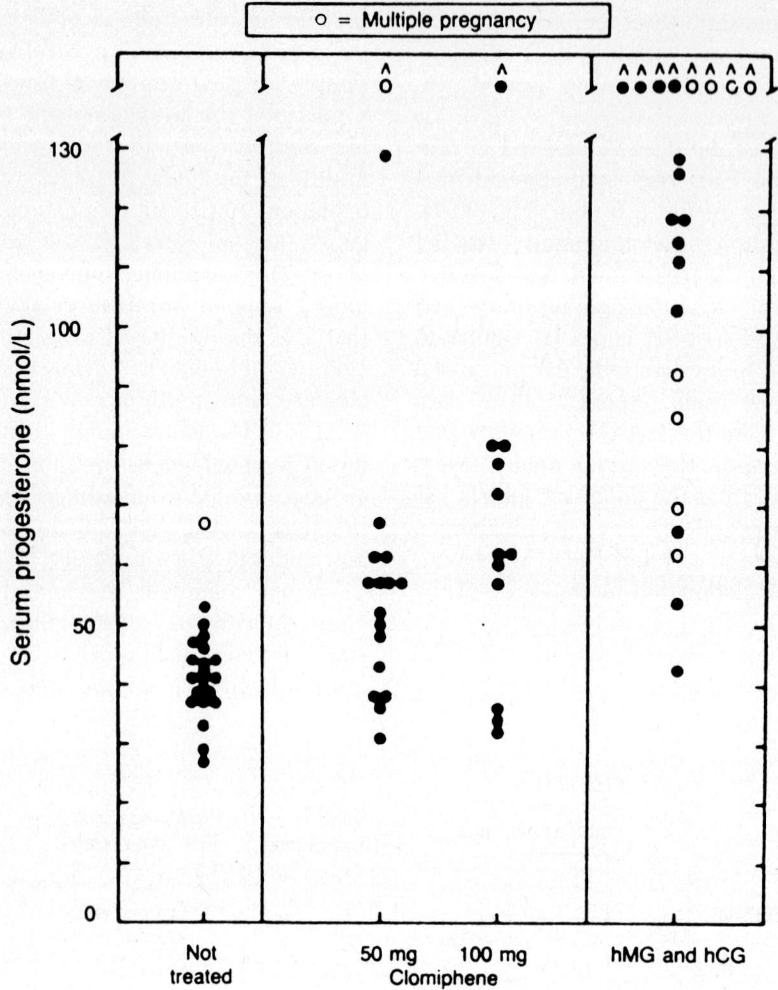

FIGURE 39-8

Midluteal serum progesterone concentration in conception cycles after treatment with clomiphene, in two different daily doses, or with gonadotrophins, compared with untreated conception cycles. (1 ng/ml = 3.18 nmol/L.) (From Hull MGR, Savage PE, Bromham DR, et al: Fertil Steril 37:355, 1982. Reproduced with permission of the publisher, The American Fertility Society.)

neous or induced menses. If presumptive evidence of ovulation occurs with this dosage, clomiphene is continued in subsequent cycles until conception occurs. If ovulation fails to occur with the initial dosage, a sequential, graduated dosage regimen has proven to be effective with a minimum of side effects. With this regimen if ovulation does not occur with the 50 mg dosage, the dosage of clomiphene is increased in the next treatment cycle to 100 mg per day for 5 days. If ovulation does not occur with 100 mg per day in subsequent cycles, the

dosage is sequentially increased to 150 mg, 200 mg, and finally 250 mg for 5 days. If ovulation is induced with any of these dosages, the patient is maintained on her individualized ovulatory dosage until conception occurs. If ovulation does not occur with 250 mg, in the next cycle 250 mg is given daily for 5 days, and 1 week after the last tablet has been ingested, 5000 IU of human chorionic gonadotrophin (HCG) is given to increase the chances of inducing ovulation by simulating the LH surge. In the 10 years' experience reported by Gysler

TABLE 39-7
Response to Clomiphene Citrate

Category	Total	Ovulated		Conceived	
		No.	%	No.	%
Oligomenorrhea	330	307	93.0	157	51.1
Amenorrhea					
Polycystic ovary disease	29	18	62.1	12	66.7
Hypothalamic-pituitary dysfunction	39	30	76.9	9	30.0
Hypothalamic-pituitary failure	10	0	0	0	0
Amenorrhea/galactorrhea					
Progesterone (+)*	10	9	90	5	55.6
Progesterone (−)†	10	1	10	0	0
All amenorrheic patients	98	58	59.1	26	44.8
TOTAL	428	365	85.3	183	50.1

Modified from Gysler M, March CM, Mishell DR Jr, et al: A decade's experience with an individualized clomiphene treatment regimen including its effect on the post-coital test. Fertil Steril 37:161, 1982. Reproduced with permission of the publisher, The American Fertility Society.
*Withdrawal bleeding after intramuscular progesterone.
†No progesterone-induced uterine bleeding.

et al. about half the patients who ovulated and those who conceived did so following treatment with the 50 mg per day regimen, and an additional one fifth did so with the 100 mg per day dosage. However, about one fourth of all women who ovulated or conceived did so following treatment with a higher dosage regimen, indicating the value of the individualized sequential treatment regimen.

With this dosage regimen of clomiphene citrate more than 90% of women with oligomenorrhea and 66% with secondary amenorrhea and progesterone-induced withdrawal bleeding (estradiol levels of 40 pg/ml or higher) will have presumptive evidence of ovulation (Table 39-7). Although only about half the patients who ovulate with this treatment will conceive, Gysler et al. reported that 85% of those with no other causes of infertility conceived after such treatment. Hammond et al. by calculating the fecundability index reported that if ovulation is induced with clomiphene citrate and no other causes of infertility are present, conception rates over time are similar to those of a normal fertile population who stop using barrier methods of contraception in order to conceive (Fig. 39-9). Using life-table analysis these investigators reported that the monthly pregnancy rate (fecundability) of patients treated with clomi-

phene who had no other infertility factor was 22%, as compared with 25% calculated for women discontinuing diaphragm use. The monthly fecundability remained constant throughout treatment. Nearly all of the anovulatory women without other infertility factors in this series as well as other women with correctable infertility factors had conceived after 10 cycles of treatment. Therefore therapy should be continued for at least 10 to 12 cycles to improve the chance of conception. These data indicate that patient discontinuation of therapy is the major reason for the reported difference in ovulation and conception rates in anovulatory women treated with clomiphene. Clomiphene citrate does not itself cause infertility, as has been stated in some reports. If other causes of infertility are found, they should be treated and clomiphene continued.

When conception occurs after ovulation has been induced with this drug, the incidence of multiple gestation is increased to about 5%, with nearly all being twin gestations. The incidence of clinical spontaneous abortion ranges between 15% and 20%, similar to the rate in the general population. The rates of ectopic gestation, intrauterine fetal death, and congenital malformation are also not significantly increased. Animal data indicate that if the drug

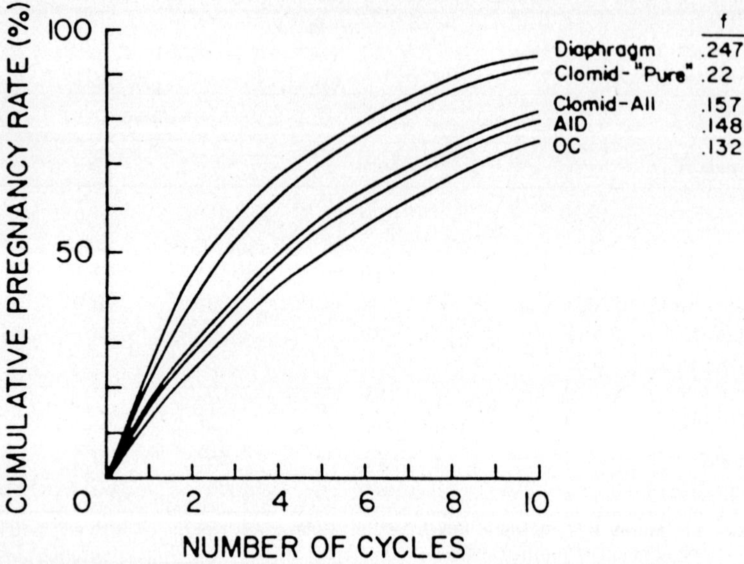

FIGURE 39-9
Life-table analysis of cumulative pregnancy rates in ovulatory patients treated with clomiphene citrate or donor insemination (artificial inseminate donor—*AID*) or in parous women discontinuing diaphragm use or oral contraceptives *(OC)* ("pure," no other infertility factors). (From Hammond MG, Halme JK, Talbert LM: Obstet Gynecol 62:196, 1983. Reprinted with permission from The American College of Obstetricians and Gynecologists.)

is given in high dosages during the time of embryogenesis, there is an increased incidence of fetal anomalies. However, limited human data indicate that if the drug is ingested during the first 6 weeks after conception has occurred, the incidence of fetal malformation, although higher (5.1%) than normal, is not significantly increased. Although no definitive data show that the drug is teratogenic in humans, it is best that the woman be reexamined before each course of treatment to be certain that she is not pregnant. It is also important to determine that the ovaries have not become enlarged, because formation of ovarian cysts is the major side effect of clomiphene treatment.

If cysts are present, they will regress spontaneously without therapy, but if clomiphene is given and further gonadotrophin release is induced, stimulation and further enlargement of the cyst may occur. Clinically palpable ovarian cysts occur in about 5% of patients treated with clomiphene but in less than 1% of treatment cycles. The cysts usually range in size from 5 to 10 cm and do not require operation. Cysts can occur in any treatment cycle with any dos-

age, and the incidence is not increased with the higher dosages of drug. Recurrence of cyst formation with the same dosage is uncommon. Other side effects, which occur in less than 10% of women treated with this drug, include vasomotor flushes, blurring of vision, abdominal pain or bloating, urticaria, and a slight degree of hair loss.

About 5% to 10% of women treated with the individually graduated, sequential regimen of clomiphene citrate fail to ovulate with the highest dosage. Because treatment with HMG and GnRH is expensive and time consuming, other treatment regimens have been used with success. For the patient with evidence of adrenal hyperplasia as determined by the finding of an elevation of dehydroepiandrosterone sulfate (DHEA-S) (>2.8 mg/ml), Lobo et al. report an ovulation rate of approximately 50% when clomiphene is given after adrenal suppression has been achieved by administration of 0.5 mg dexamethasone nightly for 2 weeks. Withdrawal bleeding is then induced with 100 mg progesterone in oil given intramuscularly. Dexamethasone is continued nightly, and the high dose

HUMAN MENOPAUSAL GONADOTROPHIN: TREATMENT PROTOCOL

1. Perform baseline estradiol determination and ultrasound.
2. Administer HMG, two ampules per day for 3 days.
3. Repeat estradiol. If it is doubled, monitor HMG dosage; if not, increase HMG by 50% for 3 days.
4. Repeat step 3 until estradiol doubles.
5. Perform ultrasound scan every 2 to 3 days until the dominant follicle is ≥14 mm.
6. Perform daily ultrasound until the follicle is ≥16 mm.
7. Stop HMG and perform PCT.
8. Twenty-four hours later give 5000 IU HCG. If the PCT result is poor, use AIH. If it is good, recommend natural intercourse.
9. Administer HCG, 3000 IU, 7 days later.

TABLE 39-8

Typical Overall Results Following Human Menopausal Gonadotrophin Therapy

Result	Incidence
Ovulation	>99%
Pregnancy	60%
Multiple gestation (75% twins)	10%
Abortion	25%
Ovarian enlargement	5%
Hyperstimulation syndrome	<0.1%
Teratogenicity	No ↑

From March CM, Mishell DR Jr: Induction of ovulation. Reproduced with permission from Infertility, contraception and reproductive endocrinology, 2nd ed, by Daniel R. Mishell, Jr., M.D., and Val Davajan, M.D. Copyright © 1986 Medical Economics Books, Oradell, N.J. 07649. All rights reserved.

of clomiphene (250 mg per day) is given for 5 days, followed 1 week later by 5000 IU of HCG. In patients with normal DHEA-S levels, Lobo et al. report that ovulation can sometimes be induced if clomiphene is given at a dosage of 250 mg per day for 8 days instead of 5 days, followed 1 week later by HCG. Others, such as O'Herlihy et al., have recommended that the higher dosage of clomiphene be administered daily until the diameter of the largest follicle measured by ultrasound reaches 1.8 cm, at which time HCG is given.

HMG and GnRH

Anovulatory women with adequate estrogen who fail to respond to these regimens, as well as amenorrheic women with low estrogen levels, need to be treated with either HMG or GnRH. Both these methods of ovulation induction are more complicated, time consuming, and expensive than treatment with clomiphene citrate. The incidence of side effects is greater and the type of side effect is more serious than occurs with clomiphene. These side effects include superovulation, multiple pregnancy, and the hyperstimulation syndrome, which includes ascites, pleural effusion, and possibly thrombosis secondary to hemoconcentration.

Because each patient responds individually to the dosage of HMG—even the same patient in different treatment cycles—it is essential to monitor treatment carefully with frequent measurement of estrogen levels and ovarian ultrasonography. Monitoring needs to take place daily, because there is little difference between the minimal degree of ovarian follicular development necessary to induce ovulation and the amount of follicular development that results in hyperstimulation. When urinary estrogen alone was used to determine the optimal time to induce ovulation with HCG, a level between 50 and 100 μg per day was used, equivalent to serum estrogen levels of 500 to 1000 pg/ml. With ultrasound monitoring, HCG is administered when the follicle reaches a diameter of at least 1.6 cm. A treatment protocol for HMG monitoring is shown in the box, above left.

This regimen should be able to consistently induce ovulation with an overall pregnancy rate of about 60% (Table 39-8). The pregnancy rate per cycle is similar to that following clomiphene therapy—22%. Therefore, with sufficient duration of treatment and no other infertility factors, pregnancy rates should be greater than 90%. The incidence of spontaneous abortion after HMG therapy is high (25% to 35%), and despite monitoring, clinically detectable ovarian enlargement occurs in about 5% to 10% of treatment cycles. There is no evidence of an increase in fetal malformation rates after HMG treatment.

Gonadotrophin-Releasing Hormone

An alternative to administration of HMG is GnRH treatment. Because continuous administration of GnRH will saturate the receptors and thus inhibit gonadotrophin release, GnRH should be administered in a pulsatile manner at intervals of 1 to 2 hours. Because GnRH is a peptide, it cannot be administered orally, and the two routes of administration in current use are intravenous and subcutaneous. A greater

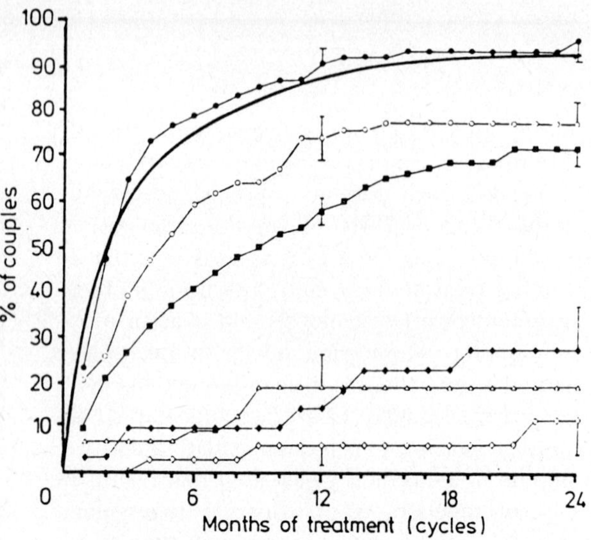

FIGURE 39-10
Cumulative rates of conception in couples with single cause of infertility managed as appropriate, excluding use of donor insemination or in vitro fertilization, compared with normal rates (highest rates reported in couples of proved fertility). Rates for couples with each cause shown as *solid line*, normal; *solid circles*, amenorrhea; *open circles*, oligomenorrhea; *solid squares*, unexplained infertility; *open triangles*, tubal damage (moderate or severe); *solid diamonds*, failure of sperm penetration of mucus (normal semen); *open diamonds*, oligospermia and failure to penetrate mucus. Standard errors of proportions are given at 12 and 24 months. (From Hull MGR, Glazener CMA, Kelly NJ, et al: Br Med J 291:1693, 1985.)

amount of drug must be administered by the subcutaneous route than by the intravenous route; however, the subcutaneous route avoids use of an intravenous catheter with its accompanying problems. The medication is administered by means of a small portable pump, which is usually worn attached to an article of clothing. Ovulation rates of about 75% to 85% and overall pregnancy rates of about 25% to 30% have been reported in the literature with both routes of administration, but most series are small, and there are no data regarding fecundability. The rates of ovulation and pregnancy reported in the literature appear to be slightly lower with GnRH than with HMG, but no comparative studies are available. One advantage of GnRH is that hyperstimulation is less common with it than with HMG, and therefore less monitoring is required.

• • •

In 1985 Hull et al. reported that of all the causes of infertility, treatment of anovulation results in the greatest success. In their study treatment of women with anovulation accompanied by amenorrhea (excluding ovarian failure) by one of the methods discussed above resulted in a 96% pregnancy rate after 2 years, with a fecundability curve nearly identical to the rates of normal fertile couples (Fig. 39-10). In a group of women with oligomenorrhea the 2-year pregnancy rate was 78%—significantly lower, mainly because of failure of ovulation induction in some women with polycystic ovarian syndrome. Newly developed gonadotrophin preparations that contain three to nine times as much FSH as LH may prove to be more successful for such patients.

Abnormal Postcoital Test

Although some authorities have questioned the clinical validity of the prognostic value of the PCT, a 1982 study by Hull et al. using life-table analysis demonstrated a highly significant difference in cumulative conception rates between couples with a normal PCT and couples with an abnormal PCT (Fig. 39-11). At the end of 2 years, 84% of the couples with a normal PCT had conceived, but only 16% of the couples with an abnormal PCT had become pregnant. Thus an abnormal PCT, without treatment, represents a poor prognosis for conception.

Treatment initiated because of an abnormal PCT depends on the cause. If the amount of mucus is small or the mucus is not thin and watery with good spinnbarkeit, some success has been achieved by administration of low-dose estrogen (diethylstilbestrol [DES] 0.1 mg or estrone sulfate 0.3 mg) daily from day 5 of the cycle for 10 to 12 days. This problem can also be treated by means of intrauterine insemination of sperm following their separation from the semen by centrifugation, a technique called *washed intrauterine insemination.* If the mucus is adequate in amount and quality but no sperm are found in the semen, it is essential to determine that sperm are being deposited in the vagina. If they are not, sexual counseling is warranted. If sperm are found in the vagina but not in the mucus, or if sperm are found in the mucus but they are nonmotile or do not exhibit good forward motility, either cervical insemination with a plastic cup or washed intrauterine insemination should be performed. Intrauterine insemination is also of benefit to women with cervical stenosis, such as that sometimes found following cervical conization. This technique is also useful for men with oligospermia

or those whose volume of semen is small (<2 ml) or large (>8 ml) or whose semen has a high viscosity. Ideally, insemination should take place 1 or 2 days before ovulation. If timing is done by the calendar or BBT, it may be necessary to repeat the procedure at 2-day intervals until the BBT increases. Urinary LH ELISA kits provide a more precise method to determine the optimal date to perform insemination.

The technique of cervical cup insemination with the husband's sperm is illustrated in Fig. 39-12. The semen sample should be placed into the woman as soon as possible after it liquefies. The cup should be left on the cervix for 2 to 3 hours, after which the woman can remove it herself. Following the first cup insemination, another PCT should be done at the time the cup is removed to determine whether the technique has improved the mucus penetration by sperm. If improvement is observed, the insemination should be repeated in subsequent cycles until conception occurs.

The technique of washed intrauterine insemination allows insemination of only sperm into the uterine cavity. Intrauterine insemination of seminal fluid can produce severe uterine cramps as a result of prostaglandin release. To separate the sperm from the semen, the semen specimen is placed in a centrifuge tube and the volume is tripled with an electrolyte and amino acid solution such as Ham's F-10. After being mixed on a vortex mixer, the specimen is centrifuged three times, with the addition of smaller volumes of diluent each time. Ultimately the sperm pellet is mixed with 0.5 ml of solute and inseminated high into the fundus through a small plastic or metal cannula (Fig. 39-13).

Techniques have also been developed to separate the sperm with the greatest motility from the remainder of sperm in the specimen, so that only the highest quality sperm are used for insemination. Separation with various gradients such as Percoll or albumin or layering a solution of Ham's F-10 over the sperm pellet and inseminating the supernate (the swim-up technique) has been utilized in an attempt to improve conception rates (Fig. 39-14).

Few data are available regarding the effectiveness of these various insemination procedures. Before the use of washed intrauterine

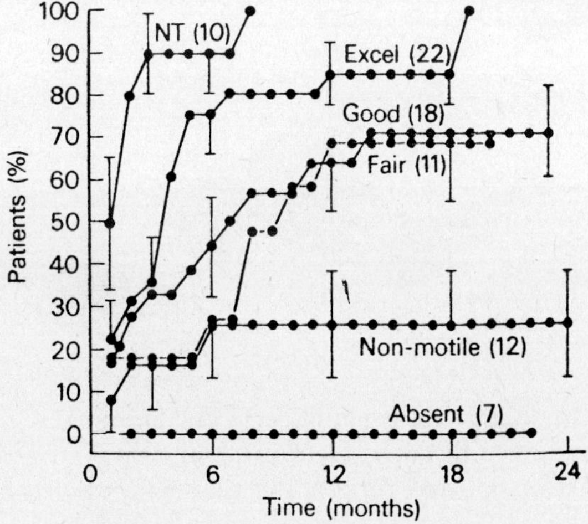

FIGURE 39-11
Cumulative conception rates related to result of postcoital test. *NT* = not tested. *Excel* = excellent. Standard error bars are shown. (From Hull MGR, Savage PE, Bromham DR: Br J Obstet Gynecol 89:299, 1982.)

insemination, Scott et al. reported pregnancy rates of about 20% with the use of estrogen and cup insemination. Pregnancy rates of 20% to 40% have been reported following washed intrauterine insemination. The only study using life-table analysis was that of Hull et al., who reported a cumulative pregnancy rate of 27% by 2 years following cervical and intrauterine insemination of women whose husbands had a normal semen analysis but abnormal PCT.

Male Factor Infertility

Most gynecologists who care for infertile couples should understand how to interpret a

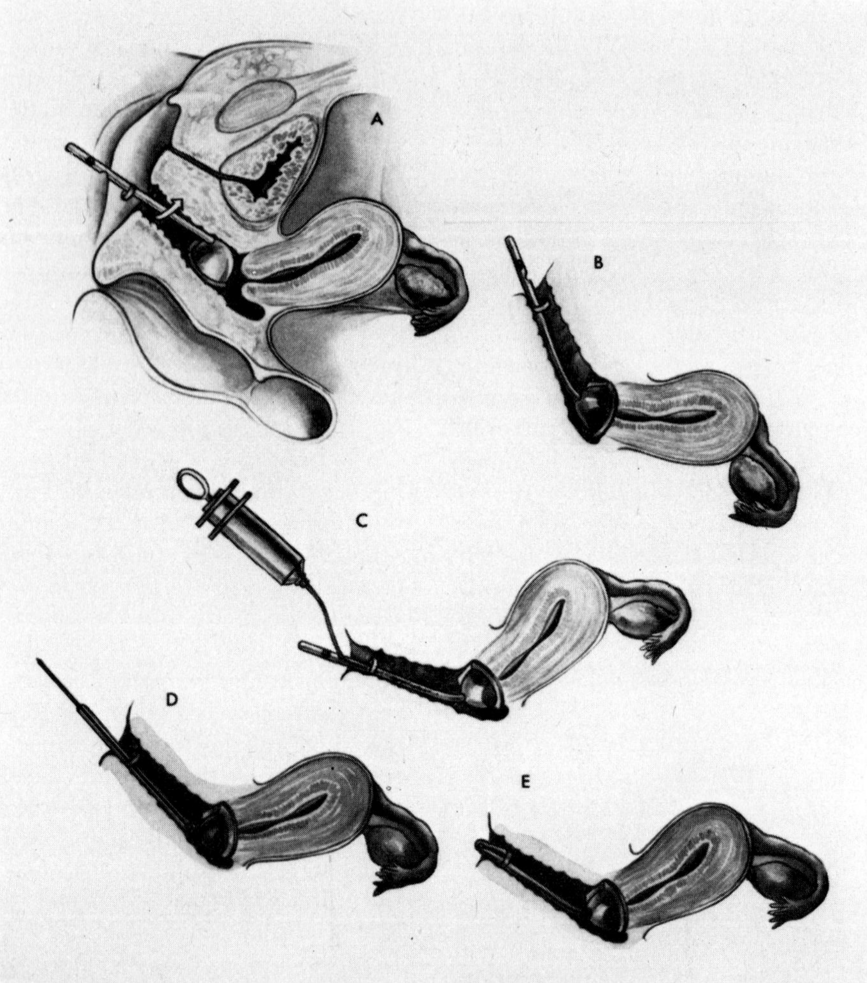

FIGURE 39-12
Use of Milex cervical cup for insemination. **A,** Before insertion of cervical cup into vagina, ball valve must be pushed past aperture to distal segment of stem. Cup is introduced into vagina with dome up. **B,** Cup is then turned 180 degrees and applied to cervix with dome pointing dorsally. **C,** Semen is injected through aperture in stem. **D,** After injection of semen, ball valve is pushed down stem to its junction with cup. **E,** Stem is folded into vagina. (From Davajan V: Postcoital testing: The cervical factor as a cause of infertility. Reproduced with permission from Infertility, contraception and reproductive endocrinology, 2nd ed, by Daniel R. Mishell, Jr., M.D., and Val Davajan, M.D. Copyright © 1986 Medical Economics Books, Oradell, N.J. 07649. All rights reserved.)

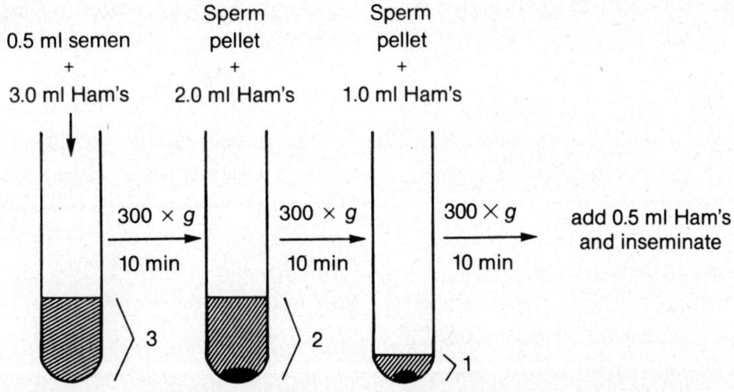

FIGURE 39-13

Sperm-washing technique (two-step wash). (From Marrs RP, Vargyas JM: Human in vitro fertilization: State of the art. Reproduced with permission from Infertility, contraception and reproductive endocrinology, 2nd ed, by Daniel R. Mishell, Jr., M.D., and Val Davajan, M.D. Copyright © 1986 Medical Economics Books, Oradell, N.J. 07649. All rights reserved.)

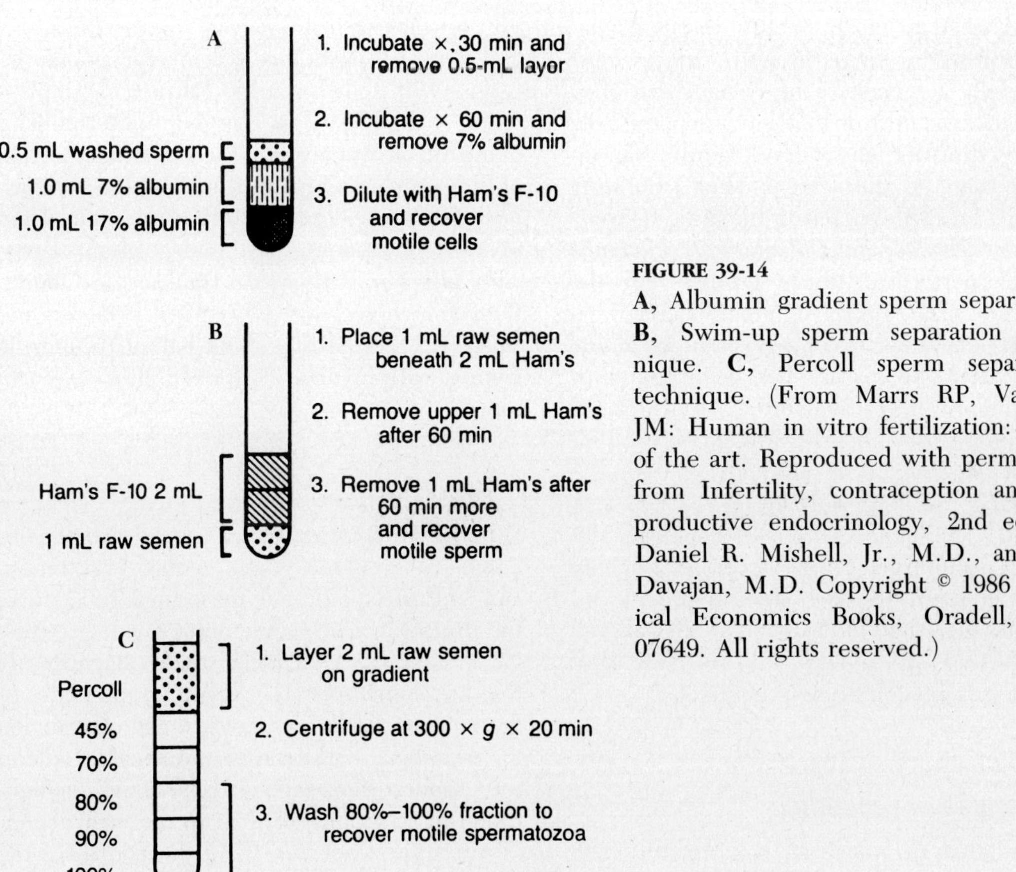

FIGURE 39-14

A, Albumin gradient sperm separation. **B,** Swim-up sperm separation technique. **C,** Percoll sperm separation technique. (From Marrs RP, Vargyas JM: Human in vitro fertilization: State of the art. Reproduced with permission from Infertility, contraception and reproductive endocrinology, 2nd ed, by Daniel R. Mishell, Jr., M.D., and Val Davajan, M.D. Copyright © 1986 Medical Economics Books, Oradell, N.J. 07649. All rights reserved.)

semen analysis as well as how to offer a prognosis for a disorder of abnormal semen. Although gynecologists usually do not perform a diagnostic evaluation or treat the male with a reproductive disorder, they should be able to provide counsel regarding the use of artificial insemination with either the husband's or a donor's semen.

AIH has been used to treat oligospermia as well as abnormalities of semen volume or viscosity. Pregnancy rates following either cervical cup insemination or intrauterine insemination have been reported to be in the 25% to 35% range in various series. In the life-table analysis study by Hull et al. the cumulative pregnancy rate at the end of 2 years was only 11%. Thus this type of treatment is not very effective, and the couple should be so advised.

Couples who fail to conceive with AIH because of azoospermia, oligospermia, or other semen abnormalities may elect to utilize donor semen insemination. The attitudes of both partners regarding AID and the stability of the marriage need to be thoroughly discussed before the procedure is performed. Donors must be carefully screened to be certain that they are in good health, do not have a potentially inherited disorder, and will not transmit an infectious agent in the semen. Thus laboratory screening for syphilis, serum hepatitis B, *Neisseria gonorrhoeae*, and *Chlamydia trachomatis* must be performed. Since cultures for the AIDS retrovirus (human immunodeficiency virus—HIV) may not become positive for 2 to 3 months after the disease has been acquired, some authorities recommend that only frozen semen of at least 2 months' storage be used for AID, at which time an antibody test for the AIDS virus can be performed on the donor. A new set of guidelines for semen donor insemination was published by the American Fertility Society in 1986. These guidelines provide information regarding indications for AID as well as suggested procedures for selection and screening of possible semen donors.

Uterine Causes of Infertility

Intrauterine Adhesions

In addition to menstrual abnormalities and recurrent abortion, some women may not be able to conceive because of the presence of intrauterine adhesions (IUA). As mentioned in Chapter 15, most women with IUA have had a previous curettage of the uterine cavity, most often during or shortly following a pregnancy. If the only abnormal finding in the infertility investigation is the presence of IUA, the prognosis for conception after hysteroscopic lysis of the adhesions is good. March reported that of 69 infertile women with IUA and no other infertility factors, 52 (75%) conceived after hysteroscopic treatment.

Leiomyoma

Congenital uterine defects rarely cause infertility, and the uterine anomalies associated with maternal ingestion of DES have not been shown in randomized studies to be a cause of infertility. It is also difficult to assess the effect of leiomyomas on conception, since so many women with leiomyomas have no difficulty conceiving. Nevertheless, it is plausible that cervical myomas cause distortion of the endocervix, interfering with normal sperm transport, and that some submucous leiomyomas may interfere with sperm transport or normal implantation of the blastocyst. Large intrauterine leiomyomas can also occlude the interstitial portion of the oviduct and prevent normal sperm transport. If no other cause of infertility is found and myomas of moderate size and position to possibly interfere with sperm transport are found, then a myomectomy is justified. Malone and Ingersol reported that about half of 75 infertile women with myomas conceived after myomectomy.

Tuberculosis

If the HSG reveals findings consistent with pelvic tuberculosis, then endometrial biopsy and culture should be performed to confirm the diagnosis. The radiographic features of pelvic tuberculosis that are virtually diagnostic of the disease include (1) calcified lymph nodes or granulomas in the pelvis, (2) tubal obstruction in the distal isthmus or proximal ampulla, sometimes resulting in a "pipe-stem" configuration of the tube proximal to the obstruction, (3) multiple strictures along the course of the tube, (4) irregularity to the contour of the ampulla, and (5) deformity or obliteration of the endometrial cavity without a previous curettage (Fig. 39-15). Appropriate chemotherapy should be initiated, but women with pelvic tuberculosis should be considered sterile, as pregnancies after chemotherapy are rare.

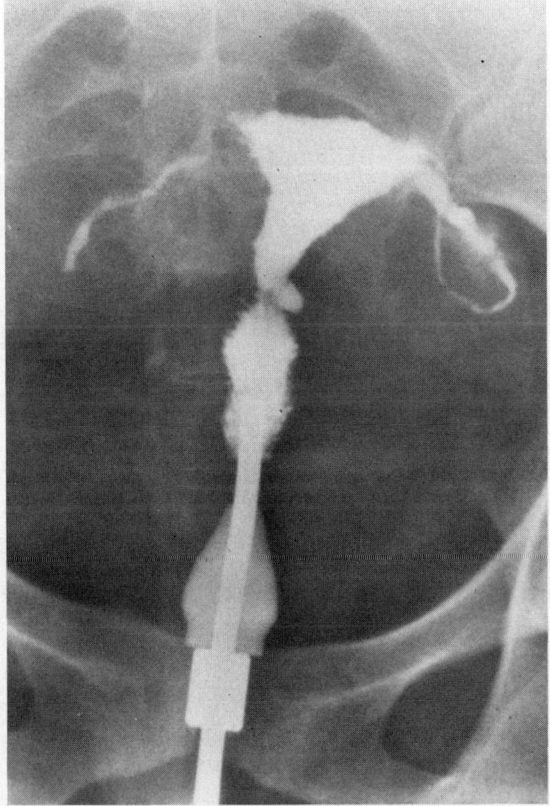

FIGURE 39-15
Tuberculous salpingitis in 37-year-old nulligravida with primary infertility for 15 years. Right tube is obstructed in zone of transition between isthmus and ampulla. Arrows indicate multiple strictures in both tubes. Nodular contour of endometrial cavity may also be related to tuberculosis and is analogous to pattern that has been found in ampulla in other cases. Small diverticulum near internal os probably represents adenomyosis. Diagnosis of tuberculosis was confirmed by endometrial culture. (From Richmond JA: Hysterosalpingography. Reproduced with permission from Infertility, contraception and reproductive endocrinology, 2nd ed, by Daniel R. Mishell, Jr., M.D., and Val Davajan, M.D. Copyright © 1986 Medical Economics Books, Oradell, N.J. 07649. All rights reserved.)

Therefore no tubal reconstructive surgical procedures should be attempted.

Tubal Causes of Infertility

During the past decade the incidence of infertility caused by damage to the oviduct has increased because of an increased incidence of salpingitis. Obstructions occur either at the distal or proximal portion of the oviduct and sometimes in both regions. The prognosis for fertility after surgical tubal reconstruction depends on the amount of damage to the oviduct as well as the location of the obstruction. If there is extensive damage, the chances for conception after tubal reconstruction are almost nil. These women have a greater chance of conceiving with an in vitro fertilization procedure, and thus the extent and location of the intrinsic and extrinsic tubal disease must be ascertained by both hysterosalpingography and laparoscopy in an effort to determine whether tubal reconstruction or in vitro fertilization offers the better prognosis. If both proximal and distal obstructions of the oviduct exist, the damage to the oviduct is usually so extensive that the oviduct can never function normally. Therefore, although it is possible to achieve tubal patency after surgical repair of a tube with both proximal and distal blockage, subsequent intrauterine pregnancy is uncommon. Therefore, surgical reconstruction should not be performed in such instances.

Distal Tubal Disease

The HSG will determine whether the tubal obstruction is complete or partial, the size of the distal sacculation, and the appearance of the mucosal folds and rugal pattern of the endosalpinx (Fig. 39-16). Laparoscopy will assist in determining the size of the hydrosalpinx, the amount of muscularis, and the thickness of the wall of the oviduct after distension with dye. Laparoscopic examination will determine whether pelvic adhesions are present and the extent of such adhesions. Women with fimbrial obstruction are not a homogeneous group, and the prognosis for intrauterine pregnancy following distal tubal reconstruction is related to the extent of the disease process. Therefore, it is important to perform both hysterosalpingog-

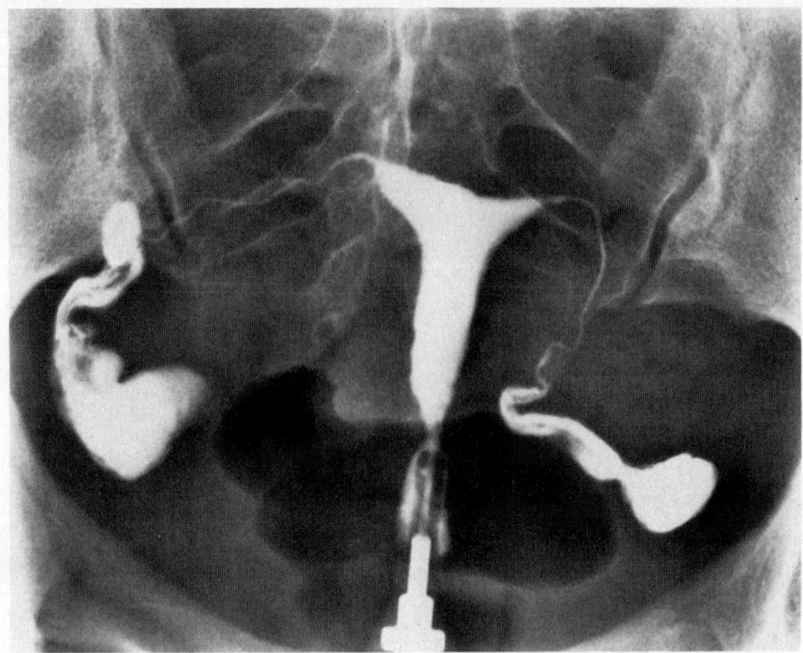

FIGURE 39-16
HSG showing bilateral hydrosalpinges with dilation, clubbing, and obstruction at fimbriated ends. Patient was 32-year-old woman with 10-year history of primary infertility. (From Richmond JA: Hysterosalpingography. Reproduced with permission from Infertility, contraception and reproductive endocrinology, 2nd ed, by Daniel R. Mishell, Jr., M.D., and Val Davajan, M.D. Copyright © 1986 Medical Economics Books, Oradell, N.J. 07649. All rights reserved.)

raphy and laparoscopy before surgical reconstruction to provide an individualized prognosis.

If the fimbriae of the distal end of the oviduct are relatively normal with only partial occlusion by adhesions or fimbrial bridges, removal of these adhesions by means of a fimbrioplasty procedure will result in higher conception rates (in the range of 60%) than if the distal end is completely occluded and a cuff salpingostomy procedure is required. Overall conception rates following salpingostomy are in the 30% range, with a high percentage (about one fourth) being tubal pregnancies. With the use of microsurgical techniques for the treatment of distal tubal disease the intrauterine pregnancy rate has not increased as compared with the results following conventional macrosurgery, but the rate of ectopic pregnancy appears to be somewhat greater following microsurgery. The incidence of ectopic pregnancy after surgical reconstruction for distal tubal dis-

ease is directly related to the amount of tubal damage existing before the operative procedure.

Boer-Meisel et al. correlated the results of tubal reconstruction with the degree of tubal damage according to the severity of five factors: (1) extent of adhesions, (2) nature of adhesions, (3) diameter of the hydrosalpinx, (4) appearance of the endosalpinx, and (5) thickness of the tubal wall. Utilizing these criteria they developed three prognostic categories: good—with a cumulative pregnancy rate of about 75%; intermediate—about 20%; and poor—less than 5%. In the good category, only 1 of 22 pregnancies was ectopic, but in the intermediate group half the pregnancies were tubal, and in the poor prognostic group six of seven pregnancies were ectopic. They concluded that if there were fixed adhesions with absent rugal folds and a thick, fixed tubal wall, distal tubal operation should not be performed.

Donnez and Casanas-Roux classified the de-

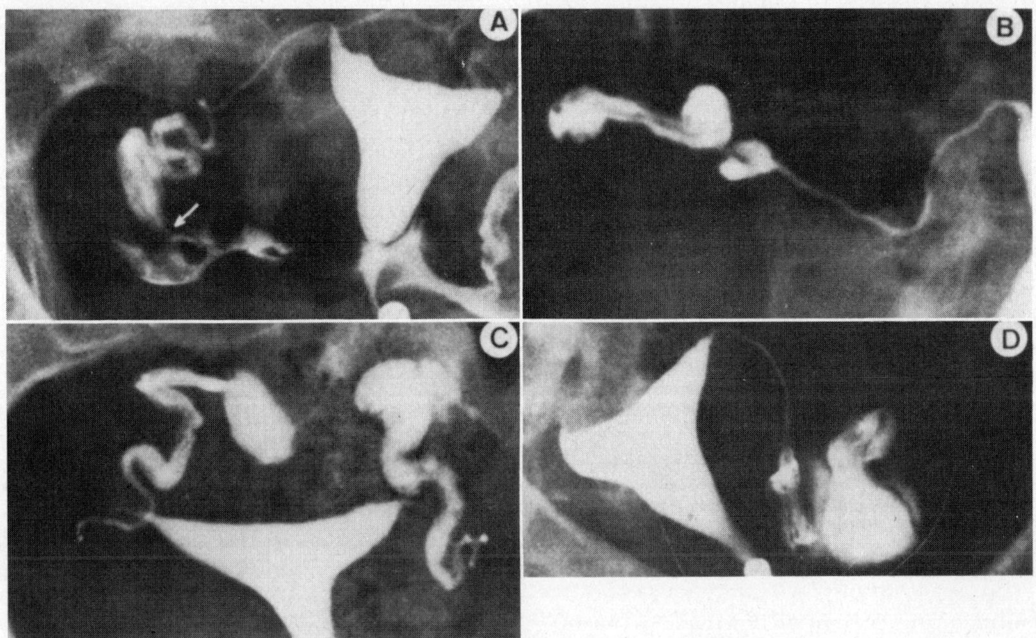

FIGURE 39-17
Classification of distal tubal occlusion based on degree of dilation seen on HSG. **A,** Degree I, conglutination of the fimbrial folds *(arrow)* with tubal patency. **B,** Degree II, complete distal occlusion with normal ampullary diameter. **C,** Degree III, complete distal occlusion with ampullary dilation 15 to 25 mm in diameter. **D,** Degree IV, occlusion with ampullary distension greater than 25 mm. (From Donnez J, Casanas-Roux F: Fertil Steril 46:200, 1986. Reproduced with permission of the publisher, The American Fertility Society.)

gree of distal tubal occlusion into four categories on the basis of hysterosalpingography (see Fig. 39-17). Following microscopic tubal reconstruction the cumulative pregnancy rate was directly related to the degree of occlusion. If the distal tubal ostium was completely normal but peritubal adhesions were present, lysis of these adhesions by a procedure called salpingolysis resulted in a 64% intrauterine pregnancy rate, similar to that obtained with a fimbrioplasty for partial obstruction. About half the women who underwent salpingostomy for degree II occlusion conceived, with no ectopic pregnancies, but only about one fourth of those with degree III or IV occlusions had subsequent intrauterine pregnancies, and the ectopic pregnancy rate was about 10% (Table 39-9). Thus following operation for more extensive distal tubal disease, nearly one third of the pregnancies that occurred were ectopic.

In both these studies the best prognostic factor was thickness of the tubal wall. If there was a hydrosalpinx greater than 2 cm in diameter with a thick tubal wall, the prognosis for a term pregnancy following distal tubal reconstruction was extremely poor. Hulka reported that when more than one half of the ovary was involved with adhesions, no patient had a term pregnancy following salpingostomy. Thus this information should be presented to the woman when she is counseled, and if the prognosis for term pregnancy is poor, she should be advised to undergo in vitro fertilization instead of surgical tubal reconstruction.

Proximal Tubal Blockage

If no dye reaches the oviduct during an HSG, the diagnosis of proximal tubal blockage should be considered. However, since spasm of

TABLE 39-9
Pregnancy Rate After Microsurgery and Ciliated Cell Percentage in Cases of Distal Tubal
Occlusion

Type of Operation	No. Patients	No. Intrauterine Pregnancies	No. Ectopic Pregnancies
Fimbrioplasty			
Occlusion of degree I	132	79 (60%)	2 (2%)
Salpingostomy			
Occlusion of degree II	27	13 (48%)	0
Occlusion of degree III	16	4 (25%)	1 (6%)
Occlusion of degree IV	40	9 (22%)	5 (12%)
TOTAL	83	26 (31%)	6 (7%)
Salpingolysis	42	27 (64%)	1 (2%)

Modified from Donnez J, Casanas-Roux F: Prognostic factors of fimbrial microsurgery. Fertil Steril 46:200, 1986. Reproduced with permission of the publisher, The American Fertility Society.

the intrauterine portion of the oviduct can occur, the diagnosis should be confirmed during laparoscopy performed with the patient under general anesthesia. Laparoscopy also allows examination of the distal portion of the oviduct. Proximal tubal blockage is most commonly due to residual damage after infection, but it can occasionally be due to endometriosis. Frequently tubal diverticula, also called salpingitis isthmica nodosa (SIN), are present.

Unlike the results of distal tubal reconstruction, the use of microsurgery has improved intrauterine rates for proximal tubal disease. Before the use of microsurgery, tubal intrauterine blockage was treated by reimplantation of the patent portion of the oviduct into the endometrial cavity. Term pregnancy rates following tubocornual implantation were in the 30% range. This procedure has now been replaced by a microsurgical tubocornual reanastomosis procedure in which the diseased portion of oviduct is excised and the patent distal oviduct is reanastomosed to the portion of the interstitial segment of the oviduct that is patent. With this technique various authors have reported term pregnancy rates of about 50%, with ectopic pregnancy rates of less than 10%.

Donnez and Casanas-Roux reported that the pregnancy rate following tubocornual reanastomosis was related to the extent of preexisting disease as determined at the time of HSG (Fig. 39-18). The best pregnancy rate—55%—was obtained when the interstitial portion of the oviduct was not damaged and less than 1.5 cm of occluded tube needed to be removed. The pregnancy rate declined to 33% when the interstitial portion of the tube was occluded and still further with the presence of some (25%) or numerous (16%) diverticular lesions. The overall ectopic pregnancy rate was 7%. Thus of patients who conceived, 15% had an ectopic pregnancy.

Adjunctive Therapy

Adjunctive procedures for surgical tubal reconstruction include prophylactic antibiotics, postoperative hydrotubation, placement of tubal stents, and methods to reduce postoperative adhesion formation, such as intraoperative instillation of high-molecular-weight dextran or corticosteroids or both, as well as systemic postoperative corticosteroid treatment. No prospective studies have shown postoperative hydrotubation to be of value, and tubal stents should not be used because they may cause mucosal damage. Intraperitoneal dextran is widely used, and some studies indicate that it may reduce adhesion formation. No randomized studies have shown that prophylactic antibiotic treatment or postoperative corticosteroid treatment is of any value, but each is widely used. Probably the most important way to reduce adhesion formation is meticulous surgical technique, including atraumatic tissue handling and small-caliber, nonreactive suture

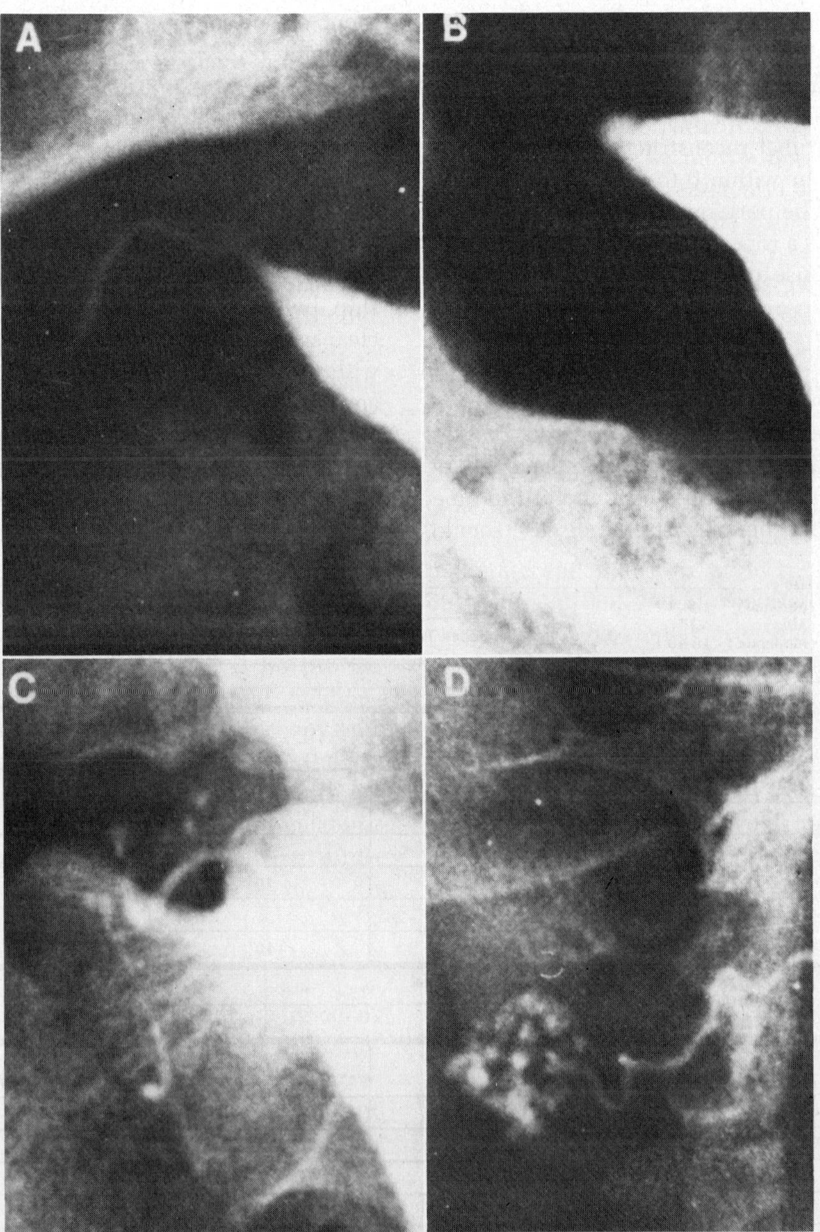

FIGURE 39-18
Types of occlusion following HSG. **A,** Undamaged intramural portion. **B,** Occluded intramural portion. **C,** Cornual occlusion with contrast extravasation in tubal wall. **D,** Occlusion with numerous diverticular lesions. (From Donnez J, Casanas-Roux F: Fertil Steril 46:1089, 1986. Reproduced with permission of the publisher, The American Fertility Society.)

<hr>

______________ KEY POINTS, cont'd ______________

- A sustained rise in BBT or a serum progesterone level greater than 5 ng/ml is presumptive evidence of ovulation.

- More than 90% of women with oligomenorrhea and 66% with secondary amenorrhea and estradiol levels of 40 pg/ml or higher will have presumptive evidence of ovulation following clomiphene therapy.

- When ovulation is induced with clomiphene citrate and no other causes of infertility are present, conception rates over time are similar to those of a normal fertile population.

- Patient discontinuation of therapy is the major reason for the reported difference in ovulation and conception rates in anovulatory women treated with clomiphene.

- When conception occurs after clomiphene treatment, the incidence of multiple gestation is increased to about 5%, with nearly all of them being twin gestations. The incidences of clinical spontaneous abortion, ectopic gestation, intrauterine fetal death, and congenital malformation are not significantly increased.

- Formation of ovarian cysts is the major side effect of clomiphene treatment.

- About 5% to 10% of women treated with the individualized, graduated, sequential regimen of clomiphene citrate fail to ovulate with the highest dosage.

- Treatment of anovulation with HMG effects an ovulatory rate of about 100% and an overall pregnancy rate of about 60%.

- The pregnancy rate per cycle with HMG treatment is similar to that following clomiphene therapy—22%.

- The incidence of spontaneous abortion after HMG therapy is high—25% to 35%—and clinically detectable ovarian enlargement occurs in about 5% to 10% of treatment cycles.

- For ovulation induction GnRH should be administered in a pulsatile manner at intervals of 1 to 2 hours.

<hr>

- Ovulation rates of 75% to 85% and overall pregnancy rates of 25% to 30% have been reported with GnRH treatment.

- Of all the causes of infertility, treatment of anovulation results in the greatest success.

- It is best to perform the postcoital test on the day before ovulation. A normal postcoital test is the presence of more than five motile sperm per high-power field.

- Pregnancy rates of 20% to 40% have been reported following washed intrauterine insemination for couples with an abnormal PCT.

- Pregnancy rates for oligospermia following either cervical cup insemination or intrauterine insemination are in the 25% to 35% range.

- Semen donors need to be carefully screened to be certain that they are in good health, do not have a potentially inherited disorder, and will not transmit an infectious agent in the semen.

- About half of infertile women with myomas conceive after myomectomy.

- Women with pelvic tuberculosis should be considered sterile, and no tubal reconstructive procedures should be attempted.

- The prognosis for fertility after tubal reconstruction depends on the amount of damage to the oviduct as well as the location of the obstruction.

- If both proximal and distal obstructions of the oviduct exist, intrauterine pregnancy is uncommon, and operative reconstruction should not be performed.

- Overall conception rates following salpingostomy are in the 30% range with a high percentage—about one fourth—being tubal pregnancies.

- The pregnancy rate after salpingolysis and fimbroplasty for partial obstruction is about 65%.

KEY POINTS, cont'd

- Unlike the results of distal tubal reconstruction, the use of microsurgery has improved intrauterine pregnancy rates for proximal tubal disease.

- With tubocornual reanastomosis for proximal tubal blockage, term pregnancy rates of about 50% have been reported, with ectopic pregnancy rates less than 10%.

- Evidence that minimal or mild endometriosis is a cause of infertility has not been established.

- Overall pregnancy rates for women with mild endometriosis, with or without treatment, are in the 60% to 75% range.

- About 65% of women with mild endometriosis and no other cause of infertility conceive without treatment. With moderate or severe disease, pregnancy rates with expectant management are 25% and 0%, respectively.

- Pregnancy rates following use of danazol for the treatment of moderate endometriosis are in the 40% to 50% range.

- Conception rates for women treated surgically have been reported to be in the 50% to 60% range for those with moderate endometriosis and 30% to 40% for those with severe endometriosis.

- The five secondary tests for infertility are measurement of serum prolactin and TSH; a late luteal phase endometrial biopsy; immunologic tests to detect sperm antibodies; bacterial culture of cervical mucus and semen; and zona-free hamster egg penetration test by husband's sperm.

- The rate of pregnancy following in vitro fertilization is related to the number of embryos placed in the uterine cavity.

- The pregnancy rate is about 13% in the first in vitro fertilization treatment cycle.

- The pregnancy rate per cycle of in vitro fertilization remains relatively constant, and after six cycles the cumulative pregnancy rate is about 60%.

- There is a high spontaneous abortion rate (about 30%) for pregnancies after in vitro fertilization.

- If an infertile couple fails to conceive after 2 years or with unexplained infertility 3 years after laparoscopy, they should be informed the chances for conception are remote.

BIBLIOGRAPHY

Alper MM, Garner PR, Spence JEH, et al: Pregnancy rates after hysterosalpingography with oil- and water-soluble contrast media. Obstet Gynecol 68:6, 1986.

Andrews WC, Buttram VC, Behrman SJ, et al: Revised American Fertility Society classification of endometriosis: 1985. Fertil Steril 43-351, 1985.

Asch RH, Balmaceda JP, Ellsworth LR, et al: Preliminary experiences with gamete intrafallopian transfer (GIFT). Fertil Steril 45:366, 1986.

Barbieri RL, Evans S, Kistner RW: Danazol in the treatment of endometriosis: Analysis of 100 cases with a 4-year follow-up. Fertil Steril 37:737, 1982.

Bartin D, Vargyas JM, Sato F, et al: The correlation between in vitro fertilization of human oocytes and semen profile. Fertil Steril 44:835, 1985.

Berger T, Marrs RP, Moyer DL: Comparison of techniques for selection of motile spermatozoa. Fertil Steril 43:268, 1984.

Berger T, Marrs R, Saito H, et al: Factors affecting human sperm penetration of zona free hamster ova. Am J Obstet Gynecol 145:397, 1983.

Bernstein GS: Male factor in infertility. In Mishell DR Jr, Davajan V, eds: Infertility, contraception and reproductive endocrinology, 2nd ed. Oradell, N.J., Medical Economics Books, 1986.

Bernstein GS: Occult genital infection. In Mishell DR Jr, Davajan V, eds: Infertility, contraception and reproductive endocrinology, 2nd ed. Oradell, N.J., Medical Economics Books, 1986.

Boer-Meisel ME, te Velde ER, Habbema JDF, et al: Predicting the pregnancy outcome in patients treated for hydrosalpinx: A prospective study. Fertil Steril 45:23, 1986.

Buttram VC Jr: Conservative surgery for endometriosis in the infertile female: A study of 206 patients with implications for both medical and surgical therapy. Fertil Steril 31:117, 1979.

Buttram VC Jr: Surgical treatment of endometriosis in the infertile female: A modified approach. Fertil Steril 32:635, 1979.

Buttram VC Jr: Evolution of the revised American Fertility Society classification of endometriosis. Fertil Steril 43:347, 1985.

Buttram VC Jr, Reiter RC, Ward S: Treatment of endometriosis with danazol: Report of a 6-year prospective study. Fertil Steril 43:353, 1985.

Clarke GN, Lopata A, Johnston WIH: Effect of sperm antibodies in females on human in vitro fertilization. Fertil Steril 46:435, 1986.

Collins JA, Wrixon W, Janes LB, et al: Treatment-independent pregnancy among infertile couples. N Engl J Med 309:1201, 1983.

Cook CL, Rao CV, Yussman MA: Plasma gonadotropin and sex steroid hormone levels during early, midfollicular, and midluteal phases of women with luteal phase defects. Fertil Steril 40:45, 1983.

Cruz RI, Kemmann E, Brandeis VT, et al: A prospective study of intrauterine insemination of processed sperm from men with oligoasthenospermia in superovulated women. Fertil Steril 46:673, 1986.

Daly DC, Walters CA, Soto-Albors CE, et al: A randomized study of dexamethasone in ovulation induction with clomiphene citrate. Fertil Steril 41:844, 1984.

Daniell JF, Herbert CM: Laparoscopic salpingostomy utilizing the CO_2 laser. Fertil Steril 41:558, 1984.

Davajan V: Postcoital testing: The cervical factor as a cause of infertility. In Mishell DR Jr, Davajan V, eds: Infertility, contraception and reproductive endocrinology, 2nd ed. Oradell, N.J., Medical Economics Books, 1986.

Davajan V, Mishell DR Jr: Evaluation of the infertile couple. In Mishell DR Jr, Davajan V, eds: Infertility, contraception and reproductive endocrinology, 2nd ed. Oradell, N.J., Medical Economics Books, 1986.

Dellenbach P, Nisand I, Moreau L, et al: Transvaginal sonographically controlled follicle puncture for oocyte retrieval. Fertil Steril 44:656, 1985.

Dmowski WP, Cohen MR: Antigonadotropin (danazol) in the treatment of endometriosis: Evaluation of posttreatment fertility and 3-year follow-up data. Am J Obstet Gynecol 130:41, 1978.

Donnez J, Casanas-Roux F: Prognostic factors influencing the pregnancy rate after microsurgical cornual anastomosis. Fertil Steril 46:1089, 1986.

Donnez J, Casanas-Roux F: Prognostic factors of fimbrial microsurgery. Fertil Steril 46:200, 1986.

Eliasson R: Parameters of male fertility. In Hafez ESE, Evans TN, eds: Human reproduction. New York, Harper & Row, Publishers, 1973.

Eliasson R: Semen analysis and laboratory work-up. In Cockett ATK, Urry RL, eds: Male infertility: Work-up, treatment, and research. New York, Grune & Stratton, 1977.

Fayez JA, Jobson VW, Lentz SS, et al: Tubal microsurgery with the carbon dioxide laser. Am J Obstet Gynecol 146:371, 1983.

Filmar S, Gomel V, McComb P: The effectiveness of CO_2 laser and electromicrosurgery in adhesiolysis: A comparative study. Fertil Steril 45:407, 1986.

Friberg J, Gnarpe H: *Mycoplasma* and human reproductive failure. III. Pregnancies in "infertile" couples treated with doxycycline for T-mycoplasmas. Am J Obstet Gynecol 116:23, 1973.

Garcia CR, David SS: Pelvic endometriosis: Infertility and pelvic pain. Am J Obstet Gynecol 129:740, 1977.

Guzick DS, Wilkes C, Jones HW Jr: Cumulative pregnancy rates for in vitro fertilization. Fertil Steril 46:663, 1986.

Gysler M, March CM, Mishell DR Jr, et al: A decade's experience with an individualized clomiphene treatment regimen including its effect on the postcoital test. Fertil Steril 37:161, 1982.

Haas GG Jr, Beer AE: Immunologic influences on reproductive biology: Sperm gametogenesis and maturation in the male and female genital tracts. Fertil Steril 46:753, 1986.

Hammond MG: Monitoring techniques for improved pregnancy rates during clomiphene ovulation induction. Fertil Steril 42:499, 1984.

Hammond MG, Halme JK, Talbert LM: Factors affecting the pregnancy rate in clomiphene citrate induction of ovulation. Obstet Gynecol 62:196, 1983.

Hammond MG, Talbert LM: Clomiphene citrate in the management of infertile women with low luteal phase progesterone levels. Am J Obstet Gynecol 59:275, 1982.

Harrison RF, DeLouvois J, Blades M, et al: Doxycycline treatment and human infertility. Lancet 1:605, 1975.

Hendershot GE, Mosher WD, Pratt WF: Infertility and age: An unresolved issue. Fam Plann Perspect 14:287, 1982.

Holtz G, Kling OR: Effect of surgical technique on peritoneal adhesion reformation after lysis. Fertil Steril 37:494, 1982.

Horton R, Lobo R: Peripheral androgens and the role of androstanediol glucuronide. Clin Endocrinol Metab 15:293, 1986.

Howe G, Westhoff C, Vessey M, et al: Effects of age, cigarette smoking, and other factors on fertility: Findings in a large prospective study. Br Med J 290:1697, 1985.

Hulka JF: Adnexal adhesions: A prognostic staging and classification system based on a five-year survey of fertility surgery results at Chapel Hill, North Carolina. Am J Obstet Gynecol 144:141, 1982.

Hull MGR, Glazener CMA, Kelly NJ, et al: Population study of causes, treatment, and outcome of infertility. Br Med J 291:1984, 1985.

Hull MGR, Savage PE, Bromham DR: Prognostic value of the postcoital test: Prospective study based on time-specific conception rates. Br J Obstet Gynecol 89:299, 1982.

Hull MGR, Savage PE, Bromham DR, et al: The value of a single serum progesterone measurement in the midluteal phase as a criterion of a potentially fertile cycle ("ovulation") derived from treated and untreated conception cycles. Fertil Steril 37:355, 1982.

Hurley DM, Brian R, Outch K, et al: Induction of ovulation and fertility in amenorrheic women by pulsatile low-dose gonadotropin-releasing hormone treatment of anovulatory infertility. Fertil Steril 40:575, 1983.

Isojima S, Li TS, Ashitaka Y: Immunologic analysis of sperm-immobilizing factor found in sera of women with unexplained sterility. Am J Obstet Gynecol 101:677, 1968.

Israel R, March CM: Diagnostic laparoscopy: A prognostic aid in the surgical management of infertility. Am J Obstet Gynecol 125:969, 1976.

Jones GES, Delfs E: Endocrine patterns in term pregnancies following abortion. JAMA 146:1212, 1951.

Jones HW, Acosta AA, Andrews MC, et al: Three years of in vitro fertilization at Norfolk. Fertil Steril 42:826, 1984.

Jones WR: Immunologic infertility: Fact or fiction? Fertil Steril 33:577, 1980.

Kovacs GR, Rogers P, Leeton JF, et al: In-vitro fertilization and embryo transfer. Med J Aust 144:682, 1986.

Kurachi K, Aono T, Minagawa J, et al: Congenital malformations of newborn infants after clomiphene-induced ovulation. Fertil Steril 40:187, 1983.

Lauritsen JG, Pagel JD, Vangsted P, et al: Results of repeated tuboplasties. Fertil Steril 37:68, 1982.

Lenz S, Lauritsen JG: Ultrasonically guided percutaneous aspiration of human follicles under local anesthesia: A new method of collecting oocytes for in vitro fertilization. Fertil Steril 38:673, 1982.

Lewin A, Laufer N, Rabinowitz R, et al: Ultrasonically guided oocyte collection under local anesthesia: The first choice method for in vitro fertilization—a comparative study with laparoscopy. Fertil Steril 46:257, 1986.

Lipshultz LI, Howards SS, eds: Infertility in the male. New York, Churchill Livingstone, 1983.

Lobo RA, Granger LR, Davajan V, et al: An extended regimen of clomiphene citrate in women unresponsive to standard therapy. Fertil Steril 37:762, 1982.

Lobo RA, Paul W, March CM, et al: Clomiphene and dexamethasone in women unresponsive to clomiphene alone. Obstet Gynecol 60:497, 1982.

Luciano AA, Hauser KS, Benda J: Evaluation of commonly used adjuvants in the prevention of postoperative adhesions. Am J Obstet Gynecol 146:88, 1983.

Malone MJ, Ingersol FM: Myomectomy in infertility. In Behrman SJ, Kistner RW, eds: Progress in infertility, 2nd ed. Boston, Little, Brown & Co., 1975.

March CM: Luteal phase defects. In Mishell DR Jr, Davajan V, eds: Infertility, contraception and reproductive endocrinology, 2nd ed. Oradell, N.J., Medical Economics Books, 1986.

March CM: Improved pregnancy rates with monitoring of gonadotropin therapy by three modalities. Am J Obstet Gynecol. In press.

March CM, Israel R: Gestational outcome following hysteroscopic lysis of adhesions. Fertil Steril 36:455, 1981.

March CM, Mishell DR Jr: Induction of ovulation. In Mishell DR Jr, Davajan V, eds: Infertility, contraception and reproductive endocrinology, 2nd ed. Oradell, N.J., Medical Economics Books, 1986.

Marrs RP, Vargyas JM: Human in vitro fertilization: State of the art. In Mishell DR Jr, Davajan V, eds: Infertility, contraception and reproductive endocrinology, 2nd ed. Oradell, N.J., Medical Economics Books, 1986.

Marrs RP, Vargyas JM: Pelvic endometriosis. In Mishell DR Jr, Davajan V, eds: Infertility, contraception and reproductive endocrinology, 2nd ed. Oradell, N.J., Medical Economics Books, 1986.

Marrs RP, Vargyas JM, Gibbons WE, et al: A modified technique of human in vitro fertilization and embryo transfer. Am J Obstet Gynecol 147:318, 1983.

Mason P, Adams J, Morris DV, et al: Induction of ovulation using pulsatile luteinizing hormone–releasing hormone. Br Med J 288:181, 1984.

Matthews CD, Clapp KH, Tansing JA, et al: T-mycoplasma genital infection: The effect of doxycycline therapy on human unexplained infertility. Fertil Steril 30:98, 1978.

Meldrum DR, Chang RJ, Lu J: "Medical oophorectomy" using a long-acting GnRH agonist—a possible new approach to the treatment of endometriosis. J Clin Endocrinol Metab 54:1081, 1982.

Menge AC, Medley NE, Mangione CM, et al: The incidence and influence of antisperm antibodies in infertile human couples on sperm–cervical mucus interactions and subsequent fertility. Fertil Steril 38:439, 1982.

Moghissi KS, Sacco AG, Borin K: Immunologic infertility.

I. Cervical mucus antibodies and postcoital tests. Am J Obstet Gynecol 136:941, 1980.

Moore EE, Harger JA, Rock JA, et al: Management of pelvic endometriosis with low-dose danazol. Fertil Steril 36:15, 1981.

Mosher WD: Infertility trends among U.S. couples: 1965-1976. Fam Plann Perspect 14:22, 1982.

Muse KN, Wilson EA: How does mild endometriosis cause infertility? Fertil Steril 38:145, 1982.

Newill RG, Katz M: The basal body temperature chart in artificial insemination by donor pregnancy cycles. Fertil Steril 39:431, 1982.

Noyes RW, Hertig AT, Rock J: Dating the endometrial biopsy. Fertil Steril 39:277, 1983.

O'Herlihy C, Pepperell JR, Brown JB, et al: Incremental clomiphene therapy: A new method for treating persistent anovulation. Obstet Gynecol 58:535, 1981.

Olive DL, Stohs GF, Metzger DA, et al: Expectant management and hydrotubations in the treatment of endometriosis-associated infertility. Fertil Steril 44:35, 1985.

Ory SJ: Clinical uses of luteinizing hormone–releasing hormone. Fertil Steril 39:577, 1983.

Patton GW Jr: Pregnancy outcome following microsurgical fimbrioplasty. Fertil Steril 37:150, 1982.

Richmond JA: Hysterosalpingography. In Mishell DR Jr, Davajan V, eds: Infertility, contraception and reproductive endocrinology, 2nd ed. Oradell, N.J., Medical Economics Books, 1986.

Rogers BJ: The sperm penetration assay: Its usefulness reevaluated. Fertil Steril 43:821, 1985.

Rosenberg SM, Luciano AA, Riddick DH: The luteal phase defect: The relative frequency of, and encouraging response to, treatment with vaginal progesterone. Fertil Steril 34:17, 1980.

Rousseau S, Lord J, Lepage Y, et al: The expectancy of pregnancy for "normal" infertile couples. Fertil Steril 40:768, 1983.

Schenken RS, Malinak LR: Conservative surgery versus expectant management for the infertile patient with mild endometriosis. Fertil Steril 37:183, 1982.

Schwarz D, Mayaux MJ: Female fecundity as a function of age: Results of artificial insemination in 2193 nulliparous women with azoospermic husbands. Fédération des Centres d'Etude et de Conservation du Sperme Humain. N Engl J Med 306:404, 1982.

Scott JZ, Nakamura RM, Mutch J, et al: The cervical factor in infertility. Diagnosis and treatment. Fertil Steril 28:1289, 1977.

Seibel MM, Berger MJ, Weinstein FG, et al: The effectiveness of danazol on subsequent fertility in minimal endometriosis. Fertil Steril 38:534, 1982.

Seiler JC, Gidwani G, Ballard L: Laparoscopic cauterization of endometriosis for fertility: A controlled study. Fertil Steril 46:1098, 1986.

Stenchever MA, Spadoni LR, Smith WD, et al: Benefits of the sperm (hamster ova) penetration assay in the evaluation of the infertile couple. Am J Obstet Gynecol 143:91, 1982.

Stumpf PG, March CM: Febrile morbidity following hysterosalpingography: Identification of risk factors and recommendations for prophylaxis. Fertil Steril 33:487, 1980.

Tredway DR, Settlage DS, Nakamura RM, et al: The significance of timing for the postcoital evaluation of cervical mucus. Am J Obstet Gynecol 121:387, 1975.

Tulandi T: Salpingo-ovariolysis: A comparison between laser surgery and electrosurgery. Fertil Steril 45:489, 1986.

Weinstein FG, Seibel MM, Taymor ML: Ovulation induction with subcutaneous pulsatile gonadotropin-releasing hormone: The role of supplemental human chorionic gonadotropin in the luteal phase. Fertil Steril 41:546, 1984.

Wikland M, Nilsson L, Hansson R, et al: Collection of human oocytes by the use of sonography. Fertil Steril 39:603, 1983.

Wilkes CA, Rosenwaks Z, Jones DL, et al: Pregnancy related to infertility diagnosis, number of attempts, and age in a program of in vitro fertilization. Obstet Gynecol 66:350, 1985.

Winston RM: Microsurgical tubocornual anastomosis for reversal of sterilization. Lancet 1:284, 1977.

Winston RM: Microsurgery of the fallopian tube: From fantasy to reality. Fertil Steril 34:521, 1980.

Yanagimachi R, Yanagimachi H, Rogers BT: The use of zona-free animal ova as a test system for the assessment of the fertilizing capacity of human spermatozoa. Biol Reprod 15:471, 1976.

Menopause

Atrophic Vaginitis. Inflammation of the vaginal mucosa due to atrophy secondary to decreased estrogen level.

Climacteric. The physiologic period in a woman's life during which there is regression of ovarian function.

Hot Flush. Pathognomonic symptom of the menopause; a sudden, explosive physiologic phenomenon lasting 3 to 4 minutes accompanied by increased digital perfusion and increased peripheral skin temperature.

Menopause. Cessation of menstruation for at least 6 months due to depletion of ovarian follicles.

Osteoporosis. Reduction of the quantity of structural material in trabecular bone.

Premature Ovarian Failure. Cessation of menstruation due to depletion of ovarian follicles before the age of 40. It is also called premature menopause.

The decline of ovarian function occurs gradually, and the cessation of menses is only one facet of the climacteric process. In practice the terms *menopause* and *climacteric* are used interchangeably. The mean age of menopause in the United States is about 51 years, with a normal distribution curve and 95% confidence limits between ages 45 and 55 years (Fig. 40-1). If a woman stops menstruating before age 40, the condition should be called premature ovarian failure instead of premature menopause because of the severe psychologic connotations of the latter term. If a woman continues to menstruate after the age of 55, there is an increased possibility that the endometrium will be hyperplastic or malignant. Therefore, it is advisable to biopsy the endometrium of any woman who continues to menstruate after the age of 55.

The age at which the menopause occurs is genetically predetermined, unlike the age of menarche, which is related to body mass. The age at menopause is not related to the number of prior ovulations, that is, is not affected by pregnancy, lactation, use of oral contraceptives, or failure to ovulate spontaneously. It is also not related to race, socioeconomic conditions, education, height, weight, age at menarche, or age at the last pregnancy. The age at menopause may be affected by smoking, as it has been reported that cigarette smokers experience an earlier spontaneous menopause than do nonsmokers. About 100 years ago the mean age of the menopause was approximately 40 years, but now it is about 50 years because women are living longer, and those who genetically would have a later menopause are now living past that age (Fig. 40-2).

In the United States the average life expectancy for a woman is about 78 years. About 28 years, or more than one-third of a woman's life, will be spent after the menopause, a time when many women will be seeking medical care. Thus a large proportion of all physicians' time (gynecologists, internists, and family practitioners) will be spent taking care of postmenopausal women. In 1980 there were 113 million women in the United States, with about 32 million women over 50 years of age, an increase in both numbers from the 1970 census.

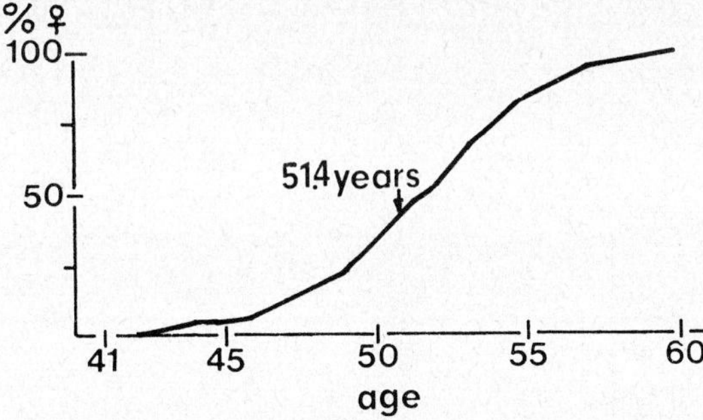

FIGURE 40-1
Frequency distribution of age at menopause. (From Jaszmann LJB: Epidemiology of the climacteric syndrome. In Campbell S, ed: Management of the menopause and post-menopausal years. Lancaster, England, MTP Press Ltd., 1976, p. 12.)

ENDOCRINOLOGY

The basic feature of menopause is depletion of ovarian follicles with degeneration of the granulosa and theca cells. As theca cells degenerate, they fail to react to endogenous gonadotrophins. As a result less estrogen is produced, and there is a decrease in the negative feedback on the hypothalamic-pituitary axis. With less inhibition, gonadotrophin production increases in an attempt to stimulate the ovary. As reported by Sherman et al., this process begins about 5 years before the actual menopause. At this time, follicle-stimulating hormone (FSH) levels increase and estradiol levels decrease, while luteinizing hormone (LH) and progesterone levels remain unchanged, indicating that the cycles probably remain ovulatory (Fig. 40-3). As estrogen concentrations decline, there is an associated decrease in prolactin levels. The decrease in estradiol before the actual menopause accounts for the fact that some women will have hot flushes during the 5 years or so before menstruation stops completely. Patients over 40 who are having regular menstrual cycles and are also having hot flushes should be treated with low doses of oral estrogen to relieve these symptoms, that is, 0.3 mg of conjugated equine estrogen or 0.3 mg of estrone sulfate from the fifth day after menstruation begins until the onset of the next menses.

In contrast to the follicular cells, the stromal cells of the ovary continue to produce androgens, androstenedione and testosterone, as the result of increased LH stimulation after the menopause. The adrenal glands also secrete

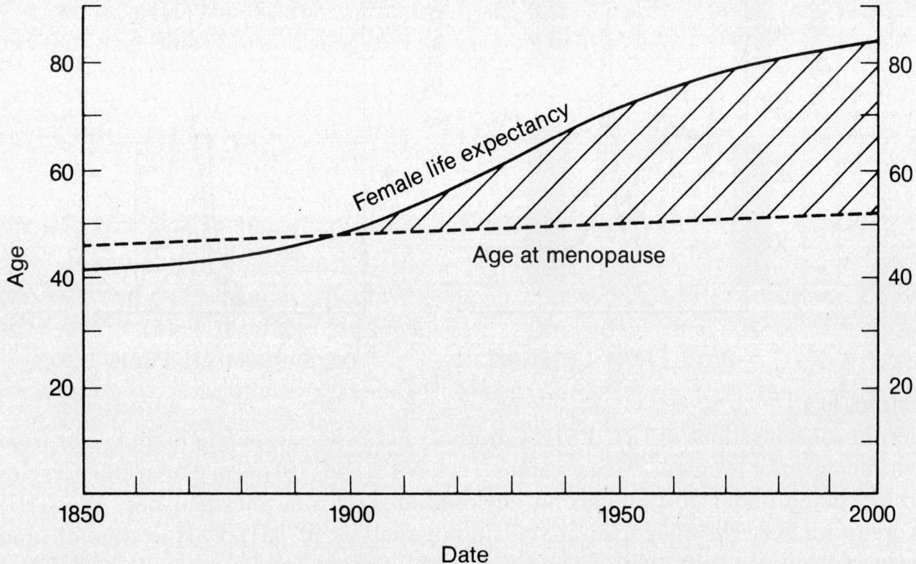

FIGURE 40-2
Female life expectancy. (From Cope E: Physical changes associated with the post-menopausal years. In Campbell S, ed: Management of the menopause and post-menopausal years. Lancaster, England, MTP Press Ltd., 1976, p. 33.)

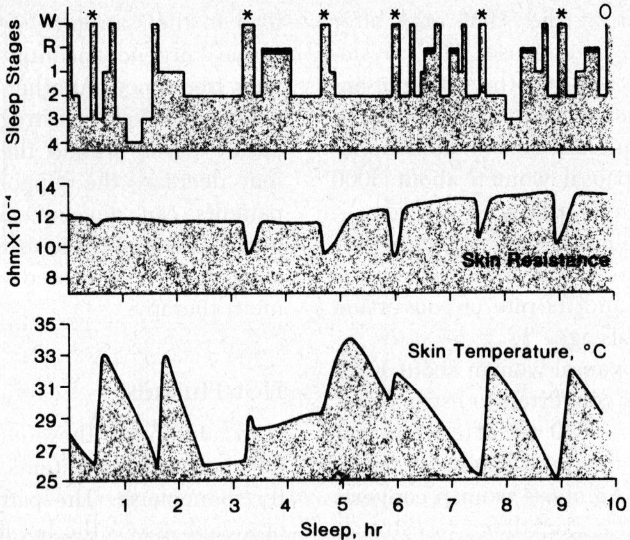

FIGURE 40-5

Sleepgram and recordings of skin resistance and temperature in postmenopausal subject with severe hot flushes. Asterisk indicates an objectively measured hot flush. (From Erlik Y, Tataryn IV, Meldrum DR, et al: JAMA 245:1741, 1981. Copyright 1981, American Medical Association.)

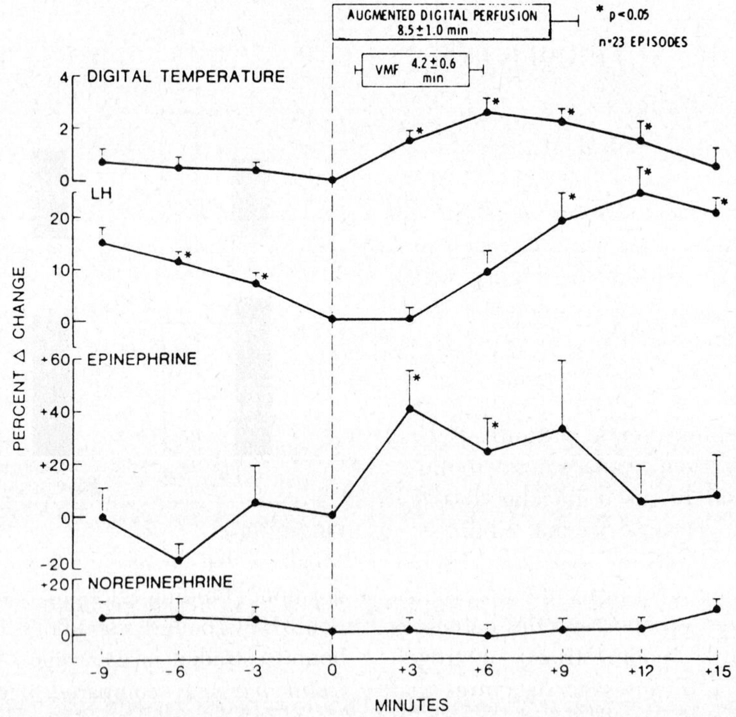

FIGURE 40-6

Composite graph of objective parameters obtained in five symptomatic postmenopausal women. Data are normalized to beginning of augmented digital perfusion (*0 time*). (From Mashchak CA, Kletzky OA, Artal R, Mishell DR Jr: Maturitas 6:301, 1984.)

is stopped. The change in estrogen levels leads to alterations in the hypothalamus that are probably mediated through the central nervous system. When the change in estrogen levels is not gradual but sudden, such as occurs after castration, the individual is more likely to develop symptomatic hot flushes.

About 75% of all women going through menopause develop hot flushes. Obese individuals are less likely to develop flushes, as they do not have as great a decrease in estrogen levels. Erlik et al. have shown that postmenopausal women with hot flushes have lower circulating estrone and estradiol levels as well as less sex hormone–binding globulin (SHBG) bound estradiol than postmenopausal women without hot flushes (Fig. 40-4). These investigators reported that women with hot flushes had less total body weight and a lower percentage of ideal body weight as compared with those without hot flushes. About one third of women with hot flushes have sufficiently severe symptoms to require medical assistance. About one half of the patients with flushes have at least one a day, and about 20% have more than one a day. These flushes frequently occur at night, awaken the individual, and then produce insomnia (Fig. 40-5). Hot flushes do not persist in most women for more than 2 to 3 years, and it is uncommon for a woman to have

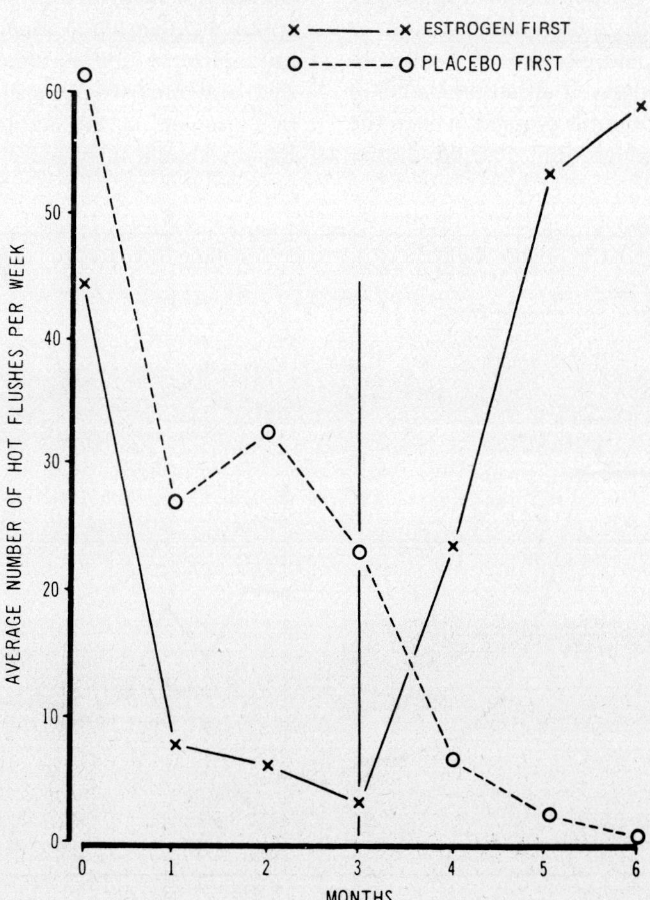

FIGURE 40-7
Average number of hot flushes per week in randomized, double-blind, 6-month crossover study of estrogen and placebo therapy. (From Coope J: Double-blind crossover study of estrogen replacement therapy. In Campbell S, ed: Management of the menopause and post-menopausal years. Lancaster, England, MTP Press Ltd., 1976, p. 167.)

hot flushes that last more than 5 years after menopause. A hot flush is a sudden, explosive systemic physiologic phenomenon that takes place over a period of 30 seconds to 5 minutes. The flush is preceded by an increase in digital perfusion, which is followed by increases in peripheral skin temperature, circulating norepinephrine and LH levels, and heart rate (Fig. 40-6). With each flush there are increases in LH, adrenocorticotropic hormone (ACTH), and cortisol but not FSH or estradiol. The LH increase is an effect of the change in the hypothalamic-pituitary axis and not a cause of the hot flush, because patients without a pituitary gland also have hot flushes.

The most effective treatment for the hot flush is estrogen, as Coope demonstrated in an excellent randomized, double-blind cross-over study with estrogen and placebo. Women with hot flushes initially received either a placebo or estrogen and after 3 months crossed over to the other therapy. Although the placebo dimin-

ished the frequency of hot flushes, when the patients receiving placebo were crossed over to estrogen therapy, their hot flushes disappeared (Fig. 40-7). Those who were treated with estrogen first had a marked diminution of hot flushes, significantly more than with the placebo, and when they were crossed over to placebo, the incidence of hot flushes returned to prestudy levels. This study demonstrates that for treatment of hot flushes, estrogen is more effective than placebo. Since so many of the hot flushes occur at night, it is advisable for the patient to ingest the estrogen tablet before bedtime. Some patients, such as those with a history of cancer of the breast or a recent (less than 2 years) cancer of the endometrium, should not take estrogen. The next best therapy is a progestogen. Schiff et al. showed in a randomized, double-blind, cross-over study that oral medroxyprogesterone acetate (MPA) in a dosage of 20 mg per day relieves hot flushes significantly more effectively than pla-

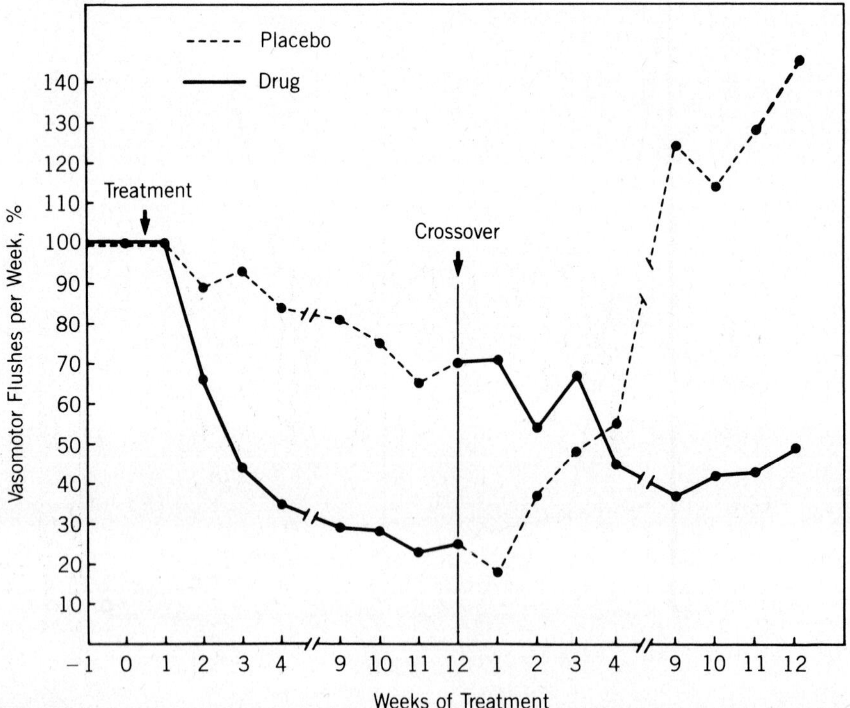

FIGURE 40-8

Mean number of vasomotor flushes as percentage change from pretreatment. Change of treatment regimen (crossover) occurred at 12 weeks. (From Schiff I, Tulchinsky D, Cramer D, Ryan KJ: JAMA 244:1443, 1980. Copyright 1980, American Medical Association.)

cebo (Fig. 40-8). Unfortunately, MPA does not prevent vaginal or urethral atrophy, but it will diminish hot flushes in patients who cannot take estrogen. Oral MPA 20 mg per day is expensive. Several investigators have shown that injections of Depo-Provera (DMPA) in a dosage of 150 mg once every 3 months relieves hot flushes very well. Lobo et al. compared DMPA with conjugated equine estrogens in the treatment of hot flushes and found that DMPA was as effective as estrogens in relieving the symptoms of the hot flush (Fig. 40-9). In addition, DMPA decreased markers of bone resorption—urinary calcium and hydroxyproline urinary excretion—to an extent similar to that

when 0.625 mg of conjugated equine estrogen (Fig. 40-10) was given. Other agents shown to significantly reduce hot flushes include clonidine, naloxone, and methyldopa (Aldomet), but these drugs are not usually prescribed for this purpose.

Other Systemic Symptoms

Symptoms such as anxiety, depression, irritability, and fatigue increase after. menopause. Controversy exists as to whether estrogen relieves these symptoms directly or whether because estrogen prevents hot flushes and allows the patient to sleep better, the other symptoms

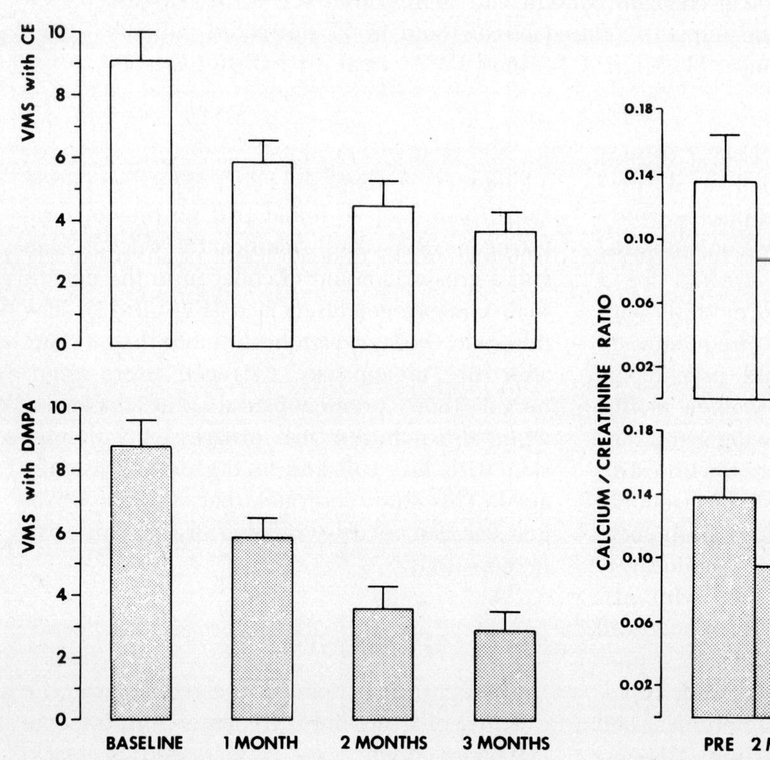

FIGURE 40-9
Vasomotor symptoms (mean ± SE) experienced before treatment (baseline) and after 1, 2, and 3 months of treatment in 23 women receiving conjugated estrogens *(open bars)* and 21 women treated with depomedroxyprogesterone acetate (DMPA; *shaded bars*). (From Lobo RA, McCormick W, Singer F, Roy S: Obstet Gynecol 63:1, 1984. Reprinted with permission from The American College of Obstetricians and Gynecologists.)

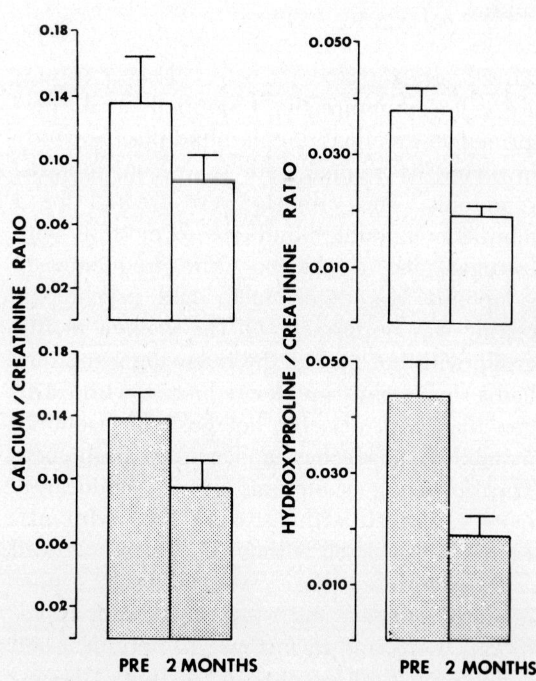

FIGURE 40-10
Calcium-creatinine and hydroxyproline-creatinine ratios (mean ± SE) before and after 2 months of treatment with either conjugated estrogens *(open bars)* or depomedroxyprogesterone acetate (DMPA; *shaded bars*). (From Lobo RA, McCormick W, Singer F, Roy S: Obstet Gynecol 63:1, 1984. Reprinted with permission from The American College of Obstetricians and Gynecologists.)

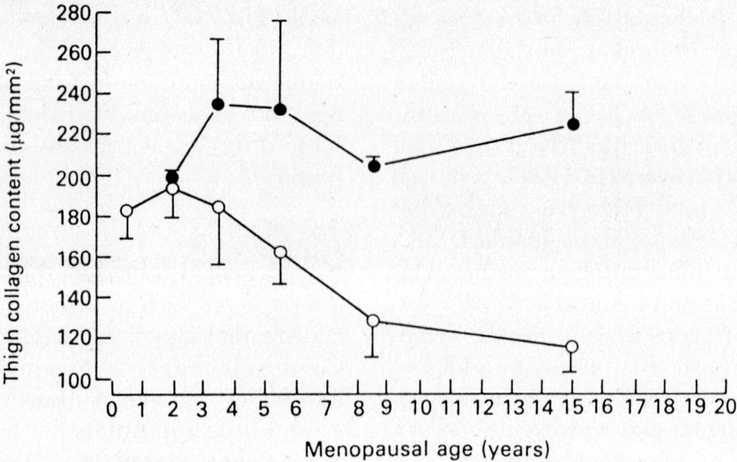

FIGURE 40-11
Relation between thigh skin collagen content and menopausal age in 52 patients treated with sex hormone implants *(closed circles)* and in 77 untreated patients *(open circles)*. (From Brincat M, Moniz CJ, Studd JWW, et al: Br J Obstet Gynaecol 92:256, 1985.)

are relieved indirectly. Campbell et al. performed an excellent double-blind placebo study involving 64 women with severe menopausal symptoms. The subjects were treated for 4 months in a double-blind cross-over study with estrogen and a placebo. The frequency of symptoms was determined, and psychologic testing was performed. Of the women in this group with hot flushes the following symptoms had a significantly greater reduction with estrogen than with placebo: hot flushes, insomnia, irritability, headaches, and urinary frequency. The following symptoms were significantly more improved with estrogen than with placebo in the women without hot flushes as well as those with hot flushes: vaginal dryness, poor memory, anxiety, and worry about self. In addition, there was an increase in optimism and good spirits with psychologic testing. Thus estrogen improves many psychological symptoms in addition to relieving the hot flush and allowing the patient to sleep better. Nevertheless estrogen is not a panacea for all the problems of aging. The Campbell et al. study found that there was no significant difference between the improvement of some symptoms with this short-term use of estrogen and with the placebo. These symptoms included arthralgias, backache, skin conditions, vaginal discomfort, coital satisfaction, and frequency of orgasm. In

a long-term study of the effect of estrogen upon skin, Brincat et al. found that postmenopausal estrogen users had significantly thicker skin and a greater amount of collagen in the dermis than nonestrogen users had (Fig. 40-11). The difference became significant more than 3 years after the menopause. Estrogen users maintained their premenopausal skin thickness, while the nonusers had progressively thinner skin with less collagen in the dermis as they aged. This study indicates that systemic estrogen use can retard wrinkling of the skin postmenopausally.

OSTEOPOROSIS

Osteoporosis is defined as a reduction in the quantity of structural bony material in trabecular bone. Bone mass is increased in black, obese, and tall women and is decreased in short, frail, thin-skinned, sedentary women. Thus, women in the former group usually do not develop osteoporosis, while women in the latter group are at greater risk for developing the disorder. In the latter group of women about 1% to 1.5% of bone mass is lost each year after menopause. Osteoporosis is an asymptomatic disease, and its presence usually is not detected until a fracture occurs many years later. At least 25% of the bone needs to be lost before osteoporosis is diagnosed by routine x-ray examination. At present the methods now available for establishing the early diagnosis of osteoporosis in trabecular bone, specifically bone density studies and computerized tomography (CT) scans, are complicated and expensive. Although dual photon absorptiometry and CT scans effectively measure bone density in trabecular bone, the equipment necessary to perform these procedures is expensive and needs to be located in institutions. The technique of single photon absorptiometry is much easier to perform, and the equipment is portable and less expensive and can be used in an office or clinic setting. Nevertheless this technique can only be used to measure the density of structures composed primarily of cortical bone—the bone in the axial skeleton such as the radius, femur, or os calcis. Since postmenopausal osteoporosis affects trabecular bone more rapidly than it does cortical bone, utilization of single photon absorptiometry on bones in the limbs can fail to detect the presence of loss of trabecular bone in the thoracic spine because the density of the bone being measured may remain within the normal range. Thus as stated in a recent review by Davis, neither of the photon absorptiometry techniques should be utilized for routine screening of postmenopausal women. A careful history and physical examination will determine whether risk factors for development of osteoporosis are present. Factors known to increase the risk of osteoporosis are as follows:

- Race: white or Oriental
- Reduced weight for height
- Early spontaneous menopause
- Early surgical menopause
- Family history of osteoporosis
- Diet: low calcium intake, low vitamin D intake, high caffeine intake, high alcohol intake, and high protein intake
- Cigarette smoking
- Sedentary life-style

In women undergoing a normal menopause, fractures begin to occur about age 60 in structures composed mainly of trabecular bone, such as the vertebral spine. By age 60, 25% of white and Oriental women develop spinal compression fractures. Loss of bone mass in cortical bone occurs at a much slower rate, so osteoporotic fractures of the femur usually do

not begin to occur until about age 70 or 75 (Fig. 40-12). By age 80, 20% of all white women will develop hip fractures, and about 10% will die from the fracture itself or from complications within 6 months. In the United States it has been estimated that annually there are about 300,000 hip fractures, about 100,000 radius fractures, and about 400,000 other fractures (mainly thoracic vertebral fractures). About 15,000 women die of osteoporosis or its complications annually in the United States, and femoral neck fractures are the twelfth leading cause of death in women in the United States. The total annual acute health care cost from osteoporosis is in excess of $4 billion. An additional $2 billion is spent for long-term convalescent care for women who have suffered a hip fracture.

Although the mechanism whereby estrogen prevents a decrease in bone density is not precisely known, it has been determined that postmenopausal serum levels of calcium and phosphorus are slightly increased and serum levels of parathyroid hormone and the active form of vitamin D (1,25-dihydroxyvitamin D) are decreased, as is calcium absorption. In addition, calcitonin levels are lowered. Serum calcium levels are maintained within a fairly narrow range and regulated in part by parathyroid hormone production. Parathyroid hormone increases serum calcium levels by three mechanisms: bone resorption, tubal resorption of calcium in the kidney, and production of an enzyme (1-alpha-hydroxylase) that changes vitamin D from its inactive form (which occurs in the diet or sunlight) to its active form and thereby increases calcium absorption from the gut. It has been postulated that sex steroids, including estrogen, androgens, and progestins, block the action of parathyroid hormone on bone, reducing the amount of calcium resorbed from bone (Fig. 40-13). After menopause, as estrogen levels decline, there is less inhibition of the action of parathyroid hormone on bone resorption, so serum calcium levels increase, serum parathyroid hormone levels decrease, and there is less tubular reabsorption of calcium. There is less formation of 1-alpha-hydroxylase, reducing the amount of active vitamin D and leading to less absorption of dietary calcium from the gut (Fig. 40-14). Most of the serum calcium is then derived from bone,

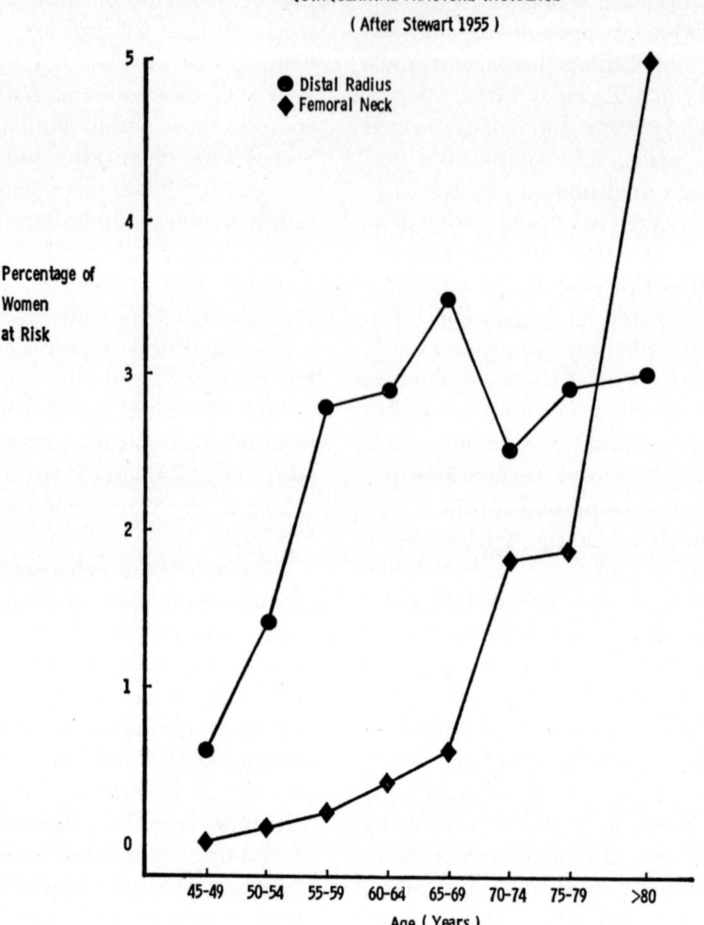

FIGURE 40-12
Relationship between incidence of distal radius and femoral neck fractures and age
in women. (From Aitken JM: Bone metabolism in postmenopausal women. In
Beard RJ, ed: The menopause: A guide to current research and practice. Lancaster,
England, MTP Press Ltd., 1976, p. 99.)

which causes the steady loss of about 1.5% of
bone mass each year after menopause. Data in
support of this mechanism were provided by
Riggs et al., who took biopsy specimens from
patients with postmenopausal osteoporotic fractures and measured bone resorption and formation before and after estrogen therapy. Patients with osteoporosis had a higher bone
resorption rate than normal (Fig. 40-15). With
a few months of estrogen treatment, bone resorption rates returned to normal. Bone formation in patients with osteoporosis was normal before and after the estrogen therapy.
Since there are no estrogen receptors in bone,
estrogen cannot inhibit the action of parathy-

roid hormone directly. However, estrogen increases calcitonin levels, and calcitonin prevents bone resorption. Therefore this action of
estrogen may be the mechanism whereby it
prevents bone loss. The best way to prevent
loss of calcium from bone in postmenopausal
women or castrated women is to administer exogenous estrogens.

Both prospective (cohort) and several retrospective (case control) studies have shown that
estrogen therapy reduces the amount of postmenopausal bone loss as well as the incidence
of fracture. Lindsay et al. studied a group of
young Scottish women who had undergone oophorectomy. Half of them were treated with 20

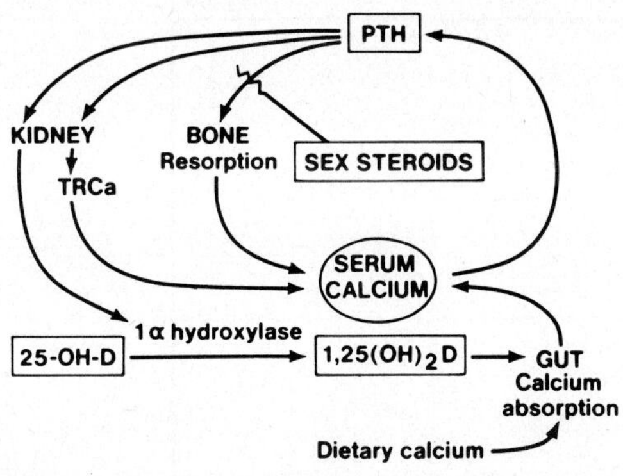

FIGURE 40-13
Hormonal control of calcium hemostasis in normal premenopausal women. Parathyroid hormone *(PTH)* increases bone resorption, renal tubular reabsorption of filtered calcium *(TR Ca)*, and conversion of 25-hydroxyvitamin D to 1,25-dihydroxyvitamin D. (From Riggs BL, Gallagher JC: Evidence for bihormonal deficiency state (estrogen and 1,25-dihydroxyvitamin D) in patients with postmenopausal osteoporosis. In Norman AW, Schaefer K, Herrath Dv, et al, eds: Vitamin D: Biochemical, chemical and clinical aspects related to calcium metabolism. Berlin, Walter de Gruyter & Co., 1977, p. 643.)

μg of mestranol and half with placebo; bone density was measured at yearly intervals. After 10 years the group receiving estrogen had no decrease of bone density, whereas those who received the placebo had a steady decline in bone density (Fig. 40-16), and some in this group developed loss of anterior vertebral height, indicating that compression fractures had occurred. One group of women received the estrogen for 4 years and then stopped taking it. Although they did not lose bone mass in the 4 years they took estrogen, once they stopped taking it they started losing bone at the same rate as the placebo group (Fig 40-17). These data indicate that estrogen replacement therapy should be maintained as long as the woman is ambulatory.

In addition to this prospective study, several retrospective epidemiologic studies have shown that estrogens reduce the incidence of fractures. Weiss et al. reported that a reduction in fractures occurred mainly in those women who had taken estrogen for more than 5 years

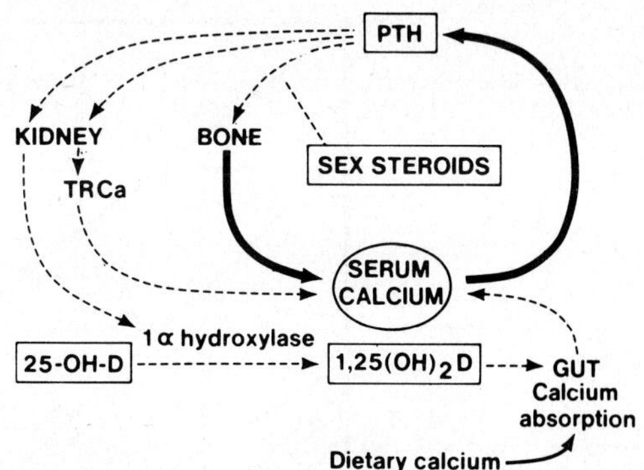

FIGURE 40-14
Postulated changes in hormonal control of calcium hemostasis in postmenopausal women with osteoporosis. Bone-resorbing cells have increased sensitivity to parathyroid hormone *(PTH)* action. Bone resorption increases despite decreased PTH. Decreased PTH results in decreased production of 1,25-dihydroxyvitamin D, leading to increased intestinal calcium absorption. (From Riggs BL, Gallagher JC: Evidence for bihormonal deficiency state (estrogen and 1,25-dihydroxyvitamin D) in patients with postmenopausal osteoporosis. In Norman AW, Schaefer K, Herrath Dv, et al, eds: Vitamin D: Biochemical, chemical and clinical aspects related to calcium metabolism. Berlin, Walter de Gruyter & Co., 1977, p. 643.)

(Table 40-1). In this study, women who took estrogen for more than 5 years had less than half the number of fractures as the control subjects. Paganini-Hill et al. reported similar results among women undergoing a natural menopause. After 5 years of using estrogen the users had only 35% as many chances of developing a hip fracture as nonusers did. However, even less than 5 years' use of estrogen reduced the incidence of hip fractures by 50% in women who had had a premenopausal oophorectomy, and more than 5 years of use resulted in a 90% lower incidence of fracture compared with nonusers. Two studies in which bone density was recorded have shown the minimum dosage of estrogen needed to prevent osteoporosis to be 0.625 mg of conjugated equine estrogens. Bone density studies with other estrogen formulations have not been published. In addition to estrogen replacement, calcium sup-

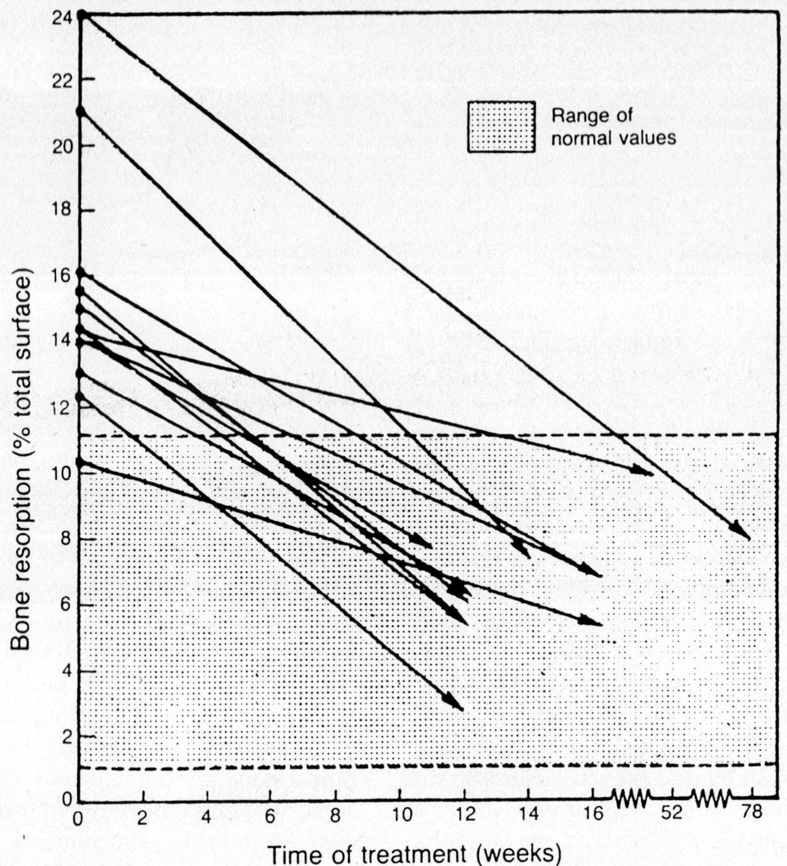

FIGURE 40-15

Effect of sex hormone on bone resorption. (Reproduced from Riggs BL, Jowsey J, Kelley PJ, et al: J Clin Invest 48:1065, 1969, by copyright permission of The American Society for Clinical Investigation.)

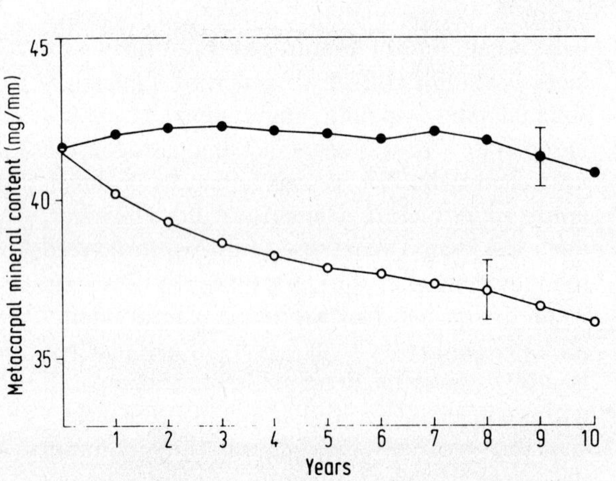

FIGURE 40-16

Bone mineral content (± maximum SE) in those treated with estrogen *(upper line)* and placebo *(lower line)*. (From Lindsay R, Hart DM, Forrest C, Baird C: Lancet 2:1151, 1980.)

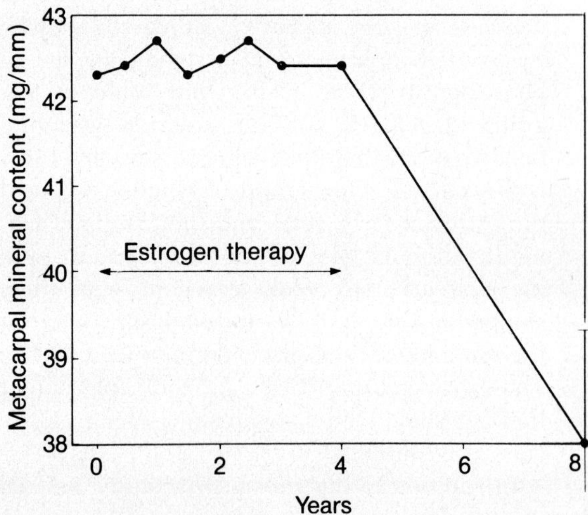

FIGURE 40-17

Effects of withdrawal of estrogen therapy on bone mineral content after 4 years of active treatment. (From Lindsay R, Hart DM, MacLean A, et al: Lancet 1:1325, 1978.)

TABLE 40-1

Menopausal Estrogen Use and Osteoporotic Fractures

Duration of Use (Years)	Cases (%)	Controls (%)	Relative Risk*	95% Confidence Limit†
None‡	66	48	1.0	—
1-2	10	9	0.84	0.51-1.4
3-5	9	10	0.89	0.54-1.4
6-9	5	12	0.38	0.22-0.66
≥10	11	21	0.46	0.30-0.69

From Weiss NS, Ure CL, Ballard JH, et al: Decreased risk of fractures of the hip and lower forearm with postmenopausal use of estrogen. N Engl J Med 303:1195, 1980. Reprinted by permission of The New England Journal of Medicine.
*Standardized for age group (50 to 59, 60 to 69, and 70 to 74 years), history of hysterectomy, and current use versus past use of estrogens, by the method of Mantel and Haenszel.
†Approximate values, by the method of Miettinen.
‡Includes women using estrogens for less than 1 year.

plementation and weight-bearing exercise are of ancillary benefit in preventing postmenopausal osteoporosis. It is recommended that in addition to estrogen, 1 to 1.5 g of elemental calcium should be ingested daily. Calcium supplementation can be in any form such as three glasses of low-fat milk per day or four 500 mg calcium carbonate tablets. Calcium supplementation alone, even with weight-bearing exercise, will not prevent osteoporosis. However, Genant et al. have shown that with calcium supplementation the dosage of estrogen supplement may be reduced to 0.3 mg conjugated equine estrogen (Fig. 40-18). It is not necessary for postmenopausal women to receive vitamin D, because Riggs and Gallagher showed

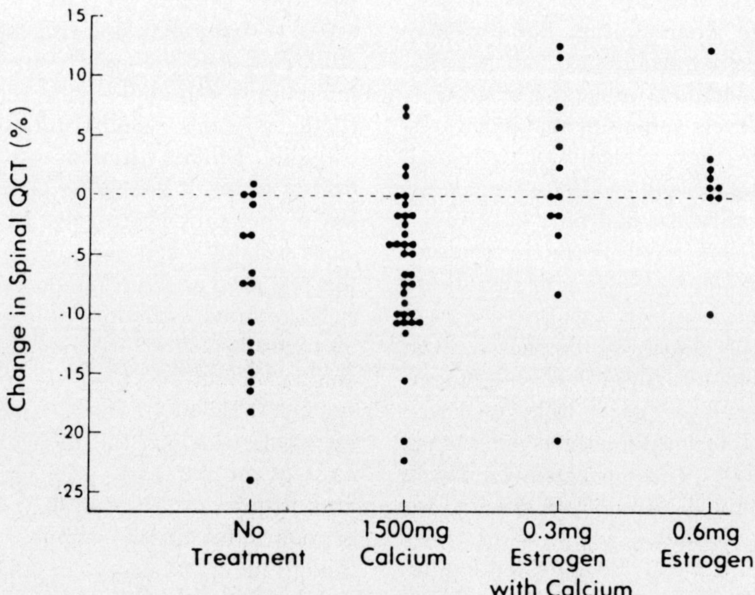

FIGURE 40-18
Vertebral trabecular bone loss following menopause. The change in spinal quantitative CT over 12 months is shown as a function of treatment. (From Genant HK, Cann CE, Ettinger B, et al: Quantitative computed tomography for spinal mineral assessment in osteoporosis. Proceedings of the Copenhagen International Symposium on Osteoporosis. Aalborg Stiftsbogtrykkeri, 1984.)

that women with osteoporosis treated with various regimens with and without vitamin D had no difference in incidence of osteoporotic fractures.

In summary, estrogen increases calcium absorption and reduces the rate of bone resorption. It will not stimulate new bone growth but will stabilize osteoporosis if it is present and, most important, will prevent osteoporosis if therapy is started at the time of menopause. For women at risk to develop osteoporosis, specifically nonobese white or Oriental women, estrogen replacement is the keystone to the triad approach of estrogen, calcium supplementation, and weight-bearing exercise as a method to prevent this debilitating and painful disease.

Effects of Estrogen Replacement

Metabolic Effects

With any drug there is a benefit-risk ratio, but the risks of estrogen replacement therapy are minimal. Exogenous estrogen administration produces effects on serum proteins, specifically an increase in serum globulins. One of these globulins, angiotensinogen, can be converted to angiotensin and produce an increase in blood pressure, whereas other globulins may produce a hypercoagulable state and possibly thrombosis. In addition, exogenous estrogens may alter lipid levels and other metabolic processes. However, these metabolic changes are related to the dosage and type of estrogen administered, and the dose and type of estrogen given for postmenopausal hormone replacement therapy are much less potent than those used in oral contraceptives. For prevention of osteoporosis, bone density studies have shown that at least the equivalent of 0.625 mg of conjugated equine estrogen needs to be ingested. Patients with hot flushes sometimes need to receive a higher dose, the equivalent of 1.25 mg of conjugated equine estrogen or greater, for relief of these symptoms.

However, even 2.5 mg of conjugated equine estrogen causes less of an increase in the liver-binding globulins than does 30 μg of ethinyl estradiol (Fig. 40-19). The estrogen used in oral contraceptives, ethinyl estradiol, because of the presence of the ethinyl group on the 17 position of the steroid molecule, causes a much

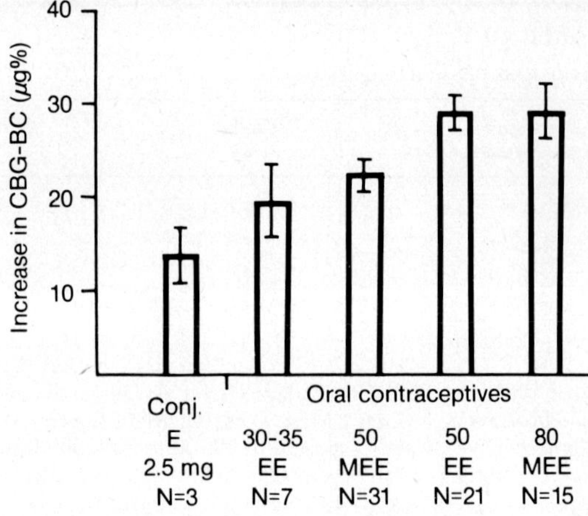

FIGURE 40-19

Increase in corticosteroid-binding-globulin binding capacity (CBG-BC) (μg/dl) in relation to dose of synthetic estrogen. *Conj E*, conjugated equine estrogen; *EE*, ethinylestradiol; *MEE*, mestranol. (From Moore DE, Kawagoe S, Davajan V, et al: Am J Obstet Gynecol 130:482, 1978.)

greater increase in liver globulin production than does estrone sulfate. Mashchak et al. compared the potency of various doses of three types of natural oral estrogens—estrone sulfate, conjugated equine estrone sulfate, and micronized estradiol—with that of two synthetic estrogens—diethylstilbestrol and ethinyl estradiol. Ethinyl estradiol was much more potent in terms of increasing globulin levels than any of the natural estrogens. In terms of equivalent weight, when an increase in liver globulins was used as the parameter of estrogenic activity, ethinyl estradiol was found to be about 90 times as potent as conjugated equine estrogen and about 200 times as potent as estrone sulfate (Table 40-2). Thus 30 or 35 μg of ethinyl estradiol, which is the dosage of estrogen in most of the currently used oral contraceptive formulations, is the equivalent of about 2.5 mg of conjugated equine estrogens. Therefore, although the usual dosage of 0.625 mg of conjugated estrogen is 20 times greater than the minimum weight of estrogen used in oral contraceptives, it is only about one-fifth as potent in terms of effects on liver globulins. Estrogen appears to have little effect on glucose metabolism, as several recent studies have shown no

TABLE 40-2

Relative Potency According to Four Specific Parameters of Estrogenicity

Estrogen Preparation	Serum FSH	Serum CBG-BC	Serum SHBG-BC	Serum Angiotensinogen
Piperazine estrone sulfate	1.0	1.0	1.0	1.0
Conjugated estrogens	1.4	2.5	3.2	3.5
Micronized estradiol	1.3	1.9	1.0	0.7
Diethylstilbestrol	3.8	70.0	28.0	13.0
Ethinyl estradiol	(80-200)*	(1000)*	614	232

From Mashchak CA, Lobo RA, Dozono-Takano R, et al: Comparison of pharmacodynamic properties of various estrogen formulations. Am J Obstet Gynecol 144:511, 1982.
FSH, follicle-stimulating hormone; *CBG-BC*, corticosteroid-binding globulin–binding capacity; *SHBG-BC*, sex hormone–binding globulin–binding capacity.
*Estimate in absence of parallelism.

TABLE 40-3

Systolic and Diastolic Blood Pressure According to Age and Postmenopausal Estrogen Use*

Age	Systolic Blood Pressure (mm Hg)		Diastolic Blood Pressure (mm Hg)	
	Users	Nonusers	Users	Nonusers
55-59	130.8 ± 18.8	135.0 ± 25.1	79.4 ± 9.6	81.3 ± 12.0
60-64	134.1 ± 18.9	136.5 ± 19.2	79.4 ± 9.4	81.6 ± 9.8†
65-69	139.3 ± 20.3	140.4 ± 21.4	81.9 ± 10.8	82.6 ± 12.2
70-74	147.9 ± 25.9	147.8 ± 20.9	82.0 ± 10.3	83.8 ± 22.7

From Barrett-Connor E, Brown WV, Turner J, et al: Heart disease risk factors and hormone use in postmenopausal women. JAMA 241:2167, 1979. Copyright 1979, The American Medical Association.
*All data adjusted for obesity. Means and standard deviations are given.
†$P \leq .05$.

decrease in glucose tolerance in patients treated with doses of estrogen equivalent to 1.25 mg of conjugated equine estrogen. Although some studies have shown a statistically increased risk of gallbladder disease in postmenopausal estrogen users, others have reported no such risk. Estrogens may accelerate the formation of cholelithiasis in susceptible individuals.

Cardiovascular Effects

Oral contraceptives increase the blood pressure of some women, but there is no evidence that the doses of natural oral estrogens used to treat menopausal women cause an increase in blood pressure.

In contrast to the increase in blood pressure that has been reported in some women using oral contraceptives, no such increase has been observed with use of estrogen replacement therapy. In a cross-sectional study reported by Barrett-Connor et al., although mean systolic and diastolic blood pressure increased with age, there was no significant difference between estrogen users and nonusers (Table 40-3). In a longitudinal prospective study Wren and Routledge reported that women ingesting piperazine estrone sulfate actually had a significant decrease in systolic and diastolic blood pressure, whether or not they were receiving antihypertensive therapy (Table 40-4). These data indicate that it is safe to prescribe estrogen replacement for postmenopausal women with hypertension, and if blood pressure increases while they are receiving this treatment,

TABLE 40-4

Piperazine Estrone Sulfate—On and Not On Antihypertensives

	Mean	SD	t*	P	N
On antihypertensives (N = 34)					
Systolic visit 1	151.26	22.75	—	—	34
Systolic visit 2	143.03	16.45	—	—	34
Mean change	−8.23	17.21	2.79	< 0.01	34
Diastolic visit 1	91.82	9.69	—		34
Diastolic visit 2	86.53	10.72	—		34
Mean change	−5.29	9.29	3.32	< 0.01	34
Not on antihypertensives (N = 150)					
Systolic visit 1	134.77	16.35	—	—	150
Systolic visit 2	130.41	15.42	—	—	150
Mean change	−4.36	15.35	3.48	< 0.001	150
Diastolic visit 1	84.37	9.83	—	—	150
Diastolic visit 2	81.08	9.32	—	—	150
Mean change	−3.29	9.49	4.25	< 0.001	150

From Wren BG, Routledge AD: The effect of type and dose of oestrogen on the blood pressure of post-menopausal women. Maturitas 5:135, 1983.
*Student's t test.

it is unlikely that the estrogen is the cause of the blood pressure elevation.

In addition, Aylwood showed that the natural estrogens in the dosages used for hormonal replacement do not increase clotting factors, but ethinyl estradiol did produce a hypercoagulable state. There is no epidemiologic evidence of an increased incidence of thrombophlebitis or thromboembolism in postmenopausal estrogen users as compared with control subjects. Several epidemiologic studies have reported no increased incidence of these disorders in postmenopausal women taking estrogen in comparison to the increased incidence found in oral contraceptive users. Furthermore there is no evidence that postmenopausal women with a past history of thrombophlebitis have an increased incidence of thrombophlebitis with estrogen replacement therapy.

In contrast to the increased risk of myocardial infarction found in women over 35 who smoke and ingest high dosages of oral contraceptives, use of estrogen replacement has been shown to reduce the risk of myocardial infarction. A retrospective study by Ross et al. showed that diabetes, hypertension, and smoking increased the chance of dying from ischemic heart disease but that estrogens decreased the chance of dying from ischemic

TABLE 40-5

Matched Risk Ratios for Death from Ischaemic Heart Disease

	Living Controls		Deceased Controls	
Variable	Discordant Pairs (No.)	Risk Ratio	Discordant Pairs (No.)	Risk Ratio
Stroke	31	3.43*	32	2.20†
Hypertension	72	3.24‡	80	2.33‡
Angina pectoris	53	6.57‡	42	2.50*
Myocardial infarction	50	7.33‡	44	3.89‡
Diabetes before age 65	11	2.67	14	2.50
Family history of myo-cardial infarction	37	2.29	23	0.95
Cholesterol ≥ 300 mg/dl	25	1.27	24	3.00*
Cigarettes > 1 pack/day	13	3.33†	20	1.00
Alcohol	33	0.38*	45	0.88
Conjugated estrogens	57	0.43*	55	0.57†

From Ross RK, Mack TM, Paganini-Hill A, et al: Menopausal oestrogen therapy and protection from death from ischaemic heart disease. Lancet 1:858, 1981.
*P ≤ 0.01.
†P ≤ 0.05.
‡P ≤ 0.001.

TABLE 40-6

Case Control Studies of Estrogen Replacement Therapy and Coronary Heart Disease

Investigator/Year	Data Source	Endpoint*	Crude Relative Risk		"Adjusted" Relative Risk	
			Ever Use	Current Use	Ever Use	Current Use
Rosenberg et al., 1976	Interviews	Nonfatal MI	Not reported	0.5	Not reported	1.0
Pfeffer et al., 1978	Pharmacy records	Fatal or nonfatal MI	0.9	0.6	0.9	0.7
Jick et al., 1978	Interviews	Nonfatal MI	Not reported	4.2	Not reported	Not reported
Rosenberg et al., 1980†	Interviews	Nonfatal MI	0.7 1.5	0.5 0.9	Not reported	Not reported
Ross et al., 1981‡	Medical records	Fatal IHD	0.4 0.6	Not reported	0.4 0.6	Not reported
Bain et al., 1981	Mailed survey	Nonfatal MI	0.9	0.7	0.8	0.7
Adam et al., 1981	Doctors	Fatal MI	0.6	0.8	0.6	0.8
Szklo et al., 1984	Interviews	Nonfatal MI	0.5	0.4	0.4	0.4

From Ross RK, Paganini-Hill A, Mack TM, Henderson BE: Estrogen use and cardiovascular disease. In Mishell DR Jr, ed: Menopause: Physiology and pharmacology. Chicago, Year Book Medical Publishers, 1987. Reproduced with permission.
*MI, myocardial infarction; IHD, ischemic heart disease.
†Rosenberg et al. reported the data on women aged 30 to 44 years separately from those on women aged 45 to 49 years. "Adjusted" relative risks for postmenopausal women only were not reported.
‡Ross et al. used two control groups for comparison: living controls *(top)* and decreased controls.

TABLE 40-7

Cohort Studies of Estrogen Replacement Therapy and Coronary Heart Disease

Investigator/Year	Study Population	Description of Cohort	Endpoint*	Relative Risk
Burch et al., 1974	Surgical Practice Nashville, Tenn.	737 hysterectomized women	CHD	0.4
Hammond et al., 1974	Duke Medical Center	610 hypoestrogenic inpatients and outpatients	CHD	0.3
Petitti et al., 1979	Walnut Creek, Cal. Kaiser Permanente	1675 white women	MI	1.2
Bush et al., 1983	Lipid Research Clinics, USA	2269 white women	Fatal CHD	0.3
Wilson et al., 1985	Framingham, Mass.	1234 postmenopausal residents	CHD	1.9
Stampfer et al., 1985	Nurses Health Study, USA	32,317 postmenopausal women	CHD	0.5

From Ross RK, Paganini-Hill A, Mack TM, Henderson BE: Estrogen use and cardiovascular disease. In Mishell DR Jr, ed: Menopause: Physiology and pharmacology. Chicago, Year Book Medical Publishers, 1987. Reproduced with permission.
*CHD, coronary heart disease; MI, myocardial infarction.

TABLE 40-8

Concentrations of Lipids and Lipoproteins in Users and Nonusers of Estrogen

	Mean ± SD (Median)	
Lipid Profile	Nonuser	Equine Estrogen
Cholesterol	230 ± 44.3 (226)	219 ± 33.9 (218)*
Triglyceride	174 ± 66.9 (100)	141 ± 71.5 (126)*
HDL Cholesterol	61 ± 15.6 (61)	69 ± 17.7 (67)*
LDL Cholesterol	154 ± 43.8 (147)	133 ± 33.9 (131)*
VLDL Cholesterol†	16 ± 13.8 (13)	18 ± 12.5 (16)

From Wahl P, Walden C, Knopp R, et al: Effect of estrogen/progestin potency on lipid/lipoprotein cholesterol. N Engl J Med 308:862, 1983. Reprinted by permission of The New England Journal of Medicine.
VLDL, very low density lipoprotein.
*Significantly different from nonusers at the 0.05 level.

heart disease (Table 40-5) and thus demonstrated a protective effect of estrogens against myocardial infarction, even in women who smoked. Several other retrospective studies have also demonstrated a reduction in risk of coronary heart disease in estrogen users (Table 40-6).

In addition, many prospective studies also demonstrated that there is about a 50% reduction in myocardial infarction in estrogen users (Table 40-7). The large, nationwide study of Stampfer et al. has been confirmed by a recent study reported by Henderson et al. The Framingham study by Wilson et al. that found an increased risk of myocardial infarction in postmenopausal estrogen users utilized a small cohort of women and adjusted the risk ratio with statistical techniques that corrected for the changes in lipids produced by estrogen.

Levels of low-density-lipoprotein (LDL) cholesterol have a positive correlation with coronary heart disease, while levels of high-density lipoprotein (HDL) cholesterol have an inverse relation. Thus individuals with naturally high LDL cholesterol and low HDL cholesterol levels are at greater risk of having coronary heart disease. The results of a Lipid Research Clinical Program revealed that in contrast to some

TABLE 40-9

Age-Adjusted All-Cause Mortality Rates (per 1000 per year) by Hysterectomy Status and Estrogen Use*

	Estrogen Use		
Hysterectomy Status	Nonuser	User	Total
Intact uterus and ovaries	9.0 (6.5-12.0)	4.9 (1.8-10.7)	8.2 (6.1-10.8)
Hysterectomy	8.2 (3.3-16.8)	2.8 (0.3-10.0)	5.7 (2.6-10.8)
Oophorectomy	11.8 (5.9-21.2)	1.4 (0.0-7.6)	7.2 (3.7-12.6)
TOTAL	9.3 (7.2-11.9)	3.4 (1.5-6.4)	

From Bush TL, Cowan LD, Barrett-Connor E, et al: Estrogen use and all-cause mortality. Preliminary results from the Lipid Research Clinics Program Follow-Up Study. JAMA 249:903, 1983. Copyright 1983, American Medical Association.
*Ninety-five percent confidence limits on rate.

oral contraceptive users who had increased levels of LDL cholesterol, postmenopausal estrogen users had decreased levels of LDL cholesterol as well as increased levels of HDL cholesterol as compared with postmenopausal nonestrogen users (Table 40-8). Although it has not been determined that this is the mechanism whereby estrogen prevents myocardial infarction, the demonstrated reduction in this major cause of mortality in women is a major beneficial effect of estrogen. Additional age-adjusted data from the Lipid Research Program revealed that all causes of mortality were significantly lower in estrogen users than in nonusers regardless of whether the uterus or ovaries were intact or had been removed (Table 40-9).

Neoplastic Effects

Much concern has been raised about the neoplastic risks of postmenopausal estrogen replacement therapy, particularly breast and endometrial cancer, since these areas are estrogen target tissues. Despite the fact that only a few of many epidemiologic studies investigating the relation of estrogen use and breast cancer have shown an increased risk of breast cancer in some postmenopausal estrogen users, the possibility exists that estrogen can stimulate a nonpalpable breast cancer. Carcinoma of the breast may exist in the preclinical state for as long as 8 years before it is palpable. Thus it

is advisable to obtain a mammogram to rule out subclinical breast cancer on all patients before initiating estrogen therapy. However, if no tumor is found, current evidence indicates that oral estrogen use will not increase the risk of developing breast cancer (Table 40-10).

Many epidemiologic studies have reported that there is a significantly increased risk of developing endometrial cancer in postmenopausal women who are ingesting estrogen without progestins as compared with nonestrogen users. The risk increases with increasing duration of use of estrogen as well as with increased dosage (Table 40-11). A study of three large series of routine autopsies during the last 30 years in New England revealed that about 1 in 300 women who died of other causes had undiagnosed and unsuspected endometrial cancer. Therefore it appears that a certain number of women of the control group of the epidemiologic studies linking endometrial cancer with estrogen use had an undiagnosed endometrial cancer that may have become manifest by uterine bleeding if the women had received exogenous estrogen, thus spuriously increasing the risk ratio. Therefore the risk of developing endometrial cancer with estrogen treatment is probably substantially overestimated. Furthermore, in terms of actual risk the increased risk for a woman developing endometrial cancer even if the relative risk was sevenfold is only about 1 in 500.

The endometrial cancer that develops in es-

TABLE 40-10
Case Control Studies of Exogenous Estrogen and Breast Cancer

Author	Year of Diagnosis	No. of Cases	No. of Controls	Relative Risk*
Wydner	1969-1975	785	2231	1.1
Sartwell	1969-1972	284	367	0.8
Boston	1972	51	774	1.0
Brinton	1973-1977	405	1156	1.0
Henderson	1969-1972	308	308	0.8
Casagrande	1972-1973	47	31	3.1
Craig	1949-1967	134	260	1.0
Mack	1971-1975	111	444	1.6
Ross	1971-1977	67	128	1.1

From Hulka BS: Effect of exogenous estrogen on postmenopausal women: The epidemiologic evidence. Obstet Gynecol Surv 35:389, 1980. © by Williams & Wilkins, 1980.
*Relative risk for "ever use" of estrogen.

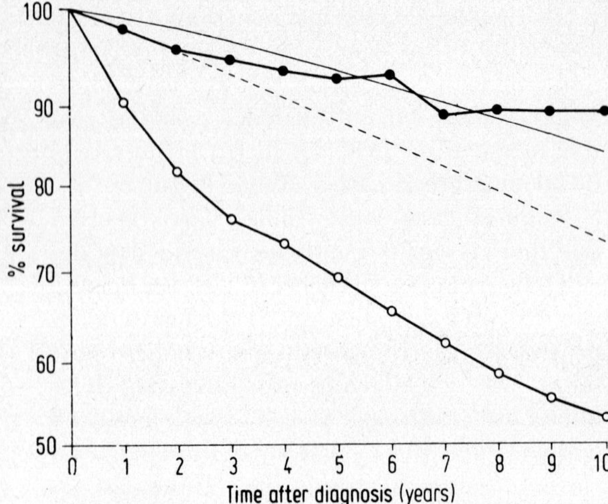

FIGURE 40-20

Survival of women with endometrial cancer and history of estrogen use *(solid circles)* compared with estrogen-user controls (age-adjusted mortality) *(solid line)*, with women with endometrial cancer who were not estrogen users *(open circles)*, and with non-estrogen-user controls (age-adjusted mortality) *(dashed line)*. (From Collins J, Donner A, Allen LH, Adams O: Lancet 2:961, 1980.)

TABLE 40-11

Risk Estimates from Case-Control Studies of Estrogen Replacement Therapy and Endometrial Cancer

Study		Relative Risks*	
Author	Year	Ever Users	Long-Term Users
Smith	1975	4.5	—
Ziel	1975	7.6	13.9
Mack	1976	5.6	8.8
Gray	1977	3.1	11.6
McDonald	1977	2.0	7.9
Wigle	1978	2.2	5.2
Horwitz	1978	12.0	—
Hoogerland	1978	2.2	6.7
Antunes	1979	6.0	15.0
Weiss	1979	7.5	8.2
Hulka	1980	—	4.2
Shapiro	1980	3.9	6.0
Jelovsek	1980	2.4	4.8
Spengler	1981	3.2	8.6
Stavraky	1981	4.2	14.4
Kelsey	1982	—	8.2
LaVecchia	1982	2.7	—
Henderson	1983	1.4	3.1

From Peterson HB, Lee MC, Rubin GL: Genital neoplasia. In Mishell DR Jr ed: Menopause: Physiology and pharmacology. Chicago, Year Book Medical Publishers, 1987.
*Risk relative to never-users

trogen users is nearly always well differentiated and is usually cured by performing a simple hysterectomy. Collins et al. showed that women who had endometrial cancer and were not receiving estrogen had a 10-year survival rate of about 50%, and a control population without cancer matched for age and lack of estrogen had about an 80% survival rate at the end of 10 years (Fig. 40-20). A group of patients who had endometrial cancer and were also taking estrogen had a survival rate about the same as a control population taking estrogen (90%), indicating that the well-differentiated endometrial carcinoma occurring with estrogen treatment can be adequately treated by performing a hysterectomy and is usually not lethal. The risk of developing endometrial carcinoma for women receiving estrogen replacement can be markedly reduced by giving the patient progestogens. Estrogen acts only if a specific receptor is present within the target cell. The estrogen receptor complex activates messenger RNA, which then changes DNA to produce cell division and also synthesize new estrogen receptors. Progesterone, which normally is produced in the last half of the normal menstrual cycle, blocks receptor synthesis so no new receptors are formed. Therefore the endometrium does not proliferate in the latter half of the menstrual cycle because progesterone prevents receptor synthesis and further growth and division of the cells despite continued estrogen production. To summarize, estrogen increases the synthesis of both estrogen and progesterone receptors in the endometrium; progesterone and synthetic progestins decrease the synthesis of both these receptors and thus have an antiproliferative action.

Progestins have been shown to prevent endometrial hyperplasia. Sturdee et al. performed endometrial biopsies annually in women receiving sex steroids. Twenty-three percent of the women receiving continuous estrogen alone and 12% of patients taking cyclic estrogen alone developed endometrial hyperplasia. When progestins were added for 5 days each month in addition to estrogen, the incidence of hyperplasia decreased to 8%. When progestins were added to treatment for more than 10 days each month for more than 200 women for 4 years, no hyperplasia developed. These and other studies have shown that the duration of progestin therapy is more important than the dosage. Small amounts of progestin administered for more than 10 days each month have also been shown to reduce the incidence of endometrial carcinoma in studies performed by Gambrell et al. and Hammond et al. Thus there is evidence that use of progestins lowers the chances of postmenopausal estrogen users' developing cancer of the endometrium, and therefore progestins should be given to postmenopausal women receiving estrogen if they have a uterus. The addition of a progestin to estrogen therapy does not appear to cause an increase of any other systemic disease and acts synergistically with estrogen to cause a slight increase in bone density. The use of synthetic progestins may reverse the beneficial effect of estrogen upon serum lipids. Ottoson et al. reported that daily ingestion of 10 mg of MPA in addition to the estrogen reduced HDL cholesterol levels to those present prior to the ingestion of estrogen. The epidemiologic data showing a reduction in heart attacks in estrogen users was derived from women taking estrogen without a progestin. Whether the addition of a progestin to the regimen will reverse the beneficial action of estrogen upon cardiovascular disease remains to be determined. Nevertheless until oral micronized progesterone, which does not lower HDL cholesterol, becomes available, it would appear prudent to use the lowest dose of progestin that will prevent the endometrial proliferation produced by estrogen.

Treatment Regimens

The minimum dosage and type of progestin necessary to prevent endometrial cancer have not been determined. Whitehead et al. showed that in patients receiving 0.625 mg of conjugated estrogens, as little as 1 mg of norethindrone and 150 µg of levonorgestrel was sufficient to decrease the receptor and DNA

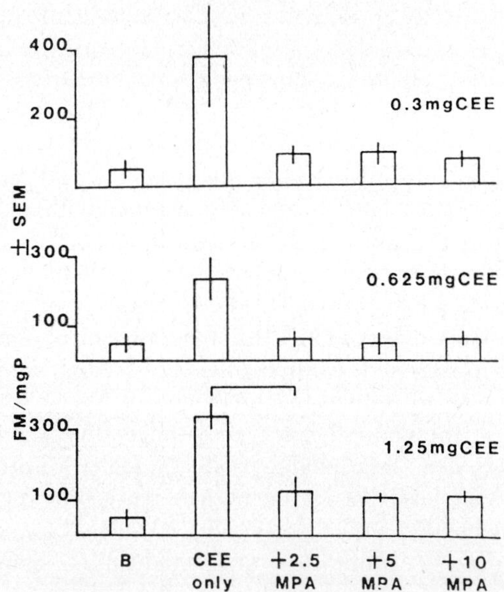

FIGURE 40-21
The concentrations of nuclear estrogen receptor in the three groups of postmenopausal women receiving no therapy *(B)*, estrogen only *(CEE)*, and estrogen plus various doses of medroxyprogesterone acetate *(MPA)*. * = *P*< 0.001. (From Gibbons WE, Moyer DL. Lobo RA, et al: Am J Obstet Gynecol 154:456, 1986.)

activity in endometrial cells to a level similar to the secretory phase of the normal cycle. A study by Gibbons et al. showed that in patients receiving 0.625 mg of conjugated estrone, 2.5 mg of MPA reduced nuclear estrogen receptor levels to those found in the secretory phase of the normal cycle (Fig 40-21). With 1.25 mg of conjugated estrogen, 5 mg of MPA was necessary to decrease receptor synthesis.

The treatment regimen most commonly used in the United States is 0.625 mg of conjugated equine estrogen or estrone sulfate for the first 25 days of each month. Beginning on days 12 to 15 of estrogen treatment, 5 to 10 mg of MPA is added daily for 10 to 13 days. With this regimen about half the women have regular withdrawal bleeding, an annoying problem for the postmenopausal woman. Other therapeutic regimens are also used. For example, a treatment regimen of 0.625 mg of conjugated equine estrone or estrone sulfate together with 2.5 to 5 mg of MPA administered daily or every day Monday to Friday reduces the chance of developing breakthrough bleeding as well as avoids a week off treatment during which symptoms may appear. Preliminary data indicate that most women do not bleed with this regimen, and their endometrium remains atrophic. Several authorities recommend that progestins not be given to women without a uterus because of the adverse effects on lipids. There are no well-controlled epidemiologic studies that provide evidence that use of progestins reduces the risk of breast cancer, and long-term oral contraceptive use has not been shown to reduce the incidence of breast cancer. Intramuscular as well as once-a-week oral estrogen treatments produce higher initial blood levels of estrogen than daily oral regimens do, and theoretically it would appear safer to administer oral medication daily. Transdermal and subdermal estradiol administration provides a relatively constant level of estrogen and may be preferred by some women. However, administration of transdermal estrogen has not been shown to alter serum lipid levels. If the woman has a uterus, oral progestins should be added to these regimens. A routine pretreatment endometrial biopsy is unnecessary, as it is not cost effective, and routine annual endometrial biopsies are not necessary unless breakthrough bleeding occurs.

To summarize, indications for estrogen therapy in menopause include the presence of vasomotor symptoms as well as prevention of atrophic vaginitis, atrophic urethritis, and osteoporosis. Estrogen also appears to retard the onset of myocardial infarction. If these data are confirmed, then estrogen replacement therapy is indicated for nearly all postmenopausal women. Contraindications to estrogen replacement are uncommon. These include a history of breast cancer, recent history of endometrial cancer, active liver disease, or thrombophlebitis.

KEY POINTS

- The mean age of menopause is about 51 years.

- Age at menopause is genetically predetermined and is not related to the number of ovulations, race, socioeconomic conditions, education, height, weight, age at menarche, or age at last pregnancy.

- The basic feature of menopause is depletion of ovarian follicles with degeneration of the granulosa and theca cells while stromal cells continue to produce the androgens androstenedione and testosterone.

- Androstenedione is converted to estrone in the peripheral body fat, and its rate of conversion increases as women age.

- Postmenopausal women with hot flushes have lower circulating estrone and estradiol levels, less total body weight, and a lower percentage of ideal body weight as compared to those without hot flushes.

- About 1% to 1.5% of bone mass is lost each year after menopause in nonobese white and Oriental women. Fractures begin to occur about age 60 to 65 in trabecular bone, such as the vertebral spine, and by age 60, 25% of these women develop spinal compression fractures.

- By age 80, 20% of all white women will develop hip fractures, and 10% of these fractures are fatal within 6 months. In the United States each year osteoporosis causes about 300,000 hip fractures, 100,000 radius fractures, and 400,000 other fractures. About 15,000 women die of osteoporosis or its complications annually in the United States.

- Patients with postmenopausal osteoporosis have a higher bone resorption rate than normal, while bone formation in patients with osteoporosis is normal.

- After menopause, 1.5 g of elemental calcium should be ingested daily.

- For prevention of osteoporosis, at least the equivalent of 0.625 mg of conjugated equine estrone needs to be ingested.

- In terms of equivalent weight, when an increase in liver globulins is used as the parameter of estrogenic activity, ethinyl estradiol is about 90 times as potent as conjugated equine estrogen.

- Levels of LDL cholesterol have a positive correlation with coronary heart disease, while levels of HDL cholesterol have an inverse relation to coronary heart disease. Postmenopausal estrogen users have decreased levels of LDL cholesterol as well as increased levels of HDL cholesterol as compared with postmenopausal nonestrogen users.

- The risk of developing endometrial cancer is 3 to 7 times greater in postmenopausal women who are ingesting estrogen without progestins as compared with nonestrogen users.

- Estrogen increases the synthesis of both estrogen and progesterone receptors in the endometrium; progesterone and synthetic progestins decrease the synthesis of both these receptors and thus have an antimitotic, antiproliferative action.

- Indications for estrogen therapy in menopause include the presence of vasomotor symptoms as well as prevention of atrophic vaginitis, atrophic urethritis, and osteoporosis.

KEY POINTS, cont'd

- Before estrogen therapy is instituted, a pretreatment mammogram should be performed.

BIBLIOGRAPHY

Aitken JM: Bone metabolism in postmenopausal women. In Beard RJ, ed: The menopause: A guide to current research and practice. Lancaster, England, MTP Press Ltd., 1976, p. 99.

Aylwood M, Maddock J, Lewis PA, et al: Oestrogen replacement therapy and blood clotting. Curr Med Res Opin 4(suppl 3):83, 1971.

Barrett-Connor E, Brown WV, Turner J, et al: Heart disease risk factors and hormone use in postmenopausal women. JAMA 241:2167, 1979.

Brincat M, Moniz CJ, Studd JWW, et al: Long-term effects of the menopause and sex hormones on skin thickness. Br J Obstet Gynaecol 92:256, 1985.

Campbell S, Beard RJ, McQueen J, et al: Double blind psychometric studies on the effects of natural estrogens on post-menopausal women. In Campbell S, ed: Management of the menopause and post-menopausal years. Lancaster, England, MTP Press Ltd., 1976, p. 152.

Collins J, Donner A, Allen LH, Adams O: Oestrogen use and survival in endometrial cancer. Lancet 2:961, 1980.

Coope J: Double-blind cross-over study of estrogen replacement therapy. In Campbell S, ed: Management of the menopause and post-menopausal years. Lancaster, England, MTP Press Ltd., 1976, p. 167.

Cope E: Physical changes associated with the postmenopausal years. In Campbell S, ed: Management of the menopause and post-menopausal years. Lancaster, England, MTP Press Ltd., 1976, p. 33.

Davis MR: Screening for postmenopausal osteoporosis. Fertil Steril 156:1, 1987.

Erlik Y, Meldrum DR, Judd HL: Estrogen levels in postmenopausal women with hot flashes. Obstet Gynecol 59:403, 1982.

Erlik Y, Tataryn IV, Meldrum DR, et al: Association of waking episodes with menopausal hot flushes. JAMA 245:1741, 1981.

Gambrell RD Jr, Massey FM, Castaneda TA, et al: Reduced incidence of endometrial cancer among postmenopausal women treated with progestogens. J Am Geriatr Soc 27(9):389, 1979.

Genant HK, Cann CE, Ettinger B, et al: Quantitative computed tomography for spinal mineral assessment in osteoporosis. Proceedings of the Copenhagen International Symposium on Osteoporosis. Aalborg Stiftsbogtrykkeri, 1984.

Gibbons WE, Moyer DL, Lobo RA, et al: Biochemical and histologic effects of sequential estrogen/progestin therapy on the endometrium of postmenopausal women. Am J Obstet Gynecol 154:456, 1986.

Hammond CB, Jelovsek FR, Lee KL, et al: Effects of long-term estrogen replacement therapy. II. Neoplasia. Am J Obstet Gynecol 133:537, 1979.

Henderson BE, Ross RK, Paganini-Hill A, Mack TM: Estrogen use and cardiovascular disease. Am J Obstet Gynecol 154:1181, 1986.

Hulka BS: Effect of exogenous estrogen on postmenopausal women: The epidemiologic evidence. Obstet Gynecol Surv 35:389, 1980.

Jaszmann LJB: Epidemiology of the climacteric syndrome. In Campbell S, ed: Management of the menopause and post-menopausal years. Lancaster, England, MTP Press Ltd., 1976, p. 12.

Lind T, Cameron EC, Hunter WM, et al: A prospective, controlled trial of six forms of hormone replacement therapy given to postmenopausal women. Br J Obstet Gynaecol 86(suppl 3):1, 1979.

Lindsay R, Hart DM, Forrest C, Baird C: Prevention of spinal osteoporosis in oophorectomized women. Lancet 2:1151, 1980.

Lindsay R, Hart DM, MacLean A, et al: Bone response to termination of oestrogen treatment. Lancet 1:1325, 1978.

Lobo RA, McCormick W, Singer F, et al: Depomedroxyprogesterone acetate compared with conjugated estrogens for the treatment of postmenopausal women. Obstet Gynecol 63:1, 1984.

Mashchak CA, Kletzky OA, Artal R, Mishell DR Jr: The relation of physiological changes to subjective symptoms in postmenopausal women with and without hot flushes. Maturitas 6:301, 1984.

Mashchak CA, Lobo RA, Dozono-Takano R, et al: Comparison of pharmacodynamic properties of various estrogen formulations. Am J Obstet Gynecol 144:511, 1982.

Moore DE, Kawagoe S, Davajan V, et al: An in vivo system in man for quantitation of estrogenicity. II. Pharmacologic changes in binding capacity of serum corticosteroid–binding globulin induced by conjugated estrogens, mestranol, and ethinyl estradiol. Am J Obstet Gynecol 130:482, 1978.

Nordin BEC, Gallagher JC, Aaron JE, et al: Postmenopausal osteopenia and osteoporosis. Estrogens in the postmenopause. Front Horm Res 3:133, 1975.

Notelovitz M, Kitchens C, Ware M, et al: Combination estrogen and progestogen replacement therapy does not adversely affect coagulation. Obstet Gynecol 62:596, 1983.

Ottosson UB, Johansson BG, Von Schoultz B: Subfractions of high-density lipoprotein cholesterol during estrogen replacement therapy: A comparison between progestogens and natural progesterone. Am J Obstet Gynecol 151:746, 1985.

Paganini-Hill A, Ross RK, Gerkins VR, et al: A case control study of menopausal estrogen therapy and hip fractures. Ann Intern Med 95:28, 1981.

Peterson HB, Lee NC, Rubin GL: Genital neoplasia. In Mishell DR Jr, ed: Menopause: Physiology and pharmacology. Chicago, Year Book Medical Publishers, 1987.

Pfeffer RI: Estrogen use, hypertension and stroke in postmenopausal women. J Chronic Dis 31:389, 1978.

Pfeffer RI, Whipple GH, Kurosaki TT, Chapman JM: Coronary risk and estrogen use in postmenopausal women. Am J Epidemiol 107:479, 1978.

Riggs BL, Gallagher JC: Evidence for bihormonal deficiency state (estrogen and 1,25 dihydroxyvitamin D) in patients with postmenopausal osteoporosis. In Norman AW, Schaefer K, Herrath Dv, et al, eds: Vitamin D: Biochemical, chemical and clinical aspects related to calcium metabolism. Berlin, Walter de Gruyter & Co., 1977, p. 643.

Riggs BL, Jowsey J, Kelley PJ, et al: Effects of sex hormones on bone in primary osteoporosis. J Clin Invest 48:1065, 1969.

Ross RK, Mack TM, Paganini-Hill A, et al: Menopausal oestrogen therapy and protection from death from ischaemic heart disease. Lancet 1:858, 1981.

Ross RK, Paganini-Hill A, Mack TM, Henderson BE: Estrogen use and cardiovascular disease. In Mishell DR Jr, ed: Menopause: Physiology and pharmacology. Chicago, Year Book Medical Publishers, 1987.

Schiff I, Tulchinsky D, Cramer D, Ryan KJ: Oral medroxyprogesterone in the treatment of postmenopausal symptoms. JAMA 224:1443, 1980.

Sherman BM, West JH, Korenman SG: The menopausal transition: Analysis of LH, FSH, estradiol, and progesterone concentrations during menstrual cycles of older women. J Clin Endocrinol Metab 42:629, 1976.

Sturdee DW, Wade-Evans T, Paterson ME, et al: Relations between bleeding pattern, endometrial histology, and oestrogen treatment in menopausal women. Br Med J 1(6127):1575, 1978.

Wahl P, Walden C, Knopp R, et al: Effect of estrogen/progestin potency on lipid/lipoprotein cholesterol. N Engl J Med 308:862, 1983.

Weiss NS, Ure CL, Ballard JH, et al: Decreased risk of fractures of the hip and lower forearm with postmenopausal use of estrogen. N Engl J Med 303:1195, 1980.

Whitehead MI, Townsend PT, Pryse-Davies J, et al: Effect of estrogens and progestins on the biochemistry and morphology of the postmenopausal endometrium. N Engl J Med 305:1599, 1981.

Wren BG, Routledge AD: The effect of type and dose of oestrogen on the blood pressure of post-menopausal women. Maturitas 5:135, 1983.

Gamma rays, 711
  as photon radiation source, 713
Ganglionic blockers, bladder function and, 564*t*
Gardnerella vaginalis, vaginitis from, 594-596
Gartner's duct
  cysts of, 48
    definition of, 440
  definition of, 3
Gastric restriction operations for severe obesity,
      173-174
Gastrointestinal tract
  endometriosis of, 507-508
  postoperative problems with, 689-693
    ileus as, 689-690
    intestinal obstruction as, 690-692
    rectovaginal fistula as, 692-693
  preoperative management of, 655-656
Gelastic seizures, definition of, 247
Gene(s)
  definition of, 23
  and gene action, 24
  mutation of, 24-25
Genetic code, 24
  mutations and, 24-25
Genetic predisposition, endometriosis from, 495
Genetics, 23-40
Genital duct system
  embryonic development of, 12-18
  external genitalia of, embryonic development of,
      14-15, *17*, 18
  female, embryonic development of, 14, *16*
  male, embryonic development of, 12, 14, *16*
Genital herpes, 577-581
  abortion and, 390
Genital papilloma infection, intraepithelial neoplasia
      and, 741-750; *see also* Intraepithelial
      neoplasia of cervix genital papilloma
      infection and
Genital tract
  lower; *see also* Cervix; Vagina
    infections of, 567-610
  upper; *see also* Fallopian tube(s); Ovary(ies);
      Uterus
    infections of, 614-641
      Actinomyces, 637
      endometritis as, 614-615
      pelvic inflammatory disease as, 614-637; *see
        also* Pelvic inflammatory disease (PID)
      tuberculous, 637-639
Genital trauma in childhood, 255-256
Genital ulcers, 577-587
  in chancroid, 583-584
  in genital herpes, 577-581
  in granuloma inguinale, 581-582
  in lymphogranuloma venereum, 582-583
  in syphilis, 584-587
Genital warts, 573, 575-577

Genitalia
  ambiguous, definition of, 231
  congenital defects of, 232-238
  external
    anatomy of, 43-46
    embryonic development of, 14-15, *17*, 18
    innervation of, 65-66
  internal, innervation of, 64-65
Genitocrural fold, definition of, 42
Genitourinary system
  changes in, in menopause, 1085
  embryonic development of, 11-18
    bladder in, 12, *13*
    excretory system in, 11-12
    genital duct system in, 12-18
    urethra in, 12, *13*
Genome, definition of, 23
Genotype, definition of, 23
Genuine stress incontinence, 551-557; *see also*
      Stress incontinence, genuine
Germ cell sex cord-stromal tumors, 866
Germ cell tumors, 857-866
  carcinoids as, 863
  choriocarcinomas as, 865-866
  classification of, 857-858
  definition of, 833
  dysgerminomas as, 863-864
  embryonal carcinomas as, 866
  endodermal sinus tumors as, 864-865
  histogenesis of, 858, *859*
  mixed, 866
  polyembryomas as, 866
  specialized, 863
  struma ovarii as, 863
  teratomas as, 858-863; *see also* Teratoma(s),
      ovarian
  yolk sac tumors as, 864-865
Germinal vesicle, definition of, 76
Gestagen(s), 269
  synthetic, in oral contraceptives, 275-293; *see
      also* Oral contraceptives
Gestation, tubal, unruptured, definition of, 406
Gestational trophoblastic disease (GTD), 923-935
  characteristics of, 923
  clinical aspects of, 929-935
  clinical classification of, 928-929
  definition of, 923
  epidemiology of, 926-927
  incidence of, 927-928
  morphology of, 923-926
Gestational trophoblastic neoplasia (GTN), 933-935
  definition of, 923
  diagnosis of, 933
  fertility after treatment for, 935
  incidence of, 933
  management of, 934-935
  prognosis of, 934